麻醉并发症

Complications in Anesthesia

（第 3 版）

原著主编　Lee A. Fleisher
　　　　　Stanley H. Rosenbaum
主　　译　卞金俊　薄禄龙
主　　审　邓小明

北京大学医学出版社

MAZUI BINGFAZHENG（DI 3 BAN）

图书在版编目（CIP）数据

麻醉并发症：第 3 版 /（美）李·弗莱舍（Lee A. Fleisher），（美）斯坦利·罗森鲍姆（Stanley H. Rosenbaum）原著；卞金俊，薄禄龙主译．—北京：北京大学医学出版社，2021.1

书名原文：Complications in Anesthesia，3rd edition

ISBN 978-7-5659-2343-2

Ⅰ．①麻…　Ⅱ．①李…②斯…③卞…④薄…　Ⅲ．①麻醉－并发症－处理　Ⅳ．① R614

中国版本图书馆 CIP 数据核字（2020）第 247757 号

北京市版权局著作权合同登记号：图字：01-2020-7225

ELSEVIER

Elsevier (Singapore) Pte Ltd.
3 Killiney Road, #08-01 Winsland House I, Singapore 239519
Tel: (65) 6349-0200; Fax: (65) 6733-1817

Complications in Anesthesia, 3rd edition

ISBN-13: 978-1-4557-0411-8

This translation of Complications in Anesthesia, 3rd edition by Lee A. Fleisher and Stanley H. Rosenbaum, was undertaken by Peking University Medical Press and is published by arrangement with Elsevier（Singapore）Pte Ltd.
Complications in Anesthesia, 3rd edition by Lee A. Fleisher and Stanley H. Rosenbaum 由北京大学医学出版社进行翻译，并根据北京大学医学出版社与爱思唯尔（新加坡）私人有限公司的协议约定出版。

《麻醉并发症》（第 3 版）（卞金俊，薄禄龙主译）
ISBN：978-7-5659-2343-2

麻醉并发症（第 3 版）

主　　译：卞金俊　薄禄龙
出版发行：北京大学医学出版社
地　　址：（100083）北京市海淀区学院路 38 号　北京大学医学部院内
电　　话：发行部 010-82802230；图书邮购 010-82802495
网　　址：http://www.pumpress.com.cn
E-mail：booksale@bjmu.edu.cn
印　　刷：中煤（北京）印务有限公司
经　　销：新华书店
策划编辑：王智敏
责任编辑：袁帅军　　**责任校对**：靳新强　　**责任印制**：李　啸
开　　本：889 mm×1194 mm　1/16　　**印张**：58.5　　**字数**：1720 千字
版　　次：2021 年 1 月第 1 版　2021 年 1 月第 1 次印刷
书　　号：ISBN 978-7-5659-2343-2
定　　价：320.00 元

资深教育者皆知，我们所教之人也是最热心、最投入的老师。
由此，本书敬献给宾夕法尼亚大学和耶鲁大学的住院医师
——他们曾是我们的学生、老师和同事。

原著前言

“并发症是追求完美的天然副产品。”

与前两版一样,《麻醉并发症》(第 3 版)旨在为麻醉学和重症医学从业人员应对临床实践中可能出现的大量并发症，提供一个全面、可靠的信息来源。本书前两版由 John L. Atlee 医师主编，他为本书搭建了处理并发症时高度结构化的框架，包括病例概要、问题分析、管理和预防。在本书第 3 版中，所有章节已被归类为术前病情、手术相关并发症、术中药物和潜在并发症、设备相关并发症、围术期事件和小儿围术期事件。

这些单独的章节主题在以前版本中已多有涉及，但本书绝大部分作者都有变化，并增加了新的主题。编者在此感谢 Atlee 医师和上一版的所有作者。本书部分章节的编写正是基于他们对上一版的贡献。

我们希望，这种处理麻醉和重症领域并发症的方法，能为当前临床实践提供参考，能成为住院医师学习如何处理并发症并为之做好准备的有益工具。

Lee A. Fleisher

Stanley H. Rosenbaum

译者前言

随着麻醉学理论与技术的完善与成熟，麻醉学科在保障患者围术期安全中发挥了无可替代的关键作用。保障临床麻醉的安全，避免或降低各类并发症的发生，是确保临床麻醉质量的核心指标之一，也是麻醉科医师围术期工作的重要目标之一。当前，随着麻醉安全意识与文化的普遍树立，各类规章制度的严格规范执行，麻醉医护人员培训质量的全面提高，各类临床设备和技术的有效运用，患者围术期安全得到了确实的保障。

随着医疗技术水平的进步，我国人口结构的变化，以及患者医疗及健康需求的不断增长，高龄、危重、复杂、疑难手术的比例日渐增加，这也对麻醉科医师的工作提出了前所未有的挑战。如何更有效地避免或防范围术期各类并发症的发生？如何构建更系统的围术期并发症及危急事件的应对策略？如何基于制度和教学提升麻醉科医师应对围术期各类并发症的管理能力和水平？

为进一步更新有关麻醉并发症的围术期处置应对的新知识、新理念，我们组织团队翻译了这本书。全书共有六部分203个章节，涵盖患者术前病情、手术及设备相关并发症、术中药物和潜在并发症、成人及小儿围术期事件等内容，可谓面面俱到。与其他麻醉学专著相比，本书主题明确，体例独特，聚焦于麻醉并发症，采用问题解决式的临床路径，由表及里，步步为营，让读者可直接获取处置某一麻醉并发症的有效方案。在编写上，每个章节均从病例概要引入，随后提出临床问题。通过结构化的框架予以问题分析，阐明相应并发症的定义和识别，对管理和预防策略予以基于证据的最新建议。

本书既有基于最新证据的坚实理论支撑，也有融汇于临床实践的具体方案，还包含了大量图片、表格及流程图，对各级麻醉科医师而言都是一部便捷实用的学习参考书。对正在接受麻醉科规范化培训住院医师和专科医师，本书更是一本难得的“掌中宝”。本书列举的大量麻醉并发症的临床处置与防范，对参与医疗抢救的各个临床专科医师也大有裨益，相信他们在阅读本书后也将有所收获。

诚如本书主编 Lee A. Fleisher 教授在 2020 年 12 月份 Anesthesiology Clinics 杂志的一篇编者按中所言:“应对危急事件的能力塑造了麻醉科医师。我们学着应对麻醉并发症的方法，将不断拓宽我们的认知。”我们相信，这本以麻醉并发症为主题的专著，必将开拓广大麻醉科医师的视野，也期望能有助于中国麻醉科医师的知识更新，提高专业理论和技能水平，促进麻醉学科的向前发展，在促进并改善患者围术期预后中继续发挥领导性角色，更好地服务于患者、服务于临床。

在此，感谢中国人民解放军海军军医大学第一附属医院（上海长海医院）麻醉学部的所有医护人员，他们参与了本书的翻译和审校工作，在繁忙的临床工作中依旧辛勤付出，为本书的顺利出版提供了保障。感谢邓小明教授承担本书的主审工作，作为国内知名的麻醉学专家，他主持国内多部教材和重要麻醉学专著的编写，主译国外多部麻醉学重要专著，他严谨求实的学者风范、孜孜以求的专业精神值得我们学习。本书的引进、翻译和出版，得到了北京大学医学出版社的大力支持。特别感谢王智敏编审严谨、求实、细致的工作，使本书顺利出版，及早与读者见面。

卞金俊

2020 年 12 月

译校者名单

主　审　邓小明

主　译　卞金俊　薄禄龙

副主译　赵珍珍　孟 岩　刘 毅

译　者（按姓名汉语拼音排序）

常馨宁	常永青	陈 君	陈丽茹	陈文颖	成天华	成雨彤	程 芳	戴柠宇	邓 瑜
董 朋	杜兆宁	段盼盼	凡丽华	范翠翠	范丰启	方 亚	封莉莉	耿长振	顾姣姣
顾士杰	郭品豪	郭 玉	韩风瑞	胡琍琍	黄 成	黄 捷	黄 婷	姜 静	蒋政宇
解 健	金培培	李海莲	李金泰	李路路	李露茜	李盼盼	李荣岩	李 岩	李之娥
林安琪	林省伟	刘洪君	刘洪伟	卢凌宇	卢文斌	鲁 璐	陆梁梁	栾延敏	罗金华
孟庆元	蒲君洿	钱 爽	钱晓春	饶苗苗	仁泽锋	阮林星	沈 玲	沈怡佳	石亚平
时 鹏	孙 莉	孙媛媛	谭可哲	王昌理	王 春	王 翰	王家强	王靖云	王丽珍
王树欣	王 委	王 晓	王月影	王云鹏	王 芷	魏 玲	文 岑	吴 巧	吴 玮
吴 昱	夏博洋	项 前	谢 芳	谢 韬	徐 冰	徐 航	徐业好	薛改改	杨迪迪
杨 锴	杨心月	姚 寒	叶偲敏	尹光敏	袁宁平	袁 炜	翟学花	张程程	张 平
张 婉	张晓秀	张莹莹	赵晗燚	赵景昕	赵 莉	郑 敏	周 艳	朱 洁	朱立鹏

校　者（按姓名汉语拼音排序）

包 睿	卞金俊	薄禄龙	卜 岚	曹 霞	陈 芳	陈 辉	陈 玲	陈元杰	代元强
樊玉花	范晓华	费苗苗	韩文军	韩 烨	侯 炯	吉 栋	季 锋	李斌本	李 博
李 黛	李晓菲	刘 佳	刘 毅	刘 征	陆 军	马 宇	孟 岩	倪丽亚	倪 文
潘 科	沈 镀	盛睿方	盛 颖	石亚平	唐念中	万小健	汪 惠	王恒跃	王嘉锋
王 薇	王晓琳	文平山	吴 倩	席 鹏	熊源长	许 华	许 涛	严姝姝	杨 涛
杨宇光	姚 滢	余喜亚	查燕萍	张丽君	赵珍珍	周 懿	朱科明	朱文忠	

原著者名单

Devon Aganga, MD
Instructor in Anesthesiology and Pediatrics
Department of Anesthesiology
Mayo Clinic
Rochester, Minnesota
Anterior Mediastinal Mass

Bryan S. Ahlgren, MD
Assistant Professor
Department of Anesthesiology
University of Colorado, Anschutz Medical Campus
Aurora, Colorado
Hemodilution and Blood Conservation

Lourdes Al Ghofaily, MD
Assistant Professor of Clinical Anesthesiology
Department of Anesthesiology and Critical Care
University of Pennsylvania
Philadelphia, Pennsylvania
Postobstruction Pulmonary Edema in Pediatric Patients

Maurice S. Albin, MD (deceased)
Professor of Anesthesiology
Department of Anesthesiology and Perioperative Medicine
University of Alabama at Birmingham
Birmingham, Alabama
Venous Air Embolism

Laura J. Alexander, MD
Obstetric Anesthesiology Fellow
Department of Anesthesiology, Perioperative and Pain Medicine
Brigham and Women's Hospital
Boston, Massachusetts
Pulmonary Aspiration in the Parturient

Nicolas N. Algarra, MD
Assistant Professor
Department of Anesthesiology
University of Florida College of Medicine
Gainesville, Florida
Barbiturates: Porphyrias

Maged Argalious, MD, MSc, MBA, MEd
Professor of Anesthesiology
Cleveland Clinic Lerner College of Medicine
Director, Center for Anesthesiology Education
Residency Program Director, Anesthesiology Institute
Cleveland Clinic
Cleveland, Ohio
Complications of Trauma Surgery

Lori A. Aronson, MD
Associate Professor of Clinical Anesthesia and Pediatrics
Director of Liver Transplant Anesthesia
Department of Anesthesia
University of Cincinnati College of Medicine
Cincinnati Children's Hospital Medical Center
Cincinnati, Ohio
Hypoxemia in the Pediatric Patient

Michael A. Ashburn, MD, MPH, MBA
Professor
Department of Anesthesiology and Critical Care
Director, Pain Medicine
Co-Director, Palliative Care
Hospital of the University of Pennsylvania
Philadelphia, Pennsylvania
Chronic Opioid Use

Joshua H. Atkins, MD, PhD
Associate Professor of Anesthesiology and Critical Care
Associate Professor of Otorhinolaryngology: Head and Neck Surgery (Secondary)
Perelman School of Medicine at the University of Pennsylvania
Philadelphia, Pennsylvania
Laryngoscopy and Microlaryngoscopy

Michael S. Avidan, MB BCh, FCASA
Professor of Anesthesiology and Surgery
Department of Anesthesiology
Washington University School of Medicine
St. Louis, Missouri
HIV Infection and AIDS

Hamdy Awad, MD
Associate Professor
Department of Anesthesiology
The Ohio State University
Wexner Medical Center
Columbus, Ohio
Porphyrias

Diana Ayubcha, MS, DO
Clinical Instructor
Department of Anesthesiology and Critical Care
Hospital of the University of Pennsylvania
Philadelphia, Pennsylvania
Complications of Spinal Surgery
Perioperative Hypoxia
Posterior Fossa Surgery

Ignacio Badiola, MD
Assistant Professor of Anesthesiology and Critical Care
Perelman School of Medicine at the University of Pennsylvania
Philadelphia, Pennsylvania
Celiac Plexus Block: Side Effects and Complications
Fat Embolism Syndrome
Persistent Paresthesia

Mark Bain, MD
Staff Neurosurgeon
Cerebrovascular Center
Cleveland Clinic
Cleveland, Ohio
Intracranial Aneurysms: Vasospasm and Other Issues

Kate E. Balbi, DO
Resident
New York Presbyterian, Columbia Campus
New York, New York
Pediatric Hyperthermia

Jennifer M. Banayan, MD
Assistant Professor
Department of Anesthesia and Critical Care
University of Chicago
Chicago, Illinois
Perioperative Myocardial Ischemia and Infarction

Dimitry Y. Baranov, MD
Assistant Professor of Clinical Anesthesiology and Critical Care
Department of Anesthesiology and Critical Care
Perelman School of Medicine at the University of Pennsylvania
Philadelphia, Pennsylvania
Posterior Fossa Surgery

Catherine B. Barden, MD
Associate Professor of Anesthesiology and Pain Management
University of Texas Southwestern
Dallas, Texas
Autonomic Dysreflexia

Juliana Barr, MD
Associate Professor
Department of Anesthesiology
Stanford University School of Medicine
Stanford, California
Reversal Agents: Naloxone, Flumazenil, and Sugammadex

James N. Bates, PhD, MD
Associate Professor
Department of Anesthesia
University of Iowa, Carver College of Medicine
Iowa City, Iowa
Fetal Distress

Curtis L. Baysinger, MD
Professor of Anesthesiology
Department of Anesthesiology
Vanderbilt University School of Medicine
Nashville, Tennessee
Hypertensive Disorders of Pregnancy

Joan Benca, MD
Associate Professor
Department of Anesthesiology
University of Wisconsin School of Medicine and Public Health
Madison, Wisconsin
Bronchospasm

Martin L. Birch, MD
Assistant Professor
Department of Anesthesiology
University of Minnesota School of Medicine
Minneapolis, Minnesota
Hyperthyroidism: Thyroid Storm

Alain Borgeat, MD
Senior Clinical and Research Consultant, Anesthesiology
Balgrist University Hospital
Zurich, Switzerland
Interscalene Nerve Block: Potential Severe Complications

Gwendolyn L. Boyd, MD
Professor of Anesthesiology and Perioperative Medicine
University of Alabama at Birmingham
Birmingham, Alabama
Venous Air Embolism

John Bracken, MD
Assistant Professor and Associate Program Director of Resident Education
Department of Anesthesiology
University of Kansas School of Medicine
Kansas City, Kansas
Hyperglycemia and Diabetic Ketoacidosis

Lois L. Bready, MD
Professor and Vice Chair
Department of Anesthesiology
Vice Dean for Graduate Medical Education and Designated Institutional Official
University of Texas Health Science Center at San Antonio
San Antonio, Texas
Corneal Injury

James Bromilow, BM, MRCP, FRCA, FFICM
Consultant in Intensive Care Medicine and Anaesthesia
Poole Hospital NHS Foundation Trust
Poole, United Kingdom
Perioperative Tachyarrhythmias

Yuriy S. Bronshteyn, MD
Assistant Professor
Department of Anesthesiology
Duke University School of Medicine
Durham, North Carolina
Pulmonary Artery Pressure Monitoring

Benjamin B. Bruins, MD
Assistant Professor
Department of Anesthesia and Critical Care Medicine
Children's Hospital of Philadelphia
Philadelphia, Pennsylvania
Postoperative Apnea in Infants

Casey D. Bryant, MD
Critical Care Fellow
Department of Anesthesia Critical Care
Wake Forest University Baptist Medical Center
Winston-Salem, North Carolina
Toxic Ingestion

W. Michael Bullock, MD, PhD
Assistant Professor
Department of Anesthesiology
Duke University Hospital
Durham, North Carolina
Continuous Nerve Blocks: Perineural Local Anesthetic Infusion

Kristen Burton, MD
Resident Physician
Anesthesiology and Critical Care
University of Pennsylvania
Philadelphia, Pennsylvania
Nonbarbiturate Anesthetics

Lu Fan Cai, MD
Assistant Professor
Department of Anesthesiology and Critical Care
Hospital of the University of Pennsylvania
Philadelphia, Pennsylvania
Infectious Complications of Central Neuraxial Block

William R. Camann, MD
Director of Obstetric Anesthesiology
Department of Anesthesiology, Perioperative and Pain Medicine
Brigham & Women's Hospital
Associate Professor of Anaesthesia
Harvard Medical School
Boston, Massachusetts
Pulmonary Aspiration in the Parturient

Michelle Capdeville, MD
Associate Professor
Department of Cardiothoracic Anesthesia
Cleveland Clinic
Cleveland, Ohio
Mechanical Assist Devices

Maurizio Cereda, MD
Assistant Professor
Department of Anesthesiology and Critical Care
Perelman School of Medicine at the University of Pennsylvania
Philadelphia, Pennsylvania
Postoperative Respiratory Failure

Mark A. Chaney, MD
Professor
Director, Cardiac Anesthesia
Program Director, Adult Cardiothoracic Fellowship
Department of Anesthesia and Critical Care
University of Chicago
Chicago, Illinois
Adverse Neurologic Sequelae: Central Neurologic Impairment
Hypercoagulable States: Thrombosis and Embolism
Perioperative Myocardial Ischemia and Infarction

Michael I. Chen, MD
Clinical Associate Professor
Department of Pediatric Anesthesia
Stanford University School of Medicine
Stanford, California
Air Emboli

S. Devi Chiravuri, MD
Assistant Professor
Department of Anesthesiology
University of Michigan
Ann Arbor, Michigan
Rapid Fluid and Blood Delivery Systems

Lois A. Connolly, MD
Professor
Department of Anesthesiology
Medical College of Wisconsin
Milwaukee, Wisconsin
Intracranial Aneurysms: Rebleeding
Unstable Cervical Spine: Atlantoaxial Subluxation

Scott D. Cook-Sather, MD
Assistant Professor of Anesthesia
Department of Anesthesiology and Critical Care Medicine
University of Pennsylvania School of Medicine
Associate Anesthesiologist
Children's Hospital of Philadelphia
Philadelphia, Pennsylvania
Ophthalmic Problems and Complications

John R. Cooper, Jr., MD
Clinical Professor of Anesthesiology
Department of Anesthesiology
Baylor College of Medicine
Attending Anesthesiologist
Division of Cardiovascular Anesthesia
Texas Heart Institute/Baylor St. Luke's Medical Center
Houston, Texas
Troubleshooting Common Problems During Cardiopulmonary Bypass

Douglas B. Coursin, MD
Professor
Departments of Anesthesiology and Medicine
University of Wisconsin
Madison, Wisconsin
Adrenal Insufficiency

Chad D. Courtemanche, MD
Assistant Professor of Anesthesiology
Section on Neuroanesthesiology
Wake Forest School of Medicine
Winston-Salem, North Carolina
Pituitary Tumors: Diabetes Insipidus

Joseph P. Cravero, MD
Senior Associate in Perioperative Anesthesia
Department of Anesthesiology, Perioperative and Pain Medicine
Boston Children's Hospital
Associate Professor of Anaesthesiology
Harvard Medical School
Boston, Massachusetts
Sedation of Pediatric Patients

Craig E. Cummings, MD
Assistant Professor
Department of Anesthesiology
Medical College of Wisconsin
Clement J. Zablocki Veterans Affairs Medical Center
Milwaukee, Wisconsin
Local Anesthetic Systemic Toxicity

Christopher J. Curatolo, MD, MEM
Fellow, Division of Pain Management
Department of Anesthesiology, Perioperative and Pain Medicine
The Mount Sinai Hospital
Icahn School of Medicine at Mount Sinai
New York, New York
Vaporizers

Armagan Dagal, MD, FRCA
Associate Professor
Department of Anesthesiology and Pain Medicine
Harborview Medical Center, University of Washington
Seattle, Washington
Head Injury

Joanna David, MBBS, FCAI
Consultant Anaesthetist
North West Anglia NHS Foundation Trust
Peterborough, United Kingdom
Complications of Massive Transfusion
Postpartum Hemorrhage
Respiratory Depression After Spinal Anesthesia

Andrew Davidson, MBBS, FRCA, FICM
Consultant Anaesthetist
Department of Anaesthesia
Sheffield Teaching Hospitals NHS Foundation Trust
Sheffield, United Kingdom
Pulmonary Aspiration

Anthony de la Cruz, MD
Assistant Professor
Department of Anesthesiology
Rush University Medical Center
Chicago, Illinois
Abdominal Aortic Aneurysm Repair

Martin L. De Ruyter, MD
Associate Professor of Anesthesiology
Department of Anesthesiology
Kansas University School of Medicine
Kansas City, Kansas
Hyperglycemia and Diabetic Ketoacidosis
Sarcoidosis

Ronak Desai, DO
Assistant Professor of Anesthesiology
Department of Anesthesiology
Cooper Medical School of Rowan University
Camden, New Jersey
Peripheral Vascular Surgery

Somi R. Desikan, MD, FRCA, FFICM
John Hammond Department of Anaesthesia
East Surrey Hospital
Redhill, United Kingdom
Delayed Emergence

Barbara M. Dilos, DO
Assistant Clinical Professor
Department of Anesthesiology
Icahn School of Medicine at Mount Sinai
New York, New York
Hypothermia in the Pediatric Patient
Postintubation Croup

Andrew Disque, MD, MS
Assistant Clinical Professor
Department of Anesthesiology and Perioperative Medicine
David Geffen School of Medicine at UCLA
Los Angeles, California
Hypercoagulable States: Thrombosis and Embolism

Sylvia Y. Dolinski, MD, FCCP
Professor of Anesthesiology and Critical Care
Director, Critical Care Fellowship
Medical College of Wisconsin
Milwaukee, Wisconsin
Anaphylaxis and Anaphylactoid Reactions

Catherine Drexler, MD
Assistant Professor
Department of Anesthesiology
Medical College of Wisconsin
Milwaukee, Wisconsin
Angioedema and Urticaria

Michael P. Eaton, MD
Denham S. Ward Professor and Chair
Department of Anesthesiology
University of Rochester School of Medicine
Rochester, New York
Patient Warming Systems

Roderic G. Eckenhoff, MD
Austin Lamont Professor
Department of Anesthesiology and Critical Care
University of Pennsylvania Perelman School of Medicine
Philadelphia, Pennsylvania
Alzheimer's Disease

Jan Ehrenwerth, MD
Professor
Department of Anesthesiology
Yale School of Medicine
New Haven, Connecticut
Electrical Safety
Surgical Electrocautery

James B. Eisenkraft, MD
Professor
Department of Anesthesiology, Perioperative and Pain Medicine
Icahn School of Medicine at Mount Sinai
New York, New York
Carbon Dioxide Absorbers
Scavenging Systems
Vaporizers

Nabil M. Elkassabany, MD, MSCE
Assistant Professor
Department of Anesthesiology and Critical Care
University of Pennsylvania
Philadelphia, Pennsylvania
Methylmethacrylate

Herodotos Ellinas, MD
Associate Professor
Department of Anesthesiology
Medical College of Wisconsin
Milwaukee, Wisconsin
Difficult Pediatric Airway
Fires in the Operating Room
Magnetic Resonance Imaging
Malignant Hyperthermia

Jason A. Ellis, MD
Chief Resident
Department of Neurological Surgery
Columbia University Medical Center
New York, New York
Arteriovenous Malformation: Normal Perfusion Pressure Breakthrough

Mohammad El-Orbany, MD
Professor
Department of Anesthesiology
Medical College of Wisconsin
Milwaukee, Wisconsin
Difficult Airway and Failed Extubation
Nondepolarizing Neuromuscular Block

Brenda G. Fahy, MD
Professor of Anesthesiology
Department of Anesthesiology
University of Florida
Gainesville, Florida
Disorders of Water Homeostasis: Hyponatremia and Hypernatremia

Scott A. Falk, MD
Assistant Professor
Department of Anesthesiology and Critical Care
University of Pennsylvania
Philadelphia, Pennsylvania
Adverse Events and Unanticipated Outcomes: Comprehensive Disclosure

Zhuang T. Fang, MD, MSPH
Clinical Professor
Department of Anesthesiology and Perioperative Medicine
David Geffen School of Medicine at UCLA
Los Angeles, California
Unanticipated Hospital Admission and Readmission

Ehab Farag, MD, FRCA
Professor of Anesthesiology
Cleveland Clinic Lerner College of Medicine
Case Western University
Director of Clinical Research
Department of General Anesthesia
Cleveland Clinic
Cleveland, Ohio
Intracranial Aneurysms: Vasospasm and Other Issues

Michael Feduska, MD
Assistant Professor of Clinical Anesthesiology and Critical Care
Department of Anesthesiology & Critical Care
Hospital of the University of Pennsylvania
Philadelphia, Pennsylvania
Antihistamines: H_1- and H_2-Blockers

Lynne R. Ferrari, MD
Chief of Perioperative Anesthesia
Boston Children's Hospital
Associate Professor of Anaesthesia
Harvard Medical School
Boston, Massachusetts
Adenotonsillectomy

Paul G. Firth, MBChB
Attending Anesthesiologist
Department of Anesthesia, Critical Care and Pain Medicine
Massachusetts General Hospital
Assistant Professor
Harvard Medical School
Boston, Massachusetts
Foreign Body Aspiration

Lee A. Fleisher, MD
Robert D. Dripps Professor and Chair of Anesthesiology and Critical Care
Professor of Medicine
Perelman School of Medicine at the University of Pennsylvania
Philadelphia, Pennsylvania
Preoperative Cardiac Intervention

Randall P. Flick, MD, MPH
Associate Professor
Department of Anesthesiology and Pediatrics
Mayo Clinic Children's Center
Rochester, Minnesota
Anterior Mediastinal Mass

Keith M. Franklin, MD
Assistant Professor
Department of Anesthesiology
University of Rochester
Rochester, New York
Proportioning Systems

Eugene B. Freid, MD
Anesthesiologist
JLR Medical Group, US Anesthesia Partners
Affiliated Professor
University of Central Florida College of Medicine
Clinical Professor
Florida State University College of Medicine
Maitland, Florida
Succinylcholine

Andrea Gabrielli, MD, MBA
Professor
Department of Anesthesiology and Critical Care
Hospital of the University of Pennsylvania
Philadelphia, Pennsylvania
Postoperative Hemodynamic Instability

Elizabeth Mahanna Gabrielli, MD
Clinical Associate, Anesthesiology and Critical Care Medicine
Perelman School of Medicine at the University of Pennsylvania
Philadelphia, Pennsylvania
Postoperative Hemodynamic Instability

Arjunan Ganesh, MBBS, FRCS
Associate Professor
Department of Anesthesiology and Critical Care
Perelman School of Medicine at the University of Pennsylvania
Philadelphia, Pennsylvania
Upper Respiratory Tract Infection

Jeremy M. Geiduschek, MD
Professor
Pediatric Anesthesiology Division Chief
Department of Anesthesiology and Pain Medicine
University of Washington School of Medicine
Seattle, Washington
Intraoperative Cardiac Arrest: Pediatric

J.C. Gerancher, MD
Professor of Anesthesiology
Section Head, Regional Anesthesia and Acute Pain Management
Department of Anesthesiology
Wake Forest University School of Medicine
Winston-Salem, North Carolina
Epidural Anesthesia: Unintended Intrathecal Injection

Rebecca M. Gerlach, MD, FRCPC
Assistant Professor
Director, Anesthesia Perioperative Medicine Clinic
Department of Anesthesia and Critical Care
University of Chicago
Chicago, Illinois
Adverse Neurologic Sequelae: Central Neurologic Impairment
Mediastinal Masses

David B. Glick, MD, MBA
Professor
Medical Director, Post-Anesthesia Care Unit
Department of Anesthesiology and Critical Care
University of Chicago
Chicago, Illinois
Hyperthermia (Perioperative)

Mark S. Gold, MD
Chairman, Scientific Advisory Boards
RiverMend Health
Adjunct Professor
Department of Psychiatry
Washington University in St. Louis School of Medicine
St. Louis, Missouri
Chemical Dependency: Nonopioids
Chemical Dependency: Opioids

Suneeta Gollapudy, MD
Associate Professor
Department of Anesthesiology
Director, Division of Neuroanesthesia
Director, Division of PACU Rotation (FMLH)
Medical College of Wisconsin
Milwaukee, Wisconsin
Intracranial Aneurysms: Rebleeding
Unstable Cervical Spine: Atlantoaxial Subluxation

Stuart A. Grant, MD
Assistant Professor
Department of Anesthesiology
Duke University School of Medicine
Durham, North Carolina
Continuous Nerve Blocks: Perineural Local Anesthetic Infusion

Glenn P. Gravlee, MD
Professor
Department of Anesthesiology
University of Colorado, Anschutz Medical Campus
Aurora, Colorado
Hemodilution and Blood Conservation

Philip E. Greilich, MD, FAHA
Professor
University of Texas Southwestern Medical Center
Dallas, Texas
Steroids

Nancy B. Greilich, MD
Associate Professor
University of Texas Southwestern Medical School
Dallas, Texas
Steroids

Taras Grosh, MD
Instructor
Department of Anesthesiology, Critical Care and Pain Management
Hospital of the University of Pennsylvania
Philadelphia, Pennsylvania
Chronic Opioid Use
Perioperative Hypoxia

Harleena Gulati, BComm, MD, FRCPC
Anesthesiologist
Department of Anesthesia and Perioperative Medicine
University of Manitoba
Winnipeg, Canada
Complications After Pneumonectomy

Harshad Gurnaney, MBBS, MPH
Assistant Professor
Department of Anesthesiology and Critical Care
Hospital of the University of Pennsylvania
Children's Hospital of Philadelphia
Philadelphia, Pennsylvania
Upper Respiratory Tract Infection

Jacob T. Gutsche, MD
Assistant Professor
Department of Anesthesiology and Critical Care
University of Pennsylvania
Philadelphia, Pennsylvania
Sepsis, Systemic Inflammatory Response Syndrome, and Multiple Organ Dysfunction Syndrome

Michael A. Hall, MD
Instructor of Anesthesiology
Department of Anesthesiology and Critical Care
Hospital of the University of Pennsylvania
Philadelphia, Pennsylvania
Laryngeal and Tracheal Injury

Charles B. Hantler, MD
Professor
Department of Anesthesiology and Cardiothoracic Surgery
Washington University in St. Louis School of Medicine
St. Louis, Missouri
Bradyarrhythmias

Mohammed E. Haque, MBBS, BSc, FRCA
Specialist Registrar
Central London School of Anaesthesia
London, United Kingdom
Long QT Syndromes and Torsades de Pointes

H. David Hardman, MD, MBA
Professor of Anesthesiology
Vice-Chair for Professional Affairs
University of North Carolina
Chapel Hill, North Carolina
Extremity Tourniquets

Barry A. Harrison, MB, BS
Assistant Professor of Anesthesiology
Department of Anesthesiology
Mayo Clinic College of Medicine
Jacksonville, Florida
Hyperglycemia and Diabetic Ketoacidosis
Sarcoidosis

Elizabeth Healy, MD
Cardiac Anesthesia and Critical Care Fellow
Department of Anesthesia and Critical Care
University of Chicago
Chicago, Illinois
Adverse Neurologic Sequelae: Peripheral Nerve Injury

Daryl S. Henshaw, MD
Associate Professor of Anesthesiology
Wake Forest School of Medicine
Winston-Salem, North Carolina
Psoas Compartment Block: Potential Complications

Rosemary Hickey, MD
Clinical Professor of Anesthesiology and Neurosurgery
University of Texas Health Science Center at San Antonio
San Antonio, Texas
Intracranial Hypertension

Natalie F. Holt, MD, MPH
Assistant Professor
Department of Anesthesiology
Yale School of Medicine
New Haven, Connecticut
Staff Anesthesiologist and Medical Director, Ambulatory Procedures Unit
VA Connecticut Healthcare System, West Haven Campus
West Haven, Connecticut
Hypothermia

Jiri Horak, MD
Assistant Professor of Clinical Anesthesiology and Critical Care
Department of Anesthesiology and Critical Care
Hospital of the University of Pennsylvania
Philadelphia, Pennsylvania
Postoperative Pulmonary Hypertension

Nathaniel Hsu, MD
Instructor/OB Anesthesia Fellow
Department of Anesthesiology and Critical Care
Hospital of the University of Pennsylvania
Philadelphia, Pennsylvania
Peripartum Neurologic Complications

Stephanie Huang, MD
Resident Physician
Department of Anesthesiology and Critical Care
University of Pennsylvania
Philadelphia, Pennsylvania
Infectious Complications of Central Neuraxial Block

William S. Jacobs, MD
Associate Professor
Departments of Psychiatry and Health Behavior
Director, Addiction Medicine
Medical College of Georgia
Augusta, Georgia
Chemical Dependency: Nonopioids
Chemical Dependency: Opioids

Eric Jacobsohn, MD
Professor and Head
Department of Anesthesia
University of Manitoba
Winnipeg, Manitoba, Canada
Complications After Pneumonectomy

Arul Prakash Pandian James, MBBS, MD, MRCA
Anaesthetics
Queen's Medical Centre, Nottingham University Hospitals NHS Trust
Nottingham, United Kingdom
Laser Complications

Shailendra Joshi, MD
Assistant Professor
Department of Anesthesiology
Columbia University Medical Center
New York, New York
Arteriovenous Malformation: Normal Perfusion Pressure Breakthrough

Zeev N. Kain, MD
Professor of Anesthesiology
Department of Anesthesiology
Yale University School of Medicine
New Haven, Connecticut
Perioperative Psychological Trauma

Wendy B. Kang, MD, JD
Clinical Professor of Anesthesiology
Department of Anesthesiology
University of Texas Health Science Center at San Antonio
San Antonio, Texas
Retrobulbar Block

Ravish Kapoor, MD
Assistant Professor
Department of Anesthesiology and Perioperative Medicine
University of Texas MD Anderson Cancer Center
Houston, Texas
Postoperative Nausea and Vomiting: Pediatric

Amanpreet Kaur, MD
High Risk Obstetric Anesthesiologist
Gateway Anesthesia Association, PLLC
Gilbert, Arizona
Preterm Labor

Jeffrey S. Kelly, MD
Associate Professor
Department of Anesthesiology, Critical Care Section
Wake Forest School of Medicine
Winston-Salem, North Carolina
Toxic Ingestion

Kevin J. Kelly, MD
Professor and Chair
Department of Pediatrics
Associate Dean, School of Medicine
Children's Mercy Hospital and Clinics
University of Missouri
Kansas City, Missouri
Latex Reactions in Health Care Personnel

Johnny J. Kenth, MBBS, FRCA
Department of Anaesthesia
Royal Manchester Children's Hospital
Manchester, United Kingdom
Cardioversion

Michael L. Kentor, MD
Associate Professor
Department of Anesthesiology
University of Pittsburgh School of Medicine
Pittsburgh, Pennsylvania
Chief Anesthesiologist
UPMC East
Monroeville, Pennsylvania
Medical Director
UPMC Mercy South Side
Pittsburgh, Pennsylvania
Inadequate Pain Relief

Robert E. Kettler, MD
Associate Professor
Department of Anesthesiology
Medical College of Wisconsin
Froedtert Memorial Lutheran Hospital East
Milwaukee, Wisconsin
Latex Reactions in Health Care Personnel

Jonathan T. Ketzler, MD
Associate Professor
Department of Anesthesia and Critical Care
University of Wisconsin
Madison, Wisconsin
Adrenal Insufficiency

Evan D. Kharasch, MD, PhD
Assistant Dean for Clinical Research
Professor and Research Director
Department of Anesthesiology
University of Washington School of Medicine
Seattle, Washington
Volatile Anesthetics: Organ Toxicity

Arthur Kitt, MD, MPH
Pain Management Fellow
Department of Anesthesiology and Critical Care
Hospital of the University of Pennsylvania
Philadelphia, Pennsylvania
Chronic Nonsteroidal Antiinflammatory Drug Use

Koffi M. Kla, MD
Assistant Professor, Department of Anesthesiology
Professor, Department of Anesthesiology and Neurological Surgery
Vanderbilt University School of Medicine
Nashville, Tennessee
Autonomic Hyperreflexia

Jerome M. Klafta, MD
Professor
Vice-Chair for Education and Academic Affairs
Department of Anesthesia and Critical Care
University of Chicago
Chicago, Illinois
Mediastinal Masses

Antoun Koht, MD
Professor of Anesthesiology, Neurological Surgery, and Neurology
Northwestern University Feinberg School of Medicine
Chicago, Illinois
Spinal Cord Injury

Sandra L. Kopp, MD
Consultant
Department of Anesthesiology and Perioperative Medicine
Mayo Clinic
Associate Professor of Anesthesiology
Mayo Clinic College of Medicine
Rochester, Minnesota
Supraclavicular and Infraclavicular Block: Pneumothorax

Kenneth Kuchta, MD
Clinical Professor
Department of Anesthesiology and Perioperative Medicine
David Geffen School of Medicine at UCLA
Los Angeles, California
Misidentification of a Patient

Kavitha Kuntumalla, MBBS, DA, FRCA
Registrar
Department of Anaesthesia
Ipswich Hospital
Ipswich, Great Britain
Complications of Thyroid Surgery

Madhuri S. Kurdi, MBBS, MD
Professor
Department of Anaesthesiology
Karnataka Institute of Medical Sciences
Hubli, India
Ketamine

C. Dean Kurth, MD
Professor of Anesthesia and Pediatrics
University of Cincinnati College of Medicine
Anesthesiologist-in-Chief and Chair
Institute for Pediatric Research
Cincinnati Children's Hospital Medical Center
Cincinnati, Ohio
Postoperative Apnea in Infants

Arthur M. Lam, MD, FRCPC, FNCS
Professor of Anesthesiology and Neurological Surgery and Anesthesiologist-In-Chief
Department of Anesthesiology
Co-Director, Cerebrovascular Laboratory
Harborview Medical Center
Seattle, Washington
Head Injury

Jennifer E. Lam, DO
Associate Professor of Clinical Anesthesia and Pediatrics
Pediatric Cardiac Anesthesia Fellowship Director
Department of Anesthesia
University of Cincinnati College of Medicine
Cincinnati Children's Hospital Medical Center
Cincinnati, Ohio
Hypoxemia in the Pediatric Patient

Mary Landrigan-Ossar, MD, PhD
Senior Associate in Perioperative Anesthesia
Department of Anesthesiology, Perioperative and Pain Medicine
Boston Children's Hospital
Assistant Professor of Anaesthesiology
Harvard Medical School
Boston, Massachusetts
Sedation of Pediatric Patients

Elizabeth M.S. Lange, MD
Assistant Professor
Department of Anesthesiology
Northwestern University Feinberg School of Medicine
Chicago, Illinois
Antepartum Hemorrhage

Dale W. Lanks, MSN, RN
Director of Risk Management
Office of the General Counsel
University of Pennsylvania Health System
Philadelphia, Pennsylvania
Adverse Events and Unanticipated Outcomes: Comprehensive Disclosure

Krzysztof Laudanski, MD, PhD, MA, FCCM
Assistant Professor
Department of Anesthesiology and Critical Care
University of Pennsylvania
Philadelphia, Pennsylvania
The Hostile-Combative Patient

Melissa A. Laxton, MD
Associate Professor of Anesthesiology
Section on Neuroanesthesiology
Wake Forest School of Medicine
Winston-Salem, North Carolina
Pituitary Tumors: Diabetes Insipidus

Huong Le, MD
Assistant Professor
Division of Cardiothoracic Anesthesiology, Department of Anesthesiology
University of Florida College of Medicine
Gainesville, Florida
Antibiotics

Jeffrey W. Lee, MD, MS
Assistant Professor
Section Head of Ambulatory Anesthesia
Department of Anesthesiology
University of Wisconsin Hospital and Clinics
Madison, Wisconsin
Preanesthetic Evaluation: False-Positive Tests
Preanesthetic Evaluation: Inadequate or Missing Test Result

Lorri A. Lee, MD
Professor
Chief, Division of Neuroanesthesiology
Department of Anesthesiology and Neurosurgery
Vanderbilt University Medical Center
Nashville, Tennessee
Autonomic Hyperreflexia

John T. Lemm, MD
Assistant Professor of Anesthesiology
Department of Anesthesiology
Duke University Medical Center
Durham, North Carolina
Central Venous Pressure Monitoring

Adam J. Lemmon, MD
Associate Professor
Department of Anesthesia
Indiana University School of Medicine
Indianapolis, Indiana
Postoperative Peripheral Neuropathy

Philip R. Levin, MD
Clinical Professor
Department of Anesthesiology and Perioperative Medicine
David Geffen School of Medicine at UCLA
Los Angeles, California
Postoperative Delirium

Jerrold H. Levy, MD, FAHA, FCCM
Professor of Anesthesiology and Associate Professor of Surgery
Co-Director, Cardiothoracic ICU
Duke University Hospital
Durham, North Carolina
Perioperative Hypertension

Charles J. Lin, MD
Assistant Professor
Department of Anesthesiology
University of Pittsburgh Medical Center
Pittsburgh, Pennsylvania
Inadequate Pain Relief

Regina E. Linganna, MD
Resident Physician
Department of Anesthesiology and Critical Care
Hospital of the University of Pennsylvania
Philadelphia, Pennsylvania
Postoperative Pulmonary Hypertension

Ronald S. Litman, DO
Professor and Attending Anesthesiologist
Department of Anesthesiology and Critical Care
Children's Hospital of Philadelphia
Philadelphia, Pennsylvania
Pediatric Hyperthermia

Jaibin Liu, MD, PhD
Assistant Professor
Department of Anesthesiology and Critical Care
Perelman School of Medicine at the University of Pennsylvania
Philadelphia, Pennsylvania
Fat Embolism Syndrome

Luis L. Llamas, MD
Assistant Professor
Departments of Anesthesiology and Neurosurgery
Director of Neuroanesthesia
University of Texas Health Science Center at San Antonio
San Antonio, Texas
Corneal Injury

Robert G. Loeb, MD
Clinical Professor of Anesthesiology
University of Florida School of Medicine
Gainesville, Florida
Flowmeters

Celeste M. Lombardi, MD
Physician Advisor, Office of Quality, Safety and Improvement
Director, Outpatient Interventional Pain Service
Department of Neurology/Pain Management
Baltimore VA Medical Center, VA Maryland Health Care System
Baltimore, Maryland
Chronic Nonsteroidal Antiinflammatory Drug Use

Katarzyna Luba, MD, MS
Assistant Professor
Department of Anesthesiology
Medical College of Wisconsin
Milwaukee, Wisconsin
Complications of Laparoscopic Surgery
Perioperative Management of Patients with Muscular Dystrophy
Postobstruction Pulmonary Edema
Thermally Injured Patients

Monica I. Lupei, MD
Assistant Professor
Department of Anesthesiology
University of Minnesota
Minneapolis, Minnesota
Hypothyroidism: Myxedema Coma

Stewart J. Lustik, MD, MBA
Professor of Anesthesiology
Department of Anesthesiology
University of Rochester Medical Center
Rochester, New York
Proportioning Systems

Daqing Ma, MD, PhD, FRCA
Professor of Anaesthesia
Department of Surgery and Cancer
Anaesthetics, Pain Medicine and Intensive Care
Imperial College London, Chelsea and Westminster Hospital
London, United Kingdom
Nitrous Oxide: Neurotoxicity

Alvaro Andres Macias, MD
Instructor in Anesthesia
Department of Anesthesiology, Perioperative and Pain Medicine
Brigham and Women's Hospital
Department of Anesthesia
Massachusetts Eye and Ear
Boston, Massachusetts
Open Globe Injury

Ross MacPherson, BPharm, MSc, PhD, FANZCA
Clinical Professor
Department of Anaesthesia and Pain Management
Royal North Shore Hospital
Sydney, Australia
Anesthesia for Electroconvulsive Therapy

Anuj Malhotra, MD
Assistant Professor
Department of Anesthesiology
Icahn School of Medicine at Mount Sinai
New York, New York
Complications of Transurethral Surgery

Gaurav Malhotra, MD
Assistant Professor
Department of Anesthesiology and Critical Care
University of Pennsylvania
Philadelphia, Pennsylvania
Blood and Blood Products: Infections
Nonbarbiturate Anesthetics

Vinod Malhotra, MD
Professor
Departments of Anesthesiology and Urology
Weill Cornell Medical College
New York, New York
Complications of Transurethral Surgery

Gerard R. Manecke, MD
Professor and Chair
Department of Anesthesiology
University of California San Diego Health Sciences
San Diego, California
Thromboembolic Complications

Jonathan B. Mark, MD
Professor of Anesthesiology
Duke University Medical Center
Chief, Anesthesiology Service
Veterans Affairs Medical Center
Durham, North Carolina
Central Venous Pressure Monitoring
Pulmonary Artery Pressure Monitoring

Klaus Martin, MD
Deputy Director
Department of Anesthesiology
German Heart Center Munich
Munich, Germany
Bleeding After Cardiac Surgery

Lizabeth D. Martin, MD
Assistant Professor
Department of Anesthesiology and Pain Medicine
University of Washington School of Medicine
Seattle, Washington
Intraoperative Cardiac Arrest: Pediatric

Michael R. Mathis, MD
Clinical Lecturer and Research Fellow
Department of Anesthesiology, Cardiothoracic Division
University of Michigan
Ann Arbor, Michigan
Anesthesia Circuit

Jagroop Mavi, MD
Assistant Professor
Department of Anesthesiology and Pain Management
Cincinnati Children's Hospital Medical Center
Cincinnati, Ohio
Anesthetic Complications of Fetal Surgery: EXIT Procedures

Elizabeth W. Mburu, MD
Fellow, Cardiothoracic Anesthesiology
Department of Cardiothoracic Anesthesiology
Cleveland Clinic
Cleveland, Ohio
Peripheral Vascular Surgery

Victoria L. McCormack, BScMedSci, MBChB, FRCA, FFICM
Specialist Trainee
Department of Anaesthesia and Intensive Care Medicine
North West Deanery
Manchester, United Kingdom
Complications of Radical Urologic Surgery

Thomas McCutchen, MD
Assistant Professor of Anesthesiology
Department of Anesthesiology
Wake Forest University School of Medicine
Winston-Salem, North Carolina
Epidural Anesthesia: Unintended Intrathecal Injection

David L. McDonagh, MD
Professor of Anesthesiology and Pain Management,
Neurological Surgery, and Neurology
University of Texas Southwestern
Dallas, Texas
Autonomic Dysreflexia

Nolan McDonnell, FANZCA
Clinical Associate Professor
University of Western Australia
Crawley, Western Australia
Embolic Events of Pregnancy

Marc Mecoli, MD
Assistant Professor
Department of Pediatric Anesthesiology and Pain Management
Cincinnati Children's Hospital Medical Center
Cincinnati, Ohio
Perioperative Aspiration Pneumonitis

Mohammed M. Minhaj, MD, MBA
Associate Professor
Vice Chair for Finance and Operations
Associate Chair for Faculty Development
Department of Anesthesia and Critical Care
University of Chicago Medicine
Chicago, Illinois
Adverse Neurologic Sequelae: Peripheral Nerve Injury

Constance L. Monitto, MD
Assistant Professor
Department of Anesthesiology and Critical Care Medicine
The Johns Hopkins University School of Medicine
Baltimore, Maryland
Muscle Relaxants

Richard C. Month, MD
Assistant Professor of Clinical Anesthesiology
Department of Anesthesiology and Critical Care
University of Pennsylvania Health System
Philadelphia, Pennsylvania
Magnesium

Timothy E. Morey, MD
Professor and Chair
Department of Anesthesiology
University of Florida College of Medicine
Gainesville, Florida
Antibiotics

Senthil Nadarajan, MBBS, FRCA
Department of Anaesthesia
Ipswich Hospital
Ipswich, Great Britain
Complications of Thyroid Surgery

Carsten Nadjat-Haiem, MD
Associate Clinical Professor
Department of Anesthesiology and Perioperative Medicine
David Geffen School of Medicine at UCLA
Los Angeles, California
Syringe Swaps

Mohamed Naguib, MB, BCh, MSc, FCARCSI, MD
Professor
Department of Anesthesiology
Cleveland Clinic
Cleveland, Ohio
Myasthenic Disorders

Bhiken I. Naik, MBBCh
Associate Professor of Anesthesiology and Neurosurgery
University of Virginia Health System
Charlottesville, Virginia
Intrathecal Opioids

David A. Nakata, MD, MBA
Program Director
Department of Anesthesia
Indiana University Medical Center
Indianapolis, Indiana
Intractable Nausea and Vomiting
Postoperative Peripheral Neuropathy

Patrick J. Neligan, MA, MB, FCARCSI
Department of Anaesthesia and Intensive Care
University Hospital Galway
Galway, Ireland
Metabolic Acidosis and Alkalosis

Mary Ellen Nepps, JD
Senior Counsel
University of Pennsylvania
Philadelphia, Pennsylvania
Alleged Malpractice

Myrna C. Newland, MD
Professor Emeritus
Department of Anesthesiology
Nebraska Medical Center
Omaha, Nebraska
Dental Injuries

Richard J. Novak, MD
Adjunct Clinical Associate Professor
Department of Anesthesiology, Perioperative and Pain Medicine
Stanford University
Associated Anesthesiologists Medical Group
Stanford, California
Disorders of Potassium Balance

Andrew E. Ochroch, MD
Professor
Department of Anesthesiology and Critical Care
Hospital of the University of Pennsylvania
Director, Thoracic Anesthesiology
Department of Anesthesiology and Critical Care
University of Pennsylvania
Philadelphia, Pennsylvania
Laryngeal and Tracheal Injury

Jason A. Ochroch, MD
Anesthesiology Resident
Department of Anesthesiology and Critical Care
Hospital of the University of Pennsylvania
Philadelphia, Pennsylvania
Blood and Blood Products: Infections

Christopher J. O'Connor, MD
Professor
Department of Anesthesiology
Rush University Medical Center
Chicago, Illinois
Abdominal Aortic Aneurysm Repair

Jerome F. O'Hara, Jr., MD
Professor
Department of Anesthesiology
Case Western Reserve University School of Medicine
Departments of General Anesthesiology, Urology, and
Outcomes Research
Cleveland Clinic Foundation
Cleveland, Ohio
Complications of Lithotripsy

Tyson Olds, MD
Anesthesiology Resident Physician
Department of Anesthesiology
University of Missouri
Columbia, Missouri
Emergence Agitation and Emergence Delirium

David A. Olsen, MD
Senior Associate Consultant
Department of Anesthesiology and Perioperative Medicine
Mayo Clinic
Instructor of Anesthesiology
Mayo Clinic College of Medicine
Rochester, Minnesota
Supraclavicular and Infraclavicular Block: Pneumothorax

Paul S. Pagel, MD, PhD
Staff Physician, Anesthesia Service
Clement J. Zablocki Veterans Affairs Medical Center
Milwaukee, Wisconsin
Major Organ System Dysfunction After Cardiopulmonary Bypass

Eric Pan, MD
Acting Assistant Professor
Department of Anesthesiology and Pain Medicine
University of Washington
Seattle, Washington
Postoperative Urinary Retention

Jaideep J. Pandit, MA, BM, DPhil, FRCA, FFPMRCA, DM
Consultant Anaesthetist
Nuffield Department of Anaesthetics
Oxford University Hospitals NHS Foundation Trust
Professorial Fellow
St. John's College
Oxford, United Kingdom
Awareness Under Anesthesia

Komal Patel, MD
Associate Professor of Anesthesiology
Department of Anesthesiology and Perioperative Medicine
David Geffen School of Medicine at UCLA
Los Angeles, California
Hypercoagulable States: Thrombosis and Embolism

Vijal N. Patel, MD
Resident and Fellow
Department of Anesthesiology and Critical Care
University of Chicago
Chicago, Illinois
Hyperthermia (Perioperative)

D. Janet Pavlin, MD
Professor
Department of Anesthesiology
University of Washington
Seattle, Washington
Postoperative Urinary Retention

Seth Perelman, MD
Clinical Assistant Professor
Department of Anesthesiology, Perioperative Care, and Pain Medicine
New York University Langone Medical Center
New York University School of Medicine
New York, New York
Blood and Blood Products: Transfusion Reactions and Complications

Adam Pichel, MBChB, FRCA
Department of Anaesthesia
Manchester Royal Infirmary
Manchester, United Kingdom
Complications of Radical Urologic Surgery

Adrian Pichurko, MD
Fellow and Clinical Lecturer
Department of Anesthesiology
University of Michigan Health System
Ann Arbor, Michigan
Intracranial Pressure Monitoring

L. Kareen Porter, MD
Pediatric Anesthesiologist
Valley Anesthesiology Consultants
Phoenix, Arizona
Rapid Fluid and Blood Delivery Systems

Joseph Previte, MD, FAAP
Associate Professor of Pediatric Anesthesiology
Cincinnati Children's Hospital Medical Center
Cincinnati, Ohio
Complications of Fetal Surgery: EXIT Procedures
Perioperative Aspiration Pneumonitis

Richard C. Prielipp, MD, MBA, FCCM
Professor
Department of Anesthesiology
University of Minnesota
Minneapolis, Minnesota
Hyperthyroidism: Thyroid Storm
Hypothyroidism: Myxedema Coma

Donald S. Prough, MD
Professor and Chair
Department of Anesthesiology
University of Texas Medical Branch
Galveston, Texas
Perioperative Fluid Management

Bridget Perrin Pulos, MD
Consultant
Department of Anesthesiology and Perioperative Medicine
Mayo Clinic
Rochester, Minnesota
Methylmethacrylate

Jesse M. Raiten, MD
Assistant Professor
Department of Anesthesiology and Critical Care
University of Pennsylvania
Philadelphia, Pennsylvania
Sepsis, Systemic Inflammatory Response Syndrome, and Multiple Organ Dysfunction Syndrome

Satya Krishna Ramachandran, MD, FRCA
Assistant Professor
Department of Anesthesiology
University of Michigan
Ann Arbor, Michigan
Anesthesia Circuit

Mohamed Ehab Ramadan, MBBCh
Research Fellow
Department of Anesthesiology
The Ohio State University, Wexner Medical Center
Columbus, Ohio
Research Assistant
Department of Anesthesiology
Theodor Bilharz Research Institute
Giza, Egypt
Porphyrias

Mallikarjun G. Reddy, MD, MPH
Clinical Instructor of Anesthesiology
Department of Anesthesiology
Weill Cornell Medical College
Assistant Attending Anesthesiologist
New York Presbyterian Hospital
New York, New York
Cardiomyopathies

Clare H. Ridley, MD
Assistant Professor
Washington University in St. Louis
St. Louis, Missouri
Bradyarrhythmias

David Roberts, MD
Resident Physician
Department of Anesthesiology
Vanderbilt University
Nashville, Tennessee
Postoperative Acute Kidney Injury

Michael Robinson, MBChB, FRCA
Consultant Anaesthetist
Department of Anaesthetics
Sheffield Teaching Hospitals NHS Foundation Trust
Sheffield, United Kingdom
Pulmonary Aspiration

Andrew Roscoe, MBChB
Consultant in Anaesthesia and Intensive Care
Papworth Hospital
Cambridge, United Kingdom
Pulmonary Hypertension

John B. Rose, MD
Professor
Department of Anesthesia and Pediatrics
University of Cincinnati, College of Medicine
Department of Anesthesia, Division of Pain Management
Cincinnati Children's Hospital Medical Center
Cincinnati, Ohio
Delayed Emergence in Pediatric Patients

Cody Rowan, MD
Assistant Professor
Department of Anesthesiology
University of North Carolina
Chapel Hill, North Carolina
Extremity Tourniquets

Marc A. Rozner, PhD, MD (deceased)
Professor of Anesthesiology and Perioperative Medicine
Professor of Cardiology
University of Texas MD Anderson Cancer Center
Houston, Texas
Patients with a Cardiovascular Implantable Electronic Device Undergoing Surgery

Mashhood Salahuddin, BS
Medical Student
Atlantic University School of Medicine
Rodney Bay, St. Lucia
Department of Anesthesiology
The Ohio State University, Wexner Medical Center
Columbus, Ohio
Porphyrias

Reza Salajegheh, MD
Assistant Professor of Anesthesiology and Pain Medicine
University of Virginia Medical Center
Charlottesville, Virginia
Intrathecal Opioids

Nancy B. Samol, MD
Assistant Professor of Anesthesiology
University of Cincinnati College of Medicine
Cincinnati Children's Hospital
Cincinnati, Ohio
Pediatric Laryngospasm

William J. Sauer, MD
Critical Care Fellow
Department of Anesthesia and Critical Care
Stanford University
Stanford, California
Reversal Agents: Naloxone, Flumazenil, and Sugammadex

R. Alexander Schlichter, MD
Assistant Professor of Clinical Anesthesiology and Critical Care
Department of Anesthesiology and Critical Care
Perelman School of Medicine at the University of Pennsylvania
Philadelphia, Pennsylvania
Patients With Seizure Disorders

Jay Schoenherr, MD
Assistant Professor
Department of Anesthesiology
University of North Carolina
Chapel Hill, North Carolina
Extremity Tourniquets

Peter M. Schulman, MD
Associate Professor
Department of Anesthesiology and Perioperative Medicine
Oregon Health and Science University
Portland, Oregon
Patients With a Cardiovascular Implantable Electronic Device Undergoing Surgery

Jeffrey J. Schwartz, MD
Associate Professor
Department of Anesthesiology
Yale University School of Medicine
New Haven, Connecticut
Electrical Safety
Surgical Electrocautery

Rajamani Sethuraman, MD, DNB, FRCA, FICM
Consultant in Anaesthesia and Intensive Care
Princess Alexandra Hospital
Harlow, United Kingdom
Intravenous Drug Delivery Systems
Long QT Syndromes and Torsades de Pointes

Christoph N. Seubert, MD, PhD, DABNM
Professor of Anesthesiology and Neurosurgery
Department of Anesthesiology
University of Florida College of Medicine
Gainesville, Florida
Barbiturates: Porphyrias

Danielle Shafiepour, MDCM, FRCPC
Thoracic Anesthesiologist
Montreal General Hospital
Montreal, Canada
One-Lung Ventilation

Jack S. Shanewise, MD, FASE
Professor of Anesthesiology at CUMC
Chief, Division of Cardiothoracic Anesthesiology
Columbia University College of Physicians and Surgeons
New York, New York
Transesophageal Echocardiography

Andrew Shaw, MB, FRCA, FCCM, FFICM
Professor of Anesthesiology
Division of Cardiothoracic Anesthesiology
Executive Vice Chair
Department of Anesthesiology
Vanderbilt University Medical Center
Nashville, Tennessee
Postoperative Acute Kidney Injury

Marc Sherwin, MD
Resident
Department of Anesthesiology, Perioperative and Pain Medicine
Icahn School of Medicine at Mount Sinai
New York, New York
Carbon Dioxide Absorbers
Scavenging Systems

Peter D. Slinger, MD, FRCPC
Professor
Department of Anesthesia
University of Toronto
Staff Anesthesiologist
Toronto General Hospital
Toronto, Canada
One-Lung Ventilation

Tod B. Sloan, MD, MBA, PhD
Professor Emeritus
Department of Anesthesiology
University of Colorado School of Medicine
Aurora, Colorado
Spinal Cord Injury

Andrew F. Smith, MBBS
Professor
Department of Anaesthesia
Lancaster Royal Infirmary
Lancaster, United Kingdom
Cardioversion

David S. Smith, MD, PhD
Associate Professor
Department of Anesthesiology and Critical Care
University of Pennsylvania
Philadelphia, Pennsylvania
Alleged Malpractice

Paul Smythe, MD
Assistant Professor
Department of Anesthesiology
University of Michigan Health System
Ann Arbor, Michigan
Intracranial Pressure Monitoring

Michael J. Sopher, MD
Clinical Professor
Department of Anesthesiology and Perioperative Medicine
David Geffen School of Medicine at UCLA
Los Angeles, California
Syringe Swaps

Christina M. Spofford, MD, PhD
Associate Professor
Department of Anesthesiology
Medical College of Wisconsin
Milwaukee, Wisconsin
Anticoagulants and Peripheral Nerve Block
Local Anesthetic Neurotoxicity: Cauda Equina Syndrome
Spinal Anesthesia: Post–Dural Puncture Headache

Scott R. Springman, MD
Professor of Anesthesiology
School of Medicine and Public Health
University of Wisconsin
Madison, Wisconsin
Preanesthetic Evaluation: False-Positive Tests
Preanesthetic Evaluation: Inadequate or Missing Test Result

Michael J. Stentz, MD, MS
Critical Care Fellow
Department of Anesthesiology and Critical Care
University of Pennsylvania
Philadelphia, Pennsylvania
Postoperative Respiratory Failure

Alexander Michael Stewart, BSc (Hons), MPhil, MRCP, FRCA
Department of Anaesthetics
University Hospital Southampton
Southampton, United Kingdom
Perioperative Tachyarrhythmias

Jennifer L. Stewart, DO
Assistant Professor
Department of Anesthesiology
Indiana University School of Medicine
Indianapolis, Indiana
Intractable Nausea and Vomiting

Mark D. Stoneham, MA, FRCA
Consultant Anaesthetist and Senior Clinical Lecturer
Nuffield Division of Anaesthetics
John Radcliffe Hospital
Oxford, United Kingdom
Carotid Endarterectomy

Laura Stover, MD
Assistant Clinical Professor
Department of Anesthesiology
McMaster University Faculty of Health Sciences
Staff Anesthesiologist
Hamilton Health Sciences
Hamilton, Canada
Drugs Affecting the Renin-Angiotensin System

Rajeshwari Subramaniam, MBBS, MD
Professor of Anesthesiology, Pain Medicine and Critical Care
All India Institute of Medical Sciences
New Delhi, India
Complications of Adrenal Surgery

Ka Chun Suen, BSc
Fellow in Anaesthetics, Pain Medicine and Intensive Care
Department of Surgery and Cancer
Imperial College London, Chelsea and Westminster Hospital
London, United Kingdom
Nitrous Oxide: Neurotoxicity

Christer H. Svensén, MD, PhD, MSc, DESA
Associate Professor
Department of Clinical Science and Education
Section of Anesthesiology and Intensive Care
Karolinska Institutet/Södersjukhuset
Stockholm, Sweden
Perioperative Fluid Management

BobbieJean Sweitzer, MD
Professor of Anesthesiology
Northwestern Feinberg School of Medicine
Chicago, Illinois
Perioperative Myocardial Ischemia and Infarction

Alexandra Szabova, MD
Associate Professor
Department of Anesthesiology
University of Cincinnati, College of Medicine
Department of Anesthesia, Division of Pain Management
Cincinnati Children's Hospital Medical Center
Cincinnati, Ohio
Delayed Emergence in Pediatric Patients

James F. Szocik, MD
Associate Professor
Department of Anesthesiology
University of Michigan
Ann Arbor, Michigan
Pipeline Source Failure

Perumal Tamilselvan, MBBS, MD, FRCA
Consultant Anaesthetist
Princess Alexandra Hospital
Harlow, United Kingdom
Complications of Massive Transfusion
Postpartum Hemorrhage
Respiratory Depression After Spinal Anesthesia

Peter Tassani-Prell, MD
Chairman
Department of Anesthesiology
German Heart Center Munich
Munich, Germany
Anticoagulation Initiation and Reversal for Cardiac Surgery
Bleeding After Cardiac Surgery

Justin Tawil, MD
Assistant Professor
Department of Anesthesiology and Critical Care
Medical College of Wisconsin
Milwaukee, Wisconsin
Thoracic Aortic Aneurysm

Paloma Toledo, MD, MPH
Assistant Professor
Department of Anesthesiology
Center for Healthcare Studies
Northwestern University Feinberg School of Medicine
Chicago, Illinois
Antepartum Hemorrhage

Klaus D. Torp, MD
Assistant Professor
Department of Anesthesiology
Mayo Clinic
Jacksonville, Florida
Dialysis-Dependent Patients

Arturo G. Torres, MD
Clinical Assistant Professor of Anesthesiology
Division of Critical Care Medicine
University of Florida
Gainesville, Florida
Disorders of Water Homeostasis: Hyponatremia and Hypernatremia

Gail A. Van Norman, MD
Professor of Anesthesiology and Pain Medicine
Adjunct Professor of Bioethics
University of Washington
Seattle, Washington
Do-Not-Resuscitate Orders in the Operating Room
The Jehovah's Witness Patient
Patient Confidentiality

Gina Votta-Velis, MD, PhD
Associate Professor of Anesthesiology/Pain
Program Director, Pain Medicine Fellowship
Program Director, Acute Pain and Regional Anesthesia Fellowship
Department of Anesthesiology
University of Illinois at Chicago College of Medicine
Chicago, Illinois
Interscalene Nerve Block: Potential Severe Complications

Mahmoud I. Wagih, MBChB, MSc, FFICM, FRCA
Consultant in Anaesthesia and Intensive Care
Princess Alexandra Hospital
Harlow, United Kingdom
Antiemetics
Latex Allergy
Spinal Hematoma

Kerri M. Wahl, MD, FRCP(C)
Professor
Department of Anesthesiology
Duke University
Durham, North Carolina
Complications of Carcinoid Tumors
Postoperative Hepatic Dysfunction
Postoperative Visual Loss

Jason D. Walls, MD
Assistant Professor
Department of Anesthesiology and Critical Care
Hospital of the University of Pennsylvania
Philadelphia, Pennsylvania
Complications of Spinal Surgery

Mehernoor F. Watcha, MD
Associate Professor
Department of Anesthesiology
Baylor College of Medicine, Texas Children's Hospital
Houston, Texas
Postoperative Nausea and Vomiting: Pediatric

Ari Y. Weintraub, MD
Attending Anesthesiologist
Children's Hospital of Philadelphia
Assistant Professor of Clinical Anesthesiology and Critical Care
Perelman School of Medicine at the University of Pennsylvania
Philadelphia, Pennsylvania
Hypoglycemia and Hyperglycemia

B. Craig Weldon, MD
Professor
Department of Anesthesiology and Pediatrics
University of Missouri
Columbia, Missouri
Cardiomyopathies
Emergence Agitation and Emergence Delirium

Robert S. Weller, MD
Professor of Anesthesiology
Section Head, Regional Anesthesia and Acute Pain Management
Wake Forest School of Medicine
Winston-Salem, North Carolina
Psoas Compartment Block: Potential Complications

Robert A. Whittington, MD
Professor of Anesthesiology
Department of Anesthesiology
Columbia University Medical Center
New York, New York
Alzheimer's Disease

Brian A. Williams, MD, MBA
Professor
Department of Anesthesiology
University of Pittsburgh School of Medicine
Director of Outpatient Regional Anesthesia Service
Department of Anesthesiology
University of Pittsburgh Medical Center
Pittsburgh, Pennsylvania
Inadequate Pain Relief

Lisa Wise-Faberowski, MD, MS
Assistant Professor, MCL
Department of Anesthesiology
Stanford University
Palo Alto, California
Air Emboli

Alex M. Witek, MD
Resident, Neurological Surgery
Department of Neurosurgery and Cerebrovascular Center
Cleveland Clinic
Cleveland, Ohio
Intracranial Aneurysms: Vasospasm and Other Issues

Eric P. Wittkugel, MD
Associate Professor of Anesthesia and Pediatrics
University of Cincinnati College of Medicine
Cincinnati Children's Hospital
Cincinnati, Ohio
Pediatric Laryngospasm

David Wlody, MD
Professor of Clinical Anesthesiology and Vice Chair for Education
State University of New York Downstate Medical Center
New York, New York
Postpartum Headache Other Than Post-Dural Puncture Headache

Brian J. Woodcock, MD
Assistant Professor of Anesthesiology
Department of Anesthesiology
University of Michigan Medical School
Ann Arbor, Michigan
Mechanical Ventilators

Miguel A. Yaport, MD
Resident
Department of Anesthesiology and Critical Care
University of Pennsylvania
Philadelphia, Pennsylvania
Persistent Paresthesia

Peter K. Yi, MD
Assistant Professor of Clinical Anesthesiology and Critical Care
Attending Anesthesiologist
Hospital of the University of Pennsylvania
Director of Anesthesiology
Tuttleman Surgical Center, Pennsylvania Hospital
Philadelphia, Pennsylvania
Uncontrolled Acute Postoperative Pain

Paul B. Zanaboni, MD, PhD
Associate Professor
Department of Anesthesiology
Washington University in St. Louis School of Medicine
St. Louis, Missouri
Bradyarrythmias

Ronnie H. Zeidan, MD
Assistant Professor
Department of Anesthesiology
University of Kentucky
Lexington, Kentucky
Uncontrolled Acute Postoperative Pain

Katharine H. Zentner, MD
Resident
Department of Anesthesiology
University of Texas Health Science Center at San Antonio
San Antonio, Texas
Corneal Injury

M. Tracy Zundel, MD
Assistant Professor
Department of Anesthesiology
Medical College of Wisconsin
Milwaukee, Wisconsin
Major Organ System Dysfunction After Cardiopulmonary Bypass

目　　录

第一部分

术前病情

第 1 章 肾上腺功能不全

Jonathan T. Ketzler，Douglas B. Coursin

病例概要

患者，男性，68 岁，身高 178 cm，体重 100 kg，因反复性憩室炎、可疑憩室周围脓肿，行左半结肠切除术，手术结束前出现顽固性低血压。术毕，患者保留气管导管转运至重症监护病房（intensive care unit，ICU），行肺动脉导管置入术及经胸超声心动图（transthoracic echocardiogram，TTE）检查。肺动脉楔压为 6 mmHg，体循环阻力为 475 dynes/cm^5，心排血量为 10 L/min，心脏指数为 6 L/（min·m^2）。TTE 表现为高动力性左心室伴收缩末期室腔闭塞，右心室收缩性轻度增强，下腔静脉管径缩小，且具有显著的呼吸变异度。给予患者机械通气，去甲肾上腺素 0.1 μg/（kg·min），肾上腺素 0.1 μg/（kg·min），血管加压素 0.03 U/min，维持窦性心律，心率 128 次 / 分，血压 88/42 mmHg。患者既往高血压病、2 型糖尿病病史，分别服用赖诺普利、二甲双胍控制病情。两种药物均在手术当天停止服用。患者转入 ICU 后立即进行诊断性试验并在治疗方案中增加药物。几小时后，患者血流动力学平稳，停用血管升压药。

问题分析

定义

肾上腺功能不全（adrenal insufficiency，AI）是一种相对罕见但可能危及生命的疾病，可能并无症状，但在诸如脓毒症、创伤性损伤、出血性休克或外科手术应激时表现出来。

1855 年，Thomas Addison 提出原发性 AI。大约一个世纪后，Harvey Cushing 提出了继发性 AI 的概念。原发性和继发性 AI 的病因见框 1.1。

下丘脑–垂体–肾上腺皮质（hypothalamic-pituitary-adrenocortical, HPA）轴（图 1.1）调节肾上腺释放皮质醇的量。该循环始于下丘脑释放促肾上腺皮质激素释放因子（corticotropin-releasing factor，CRF），CRF 刺激腺垂体（垂体前叶）释放促肾上腺皮质激素（adrenoco-rticotropic hormone，ACTH）。随后 ACTH 刺激肾上腺皮质以每天 20 mg 的速度释放皮质醇。皮质醇（或合成类似物）抑制下丘脑释放 CRF，抑制垂体前叶释放 ACTH。皮质醇释放有昼夜节律性，上午和午后达峰值，随后逐渐下降，夜间达低谷。尽管成人皮质醇（或氢化可的松）的正常分泌量为 5 ～ 10 mg/m^2，但在急性应激期间，肾上腺皮质 24 h 分泌量可高达 100 mg/m^2。

原发性 AI 比较罕见，由肾上腺破坏或手术切除引起。病因包括自身免疫性原因、创伤、出血、感染、浸润性疾病或手术切除。继发性 AI 继发于任何影响下丘脑或垂体功能及干扰 CRF 和（或）ACTH 的分泌的因素。急性或慢性糖皮质激素治疗后，肾上腺萎缩可能导致三发性肾上腺功能不全。肾上腺萎缩的患者可能无肾上腺功能不全的症状；然而，当患者处于即使是在轻度手术或急性疾病的应激状态，可能会出现危及生命的 AI 症状。

AI 除了分为原发性和继发性，又可分为绝对性或相对性。例如，肾上腺自身免疫破坏引起的典型艾迪生病是原发性、绝对性 AI。相反，由于相对性 AI，某些患者在致命性疾病（如脓毒症）时由正常应激引起的皮质醇生成增加的反应则可能被削弱。或者，尽管正常应激诱导的类固醇生成增加，但与皮质醇结合和肾上腺素能受体可能下调，这是相对

框 1.1 肾上腺功能不全的病因

原发性肾上腺功能不全
- 自身免疫性

多腺体自身免疫综合征 I 或 II
- 感染性
- 结核
- 组织胞浆菌病
- 芽生菌病
- 球孢子菌病
- 隐球菌病
- 人免疫缺陷病毒
- 巨细胞病毒
- 鸟-胞内分枝杆菌
- 隐球菌
- 弓形体病
- Kaposi 肉瘤

纤维化

梗死

肾上腺出血
- 沃-弗综合征
- 狼疮抗凝物
- 抗磷脂抗体
- 免疫性血小板减少性紫癜
- 肝素诱导
- 血小板减少症
- 抗凝剂

肿瘤转移
- 肺
- 胃
- 乳腺
- 恶性黑色素瘤
- 淋巴瘤

药物
- 类固醇合成抑制剂
  - 美替拉酮
  - 氨鲁米特（氨苯哌酮）
  - 米托坦
  - 依托咪酯*
  - 酮康唑
- 促类固醇分解代谢剂
  - 利福平
  - 苯妥英钠
  - 苯巴比妥钠

家族遗传
- 家族性糖皮质激素缺乏
- 肾上腺脑白质营养不良
- 肾上腺脊髓神经病

医源性
- 双侧肾上腺切除
- 双侧肾上腺栓塞

继发性肾上腺功能不全

外源性补充类固醇（通常称为三发性或医源性）

垂体或下丘脑疾病
- 浸润性肿瘤（腺瘤）
- 肉瘤
- 出血
- 自身免疫

孤立性 ACTH 缺乏

手术
- 垂体手术
- 肾上腺功能性腺瘤切除术

* 尚未证实，为推测性的

ACTH，促肾上腺皮质激素

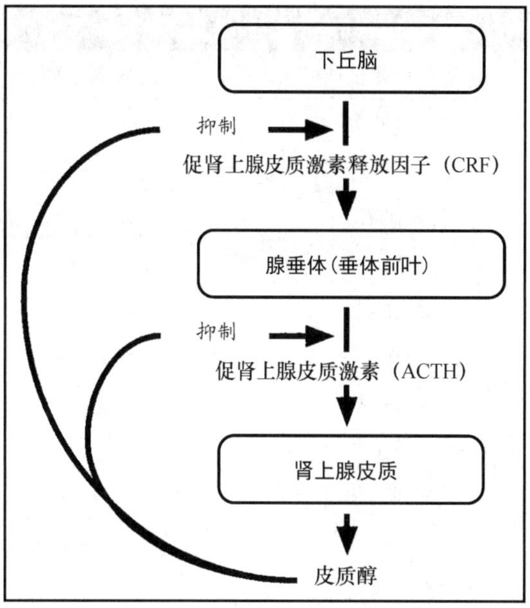

图 1.1 下丘脑-垂体-肾上腺皮质轴

性 AI 的另一个解释。依托咪酯可短暂抑制正常肾上腺皮质激素的生成（框 1.1），可能会导致危重患者发生相对性 AI。鉴于其对危重患者生存率存在有害影响，依托咪酯持续输注不再应用于危重患者的镇静。最后，如本病例概要所述，相对性 AI 可能会引起危及生命的血流动力学不平稳。然而，如果正确诊断并给予应激剂量的糖皮质激素，此过程可能会被逆转。

识别

急性 AI 的表现多样，可为患者无应激状态时几天内逐渐起病，或在重大应激状态下，如手术、创伤或感染时发生突然性血压下降。与 AI 相关的低血压可表现为严重难治性低血压。慢性 AI 发病过程中，症状隐匿，非特异性，通常数月内无明确诊断。AI 的症状、体征详见表 1.1。原发性 AI 最明显的症状为皮肤和黏膜表面色素沉着，这是由皮质醇降低反馈性导致的促肾上腺皮质激素水平过高所致。

由于原发性 AI（艾迪生病）是肾上腺自身功能衰竭所致，因此存在糖皮质激素和盐皮质激素均缺乏的证据。继发性 AI 是由于刺激肾上腺分泌皮质醇的 HPA 轴中断所致，而与肾上腺自身无关，表现为单纯的糖皮质激素缺乏。本病例中患者可能存在低钠血症；这与钠排泄无关，而与因抗利尿激素升高而引起的水中毒及糖皮质激素缺乏相关的原发性游离水排泄障碍有关。

表 1.1 慢性肾上腺功能不全症状和体征的患病率

症状和体征	患病率（%）
虚弱和疲劳	74 ～ 100
体重减轻	56 ～ 100
色素沉着	92 ～ 96
高血压	59 ～ 88
低钠血症	88 ～ 96
高钾血症	52 ～ 64
胃肠道症状	56
体位性头晕	12
肾上腺钙化	9 ～ 33
高钙血症	6 ～ 41
肌肉和关节疼痛	6
白癜风	4

Dafa from De Rosa G，Corsello SM，Cecchin L，et al：Clinical study of Addison's disease. *Exp Clin Endocrinol* 90：232-242，1987.

低血压是慢性和急性 AI 常见症状。据报道，急性 AI 所致的低血压表现为高排血量循环衰竭，其特点是心排血量和心指数升高，肺动脉楔压降低或正常，体循环阻力降低。这种低血压的发病机制尚不清楚，但可能包括三种作用机制：①糖皮质激素对血管平滑肌直接作用的损害；②糖皮质激素对儿茶酚胺合成和作用的“允许作用”消失；③糖皮质激素对血管活性肽的作用减弱。脱水也是急性和慢性 AI 相关性低血压的一个因素。

风险评估

患者合并诸如哮喘、炎症性肠病、胶原血管疾病和类风湿性关节炎等疾病，1 年内可能接受类固醇治疗，相对小剂量外源性类固醇应用 7 ～ 10 天可抑制 HPA 轴。除了小剂量强的松（<5 mg/d）和隔日方案外，长期服用皮质类固醇会抑制 HPA 轴，其功能恢复可长达 12 个月。垂体功能首先恢复正常，然后肾上腺皮质功能逐渐恢复。

有文献报道围术期 AI 的发生率为 0.01% ～ 0.7%。Rivers 等报道老年患者合并相对性 AI 的风险更大。脓毒性休克合并 AI 的发生率也较高，类固醇替代疗法能显著改善某些患者的预后。2013 年脓毒症救治指南指出，在成人脓毒性休克的治疗中，如果足够的液体复苏和升压药物可以恢复血流动力学的稳定性，不建议静脉使用氢化可的松；如果不能维持血流动力学稳定，建议单独静脉使用氢化可的松每天 200 mg，无需进一步测试。

尽管有大量的病例报告 AI 可导致低血压甚至是死亡，但也有许多文献报道长期接受糖皮质激素治疗的患者，在围术期没有接受超应激剂量糖皮质激素的情况下接受各种手术。大部分患者围术期无异常，可能是因为其围术期 HPA 功能生化指标正常。这表明仅以据糖皮质激素用药史进行病史评估并不可靠。

既往观点认为，对怀疑肾上腺功能衰竭的患者必须进行内分泌评估。急诊应激情况下，随机筛查皮质醇水平 <25 μg/dl 被认为不正常。疾病性应激或手术性应激时低水平皮质醇（<25 μg/dl）需要进一步评估。严重创伤和手术应激时血浆皮质醇水平通常升高 2 ～ 3 倍，应激后 4 ～ 5 天恢复正常水平。如果出现并发症，皮质醇水平可能会持续升高。

一直以来，促肾上腺皮质激素刺激试验是评估危重患者肾上腺功能的“金标准”。然而，如果怀疑存在危及生命的 AI，特别是在难治性脓毒性休克中，可不进行试验即开始治疗。静脉注射 ACTH 250 μg 30 min、60 min 后，检测皮质醇水平并与基础水平进行比较。对于这些试验的解读及试验中使用 ACTH 的剂量均存在争议。正因如此，许多专家认为，如果强烈怀疑存在危及生命的 AI，则不应因诊断试验而延迟治疗。应用地塞米松进行糖皮质激素覆盖时，不影响 ACTH 的试验。

启示

急性肾上腺危象可以自发发生，也可以在重大情绪或生理应激下发生。应激源可能包括极度的心理应激、创伤、酒精或阿片类药物戒断、感染、全身麻醉或手术。在这些应激下，患者无法分泌足量的皮质醇来维持血流动力学的平稳。

管理

由于 AI 进展迅速，因此早诊断早治疗对于改善预后至关重要。肾上腺危象是一种内科急症，不能因大量的诊断性检查而延迟治疗。治疗的方向是迅速增加循环中的皮质醇水平。如果没有这样的治疗，即使针对血容量不足和电解质失衡进行对症治疗也是无效的。

如果怀疑存在 AI，则分析血清电解质、全血细胞计数、血糖、血尿素氮和肌酐，以评估是否存在低钠血症、高钾血症和低血糖。

肾上腺危象期间，患者可失去 20% 的循环血管内容量。这可能导致低血容量休克和组织低灌注，这两者都会导致乳酸酸血症。因此，应开始快速静脉输液以纠正脱水和低血容量。生理盐水是首选的液体。随后可通过实验室检查及患者对治疗的反应来指导电解质失衡、容量不足和低血糖的治疗。

如果已知患者存在 AI，应根据手术大小及医源性应激对患者进行个体化替代治疗。对于拟行重大手术或有危及生命的创伤或疾病的高危患者，可给予氢化可的松 100 mg，每 6 ～ 8 h 静脉追加剂量为 50 ～ 100 mg（见第 25 章）。随着患者临床状况改善，通常剂量会迅速减小。如果患者没有明确 AI 病史，可静脉给予地塞米松 4 ～ 10 mg。地塞米松不影响血清皮质醇水平的测定，因此仍可进行诊断试验。然而，由于地塞米松没有醛固酮活性，可能需应用氟氢可的松，一种口服盐皮质激素，但它可能干扰血清皮质醇测定准确性。

患者通常对最初的治疗反应迅速，通常在几小时内得到改善。高达 70% 的脓毒性休克患者存在肾上腺功能障碍，20% 的患者的预后会因替代治疗明显改善。最后，40% ～ 65% 的危重症患者血浆肾素活性较高，既往建议不包括使用盐皮质激素。根据最近的数据，目前专家建议脓毒症诱发的相对性 AI 患者可给予氟氢可的松≥ 50 μg/d 口服或纳肛。

预防

疑似肾上腺功能受抑制的应激患者有多种治疗方法。有研究建议根据应激大小调整氢化可的松的剂量。其他研究则主张对 AI 高危患者进行 HPA 轴试验。可应用 ACTH 刺激试验来完成的，既简单又安全。然而，关于试验解读及 ACTH 应用剂量存在争议。有人主张使用生理剂量（例如 1 μg），而不是目前推荐的 250 μg。大多数应激患者应用类固醇的风险很小，因此建议任何 AI 高危患者均应使用应激剂量类固醇。因为极度应激下的皮质醇分泌量可高达每天 200 mg，可每 6 h 静脉注射氢化可的松 50 mg，持续 2 天，或静脉持续输注氢化可的松每天 200 mg，持续 2 天（见第 25 章）。在没有持续应激的情况下，氢化可的松剂量可减为每 8 h 50 mg，持续 1 ～ 2 天，随后停药；或继续每 8 h 25 mg，持续 1 ～ 2 天，然后停药。必须根据患者具体情况来确定类固醇如何减量，这取决于可能出现肾上腺功能抑制患者的应激程度及持续时间。最后，有报告指出，长期 AI 治疗时根据体重使用药物剂量预后较好。

（蒲君涔　译　樊玉花　校）

延伸阅读

Bancos I, Hahner S, Tomlinson J, et al.: Diagnosis and management of adrenal insufficiency, *Lancet Diabetes Endocrinol* 3:216–226, 2015.

Boonen E, Bornstein SR, Van den Berghe G: New insights into the controversy of adrenal function during critical illness, *Lancet Diabetes Endocrinol* 10:805–815, 2015.

Connery LE, Coursin DB: Assessment and therapy of selected endocrine disorders, *Anesthesiol Clin North Am* 22:93–123, 2004.

Coursin DB, Wood KE: Corticosteroid supplementation in adrenal insufficiency, *JAMA* 287:236–240, 2002.

Eichacker PQ, Parent C, Kalil A, et al.: Risk and the efficacy of anti-inflammatory agents: retrospective and confirmatory studies of sepsis, *Am J Respir Crit Care Med* 9:1197–1205, 2002.

Garcia JE, Hill GE, Joshi GP: Perioperative stress dose steroids: is it really necessary? *Am Soc Anesthesiologists Newsletter* 77(11):32–35, 2013.

Holmes CL, Walley KK: The evaluation and management of shock, *Clin Chest Med* 24:775–789, 2003.

Mah PM, Jenkins RC, Rostami-Hodjegan A: Weight-related dosing, timing and monitoring hydrocortisone replacement therapy in patients with adrenal insufficiency, *Clin Endocrinol* 61:367–375, 2004.

Minneci PC, Deans KJ, Banks SM, et al.: Meta-analysis: the effect of steroids on survival and shock during sepsis depends on the dose, *Ann Intern Med* 1:47–56, 2004.

Oelkers W: Adrenal insufficiency, *N Engl J Med* 335:1206–1211, 1996.

Rivers EP, Gaspari M, Saad GA, et al.: Adrenal insufficiency in high-risk surgical ICU patients, *Chest* 119:889–896, 2001.

第2章 阿尔茨海默病

Robert A. Whittington，Roderic G. Eckenhoff

病例概要

患者，女性，78岁，在家里独立生活时摔倒并造成髋部骨折被收治入院，既往病史仅有高血压，服用氢氯噻嗪。择期髋关节置换术，手术时间3 h，异氟烷气管插管全身麻醉，无手术相关并发症。术中中度失血（900 ml），但没有发生低血压或低氧血症。拔管后，在术后麻醉恢复室（PACU）被发现发生谵妄。在接下来的24～36 h里，谵妄时有发生，并在术后第5天出院进入康复机构。患者康复治疗困难，工作人员记录到其患有抑郁、健忘和注意力不集中。患者家人形容其与摔倒前"非常不同"，尽管他们承认患者似曾"有一点健忘"。目前患者已出院回家，日常生活无法自理，并被转移到一家辅助护理机构。6个月后这种情况依然没有任何改善，经一位老年神经内科医师的正式评估，包括行腰椎穿刺脑脊液（cerebrospinal fluid，CSF）测生物标志物，患者被诊断为阿尔茨海默型痴呆症。

问题分析

识别

认知功能问题是老年患者在接受手术时常见的并存疾病，其中最常见的是与年龄有关的神经退行性疾病。此类疾病有很多，且存在神经病理学和症状学的重叠，但阿尔茨海默病（Alzheimer's disease，AD）最为常见。65岁以上的美国人中约有10%患有AD，其中30%是85岁以上的老年患者。目前认为，这种疾病的神经病理学改变在疾病被诊断前20多年即已开始。例如，在早期阶段，淀粉样β蛋白开始在大脑特定区域细胞外聚集。这可能会在数年内缓慢发生，并逐渐耗尽CSF循环中的水平，从而构成AD主要诊断检测的依据之一。在某些阶段，淀粉样病变开始促进tau蛋白从微管脱离，聚集成细胞内的细丝，称为神经纤维缠结。后一个过程似乎比淀粉样病变更具有细胞毒性，并与神经炎症增强和细胞丢失（神经退行性变）有关。过量的tau蛋白，可能是从濒临死亡的神经元中释放出来的，最终在CSF中形成了CSF诊断检测的其他特征。只有在此后期，当有明显的tau蛋白病变和大量的细胞丢失时，磁共振扫描显示皮质和海马灰质层变薄，认知能力的变化才能表现得明显。

认知功能的变化最初发生在记忆和执行功能上，但随着神经退行性变的进展，可扩展到其他范围和感觉功能。临床上，AD分为两个主要阶段：轻度认知损害（mild cognitive impairment，MCI）（DSM-5中称为**轻度神经认知障碍**）和阿尔茨海默病（AD）或痴呆（DSM-5中称为**严重神经认知障碍**）。这些阶段中的每一个阶段在很大程度上都是基于生物标志物的最新进展而进一步划分的。目前诊断和分期的依据有三种主要模式：神经心理学测试、CSF生物标志物和淀粉样正电子发射断层扫描（positron emission tomography，PET）。在不久的将来，新的成像形式（如tau）和基于血液的生物标记物也有可能将大大促进诊断和分期。

该病例描述了"迟发型"或偶发型AD的进展，但在30～50岁的人群中观察到一种更为罕见的形式，大多数是由于淀粉样蛋白通路中一些元素的特定突变。散发型AD的早期加速还存在其他遗传危险因素，最显著的是ApoE ε4等位基因。

对于神经退行性疾病在围术期主要存在两种担忧。第一种是神经退行性变患者所需管理方式的改变，第二种是围术期对疾病神经病理学轨迹的影响。

管理

术前

第一个问题涉及知情同意。如果患者已经被诊断为 AD 或严重神经认知障碍（major neurocognitive disorder，NCD），则须征得配偶、家庭成员或其他授权照顾者的同意。然而，大量的患者会被诊断为 MCI 或轻度 NCD，或者是仅仅为未确诊。在试图获得 AD 患者的知情同意之前，麻醉科医师必须确保此操作之前所有容易纠正的听力和视力缺陷已得到治疗。可以考虑对所有 65 岁以上的患者进行筛查评估，尽管目前很少这样做。如诊断所示，对未通过筛检的患者应进行更全面的评估，并按照诊断指示取得同意。关于之前的认知功能的信息也是至关重要的，因为它已经被发现是谵妄和术后 NCD 最强有力的预测指标。如果时间允许，**预适应训练**的概念（锻炼、营养和社会化的项目）可能对优化认知和功能结果均有益。应继续使用包括胆碱酯酶抑制剂（多奈哌齐、加兰他敏和卡巴拉汀）和（或）美金刚胺在内的药物。

此外，许多这样的患者接受各种抗抑郁药、抗精神病药、抗痉挛药和情绪稳定药物治疗并不少见。因此，鉴于这些患者多重用药的可能性很高，麻醉科医师必须考虑这些药物与围术期使用的各种麻醉药、镇静药和其他辅助药物之间的相互作用。

术中

在手术中，尽管有证据表明全凭静脉麻醉导致认知功能障碍的风险更小，但关于最佳麻醉方案的证据尚不足。AD 患者被认为对所有麻醉药都比较敏感，尽管几乎没有设计严谨的研究。脑电图对镇静深度的监测意义仍有争议，但许多研究表明，避免麻醉过深可减少谵妄和术后神经认知障碍。应避免使用的药物包括苯二氮䓬类、苯海拉明、某些精神药物（如氟哌啶醇）和中枢抗胆碱能药物。如果需要使用镇静药，α_2 肾上腺素激动剂右美托咪啶可能更佳。由于神经退行性变发生机制可能是神经性炎症，因此已有临床试验测试过地塞米松等抗炎药物，但没有任何有益的证据。

因为这些患者缺乏储备和代偿能力，所以避免异常生理状态（血流动力学、气体交换、代谢、低温）可能更为关键。一些研究者主张为此类患者使用脑氧饱和度或血流动力学监测直至手术结束。应避免发生低体温，因为其可增强麻醉的中枢神经系统抑制作用；临床前研究表明，低温可以增加 tau 蛋白磷酸化，甚至可能加速神经原纤维的病变。

术后

术后积极运动、恢复感觉（如眼镜、助听器）、恢复社交活动（如家庭成员）、保证睡眠和营养被认为能加速恢复正常的功能和认知活动。有术前认知障碍的患者最需要此类干预。除恢复术前生活规则外，其他有益的药理学干预措施尚未见报道。目前已有尽量减少谵妄的治疗方案，并应尽可能遵循。

围术期对神经退行性变轨迹的影响

前面的讨论主要涉及对神经退行性疾病患者的围术期管理。另一个需要讨论的方面：围术期本身是否是加速 AD 随后进展的风险因素？这仍然是一个存在争议的公开话题。在过去的十年里，有持续增加的在体和离体临床前试验证据表明，麻醉和手术均能独立地影响前文提到的淀粉样蛋白、tau 蛋白和凋亡途径。

尽管有这些临床前证据，目前还没有明确的高水平流行病学证据表明麻醉和外科手术会实际导致人群中 AD 随后的进展。事实上，关于这一话题的文献主要为多项回顾性研究，这些研究既支持又否定了手术和麻醉与随后的 AD 之间的关联。应谨慎地解读这些临床数据，因为这些研究中有许多研究统计效能低、缺乏随机性、数量充足、匹配良好的对照组。

尽管如此，仍有一些小规模的前瞻性临床研究显示了术后 CSF 中 Aβ 和 tau 蛋白水平的变化；此外，其中一些生物标志物的改变已被证明类似于已知 AD 患者的水平。当然，这些研究与前文提到的研究存在相同的不足，因此临床相关性仍然不确定。尽管如此，可预期的生物标记技术的进步将使麻醉和手术暴露对 AD 进展的影响得以确定。

除了之前提及的知情同意问题，还有一个额外的问题是，是否要告知患者和他们的家人，经历围术期实际上可能会使他们的认知能力恶化。虽然持续的（超过 3 个月）认知能力下降的证据并不充分，但它可能比许多患者通常被告知的风险更有可能发生，例如卒中、心肌梗死和死亡。因此，我们认为应预先告知患者及其家属术后认知能力可能下降，原因是多因素的且尚不清楚，但在大多数情况下，它会在数周到数月内好转。

总之，MCI 或阿尔茨海默病患者对围术期管理是重大挑战。至少应常规对 65 岁以上的患者进行认知筛查评估，并应告知所有患者术后发生认知障碍的风险。患有神经退行性疾病的患者，易受围术期管理的许多方面的影响，尤其易产生术后谵妄和其他认知障碍，应在术后积极让患者恢复运动和再定向。尚无特异性的术中措施或药物被 1 级证据证实为最佳做法。

（王 春 译 刘 征 校）

延伸阅读

Berger M, Burke J, Eckenhoff RG, Mathew J: Alzheimer's disease, anesthesia, and surgery: a clinically focused review, *J Cardiothorac Vasc Anesth* 28(6):1609–1623, 2014.

Papon MA, Whittington RA, El-Khoury NB, Planel E: Alzheimer's disease and anesthesia, *Front Neurosci* 4:272, 2011.

Terrando N, Eriksson L, Eckenhoff RG: Perioperative neurotoxicity in the elderly: report of the 4th International Workshop, *Anesth Analg* 120(3):649–652, 2015.

Whittington RA, Bretteville A, Dickler MF, et al.: Anesthesia and tau pathology, *Prog Neuropsychopharmacol Biol Psychiatry* 47:147–155, 2013.

药物依赖：非阿片类药物 第3章

Mark S. Gold，William S. Jacobs

病例概要

酒精

P医生，男性，60岁，白人麻醉科医师，有40年酗酒史。5年前的一天，在早上8：00工作开始前，同事质疑他呼吸中有酒精气味。他随即做了血液酒精浓度测定，结果低于可检测到的范围，他继续工作。2年后，手术室同事再次闻到他的呼吸中有酒精气味，这次他的血液酒精浓度值为0.12。P医生否认午夜后喝酒，只承认晚上之前喝了含伏特加的汤尼水。根据医生健康项目（physician's health program，PHP）规定，他接受了一名美国成瘾研究会授权的医师评估。P医生顺利地完成了门诊检查流程，并与PHP签订监管协议。他积极参加促进康复的团队会，也参加了12-步骤的见面会（12-step meetings），但没有得到一名保证人的帮助，未能按照这12-步骤要求去做。直到1个月前他的随机尿检均为阴性。在他妻子辞职的那个晚上，P医生喝了三杯酒，第二天早上他被随机抽查做尿检。在阳性结果出来之前他就告知了PHP他戒酒失败。

烟草

K医生，男性，62岁，白人麻醉科医师，抽烟100年包。他从12岁开始每天抽烟2包，至少在12年前他就被诊断为慢性支气管炎和慢性阻塞性肺疾病。他做了大量的尝试来戒烟，包括突然戒烟、催眠和尼古丁补充法，结果都失败了。现在他认为自己年龄太大了，不能完成戒烟这件事。上个星期他在手术室的湿滑地面上摔了一跤，并撞在了麻醉机上。他的左侧胸壁撞击部位疼痛，胸片上显示右肺上叶有一个空洞损伤。

大麻

B医生，男性，28岁，黑人麻醉科医师，通过了大学常规的麻醉科医师培养计划，在完成了住院总培训后，就职于一家有名的私人诊所。他很快成为外科医师和手术室同事中受欢迎的人。很多次有人看见他在下班的路上抽雪茄。工作了6个月后，他买了一台价值10万美金的新车。周五他完成工作后离开医院，警察看到他的车停在了路边，车中发现大麻和吸毒工具，他因行为失检而被逮捕。B医生被查获了6支大麻烟卷。通过调查他的伴侣，事情在24 h后弄清，他有两个选择，要么自己向州PHP汇报，要么由他的伴侣向州医学委员会汇报。他被确定为长期多种药物依赖史，进展为大麻依赖和酗酒。他将进行一个长期住院治疗，并签订为期5年的PHP监管协定。他的行医资格在治疗后被暂停了2年，之后才恢复到正常状态。在完成住院治疗之后他回到私人诊所继续工作。

可卡因

W医生，男性，44岁，白人麻醉科医师，有人看见他在医院圣诞派对期间，在洗手间吸食疑为可卡因的白色粉状物，并上报了PHP。在派对后两天的约谈中，他否认吸毒。他被要求立即做尿液药检，他勉强同意。结果苯甲酮阳性，这是可卡因代谢产物。从报告至PHP起，他就被停职，在由戒毒医师做了评估后，他被收入院进行戒毒治疗。在成功地完成正规治疗方案后，他获得州PHP为期5年的监管和申辩协议。

问题分析

定义

非阿片类药物滥用和依赖常见于医务人员，其中酒精和烟草是最常见的滥用物，但在普通人群中最常见的违禁品却是大麻。

众所周知，烟草、酒精和大麻是医生中最常见的滥用物。医师酒精依赖的发生率与和他们年龄、性别、社会经济地位相匹配的人群一样。烟草滥用常见于医学院的大学生和低年资医师，不过，随着婴儿潮这一代人的年龄增大，以及近期烟草相关州法律改变，年长医师抽烟比例上升。酒精依赖在年长医师中更常见。尽管滥用其他违禁品、非违禁品（例如可卡因）不是那么流行，但可导致明显的损害，并对医疗卫生行业从业者、他们的患者及其家庭产生不良影响。尽管医生和其他医疗卫生从业人员吸毒、滥用处方药也是个问题，但在此不展开讨论。

药物依赖可导致大量不良影响，包括严重的医疗和法律上的问题。化学物质依赖会产生与急性中毒、觅毒行为、慢性依赖和戒断反应相关的功能损害。本章节，我们重点讨论非阿片类药物依赖，主要为酒精、烟草、大麻和可卡因，我们也谈谈与药物依赖相关的行为表现、诊断及其启示，以及对药物依赖的预防和治疗。

识别和风险评估

诊断

数项实验室检查用于诊断药物成瘾，比如检测酒精成瘾的CAGE和AUDIT项目，这些现在被修改后也用于检测大麻成瘾。药物成瘾的临床诊断常常很困难，因为否认和欺骗是成瘾表现之一，病史采集时“否认”具有标志性意义。医师承认用过某些物质，但只是偶尔使用。他们会引用《纽约日报》《时代周刊》上的报道为自己辩解，对权威的医学、药物成瘾及精神病学书籍和期刊上的内容却持反对意见。他们可能辩解吸食大麻对身体无害，吸食大麻与抽烟和吸二手烟不同。医疗卫生行业从业人员，被人发现吸食药物、持有药物、不当获取药物、出现中毒或戒断症状和体征可有助于对其做出诊断。药物成瘾的诊断要根据《精神疾病诊断和统计手册（第5版）》（DSM-5）。病史、体格检查和实验室确诊有助于诊断。尽管有很多其他因素，如个性、家庭问题、不育（男性）、不参加社交活动以及没有行使个人职责的能力都会引起类似于药物依赖的临床表现，但实验室检测结果阳性将药物滥用列于鉴别诊断的首位。

医师自己很少会因药物滥用或依赖问题向药物成瘾专家汇报。实验室检查是诊断成瘾的金标准并且对治疗过程也有帮助。然而药物检查并不能检查出所有大麻、可卡因及其他违禁药物使用者。随机抽查也不能查出所有药物滥用以及较少使用者。例如，对每天都使用违禁药物的人每年八次尿检，任何一个月尿检阳性率也只有约50%。尿检是评估和治疗药物滥用的标准，常用药物尿液检出时间见表3.1。现在还可检测其他身体物质，比如头发、指甲、汗液和唾液。薄层色谱法和酶联抗体法检测最全面，又便宜，已广泛应用于药物筛选检查，而气相色谱法和质谱法是确定化学药物种类的金标准。大麻损害的诊断必须通过检测血液中四氢大麻酚（tetrahydrocannabinol，THC）浓度来确定，因为通常对大麻制品的筛查是通过检测THC代谢物，此代谢物在规律吸食大麻后数周仍可呈阳性。酒精检出时间窗从数小时到数天，是通过检测尿液中的酒精代谢物乙基葡萄糖醛酸酐和硫化乙烷来完成的。随机尿检应当成为医务工作者健康计划的强制执行部分。

实验室检查亦可有助于对慢性药物依赖问题的诊断，但常常是在病程晚期才做。严重酗酒（如一天一瓶葡萄酒）连续几个月便可导致巨红细胞症（平均红血球体积在100～110 fl），可先于贫血发生。酒精相关的肝损害表现为异常的血浆γ-谷氨酰转移酶、天冬氨酸转氨酶和丙氨酸转氨酶。事实上，和其他肝疾病不同，发生酒精性肝炎时天冬氨

表3.1 药物在尿液中的检出时间

药物	检出时间
安非他命	24 h内
巴比妥类药物	5～10天
苯二氮䓬类药物	5～7天
大麻素类	1～3天；长期使用者时间更久
可卡因	1～3天
阿片类	1～3天
苯环己哌啶	3天内

酸转氨酶是丙氨酸转氨酶的两倍以上。食品药品管理局批准了通过检测血浆碳水化合物缺乏转铁蛋白以确定长期过量饮酒。

酒精和烟草

以下是酒精和烟草成瘾症状：

- 药物使用的自制力受损。
- 对获得药物的渴望。
- 虽然知道不良结果，但仍继续使用。
- 思维扭曲，特别表现为否认成瘾。
- 对药效出现耐受。
- 停药出现戒断症状。

尚无特异性的症状用于酗酒的明确诊断，与酗酒相一致的体格检查结果包括血压增高、摔倒或意外的身体伤害证据、震颤、阻塞性肺部疾病（同时有抽烟）、不明原因的心动过速、肝脾大以及外周神经疾病。与酒瘾相比较，烟瘾对身体的影响通常要积累多年，与原发肺癌和慢性肺部疾病有关。戒烟对身体的益处立竿见影，并随着时间推移进一步降低其产生的不良影响，并延长预期寿命（详见 http://www.cancer.org）。

可卡因

服用可卡因的大量临床和行为学的症状体征通常很明显，其中一些与急性中毒相关，另一些要到慢性期或戒毒时才会表现出来（表 3.2）。尽管可卡因是常见滥用药物，被称之为“街售滥用药物”，但是在医学上也用作表面麻醉剂和血管收缩剂（比如用于耳、鼻、喉的手术时行清醒经口或经鼻气管插管，或者极少用于复合丁卡因和肾上腺素行局部表面麻醉）。因此，与芬太尼及其他强效麻醉药一样，医务工作者更容易获得纯的可卡因。街头可卡因常常不纯，或者混入可能导致其他损害的成分。

大麻

20 世纪 60 年代和 70 年代，大麻被认为是安全、天然的药物，可以产生“欣快感”，但没有副作用和成瘾的风险。一些年轻医生也不相信大麻有成瘾可能，抽大麻多于抽香烟。大麻的成瘾与大麻烟中的四氢大麻酚（THC）浓度和抽大麻时间有关，大麻戒断症状可以通过服用 THC 拮抗剂引出。现在大麻中 THC 浓度提高后产生的欣快感更强烈，诱惑人们再次使用。哈佛大学和哥伦比亚大学的研究者发现效能增强后，长期吸食大麻者会产生耐受、依赖（甚至非人类的动物也会产生 THC 依赖）和明确的戒断症状，这些症状的高峰在停止吸食后数周才会出现。现在大麻被认为是对人类具有成瘾、需对其成瘾进行治疗的物质。

DSM-5 定义，大麻中毒首先有“欣快感”，表现多样，通常包括夸大、欣快和傻笑。吸食大麻急性期表现为专注和复杂思维困难、感觉和时间知觉错乱、漠然和镇静、判断力受损、记忆（特别是近期记忆）以及运动行为受损。吸食大麻有时会引起焦虑和惊恐，这是需要治疗的。在中毒期和中毒期之后，常有食欲增强、红眼、口干和心率增快。高效能的大麻被认为与第一次精神病的发生有关，也明显增加一生中发生精神疾病的风险。随着这些作用退去，吸食者常常出现情绪抑郁、发怒、暴躁甚至脱离社会。在临床试验中，大麻油对顽固性的小

表 3.2 急性可卡因中毒和慢性滥用及依赖的症状和体征

急性可卡因中毒		慢性可卡因滥用或依赖	
表现	临床症状	体格和精神症状	行为和社会性行为
社交能力：低剂量时多	血压改变	焦虑、谵妄、抑郁、幻觉、失眠、记忆减退、精神错	车船意外
表现为过于爱“说话”	呼吸困难	乱、言语不清、生理反射改变、一过性黑矇、急性视	家庭或工作出现问题
过于警觉	瞳孔扩大	力改变，共济失调、眩晕、震颤、阳痿	（如：办事拖拉、旷工）
判断力受损	精神错乱	高血压、心律不齐、心动过缓	法律或财务问题
想法和计划极度夸大	肌无力	支气管炎、迁延不愈的感冒和流感症状、频繁的呼吸	对毒品依赖增加
过度焦虑、紧张	心动过速、胸痛	道感染	被动攻击行为、自杀
情绪变化快	恶心或呕吐	因摔倒而导致的肿块和擦伤	的想法或姿势、暴力
性欲增强	精神运动性激躁或	寻找或回避毒品、食欲减退、营养不良、肝脏肿大	或攻击行为、多疑
	迟缓，癫痫	酒精或毒品的耐受力增强或减弱	
	出汗或战栗	脸部红肿；鼻黏膜红肿	

儿癫痫发作和精神病治疗有效。吸食大麻对健康的长期影响难以确定，因为吸食大麻的人经常同时也使用烟草产品。近期研究表明，大麻烟中有大量致癌物，其焦油和致癌物水平都要高出烟草 50%。病例对照研究也指出头颈部肿瘤与吸食大麻有关。

依赖大麻的人一般每天都吸食，持续几个月或几年。尝试停吸常常超不过 30 天。若被问到大麻问题他们很容易发怒，因为他们已经患有毒品所致的精神疾病。通常这对他们的健康、家庭和事业都有不良影响。另外，他们会以可以得到大麻为基础选择派对、社交或朋友，每天都会用大量的时间考虑吸食大麻以及从其作用中恢复过来。他们还试图通过抽烟和使用神经兴奋药来逆转大麻对记忆和行为的影响。药物依赖妨碍了家庭生活和工作，虽然会导致一些长期问题的出现，比如吸烟者的咳嗽和心理问题（例如，反复使用大剂量毒品导致过度镇静、焦虑或惊恐、甚至精神异常），以及社会和法律问题，但仍会继续使用这些药品。

启示

药物依赖常首先表现为不良行为问题。但是直到药物成瘾被确定，不良行为才被认为是由于药物滥用所致。医务人员常常比其他行业的人更善于隐藏和否认药物滥用情况。更多见的是，与吸毒相关的家庭、社会问题的发生远早于在工作中出现的问题。滥用药物的医务人员常出现情绪、体能和专注能力的改变。他们会耽误工作或迟到。他们会经常使用药物，在不恰当的时间，或更加频繁地要求休息。另外，他们呼出气体中常有酒精味，或者烟草或大麻的味道。通常其家人和朋友比患者和同事更早发现医务工作者觅毒、取毒和吸毒行为。

药物依赖的医务人员常常在人际关系方面出现问题，他们在医疗资质和许可以及犯罪调查方面具有较高的职业风险。他们常因非法性交易或与赌博、买毒相关的经济问题而被注意。但是这些是后期的行为。想要早期发现药物依赖的医务人员需要在工作场所和家庭高度怀疑他们的行为。药物依赖者的工作表现越来越差在最后才表现出来，医务人员凭借此否认他们存在药物依赖的问题。药物滥用常见严重影响包括交通事故、头部损伤、记忆力衰退、财务危机、性传播疾病、癫痫、抑郁、冲动、自杀念头以及自杀企图。

几乎所有药物滥用停药时都有不良影响（如兴趣缺失）、抑郁以及焦虑。某种药物特有的戒断症状可能是另一种药物长期使用、依赖的表现。戒断期间对药物的渴望是最强烈的，因为成瘾的人希望减轻难受的戒断症状。滥用或者已有依赖性的医务人员发生抑郁的概率较高，如果不进行干涉或治疗会导致自杀。

酒精和烟草

酒精和烟草是使用最普遍的成瘾物。酒精常被认为是安全的，适度饮用甚至对身体有益。而对于烟草却没有明确的适度与安全的说法。抽烟的人常常也饮酒，酗酒的人常常也抽烟，因此常常见到对酒精和烟草都依赖的人。抽烟是酒精中毒的人死亡的主要原因。酒精也有很强的影响力和危险性，饮酒比烟草以外的其他违禁品更易导致死亡和个人毁灭。每年，酗酒导致 10 万以上的人死亡，超过 200 万人受伤；每年因烟草直接致死的人数超过 40 万。

可卡因

对可卡因的病态需求极其强烈，许多专家一致认为它是违禁品中诱惑力最强的。针对戒断症状，医疗措施常常无效，临床表现为治疗中断，或者离开医院或其他严格管理的环境后就很难控制。渴求可卡因、快感缺失、无助的感觉、毒品趋向性可能导致复吸。动物自身给药模型显示，为了获得可卡因，动物能够承受并忍耐大量的工作和惩罚，这个现象在可卡因超过其他多数违禁品。

一旦成瘾的医生停止使用可卡因，就可开始治疗。我们已经报告了医生中有采取鼻吸可卡因、注射可卡因，甚至吸食可卡因的。可卡因成瘾性强，复吸很常见，因此 DSM 不得不修改诊断标准以在吸食者还没有明显的耐受和身体依赖的症状体征时就能及时诊断。医生成瘾者常要签署同意书，同意接受随机、至少两周一次的尿液检查，并住院治疗。

大麻

持有、吸食、种植以及购买大麻都是违反美国联邦法律的行为。打一两个电话就能让这样做的医生丢掉行医执照。但这很少发生。他们的配偶、儿女或愤怒的患者可能会打匿名举报电话报告他们的行为。吸食大麻的医生常常会进一步接触到其他违禁品，导致进一步的涉险。有时吸食大麻或使用其他违禁品会让医生牵涉到毒品交易或其他犯罪。不谙世事的医务人员在违禁品交易中常被勒索或抢劫。

管理

思维和行为的改变同时药检阳性，常是医院工作人员、医疗团体、州医生健康监测项目用来确诊药物滥用的确切依据。对于药物成瘾的医务人员来说，先用解毒剂治疗戒断症状，然后进入 12- 步骤见面会和治疗团体是首选的治疗方法。必须指出的是解毒或戒毒治疗并不够。针对药物成瘾的医务人员，还有许多特殊治疗方案。还有大量的药物可用于治疗酒精、烟草、大麻和可卡因依赖（表 3.3）。当成瘾的医生进行长期的随访同时接受应急管理、随机尿检、参加 12- 步骤见面会，以及针对个人的精神科医师和治疗辅助师的治疗，他才会获得最佳的治疗结局。

酒精和烟草

社会心理学和药物学治疗均可有助于克服酒精和烟草成瘾。其中一些药物可以在药店买到（比如尼古丁替代物），但是其他药物需要开处方。在美国有大量的药物被批准用于酒精成瘾药物治疗，包括戒酒硫（安塔布司）、纳曲酮和阿坎酸。

可卡因

可卡因依赖的治疗包括住院和门诊两种途径。

表 3.3 针对非阿片类药物成瘾的药物治疗

名称	药物治疗
酒精	戒酒硫（antabuse）——通过喝酒后产生疼痛症状来阻止喝酒
	纳曲酮——可能减少对酒精的渴望，可以降低饮酒后的愉悦感
	阿坎酸——减少对酒精的渴望和预防复发
烟草	尼古丁替代：口胶剂、贴剂、吸入剂、喷雾
	解毒剂：安非他酮（载班、丁氨苯丙酮）——最初用于抗抑郁，现在主要用于戒烟
大麻	治疗维持：屈大麻酚——在临床试验中
	拮抗剂：Rimonblat——在临床试验中
可卡因	确定性治疗药物：目前没有
	支持性药物：抗抑郁药、情绪稳定剂（如锂剂）

一种基本方法是行为干预。稳定以后，康复从学习改变旧的习惯，不再与吸毒的朋友联系，识别引起毒瘾发作的“触发点”做起，当识别了这些触发点后，患者就有信心重新建立生活方式来避开它们。认知-行为配合训练是另一种治疗，这能在短期内通过学习帮助成瘾者禁欲。这种治疗可以和一系列的其他治疗同时进行，比如药物治疗。积极地参加 12- 步骤计划，如麻醉品匿名者协会和可卡因匿名者协会，是使成瘾者远离可卡因或其他药物的最有效方法之一。对于药物成瘾的医务人员，经常接受随机药物检查，长期随访将有助于治疗的成功。任何药检阳性结果必须立即明确，并且要立即对治疗方案进行调整。等待只会导致治疗迅速、完全地失败。最后，可卡因禁用和长期使用可卡因都会导致抑郁、自杀倾向、自杀行为，因此可卡因依赖的医生必须被严密看护。

大麻

治疗的研究包括使用合成大麻碱类（屈大麻酚）。这类似于给海洛因成瘾者使用美沙酮。大麻二酚可能对缓解戒断症状有效。大麻成瘾者治疗成功的一个重要因素是复吸的预防。复吸的成瘾者必须改变他们的行为，并且能够抵制社会和环境中再次吸毒的诱惑。社会心理学治疗，比如认知行为治疗可能有效。研究中的药物治疗也可能是有效的维持治疗。

预防

预防药品滥用和依赖从停用开始，这是无需证明的事情。医生都受过良好教育，因此医生药物成瘾被作为防止成瘾教育失败的范例。药物使用、滥用及依赖现在不仅存在于年长的医生中，也存在于医学生和住院医生中。已学会平衡生活和管理压力、焦虑和工作上问题且已停药的医生可以指导医学生，帮助他们做到同样的事情。医务工作中的成瘾者是需要解决的一项严重的公共健康问题。医务人员被看做是从事一项重要的安全性职业的人员，类似于飞机驾驶员。如果不治疗，成瘾者会伤害他们自己、家庭和患者。至少 15% 的医生在他们职业生涯中的某个时间经历过明显的挫折，但是关于医务人员初次药物滥用和依赖的研究还不足。

最好的预防药物依赖的方法是防止成瘾药物的第一次使用。比如，对于有喝酒习惯，特别是直系亲属喝酒的家庭，酒精成瘾就有很大的基因风险。这样的人应该避免饮酒。从儿童早期和青少年期就要防止暴露于药品环境或使用违禁药物，这是减少以后药物成瘾的关键。医科大学和其他医学职业教育计划努力预防和恰当的培养也是降低医务人员未来药物依赖问题的重要环节。如果第一步预防失败了，早期干预还有机会。即使医务人员还处于培训阶段，随机药检也具有威慑作用，就像在军队或交通部中其发挥的作用一样。一些在这方面处于领先的机构，如麻省总医院，已将随机药检项目纳入预防药物滥用的方案中，现在常常检查住院医生和工作人员。

即使药物依赖已发生，治疗也可有效，特别是对于医生成瘾，其有较高的5年治愈率。治疗可以预防或大大降低一些对身体的不良影响。

（范翠翠　译　盛睿方　校）

延伸阅读

Aach RD, Girard DE, Humphrey H, et al.: Alcohol and other substance abuse and impairment among physicians in residency training, *Ann Intern Med* 116:245–254, 1992.

American Psychiatric Association: *Diagnostic and statistical manual of mental disorders*, ed 5, Washington, DC, 2013, American Psychiatric Press. [DSM-5].

Bohigian GM, Croughan JL, Sanders K: Substance abuse and dependence in physicians: an overview of the effects of alcohol and drug abuse, *Mo Med* 91:233–238, 1994.

Gold MS, Aronson MD: *Screening and diagnosis of patients with alcohol problems, and treatment of alcohol abuse and dependence*, Harvard University's UpToDate Website and CD-ROM Educational Program, 2005.

Gold MS, Frost-Pineda K: Substance abuse and psychiatric dual disorders: focus on tobacco, *J Dual Diagnosis* 1:15–36, 2005.

Gold MS, Frost-Pineda K, Jacobs WS: Cannabis. In Galanter M, Kleber HD, editors: *The American Psychiatric Publishing textbook of substance abuse treatment*, ed 3, New York, 2004, American Psychiatric Press, pp 167–188.

Gold MS, Jacobs W: Cocaine (and crack): clinical aspects. In Lowinson JH, Ruiz P, Millman RB, editors: *Substance abuse: a clinical textbook*, ed 2, Baltimore, 2004, Williams & Wilkins, pp 218–251.

Herridge P, Gold MS: Pharmacological adjuncts in the treatment of opioid and cocaine addicts, *J Psychoactive Drugs* 20:233–242, 1988.

Jacobs WS, Hall JD, Pomm R, et al.: Prognostic factors for physician addiction: outcomes at five years, *J Addict Dis* 22:140, 2003.

Jacobs WS, Repetto M, Vinson S: Random urine testing as an intervention for drug addiction, *Psych Ann* 34:781–785, 2004.

Koob GF: Neuroadaptive mechanisms of addiction: studies on the extended amygdala, *Eur Neuropsychopharmacol* 13:442–452, 2003.

Miller NS, Mahler JC, Gold MS: Suicide risk associated with drug and alcohol dependence, *J Addict Dis* 10:49–61, 1991.

Repetto M, Frost-Pineda K, Gold MS: Pharmacological therapeutics for alcohol, cocaine and opioid intoxication and detoxification. In Miller NS, Wadland WC, editors: *Addictions in medicine: principles and practice.* Hoboken, NJ, John Wiley & Sons, 2004.

Repetto M, Gold MS: Cocaine (and crack): neurobiology. In Lowinson JH, Ruiz P, Millman RB, editors: *Substance abuse: a clinical textbook*, ed 2, Baltimore, 2004, Williams & Wilkins, pp 195–218.

Robinson TE: Addicted rats, *Science* 305:951–953, 2004.

Talbott GD, Richardson Jr AC, Mashburn JS, et al.: The Medical Association of Georgia's Disabled Doctors Program—a 5-year review, *J Med Assoc Ga* 70:545–549, 1981.

Vaillant GE, Brighton JR, McArthur C: Physicians' use of mood-altering drugs: a 20-year follow-up report, *N Engl J Med* 282:365–370, 1970.

药物依赖：阿片类药物　第 4 章

Mark S. Gold，William S. Jacobs

病例概要

患者，男性，38 岁，麻醉科医师，在完成一例颅内肿瘤的麻醉之后，在值班室内休息时，被发现其对外界刺激无应答，发绀，在其左前臂处发现新的注射针孔以及 1 ml 胰岛素注射器和橡皮止血带。

问题分析

定义

美国医学会将医生的职业损害定义为“由于精神疾病、酒精中毒或药物依赖而无法履行专业或个人责任”。这与职业运动员或飞行员中的定义不同，在这些领域中，往往将职业损害定义为“无法完成任务、影响工作或是留下后遗症”。

识别

虽然在《精神障碍诊断与统计手册（第 5 版）》（DSM-5）中没有提到药物检测，但它常被医生用来辅助临床诊断，这是因为在成瘾性疾病中，患者提供的病史往往是不可靠的。药物依赖性疾病的诊断需要可靠的病史、体格检查以及实验室检查的结果三者相结合。直接看到医务人员使用药物、明显酒醉样、不当持有或获取令人欣快的药物或具有戒断症状时应当启动此类评估。对于阿片类药物，其停药的剂量和时机取决于特定阿片类药物使用的剂量和频率，突然停用阿片类药物通常会导致打哈欠、流涕流泪、焦虑、全身疼痛、睡眠障碍、恶心、呕吐、腹泻、寒战、瞳孔放大、出汗、生命体征（脉搏、呼吸频率、血压）升高，甚至会使患者产生濒死感。产生这些症状主要是因为患者对于药物的强烈依赖。一些麻醉科医师在自身开始使用阿片类药物时先采取口服或喷雾的方式，但通常很快会发展为使用静脉注射的方式。在对药物依赖的麻醉科医师检查过程中，检查人员发现他们使用肠外途径给药，并且他们擅长使用小号针头在合适的位置进行注射，从而不易被其他人发现。为了不被发现，这些医生都刻意否认其异常的行为是因阿片类药物成瘾而引起的，这就导致他们直到过量服用药物、无法用其他理由去掩盖其异常行为时才被发现。长期成瘾的患者突然停药往往会引起顽固的戒断综合征，可能会持续数月之久，包括出汗、夜惊、烦躁不安、渴求药物以及心神不宁等，通常发生于急性戒断期后且症状强烈。

实验室诊断被认为是判断是否滥用阿片类药物的金标准。在使用正确的检测方法和合适的样本的前提下，实验室诊断的结果比较可信，目前使用较多的样本是受试者的尿液。在检测方法方面，现在有较多选择，床旁免疫检测是最快的筛查方法，薄层色谱法最经济、最常用，而气相色谱质谱法是目前最精确的验证性检测方法。而对于那些尿液检测阴性，但仍有服药嫌疑的受试者，头发或指甲可提供更多的检测结果。值得注意的是，对合成类阿片类药物如芬太尼及其类似物，需要进行更特异性的检测，因为通常的药物测试仅对吗啡、可待因、氢可酮和氢吗啡酮有效。

风险评估

几个世纪以来，阿片制剂一直是重要的镇痛剂，但也是滥用最多的药物之一。而由于皮下注射器的发明，阿片制剂不再局限于口服给药，这也导致美国在南北战争之后，士兵的药物成瘾及戒断综合征成了非常棘手的问题。这种药物成瘾的情况甚至被称为军人病，并且从 20 世纪 90 年代中期开始，由于美国对于口服阿片类药物的处方模式进行修改，导致了这类药物在美国国内的流行。现在药物成瘾普遍被认为是由于强烈渴望服药引起的精神障碍，患者尽管清楚其不良后果仍无法克制这种渴望，并且无法忍受停药时引起的戒断综合征并再次服用该药物，这种情况在阿片类药物中更常见。

药物耐受的概念最初是在一些服用阿片类药物的患者身上发现的，因为在其反复服用该药物之后，无法获得应有的疗效。而随着耐受性的升高，需逐渐加大剂量以达到最初体验到的欣快感。在精神药理学背景下，药物耐受性是机体对外源性物质的超生理水平的适应性反应。这种适应的一个主要结果是，在停止使用药物时，机体的生理水平并没有恢复，这也导致出现特定于该类药物的生理戒断综合征。对于长期使用阿片类药物的人群，停止使用会导致严重的身体戒断综合征，包括腹泻、高血压、心动过速、呕吐和肌肉痉挛，此外抑郁、烦躁不安或消极情感症状（如快感缺乏症）与几乎所有滥用药物（包括阿片类药物）的停药有关。而在被干预之后，抑郁和自杀倾向是药物滥用和依赖的常见并发症。对于麻醉科医师来说，这种情况更加危险，因为他们往往具备医学知识和手段以成功完成自杀尝试，因此需要制订一项安全计划，减少从干预到收治入院进行成瘾治疗期间的自杀危险。

医务人员的成瘾问题是一个重大的公共卫生问题，他们处在安全性敏感的岗位，如果没有得到干预和治疗，这部分人群可能会对其自身、家人和患者造成伤害。虽然对于医生的治疗效果良好，但是关于药物滥用和成瘾的初级预防的研究还很缺乏。有研究者对一些阿片类药物成瘾的医生进行了数十年的研究，报道了这些人群中可乐定及纳屈酮的使用情况，并且在这些人接受了治疗后进行了多年的随访。研究表明虽然医生在处方药成瘾方面比例较高，但他们酒精滥用和依赖的比例与对照组无明显差异。

几乎所有的医学院及医院中都有医生滥用药物甚至成瘾的情况发生，但是他们都将这些现象归因于自控性差或药物易获取。这些情况表明药物滥用和成瘾已经成为了医生，尤其是麻醉科医师的一种职业危害。而目前的社会中，要想成为一名医生，人们需要在高中及大学取得优异的成绩并通过医学院的入学考试，并且在医学院中也需要表现突出才能获得实习生和住院医生的机会，最终才可能成为合格的医生。

在一般人看来，医生不像是会滥用药物的人群，然而他们药物成瘾的可能性是普通人的 30～100 倍。有研究表明，12.5% 的男性医生会有药物依赖的情况，比普通男性要高出不少，普通男性为 0.1%。在哈佛大学的毕业生中，尽管医生和其他职业人群的酗酒率和吸烟率相当，但其药物滥用率、抑郁症、自杀率等均高于对照组人群，至少有 15% 的医生会在其职业生涯中受到明显影响。目前普遍接受的理论是由于过大的压力以及更易获取药物的原因使医生滥用阿片类药物，但也有研究表明从事可卡因或麻醉剂研究的基础科学家自身不会使用这些药物。药物滥用的情况在不同专科中也不一样（图 4.1）。麻醉科医师需要给患者使用包括阿片类药物在内的强效麻醉剂，在患者头部周围限定的区域工作，暴露于废弃药物如阿片类药物、丙泊酚、苯二氮䓬类，这些药物会对医生的大脑、情绪及行为产生影响，并且会使他们的大脑对这些药物更加敏感，如果其

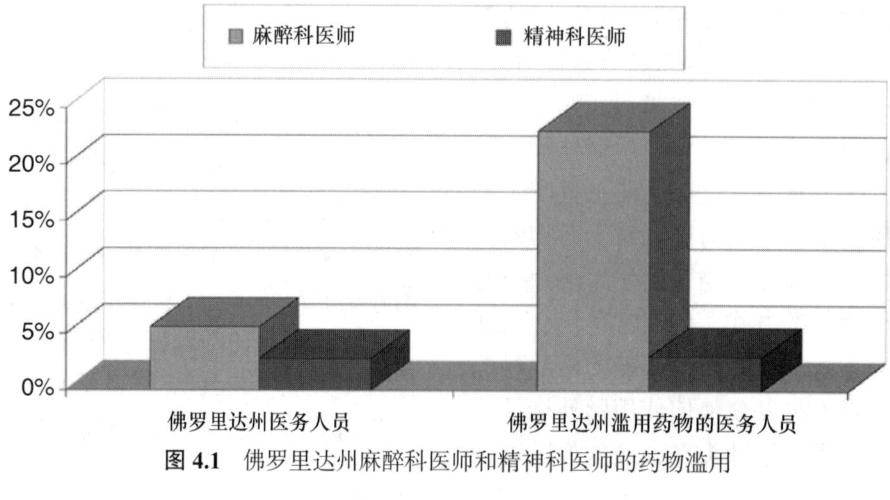

图 4.1 佛罗里达州麻醉科医师和精神科医师的药物滥用

服用这些药物，比正常人群更易上瘾。

芬太尼及其类似物需要麻醉科医师的特别注意。多年来，芬太尼的滥用及其导致的成瘾甚至死亡现象主要发生在医务人员中，因为他们是接触芬太尼的主要人群。芬太尼是 20 世纪 60 年代早期由比利时 Janssen 制药公司开发的一种麻醉性镇痛药，其药理作用与吗啡一样，也是一种阿片受体激动剂，优先与 μ 阿片受体结合，但由于化学结构与吗啡类似物稍有不同，导致其无法通过尿液试纸检测出来。此外，芬太尼的药效是吗啡的 50 ～ 100 倍，而且新的芬太尼类似物已经研发出来，其中最有效的是 3-甲基芬太尼，其药效是吗啡的 6000 倍、海洛因的 600 倍。不幸的是，这些强效镇痛药也有极高的滥用率并与药物过量导致死亡有关。1979—1988 年间，仅加州就有 108 例药物过量致死与芬太尼类似物有关，其主要原因是芬太尼对呼吸有很强的抑制作用。据报道，因芬太尼服用过量导致死亡的患者体液中，芬太尼浓度在 1 ～ 10 ng/ml 之间，与其他阿片类药物过量死亡者相比，芬太尼致死浓度非常低。例如，由于服用海洛因过量死亡者体液中游离吗啡浓度在 462 ～ 1350 ng/ml。2004 年在佛罗里达州，美沙酮、奥施康定和芬太尼比海洛因更容易导致过量死亡。

启示

在开始治疗之前，对患者进行全面的医学和精神病学评估可有助于预测长期结局。静脉药物滥用与许多疾病有关，包括细菌性或病毒性心内膜炎、肝炎、获得性免疫缺陷综合征、结核、蜂窝织炎、脑炎、伤口脓肿、脓毒症、动脉血栓、肾梗死和血栓性静脉炎。最常见的严重并发症是事故、头部损伤、记忆障碍、性传播疾病、癫痫、抑郁、自杀念头甚至自杀企图等。因此阿片类药物成瘾的人群有很高的死亡率，在未经治疗的人群中，每年每 1000 人中约有 10 人死亡。致死的原因主要是服药过量、意外、受伤，一般医疗并发症。不过在某些地域药物成瘾导致的暴力冲突是致死的主要原因。除了这些医学相关问题之外，医生当中的成瘾者还面临着医疗证书和执照的职业风险，以及婚姻和其他个人问题。

管理

经过适当的干预和治疗后，这些医生须接受戒除成瘾性治疗，替代治疗或维持治疗（如使用美沙酮或丁丙诺啡）并不适用于这类成瘾人群。戒毒阶段，可乐定不仅可提供有效的非阿片制剂治疗戒断综合征，还可以加速从对阿片制剂的依赖到维持治疗阶段的进程，尤其是使用可乐定联合阿片受体阻滞剂纳屈酮可有效地控制成瘾性。两药联用可使解毒过程缩短至数天。这种联合用药的方法，与应用纳屈酮维持，12- 步骤见面会，社区性治疗，个人和团体与康复中的同龄人一起治疗，管理并发的精神和医疗病情，以及初始正规治疗后维持 5 年的随访监测，已经成为治疗阿片类药物成瘾的新标准。

药物成瘾有类似于慢性病的特征以及较低的长期恢复概率，但在医生当中的治疗效果显著优于一般群体。成瘾者的多数治疗项目已持续缩短，而对于医务人员的治疗项目则延伸至包括院内治疗、出院后治疗以及康复等阶段。使用这些技术，医生的长期治疗结局远好于普通人群同样诊断的成瘾者。最新一项称为随机选择医生康复的研究表明，阿片类药物成瘾 5 年以上的医生当中，有 91.4% 的人在治疗后重返工作岗位，这一比例与其他关于医生群体的研究结果很接近。在麻醉科医师中这种情况也是类似的，在之前曾建议有静脉阿片类药物成瘾史的麻醉科医师不适合回到原来的岗位上，但随着纳屈酮的常规使用，目前已改变这种观点。总之，麻醉科医师可在治疗后重返岗位。综上所述，对于阿片类药物成瘾的医生（尤其是麻醉科医师），良好的管理设置可以使他们得到有意义的恢复并回到自己的专业职责和职业岗位。

预防

我们的研究证实了其他研究的发现，即麻醉科医师阿片类药物滥用的发生率更高，如果不加以治疗，成瘾会给麻醉科医师及其患者和家人带来许多不良的后果。早期发现是防止过量死亡和使治疗更加成功的关键。为预防和早期发现，应强烈考虑对所有麻醉从业人员进行随机抽查检测。

致谢

感谢 Adrie Bruijnzeel 医生对本章上一版的贡献。

（栾延敏　译　倪丽亚　校）

延伸阅读

Aach RD, Girard DE, Humphrey H, et al.: Alcohol and other substance abuse and impairment among physicians in residency training, *Ann Intern Med* 116:245–254, 1992.

American Psychiatric Association: *Diagnostic and statistical manual of mental disorders*, ed 5, Washington, DC, 2013, American Psychiatric Press. [DSM-5].

Bohigian GM, Croughan JL, Sanders K: Substance abuse and dependence in physicians: an overview of the effects of alcohol and drug abuse, *Mo Med* 91:233–238, 1994.

Gold MS: Opiate addiction and the locus coeruleus, *Psychiatr Clin North Am* 16:61–73, 1993.

Gold MS, Frost-Pineda K, Pomm R: Is addiction an occupational hazard for anesthesiologists? *College on Problems of Drug Dependence*, 2004.

Gold MS, Miller NS: Intoxication and withdrawal from opiates and inhalants. In Miller NS, Gold MS, Smith DE, editors: *Manual of therapeutics for addictions*, New York, 1992, Wiley-Liss, pp 72–86.

Gold MS, Redmond Jr DE, Kleber HD: Clonidine may relieve opiate withdrawal symptoms, *JAMA* 240:25–27, 1978.

Goldberger BA, Merves ML, Frost-Pineda K, et al.: Use, misuse and diversion of methadone and hydrocodone: the deaths continue to increase, *J Clin Pharmacol* 43:83, 2003.

Henderson GL: Blood concentrations of fentanyl and its analogs in overdose victims, *Proc West Pharmacol Soc* 26:287–290, 1983.

Henderson GL: Designer drugs: past history and future prospects, *J Forensic Sci* 33:569–575, 1988.

Herridge P, Gold MS: Pharmacological adjuncts in the treatment of opioid and cocaine addicts, *J Psychoactive Drugs* 20:233–242, 1988.

Jacobs WS, Hall JD, Pomm R: Prognostic factors for physician addiction outcomes at five years, *J Addict Dis* 22:140, 2003.

Janssen PAJ: 1-Aralkyl-4-(n-aryl-carbonyl-amino)-piperidines and related compounds, *US Patent Office No. 3,164,600*, 1965.

Koob GF: Neuroadaptive mechanisms of addiction: studies on the extended amygdala, *Eur Neuropsychopharmacol* 13:442–452, 2003.

Maguire P, Tsai N, Kamal J, et al.: Pharmacological profiles of fentanyl analogs at mu, delta and kappa opiate receptors, *Eur J Pharmacol* 213:219–225, 1992.

Miller NS, Mahler JC, Gold MS: Suicide risk associated with drug and alcohol dependence, *J Addict Dis* 10:49–61, 1991.

Moriya F, Hashimoto Y: Distribution of free and conjugated morphine in body fluids and tissues in a fatal heroin overdose: is conjugated morphine stable in postmortem specimens? *J Forensic Sci* 42:736–740, 1997.

Repetto M, Frost-Pineda K, Gold MS: Pharmacological therapeutics for alcohol, cocaine and opioid intoxication and detoxification. In Miller NS, Wadland WC, editors: *Addictions in medicine: principles and practice*, Hoboken, NJ, 2004, John Wiley & Sons.

Shook JE, Watkins WD, Camporesi EM: Differential roles of opioid receptors in respiration, respiratory disease, and opiate-induced respiratory depression, *Am Rev Respir Dis* 142:895–909, 1990.

Talbott GD, Richardson Jr AC, Mashburn JS, et al.: The Medical Association of Georgia's Disabled Doctors Program—a 5-year review, *J Med Assoc Ga* 70:545–549, 1981.

Vaillant GE, Brighton JR, McArthur C: Physicians' use of mood-altering drugs: a 20-year follow-up report, *N Engl J Med* 282:365–370, 1970.

Van Bever WF, Niemegeers CJ, Janssen PA: Synthetic analgesics: synthesis and pharmacology of the diastereoisomers of N-(3-methyl-1-(2-phenylethyl)-4-piperidyl)-N-phenylpropanamide and N-(3-methyl-1-(1-methyl-2-phenylethyl)-4-piperidyl)-N-phenylpropanamide, *J Med Chem* 17:1047–1051, 1974.

阿片类药物长期使用

第5章

Taras Grosh，Michael A. Ashburn

病例概要

患者，女性，38 岁，因机动车碰撞后由救护车转运至急诊科。既往有甲状腺功能减退病史，25 岁时被发现有静脉滥用阿片类药物史。因为滥用阿片类药物，十年前，患者开始接受药物辅助治疗（medication-assisted treatment，MAT）。目前的治疗方案是口服丁丙诺啡 / 纳洛酮 8 mg/2 mg，每日两次。在急诊科对她进行评估后，她被诊断为股骨骨折，拟行急诊矫正手术。

问题分析

定义

尽管记录阿片类药物的安全性和有效性的证据极其有限，在过去的 15 年中，阿片类药物在慢性非癌性疼痛的治疗应用已经有了明显的增长。随着阿片类处方药物的使用增加，阿片类药物的滥用和误用率也正在增加。对处方药的成瘾，多数通常为阿片类药物正在激增，很多人因阿片类药物的不良反应而死亡。目前海洛因滥用的现象呈现急剧上升的态势，并且因海洛因过量致死的案例层出不穷，这些都与处方药物的误用和滥用密切相关。

许多长期使用的药物，包括阿片类药物都会产生耐药性。**耐药性**是指患者长时间使用某一药物而产生依赖，以至于需要增加剂量来达到相同的效果。由于对阿片类药物不同作用（即镇痛、呼吸抑制、镇静、便秘）的耐受性以不同的速度和不同的程度发生，阿片类药物的耐受性也有所差别。对镇痛作用的耐受可迅速出现，而阿片类药物对通气影响的耐受则发生缓慢，比观察到的对镇痛耐受的程度较轻。因此，与从未接触过阿片类药物的患者相比，对阿片类药物耐受的患者积极地增加药量则会**增加**呼吸相关并发症的风险。美国食品药品监督管理局（FDA）关于阿片类药物耐受的定义是：当患者接受了至少每天 60 mg 的吗啡或与其等效剂量的其他阿片类药物至少 1 周。

尽管《精神疾病诊断与统计手册（第 5 版）》（DSM-5）中已不再使用“**成瘾**”一词，而用“**物质使用障碍**”替代，但人们仍习惯使用“**成瘾性**”。根据美国成瘾医学协会的定义，**成瘾**是一种原发的、慢性的神经生理疾病，其发生及临床表现受遗传、社会心理及环境因素的影响。它包括以下行为学特征：**对药物使用的控制能力受损，渴求药物，明知有危害但仍强迫和持续使用药物**。

DSM-5 中修订了阿片类药物使用障碍的诊断标准（见第 4 章框 4.1）。新的诊断标准试图抓住成瘾的本质，同时避免将那些在医生指导下长期规范化使用阿片类药物的患者归为成瘾患者。

对长期接受阿片类药物治疗的讨论中，需要理解的一个重要概念是如何正确量化每日阿片类药物的剂量。目前普遍采用的方法是“吗啡等效剂量”（morphine equivalent dose，MED）。确定每天摄入阿片类药物的总剂量，然后通过阿片类药物换算表转化为 MED。患者的 MED 可以指导医生合理开具阿片类药物的处方，并能预估患者术后疼痛的体验情况。

识别

详细询问病史和体格检查对于指导临床决策至关重要。仔细了解患者服用何种药物亦很重要。同时，医生必须仔细确定目前的阿片类药物剂量，以及该剂量是最近刚开始服用还是长期服用。

慢性疼痛患者和药物使用障碍患者均有精神健康障碍的高风险，包括抑郁症和焦虑症。此外，药物使用障碍的患者较普通人群出现创伤后应激障碍和第Ⅱ轴人格碍可能性大。这些病情的出现可能会影响围术期治疗，也会影响到这些病情的药物治疗。

风险评估

长期接受阿片类药物治疗的手术患者更可能出现术后疼痛控制不佳。由于长期应用阿片类药物出现的差异性耐受，再加上主诉镇痛效果不佳，可能会增加呼吸相关并发症的风险，包括全身性大量应用阿片类药物治疗疼痛所致的呼吸停止和死亡。如果阿片类药物和苯二氮䓬类药物联合使用，损害风险也显著增加。

呼吸睡眠功能紊乱包括阻塞性睡眠呼吸暂停（obstructive sleep apnea，OSA）和中枢性睡眠呼吸暂停（central sleep apnea，CSA），这类患者全身应用阿片类药物后存在通气功能受损的风险。如果患者每天服用阿片类药物 MED 大于 100 mg，则 CSA 的风险将增加。OSA 虽然比较常见，但未得到及时诊断和正确治疗。因此很多人主张对 OSA 进行围术期筛查，并对高危患者加强监测和干预，确保适当的氧合和通气。同样，早期识别出大剂量服用阿片类药物的患者（大于 80 ～ 100 mg MED），在有指征时可对其建立监测和早期干预。

启示

越来越多的文献证据证实，长期接受大剂量阿片类药物治疗的患者行择期手术时，预后可能受到影响。例如，长期使用阿片类药物大于 80 mg MED 的患者，接受关节假体置换手术时，常报告急性和慢性疼痛控制不佳，且其生理功能无改善或有限的改善。因此早期识别出长期应用阿片类药物的患者并考虑尽量减少术前阿片类药物的处方剂量可以改善术后预后。

长期接受阿片类药物治疗的患者如果突然停药，会存在发生阿片类药物戒断症状的高风险。戒断症状的发作时间因使用阿片类药物的药代动力学不同而有所不同（表 5.1）。虽然阿片类药物的戒断症状通常不会危及生命，但它使患者非常痛苦。当术后出现症状时，如果不能识别则会导致大量的不必要

表 5.1 阿片类药物戒断症状的时程

阿片类药物	发作时间	最强时间	持续时间
哌替啶	2 ～ 6 h	6 ～ 12 h	4 ～ 5 天
芬太尼			
吗啡	6 ～ 12 h	36 ～ 72 h	7 ～ 10 天
海洛因			
美沙酮	24 ～ 48 h	3 ～ 21 天	6 ～ 7 周

Modified from Mitra S，Sinatra R：Perioperative management of acute pain in the opioid-dependent patient. *Anesthesiology* 101（1）：212-227, 2004.

的医学评估。长期应用阿片类药物的患者，如果术后未继续用药，术后将会产生严重的疼痛。因此，术前识别出长期应用阿片类药物的患者很重要，可以主动地制订方案，以避免出现阿片类药物戒断症状，并尽可能地治疗预期的疼痛。

丁丙诺啡是 μ 受体部分激动剂，能紧密结合 μ 受体。尽管它可提供阿片类镇痛作用，但这种作用可能会有天花板效应。丁丙诺啡还可能限制其他阿片类镇痛药的有效性，因此，如果患者已经服用了丁丙诺啡，使用其他阿片类药物的疗效会被削减。据报道，接受丁丙诺啡 MAT 的患者，如果术前将丁丙诺啡换成美沙酮或其他短效阿片类药物，则可改善围术期镇痛效果。

管理

术前管理

确定当前阿片类药物剂量并计算 MED

患者的自述（例如，根据需要我每 4 h 服用羟考酮 15 mg）不足以帮助确定 MED，医生必须明确实际使用的阿片类药物剂量。医生可能无法从患者及其家属那里获取真实信息，可能需要通过其他途径来确认阿片类药物的使用剂量。阿片类药物剂量可能通过查询医疗记录或州处方药物监测项目（prescription drug monitoring program，PDMP），或联系患者取药的药房来获得。在确定 MED 时，确定每日使用的阿片类药物剂量至关重要，再根据阿片类药物换算表仔细计算 MED。

明确合用其他镇静药引起呼吸功能受损的风险

阿片类药物与其他中枢性镇静药合用时，呼吸

功能受损的风险显著增加。许多医生常给患者同时开具阿片类药物和苯二氮革类药物的处方。由于突然停用苯二氮革类药物会引起威胁生命的戒断症状，如果这些药物可在择期手术之前逐渐减量并停用，苯二氮革类药物可能需要在围术期继续使用。

乙醇是强效中枢神经系统抑制剂，如果与阿片药物联合使用，可导致比单用其中任何一种都更强的呼吸抑制作用。如同预期的一样，这种抑制程度在老年人中更显著。因此对于有酒精滥用史的患者，医生开具阿片类药物处方时应格外谨慎。

确定应用阿片类药物同时存在 OSA 或 CSA 引起的呼吸功能受损的风险

筛查 OSA 患者，对于每日阿片类药物 MED 大于 100 mg 的患者，应考虑其存在 OSA 的风险，除非对其进行大剂量阿片应用下的睡眠监测，且已排除呼吸睡眠障碍。

确定患者是否需要进行预防性治疗（详见后面讨论）。

作为麻醉计划的一部分制定疼痛治疗方案，尽可能应用多模式镇痛（表 5.2）

如有指征，请尽早咨询疼痛专家。疼痛治疗的注意事项包括以下内容：

- 除禁忌证外，按计划使用对乙酰氨基酚。
- 除禁忌证外，按计划使用非甾体抗炎药（适当监测）。
- 考虑使用加巴喷丁和普瑞巴林。
- 尽可能积极使用区域麻醉和镇痛技术，包括硬膜外或周围神经置管。
- 继续使用与长期应用相匹配的 MED 剂量的阿片类药物，避免阿片类药物戒断症状。
- 制订计划，包括患者术后合理安置和术后监测通气是否充足。

表 5.2 多模式镇痛的药物使用

药物	常规给药剂量
对乙酰氨基酚	650 mg ～ 1 g q6 ～ 8 h PO/IV
NSAIDs（COX-2，布洛芬，酮咯酸）	塞来昔布 200 mg q12 h PO
	布洛芬 800 mg q6 h PO
	布洛芬 400 mg q6 h IV
	酮咯酸 15 ～ 30 mg q6 h PO 5 d
抗惊厥药	加巴喷丁每天 900 ～ 1200 mg PO
	普瑞巴林每天 300 ～ 600 mg PO
NMDA 拮抗剂	氯胺酮 0.1 ～ 0.5 mg/kg IV
	氯胺酮 125 ～ 500 ug/（kg·h）IV

COX-2，环氧化酶 -2；NMDA，N- 甲基 -D- 门冬氨酸；NSAIDs，非甾体抗炎药

注意：应每周以及减药 / 停药时对患者进行再评价，只要症状不再持续，药物用量尽可能减至最低

为患者、家庭、外科和护理确立合理预期

长期接受阿片类药物治疗的患者应了解，术后他们可能会出现疼痛增加，增加药物剂量也不大可能会改善止痛效果，反而可能会加大损害风险。跟患者保证，他们的治疗会得到尊严和尊重，并尽可能全力去治疗其疼痛，但最终他们会更可能不可避免地经历疼痛增加的阶段。

阿片类药物使用障碍的患者需要与其成瘾治疗团队认真咨询和沟通其疼痛治疗计划。至关重要的是，该治疗计划应清晰标明在出院时开具阿片类药物处方，并提前规划去成瘾治疗团队进行复诊。

术中管理

尽可能考虑将区域麻醉技术作为麻醉方法的一部分。确保阿片类药物按正确的 MED 使用，以避免术中出现阿片类药物戒断症状。

考虑使用以下方法：

- 伤口用长效局麻药浸润。
- 静脉输注利多卡因 [首次 1 mg/kg 推注，然后以 2 mg/（kg·h）输注]。
- 静脉输注氯胺酮 [诱导 0.5 mg/kg 推注，然后以 10 μg/（kg·min）输注]。

术后管理

- 持续使用合理 MED 的阿片类药物，避免戒断反应。
- 若需要，按计划使用对乙酰氨基酚、非甾体抗炎药和加巴喷丁。
- 术后即刻阶段性尽可能长的时间进行持续区域镇痛。
- 对全身使用阿片类药物的患者，特别是确诊为睡眠呼吸紊乱或者高风险的患者，适当监测通气是否充分。
- 全身使用阿片类药物镇痛时应谨慎，应充分认识

到，由于耐受差异，不可能单独使用阿片类药物既能达到充分镇痛又不影响呼吸。

- 对未治疗的药物使用障碍患者，在其出院前应即刻进行精神评估并针对药物使用障碍提供合理的诊疗方案。
- 出院时制订并实施阿片类处方计划。计划应包括：有限天数内的阿片类处方药物，然后患者转诊至疼痛专家或成瘾专家处，由他们接管和监控后续的阿片类处方。

预防

在计划择期手术前，邀请疼痛专家进行术前会诊指导，可以充分改善围术期治疗和患者预后。成瘾专家认真计算MAT，仔细调整治疗方案，必要时将丁丙诺啡换成美沙酮或其他阿片类药物，逐渐减少慢性非癌性疼痛患者的阿片类药物剂量。通过创建围术期疼痛治疗计划并记录下来，可用于指导手术中的临床决策，并可讨论患者及其家庭的合理期望。

纵观全球，医疗机构可能希望为拟行手术的使用丁丙诺啡或长期使用阿片类药物的患者创建标准化治疗流程（图5.1）。该治疗流程可用于对治疗团队的宣教，并制定标准化治疗过程以用于手术中新用药物的输注（如氯胺酮），同时制定和实施监测术后易发生通气障碍的高危患者的流程。

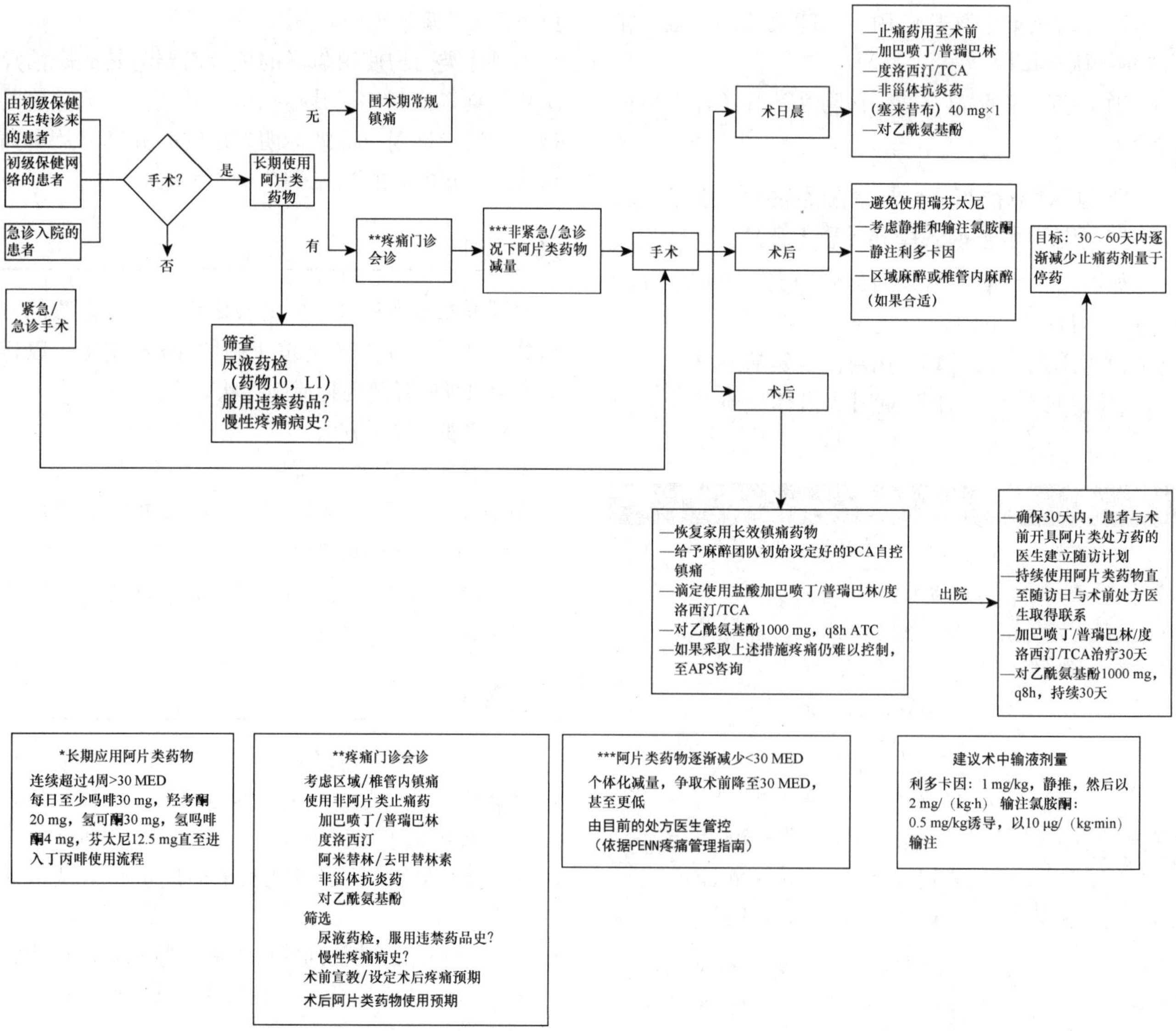

图 5.1 宾夕法尼亚大学拟行择期脊柱手术的阿片类药物耐受患者的疼痛治疗流程

（杨　锴　译　李晓菲　校）

延伸阅读

Alford DP, Compton P, Samet JH: Acute pain management for patients receiving maintenance methadone or buprenorphine therapy, *Ann Intern Med* 144(2):127–134, 2006.

Bailard NS, Ortiz J, Flores RA: Additives to local anesthetics for peripheral nerve blocks: evidence, limitations, and recommendations, *Am J Health Syst Pharm* 71(5):373–385, 2014.

Bisgaard T, Klarskov B, Rosenberg J, Kehlet H: Characteristics and prediction of early pain after laparoscopic cholecystectomy, *Pain* 90:261–269, 2001.

Brummett CM: Dexmedetomidine as a novel therapeutic for postoperative pain in a patient treated with buprenorphine, *J Opioid Manag* 5(3):175–179, 2009.

Carroll IR, Angst MS, Clark JD: Management of perioperative pain in patients chronically consuming opioids. *Reg Anesth Pain Med* 29(6):576–591.

Caumo W, Schmidt AP, Schneider CN, et al.: Preoperative predictors of moderate to intense acute postoperative pain in patients undergoing abdominal surgery, *Acta Anaesthesiol Scand* 46:1265–1271, 2002.

Center for Substance Abuse Treatment: Clinical guidelines for the use of buprenorphine in the treatment of opioid addiction: pharmacology. Rockville, MD, 2004, Substance Abuse and Mental Health Services Administration (US). Treatment Improvement Protocol (TIP) Series, No. 40.

Chapman CR, Davis J, Donaldson GW, et al.: Postoperative pain trajectories in chronic pain patients undergoing surgery: the effects of chronic opioid pharmacotherapy on acute pain, *J Pain* 12(12):1240–1246, 2011.

Daubresse M, Chang HY, Yu Y, et al.: Ambulatory diagnosis and treatment of nonmalignant pain in the United States, 2000–2010, *Med Care* 51:870–878, 2013.

de Leon-Casasola OA, Lema MJ: Epidural sufentanil for acute pain control in a patient with extreme opioid dependency, *Anesthesiology* 76(5):853–856, 1992.

Garg N, Panda NB, Gandhi KA, et al.: Comparison of small dose ketamine and dexmedetomidine infusion for postoperative analgesia in spine surgery—a prospective randomized double-blind placebo controlled study, *J Neurosurg Anesthesiol* 28(1):27–31, 2016.

Gonzalez JP, Brogden RN: Naltrexone. A review of its pharmacodynamic and pharmacokinetic properties and therapeutic efficacy in the management of opioid dependence, *Drugs* 35(3):192–213, 1988.

Goyal R, Khurana G, Jindal P, Sharma JP: Anesthesia for opioid addict: challenges for perioperative physician, *J Anaesthesiol Clin Pharmacol* 29(3):394–396, 2013.

Gust R, Pecher S, Gust A, et al.: Effect of patient-controlled analgesia on pulmonary complications after coronary artery bypass grafting, *Crit Care Med* 27:2218–2223, 1999.

Gustin HB, Akil H: Opioid analgesics. In Hardman JG, Limbird LE, editors: *Goodman and Gilman's the pharmacological basis of therapeutics*, ed 10, New York, 2001, McGraw-Hill, pp 569–619.

Harden RN, Bruehl S, Stanos S, et al.: Prospective examination of pain-related and psychological predictors of CRPS-like phenomena following total knee arthroplasty: a preliminary study, *Pain* 106(3):393–400, 2003.

Howard LA, Sellers EM, Tyndale RF: The role of pharmacogenetically-variable cytochrome P450 enzymes in drug abuse and dependence, *Pharmacogenomics* 3(2):85–99, 2002.

Inacio MC, Hansen C, Pratt NL, et al.: Risk factors for persistent and new chronic opioid use in patients undergoing total hip arthroplasty: a retrospective cohort study, *BMJ Open* 6(4):e010664, 2016.

Ip HY, Abrishami A, Peng PW, et al.: Predictors of postoperative pain and analgesic consumption: a qualitative systematic review, *Anesthesiology* 111(3):657–677, 2009.

Joels CS, Mostafa G, Matthews BD, et al.: Factors affecting intravenous analgesic requirements after colectomy, *J Am Coll Surg* 197:780–785, 2003.

Kain ZN, Sevarino F, Alexander GM, et al.: Preoperative anxiety and postoperative pain in women undergoing hysterectomy: a repeated-measures design, *J Psychosom Res* 49:417–422, 2000.

Kalkman CJ, Visser K, Moen J, et al.: Preoperative prediction of severe postoperative pain, *Pain* 105:415–423, 2003.

Kim SH, Stoicea N, Soghomonyan S, Bergese SD: Intraoperative use of remifentanil and opioid induced hyperalgesia/acute opioid tolerance: systematic review, *Front Pharmacol* 5:108, 2014.

Kipping K, Maier C, Bussemas HH, Schwarzer A: Medication compliance in patients with chronic pain, *Pain Physician* 17(1):81–94, 2014.

Levy B, Paulozzi L, Mack KA, Jones CM: Trends in opioid analgesic-prescribing rates by specialty, U.S., 2007–2012, *Am J Prev Med* 49:409–413, 2015.

Martin BC, Fan M-Y, Edlund MJ, et al.: Long-term chronic opioid therapy discontinuation rates from the TROUP study, *J Gen Intern Med* 26(12):1450–1457, 2011.

McCormick Z: Acute pain control challenges with buprenorphine/naloxone therapy in a patient with compartment syndrome secondary to McArdle's disease: a case report and review, *Pain Med* 14(8):1187–1191, 2013.

Mitra S, Sinatra R: Perioperative management of acute pain in the opioid-dependent patient, *Anesthesiology* 101(1):212–227, 2004.

Paulozzi LJ, Mack KA, Hockenberry JM: Vital signs: variation among states in prescribing of opioid pain relievers and benzodiazepines—United States, 2012, *MMWR Morb Mortal Wkly Rep* 63:563–568, 2014.

Puntillo K, Weiss SJ: Pain: its mediators and associated morbidity in critically ill cardiovascular surgical patients, *Nurs Res* 43:31–36, 1994.

Rice JB, White AG, Birnbaum HG, et al.: A model to identify patients at risk for prescription opioid abuse, dependence, and misuse, *Pain Med* 13(9):1162–1173, 2012.

Riley III TR: Predictors of pain medication use after percutaneous liver biopsy, *Dig Dis Sci* 47:2151–2153, 2002.

Saberski L: Postoperative pain management for the patient with chronic pain. In Sinatra RS, Hord AH, Ginsberg B, Preble LM, editors: *Acute pain: mechanisms and management*, St. Louis, 1992, Mosby Yearbook, pp 422–431.

Sapira JD: The narcotic addict as a medical patient, *Am J Med* 45:555–588, 1968.

Schrier R, Roozekranz M, Olofsen E, et al.: Influence of ethanol on oxycodone-induced respiratory depression. A dose escalating study in young and elderly individuals, *Pain Med* 126(3):534–542, 2017.

Shea RA, Brooks JA, Dayhoff NE, Keck J: Pain intensity and postoperative pulmonary complications among the elderly after abdominal surgery, *Heart Lung* 31:440–449, 2002.

Thomas T, Robinson C, Champion D, et al.: Prediction and assessment of the severity of post-operative pain and of satisfaction with management, *Pain* 75:177–185, 1998.

Tsui SL, Law S, Fok M, et al.: Postoperative analgesia reduces mortality and morbidity after esophagectomy, *Am J Surg* 173:472–478, 1997.

Yi P, Pryzbylkowski P: Opioid induced hyperalgesia, *Pain Med* 16(Suppl 1):S32–S36, 2015.

第6章 透析依赖患者

Klaus D. Torp

病例概要

患者，男性，43岁，非裔美国人，职业为加油工人，因在一次抢劫未遂中腹部被刺伤拟行急诊剖腹探查术。该患者长期接受透析治疗并且一直在等待肾移植，最后一次血液透析是52 h之前。患者神志清楚且警醒，血压102/90 mmHg，心率114次/分；呼吸频率24次/分；在输注3U的红细胞后血红蛋白达到82 g/L，输血前血钾为6.0 mEq/L。使用依托咪酯、芬太尼、罗库溴铵行麻醉诱导，同时给予环状软骨压迫。手术开始后不久，外科医师抱怨止血困难，监护仪显示T波高尖。

问题分析

定义

美国国家肾基金会将慢性肾疾病（chronic kidney disease，CKD）定义为肾损伤（定义为影像学或实验室检查异常）或肾小球滤过率降低至60 ml/（min·1.73 m^2）以下，在疾病早期常不易发现。尿白蛋白检查可计算出白蛋白/肌酐比值（albumin/creatinine ratio，ACR），常作为肾损害的一个标志，CKD的分期见表6.1。

2012年，在美国约有637 000名患者受到终末期肾病（end-stage renal disease，ESRD）的影响，在统计范围覆盖66%美国地区的发病率约为353/100万人口，较2009年略低，而在统计范围覆盖33%的美国地区患病率为1943/100万人口，较2011略有增加。非洲裔美国人的患病率约为白种人的4倍，西班牙裔的患病率则比非西班牙裔高出60%。各年龄组的发病率都比较稳定，但在65岁以上的老年人群中发病率则显著下降，而同时各年龄组患病率却是增加的，特别是年龄超过65岁的人群（30%～50%），提示ESRD患者生存时间越来越长。在最初接受血液透析患者中，约有45%的主要诊断为糖尿病，其次是高血压（30%）和肾小球肾炎（7%），其余的患者则患有较为罕见的疾病，如多囊肾病、免疫球蛋白A（IgA）和IgM肾病、系统性红斑狼疮、Wegener肉芽肿、多发性骨髓瘤、淀粉样变和艾滋病肾病等，这些患者往往较年轻，较少发生透析患者的典型并存疾病。在2012年约100 000名患者开始用血液透析或腹膜透析治疗ESRD，其中2800例患者优先接受了肾移植。通常当肾小球滤过率（glomerular filtration rate，GFR）降至20 ml/min以下时需要进行长期透析，其适应证为：利尿剂治疗无效的容量超负荷、严重的代谢性酸中毒、高钾血症、癫痫或其他神经症状以及心包炎，通常在血尿素氮超过100 mg/ml或肌酐接近100 mg/L时进行。不管何种病因导致的ESRD都会导致几乎所有的脏器或系统的功能异常，对接受手术的该类患者影响重大（框6.1）。脏器或系统的功能异常是由于肾不能排出尿素和其他代谢终产物，以及肾主导的代谢和内分泌功能的丧失所致。

表6.1 慢性肾疾病的分类

CKD分期	异常
1	eGFR ≥ 90 ml/（min·1.73 m^2）ACR ≥ 30 mg/g
2	eGFR 60～89 ml/（min·1.73 m^2）ACR ≥ 30 mg/g
3	eGFR 30～59 ml/（min·1.73 m^2）
4	eGFR 15～29 ml/（min·1.73 m^2）
5	eGFR ≤ 15 ml/（min·1.73 m^2）

eGFR，估算肾小球滤过率；ACR，白蛋白/肌酐比值

框 6.1 终末期肾病的异常临床表现

神经系统
- 睡眠障碍
- 运动无力
- 多发性神经炎
- 扑翼样震颤
- 惊厥
- 昏迷

血液系统
- 贫血
- 红细胞脆性增加
- 血小板凝血功能障碍
- 血栓形成

代谢和内分泌系统
- 葡萄糖耐受
- 甲状旁腺功能亢进
- 性腺功能减退

免疫系统
- 感染易感性增加

体表系统
- 瘙痒

心血管系统
- 高血压
- 低血压
- 心肌病
- 舒张功能障碍
- 左心室肥厚
- 充血性心力衰竭
- 心包炎

胃肠系统
- 消化道出血
- 胰腺炎

酸碱平衡和电解质
- 阴离子间隙代谢性酸中毒
- 高钾血症
- 低钠血症
- 高镁血症或低镁血症
- 高磷血症

肌肉骨骼系统
- 肾性骨营养不良（骨质疏松，骨软化症）

识别

ESRD 围术期并发症列于框 6.2。ESRD 常见的急性危及生命的围术期并发症之一是高钾血症，它往往与酸中毒以及创伤后损伤组织和血肿释放钾有关。高钾血症可导致进行性心脏传导异常，最终导致心室颤动甚至心脏停搏（表 6.2）。心电图的改变也取决于发病时长以及血清钾升高的速率。

框 6.2 终末期肾病围术期并发症

- 高钾血症
- 出血
- 心血管功能障碍
- 高血压 / 低血压
- 充血性心力衰竭
- 缺血
- 脓毒症
- 植入物血栓形成

表 6.2 进行性高钾血症的心电图改变

K^+（mEq/L）	心电图异常
5.0	通常无 T 波或 T 波抬高
6.0	T 波高尖
7.0	ST 段压低伴 PR 间期延长
8.0	心房停搏伴“正弦波”QRS 波群
9.0	心室颤动

由于初期止血的获得性缺陷，尿毒症患者常有出血倾向，但他们的凝血因子检测通常是正常的，血小板计数可能略有下降，其出血机制比较复杂，主要是由于血小板与血管壁的黏附能力减弱，以及血小板对肾上腺素、二磷酸腺苷、胶原和纤维蛋白原反应不敏感导致血小板凝集障碍。尿毒症患者血小板释放的三磷酸腺苷和血清素减少，环氧合酶活性降低，同时尿毒症时糖蛋白Ⅱ b- Ⅲ a 复合物激活依赖的受体功能存在缺陷，导致血管性血友病因子（von Willebrand factor，vWF）和纤维蛋白原与血小板的结合减少，一氧化氮（nitric oxide，NO）和前列环素也限制了血小板的活化。

血小板功能下降的检测方法较多，从作为金标准的劳动密集型的光学密度比浊法（light transmission aggregometry，LTA）到检测周期较短的自动分析仪，如血小板功能分析仪（PFA-100，Siemens Medical Solutions，Erlangen，Germany），多板全血小板聚集检测（Roche，Switzerland），或血栓弹力图检测，如 TEG 血小板图谱（Haemonetics，Braintree，MA，USA）或 ROTEM（TEM Intl，Munich Germany）等。虽然皮肤出血时间检测简单易获得，但由于其对出血风险的预测不准确以及操作者操作技术差异性大，许多机构已经放弃这项检测。尽管 ESRD 患者有出血倾向，但其高凝状态的标志物，如 vWF 活性和血栓弹力图振幅升高却常显而易见。事实上，ESRD患者常服用抗血小板药物治疗心血管疾病，或预防房室植入物血栓形成，这也是导致出血倾向的原因之一。

心血管功能障碍在ESRD患者中很常见，因为慢性透析患者高血压、左心室肥厚和冠状动脉疾病发病率很高。此外，心脏自主神经功能障碍导致心脏 α 受体和 β 受体反应性降低，导致患者对急性血流动力学变化的代偿能力下降。高达40%的ESRD和动静脉瘘患者存在肺动脉高压。

低氧血症和平衡失调综合征是本病的常见的并发症，麻醉科医师应警惕在透析过程中或透析后不久均可能发生这两种情况。在透析液使用醋酸盐时，低氧血症发生概率较使用碳酸氢盐高，这与透析时继发的 CO_2 丢失，醋酸盐代谢所致 CO_2 产生减少，氧耗增加，以及ESRD患者补体激活诱发的肺部炎症相关，但是低氧血症通常是一过性的。不平衡综合征是由于尿素和其他渗透活性物质的快速清除所致，因为血脑屏障为了阻止这些物质从脑细胞中迅速清除，脑细胞变得相对高渗，液体沿渗透梯度进入脑细胞，从而可能出现脑水肿。

风险评估

长期透析并接受大手术的患者，围术期死亡率高于肾功能正常的患者，尤其是接受心脏直视手术的患者（约为12%，而非透析人群的2.9%）。大手术的风险与ESRD导致的异常相关，也与患者的基础疾病病程有关，如高血压。心脏舒张功能障碍与扩张型心肌病均是导致透析患者充血性心力衰竭的常见原因，因此在ESRD患者中，即使是摄入轻微过量的食盐和水可也可导致左心室舒张末期压大幅升高，从而导致肺水肿。透析患者每年因心绞痛或心肌梗死住院治疗的概率为10%，心脏疾病约占透析患者死亡原因的45%。贫血和高血压是死亡率的独立预测因素。虽然ESRD患者的全因死亡率在过去几年有所改善，但30～50岁的透析患者的预期寿命仍然只有普通人群的1/3左右。

琥珀胆碱等可导致血钾升高的麻醉药物，其插管剂量可增加死亡的风险；然而，在手术前血钾水平正常的ESRD患者中，这一风险似乎并不高，如有指征则不必禁用此药。多次输血（1 U全血可含有高达70 mEq/L的钾），以及由于低灌注期间或无法通过增加分钟通气量来充分代偿增加的代谢性酸中毒而引起的酸中毒都会提高血钾水平。药物蓄积和过量主要是由于药物本身及其活性代谢产物的肾清除率下降所致，这是重复给药时的主要顾虑。另外，由于血浆蛋白减少，药物蛋白未结合率增加也会导致药物相对过量，因此对于需要高度蛋白结合的药物，如咪达唑仑、阿芬太尼或巴比妥酸盐，需要降低初始剂量。

中性粒细胞和单核细胞功能改变，以及淋巴细胞激活受损，可能会增加ESRD患者感染的风险，由于常常出入医疗机构，这些患者感染细菌病原体的风险也很高。

所有的全麻技术都可能减少肾灌注，并可能对患者残留肾功能产生不利影响，这些残留肾功能对患者的健康仍极为重要。尚无一种吸入麻醉剂显示优于其他吸入药物，或优于全凭静脉麻醉。

启示

对于ESRD患者，始终潜在发生与电解质、凝血和酸碱平衡相关的严重威胁生命问题的可能，而患者共存的疾病，特别是严重的心血管异常，使这种可能性进一步加剧。

管理

框6.3列出了治疗接受手术的ESRD患者的一般原则，不论其病因如何。

长期透析患者的血管通路

由于ESRD手术患者常存在多种并存疾病，因

框 6.3 ESRD 手术患者的一般管理

- 手术后24 h内透析
- 血清钾在正常范围
- 血清碳酸氢盐浓度≥20 mEq/L
- 术前尽可能维持血容量正常或轻微低血容量
- 血细胞比容在30%左右
- 无钾液体；洗涤红细胞以最大限度地减少输入的钾负荷
- 谨慎使用琥珀胆碱
- 选择不依赖于肾排泄的药物；调整（减少）依赖于肾代谢或高度蛋白结合的药物剂量
- 放置血管内装置时严格无菌操作
- 术中识别并充分保护功能性分流
- 注意压力支点的衬垫

此这类患者常需要进行有创血流动力学监测，另外，患者可能还需要静脉输血和使用血管活性药物。外周静脉通路可能很难开放，而中心静脉通路建立也同样具有挑战，因为在多次放置透析导管后常有血管血栓形成，因此在穿刺消毒铺单前使用超声评估血管通畅度，以及在操作时使用超声实时引导很有必要，超声已成为临床上极具价值的工具。在紧急情况下，谨慎使用动静脉瘘或透析导管，使用前有必要权衡移植物或导管血栓的形成或感染的风险及其严重后果。

高钾血症的处理

急性高血钾的处理可分为三个步骤：第一步治疗是给予钙剂来拮抗钾的不良影响；第二步通过刺激 Na-K-ATP 酶或跟随电流梯度将血清钾转移到细胞内；第三步包括通过透析或使用离子交换树脂去除多余的血钾（表 6.3）。

尿毒症患者出血的治疗

使用促红细胞生成素和（或）输注洗涤红细胞治疗使血细胞比容升高到 30% 以上，可明显缩短尿毒症患者的出血时间。红细胞通过释放二磷酸腺苷，使血小板远离轴流并向血管壁靠近而增加血小板与血管壁的接触，以及通过使前列环素和一氧化氮等血小板聚集抑制剂失活，从而增强血小板的功能。输注去氨加压素（1-deamino-8-D-arginine vasopressin，DDAVP）的升压作用比血管升压素小，它可以能刺激内皮细胞释放 vWF，这可能是其用于治疗尿毒症的原因之一。持续静脉或皮下注射 0.3 μg/kg DDAVP（稀释至 50 ml 生理盐水）15 ～ 30 min，可使尿毒症患者出血时间缩短 50% ～ 100%，30 ～ 60 min 起效，持续时间约为 4 h，该效应与血浆中 vWF 浓度升高以及 vWF 中高分子量多聚体比例的增加有关。在应用 DDAVP 的第二个剂量之后可发生快速耐药，可能是由于内皮细胞多聚体损耗所致。冷沉淀含有丰富的Ⅷ /vWF 因子，初始应用剂量 10 ～ 20 U，起效时间与去氨加压素相似，但有效作用时间可持续 24 ～ 36 h。

择期大手术前使用结合雌激素 [普罗马林 0.6 mg/（kg · d），连续 5 天] 是有效的，有效时间持续 3 ～ 4 周。

血液透析可显著改善血小板功能障碍，如有必要，应在择期手术后 24 h 内使用。然而研究表明，血液透析可能会一过性地恶化血小板功能，但这一作用似乎在透析后的第二天就可以逆转。氨甲环酸也可以在这些治疗无效时使用，然而，在肾衰竭时它可能产生蓄积。

表 6.3 急性高钾血症的治疗

机制	干预
钾离子的拮抗作用	氯化钙或葡萄糖酸钙 1 ～ 2 g 缓慢静脉推注
钾离子细胞内转移（30 min 内有效）	中度过度通气 胰岛素 20 单位 / 葡萄糖 50 g 静脉输注 20 ～ 30 min 碳酸氢钠，50 ～ 100 mEq Ⅳ 沙丁胺醇，10 mg（雾化） 肾上腺素，0.01 μg/（kg · min）Ⅳ
体内除钾	聚苯乙烯磺酸钠（kayexate）（100 ml 20% 山梨醇中 30 g 聚苯乙烯磺酸钠），通过鼻胃管（30 g）或直肠（30～60 g）给予（钾交换钠，可能导致肺水肿） 紧急血液透析（必要时在术中）；低血压、出血风险

预防

与治疗该患者的肾内科医师的沟通是预防 ESRD 围术期并发症最好的方法，在他们的帮助下，为患者在手术前一天安排透析，并在术后即刻或术中必要时安排透析。越来越多的证据表明，在透析开始之前对高血压的积极治疗是一种有效的干预措施，可以降低随后的心血管事件相关的死亡率。同样，推荐在早期治疗贫血，因其可延迟或防止左心室肥厚，并且可以减少出血问题。预防和治疗酸中毒，使血清碳酸氢盐大于 20 mEq/L，可建立酸性缓冲体系，有助于降低发生高钾血症的风险。在大手术后，这些措施的应用在未来有利于降低 ESRD 相关的严重发病率和死亡率，并改善患者的预后。

（陆梁梁　译　许　华　校）

延伸阅读

Aniskevich S, Pai SL, Shine TS: Anesthetic pharmacology for kidney transplant patients, *Curr Clin Pharmacol* 10(1):47–53, 2015.

Brugnara C, Eckardt K-U: Hematologic aspects of kidney disease. In Taal

MW, Chertow GM, Marsden PA, et al.: *Brenner and Rector's the kidney*, ed 9, Philadelphia, 2012, Elsevier, pp 2081–2121.
Hakeem A, Bhatti S, Chang SM: Screening and risk stratification of coronary artery disease in end stage renal disease, *JACC Cardiovasc Imaging* 7(7):715–728, 2014.
National Kidney Foundation: K/DOQI clinical practice guidelines for chronic kidney disease: evaluation, classification and stratification, *Am J Kidney Dis* 39(Suppl 1):S1–S266, 2002.
Saran R, Li Y, Robinson B, et al.: US Renal Data System 2014 annual data report: epidemiology of kidney disease in the United States, *Am J Kidney Dis* 66(1 Suppl 1), 2015. Svii, S1–S305.
Schoorl M, Grooteman MP, Bartels PC, et al.: Aspects of platelet disturbances in haemodialysis patients, *Clin Kidney J* 6(3):266–271, 2013.
Svenson PJ, Bergqvist PB, Juul KV, et al.: Desmopressin in treatment of haematological disorders and in prevention of surgical bleeding, *Blood Rev* 28(3):95–102, 2014.
Trainor D, Bothwick E, Ferguson A: Perioperative management of the hemodialysis patient, *Semin Dial* 24(3):314–326, 2011.

手术室内不接受复苏的患者 第 7 章

Gail A. Van Norman

病例概要

患者，女性，86 岁，在某个下午晚些时候在家中摔倒致髋部骨折，拟急诊行手术治疗。患者平时生活自理，家中有护工照料，意识清楚，表达清晰。她是一位“DNR”患者，申明如果在手术室发生“心脏停搏”，不接受复苏治疗措施。她解释说，心脏停搏后即便是接受复苏治疗，自己能够继续独立生活的概率也非常小，她不愿意冒着长期残疾的风险接受复苏。麻醉科医师和矫形科医师劝她为了手术最好先搁置“DNR”协议，但被患者拒绝。随后，麻醉科医师声明，复苏是“麻醉的必要组成部分”，除非她先搁置她的“DNR”协议，否则不会为她实施麻醉。最终，患者“愤怒地”同意搁置“DNR”协议，手术顺利完成。

问题分析

定义

1960 年，Kouwenhoven 等首先描述了使用胸外心脏按压抢救呼吸心搏骤停患者，该急救方法迅速被医疗卫生行业广泛接受。尽管在 Kouwenhoven 的报告中心肺复苏（cardiopulmonary resuscitation，CPR）的存活率达到了 70%，但是后续研究却表明生存率令人沮丧。并且，在住院患者中普遍应用 CPR 会增加住院治疗以及重症监护病房（intensive care unit，ICU）治疗的费用。同时，公众也对复苏后的生活质量表示担忧。

20 世纪 70 年代初，美国最高法院开创了法律先例（如昆兰、南希布鲁赞事件）并发表了后续声明：达到法定年龄且心智健全、有自主决定能力的患者，有权利拒绝任何的医学治疗，包括生命支持治疗。1990 年，美国《患者自决权法》确立了联邦法律来保护患者拒绝生命支持治疗的权利，并以撤回联邦对所在医疗机构的资金支持为威胁，强迫医疗机构尊重并实施这项法案（框 7.1）。

尽管明确规定了患者拒绝复苏的法律权利，许多医师面对麻醉和手术的患者提出不接受复苏（do-not-resuscitate，DNR）的要求时，还是会感到矛盾。

框 7.1　第 4449 号决议——1990 年《患者自决权法》第 1395 条规定

“预先指令”定义为：州法律认可的书面指示（例如，生前遗嘱或卫生保健机构签署的永久授权书），并提及在个人丧失行为能力时提供照护的相关内容。

医疗工作者必须维护有关成人预先指令的政策和程序。

每位患者必须收到以下书面信息：

- 他们有接受或拒绝治疗的权利
- 他们有权制定预先指令
- 相关机构关于落实患者权利的书面政策

医院、专业护理机构和收容所在患者入院时必须提供以上信息。

每个患者的病历中必须有关于预先指令的文件。

相关机构不能因存在预先指令而对患者的照护加以限制或歧视。

相关机构必须确保遵守有关预先指令的州法律。

相关机构必须就预先指令的相关问题向工作人员和社区提供宣教。

心搏呼吸骤停和复苏措施在手术室与在医院其他区域有着不同的医学意义。例如，发生在医院病房的呼吸骤停可能是一个“最终事件”。为了防止死亡或永久伤害，心搏骤停需要立即识别和有效干预，包括可能的气管插管和机械通气。心脏停搏的治疗可包括心血管药物支持、直流电击、心肺复苏和机械循环支持。但是在没有其他说明时，DNR 意味着许多抢救措施（即使不是全部）不能实施。

然而，在手术室中，这些干预措施的某些组成部分是常规麻醉管理的一部分。麻醉药物可以抑制呼吸，需要呼吸辅助，包括插管和机械通气。血流动力学中常见的和可预见的变化可能需要药物支持。确实，这些干预措施正是麻醉管理的本质。

麻醉科医师提出了取消手术室患者 DNR 要求的几个常见理由是：①在手术室内 CPR 的结局比在医院其他地方更好；②麻醉“不是别的，而是进行中的复苏”，不能与其他复苏措施明确区分；③不接受复苏要求的患者也应放弃侵入性手术，因为对要求被允许死去的患者进行侵入性手术是没有意义的。

尽管经过几十年的努力，CPR 的结局仍然不尽如人意。医院外心脏停搏的出院生存率只有 6% 左右。多项研究表明，医院内心脏停搏后，只有不到一半的患者能在初期存活下来，总体的出院存活率为 6% ～ 26.5%，但是存活率的提高在一定程度上被出院后接受临终关怀或长期护理的比例上升所抵消。医院内心脏停搏的幸存者有相当比例都合并严重的神经损伤。某研究显示，总体看来，大约 42% 的幸存者都发生了明显的神经损伤。

心脏停搏在非心脏、非创伤手术中相对罕见，大约 10 000 例接受手术麻醉的患者中有 3 例发生。当我们统计在非心脏手术中发生心脏停搏的结局时，发现较在其他地方发生心脏停搏的结局要稍好些，但依然严峻。在手术室内大约 60% 的患者心脏停搏后的 1 h 内存活。至少有一项研究发现，46% 的即时生存者（约占总数的 36%）将在住院期间死亡，通常是在 ICU 内。只有 37% 的出院生存者大脑功能“良好”。简言之，与医院其他地方相比，手术室内行非心脏手术发生心脏停搏的患者长期预后较好（尽管仍然很差）。Kalkman 最近的关于与麻醉相关的心脏停搏和 CPR 的回顾报告显示，患者预后稍好，但仍然远达不到人们的期望：即时生存率约为 41.6%，1 ～ 24 h 内生存率为 32% ～ 55.7%，出院后随访时生存率为 45.3% ～ 66.8%。这篇综述的作者认为，麻醉相关心搏骤停后长期存活率实际约为 25%。该项报告还未将患者的生存**质量**纳入研究范围。我们可以得出结论，手术室内心脏停搏后的生存率要高于发生在医院外的心脏停搏，甚至比在医院的其他地方要高，但仍然是很低。

然而，关于麻醉“不是别的，而是进行中的复苏”的说法是很难令人信服，因为它实际上是对“复苏”这一术语的借用和误导。医师和患者用“复苏”这个术语来描述完全不同的事件，医师口中“复苏”的含义是多种多样，通常在不同情况下代表的意义明显不同。例如，“液体复苏”与 CPR 是差别很大的治疗措施。因此说麻醉“不是别的，而是进行中的复苏”错误地暗示“麻醉过程是一种不可控、接近濒死的体验，麻醉科医师要一直对患者进行复苏，心脏停搏在麻醉中常见，CPR 是麻醉中的常规治疗措施”，而事实上心脏停搏是麻醉科医师在工作中积极预防、避免发生的极端事件。

患者提出不接受 CPR 的要求时，他们通常指的是一个非常具体的事件，即心脏完全停止跳动，并且通常将其清楚地描述为“当我的心脏停止跳动时”。他们认为心脏停搏通常是一种终末事件，恢复原有功能的可能性是有限的。显然，他们是正确的。我们知道，大多数在手术室内发生心脏停搏的患者实际上不能活到出院，而且许多人即使能活到出院时也并存严重后遗症。

最后，仅仅因为患者不愿接受很少用到的侵入性和具有潜在伤害性的治疗措施（如 CPR），就拒绝给予患者能改善其余生质量的合理治疗是不恰当的，即使患者剩余的生存时间很短。这样做不仅违背了医学减轻痛苦的基本原则，更是对患者的胁迫。

伦理方面的考虑

西方医学伦理的基本原则是尊重和帮助患者行使自主权，“做好事”（行善）和“避免伤害”（无害原则）。过去，医学伦理强调，保全患者生命是最重要的伦理原则，为达到这一目的，医师有责任强制患者接受治疗。

尊重患者自主权的原则要求，一旦充分知情和有决定能力患者被告知有关治疗信息，他（她）同意或拒绝各种治疗的决定都应得到准许。CPR 在手术室中的结果与其他情形下有显著差异，这一事实需要与患者一起讨论，根据手术室的特殊情况让患者做出决定。然而，放弃复苏治疗的决定权仍在患者手中。医师对复苏的看法可能会受到个人价值观、过高的期望、人际关系的冲突、无意识的动机、对职业失败的恐惧以及对法律惩罚的恐惧等因素的影响，而所有这些几乎都与患者的需求无关。**在道德**

层面和法律层面，只有患者或患者指定的代理人才有权做出同意或拒绝治疗的决定。

法律上的考虑

尽管法律早已规定患者有权做出包括拒绝或停止生命支持治疗在内的医疗决定，但研究一再表明，医师仍对患者的预先决定知之甚少，而且在半数以上的病例中，医师的做法与患者的预先决定相违背。

许多医师没有意识到患者拒绝生命支持治疗的权利受联邦法律保护，甚至更少的医师意识到，违背患者事先已有的DNR要求而对患者实施复苏可能会使他们处于违法的境地。在一些案件中，法庭上原告有理由以“殴打”——一种未经同意、直接或间接有害或冒犯性的接触行为，提起诉讼。值得注意的是，“殴打”并不需要有任何直接的敌意，甚至不需要存在身体伤害就能成立。还要注意的是，殴打是一种犯罪。

治疗侵犯了患者拒绝治疗的权利，导致患者“不想要的寿命延长”时，这种“错误的生存”（wrongful living）案例涉嫌民事侵权。由于法院不愿意将继续生存视为“可补偿的损害”，在一些这类案件中，原告有权获得的损害赔偿迟迟未得到，而近期该问题得到重新关注。此外，遵守1990年《联邦患者自决权法》（也见第24章）是参加联邦医疗保险和医疗补助项目的一个条件（见框7.1）。不执行法律要求的医疗机构可能会受到惩罚和（或）被排除在医疗保险和医疗补助之外。在过去10年里，至少有两家医疗机构被医疗保险和医疗补助服务中心（Centers for Medicare and Medicaid Services）判定为违反上述法规。执行法官支持国家纪律委员会对不遵守患者事先要求的医疗服务者做出制裁，直至吊销执业医师执照。此外，法院还决定，因这种不必要的治疗而产生不利影响，患者有权要求赔偿。2011年，在俄克拉荷马州的Callsion起诉Hillcrest医联体一案中，一家医院违背患者的事先要求和家属意愿，继续对患者进行插管，法院拒绝驳回患方对院方“殴打”的指控。最终双方在庭外达成和解。其他一些法庭案例也表明，对于具有法律效力的DNR要求，原告具有法律赋予的权利获得赔偿。另一个案例是2006年美国公民自由联盟（American Civil Liberties Union）起诉一家骨科手术中心，因为该中心要求患者签署的一份文件中明确告知患方该机构“不遵循‘DNR’指令和（或）预先指令、生前遗嘱”。该案件最终在庭外和解，但其表明当医师使用强制手段（如拒绝麻醉和手术）违反DNR要求和其他预先指令时，将承担重大的法律风险。此外，在违反患者预先指令（包括DNR要求）的案件中，法院也做出了给予原告大量金钱赔偿的判决，尽管这种情况并不常见。Brenda Young就是一个例子，她在接受了“不愿意”的复苏后出现了严重的神经损伤，她的家人获得了1650万美元的赔偿（后来医院上诉，该赔偿减少到140万美元）。

1993年，美国麻醉科医师协会制定并发布了《管理不复苏要求和其他限制医疗治疗要求的患者的伦理指南》。他们建议麻醉科医师与患者或其授权者就手术室治疗的预后进行知情讨论，并尊重患者对此类治疗的决定。因个人原因不能接受患者意愿的医疗工作者应退出治疗过程，并寻找能够提供服务的替代者。1994年，美国外科医师协会和手术室护士协会也效仿了美国麻醉科医师协会的指导方针。此外，联合委员会要求实施适当的政策和程序，以便能最大限度地尊重患者拒绝复苏的意愿。

识别

确定手术室内的患者有无DNR非常重要，对于所有将进行麻醉和手术的患者，应常规询问是否签署过预先指令的相关文件。每一次麻醉操作都应该有程序和规定来确定手术室DNR将如何处理。这些规定必须与医学伦理标准和法律相一致，要记住，如果患者和（或）他的授权者已经被恰当地告知相关的预后情况，即使是在手术室内，联邦法律、法律判例和专业指南都支持患者DNR的权利。

解决办法

在本例中，我们面对的一位有明确心智决策能力的患者，她希望在手术室中遵循她的DNR要求。不幸的是，医师们错误地认为可以要求患者撤销她的要求，甚至采取胁迫手段（威胁拒绝为她做改善她生活质量的手术）来达到他们的目的。强迫患者违背自己的意愿撤销她的要求，医师们违反了尊重患者自主决定权这一医学伦理学的基本原则。不仅这种要求撤销DNR的做法在伦理和法律上是错误的，而且这也造成人们对手术同意本身的质疑，因为患者可能是在被强迫的情况下才签署了在手术室内接受某些潜在治疗的同意书。

有时患者的拒绝确实降低了手术操作标准或使手术无法进行，这种情况与我们上述讨论的并不是一回事。例如患者拒绝插管，那么医师拒绝开胸手术就是合情合理的，因为气管插管是每次开胸手术的必要和基本部分。

这个病例更可悲的是，医师们坚持认为自己有权对患者实施可能极其不利、极有可能造成巨大伤害的操作（CPR）。事实上，患者已经做出了符合现实的评估——从既往研究看，即使有必要行 CPR，她活着出院的可能性很小，即便她幸存下来，也很可能会残留神经损伤，无法独立生活。

伦理原则要求医师在医疗决策中尊重患者的自主权。美国法院的判例（包括最高法院）一再强调，患者有权拒绝任何医疗服务，包括生命支持治疗。在这种情况下，恰当的做法是麻醉科医师和外科医师向患者说明在手术室内 CPR 预后会较好，并告知患者，如果“心脏停止跳动”，患者会接受什么样的治疗措施（如果有的话）。经过这样讨论后，如果患者仍要求 DNR，就应当在病历中做出记录。如果患者决定手术前搁置她的 DNR 要求，则应制定术后恢复该指令的计划（通常在患者出麻醉恢复室后）。

预防

这一病例揭示了理论和实践上存在的差距，涉及的个别医师也可能并不是唯一对伦理和法律“知识”缺乏了解的医师。这个案件后有关部门不仅是应对相关医疗工作者进行教育，而且要针对整个医疗群体进行教育，指导所有医师在遇到类似情况时应采取何种符合伦理和法律的办法。此外，还应制定发布相关规定和章程，并向从业人员公布，规范对 DNR 患者实施麻醉和手术的管理方法。

规章制度应包括以下方面：

- 确定将行麻醉和手术的患者是否有预先指令，如 DNR。
- 与患者和（或）患者的合法授权者讨论复苏的原则，包括手术室内复苏的风险和益处。
- 如果 DNR 有任何变化，应当记录在患者病历中。
- 告知手术室团队中其他成员 DNR 的存在，并讨论在手术室如何管理患者。
- 如果对 DNR 的有效性产生疑问，机构伦理委员会或法律顾问可以提供帮助。
- 如果医疗工作者不能认同患者希望在围术期坚持 DNR 的意愿，那么相关医疗工作人员应当退出该患者的治疗过程，并将患者转交给能接受这种情况的同事。
- 在紧急情况下，尽可能确认是否存在预先指令。如果不存在任何指示，或该指示的有效性存在疑问，则应在尽可能尊重患者意愿的情况下，进行最好的医疗护理。
- 如果患者希望在围术期中止 DNR，应在术后恢复 DNR，通常是在患者出麻醉恢复室后。

（赵晗燚　译　刘　毅　校）

延伸阅读

American Civil Liberties Union of New Mexico (Press release): ACLU of New Mexico defends patients' end-of-life wishes. Available at http://www.aclu.org/technology-and-liberty/aclu-new-mexico-defends-patients-end-life-wishes, June 9, 2005 Accessed November 12, 2015.

American College of Surgeons: Statement on advance directives by patients; do not resuscitate in the operating room, *Bull Am Coll Surg* 79(9):29, 1994.

American Society of Anesthesiologists: *Committee on Ethics: Ethical guidelines for the anesthesia care of patients with do-not-resuscitate orders or other directives that limit treatment. Last amended October 15, 2013*, Park Ridge, IL, 2013, ASA. Available at http://www.asahq.org. Accessed November 12, 2015.

Anderson v. St Francis–St George Hosp, Inc, 671 N.E.2d 225, 227 (Ohio 1996).

Association of Operating Room Nurses (AORN) Position Statement: *Perioperative care of patients with do-not-resuscitate orders*, Denver, 1995, AORN.

Bloom HL, Shukrullah I, Cuellar JR, et al.: Long-term survival after successful inhospital cardiac arrest resuscitation, *Am Heart J* 153:831–836, 2007.

Callision v. Hillcrest Healthcare Sys., No. CJ-2010-3197, 2011 WL, 7990001 (Okla. Dist. Ct. Tulsa Cty Apr 14, 2011).

Collins LG, Parks SM, Winter L: The state of advance care planning: one decade after SUPPORT, *Am J Hosp Palliat Care* 23:378–384, 2006.

Cruzan v. Director, Missouri Department of Health, 497 U.S. 261, 1990.

Elshove-Bolk J, Guttormsen AB, Austlid I: In-hospital resuscitation of the elderly: characteristics and outcome, *Resuscitation* 74:372–376, 2007.

Girotra S, Nallamothu BK, Spertus JA, et al.: Trends in survival after in-hospital cardiac arrest, *N Engl J Med* 367:1912–1920, 2012.

Gragg v. Calandra 696 N.E. 2nd 1281, 1286 (Ill. App. Ct. 1998).

HR4449—The Patient Self Determination Act of 1990, an amendment to the Omnibus Budget Reconciliation Act of 1990. Available at http://thomas.loc.gov/cgi-bin/query/z?c101:H.R.4449.IH. Accessed November 12, 2015.

In re Quinlan (70 N.J. 10, 355 A.2d 647 [NJ 1976]).

Joint Commission on Accreditation of Healthcare Organizations: *Patient rights*. In *Manual of the Joint Commission on Accreditation of Health Care Organizations*, Chicago, 1994, JCAHO.

Kalkman S, Hooft L, Meijerman JM, et al.: Survival after perioperative cardiopulmonary resuscitation: providing an evidence base for ethical management of do-not-resuscitate orders, *Anesthesiology* 124(3):723–729, 2015.

Kazaure HS, Roman SA, Sosa JA: Epidemiology and outcomes of in-hospital cardiopulmonary resuscitation in the United States, 2000–2009, *Resuscitation* 84:1255–1260, 2013.

Kouwenhoven WB, Jude JR, Knickerbocker GG: Closed-chest cardiac mas-

sage, *JAMA* 173:1064–1067, 1960.
Lynch HF, Mathes M, Sawicki NN: Compliance with advance directives: wrongful living and tort law incentives, *J Leg Med* 19:133–178, 2008.
Mahmood Yoonessi, M.D., BPMC 02-188, 2002 WL 33840948 (N.Y. Dep't of Health Bd. for Prof'l Med. Conduct June 5, 2002).
Peberdy MA, Kaye W, Ornato J, et al.: Cardiopulmonary resuscitation of adults in the hospital: a report of 14,720 cardiac arrests from the National Registry of Cardiopulmonary Resuscitation, *Resuscitation* 58:297–308, 2003.
Reisfield GM, Wallace SK, Munsell MF, et al.: Survival in cancer patients undergoing in-hospital cardiopulmonary resuscitation: a meta-analysis, *Resuscitation* 71:152–160, 2006.
Sawicki N: *A new life for wrongful living. LAW eCommons. Faculty Publications and Other Works*, Chicago, 2014, Loyola University of Chicago School of Law. Available at http://lawecommons.luc.edu/cgi/viewcontent.cgi?article=1472&context=facpubs. Accessed November 12, 2015.
Sprung J, Warner M, Contreras M, et al.: Predictors of survival following cardiac arrest in patients undergoing noncardiac surgery: a study of 518,294 patients at a tertiary referral center, *Anesthesiology* 99:259–269, 2003.
Strasser M: A jurisprudence in disarray: on battery, wrongful living, and the right to bodily integrity, *36 San Diego L. Rev.* 997(1999):1021, 1999.
Strategies to improve cardiac arrest survival: a time to act. A report of the Institute of Medicine, Washington, DC, June 2015, National Academy of Sciences. Available at http://iom.nationalacademies.org/Reports/2015/Strategies-to-Improve-Cardiac-Arrest-Survival.aspx. Accessed November 12, 2015.

第 8 章 影响肾素-血管紧张素系统的药物

Laura Stover

病例概要

患者，男性，70 岁，体重 95 kg，拟行左侧颈内动脉内膜切除术。既往服用氨氯地平（每天 5 mg）和血管紧张素Ⅱ受体拮抗剂-厄贝沙坦（每天 150 mg）治疗高血压，手术日晨常规服用上述两种常规药物。术前检查：经胸超声心动图显示左心室收缩功能正常、室间隔肥厚。麻醉诱导前血压 150/70 mmHg，心率 56 次/分。静脉滴注 900 ml 晶体液后，用舒芬太尼（10 μg）、丙泊酚（150 mg）和罗库溴铵（50 mg）诱导，随后气管插管，吸入地氟烷［0.7 最低肺泡有效浓度（minimum alveolar concentration，MAC）］和空氧混合气（氧气：空气 =40：60）维持麻醉。诱导后 2 min，血压降至 80/44 mmHg。反复静注麻黄碱（共 50 mg），诱导后 4 min，血压降至 47/30 mmHg。

问题分析

定义与识别

肾素-血管紧张素系统（renin-angiotensin system，RAS）拮抗剂，包括血管紧张素转换酶（angiotensin-converting enzyme，ACE）抑制剂和血管紧张素Ⅱ受体拮抗剂。这类药物通常用于治疗特定择期手术患者的高血压和心力衰竭。ACE 抑制剂和血管紧张素Ⅱ受体拮抗剂阻断 RAS，可对麻醉和手术过程中的血流动力学产生不良影响。尽管麻醉并非总是与 RAS 阻滞的患者血流动力学不稳定相关，但仍有意外发生的难治性低血压的报道。而且，RAS 拮抗剂，特别是 ACE 抑制剂，还与潜在危及生命的头颈部血管性水肿有关。

RAS 在调节血管张力和细胞外液方面起着重要作用。如图 8.1 所示，通过 β_1-肾上腺素能受体兴奋交感、肾动脉低血压和向远端肾小管输送的钠离子减少，都可刺激肾释放肾素。肾素是一种蛋白水解酶，能裂解循环中的血管紧张素原形成血管紧张素Ⅰ，而血管紧张素Ⅰ几乎没有内在的药理活性。血管紧张素Ⅰ通过存在于血管内皮和肺组织中的 ACE 催化作用立即转化为血管紧张素Ⅱ。

在短时间期内（即术中），血管紧张素Ⅱ通过增加血管（特别是小动脉）张力来保持血管稳态。它一方面直接作用于血管紧张素Ⅱ受体，另一方面间接通过增强交感神经肾上腺素能功能来增加血管张

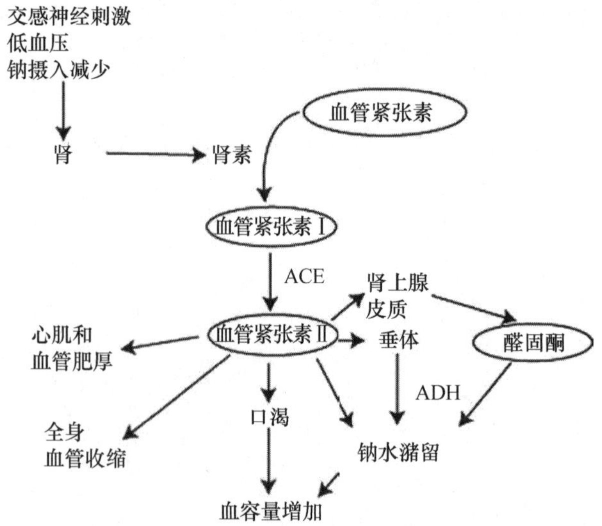

图 8.1 肾素-血管紧张素系统。ACE，血管紧张素转换酶；ADH，抗利尿激素

力，这对存在低血容量或心排血量减少的患者维持足够的灌注压是必需的。长期来看（例如几小时至数天），血管紧张素Ⅱ通过影响细胞外液容量而保持血管稳态。其促进肾上腺皮质释放醛固酮，醛固酮是一种作用于肾的激素，可增加水钠潴留。血管紧张素Ⅱ还刺激垂体后叶释放血管加压素（即抗利尿激素），使肾增加水潴留。长期接受 RAS 拮抗剂治疗的患者，由于血管紧张素Ⅱ介导增加的血管张力被阻断、血管内容量相对减少，可导致麻醉诱导后难治性低血压。

口咽部或喉部血管性水肿已被确认为 ACE 抑制剂治疗的一种少见并发症。ACE 抑制剂诱发的血管性水肿，通常在开始治疗后数小时至数天内自发表现出来，且被认为与麻醉和气管插管相关时已有相关描述。舌水肿是常出现的症状，水肿累及脸、唇、口底、咽、声门或者喉也比较常见。

血管性水肿形成的确切机制尚未确定。因其可能是由激肽释放酶–缓激肽系统介导的，所以它可能是一种生化而非免疫学现象。缓激肽是一种强效的血管扩张剂，可增加血管通透性并产生组织水肿。激酶Ⅱ（等同于 ACE）是缓激肽分解的主要组织酶。ACE 抑制剂通过抑制激酶Ⅱ阻止缓激肽分解。因此，与 ACE 抑制剂治疗相关的血管性水肿，可能是通过抑制激酶Ⅱ阻止缓激肽失活的结果。

识别

低血压

要识别低血压是否是由于 RAS 拮抗剂治疗所致，术中就要排除其他可能导致低血压的事件。对于长期使用 RAS 拮抗剂治疗的患者，尤其是左心室舒张功能不全的患者，则高度怀疑其低血压是 RAS 拮抗剂所致。长期接受 RAS 拮抗剂治疗的患者麻醉诱导时常出现心血管不稳定，以及常规剂量麻黄素和去氧肾上腺素难以纠正的低血压，RAS 拮抗剂是可能的主要原因。

血管性水肿

要识别血管性水肿是 ACE 抑制剂所致，就要排除与头颈部肿胀相关的其他围术期事件（例如变态反应、过敏反应），以及了解 ACE 抑制剂导致血管性水肿的可能性（尽管很少）。当血管性水肿发生时，通常暂时认为其与启用 ACE 抑制剂治疗有关。

风险评估

低血压

接受 RAS 拮抗剂治疗的患者，有许多因素可以影响麻醉诱导相关严重低血压的风险。接受其他抗高血压药物联合 RAS 拮抗剂治疗的患者，在诱导时更可能出现难治性低血压。同样，RAS 拮抗剂与其他扩血管药物（如胺碘酮）合用会增加低血压的风险。与高剂量和近期给药相关的 RAS 完全阻滞的患者，诱导时更可能出现血压不稳定。有严重高血压病史的患者，尤其是左心室舒张功能不全的患者（增加了心排血量对前负荷的依赖性），亦会增加难治性低血压的风险。术前短期使用 RAS 拮抗剂（1 ～ 2 天）的血压正常或者轻度高血压患者，诱导时不太可能发生难治性低血压。但 RAS 拮抗剂治疗直至手术当天的患者，低血压风险增加。有文献回顾发现，严重高血压病史的患者 ACE 抑制剂持续用至手术当天，麻醉诱导时低血压的发生率为 75% ～ 100%。

血管性水肿

累及口咽部或喉部的血管性水肿是 ACE 抑制剂治疗的少见并发症，在服用卡托普利、赖诺普利或依那普利患者中平均发生率为 0.1%，服用依那普利的患者发病率可能略高于服用其他两种药物的患者（0.2%）。患者在开始使用 ACE 抑制剂的第 1 周内风险最高，一项对 36 000 例接受依那普利治疗的患者进行的回顾性研究显示，发生血管性水肿病例中的 60% ～ 70%，都发生在此期间。然而，血管性水肿在治疗数月至数年后可突然发生，已知这种情况下发生的血管性水肿病例中约 20% 可能发生严重症状（如呼吸困难、喘鸣、喉痉挛）。不幸的是，尚无任何特征可以预测哪些患者会发展到危及生命的气道损害。

启示

关于 RAS 拮抗剂用于麻醉诱导时发生顽固性低血压的风险，目前尚未就术前继续或停止使用该药物达成共识。对于这类药物，消除半衰期不一定能预测作用持续时间，因而很难对围术期给药提出建议。

治疗

低血压

如果 RAS 阻滞明显导致麻醉诱导后难治性低血压，治疗依赖于及时恢复足够的全身血管阻力和用去氧肾上腺素与垂体加压素维持静脉张力，以及加快静脉输液。处理 RAS 拮抗剂相关低血压的其他措施包括，停用或少用可能导致低血压的其他药物。一旦出现循环虚脱，应立即启用高级心血管生命支持方案。

血管性水肿

大多数 ACE 抑制剂诱导的血管性水肿程度较轻，停药后可自行消退。然而，水肿可能会迅速进展到包括咽后部或喉部，导致上呼吸道部分或完全阻塞。即使积极治疗，症状也可能会加剧，并可能在明显缓解数小时后复发。ACE 抑制剂引起的血管性水肿可能是致命性的。

处理措施包括从简单停用 ACE 抑制剂至气管插管或气管切开术。水肿局限于舌前部或嘴唇的轻度病例，通常会在停用 ACE 抑制剂或静注苯海拉明和类固醇药物后得到缓解。水肿累及咽部和引起吞咽困难的严重病例，可能需要皮下注射肾上腺素和（或）气管插管。与任何累及气道的病程进展一样，危及生命的气道阻塞的可能性，要求临床密切观察和及时干预。急性病情缓解后，应在患者的病历中记录这种可能危及生命的 ACE 抑制剂治疗的不良反应，患者应接受适当的医疗会诊。

预防

如前所述，对于术前 RAS 拮抗剂治疗是否应用至手术当日目前尚无达成共识。如果有足够的时间恢复 RAS 活性，术前停用 RAS 拮抗剂可降低麻醉诱导时发生低血压的风险。然而，任何风险的降低都可能以高血压或心力衰竭的优化治疗为代价。确认那些发生严重低血压风险最高的患者（严重高血压，或接受高剂量 RAS 拮抗剂，或接受 RAS 拮抗剂联合其他抗高血压药或长期应用 RAS 拮抗剂的患者），在麻醉诱导前给予一定的静脉输液量，可降低顽固性低血压的风险。这种预处理结合早期使用血管升压药治疗可以缩短因 RAS 阻滞导致的低血压的持续时间。与前述一致，诱导后即刻勤测血压（可能有必要进行直接有创动脉测压）有助于早期发现严重低血压。

（项　前　译　朱科明　校）

延伸阅读

Bjerregaard J, Jaffe RA: Intraoperative cardiac arrest: was it the ACE inhibitor? *J Clin Anesth* 26:62–64, 2014.

Colson P, Ryckwaert F, Coriat P: Renin angiotensin antagonists and anesthesia, *Anesth Analg* 89:1143–1155, 1999.

Coriat P, Richer C, Douraki T, et al.: Influence of chronic angiotensin-converting enzyme inhibition on anesthetic induction, *Anesthesiology* 81:299–307, 1994.

Dean DE, Shultz DL, Powers RH: Asphyxia due to angiotensin converting enzyme (ACE) inhibitor mediated angioedema of the tongue during the treatment of hypertensive heart disease, *J Forensic Sci* 46:1239–1243, 2001.

Kharash ED: Angiotensin-converting enzyme inhibitor-induced angioedema associated with endotracheal intubation, *Anesth Analg* 74:602–604, 1992.

HIV 感染和 AIDS

第 9 章

Michael S. Avidan

病例概要

患者，女性，34 岁，已知有人类免疫缺陷病毒（human immunodeficiency virus，HIV）感染，近期被诊断为获得性免疫缺陷综合征（acquired immunodeficiency syndrome，AIDS）合并肺孢子菌（既往称为卡氏肺孢子虫）肺炎，孕 38 周，拟行择期剖宫产术。患者怀孕期间未接受过保健医师的随访，也未接受过抗逆转录病毒治疗。患者气促，干咳，吸空气外周动脉血氧饱和度为 84%；体重 62 kg，身高 164 cm，鼓膜温 37.2℃。患者精神警觉，定向正常，且无神经定位征象。血压 90/50 mmHg，心率 115 次 / 分，且不随呼吸变异；呼吸频率 26 次 / 分。最近的实验室检查显示 CD4 T 细胞计数 186 cells/ml，HIV 病毒载量为 240 000 copies/ml。

问题分析

定义

AIDS 于 1981 年在美国首次被描述。尽管近年来在 HIV 的治疗方面取得了重大进展，但 AIDS 的流行仍然对全球健康构成重大威胁。据估计，全球有超过 4 000 万人感染 HIV，迄今已造成 2 000 多万人死亡。而且感染正迅速蔓延，在非洲南部和中部以及南亚增长最快。包括在发达国家，HIV 的主要传播方式是异性性行为，女性在新感染病例中所占比例很高。

越来越多的手术患者呈 HIV- 血清学阳性或患有 AIDS。麻醉科医师应熟悉此疾病，并了解 HIV 对麻醉的影响。了解 HIV 的发病机制和了解 HIV 治疗可能发生的药物相互作用有助于指导麻醉技术的选择。医院内传播 HIV 的可能性突出了麻醉科医师需严格执行感染控制制度，以保护自己、其他医护人员和患者。抗逆转录病毒治疗可降低疾病进展速度，但目前尚无治愈方法，在可预见的将来也无疫苗。随着治疗的显著进步，重点已转移到疾病早期不论免疫状态如何均应开始多种药物联合治疗，及后续持续治疗以实现 HIV 病毒终生抑制。

识别

HIV 属于逆转录病毒科、慢病毒属。该属的成员可致细胞病变（细胞损伤），有很长的潜伏期，并介导慢性病程。当 AIDS 病例第一次出现时，其发病机制难以确定，因为该疾病不会在感染 HIV 后立即出现。这是一个可变期，在此期间患者保持健康状态，但有病毒血症。

在感染后不久出现高病毒载量即可导致急性血清转换。几个月后，随着免疫反应的发生，病毒血症逐渐缓解。病毒载量通常处于稳定状态，此时病毒产生率等于破坏率。淋巴结是病毒复制和 T 细胞破坏的主要部位，多达 98% 的 T 辅助淋巴细胞（CD4 T 细胞）位于此处。因为 AIDS 的持续发作，淋巴结逐渐退化并伴随着 CD4 T 细胞的减少和病毒载量的增加（图 9.1）。

1995 年以前，HIV 治疗的前景黯淡。随后，四个因素导致情况发生了巨大变化：

1. 对 HIV 感染发病机制认识的提高。
2. 免疫功能和血浆病毒负荷替代指标的可用性。
3. 开发了新型、更强大的药物，如蛋白酶抑制剂、非核苷类逆转录酶抑制剂。
4. 完成了几项大型临床终点试验，最终证明抗逆转录病毒联合治疗显著延缓了 HIV 疾病向 AIDS 的

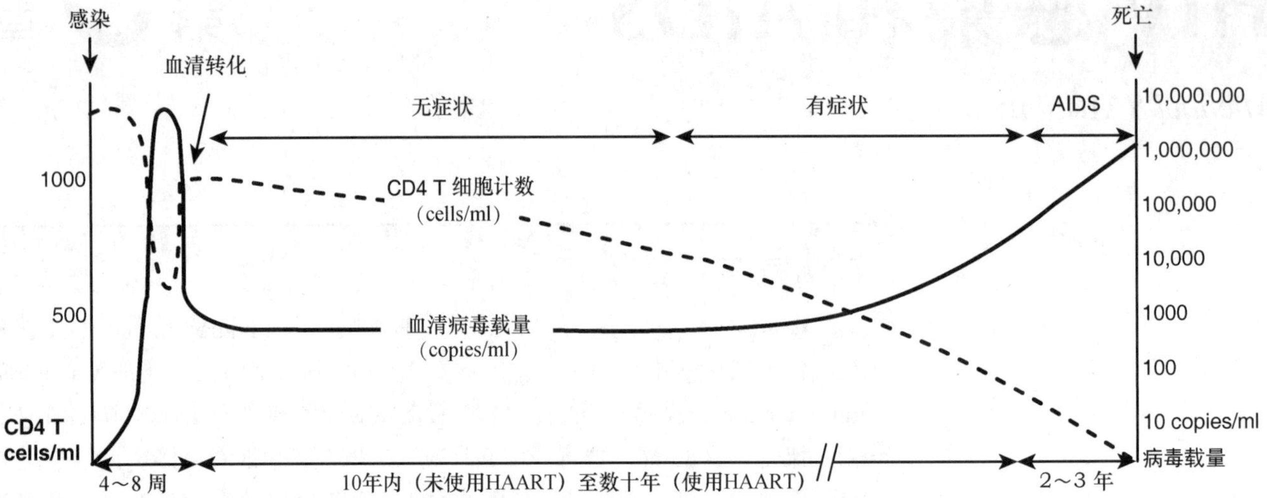

图 9.1 人类免疫缺陷病毒（HIV）感染者进展为获得性免疫缺陷综合征（AIDS）。请注意，高效抗逆转录病毒治疗（HAART）大大延缓了临床 AIDS 的发展

进展，提高了生存率。

近年来，随着治疗药物增多、副作用减少、毒性降低和载药负担下降，HIV 的治疗方法得到了进一步改变。已经证实，无论宿主 CD4 T 细胞计数如何，早期开始治疗都会使病毒几乎消失，使免疫功能恢复，可改善生活质量，防止传播，降低 HIV 相关发病率，延长生存期；事实上，有可能阻止其流行，甚至有可能根除 HIV 这种重大传染病威胁。

风险评估

HIV 是一种主要存在于 CD4 T 细胞、巨噬细胞和单核细胞中的病毒，其传播需要很大的感染剂量。从血液、脑脊液、泪液、唾液、精液、滑膜液、胸膜液、腹膜液、心包液、羊水、阴道分泌物和乳汁中均可分离出 HIV。传播方式有通过口腔、直肠和阴道性交，血液制品输血，共用静脉注射针，职业感染和母婴垂直传播。对血液制品进行 HIV 抗体筛查降低了输血相关感染的风险（每 750 000 个供体单位少于 1 个）。然而，确切的风险是难以量化的。抗体筛查在抗体形成前即所谓窗口期未能检测到病毒，此阶段持续约 3 个月。此外可选用核扩增作为替代技术，可用于早期病毒检测。

启示

普遍预防措施

疾病控制中心于 1987 年提出了预防血源性病毒传播的普遍预防措施。这些措施建议将所有患者都视为血源性病毒潜在感染者。

暴露后预防

在意外暴露于高感染风险体液后，如（空心）针刺伤，建议医护人员进行暴露后预防（postexposure prophylaxis，PEP）。预防应在伤后尽早开始，最好在 1 ～ 2 h 内，但至伤后 1 ～ 2 周内均应考虑实施。极高感染风险的暴露即使超过这个时间仍应给予处理，以期改变感染而非预防感染。持续 4 周的经典暴露后预防方案是替诺福韦 + 恩曲他滨 / 拉米夫定 + 拉替拉韦 / 度鲁特韦。此治疗方案因具有极好的耐受性，对 HIV 感染预防效力强且易于给药，是 PEP 极佳的选择。

管理

抗逆转录病毒药物治疗

目前正在使用的抗逆转录病毒药物有六大类（表 9.1）：

1. 核苷类似物逆转录酶抑制剂（nucleoside analog reverse transcriptase inhibitor，NRTI；1987 年批准）与展开的病毒 DNA 结合，阻止逆转录的完成。
2. 蛋白酶抑制剂 [（protease inhibitor，PI），1996] 抑制 HIV 蛋白酶，它能裂解最终构成成熟病毒体核心蛋白的多蛋白前体。PI 与活性剪切位点特异性结合。
3. 非核苷类逆转录酶抑制剂（nonnucleoside reverse transcriptase inhibitor，NNRTI；1998）通过在活

表 9.1 目前使用的抗逆转录病毒药物的主要类别

药物名称	给药方式	常见副作用
核苷类似物逆转录酶抑制剂		
齐多夫定（AZT/ZDV）	口服 / 静脉注射（每日 2 次）	明显的毒性，骨髓抑制（中性粒细胞减少症），胃肠不适，头痛
去羟肌苷（DDI）	口服	周围神经病变，胰腺炎，腹泻
扎西他滨（DDC）	口服	周围神经病变，胰腺炎，口腔溃疡
司他夫定（D4T）	口服	周围神经病变
拉米夫定（3TC）	口服	贫血，胃肠不适
阿巴卡韦	口服	胃肠道不适，可能致命的急性超敏反应（与 HLA-B*5701 的存在相关）
替诺福韦	口服（每日 1 次）	肾功能不全，骨软化
恩曲他滨	口服	头痛，胃肠道症状
非核苷类似物逆转录酶抑制剂		
奈韦拉平	口服	皮疹，肝炎，肝酶升高
地拉夫定	口服	皮疹，肝酶升高
依法韦仑	口服（每日 1 次，空腹）	头晕，皮疹，烦躁不安，肝酶升高，精神障碍
利匹韦林	口服（每日 1 次，随餐服用）	皮疹，肝炎
蛋白酶抑制剂		
沙奎那韦	口服	腹泻，转氨酶升高，高脂血症，细胞色素 P450 抑制，心律失常
茚地那韦	口服，24 h 饮水量≥ 1.5 L	肾结石，高胆红素血症，高脂血症，脂质代谢异常，细胞色素 P450 抑制
利托那韦	口服	胃肠道不适，口周感觉异常，高脂血症，脂质代谢异常，细胞色素 P450 抑制
奈非那韦	口服	腹泻，高脂血症，脂质代谢异常，细胞色素 P450 抑制
阿扎那韦	口服（需要酸性 pH 才能吸收）	血脂异常，胰岛素抵抗，高血糖，脂质代谢异常，细胞色素 P450 抑制，PR 间期延长
地瑞那韦	口服（随餐服用；可被利托那韦增强）	血脂异常，胰岛素抵抗，高血糖，脂质代谢异常，细胞色素 P450 抑制，胃肠道症状，肝毒性
福沙那韦	口服（可被利托那韦增强）	血脂异常，胰岛素抵抗，高血糖，脂质代谢异常，细胞色素 P450 抑制，皮疹，胃肠道症状
洛匹那韦	口服（每日 1 次，与利托那韦配伍）	血脂异常，胰岛素抵抗，高血糖，脂质代谢异常，细胞色素 P450 抑制，胃肠道症状，心律失常，肝毒性
替拉那韦	口服（高载药负担；需利托那韦增强）	血脂异常，胰岛素抵抗，高血糖，脂质代谢异常，细胞色素 P450 抑制，P 糖蛋白诱导，肝毒性，皮疹，胃肠道症状
CCR5 拮抗剂		
马拉韦罗	口服（每日 2 次）	肝毒性，上呼吸道感染，发热，体位性低血压
融合抑制剂		
恩夫韦地	注射（皮下，每日 2 次）	疼痛，红斑，硬结，结节，淤斑，过敏
整合酶抑制剂		
雷特格韦	口服（每日 2 次）	头痛，恶心，疲劳，横纹肌溶解，肌病
埃替拉韦	口服（与食物同服可增效）	仅被 CYP3A4 系统 INSTI 代谢，很多药物与之有关
度鲁特韦	口服（每日 1 次）	头痛，失眠

即使是同一类的多药联用，在发生耐药时也有益处

性催化位点下游直接与逆转录酶结合来干扰逆转录酶的转录活性。

4. 病毒融合抑制剂（2003）恩夫韦肽干扰与病毒包膜糖蛋白 gp41 中的第一个七肽重复序列（first heptad-repeat，HR1）的结合，并阻止病毒与人 CD4 T 淋巴细胞的细胞膜融合所必需的构象变化。
5. CCR5 拮抗剂（2007）马拉韦罗与 CD4 T 淋巴细胞膜上的人 CCR5 受体结合，从而阻断 HIV gp120 与 CCR5 受体的相互作用，但只针对嗜 CCR5 HIV。它不阻止 CXCR4 热带 HIV 病毒的进入，因此有必要在使用该药物之前确定感染的 HIV 是嗜 CCR5 毒株。
6. 整合酶（链转移）抑制剂 [integrase（strand transfer）inhibitor，INSTI；2007] 阻断整合酶催化宿主与病毒 DNA 共价键的形成，从而阻止病毒 DNA 整合入宿主染色体。

表 9.1 列举了目前使用的这些主要类型的抗逆转录病毒药物的示例及其给药途径和常见副作用。典型的抗逆转录病毒治疗由三种药物组成。这种联合治疗被称为高效抗逆转录病毒治疗（highly active antiretroviral therapy，HAART）。在某些情况下，需四种或更多种药物的组合使用。初治患者的治疗目的是达到不可检测的病毒载量，并改善生存质量和延长生存期。基于副作用少、毒性小和疗效好的特征，对初治患者的初始治疗常包括两种：NNRTI 和 INSTI。有多种药物可供选择治疗，同时也应受基因型耐药性测试结果的指导。该蛋白酶抑制剂利托那韦通常以低剂量用作药代动力学增强剂（通过抑制细胞色素 P450）增加其他蛋白酶抑制剂的生物利用度。最近，暴露前预防（preexposure prophylaxis，PrEP）已被证明对 HIV 阴性的高危人群（如性工作者）产生有效预防。

HAART 方案的副作用

许多副作用和药物相互作用使 HAART 治疗方案复杂化并降低其依从性。患者可能会有药物超敏反应，引起发热、低血压和急性间质性肺炎伴呼吸衰竭。同时使用齐多夫定（幸运的是，其在很大程度上已被副作用较少的新药物所取代）和皮质类固醇可能导致严重的肌肉疾病和呼吸肌功能障碍。此外，有报道记录了几例与 HAART 启动和免疫重建相关的呼吸衰竭病例，导致肺孢子菌肺炎的反常恶化；将这一事件与同时发生的呼吸道感染区分开来在临床上通常具有挑战性。对麻醉科医师而言尤为重要的是，接受 HAART 治疗的患者会出现长期的代谢并发症，包括脂质异常和葡萄糖耐受不良，这可能会导致糖尿病、冠状动脉疾病和脑血管疾病的发生。

据报道，服用 NRTI 的患者可出现类似急性革兰氏阴性菌脓毒症的综合征。通常表现为乳酸酸中毒和肝脂肪变性。患者出现高热，并迅速出现神志不清和昏迷。核苷类似物药物可能抑制 DNA 聚合酶 γ，后者是线粒体 DNA 复制所需的唯一 DNA 聚合酶。这反过来导致线粒体功能障碍和细胞有氧呼吸功能受损，并导致氧化磷酸化的抑制和呼吸链酶的紊乱。核黄素已被认为是一种潜在的治疗方法。不幸的是，尽管有重症监护加强治疗病房（intensive care unit，ICU）的支持，但大部分患者仍然以死亡告终。

HAART 药物相互作用

PI 是细胞色素 P450 的抑制剂，特别是利托那韦（见表 9.1）。相反，奈韦拉平是肝微粒体酶的诱导剂。这些药物对肝酶多变的影响使药物的剂量变得复杂化，包括麻醉剂和镇痛剂，因为其中许多药物需经肝代谢。

HIV 的结局

最初 HIV 不可避免地导致 AIDS，并普遍具有致命性。随着 HAART 的出现，HIV 已转化为与感染发病率和治疗毒性相关的慢性感染。随着 HIV 治疗的进一步进展、病毒毒力和耐受性降低，且较少有接受治疗的患者表现出器官系统或感染性并发症，事实上，许多感染 HIV 的患者均能正常老龄化且最终并非死于 HIV 感染或者其治疗。

呼吸系统并发症

在 CD4 T 细胞计数小于 200 cells/ml 之前，通常不会发生肺孢子菌肺炎 [*Pneumocystis jirovecii* pneumonia，PJP；既往称为“卡氏肺孢子虫肺炎”（*Pneumocystis carinii* pneumonia，PCP）]。气促、盗汗、体重减轻是常见主诉。胸部检查可能无异常，许多情况下胸部 X 线片显示正常。并发症包括呼吸衰竭、气胸和慢性肺部疾病。

胸部 X 线片典型表现为双侧“毛玻璃”影。可有明显气胸，也可有多处肺气肿。即使在 X 线片正常的情况下，高分辨率计算机断层扫描也会出现毛玻璃样改变。肺功能检查显示肺容量减少、顺应性降低、一氧化碳弥散功能降低。运动期间的血氧饱和度测定可能比肺功能检查更有帮助。如果怀疑 PJP，应进行纤维支气管镜检查和支气管肺泡灌洗。早期诊断的优势弥补了高频率出现阴性结果的缺点。

联合大剂量磺胺甲噁唑 [100 mg/（kg·d）] 和甲氧苄啶 [20 mg/（kg·d）] 仍是首选治疗方法。对于血氧饱和度较低的患者，建议使用全身类固醇治疗，如泼尼松龙 1 mg/（kg·d），并需要呼吸支持和吸氧。在某些情况下，使用持续气道正压可以避免使用正压机械通气。辅助皮质激素治疗后仍需机械通气的患者预后较差。此外，呼气末正压的使用可能引起气胸。

空洞性肺病可由化脓性细菌性肺脓肿、肺结核（pulmonary tuberculosis，TB）、真菌感染和诺卡菌感染引起。卡波西肉瘤（Kaposi sarcoma，KS）和淋巴瘤也可侵犯肺。淋巴结肿大可导致气管支气管阻塞或压迫大血管。支气管内 KS 可能引起大咯血。HIV 也可直接感染肺部，导致类似肺气肿的破坏性肺部综合征。

播散性结核是严重呼吸衰竭的潜在原因，对合并肺部感染的 AIDS 患者应常规检查呼吸道分泌物抗酸杆菌。细菌性肺炎（肺炎链球菌、卡他莫拉菌、流感嗜血杆菌、金黄色葡萄球菌、铜绿假单胞菌）也可引起严重的急性呼吸衰竭。当怀疑有细菌存在时，应进行经验性抗菌治疗以覆盖这些微生物。HIV 感染患者和医护人员中曾发生过多重耐药结核病暴发。其通过吸入感染性气溶胶进行空气传播，因此应采取适当的隔离措施以保护医疗人员和其他患者免受结核病的侵害。

中枢神经系统并发症

从 AIDS 痴呆到感染性或肿瘤累及的神经系统疾病均可能使 AIDS 复杂化。脑局灶性病变主要由三个实质性疾病构成：脑弓形体病、原发性中枢神经系统（central nervous system，CNS）淋巴瘤和进行性多灶性白质脑病。局灶性病变可能增加颅内压力，从而禁忌椎管内麻醉。巨细胞病毒或 HIV 感染可导致脊髓病变、周围神经病变和肌病。在这种情况下给予琥珀胆碱可能有风险。新型隐球菌、HIV 和 TB 可引起脑膜炎。HIV 感染与自主神经病变有关，可表现为麻醉或在 ICU 期间血流动力学不稳定。

心血管疾病

HIV 感染过程中心脏受累很常见，但在临床上经常并无症状。多达 50% 的 HIV 患者在疾病的某一阶段有异常的超声心动图表现。大约 25% 有心包积液。心肌炎多见于进展期 HIV，可能由弓形体、播散性隐球菌、柯萨奇病毒 B、巨细胞病毒、淋巴瘤、曲霉菌属和 HIV 本身引起，可能导致心室扩张和心功能不全。对于 PI，常见葡萄糖耐受不良和脂质代谢紊乱。侵袭性全身性血管疾病，包括心脏和脑，可能是抗逆转录病毒治疗的并发症。如果患者出现不明原因的低血压，应考虑肾上腺功能不全，这可能发生于晚期 HIV 感染。

手术和麻醉

在手术后 30 天内，HIV 感染不会增加术后并发症（包括死亡）的风险。因此，手术干预不应由于 HIV 状态和对后续并发症的顾虑而受到限制。然而，在麻醉期间，心动过速更常见于 HIV 血清阳性患者。此外，这类患者术后更易出现高热、贫血和心动过速。

一些研究表明，全身麻醉和阿片制剂可能会损害免疫功能。虽然这对于健康个体可能无临床意义，但对 HIV 感染患者的影响尚不清楚。全身麻醉引起的免疫抑制发生在诱导后 15 min 内，可持续 3 ～ 11 天。固有免疫抑制的患者术后免疫抑制可能持续更长时间，且可能更易发生术后感染或促进肿瘤生长或转移。

在当前的 HAART 时代，HIV 往往与机会性感染无关，但与慢性低度炎症和衰老疾病的早期表现有关。因此，对于 HIV 阳性多年的患者，应高度怀疑其合并冠状动脉疾病、脑血管疾病、糖尿病、肾疾病和痴呆等疾病。

产科患者

HIV 和 AIDS 在育龄妇女中很常见。在一项研究中显示，齐多夫定单药治疗可将 HIV 垂直传播的发生率从 25.5% 显著降低至 8.3%。然而，由于 HIV 耐药性发展迅速，齐多夫定单药治疗的长期获益有限。因此现在认为在妊娠期间联合治疗更为可取。

通过现代治疗方案，几乎可以消除 HIV 在母婴之间的传播。

关于在妊娠期间使用 PI 的数据极为有限。最近的一项荟萃分析强烈建议剖宫产可独立降低垂直传播的发生率。联合抗逆转录病毒治疗和择期剖宫产术可将垂直传播率降低至 2%。但众所周知，剖宫产是一项具有并发症的外科干预。即使对于健康妇女，剖宫产术后并发症发病率依然高于阴道分娩，包括更持久剧烈的疼痛、卧床时间更长、失血更多、静脉血栓形成和伤口感染发生率更高。如今，许多医务人员不建议对接受抗逆转录病毒治疗且检测不到 HIV 病毒载量的 HIV 感染孕妇进行择期剖宫产。不幸的是，CD4 淋巴细胞计数低的 HIV 阳性孕妇，从理论上讲其婴儿从剖宫产分娩中获益最多，但产妇也最有可能出现明显的术后并发症。

在一项 HIV 阳性产妇接受区域麻醉的研究中，没有发现与麻醉或产科相关的传染性或神经系统并发症。在产后即刻，免疫功能测定和疾病的严重程度基本保持不变。医务人员一直对于 HIV 血清阳性患者接受硬膜外和腰椎穿刺可能使病毒进入 CNS 存在担忧，然而 HIV 的自然病程在临床病程早期即已累及 CNS，且 CNS 感染的表现差异很大。

最后，据报道在 HIV 血清阳性患者中使用硬膜外血补丁治疗腰椎穿刺后头痛是安全有效的。尽管如此，考虑到仍存在很小的将病毒引入中枢神经系统的理论风险，应优先尝试其他镇痛策略。

ICU 并发症

收治入内科 ICU 的 HIV 血清阳性患者，尤其是合并肺炎或脓毒症患者，当其总淋巴细胞计数小于 200 cells/ml 时，APACHE Ⅱ 评分明显低估了他们的其死亡风险。HIV 感染患者入 ICU 有多种适应证。从历史上看，PCP 引起的呼吸衰竭是入住 ICU 的最常见原因，占 34%。PCP 和其他肺部疾病的机械通气患者死亡率大于 50%。相比而言，非肺部疾病的 ICU 入院及机械通气患者死亡率低于 25%。在脓毒性休克患者中，HIV 感染是预后不良的独立预测因子。在 HAART 时代，极少有感染 HIV 并患有 AIDS 诱发疾病如 PJP 的患者入 ICU。事实上，许多患者均为患有不相关的危重疾病，且偶然发现其感染了 HIV。尽管如此，已知 PJP 的患者开始 HAART 治疗仍可改善预后。然而，当开始 HAART 治疗时，必须权衡这一治疗益处与免疫重建相关问题的利弊，后者可能发生于脓毒症患者。

预防

关于 HIV 血清阳性患者麻醉和手术的总体风险的具体信息很少。美国麻醉科医师协会的身体状况评估和固有手术风险可能可提供整体风险的衡量标准。这些信息与 HIV 感染的疾病控制和阶段预防中心、免疫抑制的程度，以及机会性感染或肿瘤的存在及严重程度相结合，可能为 HIV 血清阳性患者围术期整体风险提供最佳预测因子。对于麻醉技术的选择，以尽量减少并发症为原则，区域阻滞麻醉是除某些神经病变病外的首选技术。

最后，麻醉科医师和重症治疗医师与大量的患者接触，其中许多患者可能是 HIV 血清阳性的。因此，严格遵守感染控制措施势在必行。此外，所有临床医师都应及时了解有关 HIV 治疗的最新知识，以确保患者正在接受最佳治疗。

（项 前 译 孟 岩 校）

延伸阅读

Afessa B, Green B: Bacterial pneumonia in hospitalized patients with HIV infection: the Pulmonary Complications, ICU Support, and Prognostic Factors of Hospitalized Patients with HIV (PIP) Study, *Chest* 117:1017–1022, 2000.

Avidan MS, Groves P, Blott M, et al.: Low complication rate associated with cesarean section under spinal anesthesia for HIV-1-infected women on antiretroviral therapy, *Anesthesiology* 97:320–324, 2002.

Avidan MS, Jones N, Pozniak AL: The implications of HIV for the anaesthetist and the intensivist, *Anaesthesia* 55:344–354, 2000.

Casalino E, Mendoza-Sassi G, Wolff M, et al.: Predictors of short- and long-term survival in HIV-infected patients admitted to the ICU, *Chest* 113:421–429, 1998.

Casalino E, Wolff M, Ravaud P, et al.: Impact of HAART advent on admission patterns and survival in HIV-infected patients admitted to an intensive care unit, *AIDS* 18:1429–1433, 2004.

Evron S, Glezerman M, Harow E, et al.: Human immunodeficiency virus: anesthetic and obstetric considerations, *Anesth Analg* 98:503–511, 2004.

Hughes SC, Dailey PA, Landers D, et al.: Parturients infected with human immunodeficiency virus and regional anesthesia: clinical and immunologic response, *Anesthesiology* 82:32–37, 1995.

Morris A, Wachter RM, Luce J, et al.: Improved survival with highly active antiretroviral therapy in HIV-infected patients with severe *Pneumocystis carinii* pneumonia, *AIDS* 17:73–80, 2003.

Pau AK, George JM: Antiretroviral therapy: current drugs, *Infect Dis Clin North Am* 28(3):371–402, 2014.

Vincent B, Timsit JF, Auburtin M, et al.: Characteristics and outcomes of HIV-infected patients in the ICU: impact of the highly active antiretroviral treatment era, *Intensive Care Med* 30:859–866, 2004.

Warriner AH, Burkholder GA, Overton ET: HIV-related metabolic comorbidities in the current ART era, *Infect Dis Clin North Am* 28(3):457–476, 2014.

妊娠期高血压疾病

第 10 章

Curtis L. Baysinger

病例概要

患者，女性，27 岁，妊娠 37 周，目前宫颈扩张 4 cm 并因先兆子痫恶化接受引产。其目前血压（blood pressure，BP）在静注拉贝洛尔数次后维持于 150/100 mmHg，膝反射 4+，有右上腹压痛，尿蛋白 4+。入院时血小板计数 $135 \times 10^9/L$，目前降至 $95 \times 10^9/L$。现接受 1 g/h 的硫酸镁（$MgSO_4$）和催产素静注治疗。需要注意的是，其既往因先兆子痫在妊娠 35 周分娩一次。患者病态肥胖，BMI 41 kg/m^2。产科医师和患者现请求硬膜外分娩镇痛。

问题分析

定义

2000 年，国家高血压宣教项目提出了与妊娠相关的四类高血压，这一分类获得了广泛认可。美国妇产科医师学会妊娠期高血压专责小组（American College of Obstetricians and Gynecologists，ACOG）于 2013 年更新了分类内容，与之前的 4 类分法大致相同：妊娠期高血压、先兆子痫（有或无严重症状）、慢性高血压、慢性高血压合并先兆子痫（框 10.1）。

妊娠期高血压发生在妊娠 20 周后，表现为 BP 升高且不伴有先兆子痫的其他诊断特征。先兆子痫可伴或不伴典型子痫症状，通常 BP 大于或等于 140/90 mmHg 并有蛋白尿（表 10.1）。有典型症状的重度先兆子痫特点为高血压程度更重并可有其他母体器官功能障碍（见表 10.1）。子痫的定义是有先兆子痫的妇女出现癫痫又与既往的神经系统障碍无关。慢性高血压诊断为在妊娠 20 周前或分娩后 12 周内出现的血压大于或等于 140/90 mmHg。诊断慢性高血压合并先兆子痫的依据为新发蛋白尿、原有蛋白尿或血压明显升高、或出现其他器官功能损害的症状。HELLP 综合征的特点为血管内溶血，肝酶升高 [常为丙氨酸转氨酶（alanine aminotransferase，ALT）和（或）天冬氨酸转移酶（aspartate aminotransferase，AST）]，以及血小板计数降低；与其他类型的先兆子痫相比常在妊娠更早期出现。

框 10.1 妊娠期高血压疾病分类

- 妊娠期高血压
- 先兆子痫
  - 先兆子痫
  - 伴严重症状的先兆子痫
- 慢性高血压
- 慢性高血压合并先兆子痫

识别

伴严重症状的重度先兆子痫定义为 BP 超过 160/100 mmHg 或患者出现终末器官损伤症状（见表 10.1）。严重症状可包括以下方面：

表 10.1 先兆子痫诊断标准

种类	检查发现
先兆子痫	• 妊娠 20 周后 BP>140/90 mmHg • 蛋白尿（24 h 300 mg，浸渍片测量 1+ 或 2+，蛋白质 / 肌酐比值 >0.3） • BP>160/110 mmHg

伴严重症状的重度先兆子痫	• 血清肌酐 >1.1 mg/dl 或大于基础值 2 倍
	• 患者器官功能损害症状 / 体征
	  • 头痛 / 视力受损 / 癫痫
	  • 肺水肿
	  • 血小板减少（<100 000/mm^3）
	  • 肝功能异常

- 肺水肿。
- 肾功能障碍。尽管以前将大量蛋白尿作为诊断重度先兆子痫的标准之一，但最近的研究并未显示蛋白尿程度与妊娠预后存在明确关系；因此蛋白尿程度已被降至作为严重疾病的诊断性特征。
- 中枢神经系统症状，包括头痛、视力改变或癫痫。
- 肝酶升高并有右上腹压痛（继发于肝包膜扩张）。
- 血小板减少，计数少于 100×10^9/L。

之前作为判断标准之一的胎儿宫内生长受限已从标准中移除。

HELLP 综合征的出现可伴随中度 BP 上升，也有 15% 的患者 BP 正常。对于既往有慢性高血压和肾病的产妇诊断先兆子痫相当困难；尿蛋白随时间的增加可能是唯一征象。对于急性可卡因中毒的产妇，与先兆子痫鉴别也很困难，因为两者都可出现癫痫、肺水肿、蛋白尿及血小板减少。但是，对于妊娠 20 周以上的女性出现血压升高和癫痫样症状都应考虑为子痫，直到证实为其他病变引起。具有典型症状的重度先兆子痫症状可持续至产后 2 周。

框 10.2 先兆子痫的危险因素

人口因素
- 高龄妊娠（>35 岁）
- 非裔美国人

孕产妇合并有基础疾病
- 肥胖
- 既往有高血压
- 糖尿病
- 肾病
- 抗磷脂抗体综合征
- 血管或结缔组织病
- 血管紧张素基因 T235

产科情况 / 病史
- 多胎妊娠
- 羊水过多
- 葡萄胎
- 既往先兆子痫病史
- 体外授精
- 初产妇
- 既往胎盘早剥，胎儿生长受限病史
- 婴儿父亲的其他伴侣怀孕并出现先兆子痫

风险评估

妊娠期高血压可出现在约 5% 的孕妇中，这其中 50% 的患者在妊娠 30 周前发展为先兆子痫。在美国，先兆子痫出现在 6% ～ 8% 的孕妇中，25% 发展为有严重症状的重度先兆子痫。此病引起的死亡人数占美国孕产妇死亡人数的 25%。

与先兆子痫发生相关的一些危险因素见框 10.2。人口统计因素（如高龄孕产妇和非裔美国人），患病风险增加。一些与其发生风险增加的产科因素有：子宫过度扩张（如多胎妊娠，羊水过多），滋养细胞疾病，妊娠 18 ～ 24 周子宫动脉多普勒检查异常，既往有先兆子痫和胎盘早剥病史。母亲有基础疾病，如肥胖、糖尿病、慢性高血压及胶原血管疾病，同样也是先兆子痫的高危因素。

妊娠中期出现先兆子痫的孕产妇较妊娠 34 周以上出现者预后差。早期就出现先兆子痫的患者相对于晚期者更可能有慢性高血压、肾病或胶原血管疾病。预后不良的指征有：难治性的严重高血压、进行性血小板减少或肝功能异常、少尿以及胎儿宫内窘迫（决定因素为无应激试验或胎儿生理活动评估，尤其是预估胎儿体重低于同孕周百分位的 5% 以下）。脐动脉多普勒超声可以预估分娩时间。舒张期流量缺乏是紧急分娩的指征，多普勒超声表现为舒张期血流突然逆转。

如今，即使在高危人群中也没有单一廉价有效的筛选检查来评估先兆子痫的发生。尽管在评估与先兆子痫相关的生物学指标方面取得了一些进步 [可溶性 fms 样酪氨酸激酶（soluble fms-like tyrosine kinase，sFLT1）及可溶性内皮因子（soluble endoglin，sEng）上升]，但在常规筛查中，结合这些生物学指标及早期脐动脉多普勒超声对先兆子痫并没有很好的阳性评估率。

随时间推移，先兆子痫可从亚临床症状发展为症状明显的疾病。在无症状的初期，患者的子宫螺旋动脉相较于正常孕妇扩张不明显，达不到正常孕妇动脉直径扩张 4 倍的高流低阻的子宫灌注状态。胎盘灌注减少易导致症状晚期的胎儿生长受限。此外，由于促进子宫螺旋动脉扩张的免疫级联反应被破坏，因此出现抗血管生成因子释放，主要是 sFLT1 和 sEng。sFLT1 和 sEng 水平上升又可使胎盘释放血管内皮细胞生长因子及胎盘生长因子减少，进一步阻碍了正常胎盘血管的生成。这些胎盘因子异常还会阻碍母体内皮的正常修复，导致母体血管损伤和蛋白尿、高血压、脑血管痉挛，偶尔还会出现先兆子痫靶器官损伤，典型表现为肝功能障碍。额外的炎症介质释放和胎盘脂质过氧化会进一步促进母体内皮损伤。正常妊娠期间，母体血管对血管收缩剂的敏感性降低，而患病者则变得更加敏感，这可能是由于患者血栓素相较前列环素异常升高。患病母亲同时由于内皮细胞前列环素和一氧化氮合成障碍，正常的肾素、血管紧张素Ⅱ、醛固酮系统也出现异常。全身的病理生理变化是广泛的内皮损伤，这种损伤源于全身血管收缩和凝血系统激活，包括凝血因子和血小板的消耗。水肿的原因为水钠潴留，蛋白尿引起的胶体渗透压降低可加剧水肿。

启示

母婴发病率增高的因素有：高龄产妇、妊娠早期发病（尤其是妊娠 32 周前发展为先兆子痫）、合并有基础糖尿病的产妇、肾病或高凝状态。全身水肿不是诊断标准，其通常与病情严重程度相关，并且水肿对实施麻醉者意义重大，因为要评估气道及咽喉水肿程度。肺水肿风险最高的时期发生在分娩后，因为此时胶体渗透压最低，约 3% 患有先兆子痫的产妇在这一时期会发生肺水肿。先兆子痫患者最常见的死亡原因为颅内出血或肺水肿。

产妇广泛性脑水肿的发生与脑血管系统的过度兴奋和高灌注有关。当磁共振成像（magnetic resonance imaging，MRI）确诊时，预示着预后不良，患者可出现感觉异常。产妇分娩后数月的计算机断层扫描（computed tomographic，CT）和 MRI 检查可见颅内残留小的梗死灶。

心血管系统可见血管紧张度增高，对血管收缩物质敏感性增加。多数有先兆子痫的产妇较血压正常的产妇会出现血容量减少。交感神经系统的活性增加常导致重度先兆子痫患者出现高动力型血流动力学状态，心排血量增加，全身血管阻力增加。然而，肺动脉导管研究显示，部分患者血容量减少，左心室功能下降，全身血管阻力明显增加。这项研究由经胸超声心动图（transthoracic echocardiography，TTE）证实。这些病例观察研究还报道了一些其他异常，包括左心室增大、心包积液、心室舒张功能障碍，以及较少发生的心室扩张，收缩力下降。这些病变常出现在有其他心力衰竭症状的患者中。

通常很难判断先兆子痫孕产妇典型的心血管变化，因为多数观察性血流动力学研究的患者都接受了一定的治疗。例如：低血容量孕产妇的心功能受抑制，扩容常常可明显改善心功能，心排血量可较原来增加 3 ～ 4 倍，而且大多数孕产妇住院后会谨慎地立即开始补液。此外，减轻后负荷的治疗可以显著改善受抑制的心功能，许多研究中有心力衰竭迹象的妇女常已经开始了这种治疗。因此最有可能的病理过程为，自然病程开始时为高动力循环系统，体循环阻力升高，中心容量耗竭，逐渐变化为血管内容量趋于正常，而心脏失代偿。

血小板减少症继发于消耗性凝血功能障碍，发生于 11% ～ 50% 的重症先兆子痫患者。血小板计数少于 100×10^9/L 与其他类型凝血异常有关，常常与 HELLP 综合征同时出现。内生血小板功能障碍也有可能出现。然而，血小板计数确认高于 100×10^9/L 的重症先兆子痫患者一般不会出现明显的血小板减少症，除非有其他 HELLP 综合征的征象。

少尿可能是由于心脏充盈压过低引起，常常在快速输液后会有改善。另外，少尿可能与心功能抑制及体循环阻力异常升高有关，这种情况较少出现，若发生应降低心脏后负荷。

子宫动脉痉挛可引起胎盘血流减少。胎盘血流大量减少的情况见于应用大量升压药物治疗低血压时，这种情况也可能伴随椎管内阻滞时出现。

由于很多产妇会在孕早期分娩，而先兆子痫是发达国家产妇早产的常见原因之一。此外，其还是胎盘早剥和产后出血的常见原因。胎盘早剥是因为胎盘发育附着表浅；产后出血则更多是继发于预防癫痫和血压治疗的结果。

有先兆子痫病史的产妇会有心血管疾病的长期风险，包括卒中和缺血性心脏病。这种风险随先兆子痫的严重程度而上升。一些数据显示，此类患者晚年罹患实体肿瘤的风险有所降低。

管理

产科治疗

产科治疗包括适时分娩、预防癫痫、优化容量状态以及治疗血压过高。ACOG 建议，应对血压 160/110 mmHg 的患者积极处理，降低血压的 15% ～ 25%，至收缩压在 120 ～ 160 mmHg 之间，舒张压在 80 ～ 105 mmHg 之间；血压降至正常人水平可能导致子宫灌注不足。治疗的目标是减少颅内出血、胎盘早剥或心肌缺血的风险。由于收缩压高于 160 mmHg 与卒中风险增加有关，因此 ACOG 强调要降低收缩压。除此之外，有研究指出未能辨识高血压的严重程度约占先兆子痫患者死亡原因的 60%。

2011 年，ACOG 建议用拉贝洛尔或肼屈嗪作为紧急治疗高血压的一线用药；但是，最近的一项研究显示，增加口服硝苯地平的剂量比静脉应用拉贝洛尔降压更快，风险更小。尽管 ACOG 推荐一线用药，最近的一项系统性回顾却显示没有哪种药物的治疗效果明确优于其他药物，但需要注意的是二氮嗪、尼莫地平和 $MgSO_4$ 是控制血压较差的药物。$MgSO_4$ 的血管舒张作用微弱而短暂，因此没有有效的降压作用。静脉注射肼屈嗪是一种治疗高血压的传统而有效方法，每 15 min 一次，每次 5 ～ 10 mg。拉贝洛尔应递增给药，至累计剂量 0.5 ～ 1 mg/kg*。上述两种药物对新生儿心率或子宫血流没有明显影响。二氢吡啶类钙通道阻滞剂（如尼卡地平、硝苯地平）在治疗高血压同时，对分娩和新生儿影响甚微或没有影响，因此可用于拉贝洛尔和肼屈嗪不起作用时的二线治疗。但是，理论上钙通道阻滞剂与 $MgSO_4$ 同时应用时有可能造成意外的低血压。钙通道阻滞剂也禁用于有冠心病、慢性糖尿病和主动脉瓣狭窄的产妇。静滴硝酸甘油可能有效降低血压，但因其有明显的子宫平滑肌松弛作用，所以在孕妇身上应用受限。

对于有先兆子痫而无严重症状的产妇，若孕周大于 37 周应建议分娩；此时，期待观察而不做处理可能造成产科预后不良。如果高血压在治疗 24 ～ 48 h 后仍未得到控制，或伴有进行性肾功能不全、严重血小板减少、凝血功能恶化、胎儿状态异常、即将发生惊厥、肝功能值升高至正常值的 2 倍或心肺功能受损，则有严重症状的先兆子痫产妇必须分娩。如有可能，可在糖皮质激素给药后延迟 48 h 分娩，以加速胎儿肺成熟。若血压控制良好、实验室检查结果正常、胎儿宫内环境稳定，可以待产观察。当孕周达到 34 周时，疾病程度严重的产妇应当分娩，因为待产观察可引起不良产科预后。所有无严重症状的先兆子痫产妇及大部分有严重疾病的产妇，均应尝试经阴道分娩。

一些文献报道了 $MgSO_4$ 预防癫痫发生的作用。英国子痫研究合作组织约 30 年前的一项研究发现，服用 $MgSO_4$ 可减少约 52% 的癫痫发生率。在此研究中，$MgSO_4$ 优先于地西泮或苯妥英钠用于预防癫痫，尽管在美国之外的其他地区更常用苯妥英钠。$MgSO_4$ 还有改善早产儿神经系统预后的额外益处。

目前看来，$MgSO_4$ 不会影响分娩时间，干扰凝血，或显著影响硬膜外阻滞产妇的子宫血流。单次推注剂量为 4 ～ 6 g，输注量为 1 ～ 2 g/h，但对于开始治疗的最佳时间、最佳负荷和维持剂量或分娩后最佳治疗持续时间尚未达成共识。每 8 h 检测一次血清镁浓度，保证维持在 40 ～ 60 mg/L 的治疗浓度。$MgSO_4$ 毒性的在呼吸损害之前会出现深部腱反射的消失，治疗可采取呼吸支持，以及静脉推注葡萄糖酸钙 1g（推注时间超过 10 min）。

麻醉处理

分娩和经阴道娩出

对于无严重症状的先兆子痫产妇，麻醉处理与正常产妇差异很小。对于症状严重者，硬膜外镇痛可以显著缓解疼痛并且对胎盘血流有益。不仅如此，其还能迅速转变为椎管内麻醉以施行紧急剖宫产。适当的容量负荷及增加局麻药剂量可以降低严重低血压的风险。

有严重症状的先兆子痫患者中 15% ～ 20% 可发生血小板减少症。对有严重症状的先兆子痫产妇实施椎管内麻醉前应监测血小板计数。急性血小板减少症较慢性预后更差；然而，对于可增加硬膜外出血风险的具体血小板计数仍不清楚。一项回顾性研究指出，血小板计数少于 75×10^9/L 对预测不良预后并不敏感。因此，当血小板计数小于 75×10^9/L 时，尤其在有 HELLP 综合征的产妇，应谨慎考虑测量血小板活性（如血栓弹力图）。与血小板计数减少类似，出血严重程度对引起的中枢神经系统后遗症风险增加的影响尚不清楚；但是，进行常规检查常可令医务人员更为安心。麻醉科医师应该考虑对血小

* 该静脉推注拉贝洛尔剂量非常大。在此剂量下，α-肾上腺素能通路的阻断作用更加突出，因为 β 受体阻断作用已接近临床最大效果。在出现充血性心力衰竭症状和体征的产妇中禁忌用此剂量。

板减少症产妇实施硬膜外阻滞的风险和益处，平衡椎管出血的风险和疼痛缓解的优势、对血压的益处、迅速将镇痛转换麻醉阻滞以实施剖宫产的能力，以及避免在紧急分娩时可能需要进行全身麻醉气道管理。在分娩早期，血小板计数尚未低于 100×10^9/L 时置入硬膜外导管更明智；然而，这也可能会增加分娩后导管滞留时间过长的风险，因为要等待凝血功能的恢复。

剖宫产

剖宫产可以在脊髓麻醉、硬膜外麻醉或全身麻醉下完成。椎管内麻醉可以避免全身麻醉引起的血流动力学反应。在考虑合理的容量负荷后，脊髓（蛛网膜下腔）阻滞可安全应用于有严重先兆子痫患者，一些证据表明，有先兆子痫者蛛网膜下腔麻醉发生低血压的频率低于无先兆子痫者。最近的循证综述和前瞻性队列研究比较了严重先兆子痫患者蛛网膜下腔阻滞和硬膜外阻滞麻醉过程，表明两者血压变化和升压药物的用量是相似的。然而，与接受全身麻醉的产妇相比，蛛网膜下腔阻滞下剖宫产的新生儿脐动脉碱缺失更大，pH 更低（但临床意义不显著）。腰硬联合麻醉使用低剂量高比重布比卡因（7.5 mg）和芬太尼（25 μg）可能具备一定优势，如迅速扩增麻醉平面以便于手术开展以及必要时延长麻醉时间。除此之外，它与蛛网膜下腔运用大剂量局麻药麻醉相比可能减少不良的血流动力学影响。

用于蛛网膜下腔阻滞的细针较硬膜外麻醉用的粗针造成脊髓血肿的风险小。在硬膜外麻醉中谨慎地增加药量可以减少液体的用量和升压药的使用。在硬膜外麻醉中大量应用含升压药的局麻药物仍有争议。部分研究认为此法是安全的，但也有因此造成严重高血压的报道。

为应对紧急分娩，应当准备全身麻醉，而气道水肿有可能造成气管插管困难。应随时备用各种小尺寸的气管插管，同时做好应对困难气道的准备。所有患者均应做好恰当的预防以避免吸入性肺炎。由于未经治疗的高血压可能导致肺水肿、脑水肿或颅内出血，应采取措施以减少气管插管或浅麻醉引起的血压升高。硝普钠（sodium nitroprusside，SNP）在这种情况下是一种有效的选择，但必须仔细滴定以免造成严重低血压。应用 SNP 时通常需要直接动脉压监测。与之相类似，硝酸甘油的作用也是不可预测的（其为一种主要的静脉扩张剂，可能造成前负荷的下降）。静脉应用尼卡地平（15 ～ 30 μg/kg）同样可能有效。由于其选择性作用于动脉（即对静脉容量和前负荷影响小），尼卡地平相较于 SNP 或硝酸甘油不易造成血压的迅速下降。最近研究显示，瑞芬太尼 1 μg/kg 可以减少插管时引起的血压变化反应。尽管该药可以迅速被母亲和胎儿代谢掉，新生儿依然有出现短暂的呼吸抑制的可能。

丙泊酚和依托咪酯均可用作诱导药物，而一般情况下应避免应用氯胺酮。琥珀胆碱是一种良好的肌松剂选择。对于接受镁剂治疗的产妇，去极化和非去极化制剂的持续时间都可能延长。

预防

使用 $MgSO_4$ 治疗可以降低新生儿脑室内出血的风险，改善先兆子痫母亲早产儿的神经系统预后。没有证据表明胶体液比晶体液在扩容方面更有优势，一些关于液体管理的回顾性综述指出应用胶体液与产妇死亡率上升有关。产前应用地塞米松可提高血小板计数，这可以让一些有 HELLP 综合征的患者实施椎管内镇痛或麻醉。

尚无疗法被证实可以确切降低先兆子痫的发病率。一些研究使用小剂量阿司匹林治疗来调节血栓素 / 前列环素失衡，低钙饮食的妇女补充钙剂，以及应用一些其他抗氧化剂，如维生素 C 或维生素 E，但这些研究都没有取得一致的结论。然而，ACOG 推荐对于既往怀孕有先兆子痫病史并在妊娠 34 周前分娩的产妇，应在妊娠初期末开始预防性应用阿司匹林。

目前表明，肺动脉压监测并不能改善产妇的预后，并且大多数情况下也不需要在先兆子痫患者中应用。1 例对重症先兆子痫患者常规肺动脉导管监测的病例分析显示，其所提供的数据并未改变临床管理措施。尽管如此，对于有心肺功能损害或其他适应证的患者应当考虑行肺动脉压监测。中心静脉压监测通常没有益处。TTE 为监测先兆子痫产妇的血流动力学提供了一种有效的新方法，并可能通过监测心室收缩力、评估血管内容量状态和确定射血分数以区分正常还是射血分数减少的心力衰竭，可有助于对血流动力学受损的产妇进行治疗指导。

（王 翰 译 包 睿 校）

延伸阅读

American College of Obstetricians and Gynecologists: Task Force on Hypertension in Pregnancy: Hypertension in pregnancy, *Obstet Gynecol* 122:1122–1131, 2013.

American College of Obstetricians and Gynecologists: Emergent therapy of acute-onset, severe hypertension with preeclampsia or eclampsia, *Obstet Gynecol* 118:1465–1468, 2011.

Aya AG, Vialles N, Tanoubi I, et al.: Spinal anesthesia-induced hypotension: a risk comparison between patients with severe preeclampsia and healthy women undergoing preterm cesarean delivery, *Anesth Analg* 101:869–875, 2005.

Bateman BT, Mhyre JM, Ehrenfeld J, et al.: The risk and outcomes of epidural hematomas after perioperative and obstetric epidural catheterization: a report from the multicenter perioperative outcomes group research consortium, *Anesth Analg* 116:1380–1385, 2013.

Davies JR, Fernando R, Hallworth SP: Hemostatic function in healthy pregnant and preeclamptic women: an assessment using the platelet function analyzer (PFA-100) and thromboelastograph, *Anesth Analg* 104:416–420, 2007.

Dennis AT: Transthoracic echocardiography in women with preeclampsia, *Curr Opin Anesthesiol* 28:254–260, 2015.

Dennis AT: Management of preeclampsia: issues for anaesthetists, *Anaesthesia* 67:1009–1020, 2012.

Duley L, Meher S, Jones L: Drugs for treatment of very high blood pressure during pregnancy, *Cochrane Database Syst Rev* 7:CD001449, 2013.

Leffert LR: What's new in obstetric anesthesia? Focus on preeclampsia, *Int J Obstet Anesth* 24:264–271, 2015.

Magee AG, Pels A, Helewa M, et al.: Diagnosis, evaluation and management of the hypertensive disorders of pregnancy, *Pregnancy Hypertens* 4:105–145, 2014.

Martin JN, Thigpen BD, Moore RC, et al.: Stroke and severe preeclampsia and eclampsia: a paradigm shift focusing on systolic blood pressure, *Obstet Gynecol* 105:246–254, 2005.

McElrath TF, Lim KH, Pare E, et al.: Longitudinal evaluation of predictive value for preeclampsia of circulating angiogenic factors through pregnancy, *Am J Obstet Gynecol* 207:e1–e7, 2012. 407.

Melchiorre K, Sharma R, Thilaganathan B: Cardiovascular implications in preeclampsia: an overview, *Circulation* 130:703–714, 2014.

National High Pressure Education Program Working Group: Report of the National High Blood Pressure Education Program Working Group on high blood pressure in pregnancy, *Am J Obstet Gynecol* 183:S1–S22, 2000.

Orlikowski CE, Rocke DA, Murray WB, et al.: Thrombelastography changes in pre-eclampsia and eclampsia, *Br J Anaesth* 77:157–161, 1996.

Pant M, Fong R, Scavone B: Prevention of peri-induction hypertension in preeclamptic patients: a focused review, *Anesth Analg* 119:1350–1356, 2014.

Park BY, Jeong CW, Jang EA, et al.: Dose-related attenuation of cardiovascular responses to tracheal intubation by intravenous remifentanil bolus in severe pre-eclamptic patients undergoing caesarean delivery, *Br J Anaesth* 106:82–87, 2011.

Shekhar S, Sharma C, Thakur S, et al.: Oral nifedipine or intravenous labetalol for hypertensive emergency in pregnancy: a randomized controlled trial, *Obstet Gynecol* 122:1057–1063, 2013.

Young P, Johanson R: Haemodynamic, invasive, and echocardiographic monitoring in the hypertensive parturient, *Best Pract Res Clin Obstet Gynecol* 15:605–622, 2001.

甲状腺功能亢进症：甲状腺危象

第 11 章

Martin L. Birch，Richard C. Prielipp

病例概要

患者，女性，32 岁，在全身麻醉下急诊行肱骨复合骨折固定术，术中以 1.2% 异氟烷维持。术前病史表现为严重焦虑和怕热。体格检查发现患者眼眶周围肿胀、皮肤温暖潮湿伴有手心出汗，明显的下颈部中线肿块，与肿大的甲状腺相一致。诱导 30 min 后，出现窦性心动过速（128 次 / 分）伴房性早搏，高血压（195/100 mmHg）伴高热（中心温度 37.9℃，尽管手术室内温度很低）。然而，体格检查未发现肌肉强直。将异氟烷增加到 2% 以加深麻醉深度，并静脉追加舒芬太尼，但血流动力学的变化仍无改善。

问题分析

定义

甲状腺激素的正常调节和活性在甲状腺功能减退症一章中做了概述。血液循环中的甲状腺激素增加可导致高代谢状态。以下定义适用于甲状腺功能亢进症的临床综合征：

- **真性甲状腺功能亢进**（true hyperthyroidism）：是指甲状腺功能亢进，且甲状腺激素的合成和分泌增加。
- **甲状腺毒症**（thyrotoxicosis）：是指甲状腺激素过多的临床和生化表现。在普通人群中，女性占 2%，男性占 0.2%。原因包括甲状腺功能亢进、异位甲状腺激素合成和医源性因素。
- **甲状腺毒性危象**（thyrotoxic crisis）或**甲状腺危象**（thyroid storm）：是甲状腺功能亢进症中一种危及生命的并发症，其特点是甲状腺毒症突然加重恶化。接受手术治疗或外伤性的未控制性甲状腺功能亢进患者发生甲状腺毒性危象的风险相当大。因此，麻醉科医师在进行麻醉和手术前，必须仔细评估可能存在甲状腺危象风险的患者（表 11.1）。
- **人为甲状腺毒症**（thyrotoxicosis factitia）：是指无真正的甲状腺功能亢进的甲状腺毒症（例如故意摄入合成甲状腺激素、异位甲状腺激素生成），与内源性甲状腺激素合成减少有关。

识别、风险评估和启示

病史

未确诊的甲状腺功能亢进症患者通常有焦虑史（偶尔进展到精神错乱甚至昏迷），近期体重明显减轻，怕热，胃肠功能紊乱（腹泻、恶心、呕吐、腹痛），不明原因的发烧，肌肉无力和震颤。较年轻患者和老年患者的表现不同。年轻患者有典型的肾上腺素能症状（如心动过速、焦躁不安或震颤）。年龄较大的患者表现为淡漠症状，如抑郁、疲劳和体重减轻，可能没有肾上腺素能的症状或体征。甲状腺危象通常由诸如手术、分娩、感染、心肌梗死、糖尿病酮症酸中毒或严重创伤等应激性事件引发。

体格检查

支持甲状腺功能亢进诊断的体格检查结果包括以下症状（按出现的频繁程度递减顺序）：

- 精神状态的改变（紧张、兴奋、焦虑、精神错乱、可能的精神病，甚至昏迷）。
- 出汗、畏热。
- 体重减轻、疲劳、肌肉无力。

表 11.1 甲状腺危象的诊断标准

标准	分值	标准	分值
热调节功能障碍		胃肠–肝功能障碍表现	
温度（℉）			
• 99.0 ～ 99.9	5	• 无	0
• 100.0 ～ 100.9	10	• 中度（腹泻、腹痛、恶心 / 呕吐）	10
• 101.0 ～ 101.9	15	• 严重（黄疸）	20
• 102.0 ～ 102.9	20		
• 103.0 ～ 103.9	25		
• ≥ 104.0	30		
心血管系统		中枢神经系统紊乱表现	
心动过速（次 / 分）			
• 100 ～ 109	5	• 无	0
• 110 ～ 119	10	• 轻微（兴奋）	10
• 120 ～ 129	15	• 中度（谵妄，精神错乱，极度嗜睡）	20
• 130 ～ 139	20	• 严重（癫痫，昏迷）	30
• ≥ 140	25		
心房颤动			
• 无	0		
• 有	10		
充血性心力衰竭		**病史中存在应激发性突发事件状态**	
• 无	0		
• 轻度	5	• 无	0
• 中度	10	• 有	10
• 重度	20		
总分值			
>45	甲状腺危象		
25 ～ 44	可能会发生危象		
<25	不可能发生危象		

From Burch HB，Wartofsky L：Life-threatening thyrotoxicosis. Thyroid storm. *Endocrinol Metab Clin North Am* 22（2）：263-277，1993.

- 食欲增加、腹泻和其他胃肠症状。
- 眼球突出，眼睛干涩。
- 腿部肿胀。

甲状腺功能亢进的体征包括（按出现的频繁程度递减顺序）：

- 甲状腺肿——颈部肿块，可能会影响气道（图 11.1）。
- 窦性心动过速（几乎 100% 的发生率）或伴有相关的快速型心律失常（图 11.2）。

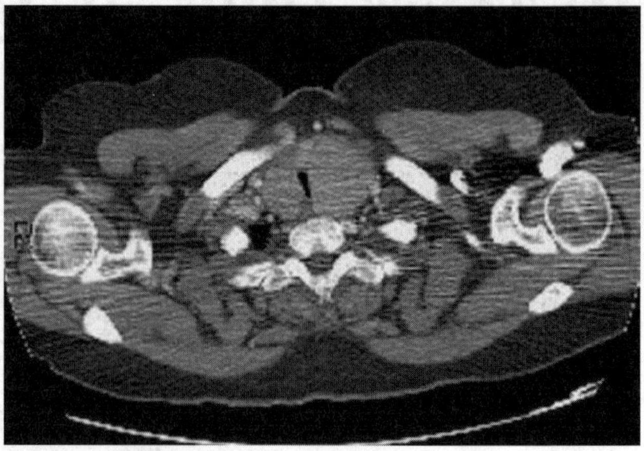

图 11.1 下颈–上胸部 CT 扫描（静脉造影剂）显示甲状腺肿大（甲状腺肿）压迫气管和食管。麻醉科医师必须认识到颈部甲状腺肿大患者在麻醉诱导过程中可能出现严重气道损害，并预计甲状腺肿可能延伸至胸骨后部。在甲状腺手术患者实施麻醉时，高达 6% 的患者会出现困难气管插管

- 皮肤湿暖。
- 肌肉震颤。
- 收缩期高血压，通常伴有脉压差增大。
- 心房颤动，常见于老年人（发病率约为 10%）。
- 甲状腺增大，可能有甲状腺杂音。
- 眼科体征，包括眼球突出、眼睑后退、眼睑退缩、眼眶周围肿胀和结膜充血。
- 胫骨前水肿。

病理生理

甲状腺毒症失代偿为甲状腺危象的确切机制知之甚少，但它最常发生在应激性突发事件之后。不管是什么原因，由此产生的综合征类似于长期过量应用 β - 肾上腺素能激动剂的严重症状。然而，尽管存在明显的高代谢状态，但实际的儿茶酚胺浓度通常仍为正常。

病因

未确诊的甲状腺功能亢进（通常是 Graves 病或中毒性结节性甲状腺肿）伴严重应激事件时是引起患者出现甲状腺危象的最常见原因。另一个原因可能是对已知的甲状腺功能亢进症患者治疗不足。与甲状腺毒症有关的疾病列于框 11.1。此外，在患者病情稳定时进行的 24 h 放射性碘摄取研究可以部分区分甲状腺毒症的多种原因（框 11.2）。

诊断

甲状腺危象在很大程度上基于临床诊断（见表

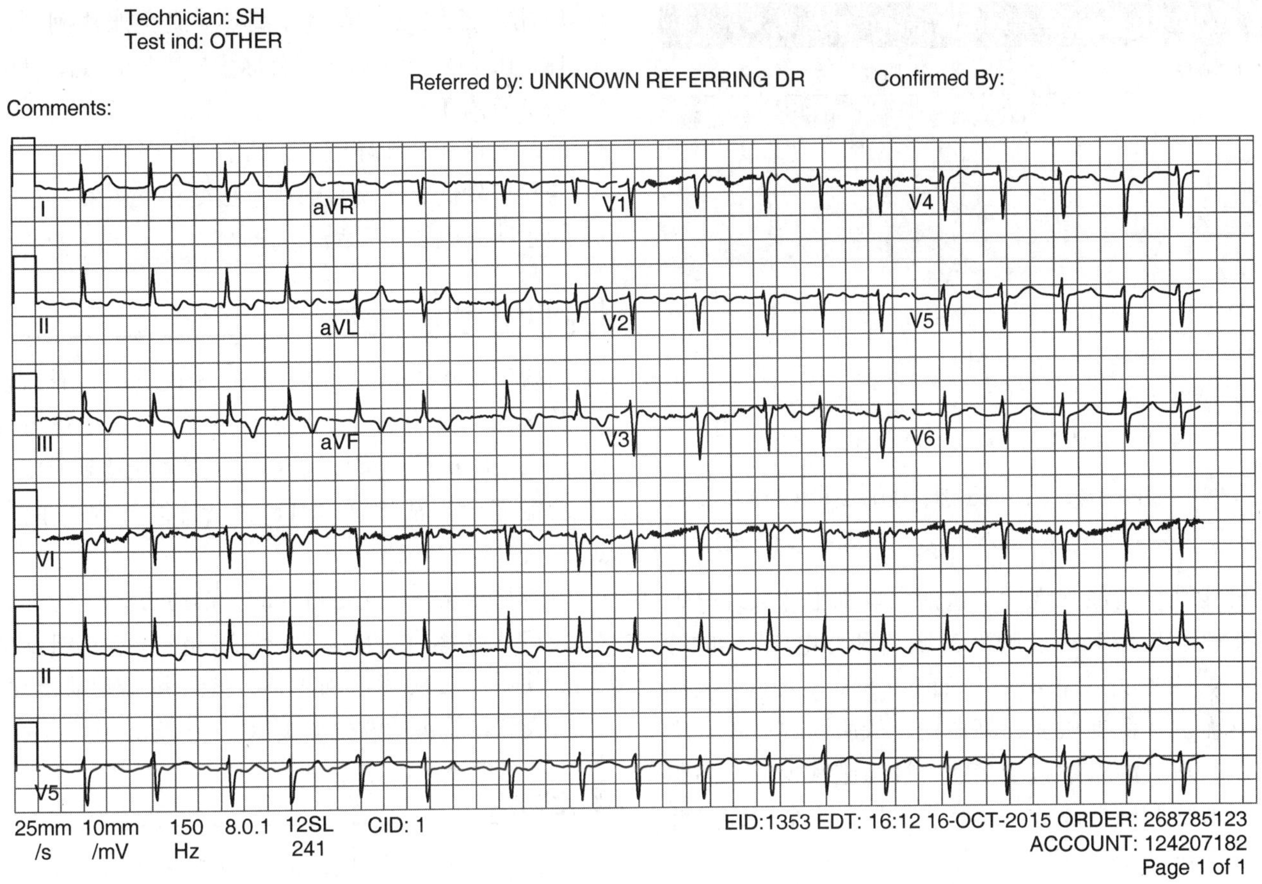

图 11.2 心电图来自一名 71 岁有甲状腺危象需要机械通气及重症监护的女性患者。心电图显示甲状腺危象的特征性改变，如心房颤动伴快速心室反应（使用艾司洛尔控制心率），非特异性 ST-T 改变，T 波倒置可能提示伴有下壁心肌缺血。在随访时，她的甲状腺功能检验结果为：FT3=9.7（正常值 =2.3 ～ 4.2 pg/ml）；FT4=3.4（正常值 =0.76 ～ 1.46 ng/dl）；TSH<0.01（正常值 =0.40 ～ 4.0 mU/L）。

框 11.1 甲状腺毒症相关疾病

Graves 病（可能占所有病例的 85%）
毒性结节性甲状腺肿
毒性腺瘤
亚急性甲状腺炎
新生儿甲状腺毒症（由母体 Graves 病引起）
分泌促甲状腺激素的垂体瘤
分娩
葡萄胎
转移性（高功能）甲状腺癌
人为的甲状腺毒症

框 11.2 放射性碘摄入鉴别甲状腺毒症的病因

颈部放射性碘摄入正常或升高的甲状腺毒症
- Graves 病
- 甲状腺腺瘤
- 滋养细胞疾病
- 产生促甲状腺激素的垂体腺瘤
- 对甲状腺激素抵抗

与几乎无颈部放射性碘摄入相关的甲状腺毒症
- 无痛性甲状腺炎
- 胺碘酮诱导的甲状腺炎
- 亚急性甲状腺炎
- 医源性甲状腺毒症
- 人为摄入甲状腺激素
- 甲状腺肿样卵巢瘤
- 急性甲状腺炎
- 甲状腺癌广泛转移

11.1）。确证和确认依靠以下甲状腺实验室检查（表 11.2）：

- 甲状腺素（T_4）升高。
- 三碘甲状腺原氨酸（T_3）升高。
- 促甲状腺激素（TSH）降低。

然而，T_4 和 T_3 浓度可能与临床症状的严重性相关性较差。事实上，Burch-Wartofsky 评分（见表 11.1）是一个仅基于临床和体检标准的分数表，它不依赖血液中甲状腺激素的浓度来评估甲状腺毒症

表 11.2 甲状腺疾病患者甲状腺功能的检验结果

检验项目	功能异常	
	甲状腺功能亢进	甲状腺功能减退
TSH	低	高
总 T_4	高	低
总 T_3	高	低
反 T_3（rT_3）	高	低至正常
游离 T_4	高	低
T_3 树脂摄取试验 *	高	低

* 甲状腺素结合球蛋白与血清激素结合的近似值（正常范围为 33%～48%）

T_3，三碘甲状腺原氨酸；T_4，甲状腺素；TSH，促甲状腺激素

的可能性。其他常规检查包括全血细胞计数、电解质水平、尿液分析、胸部 X 线片和心电图。例如，常见的相关实验室异常（目前占 5%～20%）包括高钙血症、低钾血症、高血糖、低胆固醇血症、小细胞贫血、淋巴细胞增多症、粒细胞减少症、高胆红素血症和碱性磷酸酶升高。最后，应全面检查并仔细寻找感染性病程的可能。

鉴别诊断

鉴别甲状腺危象的时间，还必须同时考虑恶性高热的可能，如果使用触发性麻醉剂且临床高度怀疑时，应立即启动治疗。尤其是患者为儿童或出现严重的高碳酸症、酸中毒、高钾血症、肌肉强直和肌酸磷酸激酶增加时。其他高代谢状态，如脓毒症、嗜铬细胞瘤，或无危象的甲状腺毒症，以及神经阻滞剂恶性综合征或 5- 羟色胺综合征，亦应予以考虑。最后，鉴别诊断必须包括严重的可卡因或苯丙胺药物中毒。

治疗

如果有足够的临床怀疑，不要等待实验室结果再开始治疗。合理的治疗包括一般支持治疗；直接抑制甲状腺激素合成和甲状腺激素释放，抑制外周 β- 肾上腺素能活性和外周 T_4 向 T_3 的转换；以及细胞内钙调节。如果经标准后仍出现难治性甲状腺危象，可特异性地尝试清除循环中的甲状腺激素。

一般支持治疗

- 静脉（IV）输液以恢复血管内容量。
- 应用对乙酰氨基酚治疗高热（避免服用阿司匹林，因为它从甲状腺结合球蛋白中取代 T_4，从而增加游离 T_4）。
- 冷却毛毯和冷却环境。
- 镁盐可降低心律失常的严重程度和发病率。
- 纠正所有电解质紊乱。

抑制甲状腺激素合成

- 丙硫氧嘧啶（propylthiouracil，PTU）——首次负荷剂量可达 1000 mg，然后每 4 h 口服或鼻胃管注入 250 mg。可能需要 6～8 周才能达到甲状腺功能完全正常状态；PTU 也会抑制外周 T_4 向 T_3 的转换。
- 甲巯基咪唑——这是目前的首选药物。每 4～6 h 经口或经鼻胃管注入 20～30 mg。它比 PTU 更快使甲状腺功能达到正常，并且粒细胞缺乏症、肝炎和血管炎的发生率更低。

碘化物治疗

碘化物抑制甲状腺激素的合成（称为 Wolff-Chaikoff 效应）。然而，在开始 PTU 或甲巯咪唑治疗后，碘化物治疗应延迟至少 4 h。

- 碘化钠——每 8 h 静脉给药 1g。
- 碘化钾（SSKI，碘化钾饱和液），如 Lugol 溶液——每 6 h 口服 10 滴。Lugol 液曾广泛应用于择期甲状腺切除术前的 7～10 天，以减少腺体的血管分布。
- 碘番酸——每天 0.5～1.0 g（也可阻断外周 T_4 向 T_3 的转化）。

抑制外周 β- 肾上腺素能活性

- β 受体阻断剂，也可阻断外周 T_4 向 T_3 的转换：
  - 普萘洛尔——0.5～1.0 mg/min 静脉注射，总剂量不超过 2～10 mg；每 3～4 h 重复一次。在使用静注药物症状得到最初控制后，每 6 h 口服 20～40 mg；因甲状腺功能亢进症患者肝代谢存在个体差异，患者有时可能需要口服高达每天 2 g 的剂量。
  - 艾司洛尔——静脉推注 0.5～0.75 mg/kg，然后静脉滴注，50 μg/（kg·min）。如果 5 min 后效果不佳，重复静脉推注，并将静脉输注

剂量增加到 100 μg/（kg·min）；甚至必要时将输注剂量增加到 300 μg/（kg·min）。
- 滴定 β 受体阻断剂以使心率达到 80～90 次 / 分。
- 如果患者有反应性气道疾病史，应谨慎使用短效心脏选择性药物，如艾司洛尔、阿替洛尔或美托洛尔。

- 如果存在 β 受体阻断剂的禁忌证，其他抑制交感药物（例如利血平是儿茶酚胺的耗竭剂，或胍乙啶可抑制儿茶酚胺释放）可为有用的二线药物。

抑制外周 T_4 向 T_3 转化

- PTU 或甲巯咪唑（剂量见上文）。
- β 受体阻滞剂（剂量见上文）。
- 氢化可的松的负荷剂量为 300 mg，然后每 8 h 静注 100 mg，或地塞米松每 6 h 静注或口服 2 mg。

细胞内钙调节剂

据案例报道，丹曲林的剂量为 1 mg/kg（相当于用于恶性高热的剂量），但其在甲状腺危象中的作用和疗效尚不明确。

清除血液循环中甲状腺激素

- 治疗性血浆置换（患者将需要多次治疗，因为每个疗程中只有 20% 的循环中的 T_4 被移除，而且 T_3 比 T_4 清除得更少）。
- 活性炭血液灌流

预防

甲状腺功能亢进症（尤其是甲状腺危象）患者并发症的预防，依赖于术前评估期间对未诊断的甲状腺功能亢进症的特征识别。此外，麻醉科医师必须预料到气管插管过程中可能出现的气道困难，其在甲状腺手术患者麻醉时的发生率为 6%（见图 11.1）。甲状腺危象的死亡率可能高达 20%，因此提高生存率依赖于早期、积极的治疗。此外，任何相关的疾病都需要进行针对性治疗，如感染或糖尿病酮症酸中毒。

致谢

感谢 Pam Roberts 博士对本章上一版的贡献。

（尹光敏　译　代元强　校）

延伸阅读

Ambus T, Evans S, Smith NT: Thyrotoxicosis factitia in the anesthetized patient, *Anesthesiology* 81:254–256, 1994.

Bahn RS, Burch HB, Cooper DS, et al.: Hyperthyroidism and other causes of thyrotoxicosis: management guidelines of the American Thyroid Association and American Association of Clinical Endocrinologists, *Thyroid* 21:593–646, 2011.

Bennett MH, Wainwright AP: Acute thyroid crisis on induction of anaesthesia, *Anaesthesia* 44:28–30, 1989.

Benua RS, Becker DV: Thyroid storm. In Bardin CW, editor: *Current therapy in endocrinology and metabolism*, 4th ed, Philadelphia, 1991, BC Decker, pp 68–70.

Burch HB, Wartofsky L: Life-threatening thyrotoxicosis, *Endocrinol Metab Clin North Am* 22:263–277, 1993.

Carroll C, Matfin G: Endocrine and metabolic emergencies: thyroid storm, *Ther Adv Endocrinol Metab* 1:139–145, 2010.

Connery LE, Coursin DB: Assessment and therapy of selected endocrine disorders, *Anesthesiol Clin North Am* 22:93–123, 2004.

Devereaux D, Tewelde SZ: Hyperthyroidism and thyrotoxicosis, *Emerg Med Clin North Am* 32:277–292, 2014.

Eckstein A, Schittkowski M, Esser J: Surgical treatment of Graves' ophthalmopathy, *Best Pract Res Clin Endocrinol Metab* 26:339–358, 2012.

Farling PA: Thyroid disease, *Br J Anaesth* 85:15–28, 2000.

Gavin LA: Thyroid crises, *Med Clin North Am* 75:179–193, 1991.

Knighton JD, Crosse MM: Anaesthetic management of childhood thyrotoxicosis and the use of esmolol, *Anaesthesia* 52:62–76, 1997.

Kreisner E, Lutzky M, Gross JL: Charcoal hemoperfusion in the treatment of levothyroxine intoxication, *Thyroid* 20:209–212, 2010.

Lacoste L, Gineste D, Karayan J, et al.: Airway complications in thyroid surgery, *Ann Otol Rhinol Laryngol* 102:441–446, 1993.

Laliberte BD, Goldenberg E, Reece-Stremtan JR: Intraoperative diagnosis and treatment of thyroid storm in a 15-year-old male, *A A Case Rep* 3:107–109, 2014.

Muller C, Perrin P, Faller B, et al: Role of plasma exchange in thyroid storm. *Ther Apher Dial* 15:522–531.

Nishiyama K, Kitahara A, Natsume H, et al.: Malignant hyperthermia in a patient with Graves' disease during subtotal thyroidectomy, *Endocr J* 48:227–232, 2001.

Pandey CK, Raza M, Dhiraaj S, et al.: Rapid preparation of severe uncontrolled thyrotoxicosis due to Graves' disease with iopanoic acid, *Can J Anaesth* 51:38–40, 2004.

Peters KR, Nance P, Wingard DW: Malignant hyperthyroidism or malignant hyperthermia? *Anesth Analg* 60:613–615, 1991.

Pugh S, Lalwani K, Awal A: Thyroid storm as a cause of loss of consciousness following anaesthesia for emergency caesarean section, *Anaesthesia* 49:35–37, 1994.

第 12 章 甲状腺功能减退症：黏液性水肿昏迷

Monica I. Lupei，*Richard C. Prielipp*

病例概要

患者，女性，53 岁，既往有甲状腺功能减退病史，吸烟多年。现因“全身乏力、嗜睡、呼吸短促、下肢水肿、便秘、言语迟缓”急诊入院。自诉 2 年前停止甲状腺替代治疗，目前仅服用丙酸氟替卡松与美达施（含车前子的膳食纤维）。体格检查示：严重低体温，嗜睡，言语迟缓；黏膜干燥，毛发粗糙易碎；心音遥远，心动过缓；双侧呼吸音减弱；腹胀，无压痛；双下肢非凹陷性水肿。实验室检查示：轻度贫血（血红蛋白 9.4 g/dl），白细胞增多（白细胞计数 17.2×10^9/L），低钾血症（3.1 mmol/L），促甲状腺激素（thyroid-stimulating hormone，TSH）水平为 120 mU/L（正常值为 0.4 ～ 4.0 mU/L）；游离甲状腺素（T_4）为 0.08 ng/dl（正常值为 0.46 ～ 0.76 ng/dl）。胸腹部及盆腔 CT 示：大量心包积液，右侧少量胸腔积液，明显腹水。就诊后，内分泌科医师迅速给予静脉注射左旋甲状腺素、甲状腺素和氢化可的松。此外，为改善心动过缓并维持血流动力学稳定，还为患者持续静脉输注多巴胺。

由于患者早期出现了轻度心脏压塞症状，对其进行了心包穿刺术。3 天后由于发生了严重的复发性心包积液，又对患者实施了心包开窗术。术前采用以下麻醉药物进行诱导：格隆溴铵 0.4 mg，氢化可的松 100 mg，依托咪酯 20 mg，芬太尼 50 μg 和琥珀胆碱 120 mg。由于气道水肿、黏膜肿胀，初次使用 7.5 号气管导管（endotracheal tube，ETT）时插管失败，随后改用 6.5 号 ETT，插管成功。术中给予 0.4 最低肺泡有效浓度（minimum alveolar concentration，MAC）异氟烷、小剂量芬太尼并间断注射顺阿曲库铵以维持适当的麻醉深度。患者于麻醉间期出现明显的低体温与心动过缓，因此静脉给予多巴胺共计 50 mg 以维持适当心率。术后患者出现苏醒延迟，随后拔管。患者于住院期间始终使用左甲状腺素治疗，使用氢化可的松并在 2 周内逐渐减量。患者于 ICU 期间，心包引流管留置 3 天后拔除。就诊 14 天后，患者转入一所长期护理机构。

问题分析

定义与生理机制

甲状腺功能减退症（简称甲减）是以甲状腺功能降低、甲状腺激素产生与分泌减少为特征的常见疾病。黏液性水肿是一种危及生命的并发症，伴随意识丧失甚至昏迷。黏液性水肿所致的昏迷是由慢性甲减或未经妥善治疗的患者在一定条件下（如感染、创伤、手术、寒冷甚至某种药物等）诱发所致。

通常，甲状腺分泌 80% 甲状腺素（thyroxine，

T_4）和 20% 三碘甲状腺原氨酸（triiodothyronine，T_3），其中 T_3 是甲状腺激素最活跃的形式。原始的 T_3 和 T_4 是由酪氨酰与甲状腺球蛋白结合并碘化后形成的，随后储存在胶质小泡中。大部分 T_3（80%）是在肝、肾、脑等非甲状腺器官中由 T_4 脱碘而成。部分 T_4 也可转化为非活跃状态的逆三碘甲状腺原氨酸（rT_3）。在血浆中，T_3 和 T_4 与蛋白（甲状腺素结合球蛋白和甲状腺素视黄质运载蛋白）结合，**只有游离的 T_3 和 T_4 才能被靶组织摄取利用**。

促甲状腺激素（thyroid-stimulating hormone，TSH）由垂体产生，促进 T_3、T_4 的合成与释放。反之，T_3、T_4 又可通过负反馈调节 TSH 的分泌。氢化可的松可抑制 TSH 的释放。TSH 的分泌具有昼夜节律性，其在夜间达到高峰。下丘脑分泌的促甲状腺激素释放激素（thyrotropin-releasing hormone，TRH）可促进 TSH 的释放。

在靶组织的细胞水平上，甲状腺激素的作用通过核酸受体进行调控。婴幼儿时期，甲状腺激素对神经系统的发育至关重要。甲状腺激素几乎作用于所有组织并对生命系统发挥重要作用，如提高基础代谢率，调节蛋白质、脂质及糖代谢，促进骨骼的生长和神经系统的发育，增强机体对儿茶酚胺的敏感性。其临床效应包括：增加心排血量，增加心率和呼吸频率，增加基础代谢率，促进脑组织发育、改善认知功能，增强全身分解代谢。

识别

临床表现与诊断

甲减的临床表现无特异性，主要取决于患者的年龄以及疾病的严重程度。一般症状包括：疲劳乏力、体重增加、认知障碍、抑郁、劳力性呼吸困难、冷漠、声音嘶哑、皮肤干燥、脱发、便秘、月经紊乱甚至不孕。实验室检查可表现为巨细胞性贫血、低钠血症、低血糖以及肌酸激酶升高。患者可能出现明显的心包积液、胸腔积液以及全身性水肿。体格检查通常发现甲状腺肿大、言语迟缓、腱反射延迟、心动过缓、舒张性高血压、自主呼吸抑制，上呼吸道水肿甚至梗阻。此外，可能出现机体对低氧及高碳酸血症的反应严重减弱，顺应性降低，血管阻力增加，血容量减少。心电图可表现为窦性心动过缓、QRS 波低电压、Q-T 间期延长、T 波改变，甚至可能出现室上性心动过速。

若怀疑发生甲减，首先应检测 TSH 水平。若 TSH 水平升高，应检测 T_4 并复查 TSH。原发性甲减表现为 TSH 升高伴游离 T_4 降低（表 12.1）。在自身免疫性甲减中，甲状腺过氧化物酶抗体的血浆浓度升高。若 TSH 升高而游离 T_4 水平正常，则为亚临床型甲减。此时治疗方案应在咨询专家后制订，以避免发生并发症。此外，分泌 TSH 的垂体腺瘤也可表现为 TSH 增加、游离 T_4 水平正常或升高。

TSH 水平降低可引起中枢性甲减，通常是由垂体分泌 TSH 减少（继发性甲减）或下丘脑分泌 TRH 减少（三发性甲减）所造成的（见表 12.1）。在中枢性甲减中，TSH 水平正常或下降，T_4 减少。甲状腺激素抵抗的特征是 TSH 升高，游离 T_4 和 T_3 的水平正常（甲状腺功能正常）或降低（甲状腺功能减退）。在非甲状腺疾病的危重症患者中，也可出现 TSH 及游离 T_4、T_3 水平降低，如心肺转流术术后或者长期禁食等（见表 12.1）。

病因学与流行病学

甲状腺疾病是仅次于糖尿病的最为常见的内分泌系统疾病。美国一项大型研究显示，在未知甲状腺疾病的人群中，4.6% 的人存在甲减症状（0.3% 有显性症状可明确诊断，4.3% 为亚临床型）。在女性中，甲减的发生率比男性高 5 ～ 8 倍，且多发于老年人。桥本慢性自身免疫性甲状腺炎是引起原发性甲减最常见的原因，其特点为甲状腺功能逐渐减退且多发于老年女性。自身免疫性甲减是引起儿童甲减最常见的原因。

妊娠期甲减的发生率与普通人群类似，但若治疗不当则可能引起流产、早产、胎儿宫内生长受限、妊娠期高血压、胎盘早剥和产后出血等并发症。

碘缺乏与碘过量均可导致甲减。碘缺乏是引起甲减及甲状腺肿大最为常见的原因。世界卫生组织

表 12.1 甲减状态的实验室诊断

评估指标	TSH	游离 T_4	游离 T_3
原发性甲减	升高	降低	降低
亚临床型甲减	升高	正常	正常
中枢性甲减	降低或正常	降低或正常	降低或正常
非甲状腺疾病	降低	降低	降低
甲状腺激素抵抗	升高	降低或正常	降低或正常

依据 1993—2003 年的数据推测，全球甲状腺肿大的发生率约为 15.8%。

甲减的病因也可能是医源性的。甲状腺全切或部分切除、甲状腺功能亢进（简称甲亢）的放射性治疗、恶性肿瘤的放疗等均可导致甲减。甲减也可继发于治疗非甲状腺疾病的药物，如锂、胺碘酮、铁、考来烯胺、干扰素 -α 和酪氨酸激酶抑制剂等（表 12.2）。对于已知的甲状腺功能正常的患者，临床医生还必须谨慎对待某些可能干扰或改变甲状腺功能检测指标的药物（表 12.3）。其他导致甲减的罕见原因包括一些炎症性疾病，如：纤维性甲状腺炎、血色素沉着病、硬皮病、白血病和结节病。无痛淋巴细胞性甲状腺炎、产后甲状腺炎、甲状腺部分切除术后或甲状腺功能正常后患者停用甲状腺激素治疗等原因，也可能引起甲减。

继发性甲减可由垂体功能减退引起，最常见于垂体腺瘤。其他原因包括：产后垂体坏死（Sheehan 综合征）、外伤和肿瘤，如颅咽管瘤。任何影响下丘脑或阻碍下丘脑-垂体血流的疾病都会导致垂体功能减退。创伤、肿瘤、脑血管意外或炎症性疾病均可导致下丘脑损伤。

甲状腺激素抵抗是一种罕见的遗传性疾病（通常是常染色体显性遗传），通常零星发病，多表现为身材矮小、骨骼发育不成熟和智力障碍。

甲减与麻醉并发症

围术期甲减患者最常出现的麻醉并发症是“苏醒延迟”。但是，麻醉后苏醒延迟的定义较为宽泛，且无明确的诊断标准。文献中病例报告显示，术前存在甲减或亚临床型甲减的患者在麻醉后出现苏醒延迟可能与低体温及药物代谢受损有关。一例黏液性水肿昏迷患者因急性肠梗阻，于硬膜外麻醉下行急诊手术。术中给予患者旋甲状腺素治疗，可使其精神状态逐渐改善。另一个病例中，一名服用舒尼替尼（酪氨酸激酶抑制剂）的患者在经历两次不同手术后均出现了苏醒延迟，随后发展为黏液性水肿昏迷。手术期间，该患者出现了低体温、心动过缓、神经肌肉阻滞延长以及麻醉后苏醒延迟。在另一个病例中，一名事先未发现甲减的患者，在平稳麻醉下的髋关节置换手术后出现了心脏停搏。该患者心肺复苏成功后，被诊断为黏液性水肿昏迷并给予甲状腺素进行治疗，之后顺利康复。一例因舌鳞状细胞癌行下颌骨部分切除术、舌骨切除术与颈部淋巴结清扫术的甲减患者的病例证实，手术与麻醉可能是诱发黏液性水肿昏迷的重要因素。在最后一个病例中，一位偶然发现肌酸激酶升高的患者麻醉后出现了苏醒延迟，随后该患者被诊断为严重甲减。最后值得警惕的是，有文献报道甲减患者于术后会出现气道梗阻。

管理与预防

大多数程度较轻或经过治疗的甲减患者手术风险并不会显著升高。病情稳定的甲减患者在围术期应继续左甲状腺素（人工合成的 T_4）的替代治疗。

黏液性水肿昏迷是一种急症，若治疗不当，则死亡率可高达 80%。因此，在等待化验及其他检查结果的同时即应给予静脉注射治疗。在围术期对黏液性水肿昏迷患者进行适当治疗至关重要，且前 24 h 是关键。建议治疗时咨询专家。其他的治疗要点包括以下内容：

- 应考虑同时使用 T_3 和 T_4，但是这种组合疗法的优越性尚不明确。
- 由于胃肠道吸收功能可能受损，静脉治疗优于口服。

表 12.2 影响服用左甲状腺素患者甲状腺功能的药物

药物作用机制	抑制吸收	增强肝代谢	降低肝代谢	抑制 5- 脱碘酶	增加甲状腺素结合蛋白
药物	铁剂	苯巴比妥	二甲双胍	丙硫脲嘧啶	雌激素
	钙剂	苯妥英		甲巯咪唑	他莫昔芬
	氢氧化铝	卡马西平		普萘洛尔	美沙酮
	考来烯胺	利福平		糖皮质激素	氟尿嘧啶
	硫糖铝			碘化物	
	雷洛昔芬（依维斯塔）				

Modified from Haugen BR：Drugs that suppress TSH or cause central hypothyroidism. *Best Pract Res Clin Endocrinol Metab* 23（6）：793-800，2009.

表 12.3 因用药导致检查指标改变的甲状腺功能正常患者

异常指标	TSH 低于正常值	TSH 升高（但 <10 U/L）	游离 T_4 升高	游离 T_4 降低
药物	糖皮质激素 地塞米松 氢化可的松 多巴胺 左旋多巴	胺碘酮 甲氧氯普胺 碘造影剂	呋塞米 非甾体类抗炎药（特别是阿司匹林）	卡马西平 苯妥英

- 30 min 内静脉给予左甲状腺素 200 ～ 400 μg（也有人推荐 500 ～ 800 μg），随后每日 1.6 μg/kg（50 ～ 100 μg）；对于可能发生心脏并发症如心肌梗死或心律失常的老年心脏病患者，建议减少剂量。
- 可同时以 5 ～ 20 μg 的剂量给予碘塞罗宁，随后每 8 h 追加 2.5 ～ 10 μg。
- 推荐持续使用 T_3 直到临床症状改善或患者病情稳定。
- 可考虑使用高剂量甲状腺激素（T_4>500 μg，T_3>75 μg），但可能引起心律失常等不良反应。
- 在测定随机皮质醇水平后，为预防肾上腺功能不全，应使用皮质类固醇：氢化可的松每 8 h 100 mg。
- 使用葡萄糖与生理盐水进行液体复苏，检查是否存在严重低钠血症（[Na] <120 mEq/L）。
- 若单纯补液无法维持血流动力学稳定，应使用血管活性药物。
- 严重通气不足或无法保护气道时，可能需要机械通气。
- 由于主动升温会促进血管扩张、加重休克，首选被动复温。
- 在正确培养后建议经验性使用抗生素治疗，因为感染可能是导致黏液性水肿昏迷的重要因素。
- 在治疗的 24 h 内，应观察到黏液性水肿缓解的积极征象。

致谢

感谢 Pan Roberts 医生对本章上一版的贡献。

（徐 冰 译 赵珍珍 校）

延伸阅读

Almandoz JP, Gharib H: Hypothyroidism: etiology, diagnosis, and management, *Med Clin North Am* 96:203–221, 2012.

Andersson M, Takkouche B, Egli I, et al.: Current global iodine status and progress over the last decade towards the elimination of iodine deficiency, *Bull World Health Organ* 83:518–525, 2005.

Benfari G, de Vincentiis M: Postoperative airway obstruction: a complication of a previously undiagnosed hypothyroidism, *Otolaryngol Head Neck Surg* 132:343–344, 2005.

Bianco AC, Kim BW: Deiodinases: implications of the local control of thyroid hormone action, *J Clin Invest* 116, 2006. 2571–2579.

Brucker-Davis F, Skarulis MC, Grace MB, et al.: Genetic and clinical features of 42 kindreds with resistance to thyroid hormone: The National Institutes of Health Prospective Study, *Ann Intern Med* 123:572–583, 1995.

Foley Jr TP, Abbassi V, Copeland KC, et al.: Brief report: hypothyroidism caused by chronic autoimmune thyroiditis in very young infants, *N Engl J Med* 330:466–468, 1994.

Haugen BR: Drugs that suppress TSH or cause central hypothyroidism, *Best Pract Res Clin Endocrinol Metab* 23:793–800, 2009.

Hollowell JG, Staehling NW, Flanders WD, et al.: Serum TSH, T(4), and thyroid antibodies in the United States population (1988 to 1994): National Health and Nutrition Examination Survey (NHANES III), *J Clin Endocrinol Metab* 87:489–499, 2002.

Jackson IM: Thyrotropin-releasing hormone, *N Engl J Med* 306:145–155, 1982.

Kohl BA, Schwartz S: How to manage perioperative endocrine insufficiency, *Anesthesiol Clin* 28:139–155, 2010.

Kumar VV, Kaimar P: Subclinical hypothyroidism: a cause for delayed recovery from anaesthesia? *Indian J Anaesth* 55:433–434, 2011.

Kwaku MP, Burman KD: Myxedema coma, *J Intensive Care Med* 22:224–231, 2007.

Larsen PR, Silva JE, Kaplan MM: Relationships between circulating and intracellular thyroid hormones: physiological and clinical implications, *Endocr Rev* 2:87–102, 1981.

Lele AV, Clutter S, Price E, et al.: Severe hypothyroidism presenting as myxedema coma in the postoperative period in a patient taking sunitinib: case report and review of literature, *J Clin Anesth* 25:47–51, 2013.

Mizuno J, Nakayama Y, Dohi T, et al.: A case of hypothyroidism found by delayed awakening after the operation, *Masui* 49:305–308, 2000.

More P, Laheri VV, Waigankar T, et al.: Delayed recovery from anaesthesia in a patient with optimised hypothyroidism and incidental hypokalemia, *J Clin Diagn Res* 9, 2015. UD06–7.

Oetting A, Yen PM: New insights into thyroid hormone action, *Best Pract Res Clin Endocrinol Metab* 21:193–208, 2007.

Ragaller M, Quintel M, Bender HJ, et al.: Myxedema coma as a rare postoperative complication, *Anaesthesia* 42:179–183, 1993.

Samuels MH, Ridgway EC: Central hypothyroidism, *Endocrinol Metab Clin North Am* 21:903–919, 1992.

Schiff RL, Welsh GA: Perioperative evaluation and management of the patient with endocrine dysfunction, *Med Clin North Am* 87:175–192, 2003.

Sherry KM, Hutchinson IL: Postoperative myxoedema. A report of coma and upper airway obstruction, *Anaesthesia* 39:1112–1114, 1984.

Shupnik MA, Ridgway EC, Chin WW: Molecular biology of thyrotropin, *Endocr Rev* 10:459–475, 1989.

Talikoti AT, Rao S, Ravi M, et al.: A case of subacute intestinal obstruction with overt hypothyroidism in stupor scheduled for emergency laparotomy, *Indian J Anaesth* 58:347–349, 2014.

Yamamoto T, Fukuyama J, Fujiyoshi A: Factors associated with mortality of myxedema coma: report of eight cases and literature survey, *Thyroid* 9:1167–1174, 1999.

第13章 机械辅助装置

Michelle Capdeville

病例概要

患者，男性，58岁，既往控制不佳的高血压病、糖尿病病史，吸烟30年包。急诊经皮冠状动脉介入术（percutaneous coronary intervention，PCI）失败后，因心源性休克入手术室（operating room，OR），经右股动脉紧急放置主动脉内球囊泵（intraaortic balloon pump，IABP）。由于患者血流动力学持续不稳定，并发肺水肿，在转入手术室前已行气管插管。进入手术室后患者心功能进一步恶化，在心肺转流术（cardiopulmonary bypass，CPB）下行三支血管的冠状动脉旁路移植术。在脱离CPB期间尝试使用IABP和大剂量强心药，但经食管超声心动图（transesophageal echocardiogram，TEE）仍显示前壁和侧壁运动缺失，估算左心室射血分数为15%～20%。

问题分析

定义

机械循环辅助装置可用来支持衰竭的心脏。多种装置可供选择，包括长期或短期支持，以及单心室或双心室支持。其中，最简单和最常用的是主动脉内球囊泵（IABP）。它根据反搏原理进行工作，并于1967年进入临床。简言之，IABP由安装在导管上的聚氨酯球囊构成，通常经皮置于胸降主动脉中，导管尖端恰好位于左锁骨下动脉远端。气囊膨胀与心动周期同步，净效应为有益于**冠状动脉灌注的舒张压增加、心脏后负荷降低**。总的结果是改善了心肌氧供需平衡。不同于心室辅助装置（ventricular assist device，VAD），IABP不提供"主动的"循环支持并需要一定程度的心脏自身的功能。一般的IABP组成包括带有引导鞘的IABP导管、控制台、触发源、气源（氦）和从属电缆（用于术中监护仪）。控制台显示心电图（electrocardiogram，ECG）、中心动脉压波形、球囊充气迹线和增强。重要控制包括触发选择、启动/待机、报警和自动/半自动/手动模式。

更复杂的用于短期或长期心脏支持的VAD包括非脉冲离心泵和轴流泵。离心泵包括体外膜肺氧合（extracorporeal membrane oxygenation，ECMO），TandemHeart经皮左心室辅助装置（PLVAD）（Cardiac Assist Technologies Inc.，Pittsburgh，PA）和HeartWare心室辅助装置（HVAD）（HeartWare International，Inc.，Miami Lakes，FL）；轴流泵包括Impella（ABIOMED，Inc.，Danvers，MA）和HeartMate Ⅱ（Thoratec Corporation，Pleasanton，CA）。

VAD支持的一般适应证可划分为四大类：①移植的过渡；②恢复期的过渡；③决策期的过渡；④目标治疗。还包括"列入移植候选名单的过渡"类别。表13.1对上述装置进行了简要的描述。ECMO的适应证是独特的，它有两种配置：静脉-动脉（V-A）和静脉-静脉（V-V）。V-A ECMO用于心力衰竭，V-V ECMO用于支持呼吸衰竭。

简言之，VAD将血液从左心输送到全身循环（LVAD），或者从右心输送到肺循环（RVAD），从而绕过衰竭的心室腔。通过LVAD的支持，血液从左心[左心房（LA）或左心室（LV）]输送到泵。泵通过流出导管或移植物推动或喷射血液到全身循环（通常吻合于升主动脉以用于长期支持）——如果主要支持来源于泵，主动脉瓣将会保持关闭；RVAD将血液从右心房（right atrium，RA）或右心

表 13.1 常用短期和长期心室辅助装置的概述

	泵类型	支持类型	流量 / 泵速	套管	适应证	一般说明
短期						
ECMO	离心	R，L	产生的流量取决于插管的大小；0 ～ 4000 rpm；高达 7 L/min	V-A ECMO 流入：股动脉、腋动脉、主动脉（中央）；流出：股静脉 / 下腔静脉、上腔静脉、右心房 V-V ECMO：股静脉-股静脉；股静脉-上腔静脉，或 V-V ECMO：Avalon 套管（双腔；下腔静脉，右心房）	心脏支持（V-A ECMO）；呼吸支持（V-V ECMO）	体外离心泵由安装在透明塑料外壳中，与马达电磁耦合的叶轮或旋转锥组成。旋转运动将血液从泵中吸出到回流套管中。连续静脉-静脉血液滤过成为可能
Impella	微轴	R，L	Impella LP 2.5，高达 2.5 L/min（最大旋转速度 50 000 rpm）；Impella LP5.0，高达 5 L/min（最大旋转速 33 000 rpm）；Impella RD 5.0，高达 5 L/min	股动脉套管 9 Fr（LVAD）；Impella LP 5.0 需要动脉切开术；Impella RD 5.0 需通过胸骨切开术插入右心房	心源性休克时的左心室支持；作为恢复期的过渡或作为长期设备的过渡；心脏术后右心室衰竭的支持	小型轴流泵。Impella LP 2.5 对高风险的 PCI 最为有效；当心脏支持所需增加时，LP 5.0 更好，如心源性休克
TandemHeart	离心	L	高达 5 L/min；3000 ～ 7500 rpm	21 Fr 股静脉经室间隔套管；12 ～ 19 Fr 股动脉套管；可经皮或在心脏手术时放置	心源性休克中的左心室支持；作为恢复期的过渡或作为长期设备的过渡	经房间隔左心房套管有 14 个侧孔进行最佳化引流。为左心室减负 80% ～ 90%，提供生理压力（90 mmHg）。六叶叶轮由磁力驱动并通过输液系统冷却和润滑
长期						
HeartMate Ⅱ	轴流	L	流量可高达 10 L/min；速度范围 6000 ～ 15 000 rpm（临床范围 8600 ～ 9800 rpm）	心室尖（流入）和升主动脉（流出）由编织涤纶制成并需要预先凝固	移植过渡；恢复期过渡；移植候选患者的过渡；目标治疗	转子位于钛泵外壳中；转子是唯一活动部分；泵壳内的电机产生能使转子转动的旋转磁场
HeartWare HVAD	离心	L	流量可高达 10 L/min；1800 ～ 4000 rpm（临床操作范围 2400 ～ 3200 rpm；较低的范围用于从 CPB 脱机）	心室尖（流入套管）和升主动脉（流出）	移植过渡；恢复期过渡；用于目标疗法等待批准	微型离心泵位于心包腔。流入套管与泵是一个整体；叶轮靠磁场和血流动力学的力量悬浮，并通过泵抽血；无摩擦旋转转速 1800 ～ 2400 rpm

L，左；PCI，经皮冠状动脉介入治疗；R，右；V-A，静脉-动脉；VAD，心室辅助装置；V-V，静脉-静脉

室（right ventricle，RV）输送至肺动脉（pulmonary artery，PA）。

理解用于描述 VAD 时使用的命名法很重要。“流入”指血液直接**流入**泵中，而“流出”指血液经泵**泵出**而进入全身循环。这不同于体外循环，其中来源于泵的全身血流进入主动脉、股动脉或腋动脉（流入），而流向泵的血液来自静脉导管（流出）进入容器。

识别

主动脉内球囊泵

IABP 既可用于危重病房，也可用于手术室，通常通过股动脉经皮置入；然而，当股动脉质量较差时，另可选择的入路有腋动脉和主动脉。可以通过胸部 X 线摄影、透视或 TEE 检查合适的定位。框 13.1 概括了使用 IABP 的适应证和禁忌证。

框 13.1 IABP 支持的适应证和禁忌证

适应证

梗死后心源性休克

梗死后机械并发症（VSD，乳头肌断裂）

心肌缺血导致的心律失常

顽固性心绞痛

高风险的心脏导管插入术 /PCI

严重 CAD 急诊（非心脏）大手术 / 缺血性右心室衰竭伴肺动脉高压

严重的脓毒性休克

对血管再梗死性心肌损伤的高风险加强溶栓

心肌挫伤

心肺转流术脱机困难

禁忌证

主动脉瓣关闭不全

严重的动脉粥样硬化性疾病（股动脉、主动脉）

主动脉夹层

主动脉瘤

插管部位感染

非移植候选者中的不可逆性心脏病

“拒绝心肺复苏”者

主动脉，髂动脉支架 / 移植物

CAD，冠状动脉疾病；PCI，经皮冠状动脉介入治疗；VSD，室间隔缺损

IABP 导管有两个腔：一个腔通向球囊，当球囊充气和放气时，里面的氦气迅速地来回穿梭；另一个腔允许经长导丝插入导管，用于监测中心动脉压。导管尖端应置于左锁骨下动脉远端 1 ～ 2 cm 处，有利于预防主要血管（即脑、肾、肠系膜）闭塞。

冠状动脉血流量取决于许多因素，包括灌注压，心肌血管外、冠状动脉内的压迫，心肌代谢率和神经体液因子。应牢记冠状动脉血流量等于舒张压减去左心室舒张末压（CBF=DBP-LVEDP），并且大部分左冠状动脉血流量来自舒张期（右冠状动脉血流来自收缩期和舒张期），这很容易理解球囊反搏增加心脏血供的原理。在收缩期推动血液进入主动脉前，球囊快速放气降低了主动脉血压，改善了前向射血，减少了心肌氧耗量（myocardial oxygen consumption，MVO_2），减少了室壁应力，并改善了心肌性能。主动脉瓣关闭时的球囊膨胀增加冠状动脉灌注，使得收缩力改善，充盈压下降，收缩性能总体改善。

心室辅助装置

短期装置

由微型轴流泵组成的 Impella 安装在导管尖端，导管经皮（Impella 2.5）或经切开（Impella 5.0）通过股动脉并逆行于胸部降主动脉，置入左心室流出道（left ventricular outflow tract，LVOT）。通过激活，血液从 LVOT 持续推入主动脉根 / 升主动脉。Impella RD 是一种微型 RVAD，通过正中胸骨切开术插入（通常在心脏手术时支持术后右心室衰竭）。流入导管直接植于右心房，并且流出导管位于主肺动脉。血流量可高达 5 L/min。

TandemHeart 推动血液从左心房（通过房间隔穿刺和股静脉通路）进入一个小离心泵，进而通过股动脉导管推动全身血液进入主动脉。它可以在 CPB 时以经皮穿刺或者手术的方式置入。

长期装置

2001 年，具有里程碑意义的 REMARCH 研究（对慢性心力衰竭治疗中机械辅助设备的随机评估）发表后，机械循环支持装置用于心力衰竭的长期支持成为现实。长期 VAD 从最初第一代容量替换搏动装置（HeartMate Ⅰ，Novacor LVAS，前 World Heart Corporation，现为 HeartWare 的一个部门；胸外体表经皮心室辅助装置 PVAD）发展到第二代（HeartMate Ⅱ，DeBakey Micromed——MicroMed Technology，Houston TX；Jarvik 2000——Jarvik Heart Inc.，New York，NY）和第三代（HeartWare，HeartMate Ⅲ）非搏动装置，使泵组件更小、动力传动系统更薄、运动零件更少、摩擦和热的产生减少，并且运行更安静。以后这些泵也可以置入更小的患者体内。第一代设备受到机械故障、血栓栓塞和与更大的动力传动系统、阀门和其他活动部件相关的感染并发症的困扰。尽管存在这些早期问题，但是 REMATCH 研究能证明，相比最大力度的内科治疗，HeartMate Ⅰ支持的移植落选的患者具有更好的结局和生活质量评价。当来自 REMATCH 研究的数据被外推和与来自 HeartMate Ⅱ目标治疗试验的结果相比较时，新一代泵显示出更好的结果和更少的并发症，最显著的是机械故障和动力传动系统相关的感染的减少。目前，大约有 25% 等待心脏移植的患者依赖 VAD 支持。框 13.2 为适应证和禁忌证。

HeartMate Ⅱ 和 HeartWare HVAD 控制台上的重要参数包括泵速（rpm）、搏动指数（取决于在主动脉瓣打开时所反映心脏原有功能对心排血量的影响）、功耗（瓦特）和心排血量估计值（L/min）。这

框 13.2 VAD 支持的适应证和禁忌证

适应证

移植过渡

可能改善在医疗监护下和死亡风险更大或等待捐献器官时间较长的 1A 状态患者的预后

恢复期过渡

一些非缺血性心肌病患者可以恢复心肌功能（即“逆向重塑”）并经历了成功的 LVAD 植入

决策过渡

ECMO、Impella 或 TandemHeart 的短期 VAD 支持可能使衰竭器官得到充分恢复，从而有更长的时间窗来确定长期机械治疗的可行性

候选资格过渡

LVAD 支持可能充分降低在之前被认为是心脏移植的非候选者的 PVR 而使他们能够符合移植条件；在心肺移植候选者中，降低 PVR 能使其移植资格状态变为仅进行心脏移植

目标疗法

无移植资格的候选者有资格获得 HeartMate Ⅱ LVAD 终身机械支持；适用于选择机械治疗代替移植的终末期心力衰竭患者

禁忌证

绝对

- 不可逆的终末器官损伤
- 持续存在的凝血功能障碍
- 神经系统状况不良
- 脓毒症
- 药物滥用
- 社会问题
- 依从性差

相对

- 机械性 AVR
- 活动期的恶性肿瘤
- 病态肥胖

AVR，主动脉瓣置换术；PVR，肺血管阻力

些参数都取决于患者的状况并提供有关泵功能的信息。基线值的变化比绝对数更重要。应设定泵速以维持一定程度的脉动，目标是室间隔无移位，降低左心室压力，达到足够的心脏指数和主动脉瓣间歇开放。

HeartMate Ⅱ 是最成功的第二代泵（图 13.1）。它于 2008 年 4 月被批准作为等待移植的过渡治疗，并于 2010 年 1 月用于目的治疗。HeartMate Ⅱ 由钛外壳内的单个转子组成。流入导管定位在左心室尖

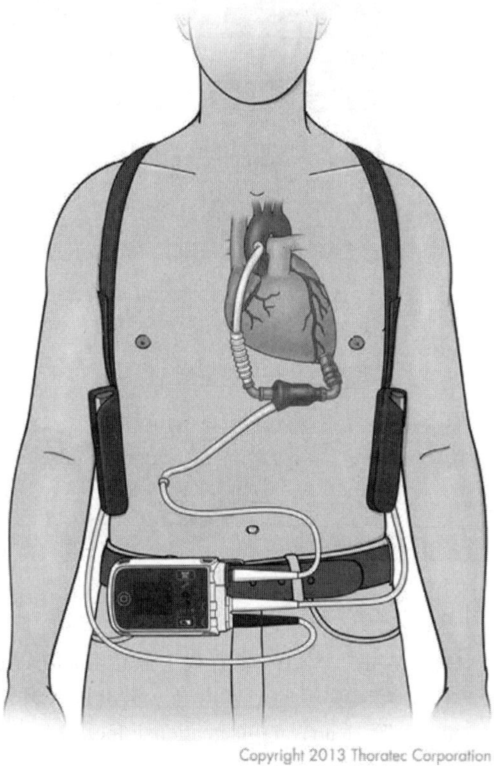

图 13.1 HeartMate Ⅱ（第二代）原位轴流 LVAD。注意左心室尖端的顶端流入套管和与升主动脉吻合的流出移植物（Image courtesy of Thoratec Corporation, Pleasanton，CA）

端并和泵链接，置于腹膜前袋中。流出导管离开泵并与升主动脉吻合。当转子旋转，血液持续从左心室尖端抽出并被推入升主动脉。隧道式经皮动力传动系统将泵连接到控制器（设备控制和电源）。泵的性能取决于转子速度和泵的压力梯度（即流量和压力呈负相关）。

HeartWare HVAD 于 2006 年在临床推广，是一种放置在心包内的泵，其中流入导管和一个小型持续流式离心泵是一个整体，而流出道与升主动脉吻合（图 13.2）。薄且灵活的动力传动系统和泵相连并从皮肤分离，它连接外部控制器和电源（转子或便携式电池组）。泵有一个运动部分，并且无机械承轴。旋转叶轮悬挂在结合了流体动力学和磁力的泵内，从而产生无摩擦运动。泵的控制台显示流量波形，搏动指数表示波形的最小值和最大值之间的差值（搏动指数应大于 2 L/min）；波形谷值应大于 2 L/min。该设备由美国食品和药物管理局（Food and Drug Administration，FDA）批准作为等待移植的过渡治疗并即将被批准用于目的治疗。

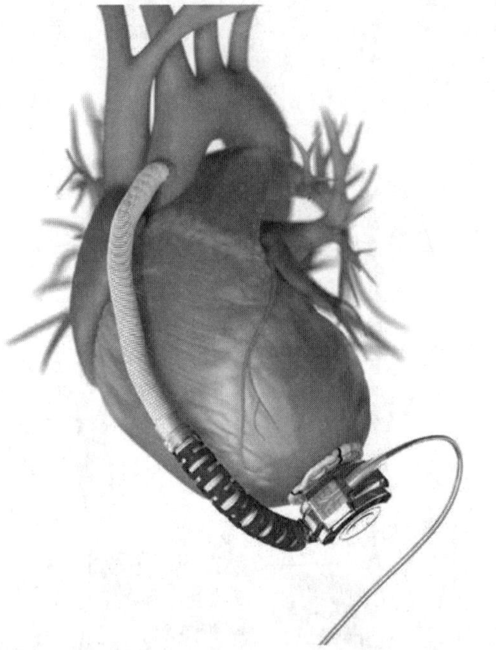

图 13.2 HeartWare HVAD（第三代）原位离心 LVAD。注意带有一体化流入套管的心包内泵。流出进入升主动脉（Image courtesy of HeartWare International, Inc., Miami Lakes FL.）

风险评估

主动脉内球囊泵

目前的球囊泵导管比早期版本更小，从而并发症明显减少，最显著的是血管损伤（主动脉夹层、假性动脉瘤、主动脉穿孔）。这些损伤在体表面积小的患者身上尤成问题，特别是在当导管型号的选择受限时。其他报道的并发症包括远心端或近心端动脉血栓（血小板性栓塞）、机械性梗阻、肢体缺血、感染、球囊漏气或破裂、截瘫、神经损伤、淋巴囊肿、导管错位、血小板减少症、出血和不适合的球囊 / 导管型号。目前的技术改善了 IABP 疗法的风险，同时精密的计算机算法提高了这种治疗方式的安全性。

心室辅助装置

风险评估对确定哪些患者将受益于 VAD 疗法非常重要。INTERMACS（机械辅助循环支持跨机构登记处）是一个选择性登记处，收集在美国、FDA 批准的需长期接受机械循环支持设备的患者的数据。这个登记处确定了患者的重要特征，并定出了启动机械支持的适当时间段（表 13.2）。其他风险评分已被用于评估 VAD 植入后的死亡风险和右心室衰竭风险。

短期 VAD

短期 VAD 对于即刻稳定的心肌梗死后心源性休克的患者有效，可采取介入或手术的方法置入。这些设备可用于可能是或不是长期 VAD 或移植候选患者的适当评估，以便这些资源能够合理分配。在心肌顿抑发生时，这些装置能让心脏从缺血性损伤中恢复时得到“休息”。

长期 VAD

非生理性的非搏动性血流的长期影响导致了在早期搏动泵中未见的一些事件，最常见的是动静脉畸形（arteriovenous malformation，AVM）引起的胃肠道出血。有趣的是，血管发育异常可见于有主动脉狭窄（Heyde 综合征）患者的小肠中，并且在瓣

表 13.2 INTERMACS（机械辅助循环支持机构间登记处）基于七个临床特征的 VAD 植入风险分级

分级 #	描述	定义	MCS 的时间
1	虚脱和烧灼感	严重的心源性休克	几小时内
2	进行性衰退	强心药依赖并持续恶化	几天内
3	稳定但依赖强心药	小至中等剂量的强心药注射可达到临床稳定（包括暂时依靠循环支持而未用强心药的稳定患者）	几周内
4	反复发作的重度心力衰竭	“复发性”而非“难治性”失代偿	几周到几月之间
5	劳动不耐受	休息可恢复	可变
6	劳动受限	能做一些轻体力活动；任何有意义的体力消耗的几分钟内就会疲劳	可变
7	进展型 NYHA Ⅲ	可做一些合理水平的舒适活动，尽管以前没有失代偿史	非 MCS 候选者

MCS，机械循环支持；NYHA，纽约心脏协会

Data from Kirklin JK, Naftel DC, Pagani FD, et al: The seventh INTERMACS annual report: 15,000 implants and counting. *J Heart Lung Transplant* 34（12）: 1495-1504, 2015.

膜置换后得以解决。这表明轴流泵的患者有相似的机制。在主动脉瓣狭窄患者和接受轴流泵支持的患者中观察到血液成分暴露在高剪切应力下，这会导致获得性血管性血友病，可通过去除主要来源的方式解决。HeartMate Ⅱ患者已被证实缺乏大型血管性血友病因子多聚体，取出装置后可恢复正常。

由于在 VAD 支持期间主动脉瓣叶连合处的融合，一些患者出现了新的主动脉瓣关闭不全。在人工瓣膜和生物瓣膜上均已出现了这种现象。如果主动脉反流量较大，这可能导致血液逆流入左心室并进入泵，导致无效的血流循环和总体前向心排血量的减少。

溶血通常是轴流的罕见后果，除非它和泵血栓形成有关。当泵功率输出增加和乳酸脱氢酶水平升高时，应怀疑溶血。

虽然报道的发生率变化很小，但是 VAD 支持能使少数特发性心肌病患者的心肌恢复（即逆向重塑），并脱离 VAD 支持。由于没有可靠的生物标志物，这种情况难以预测。机械支持期间已尝试了药理学干预，其目的是启动逆向重塑，逆转病理性肥大和恢复细胞代谢过程。在一项小型试点研究中，这些患者中的相当一部分可以不依赖泵。

使用 HeartMate Ⅱ和 HeartWare HVAD 时，泵入口处可产生高负压，这反过来可导致心室塌陷（也称为“抽吸事件”）。在使用 HeartWare HVAD 时，泵速超过 3200 rpm 会增加这种风险。低血容量、右心室衰竭、血管麻痹、心脏压塞和肺血管阻力升高会伴随抽吸事件的发生。可通过超声心动图和 HeartWare 转子上的泵流量波形来观察抽吸事件，通常显示流量低于基线。重要的是要了解泵速由操作者设定，不同于第一代 LVAD，其中充盈–排空（fill-to-empty）模式允许泵在达到阈值体积时弹出。非搏动泵是连续流动装置，并且转速不随生理需要而变化。因为这些泵是前负荷和后负荷依赖的，所以必须密切关注容量状态和血流动力学参数，特别是在植入后即刻的动态手术室环境。

启示

主动脉内球囊泵

球囊反搏具有许多独特的应用空间，但是它最大的用途是在冠心病重症监护室（coronary intensive care unit，CICU）和心脏手术室。在心脏手术室，当在 CPB 分离期，药理学支持不足以支持心排血量时，球囊反搏能改善心肌功能并利于患者脱机。

球囊反搏的净效应包括降低后负荷、增加冠状动脉血流、减少卒中、降低心率、减少壁肌张力、减少体循环阻力、降低 LVEDP、降低肺毛细血管楔压（pulmonary capillary wedge pressure，PCWP）和提高心脏整体性能。

心室辅助装置

在过去 20 年中，VAD 治疗在终末期心力衰竭和心源性休克治疗中的作用已经大大增加。适应证的范围也扩大了，包括以下内容：

- **移植的过渡**：根据最新的 INTERMACS 报告，在装置植入时，30% 的 VAD 接受者被列入心脏移植手术候选名单。当等待合适供体时间较长或血型和大小相容性成问题的情况下，推荐进行早期 VAD 治疗。
- **恢复期的过渡**：正如前文所述，相对少数的特发性心肌病患者在脱离设备前足以使心肌恢复。
- **决策期的过渡**：在患有多系统器官衰竭和难治性心源性休克的患者中，放置短期装置如 Impella、TandemHeart 或 ECMO 则须更加谨慎，因为若在植入长期设备前未使病情达到最佳化，这些患者的结局明显更差。
- **候选资格的过渡**：有 23% 的接受 VAD 植入的登记患者可能随后被列入移植手术名单。因肺动脉高压而不适合进行心脏移植手术的患者，VAD 支持能使肺血管阻力（pulmonary vascular resistance，PVR）下降，从而可进行移植手术。类似的，有 VAD 支持的心肺移植候选者可能会经历肺动脉高压逆转，其移植候选状态将变为仅进行心脏移植。
- **目标疗法（destination therapy，DT）**：2014 年 DT 中 VAD 植入物比例约为 46%。有限数量的供体心脏使得 DT 成为许多患者的可行选择。在某些情况下，因为症状和生活质量明显改善，相较等待移植的过渡治疗，患者更愿意选择 DT，因为他们倾向于避免另一种具有相关免疫抑制风险的重大外科手术。

DT 的作用意义深远，因为美国每年开展的心脏移植手术数量稳定在大约 2300 例。INTERMACS 数据库包括超过 15 000 名 VAD 患者，每年的植入物总量约为 2500 个。使用非搏动泵的 1 年和 2 年存活患者分别为 80% 和 70%。

重要的是，相当多的患者将继续需要接受非心脏手术以及 VAD 支持，包括针对消化道出血的内镜检查（发生率为 20%）、开腹手术、神经外科手术、牙科手术等。后一点强调了了解 VAD 技术的重要性，普通麻醉科医师将为大量这类患者提供照护。在许多中心，普通麻醉科医师为接受常规选择性外科手术的患者提供大部分照护，并与包括心脏外科医师、心力衰竭心脏病专家、VAD 专家 / 技师、灌注师和经过适当训练的护理人员在内的多学科团队合作。更复杂的病例通常交给心胸麻醉科医师。

管理与预防

主动脉内球囊泵

在管理 IABP 支持的患者时需要正确理解反搏原理。在开始反搏之前必须确定装置定位。如前所述，这可以通过胸部 X 线成像、透视或 TEE 来完成。球囊充气和放气将使动脉迹线具有特征性外观。球囊在重搏切迹处膨胀，在波形的收缩和舒张增强部分之间产生尖锐的“V”。相比无辅助的波形，心舒张末期的球囊放气导致低主动脉舒张期末压，以及更低的辅助收缩压。正常和不适时的 IABP 波形如表 13.3 所示。

IABP 充气的触发是指用于识别下个心动周期开始的信号，并包括心电图、中心主动脉压力波形、A 起搏、AV/V 起搏和内部模式。当前系统有触发和定时算法，能够响应心律变化并能自动评估和选择最佳触发源和 ECG 导联。反搏比例可以设置为 1∶1、1∶2 或 1∶3。后两种比例通常用于脱离支持装置。除非患者 IABP 充分肝素化（如 CPB 期间），放置入体内的 IABP 不应该停止工作；否则导管可能会形成血栓，并出现因栓塞而可能导致的破坏性后果。

原位 IABP 患者应监测以下缺血性并发症，包括

表 13.3 IABP 支持的时间问题

IABP 压力曲线	故障排除	结果
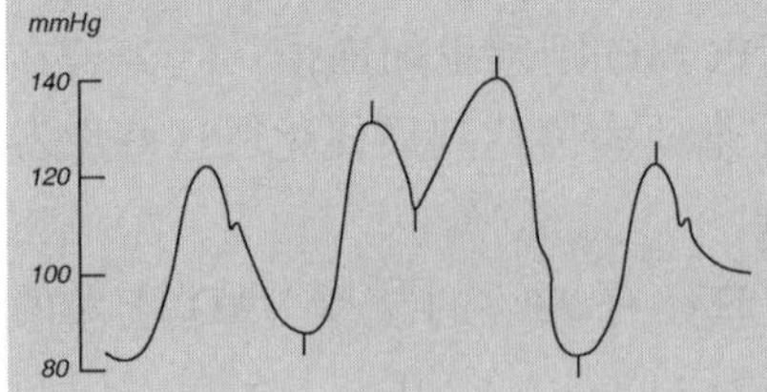	正常曲线：充气发生在舒张期之始（重搏切迹－主动脉瓣闭合）；尖锐的“V”被增强；放气发生在舒张末期；在心电图上，充气发生在 T 波（收缩末期）波峰附近，放气在 P-R 间期（舒张末期）	舒张期冠状动脉灌注增加，主动脉舒张末期压降低，减少后负荷，减少心肌耗氧量，减少心脏做功和增加心排血量
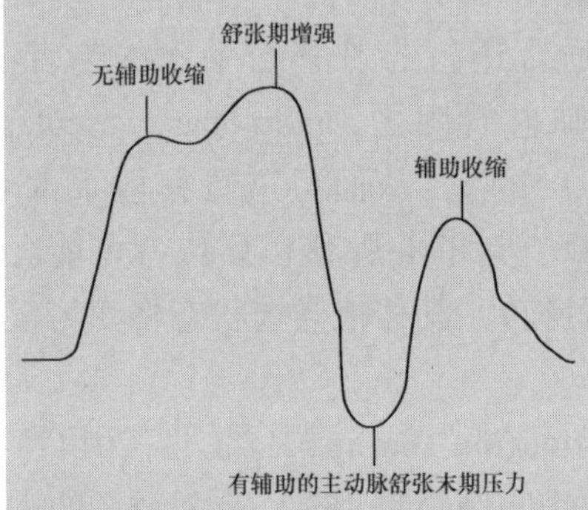	提早充气：充气发生在主动脉瓣膜关闭之前；舒张期增强波发生在收缩期左心室仍射血时	可导致 LVEDV、LVEDP 和 PCWP 的增加；增加后负荷和左心室室壁应力；增加心肌耗氧量；减少左心室射血；可能发生主动脉提前闭合，可能导致主动脉瓣关闭不全
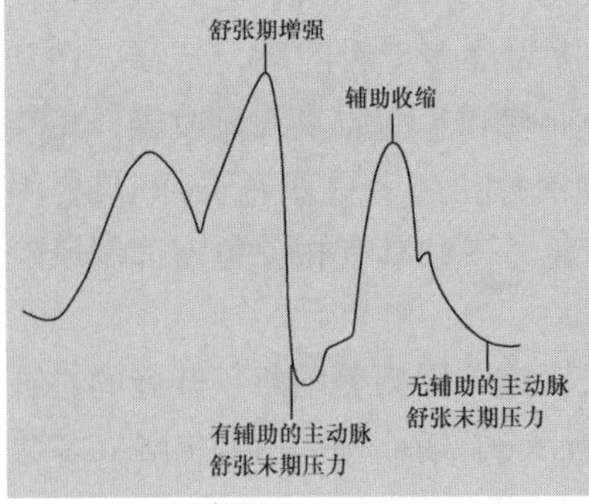	提早放气：舒张期过早发生放气会导致压力（+）在增强峰值后的急剧下降	冠状动脉灌注的舒张期增强未达最佳标准；舒张期波形的急剧下降可导致血流逆行（冠状动脉，颈动脉）；后负荷降低未达最佳；心肌耗氧量增加；有辅助的收缩压力可能增加

表 13.3 IABP 支持的时间问题

IABP 压力曲线	故障排除	结果
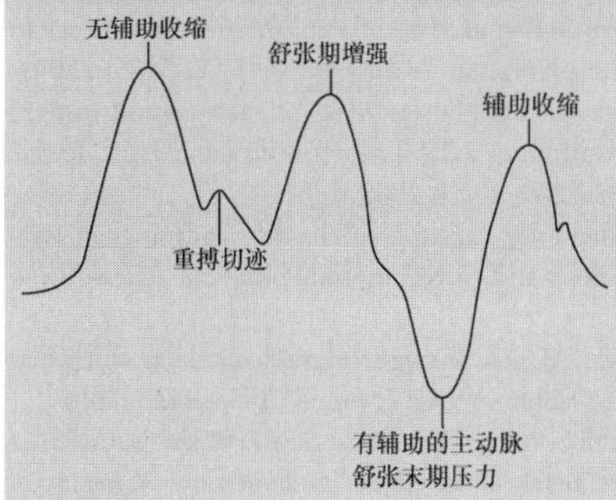	延迟充气：充气发生在主动脉瓣关闭后；舒张期增强的上升支发生在重搏切迹后（“W”形轨迹）	冠状动脉灌注的舒张期增强未最大化
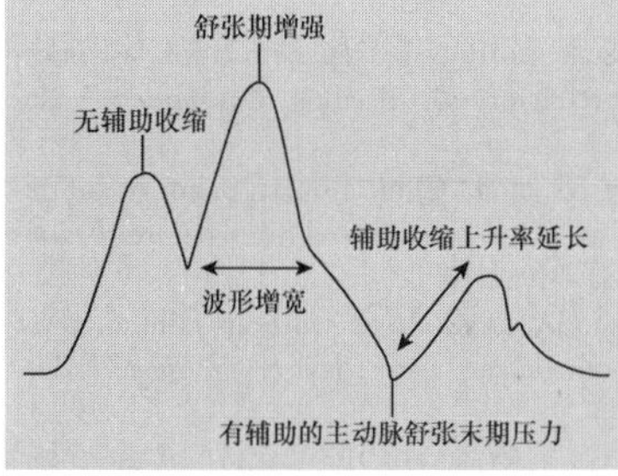	延迟放气：辅助收缩期压力上升率延长；变宽的舒张期增强波形	无后负荷减少（左心室射血以抵抗增大的后负荷）；心肌耗氧量增加；壁应变增加

压力曲线图像由 Maquet Cardiovascular，LLC，Wayne，NJ 提供

股鞘通路（肢体缺血、感染），血管损伤（夹层、假性动脉瘤），错位（每日胸部 X 线），出血和肝素诱导的血小板减少症（除非患者对肝素过敏和正在使用比卢伐定治疗）。插管技术的改进和更小导管和引导鞘的实用性（较早的导管尺寸范围在 10.5 ～ 12 Fr）使血管并发症的发生率显著降低——线性 7.5-Fr 导管可用于较小的患者。目前球囊大小在 25 ～ 50 ml。

一旦采取适当的干预措施来逆转患者心功能不全的原因，IABP 治疗就能脱机并终止。

心室辅助装置

如前所述，VAD 患者的围术期管理需要多学科团队合作。超声心动图对于 VAD 患者的实时管理必不可少，包括术中（对流入套管位置和流出植入物血流的评估，室间隔位置是否在中线，血流动力学和体积状态优化）和术后（泵速设置在合适的水平并可以进行斜坡速度测试）。

斜坡速度测试允许通过检查低端和高端范围来确定安全的操作泵速度。逐渐减速直到每次搏动时的动脉瓣开放，并且患者并未表现出可确定低端范围的心力衰竭的心电图证据。对高端范围确定，泵速逐渐增加直到主动脉瓣持续关闭，左心室舒张末期内径见效，脉压为 10 ～ 15 mmHg。通常设定的泵速出现于斜坡测试建立的低速到高速范围内。

超声心动图还允许在术后即时和之后进行故障排除。随着 LVAD 植入，许多问题早晚都会出现，包括血容量不足、心脏压塞、右心室衰竭、心律失常、低氧血症、肺栓塞和特定的机械相关问题（例如泵血栓形成、流入套管错位、流出套管扭曲）。

（黄　捷　译　王晓琳　校）

延伸阅读

Aaronson KD, Slaughter MS, Miller LW, et al.: Use of an intrapericardial, continuous-flow, centrifugal pump in patients awaiting heart transplantation, *Circulation* 125, 2012. 3191–3200.

Ambardekar AV, Buttrick PM: Reverse remodeling with left ventricular assist devices: a review of clinical, cellular, and molecular effects, *Circ Heart Fail* 4:224–233, 2011.

Aragon J, Lee MS, Kar S, Makkar RR: Percutaneous left ventricular assist device: “TandemHeart” for high-risk coronary intervention, *Cath Cardiovasc Intervent* 65:346–352, 2005.

Barbara DW, Wetzel DR, Pulido JN, et al.: The perioperative management of patients with left ventricular assist devices undergoing noncardiac surgery, *Mayo Clin Proc* 8:674–682, 2013.

Birks EJ, George RS, Hedger M, et al.: Reversal of severe heart failure with a continuous-flow left ventricular assist device and pharmacological therapy: a prospective study, *Circulation* 123:381–390, 2011.

Birks EJ, Tansley PD, Hardy J, et al.: Left ventricular assist device and drug therapy for the reversal of heart failure, *N Engl J Med* 355:1873–1884, 2006.

Capdeville M, Smedira NG: Mechanical circulatory assist: past and present, *Anesthesiol Clin* 31:321–353, 2013.

Cappell MS, Lebwohl O: Cessation of recurrent bleeding from gastrointestinal angiodysplasias after aortic valve replacement, *Ann Intern Med* 105:54–57, 1986.

Catena E, Milazzo F, Montorsi E, et al.: Left ventricular support by axial flow pump: the echocardiographic approach to device malfunction, *J Am Soc Echocardiogr* 18(1422):e7–e13, 2005.

Doi A, Marasco SF, McGiffin DC: Is a bioprosthetic valve in the aortic position desirable with a continuous flow LVAD? *J Card Surg* 30:466–468, 2015.

Estep JD, Stainback RF, Little SH, et al.: The role of echocardiography and other imaging modalities in patients with left ventricular assist devices, *J Am Coll Cardiol* 3:1049–1064, 2010.

Geisen U, Heilmann C, Beyersdorf F, et al.: Nonsurgical bleeding in patients with ventricular assist devices could be explained by acquired von Willebrand disease, *Eur J Cardiothorac Surg* 33:679–684, 2008.

Gregoric ID, Bruckner BA, Jacob L, et al.: Techniques and complications of TandemHeart ventricular assist device insertion during cardiac procedures, *ASAIO J* 55:251–254, 2009.

Heyde EC: Gastrointestinal bleeding in aortic stenosis [Letter to the editor], *N Engl J Med* 259:196, 1958.

Higgins J, Lamarche Y, Kaan A, et al.: Microaxial devices for ventricular failure: a multicenter, population-based experience, *Can J Cardiol* 27:725–730, 2011.

Holman WL, Pae WE, Teuteberg JJ, et al.: INTERMACS: Interval analysis of registry data, *J Am Coll Surg* 208:755–761, 2009.

Islam S, Cevik C, Madonna R, et al.: Left ventricular assist devices and gastrointestinal bleeding: a narrative review of case reports and case series, *Clin Cardiol* 36:190–200, 2013.

Kantrowitz A: Origins of intra-aortic balloon pumping, *Ann Thorac Surg* 50:672–674, 1990.

Kantrowitz A, Tjonneland S, Freed PS, et al.: Initial clinical experience with intra-aortic balloon pumping in cardiogenic shock, *JAMA* 203:135–140, 1968.

Kirklin JK, Naftel DC, Pagani FD, et al.: The seventh INTERMACS annual report: 15,000 implants and counting, *J Heart Lung Transplant* 34:1495–1504, 2015.

Klotz S, Danser AH, Burkhoff D: Impact of left ventricular assist device (LVAD) support on the cardiac reverse remodeling process, *Prog Biophys Mol Biol* 97:479–496, 2008.

Klovaite J, Gustafsson F, Mortensen SA, et al.: Severely impaired von Willebrand factor-dependent platelet aggregation in patients with a continuous-flow left ventricular assist device (HeartMate II), *J Am Coll Cardiol* 53:2162–2167, 2009.

Kutty RS, Parameshwar J, Lewis C, et al.: Use of centrifugal left ventricular assist device as a bridge to candidacy in severe heart failure with secondary pulmonary hypertension, *Eur J Cardiothorac Surg* 43:1237–1242, 2013.

Letsou GV, Shah N, Gergoric ID, et al.: Gastrointestinal bleeding from arteriovenous malformations in patients supported by the Jarvik 2000 axial flow left ventricular assist device, *J Heart Lung Transplant* 24:105–109, 2005.

Lietz K, Deng M, Morgan J, et al.: Selection of UNOS status 1A candidates for mechanical circulatory support as bridge-to-transplantation (BTT)—analysis of UNOS/OPTN 2000–2005, *J Heart Lung Transplant* 27(2S):S244, 2008.

Lietz K, Long JW, Kfoury AG, et al.: Outcomes of left ventricular assist device implantation as destination therapy in the post-REMATCH era: implications for patient selection, *Circulation* 116:497–505, 2007.

Mancini DM, Beniaminovitz A, Levin H, et al.: Low incidence of myocardial recovery after left ventricular device implantation in patients with chronic heart failure, *Circulation* 98:2383–2389, 1998.

Marasco SF, Lukas G, McDonald M, et al.: Review of ECMO (extra corporeal membrane oxygenation) support in critically ill adult patients, *Heart Lung Circ* 17(Suppl 4):S41–47, 2008.

Matthews JC, Koelling TM, Pagani FD, et al.: The right ventricular failure risk score: a preoperative tool for assessing the risk of right ventricular failure in left ventricular assist device candidates, *J Am Coll Cardiol* 51:2163–2172, 2008.

Meyer AL, Malehsa D, Bara C, et al.: Acquired von Willebrand syndrome in patients with an axial flow left ventricular assist device, *Circ Heart Fail* 3:675–681, 2010.

Miller LW, Pagani FD, Russell SD, et al.: Use of a continuous-flow device in patients awaiting heart transplantation, *N Engl J Med* 357:885–896, 2007.

Mudd JO, Cuda JD, Halushka M, et al.: Fusion of aortic valve commissures in patients supported by a continuous axial flow left ventricular assist device, *J Heart Lung Transplant* 27:1269–1274, 2008.

Pate GE, Mulligan A: An epidemiological study of Heyde's syndrome: an association between aortic stenosis and gastrointestinal bleeding, *J Heart Valve Dis* 13:713–716, 2004.

Rose EA, Gelijns AC, Moskowitz AJ, et al.: Long-term mechanical left ventricular assistance for end-stage heart failure, *N Engl J Med* 345:1435–1443, 2001.

Simon MA, Kormos RL, Murali S, et al.: Myocardial recovery using ventricular assist devices: prevalence, clinical characteristics, and outcomes, *Circulation* 112(Suppl 9):I32–36, 2005.

Singh P, Scoyni R, Pooran N, et al.: Aortic valve replacement: A last resort for aortic stenosis-associated refractory GI bleeding, *Gastrointest Endosc* 56:139–141, 2002.

Slaughter MS, Pagani FD, Rogers JG, et al.: Clinical management of continuous-flow left ventricular assist devices in advanced heart failure, *J Heart Lung Transplant* 29(Suppl 4):S1–39, 2010.

Slaughter MS, Rogers JG, Milano CA, et al.: Advanced heart failure treated with continuous-flow left ventricular assist device, *N Engl J Med* 361:2241–2251, 2009.

Stehlik J, Edwards LB, Kucheryavaya AY, et al.: The Registry of the International Society for Heart and Lung Transplantation: twenty-seventh official adult heart transplant report—2010, *J Heart Lung Transplant* 29:1089–1103, 2010.

Stern DR, Kazam J, Edwards P, et al.: Increased incidence of gastrointestinal bleeding following implantation of the HeartMate II LVAD, *J Card Surg* 25:352–356, 2010.

Stevenson LW, Pagani FD, Young JB, et al.: INTERMACS profiles of advanced heart failure: the current picture, *J Heart Lung Transplant* 28:535–541, 2009.

Stone M, Hinchey J, Sattler C, Evans A: Trends in the management of patients with left ventricular assist devices presenting for noncardiac surgery: a 10-year institutional experience, *Semin Cardiothorac Vasc Anesth* 20:197–204, 2016.

Teuteberg JJ, Ewald GA, Adamson RM, et al.: Risk assessment for continuous flow left ventricular assist devices: does the destination therapy risk score work? An analysis of over 1000 patients, *J Am Coll Cardiol* 60:44–51, 2012.

Thiele H, Smalling RW, Schuler GC: Percutaneous left ventricular assist devices in acute myocardial infarction complicated by cardiogenic shock, *Eur Heart J* 28:2057–2063, 2007.

Topilsky Y, Maltais S, Oh JK, et al.: Focused review on transthoracic echocardiographic assessment of patients with continuous axial flow left ventricular assist devices, *Cardiol Res Pract* 187434:2011, 2011.

Webb CAJ, Weyker PD, Flynn BC: Management of intra-aortic balloon pumps, *Semin Cardiothorac Vasc Anesth* 19:106–121, 2015.

Zimpfer D, Zrunek P, Roethy W, et al.: Left ventricular assist devices decrease fixed pulmonary hypertension in cardiac transplant candidates, *J Thorac Cardiovasc Surg* 133:689–695, 2007.

For further general and technical information about the IABP, refer to the Maquet Cardiovascular (formerly DataScope) website where a number of educational materials can be downloaded: http://ca.maquet.com/clinician-information/educational-materials/.

肌无力病

第 14 章

Mohamed Naguib

病例概要

患者，女性，22 岁，身高 154 cm，体重 44.2 kg，4 个月前表现为重症肌无力和轻度全身乏力（美国重症肌无力协会分级Ⅱ A 级）。该患者静脉注射依酚氯铵后病情迅速好转，并且乙酰胆碱受体抗体阳性（12.3 nmol/L；参考值 <0.25 nmol/L），因此其病情得到确诊。神经传导和肌电图检查正常，但是重复神经电刺激显示了肌肉动作电位的逐渐减弱。磁共振成像发现胸腺异常。患者拟行经胸骨胸腺切除术。术前口服溴吡斯的明 60 mg，一日三次，同时进行血浆置换。术前肺功能检查结果如下：用力肺活量（forced vital capacity，FVC）2.79 L/s（预计值的 79%）；50%FVC 时最大呼气流量为 3.2 L/s（预计值的 68%）；25% ～ 75% FVC 时呼气中段流速为 3.03 L/s（预计值的 77%）。芬太尼和丙泊酚诱导麻醉，胸段硬膜外阻滞复合输注丙泊酚和吸入 70% N_2O+30% O_2 维持麻醉。未使用神经肌肉阻断剂情况下在气管表面麻醉下行气管插管（4% 利多卡因 4 ml）。术后维持机械通气 12 h。

问题解析

定义

神经肌肉传导的可塑性依赖于以下机制的协同作用：①神经肌肉接头处突触前运动神经末梢乙酰胆碱的合成、贮存和释放；②乙酰胆碱与肌膜突触后膜烟碱受体结合产生动作电位；③突触间隙乙酰胆碱酯酶快速水解乙酰胆碱。

神经肌肉接头处的突触前膜、突触间隙或突触后膜的自身免疫性或遗传缺陷可能导致神经肌肉传导失败，并最终导致各种肌无力症状（图 14.1）。呈波动性的肌肉无力和易疲劳性是肌无力症的主要特征。一般来说肌无力症只影响运动系统，感觉和自主神经功能并未累及。Lambert-Eaton 综合征（Lambert-Eaton syndrome）是个例外，Lambert-Eaton 综合征是一种肌无力综合征，其中相当一小部分患者患有自主神经功能障碍。肌无力症可分为三大类：重症肌无力、先天性肌无力综合征和兰伯特-伊顿肌无力综合征（表 14.1、14.2）。

认知、风险评估和启示

重症肌无力

重症肌无力（myasthenia gravis，MG）是最常见的以肌肉无力和易疲劳为特征的肌无力症。MG 是一种 B 细胞介导的自身免疫性疾病，每年发病率为（0.25 ～ 0.5）/100 000，患病率为 5/100 000。成年患者中，女性与男性患者的比例为 3∶2。在老年患者中，男性的发病率高于女性。大约 80% ～ 85% 的 MG 患者存在抗 α 亚基 -N 乙酰胆碱受体抗体。这种抗体应答是 T 细胞依赖性的，因为调节 T 细胞（Tregs）和 $CD4^+$ T 细胞在主要组织相容性复合体Ⅱ类分子的存在下识别乙酰胆碱受体表位，并对细胞发挥辅助作用以产生抗体。在剩下的 15% ～ 20% 的患者（称为血清反应阴性患者），烟碱样乙酰胆碱受体抗体无法检测到。这些血清反应阴性的患者中大多数具有肌肉特异性受体酪氨酸激酶（muscle-specific receptor tyrosine kinase，MuSK）、脂蛋白相关蛋白 4（lipoprotein-related protein 4，LRP4）或凝集素的抗体。这些抗体不存在于血清反应阳性的患

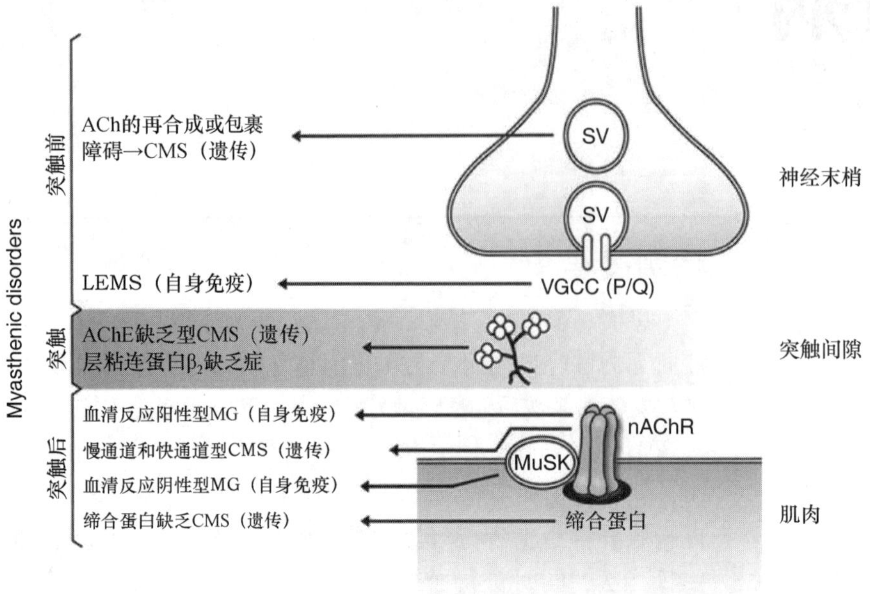

图 14.1 肌无力症。ACh，乙酰胆碱；CMS，先天性肌无力综合征；LEMS，Lambert-Eaton 肌无力综合征；MG，重症肌无力；MuSK，肌肉特异性受体酪氨酸激酶；nAChR，烟碱样乙酰胆碱受体；SV，突触小泡；VGCC（P/Q），电压门控钙离子通道（P/Q 型）

表 14.1 肌无力症

部位	疾病	分类	病因	细胞学形态	临床特点	治疗
突触前	Lambert-Eaton 肌无力综合征	自身免疫性疾病	针对运动神经末鞘电压门控钙离子通道和其他突触前成分（突触结合蛋白）的抗体，导致 ACh 释放减少	正常的 ACh 成分和 NMJ 结构	大约 60% 的患者有副瘤反应，常伴有小细胞肺癌，乏力与易疲劳	对恶性肿瘤的成功治疗可使症状明显改善 3,4- 二氨基吡啶阻断突触前钾离子通道，能够①减少钾外流，②增加动作电位时程，③延长电压门控 Ca^{2+} 通道的激活，④增加细胞内 Ca^{2+} 储存和 ACh 释放 溴吡斯的明增加 3,4- 二氨基吡啶的作用 通常，血浆置换或静脉给予免疫球蛋白可短期改善症状
	乙酰胆碱转移酯酶缺乏	遗传性疾病	乙酰胆碱转移酯酶突变导致乙酰胆碱再合成不足	nAChR 数量和终板结构正常	常染色体隐性遗传 典型的呼吸暂停发作伴随肌无力症	乙酰胆碱酯酶抑制剂
突触	AChE 缺乏	遗传性疾病	突触间隙中编码的 AChE 酶胶原末端亚基的基因突变降低了酶的表达或催化效果	AChE 活性缺失或降低（组织化学染色） nAChR 继发性消失以及突触后区域降解	常染色体隐性遗传，表型多变 常见中重度全身乏力和脊柱侧弯，合并限制性肺疾病	由于乙酰胆碱酯酶缺乏，患者不能从抗胆碱酯酶治疗中获益
	层粘连蛋白 β_2 缺乏	遗传性疾病	突变基因编码层粘连蛋白 β_2 亚基	神经末梢未成熟、再生不良，仍被 Schwann 细胞全程包裹突触后皱褶简化，终板乙酰胆碱酯酶完好	常染色体隐性遗传	麻黄碱和沙丁胺醇（而不是溴吡斯的明）可能改善神经肌肉接头的信号传递，其机制尚未阐明

表 14.1 肌无力症

部位	疾病	分类	病因	细胞学形态	临床特点	治疗
突触后	重症肌无力：血清阳性型或血清阴性型	自身免疫性疾病	抗 nAChR 抗体 抗 MuSK 抗体	终板区域皱褶更小，结构简化，nAChR 显著降低（约为正常 NMJ 的 30%）	抗 MuSK 抗体阳性患者出现肌无力症状的年龄相对较早 抗 MuSK 抗体阳性患者症状多累及颈部肌肉，抗 MuSK 抗体阴性患者症状多累及四肢肌肉	术前行血浆置换和连续的溴吡斯的明治疗改善病情 患者对 NDMR 非常敏感 对 SCh 和米库溴胺的反应依赖于丁酰胆碱酯酶的活性，这种酶的活性在血浆置换或使用溴吡斯的明后会降低
	nAChR 或结合蛋白表达减少	遗传性疾病	nAChR 或结合蛋白的突变可减少 nAChR 的表达	终板区域的变化与自身免疫性 MG 相似	常染色体隐性遗传 患者从出生时或婴儿期就表现出肌无力症状 面部畸形是结合蛋白缺乏症的常见表现	抗胆碱酯酶作用不完全 联合 3,4- 二氨基吡啶治疗有益（增加 ACh 释放）
	先天性肌无力综合征慢通道型	遗传性疾病	nAChR 的动力缺陷和（或）获得性功能突变导致 nAChR 开放时间过长，突触后退行性变使 Ca^{2+} 内流过多	突触后蜕化伴 nAChR 缺失；AChE 正常	通常为显性遗传 颈部、肩胛部和指伸肌选择性乏力；其他肌肉也出现不明确的乏力	通道开放阻滞剂（奎尼丁、氟西汀）使慢通道突变型开放时限正常 AChE 药无效 避免使用 SCh，因为它会加重兴奋毒性
	先天性肌无力综合征快通道型	遗传性疾病	nAChR 的突变显著降低了结合力，导致乙酰胆碱从结合位点迅速游离，通道开放率降低，通道关闭率增高	NMJ 结构正常 nAChRs 的浓度正常或降低	常染色体隐性遗传 出生到婴儿期症状中度 对乙酰胆碱酯酶抑制剂部分反应	3,4- 二氨基吡啶和 AChE 联合治疗

ACh，乙酰胆碱；AChE，乙酰胆碱酯酶；MG，重症肌无力；MuSK，肌肉特异性受体酪氨酸激酶；nAChR，烟碱样乙酰胆碱受体；NDMR，非去极化肌松药；NMJ，神经肌肉接头；SCh，琥珀胆碱

者中。在突触形成和发育过程中 MUSK 介导了由凝集素诱导的烟碱样乙酰胆碱受体的聚集，并在成熟的神经肌肉接头处表达。

突触后烟碱样乙酰胆碱受体的缺失会降低乙酰胆碱释放后突触后膜的兴奋性，从而导致疲劳性肌无力。为了维持突触的适应性，实际上释放的乙酰胆碱比正常的神经肌肉接头处释放的乙酰胆碱要多，用以补充 MG 中突触后乙酰胆碱受体的减少；然而，这种代偿性内稳态机制不足以恢复或维持正常的神经肌肉功能。

MG 的免疫应答触发机制尚不清楚。大约 70% 的 MG 患者胸腺淋巴滤泡生发中心增生，产生抗烟碱样乙酰胆碱受体抗体。少数 MG 患者作为副瘤综合征的一部分产生自身抗体（12% 的 MG 患者患有胸腺瘤）。有研究显示，抗烟碱样乙酰胆碱受体的抗体在胸腺以外的地方产生，因为胸腺切除术无法治愈 MG，也不能预防 MG 的发生。也有证据表明，对微生物抗原的应答产生的抗体也可能在某些患者中触发 MG。抗风湿性药物 D- 青霉胺可逆转 MG 的进程。

MG 可以发生在任何年龄。大部分患者的眼外肌肉和延髓控制的肌肉最先受到影响，导致上睑下垂、复视、吞咽困难和呼吸衰竭。随着病情的发展，颈部和骨骼肌肌无力变得明显。已有证据表明在 MG 大鼠模型中，大鼠的横膈膜功能受损。血清阳性和血清阴性患者的临床特征非常相似。肌无力母亲的新生儿会发生新生儿一过性 MG。在 MG 母亲

表 14.2 肌无力病的鉴别诊断

	重症肌无力	Lambert-Eaton 肌无力综合征	先天性肌无力综合征
病因	抗 nAChR 或抗 MuSK 的自身抗体	抗突触前电压门控（P/Q）Ca^{2+} 通道的自身抗体或抗突触结合蛋白抗体	突触前、突触或突触后蛋白的基因突变 显性或隐性遗传（无抗 nAChR、MuSK 或 P/Q 型 Ca^{2+} 通道抗体）
并发症	70% MG 患者出现胸腺淋巴滤泡增生 12% MG 患者患有胸腺瘤（副肿瘤性自身免疫反应） 相关的自身免疫性疾病包括甲状腺功能亢进、系统性红斑狼疮、类风湿关节炎和恶性贫血	60% 的 LEMS 患者有副瘤性自身免疫反应 小细胞肺癌表达电压敏感性 Ca^{2+} 通道；这些通道的抗肿瘤抗体与 NMJ 突触前电压门控 Ca^{2+} 通道发生交叉反应，减少 ACh 的释放	
发病部位	突触后	突触前	NMJ 的突触前、突触或突触后
自主神经功能障碍	无	出现在约 30% 的患者中（口干、阳痿）	无
改善肌力	休息后	运动后	休息后
抗体传递	从肌无力的母亲传递到胎儿，引起新生儿 MG 给健康的动物注射 MG IgG 会引起 MG 的症状	LEMS 患者 IgG 可阻断 Ca^{2+} 通道，抑制肌肉收缩	无抗体
肌电图检查（对 30 ～ 50 Hz 刺激的应答）	逐渐消失	易化	逐渐消失
血浆置换的效果	短暂	短暂	无效
抗胆碱酯酶药	有效控制症状	治疗价值小	治疗价值小
对 3,4- 二氨基吡啶的反应	无效	症状明显改善	对快通道型先天性肌无力综合征有效
对琥珀胆碱反应	耐药	敏感	多变，不推荐，因为在慢通道型突变中出现潜在的高钾反应
对非去极化神经肌肉阻断剂的反应	敏感	敏感	敏感

ACh，乙酰胆碱；IgG，免疫球蛋白 G；LEMS，Lambert-Eaton 综合征；MG，重症肌无力；MuSK，肌肉特异性受体酪氨酸激酶；nAChR，烟碱样乙酰胆碱受体；NMJ，神经肌肉接头

生育的新生儿中，大约 10% ～ 25% 的抗 Ach 受体的抗体或免疫细胞通过胎盘，导致新生儿神经肌肉传递的短暂受损。

Osserman 和 Genkins 提出 MG 的临床分型如下：Ⅰ型（只有眼部症状和体征），Ⅱ型（轻度全身乏力），Ⅲ型（中度全身乏力，伴或不伴有眼球受累），以及Ⅳ型（重度全身乏力，伴或不伴有眼球受累）。然而，Osserman 分类有一些局限性。例如，描述性术语用辞不明确，很难明确区分不同的分型。美国 MG 协会（Myasthenia Gravis Foundation of America，MGFA）的一个工作组制定了一种新的分类方法，可以更好地区分不同的类别（框 14.1）。

MG 是一个临床诊断。通常运动诱发的无力能为诊断提供强有力的依据，但是可能出现假阴性。静脉注射依酚氯铵（腾喜龙）后肌力的改善有助于确定 MG 的诊断。注射 1 ～ 2 mg 试验剂量后，静脉注射总剂量为 10 mg 的依酚氯铵。观察 5 min 内是否出现阳性结果。值得注意的是，依酚氯铵试验的

框 14.1 美国重症肌无力协会分级方法

Ⅰ型

任意眼部肌肉乏力；可能发生闭眼无力。其他肌肉功能都是正常的。

Ⅱ型

眼肌以外的肌肉轻度乏力；也可能出现严重的眼部肌肉乏力。

Ⅱa：主要影响四肢肌肉、躯干肌，或两者兼影响。也可能较少涉及口咽部肌肉。

Ⅱb：主要影响口咽部、呼吸肌，或两者兼影响。也可能较少或同样影响四肢肌肉、躯干肌，或两者兼影响。

Ⅲ型

眼肌以外的肌肉中度乏力；也可能出现严重的眼部肌肉乏力。

Ⅲa：主要影响四肢肌肉、躯干肌，或两者兼影响。也可能较少涉及口咽部肌肉。

Ⅲb：主要影响口咽部、呼吸肌，或两者兼影响。也可能较少或同样影响四肢肌肉、躯干肌，或两者兼影响。

Ⅳ型

眼肌以外的肌肉重度乏力；也可能出现严重的眼部肌肉乏力。

Ⅳa：主要影响四肢肌肉、躯干肌，或两者兼影响。也可能较少涉及口咽部肌肉。

Ⅳb：主要影响口咽部、呼吸肌，或两者兼影响。也可能较少或同样影响四肢肌肉、躯干肌，或两者兼影响。在不经气管插管的情况下使用鼻导管。

Ⅴ型

无论是否使用机械通气，定义为气管插管，但常规术后管理除外。

结果是非特异性的，在其他神经肌肉疾病中也可见。在依酚氯铵阳性患者血清中通常可检测到抗烟碱样乙酰胆碱受体抗体。电生理测试可用于直接评估肌肉功能，其目的在于通过对运动神经重复刺激诱发复合肌肉动作电位的递减反应。计算机断层扫描或磁共振成像可识别胸腺异常或检查出胸腺瘤。

MG 没有特异性的治疗方法。抗胆碱酯酶类药物（如溴吡斯的明和新斯的明）只能通过阻止突触间隙乙酰胆碱的降解来控制症状。其副作用包括过量的胆碱能刺激症状，如气道分泌物增加、肠蠕动增加、心动过缓，甚至无力加重、假性肌无力危象。免疫抑制剂可以通过抑制自身抗体的产生来帮助增强肌力，但它们的使用与许多潜在的不良反应有关。一些 Cochrane 的综述支持使用皮质类固醇激素，也有人提出环孢素、环磷酰胺和硫唑嘌呤改善 MG，然而其证据有限。

血浆置换和静脉注射免疫球蛋白（intravenous immunoglobulin，IVIG）可有效治疗肌无力危象和优化患者术前的状态。血浆置换与低血压或使用抗凝药物引起出血的风险有关。来自随机对照试验的有限证据表明，皮质类固醇与硫唑嘌呤或 IVIG 之间在疗效上没有任何差异。

类固醇和免疫抑制剂的非特异性免疫抑制及血浆置换常与胸腺切除术合用。胸腺切除术是年轻患者和胸腺瘤患者的标准治疗方法。胸腺切除术可改善无胸腺瘤患者的症状，并已在 50% 的病例中被证实与病程缓解有关。

先天性肌无力综合征

先天性肌无力综合征（congenital myasthenic syndrome，CMS）是一种罕见的异质性疾病，它并非由自身抗体引起，而是由突触小泡、乙酰胆碱酯酶或 N 乙酰胆碱受体的遗传突变所致，可导致乙酰胆碱反应增加（功能激活）或减弱（功能丧失）。突触后 CMS 最常见的类型是慢通道综合征。CMS 的遗传方式有常染色体显性遗传和隐性遗传。新生儿 MG 发病原因是由 MG 母亲向胎儿被动转移抗体所引起，而 CMS 患儿的母亲并未患有肌无力。CMS 的发病年龄通常在 2 岁之前。与自身免疫 MG 相比，免疫抑制和血浆置换治疗 CMS 无效，因为抗体在其发病机制中没有发挥作用。

在 MG 和 CMS 的患者中，肌电图以对重复刺激应答逐渐减弱和记录到单纤维阻滞为特点。然而，慢通道 CMS 患者在单次高频刺激下，也会出现典型的重复放电应答，即所谓的双重反应。

Lambert-Eaton 肌无力综合征

Lambert-Eaton 肌无力综合征（Lambert-Eaton myasthenic syndrome，LEMS）是由针对突触前 P/Q 电压门控钙通道的自身抗体作为目标的一种后天获得性疾病，可能还有另一种突触前成分（突触结合蛋白）的参与导致乙酰胆碱释放的减少。突触结合蛋白是一种胞外钙离子传感器，在突触小泡融合和乙酰胆碱的快速释放中发挥重要作用。在 85% 的 LEMS（血清阳性）患者中检测到抗 P/Q 型电压门控钙通道抗体。部分血清阴性的 LEMS 患者血清中存在抗突触结合蛋白抗体。在大约 60% 的 LEMS 患者中，该综合征是一种副瘤性疾病，通常与小细胞肺癌有关。在不伴有恶性肿瘤的患者中，LEMS 是一种自身免疫性疾病。LEMS 的特点是下肢和上肢近端肌无力、易疲劳和自主神经功能紊乱。延髓或呼吸肌的损害在 LEMS 患者中并不常见。

在 LEMS 患者中，肌电图通常显示低频复合肌肉动作电位与慢速刺激（2 Hz）的消退相关。在增加运动量或高频率重复刺激（30 ～ 50 Hz）后可出现促进反应。

管理与预防

胸腺切除术是一种择期手术，应在患者的病情改善后进行。MG 患者术前评估和准备应包括以下内容：①患者神经病病史回顾及神经系统检查；②术前药物治疗（如溴吡斯的明、免疫抑制剂）；③延髓症状或体征的评估，如吞咽困难、构音障碍或口咽无力（因为延髓受累的患者术后发生呼吸系统并发症的风险增加）；④检查是否存在其他自身免疫性疾病，如糖尿病、甲状腺疾病、系统性红斑狼疮、类风湿关节炎等；⑤肺功能测试的评估，包括通气-容量循环，有助于预测术后是否需要机械通气；⑥术前血浆置换或大剂量 IVIG 优化患者病情。术前继续使用溴吡斯的明治疗。

由于烟碱样乙酰胆碱受体数量的减少，肌无力患者一般对琥珀胆碱具有耐药性。然而，肌无力患者通过术前行血浆置换或服用溴吡斯的明，丁酰胆碱酯酶（血浆胆碱酯酶）活性可能会降低，这可能会导致琥珀胆碱的作用增强。在最后的分析中，当给 MG 患者使用琥珀胆碱（或米库溴铵）时，应考虑这些因素（对琥珀胆碱的抵抗与丁酰胆碱酯酶活性的降低）之间的相互作用。由于它会加重兴奋毒性慢通道，CMS 患者应避免使用琥珀胆碱。

由于突触后烟碱样乙酰胆碱受体的显著缺失，MG 患者对非去极化神经肌肉阻滞剂极其敏感。然而非去极化神经肌肉阻滞剂并不属于这些患者的使用禁忌。通过严格的滴定法及对神经肌肉功能的充分监测，非去极化药物已被安全地用于接受胸腺切除术的肌无力患者。这些患者应避免使用长效神经肌肉阻滞剂。中效的药物是更好的选择。应先将大约 1/5 的 ED_{95} 中效神经肌肉阻滞剂作为测试剂量。这有助于在定量神经肌肉监测仪的指导下估计患者的药物需要量。肌无力患者对非去极化神经肌肉阻滞剂的敏感性通常表现出明显的不同。

在肌无力患者中，拮抗术后残留阻滞剂可能无效，因为长期溴吡斯的明治疗已导致乙酰胆碱酯酶抑制作用的出现。因此，建议在维持支持性机械通气的同时，术后使患者肌松自行恢复。

肌无力患者已使用了不同的麻醉方法。虽然在不使用神经肌肉阻滞剂的情况下，仅使用强效吸入麻醉药也可提供术中肌松，但由于吸入麻醉药对神经肌肉传导的影响，这种方法可能与麻醉恢复时间延长有关。因此，使用小剂量中效非去极化神经肌肉阻滞剂辅助气管插管可能比使用深度吸入麻醉药更安全。全静脉注射丙泊酚-阿片类药物麻醉是吸入性麻醉的一种合适的替代方法。

胸部硬膜外麻醉与全身平衡麻醉相结合，在经胸骨胸腺切除术术中和术后均能提供良好的镇痛效果。区域阻滞麻醉也被成功地应用于患有 MG 产妇的分娩镇痛。然而，已知局麻药可增强神经肌肉阻滞的作用，如果溴吡斯的明治疗导致丁酰胆碱酯酶活性降低，酯类局麻药的代谢可能受到影响。

LEMS 患者对去极化和非去极化神经肌肉阻滞剂敏感。在 LEMS 患者中，新斯的明对残留的神经肌肉阻滞剂无拮抗作用。术后应继续口服 3,4- 二氨基吡啶。

所有肌无力患者术后应在外科重症监护病房密切监测神经肌无力症状。术后乏力的肌无力患者的鉴别诊断包括神经肌肉阻滞剂或麻醉药物残余的影响，干扰神经肌肉传导的药物（如氨基糖苷类抗生素、苯妥英钠、β 受体阻滞剂、奎尼丁，和锂剂）和肌无力以及胆碱能的危象。

（张 平 译 姚 滢 校）

延伸阅读

Abel M, Eisenkraft JB: Anesthetic implications of myasthenia gravis, *Mt Sinai J Med* 69:31–37, 2002.

Baraka A: Onset of neuromuscular block in myasthenic patients, *Br J Anaesth* 69:227–228, 1992.

Barohn RJ: Standards of measurements in myasthenia gravis, *Ann New York Acad Sci* 998:432–439, 2003.

Drachman DB: Myasthenia gravis, *N Engl J Med* 330:1797–1810, 1994.

Engel AG, Ohno K, Sine SM: Congenital myasthenic syndromes: progress over the past decade, *Muscle Nerve* 27:4–25, 2003.

Gajdos P, Chevret S, Toyka K: Plasma exchange for myasthenia gravis, *Cochrane Database Syst Rev*, 2002. CD002275.

Gilhus NE, Verschuuren JJ: Myasthenia gravis: subgroup classification and therapeutic strategies, *Lancet Neurol* 14:1023–1036, 2015.

Leveque C, Hoshino T, David P, et al.: The synaptic vesicle protein synaptotagmin associates with calcium channels and is a putative Lambert-Eaton myasthenic syndrome antigen, *Proc Natl Acad Sci USA* 89:3625–3629, 1992.

Lindstrom JM: Acetylcholine receptors and myasthenia, *Muscle Nerve* 23:453–477, 2000.

Naguib M, el Dawlatly AA, Ashour M, et al.: Multivariate determinants of the need for postoperative ventilation in myasthenia gravis, *Can J Anaesth* 43:1006–1013, 1996.

Naguib M, Flood P, McArdle JJ, et al.: Advances in neurobiology of the neuromuscular junction: implications for the anesthesiologist, *Anesthesiology* 96:202–231, 2002.

Takamori M, Maruta T, Komai K: Lambert-Eaton myasthenic syndrome as an autoimmune calcium-channelopathy, *Neurosci Res* 36:183–191, 2000.

Vincent A: Unravelling the pathogenesis of myasthenia gravis, *Nat Rev Immunol* 2:797–804, 2002.

Vincent A, Palace J, Hilton-Jones D: Myasthenia gravis, *Lancet* 357:2122–2128, 2001.

Whitney KD, McNamara JO: Autoimmunity and neurological disease: antibody modulation of synaptic transmission, *Annu Rev Neurosci* 22:175–195, 1999.

第15章 患者要求保密

Gail A. Van Norman

病例概要

一位医生的丈夫因左肾可疑病变在其医院行肾部分切除术。术后发生了发热和急性肾衰竭的并发症。麻醉科医师某次值夜班时，好奇朋友丈夫的病情，进入了该患者的电子病历系统。浏览该病历时，她发现该患者检测出人类免疫缺陷病毒（HIV）阳性，并要求不要告知他妻子，因为他“没做好告知妻子的准备”。这位麻醉科医师想告诉自己的朋友她丈夫的HIV检测结果。

问题分析

定义

为患者保密是医疗专业的基础。多个版本的《希波拉底誓言》明确解释为患者保密是一种道德义务，保密义务不仅限于对患者健康问题保密，还包括“不论我在行医中看到或听到了什么（即使未被发现），不论我不小心知道了什么”都要保密。换句话说，患者治疗期间的任何信息，医生都有义务为患者保密。虽然这是最基本的义务，医生通常不清楚什么是违反保密义务的行为。在一项研究中，500多位瑞士医生对7个案例进行判断，属于“重要”或“严重”违反患者保密行为，很多医生无法做出正确决断。有20年以上临床经验、接受过伦理教育、女性医生似乎更能准确地辨认违反患者保密行为。另一项研究中，71%的医生认为他们会将患者HIV阳性的病情告知外科同事，即使患者要求保密。

保密对维护医患关系的信任度至关重要。这种关系必然包括敏感信息的公开，一旦公开，患者可能因被歧视、失去社会地位及就业机会、人际关系受累、失去社会福利而受到伤害。患者就医时，是否愿意坦率地告知医生对疾病诊断和治疗至关重要的个人史或其他信息取决于患者对医生会为他完全保密的信任。通常，在保密方面三种职业受到法律保护——律师、牧师和医生，因为他们在履行义务时特殊的“社会契约”具有保密的关键性质。

保密职责禁止医生在患者未授权时泄露患者的医疗信息，广义上包括了对患者隐私权的尊重。伦理和法律均要求医务人员注意保护患者未授权的诸类信息。如，医务人员不可将患者病历放置在公众场所，不可在公众电脑中留置打开的患者电子病历。患者的医疗信息是其医疗团队所有医生共享的，团队内所有医生都有义务对患者的信息向其他无合法理由的人保密。除了一些特殊情况，医生无权获取未与其建立医患关系的患者的信息。

一般来说，如果患者没有明确允许公开信息，医生不得公开其信息，即使是对患者配偶或其他家属，要由患者自行决定。该规定存在一些特例。

警告义务

倘若患者的医疗信息或**在诊治时患者向医生主诉的任何信息**对患者配偶、家属或任意第三方可造成直接伤害，此时医生可不履行保密义务。在某些情况下，法律要求医生不得履行保密义务。

经典案例是加利福尼亚大学Tarasoff案。1969年，伯克利大学的研究生Prosinjit Podder在和Tarasoff女士几次约会后深深地迷上了她。当她断然拒绝和他继续交往，他极度抑郁并在治疗过程中向自己的心理医生Moore医生坦白了他想要杀死Tarasoff女士的意图。Moore发现这些威胁可信，于是通知了校园警察，这过程中他违背了为患者保密义务。校园警察认为Podder对Tarasoff不存在实际威胁并选择不拘留他。Podder的医生和警察都没有把Podder的威胁告知Tarasoff或她的家人，随后Podder谋杀了她。Podder被定罪并最终被驱逐出境，回到印度。随后，Tarasoff的父母向法院提出了诉讼，认为学校有提醒或保护受害者义务而不是履行为患者（Podder）保密的义务。在此案件中法院认为Moore对患者保密协议的违反程度**不充分**。只是报告和（或）调查威胁是不够的。陪审团裁定应将特定威胁告知潜在被害人和其家属以便其采取措施进行自我保护。

由于Tarasoff案，许多州颁布了“警告义务”的立法纲要。截至2014年，23个州针对医务人员采取了“警告义务”的立法，10个州的普通立法提及此义务并得到判决的支持，11个州采用宽松义务（尽管没有条例规定警告义务，但法律“允许”医务人员在这种情形下不履行保密义务）。只有6个州没有对此义务的立法（表15.1）。

法律要求的警告或保护义务为从业者带来了困扰，他们必须确定威胁的危险等级是否足够高到确立这项义务。医务人员应知晓自己从业所在地的不同规定。受害者是否有特异性或可以辨认？威胁是否紧迫？不紧迫的威胁是否严重？即使在要求对紧迫暴力威胁有公开义务的州，法律对“紧迫”也有多种解读，包括时间跨度从几天到几个月。一些法律专家建议医务人员与其担心威胁的紧迫性不如担心患者的执行能力（如，患者是否过去曾把这种威胁化为行动？他是否掌握这么做的方法？）。例如，此病例中，患者掌握了感染自己配偶的方法，证实其有紧迫性威胁，但很难证实在他已知晓自己HIV状况时，还会粗心大意地使妻子暴露在感染的危险中。对于从业者来说那些并没有明确立法和法律判例的州有巨大的法律隐患，因为一旦不履行保密义务就得不到相应的保护，而在某些州内从业者不论选择哪种应对方法都面临着民事诉讼的风险。

表 15.1　有警告义务立法的州 / 区（2014）

州立法明确警告 / 保护义务	AZ，CA，CO，ID，IN，KY，LA，MD，MA，MI，MN，MS，MO，MT，NE，NH，NJ，OH，OK，TN，UT，VA，WA
普通立法和判例支持警告 / 保护义务	AL，DE，GA，HI，IA，NC，PA，SC，SD，VT，WI
存在可信的威胁情况时“允许”医务人员不履行保密义务	AK；CT；Washington，DC；FL；IL；NY；OR；RI；TX；WV；WY
关于警告 / 保护义务无立法依据	AR，KS，ME，NV，NM，ND

公众健康和福利

州立法要求秘密信息需向合适的公共机构汇报，强调了医生的保密义务。例如，向公共卫生部门报告传染病、向多个保护机构报告可疑虐童或虐待老年人事件，和向警察局报告枪伤。这些特例也可以大致从医生警告或保护第三方不受侵害义务中推断出来，如Tarasoff案。

相反地，州立法明确提出，在特殊情况下患者有绝对保密权，如某些特殊情况，未成年人的医疗信息有权被保密。在45个州，未成年人都有权对成瘾、精神疾病和所有生殖健康问题（如节育）接受保密治疗。阿拉斯加州、爱达荷州、新墨西哥州、犹他州和怀俄明州除外。在38个州，未成年人可不经父母同意或知晓就可进行堕胎。这些特殊情况主要在于担心若没有这些权利，未成年人就不会寻求对他们的健康至关重要的医疗帮助。未成年人怀孕的案例已表明，一旦未成年人怀孕公开，青少年可能面临家人的冷落甚至暴力。

各州医生保密规则的立法情况不同，医生应始终熟悉其执业所在地区的相关规定。美国律师协会发表了未成年人诊疗的法律共识，包括50个州，哥伦比亚特区和美国境内。

在日常医疗工作中为患者保密存在许多挑战。医疗机构必须要安全、完整地保管病历。医疗团队要对电子病历负责，保护其不被有企图或无企图的不当侵犯，包括不当使用不安全邮件沟通患者私人信息。1997年，《健康信息流通和责任法案》（Health Information Portability and Accountability Act，HIPAA）被通过，将严格的医疗信息隐私条款编入联邦法律。例如，HIPAA要求患者对“治疗、费用或手术”信息公开进行授权。除外以下情况：“公益福利活动”如合法地向公共卫生机构汇报信息或向潜在受害者和有权介入 / 阻止迫害的其他人告知严重威胁。当州法和HIPAA冲突时，HIPAA规定优先以联邦法律为主。

从业者有隐性或显性的义务防止各种形式的违反保密条款，不论是有意还是无意，如在公共场所讨论患者的私人信息，如走廊、电梯这些不能保证隐私的场所，未经患者的同意向患者家属告知其私人信息。

识别

判断某一特殊情况是否需要违背保密原则的最好方法是，“倘若此信息不公开，会不会有某个人或人群处于真实严重的紧迫危险中？”如果答案是“不”，那么应按伦理及法律规则履行保密义务。如果答案是某人处于危险中，但为非紧迫性危险，那么根据职业规范医生应告知患者或他/她的监护人公开信息的重要性。在有意违背保密义务、与患者意愿背道而驰之前，医生明智之举是事先咨询当地法律专家和（或）伦理委员会。倘若有人处于紧迫危险之中，应立即联系适当的地方机构或部门（保安、警察等）。

案例分析

本案例描述了两种违反保密原则的情况。第一种是医生有意读取了与她无关的患者的病历。她意外获得的信息促使她想再次有意违背保密原则，即将患者 HIV 信息向他妻子泄密。她的理由是，担心患者妻子即她的朋友会因与丈夫接触而有 HIV 感染高度风险。

第一种情况是未经授权获取患者病历，是明显的不道德（非法）行为的例子。医生并不因为其医生的职业而赋予其查阅任何患者病历的权利。任何医生和医务人员不得获取非其参与治疗的患者的病历，除非有特殊授权，如调查危害患者安全的警讯事件或参与质量保证过程。医生这样做与黑客通过非法手段入侵普通电脑获取电子信息记录同罪。

第二种违反保密原则的情况的理由是，不论如何获取的信息，医生获取患者妻子会因与丈夫接触而处于 HIV 感染危险的信息。第二种违反保密原则的情况是否合乎伦理也更为复杂。

这位医生有“警告义务”吗？违反保密原则的可行性依赖于每个案例的细节。相关问题包括，危险是否真实、重大、紧迫。很难说 HIV 感染风险不大或一旦感染其危害不大。但是该事件紧迫性却较小：患者住院期间，处于大手术后严重并发症恢复阶段，患者配偶接触感染的概率很小。

该案例将会更复杂，这位医生决定将患者 HIV 结果告知患者妻子，首先要坦白她通过不专业不道德途径获取患者病历的事实。坦白可能会给这位医生带来严重的负面影响，即使有警告义务，她也有隐瞒倾向。然而，一旦知晓会对第三方带来巨大伤害的紧迫危险的信息，医生有责任采取措施，除非患者被说服同意自己就 HIV 结果与妻子沟通。

管理

一旦发生违背保密原则行为时，无论有意还是无意，均应告知患者泄密事宜及后续预防措施。应解决根本原因，如从业者教育及病历安全“漏洞”管理。落实医生侵犯患者隐私权后果的相关实践政策。

不管违反保密原则是否是从业者的非道德行为，泄密公开了对第三方产生伤害的真实、重要、紧迫风险，从业者有道德责任采取措施来保护第三方安全。即使为自己不道德行为冒风险，他们也不得不这么做。

本案例中，危险真实、严重但不紧迫。这种情况下，直接与患者或患者的主治医师联系尝试说服患者让他自己和妻子讨论他的 HIV 情况似乎是合理的第一步。倘若患者拒绝和妻子沟通自己 HIV 结果，下一步应当咨询汇报医院感染控制机构或当地公共卫生机构。从业者需告知患者所有后续措施及时间。

预防

未经授权获取患者病历的问题需从个体、“人文”、制度上解决。所有医生在入职培训时均应接受尊重和保护患者秘密是职业义务的教育。宣教应包括以下细节：何时为查阅病历的恰当或不恰当时间、保护患者病历不被其他未授权人员获取的责任。也应重视不同州法律法规的差异。

医疗团队应被灌输理解为患者保密原则在促进患者治疗及增进对医疗行业整体信任度中的作用。所有人都要深刻理解患者隐私信息的相关法律的要求，包括 HIPAA 规章。提醒医疗团队，即使他们觉得这些信息不具有个体识别性，也不要在公共场合谈话时涉及患者的私人信息，因为自己的猜想或许有偏差。

执行团队需采用政策和规定来处理无意和故意逾越了职责边界的人，其本质上属于“社会契约”。

应提倡一种职业“文化”即在公共场所不提及患者治疗信息。医疗机构应加强患者病历管理系统并对患者敏感信息给予充分的保障。

医疗机构政策应注明在发现患者病历安全弱点和（或）从业者违反保密原则。在保障患者病历安全方面医疗机构和个人都很重要。当今的电子病历管理员都可以设置访问权限，即时提醒管理者有人读取了特殊保密信息，并发现不直接参与患者治疗的医务人员通过不恰当的途径获取信息。

总结

医生对患者隐私权的尊重是医患关系的基石。关于保守秘密这份如此重要的责任是社会给予医生的特权，仅在特殊情形下可允许违反保密原则，如当第三方可能处于危险中。保护患者隐私要求从业者在大多数情况下积极保护患者信息，避免获取与治疗无关的信息及与自己没有医患关系患者的信息。因每个州对患者保密义务和从业者的“提醒和保护义务”都有不同的规定，因此医生应熟悉其执业当地的法律法规。

（王云鹏　译　樊玉花　校）

延伸阅读

Edelstein L: *The Hippocratic Oath: text, translation and interpretation*, Baltimore, 1943, The Johns Hopkins Press, p 56.

Elger BS: Factors influencing attitudes towards medical confidentiality among Swiss physicians, *J Med Ethics* 35:517–524, 2009.

Friedman SH, Hendrix T, Haberman J, et al.: Judicial bypass of parental consent for abortion: characteristics of pregnant minor “Jane Doe.”, *J Nerv Ment Dis* 203:401–405, 2015.

Health Information Privacy: U.S. Department of Health and Human Services: Summary of privacy rule. Available at http://www.hhs.gov/ocr/privacy/hipaa/understanding/summary/index.html. Accessed November 12, 2015.

Jonson R, Persad G, Sisti D: The Tarasoff Rule: the implications of interstate variation and gaps in professional training, *J Am Acad Psychiatry Law* 42:469–477, 2014.

Minor Consent to Medical Treatment Laws: Updated January 2013, National District Attorneys Association, Alexandria, VA. Available at http://www.ndaa.org/pdf/Minor%20Consent%20to%20Medical%20Treatment%20(2).pdf, 2013. Accessed November 12, 2015.

Moatti JP, Souville M, Obadia Y, et al.: Ethical dilemmas in care for HIV infection among French general practitioners, *Health Policy* 31:197–210, 1995.

Tarasoff v. Regents of the University of California, 17 Cal. 3d 425, 551 P.2d 334, 131 Cal. Rptr. 14 (Cal. 1976).

Weisleder P: The right of minors to confidentiality and informed consent, *J Child Neurol* 19:145–148, 2004.

第16章 心血管植入式电子设备患者的手术麻醉

Peter M. Schulman，Marc A. Rozner

病例概要

患者，男性，55岁，携带美敦力公司Micra无线起搏器（程控为VVIR），在全身麻醉下行右侧全髋关节置换术。既往有明确的心房颤动和完全性心脏传导阻滞病史。在手术室中，麻醉科医师打算用磁铁将起搏器程控为临时非同步起搏模式（即VOO模式）。在手术开始之前，护士将电刀负极贴片（如“bovie垫”）放在患者背部中央。最初，患者的血压为155/80 mmHg，100%心室起搏心律，70次/分，在使用磁铁后似乎没有变化。手术几分钟后，一旦使用单极电刀，患者就会出现心脏停搏。

问题分析

定义

美国有数百万患者植入起搏器（pacemaker，PM）或植入型心律转复除颤器（implantable cardioverter-defibrillator，ICD），并且每年植入这些植入型心血管电子设备（cardiovascular implantable electronic devices，CIED）的患者新增数十万。随着人口老龄化，这些装置适应证的更新和技术进步，CIED患者的数量可能会继续增加。因此，麻醉科医师和其他手术人员会经常遇到CIED患者，并且越来越多地为他们提供医疗服务。

经静脉CIED由一个脉冲发生器组成，其通常被植入到锁骨下胸前的囊袋中，其分为三部分，三根导线分别插入右心房（right atrium，RA）、右心室（right ventricle，RV）、和（或）冠状窦（coronary sinus，CS）。起搏器类型（如，PM或ICD）、数量以及导线的位置（RA、RV、CS）取决于患者潜在的病理状况和植入物的适应证。表16.1总结了CIED植入物的一般适应证。

经静脉CIED几乎都有RV导联，通常也有RA导联。当有指征时，另外植入CS导联以使心脏衰竭和心室内传导延迟的患者左心室起搏。在选定的患者中进行这种**心脏再同步化治疗**（cardiac resynchronization therapy，CRT）或**双心室起搏**，可改善心排血量、心力衰竭症状，并降低死亡风险。

除了提供高压电治疗，如除颤和抗心动过速起搏（antitachycardia pacing，ATP）外，经静脉ICD还能够完成经静脉起搏器的所有功能。2012年，使用皮下电极代替传统经静脉（或心外膜）导联的皮下ICD（subcutaneous ICD，S-ICD）获得了美国食品和药物管理局（Food and Drug Administration，FDA）的批准。与经静脉ICD相比，该装置功能较为有限；它没有永久性的抗心动过缓起搏能力，也不能提供ATP。2016年，FDA批准了首个经皮植入无导线起搏器，另一种无导线起搏器也有望很快在美国上市。这些装置比传统的起搏器小得多，但是它们唯一可用的起搏模式是VVI（R）（即，它们不能起搏或感测到心房）。

围术期CIED管理复杂且具有挑战性。问题包括令人困惑的命名法（参见表16.2中的起搏器代码），不断发展的技术（如无导线起搏器，皮下ICD），不同的专有功能，这些功能在不同设备类型和不同制造商之间通常是非标准化的（包括可变响应的磁铁应用），以及经常过时甚至不正确的出版文献。

另外，在手术期间经常使用的像电刀负极贴片

表 16.1 植入 CIED 的一般适应证

设备类型	左心室射血分数（%）	QRS 间期（毫秒）	心力衰竭分级	房室传导阻滞	窦房结功能障碍
经静脉 PM	>35	任何	任何	有或无	有或无
无导线 PM	>35	任何	任何	有	无
经静脉 ICD	≤ 35[a]	任何	Ⅰ，Ⅱ，Ⅲ	有或无	有或无
皮下 ICD	≤ 35[a]	任何	Ⅰ，Ⅱ，Ⅲ	无	无
双心室 PM（CRT-P）	≤ 35[b]	≥ 150[c] or ≥ 120[d]	Ⅱ，Ⅲ，非卧床Ⅳ[e]	有或无	有或无
双心室 ICD(CRT-D）	≤ 35	≥ 150[c] or ≥ 120[d]	Ⅱ，Ⅲ，非卧床Ⅳ[e]	有或无	有或无

[a] 即使左心室射血分数≥ 35%，ICD 有时也可用于二级预防。
[b] 大多数左心室射血分数≤ 35% 的患者接受 ICD。
[c] Ⅰ级推荐。
[d] Ⅱ a 级推荐。
[e] Ⅳ级心力衰竭，没有急性活动性冠状动脉综合征，没有使用正性肌力药物，也没有使用指南指导的药物治疗

Modified from Schulman PM，Rozner MA，Sera V，et al：Patients with pacemaker or implantable cardioverter-defbrillator. *Med Clin North Am* 97（6）：1051-1075，2013.

表 16.2 北美洲起搏和电生理学会 / 英国起搏和电生理学组（NASPE/BPEG）通用 PM 代码（NBG）(2002 年修订）

位置Ⅰ	位置Ⅱ	位置Ⅲ	位置Ⅳ	位置Ⅴ
起搏	感应	感应响应	可编程	多点起搏
O= 无	O= 无	O= 无	O= 无	O= 无
A= 心房	A= 心房	I= 抑制	R= 频率调整	A= 心房
V= 心室	V= 心室	T= 启动		V= 心室
D= 双（A+V）	D= 双（A+V）	D= 双（T+I）		D= 双（A+V）

Modified from Bernstein AD，Daubert JC，Fletcher RD，et al：The revised NASPE/BPEG generic code for antibradycardia，adaptive-rate，and multisite pacing. North American Society of Pacing and Electrophysiology/British Pacing and Electrophysiology Group. *Pacing Clin Electrophysiol* 25(2)：260-264，2002.

(例如，“bovie”）这样的带电设备，会产生电磁干扰（electromagnetic interference，EMI）。这些可能对 CIED 功能产生不良影响，导致 CIED 损坏和患者损伤。常见的问题包括起搏抑制（可能导致起搏依赖性患者严重的心动过缓或心脏停搏）和 ICD 患者的不适当高压电位治疗（包括除颤和 ATP）。

识别

病例概要突出了 3 个引起 CIED 相关并发症的潜在原因：①电磁干扰（EMI），②电刀负极贴片的错误位置，以及③磁铁的错误使用。

电磁干扰

CIED 的正常性能可能会被来自外部电源的电磁场破坏。虽然引起 EMI 的原因有很多，但在手术室中，最常见的罪魁祸首是单极电刀（双极电刀不太会引起 EMI）。与电切模式相比，电凝模式会产生更多的 EMI，并且当在 CIED 附近使用电刀时 EMI 的风险最高（例如，对于 CIED 植入胸腔的患者，当在患者的脐部以上使用单极电刀时，更可能出现 EMI）。

术中 EMI 最常见的后果是心室过度感知（即，该装置检测到它本应忽略的心室导联上的信号）导致①起搏抑制和起搏依赖患者的严重心动过缓或心搏停止，和（或）②通过 ICD 传递不适当的除颤或抗心动过速起搏。术中 EMI 的其他不太常见的后果包括无益的快速起搏、激活重启模式以及整个设备失灵。

电刀负极贴片定位

电刀单元（electrosurgery unit，ESU）电极版的位置应使 ESU 电流路径远离 CIED 脉冲发生器和导线（图 16.1）。因此，对于接受髋关节手术的患者（如病例），应将电极版贴在患者的腿上而不是患者的背部。

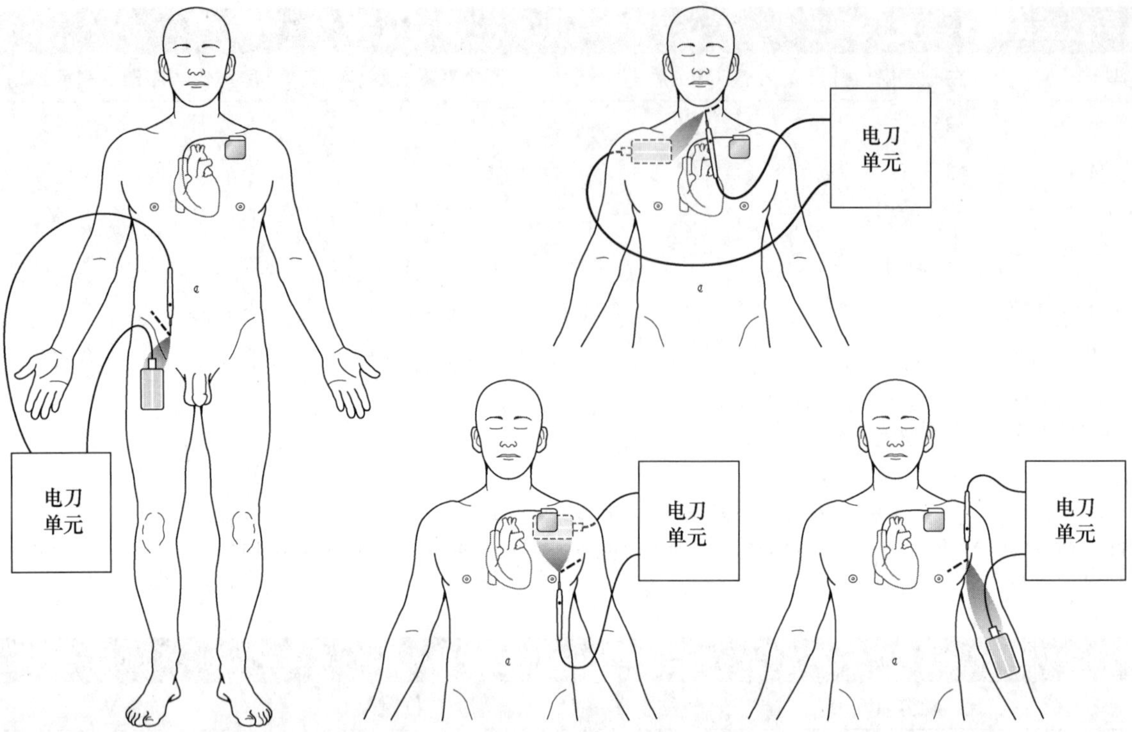

图 16.1 正确放置电刀负极贴片，使电流远离 CIED 脉冲发生器和导线

磁铁的使用

磁铁通常会暂停 ICD 的抗心动过速治疗，并且通常会导致 PM 非同步起搏。因此，当在急诊手术期间可能出现 EMI 时，磁体应用的最佳策略通常是暂停 ICD 抗心动过速治疗或在起搏依赖性 PM 患者中启用非同步起搏模式。也就是说，使用磁铁可能会产生不可预测的甚至不利的影响。一些 CIED 可以通过编程忽略磁铁，并且在许多情况下无法确认 ICD 对磁铁的反应。对于某些患者而言，磁铁产生的非同步起搏速率可能不是最佳的，并且 ICD 的起搏模式是无法用磁体改变的。此外，一些较新的 CIED（例如美敦力公司 Micra 无线起搏器）没有磁响应。因此，无论何时计划在择期手术中使用磁铁，应该知道 CIED 的磁铁反应，并且磁铁开关应该是可用的。此外，患者应保持仰卧，并且在手术期间保证磁铁可见并且可及。

风险评估

CIED 通常非常可靠；然而，有时会发生系统故障或彻底失效，可能由于 CIED 系统问题（即脉冲发生器或导线）或 EMI 等外部因素所引起的。

一项来自 FDA 的数据分析有助于深入了解这些设备一般故障的发生率。在 12 年的时间里每 1000 个植入物中，有 4.6 个 PM 和 20.7 个 ICD 因非电池耗损原因被移除。225 万个 PM 和 415 780 个 ICD 植入的患者中，30 名 PM 患者和 31 名 ICD 患者直接死于设备故障。进一步对 2003 至 2007 年间 459 000 例经静脉 ICD 和 256 000 例 CRT-D 植入物进行了分析，发现了 10 593 例（2.3%）经静脉 ICD 和 1925 例（0.8%）CRT-D 失败。

尽管数据有限，但是 CIED 可能会增加围术期的发病率和死亡率，因为在手术过程中常常会误认为设备故障或设备故障真实发生。虽然在常规情况下，真正的设备故障很少见，但手术室中经常发生的 EMI 可能会使这些患者面临更大的风险。此外，误认为的设备故障（“伪故障”）也可能导致患者受伤或设备损坏。

伪故障是多种因素共同作用的结果。因为所有经静脉 ICD 都具有抗心动过缓的起搏能力，并且设备术语经常被“不严谨”地使用（即“起搏器 / 除颤器”），所以 ICD 通常被误认为是心脏起搏器，反之亦然。所有现代 CIED 都具有复杂的功能（速率传感器，最小化右心室起搏的算法，睡眠模式等），当启用这些功能时，可能会使设备出现意外情况。ICD 处理和响应电磁干扰的方式与 PM 不同。不同制造商或不同的设备类型中，磁铁的使用效果也没有一个统一的标准。

启示

正如许多出版物所建议的那样，CIED 的存在可能会增加围术期风险，但缺乏前瞻性数据来证明。CIED 很复杂，CIED 患者的围术期处理也很复杂。包括麻醉科医师和术者在内的大多数参与手术人员，都不是 CIED 专家。

管理

为了给 CIED 的手术患者提供最佳策略，两篇重要的文献已经发表。它们分别是：美国麻醉科医师协会（American Society of Anesthesiologists，ASA）实践建议和心律协会（Heart Rhythm Society，HRS）的专家共识声明。麻醉科医师和其他手术人员应熟悉这些文件并严格遵守他们的建议。由于篇幅所限，本章并没有将上述所有建议全部罗列出来，这里总结了最重要的建议。

术前建议

1. 确定存在 CIED。
2. 识别制造商（例如，Medtronic，Boston Scientific，St.Jude Medical，Biotronik，LivaNova）和设备类型（例如，经静脉 PM，无导线 PM，双心室 PM，经静脉 ICD，皮下 ICD，双心室 ICD）。
3. 确定 CIED 运转正常（获取最近的问诊记录、与患者的 CIED 医生 / 医院取得联系）。在麻醉之前，由经验丰富的麻醉科医师对 CIED 装置情况进行询问。或者，HRS 建议择期手术需要有 ICD 6 个月且 PM 1 年之内的运行记录。
4. 确定患者的潜在心率和节律以及患者是否依赖其起搏。
5. 确定应用磁铁时 CIED 的响应方式。
6. 从 CIED 专家（HRS）那里获取明确的围术期管理计划。

术中建议

1. 关闭程控分钟通气频率响应（如果处于激活状态）。
2. 考虑关闭所有心率增强功能以防止节律错误。
3. 考虑增加起搏频率，以优化向组织输送氧气。
4. 如果可能出现 EMI：
   a. 对于 ICD 患者，禁用高电压（抗心动过速）疗法。
   b. 对于一些起搏依赖患者可以考虑非同步起搏。

   注意：磁铁通常但不总是导致经静脉的 PM 以固定频率非同步起搏。磁铁通常但不总是暂停 ICD 的高电压治疗。磁铁永远不会改变 ICD 的起搏模式。
5. 用脉搏血氧仪或动脉波形监测心律 / 外周脉搏。
6. 考虑禁用心电监护仪上的伪影过滤器。
7. 只要可行，避免使用单极电刀（monopolar electrosurgery，ESU）。如果计划使用单极电刀，电切模式导致的 EMI 低于混合模式或电凝模式。双极电刀不太可能引起 EMI。
8. 固定 ESU 的电极贴板，使其产生的电流远离脉冲发生器和导线。
9. 如果单极电刀引起诸如心室过度感知、起搏静止、不适当的心动过速或高电压治疗等问题，应立即暂停单极电刀的使用，并考虑 CIED 的重编程、磁铁的应用和（或）重新定位电刀负极贴片的位置。

术后建议

1. 强烈建议查看 CIED 以确认其功能正常（特别是在术中有血流动力学不稳定或担心 CIED 功能不正常的情况）。
2. 任何术前或术中被重新编程的 CIED 都应被重新查看，并适当地恢复其参数（可能需要重新启动速率增强，通常需要确定和编程最佳心率和起搏参数）。
3. ICD 患者必须被充分监护（在麻醉后的苏醒室或重症监护室），直到重新编程为高电压治疗模式。

预防

采取以下预防措施：

- 术前，确保 CIED 功能正常，并从 CIED 专家处获得围术期管理计划。
- 如果可能发生 EMI，应暂停 ICD 抗心动过速治疗，并使用外部除颤垫。对于那些依赖起搏的患者，都应考虑将其重新编程为非同步起搏模式。此外，一些速率增强模式可能需要禁用，对于大手术，可能需要其他编程更改（例如，增加较低的速率限制）。

- 如果计划使用磁铁，应该知道并确认磁铁的反应。
- 如果计划使用单极电刀，电刀单元电极片的放置位置应使电流的路径远离 CIED。
- 通常需要术后 CIED 的查看和编程更改。

（卢凌宇 译 万小健 校）

延伸阅读

American Society of Anesthesiologists: Practice advisory for the perioperative management of patients with cardiac implantable electronic devices: pacemakers and implantable cardioverter-defibrillators: an updated report by the American Society of Anesthesiologists Task Force on Perioperative Management of Patients with Cardiac Implantable Electronic Devices, *Anesthesiology* 114:247–261, 2011.

Bernstein AD, Daubert JC, Fletcher RD, et al.: The revised NASPE/BPEG generic code for antibradycardia, adaptive-rate, and multisite pacing. North American Society of Pacing and Electrophysiology/British Pacing and Electrophysiology Group, *Pacing Clin Electrophysiol* 25(2):260–264, 2002.

Burke MC, Gold MR, Knight BP, et al.: Safety and efficacy of the totally subcutaneous implantable defibrillator: 2-year results from a pooled analysis of the IDE study and EFFORTLESS registry, *J Am Coll Cardiol* 65:1605–1615, 2015.

Castillo JG, Silvay G, Viles-Gonzalez J: Perioperative assessment of patients with cardiac implantable electronic devices, *Mt Sinai J Med* 79:25–33, 2012.

Crossley GH, Poole JE, Rozner MA, et al.: The Heart Rhythm Society (HRS)/American Society of Anesthesiologists (ASA) Expert Consensus Statement on the perioperative management of patients with implantable defibrillators, pacemakers and arrhythmia monitors: facilities and patient management this document was developed as a joint project with the American Society of Anesthesiologists (ASA), and in collaboration with the American Heart Association (AHA), and the Society of Thoracic Surgeons (STS), *Heart Rhythm* 8:1114–1154, 2011.

Healey JS, Merchant R, Simpson C, et al.: Canadian Cardiovascular Society/Canadian Anesthesiologists' Society/Canadian Heart Rhythm Society joint position statement on the perioperative management of patients with implanted pacemakers, defibrillators, and neurostimulating devices, *Can J Cardiol* 28:141–151, 2012.

Ho JK, Mahajan A: Cardiac resynchronization therapy for treatment of heart failure, *Anesth Analg* 111:1353–1361, 2010.

Laskey W, Awad K, Lum J, et al.: An analysis of implantable cardiac device reliability. The case for improved postmarketing risk assessment and surveillance, *Am J Ther* 19:248–254, 2012.

Maisel WH, Moynahan M, Zuckerman BD, et al.: Pacemaker and ICD generator malfunctions: analysis of Food and Drug Administration annual reports, *JAMA* 295:1901–1906, 2006.

Reddy VY, Exner DV, Cantillon DJ, et al.: Percutaneous implantation of an entirely intracardiac leadless pacemaker, *N Engl J Med* 373:1125–1135, 2015.

Rozner MA, Schulman PM: Perioperative management of patients with a pacemaker or implantable cardioverter-defibrillator. In Mark JB, Link MS, editors: UpToDate, Waltham, MA. Available at https://www.uptodate.com/contents/perioperative-management-of-patients-with-a-pacemaker-or-implantable-cardioverter-defbrillator. Accessed September 30, 2016.

Schulman PM, Rozner MA: Use caution when applying magnets to pacemakers or defibrillators for surgery, *Anesth Analg* 117:422–427, 2013.

Schulman PM, Rozner MA, Sera V, Stecker EC: Patients with pacemaker or implantable cardioverter-defibrillator, *Med Clin North Am* 97:1051–1075, 2013.

癫痫患者

第 17 章

R. Alexander Schlichter

病例概要

患者，女性，33 岁，拟行部分乳腺切除术和腋窝淋巴结活检。既往有癫痫病史，服用左乙拉西坦控制良好，轻度哮喘，需偶尔使用沙丁胺醇吸入剂。体格检查正常。

问题分析

定义

癫痫是一种神经系统疾病，由大脑皮质一个（局灶）或多个（全面）位点的异常电活动引起。其症状与放电的位置和程度有关。据估计，每年的发病率为 0.5% ～ 2.3%，高达 40% 的患者发展为难治性癫痫发作（每月发作一次以上）。在美国，大约有 40 万癫痫患者药物控制不佳。每年每 1000 名患者中有 2 人猝死。诸多神经系统疾病与癫痫或抗惊厥药物的使用有关，如偏头痛、抑郁症、精神病、情绪或行为障碍以及慢性疼痛。这种情况下，抗惊厥药物的使用会影响麻醉科医师对这些患者的处理。

患者癫痫发作的类型（以及患者的过敏情况）决定医师给予何种治疗。癫痫分为局灶性或全面性。局灶性癫痫累及在一侧大脑半球，可以细分为以下类型：

- 单纯局灶性发作：意识状态无变化；
- 复杂局灶性发作：意识状态出现变化；
- 局灶性发作引发全面性发作。

全面性发作累及整个大脑皮质并影响双侧大脑半球。其往往伴随意识状态的改变并可细分为以下类型：

- 失神发作；
- 肌阵挛发作；
- 强直阵挛发作；
- 失张力性发作。

复杂局灶性发作是最常见的癫痫类型，大约占成人癫痫的 25%，占儿童癫痫的 40%。强直阵挛性发作次常见，占成人癫痫的 25%，占儿童癫痫的 19%。

癫痫的准确病因目前仍不完全清楚。癫痫与一些先天性疾病有关，如结节性硬化症、神经纤维瘤、多发性内分泌腺瘤病，以及 Jervell-Lange-Neilson 综合征。脑损伤、卒中、脑肿瘤以及阿尔兹海默病的病理改变也与癫痫有关。

失神发作常常由亮光或闪光诱发产生，被认为是由丘脑和额叶、视觉、听觉、躯体感觉皮质之间的联系发生改变导致。这种改变会导致一种分离状态，类似于清醒患者的非快速动眼睡眠阶段。丙戊酸和乙琥胺对其治疗有效提示 γ-氨基丁酸（γ-aminobutyric acid，GABA）受体（丙戊酸，苯二氮䓬类）和 T 型钙通道（乙琥胺）可能对癫痫的治疗有效。

其他有剧烈肌肉活动的全面性发作（肌阵挛，强直阵挛）被认为是由钠通道的频繁去极化引起的。随后，还研究了电压稳定钾通道数量减少与其之间的关系。

局灶性发作（单纯或复杂）可能由 GABA 受体功能障碍引起，导致相关神经元兴奋性增高，抑制性减弱。

由于在围术期与患者的接触有限，麻醉科医师应当咨询癫痫患者的管床医师，共同商讨。患者的评估应当包括以下几方面：

- 既往癫痫的诊断史；
- 癫痫可能的病因；
- 目前和既往癫痫的治疗方案；
- 目前药物治疗方案的有效性。

患者治疗的目标是使其功能达到最优化，具体包括以下几方面：

- 使癫痫发作的次数和频率降到最低；
- 脑部原发疾病（肿块、脑积水、外伤性脑损伤、卒中、出血、癫痫灶）的外科治疗；
- 平衡治疗方案和副作用；
- 遵循治疗计划。

在没有家族史、明确的医学因果关系和脑电图（electroencephalogram，EEG）检查阴性的情况下，一次癫痫发作（可能是误诊）只行保守治疗。癫痫复发的概率大约是 25%；但是，复发后再发作的概率上升至 80%，建议给予药物治疗。如果诊断为器质性病变，患者应当开始药物治疗，并可能需要进行手术干预。

合并癫痫的产妇导致以下疾病的风险增加：

- 婴儿因遗传或用药方面导致的先天性畸形；
- 妊娠期生理变化导致的现有治疗药物代谢动力学方面的变化；
- 因为产前用药可能的致畸作用，调整药物可能造成的疗效不佳；
- 早产、先兆子痫、胎盘早剥、胎儿宫内死亡的风险。

具体的药物治疗方案由患者的主诊医生决定，治疗的目标如下：

- 期待疗法；
- 单种药物治疗；
- 联合治疗（2 种或 3 种药物）。

主要的治疗方案应当对疗效与副作用进行权衡，使患者的功能状态最优，同时保证患者的依从性。如果某种治疗方案因为疗效不足或无法接受的副作用（包括过敏反应和妊娠引起）而失败，医师应当寻找一种或多种作用于可替代其作用机制的药物。

如果药物治疗无法控制癫痫，应当考虑介入治疗。迷走神经刺激（vagal nerve stimulation，VNS）、深部脑刺激（deep brain stimulation，DBS），或根据癫痫的病因，甚至可行部分或全部颞叶切除术。根据癫痫基金会的说法，VNS 也被称作“脑起搏器”。DBS 最初被推荐用于治疗帕金森，目前对药物和 VNS 治疗癫痫无效的患者显示出一定效果。最后，如果功能性磁共振成像（functional magnetic resonance imaging，fMRI）或 EEG 可以识别癫痫病灶，可以考虑行部分或全部颞叶切除术。

目前正在评估一种新的疗法，MRI 引导下激光热疗术。治疗过程包括将光纤定向放置在病灶。在 MRI 引导下，病灶被激光产生热消融。这种技术较开颅脑叶切除术创伤小很多。

识别

麻醉科医师处理癫痫患者时应当考虑到以下几点：

- 癫痫发作的频率和后遗症；
- 目前治疗方案的有效性；
- 给予治疗方案的依从性；
- 发作诱发因素。

诱发因素包括强光或闪光、噪声、饥饿、低血糖、口渴、咖啡因戒断、药品或其他物质中毒或戒断、嗜睡、疲乏、压力以及焦虑。这些诱发因素应当在围术期得到处理。

风险评估

癫痫患者的死亡风险增加了 20 倍，这还不包括患者可能患有的其他并存疾病。癫痫造成的神经系统、心血管和肺的后遗症会影响患者的围术期管理。非围术期的影响，如反复发作引起的认知功能受损、相关疾病（如脑瘫）、社交孤立、疾病的耻辱感以及小儿 / 青少年患者的婴儿化，会使知情同意、建立静脉通道和保证术后支持等工作复杂化。服用抗惊厥药物的患者常常同时服用多种药物，包括抗抑郁药物、中枢性肌松药、苯二氮䓬类药物和镇痛药物。

抗惊厥药有镇静作用，会影响麻醉的诱导、维持和苏醒。许多抗惊厥药可在肝代谢中诱导细胞色素酶，加快氨基甾类非去极化肌松药（维库溴铵、罗库溴铵）的代谢。作为补救，肌肉松弛药结合药物舒更葡糖可以减少过度松弛的发生，但其在育龄妇女和对舒更葡糖过敏的患者中应谨慎应用。

管理与预防

抗惊厥方案治疗有效的患者应维持该方案直至手术当天，包括在手术当天用少量水服用药物。实施非小脑幕上手术的患者可在围术期行静脉给药（左乙拉西坦，苯妥英钠）。如果没有肠内或肠外给药途径，应当考虑直肠、肌内或鼻内给药。有必要向神经科和药剂科咨询，以确保药物适当的生物利用度。

患者有自主发作的癫痫而麻醉科医师在场时应当做好干预的准备。根据所在地点（手术室、重症监护室或病房）和可用药物的种类，麻醉科医师可以使用苯二氮䓬类药物、巴比妥类药物、丙泊酚和（或）吸入麻醉药（异氟烷、七氟烷、地氟烷）控制癫痫发作。麻醉科医师同时也应该做好处理紧急气道的准备。这需要适当的通气和气道建立的设备。使用非去极化肌松药可以减少与其他麻醉药物联合应用时对癫痫患者造成身体伤害的风险。最后，如果患者出现血流动力学异常（高血压或休克），麻醉科医师应当备有抗高血压药物、麻醉剂或阿片类药物来应对极端高血压；或升压剂、强心剂，以及静脉补液措施应对休克。

（王　翰　译　卜　岚　校）

延伸阅读

A randomized controlled trial of chronic vagus nerve stimulation for treatment of medically intractable seizures. The Vagus Nerve Stimulation Study Group, *Neurology* 45(2):224–230, 1995.

Berman R, Negish M, Vestal M, et al.: Simultaneous EEG, fMRI and behavior in typical childhood absence seizures, *Epilepsia* 51(10):2011–2022, 2010.

Brodie MJ, Dichter MA: Antiepileptic drugs, *N Engl J Med* 334(3):168–175, 1996.

Browne TR, Holmes GL: Epilepsy, *N Engl J Med* 344(15):1145–1151, 2001.

Chang BS, Lowenstein DH: Epilepsy, *N Engl J Med* 349(13):1257–1266, 2003.

Curry DJ, Gowda A, McNichols RJ, et al.: MR-guided stereotactic laser ablation of epileptogenic foci in children, *Epilepsy Behav* 24(4):408–414, 2012.

Kofke WA: Anesthetic management of the patient with epilepsy or prior seizures, *Curr Opin Anaesthesiol* 23(3):391–399, 2010.

Lega BC, Halpern CH, Jaggi JL, Baltuch GH: Deep brain stimulation in the treatment of refractory epilepsy: update on current data and future directions, *Neurobiol Dis* 38(3):354–360, 2010.

McIntosh AM, Kalnins RM, Mitchell LA, et al.: Temporal lobectomy: long term seizure outcome, late recurrence and risks for seizure recurrence, *Brain* 127(Pt 9):2018–2030, 2004.

McNamara JC: Drugs effective in the therapy of the epilepsies. In Hardman JG, Limbird LE, editors: *Goodman and Gilman's the pharmacological basis of therapeutics*, 10th ed, New York, 2001, McGraw-Hill, pp 521–547.

Pedley TA: The epilepsies. In Goldman L, Bennett JC, editors: *Cecil textbook of medicine*, 21st ed, Philadelphia, 2000, WB Saunders, pp 2151–2163.

Rowbotham MC, Petersen KL: Anticonvulsants and local anesthetic drugs. In Loeser JD, Butler SH, Chapman CR, et al.: *Bonica's management of pain*, 3rd ed, Philadelphia, 2001, JB Lippincott–Williams & Wilkins, pp 1727–1735.

第18章 肌营养不良患者的围术期处理

Katarzyna Luba

病例概要

患儿，男性，8月龄，拟择期行鼓膜切开术。曾顺利行气管插管全身麻醉。本次静脉注射硫喷妥钠诱导，并通过面罩给氧化亚氮、氟烷和氧气维持麻醉。在鼓膜切开移除导管后，外科医师决定行腺样体切除术。此时出现气道阻塞需要紧急插管。静脉注射2 mg/kg琥珀胆碱后，患者咬肌肌张力开始增加。心电图（electrocardiogram，ECG）监测器显示增宽的复杂心动过速并且进展为心动过缓。呼气末二氧化碳（CO_2）从40～50 mmHg逐渐下降至25 mmHg，动脉血氧饱和度从100%下降至80%，然后无法测及。关闭氟烷，静脉给予氯化钙、肾上腺素和碳酸氢钠。心电图越来越紊乱，脉搏无法触及。开始胸部按压。静脉血气分析显示pH为7.13，CO_2分压（PCO_2）为73 mmHg，血清钾水平超过10 mmol/L。重复静脉给氯化钙、肾上腺素和碳酸氢钠。经心肺复苏13 min后，心电图显示阵发性室上性心动过速，收缩压升高至100 mmHg。给予琥珀胆碱20 min后，静脉血标本显示pH值为7.30，PCO_2为49 mmHg，钾水平为7.1 mmol/L。导尿管可见红色尿液。之后患者被送往儿科重症监护病房。肌酸激酶（creatine kinase，CK）水平为285 760 U/L。给予患者充足的静脉补液治疗。患者出院时情况良好。DNA研究显示肌营养不良蛋白基因缺失，符合进行性假肥大性肌营养不良（杜氏肌营养不良，duchenne muscular dystrophy，DMD）的诊断。

问题分析

定义

肌营养不良是一种临床和遗传多样性的横纹肌结构遗传性疾病，其特点是进行性肌无力和消瘦。该病诊断依据为：血清CK升高、肌病肌电图特征和肌肉活检。其形态学改变与所有的肌肉萎缩类似，肌纤维正常或肥大、坏死组织与脂肪和纤维在间质积聚随机出现。在DMD中，脂肪和纤维组织在间质的积聚导致了特征性小腿肌肉假性肥大。

对肌营养不良的分类以往主要是基于遗传模式和临床特征，最近的分类还考虑了缺陷蛋白质的类型、定位和功能，此类缺陷蛋白质参与不同肌营养不良的发病机制。

质膜相关蛋白质

质膜相关蛋白质缺陷或此类蛋白质缺乏是导致肌营养不良的最常见原因，包括DMD、贝克肌营养不良（becker muscular dystrophy，BMD）、肌肉萎缩症和其他形式的肢带型肌营养不良（limb-girdle muscular dystrophy，LGMD）。

营养不良性疾病

最常见的肌营养不良是肌营养不良蛋白基因突变引起的X连锁隐性遗传病。肌营养不良蛋白是维持肌膜完整性所必需的一种大型肌层蛋白质。病情较严重的 DMD 是由肌营养不良引起，相对轻微的等位基因形式（becker muscular dystrophy，BMD）则与截断蛋白的减少有关。DMD 的发病率为 1/3500 例活产男婴。DMD 或 BMD 表型可在具有肌营养不良蛋白基因突变和 X0 核型（特纳综合征）的女性患者中表达。该病患者一般运动发育迟缓，当他们开始学习走路时，会出现步态异常。到了 5 岁，肌无力加重，小腿逐渐发展为假性肥大。随着病情发展，肌肉力量逐渐丧失，肌腱出现挛缩，这导致了患者腰椎过度前凸和踮脚走路。到了大约 12 岁，大多数患者只能依靠轮椅来生活。16 ～ 18 岁左右，出现脊柱侧弯、胸部畸形和膈肌无力的症状，这最终导致了严重的限制性肺病的发生。呼吸衰竭是该病患者死亡最常见的原因，一般发生于 20 ～ 30 岁。另外，几乎所有患者都存在原发性心肌病，但这很少导致死亡。智力障碍在这类患者中很常见。

与 DMD 相比，BMD 发病较晚，临床病程也较轻。尽管 BMD 发病可能延迟到 30 ～ 40 岁，但是患者通常在 5 ～ 15 岁就开始表现出近端肌无力的症状。患者通常在 15 岁以后仍可以行走。小腿肿大出现在早期并且非常突出。虽然预期寿命较短，但也有许多患者可以活到 30 或 40 岁。BMD 患者一般精神发育迟缓，但与 DMD 患者相比症状稍轻微。在患有轻度或亚临床 BMD 的患者中，扩张型心肌病非常常见，心肌病带来的并发症是大多数 BMD 患者死亡的主要原因。

肌聚糖病变

这些营养不良性疾病是由编码 4 种肌糖复合物的跨膜糖蛋白基因突变引起的。4 种肌糖基因（α、β、γ 和 δ）中的任何一种突变可导致 LGMD 2D、2E、2C 和 2F。男性和女性发病率相近。小腿近端肌无力的症状一般出现在 20 ～ 30 岁，但也有可能延迟。患者还可表现为上肢受累与肩胛骨翼状发展。膈肌无力伴呼吸功能不全、心肌病、充血性心力衰竭（congestive heart failure，CHF）和心律失常也可发生，但智力功能正常。

陷窝蛋白缺乏症

这是一种罕见的常染色体显性肌营养不良。LGMD 1C 是由陷窝蛋白（一种普遍存在的质膜蛋白）缺陷引起的。

细胞外基质蛋白

细胞外基质蛋白的缺陷导致了先天性肌营养不良（congenital muscular dystrophy，CMD）的发生，这是一组常染色体隐性遗传疾病，在出生或婴儿时期即出现症状。肌张力减退和活检见营养不良的肌肉可确诊。分区蛋白质缺乏的 CMD 为该病最严重的类型。患有 CMD 的儿童最大的功能缺陷是不能维持坐姿。轻微的心肌病也可能发生。

具有酶活性的蛋白质

编码糖基转移酶的基因突变

这些有关 CMD 突变的机制是最近才发现的。编码 fukutin 相关蛋白质（FKRP，一种糖基转移酶）的基因在严重肌营养不良 CMD 1C 型以及轻度的 LGMD 2I 中发生突变。严重时将出现中枢神经系统症状，常表现为小脑囊肿、癫痫和发育迟缓。轻度心肌病也可能出现。

蛋白激酶

位于 19 号染色体上的一种蛋白激酶基因，其 3’末端翻译区域的三核苷酸重复序列（[CTG]n）扩增突变导致杂合性是强直性肌营养不良的原因，这是最常见的成人肌营养不良类型。其发病率为 1/8 000。强直性肌营养不良是一种常染色体显性遗传疾病，其特征为肌强直、缓慢加重的肌肉无力和肌萎缩、消瘦、额秃、白内障和继发于胰岛素受体表达异常的胰岛素抵抗。

其他肌蛋白

肌节蛋白

肌巨蛋白基因突变转而编码巨大的肌节蛋白，是常染色体显性先天性扩张型心肌病的基础。最近，在患有孤立性胫骨肌营养不良的患者中也发现了相同基因的突变。

核蛋白

两种核蛋白的缺陷导致了两种不同形式的 Emerry-Dreifuss 肌营养不良症（Emery-Dreifuss muscular dystrophy，EDMD）。X 连锁 EDMD 是由编码核纤蛋白的基因突变所致。常染色体显性遗传 EDMD 则由编码核纤层蛋白的核纤层蛋白 A/C 基因突变引起。该基因的突变也导致了主要累及近端的 LGMD 1B 形成和扩张型心肌病的发生。EDMD 中的骨骼肌受累通常轻微且进展缓慢。心脏受累是该疾病的主要特征。

肌营养不良性心肌病

心脏受累是肌营养不良的普遍特征，所有类型的肌营养不良患者的长期预后均取决于心脏受累的严重程度。

在 DMD 和 BMD 中，肌营养不良蛋白缺乏或缺陷已在骨骼肌和心肌中被证实。心力衰竭通常单独出现或合并呼吸衰竭成为患者死亡的主要原因。心肌损害最初是亚临床型，但通过心电图和超声心动图的轻微改变可以识别。心肌受累进展到临床上明显的肥厚阶段时会出现心律失常，表现为传导障碍（房室传导阻滞、束支传导阻滞）或严重的室上或室性心律失常，心肌广泛纤维化，并最终导致扩张型心肌病的发生。心力衰竭是 BMD 患者最常见的死亡原因。DMD 和 BMD 的女性携带者年龄渐进性心肌病的发病率为 10%。由于严重肌营养不良的长期预后不佳，患者并不适合心脏移植。最近已经报道了在具有终末期扩张型心肌病的 DMD 患者中使用左心室辅助装置的例子。

肌糖病（LGMD 2C，2D，2E，2F）可同时伴有扩张型心肌病，这是因骨骼肌和心肌中肌糖复合物被破坏所致。

LGMD 由于 *FKRP* 基因（LGMD 2I）突变可能与心肌纤维化有关，导致扩张型心肌病和复极异常。

在强直性肌营养不良中，心脏传导缺陷是导致猝死的主要原因。这些患者完全性房室传导阻滞的发生率高于一般人群。心室传导间隔的延长使患者有可能发生阵发性房室传导阻滞，因此应在疾病早期即植入起搏器。在先天性（新生儿）强直性肌营养不良中，心肌松弛异常可导致左心室舒张功能不全。

严重的心脏受累在 EDMD 中很常见。X 连锁和常染色体显性形式都有发生心动过缓（通常需要植入起搏器）和心房颤动或心房扑动的风险。心房颤动通常发生在心房停顿之前，这可能是患者在年轻时就发生栓塞性卒中的原因。对于房性心律失常或停顿的 EDMD 患者，建议进行预防性抗凝治疗。另外，虽然左心室衰竭很少见，但只要出现可能就很严重。

识别

肌营养不良患者通常需进行肌肉活检、肌腱挛缩释放、脊柱后凸侧弯畸形矫正或起搏器植入等检查和治疗。未确诊的小儿或青壮年肌营养不良症患者可进行与疾病无关的其他手术。

所有肌营养不良患者都应怀疑有呼吸和心脏功能障碍。继发于膈肌无力和脊柱侧凸的限制性肺病在肌无力的患者中发病率很高，因此所有的患者都应行肺功能检查。在诊断为肌营养不良但尚无症状的患者中，肌营养不良的具体类型和心脏受累的风险评估决定了是否有必要行进一步心脏检查。

术中 CHF 表现为心动过速和对静脉输液无反应的低血压。CHF 的体征包括自主呼吸患者出现颈静脉扩张、肺部啰音和呼吸困难。严重的 CHF 可导致急性肺水肿。经食管超声心动图或肺动脉导管的血流动力学测定可确诊。典型表现为：肺动脉闭塞压升高（>18 mmHg）、心脏指数低 [<2.2 L/（min·m^2 体表面积）] 和体循环阻力高 [>1200 dyne/（s·cm^{-5}）]。

在未确诊 DMD 的患儿中应用琥珀胆碱存在诱发高钾性心脏骤停的风险。在此类研究报告的基础上，美国食品和药物管理局建议对所有儿童在非紧急插管时不应使用琥珀胆碱。

DMD 和 BMD 患者接触挥发性麻醉剂后，氟烷、异氟烷和七氟烷可导致体温过高、肌肉僵硬、大量横纹肌溶解和高钾血症的出现。据报道，年轻患者在不使用琥珀胆碱的全身麻醉下出现高钾性心脏骤停是隐匿性 DMD 的首发表现。该临床表现类似恶性高热（malignant hyperthermia，MH），并且长期以来一直被认为是真正的 MH。然而，肌营养不良（DMD 和 BMD）和 MH 在遗传学上表现大不相同：肌营养不良是由 X 染色体突变引起的，而 MH 是由位于 19 号染色体上的雷诺丁受体（ryanodine receptor，RYR）的基因突变引起的。

风险评估

所有肌营养不良患者都存在心肌病或传导障碍的风险。术前评估时心肌功能障碍的体征和症状可能很明显，也可能因长期在轮椅上生活而被掩盖。因此，所有肌营养不良患者术前都应进行心功能评估。一般来说，出现 ECG 异常（窦性心动过速或心动过缓，P-R 间隔短，左心室肥厚征象，传导阻滞）

是很常见的。然而，超声心动图左心室收缩功能障碍的严重程度与死亡率最为相关。DMD 和 BMD 患者的心脏评估指南建议：DMD 患者确诊后，每 2 年做一次超声心动图和心电图，直到 10 岁，此后每年复查一次；BMD 患者应在诊断时进行超声心动图和心电图检查，然后每 5 年复查一次。同样的建议也适用于其他类型的肌营养不良患者。在手术前或有临床指征时应再做一次超声心动图或 ECG。

EDMD 患者在诊断时应进行 ECG 和超声心动图检查，之后每年复查一次。还应每年行 Holter 检查监测心律失常。植入式起搏器适用于有症状的患者或 ECG 显示窦房结或房室结功能障碍的无症状患者。常染色体显性遗传 EDMD 患者存在发生猝死的风险，因此，每当出现心动过缓起搏时，应考虑使用内部心律转复除颤器。而当诊断为心房颤动或心房停顿时，需要进行全身抗凝治疗。

所有成人强直性肌营养不良患者均应进行心肌传导评估。根据 ECG 的结果，筛选患者行进一步的心脏电生理学检查。

在 DMD 患者中，随着进行性肌无力和脊柱侧凸的发展，肺活量（vital capacity，VC）逐渐下降。一旦 VC 下降至预测值的 20% 以下时，呼吸衰竭就不可避免，约有 73% 的患者死于呼吸衰竭。阻塞性睡眠呼吸暂停（Obstructive sleep apnea，OSA）很常见，可导致慢性低氧血症和右心功能衰竭。术前肺功能检查和睡眠监测是评估限制性肺疾病和 OSA 严重程度的指标。

启示

肌营养不良患者围术期 CHF、心律失常和呼吸衰竭的风险增加。如果 VC 值低于预测值的 30%，患者可能需要更长时间的术后机械通气支持。OSA 和咽肌无力可增加术后早期气道梗阻和缺氧的风险。由于可发生呼吸抑制延迟，不建议在门诊行全身麻醉。此外，胃排空延迟也可增加误吸的风险。

琥珀胆碱可引起高钾性心脏骤停，因此禁忌使用。非去极化肌松药（nondepolarizing muscle relaxant，NDMR）可能有延迟作用，而新斯的明对其逆转作用尚不确切。在 DMD 或 BMD 患者中，挥发性麻醉药还可引起类似 MH 的反应（肌肉僵硬、横纹肌溶解、高钾血症和体温过高等）。

在强直性肌营养不良患者中，体温过低、颤抖、琥珀胆碱、新斯的明和直接肌肉刺激可诱发肌强直危象，其特征为骨骼肌长时间挛缩。

基于此原因，在适当的情况下，所有肌营养不良患者都应优先选择区域阻滞或局部麻醉。最后，既往使用糖皮质激素治疗的 DMD 患者需要在围术期补充类固醇。

管理

应尽量减少挥发性麻醉药物和肌肉松弛药的使用，主张行区域麻醉或静脉全麻。用于静脉全麻的药物包括丙泊酚、氯胺酮、右美托咪定和阿片类药物等。短效阿片类药物（瑞芬太尼、舒芬太尼）可降低术后呼吸抑制的风险。预先给苯二氮䓬类药物和阿片类药物可能会诱发呼吸抑制、气道阻塞和苏醒延迟，应避免使用。

气道管理应考虑误吸风险的增加。术前用药建议使用 H_2 受体阻滞剂和甲氧氯普胺（胃复安）。如果须行气管插管，应考虑使用 NDMR 改良的快速气管插管。

选择神经肌肉阻滞剂的时候应考虑琥珀胆碱的禁忌和患者对 NDMR 的敏感性增加。应使用短效 NDMR（如：顺阿曲库铵），剂量应按正常的四分之一来进行滴定。即使使用短效 NDMR，DMD 患儿也可出现恢复延迟。据报道，使用新斯的明可逆转 NDMR 并且无不良事件发生，然而如前所述，新斯的明的逆转作用尚不确切。

术中 CHF 的管理取决于血流动力学的稳定。加强利尿和保持呼气末正压可能即已足够。如出现低血压，应使用强心药（多巴酚丁胺或米力农），并监测动脉血压。对于肌营养不良患者，建议在所有的大手术中均监测动脉血压。经食管超声心动图或肺动脉导管测量来指导进一步的管理。如果前负荷足够，则收缩力和后负荷减少可能有助于增加心排血量和组织灌注。

对于强直性肌营养不良患者，麻醉目标应包括避免诱发肌强直性挛缩。严重的挛缩会导致下颌和胸壁僵硬，从而阻碍插管和机械通气。挛缩对 NDMR 无响应，可能对静脉注射奎尼丁、局部麻醉剂浸润肌肉以及复温有反应。

吸入麻醉药引起的 MH 样反应可危及生命。要求立即停止使用诱发症状的药物，使用100%氧气，主动降温，治疗相关的心律失常、高钾血症和酸中毒，并酌情持续进行心肺复苏术。高于5.5 mmol/L的高钾血症应采用静脉注射碳酸氢钠、氯化钙、50%右旋糖、胰岛素和过度通气进行治疗。为预防继发于横纹肌溶解症的急性肾衰竭，应对患者进行积极的静脉补液和甘露醇治疗。

在DMD或BMD患者中由挥发性麻醉剂引发的类似MH的发作中使用丹曲林虽然比较实际，但仍有争议。在真正的MH中，丹曲林通过与雷诺丁受体同型RYR 1结合起作用，并抑制肌质网中钙的过量释放。而吸入麻醉诱导的横纹肌溶解（anesthesia-induced rhabdomyolysis，AIR）是由肌肉破裂和肌细胞内容物释放到血液中引起的，因此丹曲林可能对AIR并没有帮助。

呼吸功能受损的患者在全身麻醉下进行重大的外科手术后，需要进入重症监护室进行长时间的通气支持。

预防

预防肌营养不良患者的围术期并发症需要彻底评估手术风险。应在DMD患者的肺功能下降至不能耐受麻醉和手术之前实施脊柱侧凸的纠正手术。了解心肌受累的严重程度对于预防CHF围术期心律失常是必要的。术前评估应包括最近的ECG、超声心动图，如ECG结果不佳应加做电生理检查。在存在严重心肌病和呼吸功能障碍的情况下，有创血流动力学监测和术后重症监护治疗应成为重大手术患者围术期管理的重要组成部分。在此群体中不鼓励进行门诊手术，由于存在延迟出现呼吸并发症的风险，不论何时手术，患者都需在全身麻醉后进行过夜留院观察。

通过预先给予H_2受体阻滞剂和胃复安以及使用适当的插管技术，可以将误吸风险降至最低。琥珀胆碱应禁忌使用。同时应避免使用吸入麻醉药，因其可能引发大量的横纹肌溶解和危及生命的高钾血症。在允许的情况下，使用区域或局部麻醉可有助于肌营养不良患者避免全身麻醉时的呼吸、心脏和代谢等并发症的发生。

（翟学花 译 陈元杰 校）

延伸阅读

Baraka A, Jalbout MI: Anesthesia and myopathy, *Curr Opin Anaesthesiol* 15:371–376, 2002.

Barresi R, Di Blasi C, Negri T: Disruption of heart sarcoglycan complex and severe cardiomyopathy caused by β-sarcoglycan mutations, *J Med Genet* 37:102–107, 2000.

Birnkrant DJ, Panitch HB, Benditt JO, et al.: American College of Chest Physicians consensus statement on the respiratory and related management of patients with Duchenne muscular dystrophy undergoing anesthesia or sedation, *Chest* 132:1977–1986, 2007.

Boriani G, Gallina M, Merlini L, et al.: Clinical relevance of atrial fibrillation/flutter, stroke, pacemaker implant, and heart failure in Emery-Dreifuss muscular dystrophy: a long-term longitudinal study, *Stroke* 34:901–908, 2003.

Buckley AE, Dean J: Cardiac involvement in Emery Dreifuss muscular dystrophy: a case series, *Heart* 82:105–108, 1999.

Corrado G, Lissoni A, Beretta S, et al.: Prognostic value of electrocardiograms, ventricular late potentials, ventricular arrhythmias, and left ventricular systolic dysfunction in patients with Duchenne muscular dystrophy, *Am J Cardiol* 89:838–841, 2002.

Do T: Orthopedic management of the muscular dystrophies, *Curr Opin Pediatr* 14:50–53, 2002.

Dubowitz V: What is muscular dystrophy? Forty years of progressive ignorance, *J R Coll Physicians Lond* 34:464–468, 2000.

Frankowski GA, Johnson J, Tobias J: Rapacuronium administration to two children with Duchenne's muscular dystrophy, *Anesth Analg* 91:27–28, 2000.

Iodice F, Testa G, Averardi M, et al.: Implantation of a left ventricular assist device as a destination therapy in Duchenne muscular dystrophy patients with end stage cardiac failure: management and lessons learned, *Neuromuscul Disord* 25:19–23, 2015.

Ishizaki M, Fujimoto A, Ueyama H, et al.: Life-threatening arrhythmias in a Becker muscular dystrophy family due to the duplication of exons 3-4 of the dystrophin gene, *Intern Med* 54:3075–3078, 2015.

Kang PB, Morrison L, Iannaccone ST, et al.: Evidence-based guideline summary: evaluation, diagnosis, and management of congenital muscular dystrophy, *Neurology* 84:1369–1378, 2015.

Le Corre F, Plaud B: Neuromuscular disorders, *Curr Opin Anaesthesiol* 11:333–337, 1998.

Mathieu J, Allard P, Gobeil G, et al.: Anesthetic and surgical complications in 219 cases of myotonic dystrophy, *Neurology* 49:1646–1650, 1997.

Melacini P, Fanin M, Danielli GA, et al.: Myocardial disease: myocardial involvement is very frequent among patients affected with subclinical Becker's muscular dystrophy, *Circulation* 94:3168–3175, 1996.

Muntoni F: Cardiomyopathy in muscular dystrophies, *Curr Opin Neurol* 16:577–583, 2003.

Parker SF, Bailey A, Drake AF: Infant hyperkalemic arrest after succinylcholine, *Anesth Analg* 80:206–207, 1995.

Politano L, Nigro V, Nigro G, et al.: Development of cardiomyopathy in female carriers of Duchenne and Becker muscular dystrophies, *JAMA* 275:1335–1338, 1996.

Poole TC, Lim TYJ, Buck J, Kong S: Perioperative cardiac arrest in a patient with previously undiagnosed Becker's muscular dystrophy after isoflurane anaesthesia for elective surgery, *Br J Anaesth* 104:487–489, 2010.

Ririe DG, Shapiro F, Sethna NF: The response of patients with Duchenne's muscular dystrophy to neuromuscular blockade with vecuronium, *Anesthesiology* 88:351–354, 1998.

Rosenberg H, Gronert GA: Intractable cardiac arrest in children given succinylcholine [letter], *Anesthesiology* 77:1054, 1992.

Schramm CM: Current concepts of respiratory complications of neuromuscular disease in children, *Curr Opin Pediatr* 12:203–207, 2000.

Segura LG, Lorenz JD, Weingarten TN, et al.: Anesthesia and Duchenne or Becker muscular dystrophy: review of 117 anesthetic exposures, *Pediatr Anesth* 23:855–864, 2013.

Stevens R: Neuromuscular disorders and anesthesia, *Curr Opin Anaesthesiol* 14:693–698, 2001.

Takagi A, Nakase H: Malignant hyperthermia-like reactions in Duchenne or Becker muscular dystrophy: review and hypothesis, *Rinsho Shinkeigaku* 48(2):101–105, 2008.

叶啉病

第 19 章

Mohamed Ehab Ramadan，*Mashhood Salahuddin*，*Hamdy Awad*

病例概要

患者，女性，36 岁，间歇性腹痛病史，拟行腹腔镜胆囊切除术。麻醉和手术都很顺利。术后第一天，患者出现烦躁不安、腹痛、呕吐等症状。生命体征：心率 124 次 / 分，血压 184/102 mmHg，体温 37.5℃，呼吸频率 20 次 / 分。护士通知值班住院医生，患者的尿液呈暗黑色。在住院医师评估过程中，患者开始抖动并发作全身抽搐，随后转入外科重症监护病房进行进一步评估和治疗。

问题分析

定义

卟啉病是一种罕见的遗传性代谢性疾病，它是由血红素生物合成过程中涉及的 8 种酶的编码基因中的任何一种突变引起的。任何一种酶的部分缺失都会导致卟啉及其前体在组织中累积，导致神经内脏和（或）皮肤表现。

卟啉病患者可能被误诊，潜在携带者可能仍然没有症状。该病最常通过常染色体显性途径传播。每个人都遗传了两个血红素合成酶基因副本。一个等位基因的突变导致酶活性下降 50%，可能完全没有症状，直到血红素合成系统在应激反应时出现严重问题（如病例概要中所述）。

识别

血红素生物合成途径的第一步和限速步骤是甘氨酸和琥珀酰辅酶 A 转化为 δ - 氨基 - γ - 酮戊酸（δ-aminolevulinic acid，ALA），ALA 由 δ - 氨基 - γ - 酮戊酸合成酶（δ-aminolevulinic acid synthase，ALAS）产生，而后者受血红素的负调节（图 19.1）。急性卟啉病是 ALAS 启动血红素合成加速，但由于其中某些酶的缺陷，卟啉及其前体在组织中累积。虽然神经病变的确切机制尚不清楚，但研究提示可能存在两种机制：卟啉累积导致神经毒性和血红素代谢紊乱影响神经元功能。

卟啉病的分类

对卟啉病提出了几种分类：

1. 根据卟啉及其前体积聚的器官不同，它们可分为**肝性**和**红细胞生成性**（骨髓）。
2. 根据其临床表现，可分为以下几类：
   a. 急性卟啉病：ALA 脱水酶（ALA dehydratase，ALAD）卟啉病，急性间歇性卟啉病（acute intermittent porphyria，AIP），遗传性粪卟啉病（hereditary coproporphyria，HC），混合性卟啉病（variegate porphyria，VP）（图 19.1）。
   b. 非急性卟啉病：先天性红细胞卟啉病（congenital erythropoietic porphyria，CEP）、迟发性卟啉病（porphyria cutanea tarda，PCT）和红细胞卟啉原卟啉病（erythropoietic protoporphyria，EP）。

在急性卟啉病中，ALAD 和 AIP 主要表现为神经内脏症状。非急性卟啉病主要表现为皮肤症状（如光敏、皮肤脆性和大疱）。HC 和 VP 可表现为急性神经内脏和皮肤表现。在所有类型中，急性卟啉病是麻醉科医师最感兴趣的。

临床表现

急性卟啉病的临床表现始于行为改变和精神异常，进而发展为感觉运动和自主神经病变：

- 烦躁不安、焦虑、失眠、抑郁；
- 疼痛：严重且不局限的腹痛，背部和四肢疼痛；
- 自主神经病变：出汗、心动过速、心律失常、高

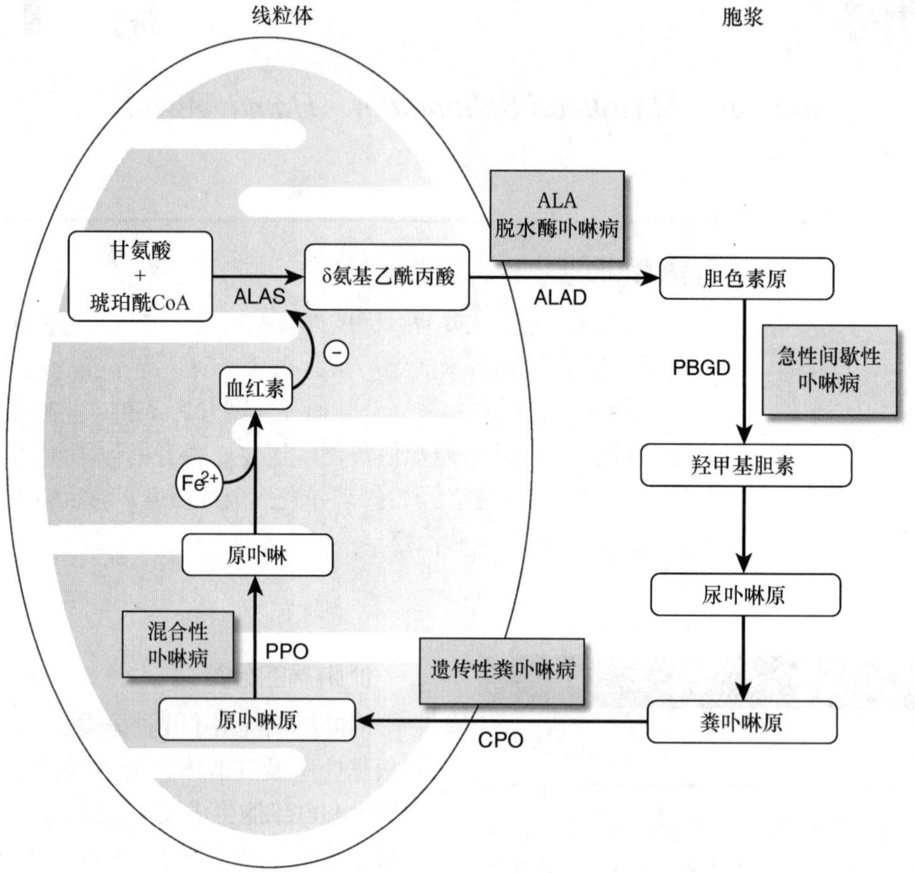

图 19.1 血红素生物合成代谢途径简化图。急性卟啉病的类型：δ-氨基-γ-酮戊酸脱水酶（ALAD）缺乏引起 ALAD 卟啉病，卟胆原脱氨酶（PBGD）缺乏引起急性间歇性卟啉病，卟啉原氧化酶（CPO）缺乏引起遗传性粪卟啉病，原卟啉原氧化酶（PPO）缺乏引起混合性卟啉病。ALA，δ 氨基-γ-酮戊酸；ALAS，δ 氨基-γ-酮戊酸合成酶；CoA，辅酶 A；Fe^{2+}，亚铁。

血压、尿潴留、恶心、呕吐、便秘（腹泻少见）；

- 运动神经病变：近端肌无力而非远端肌无力、延髓和呼吸麻痹；
- 感觉丧失：麻木和感觉异常；
- 抗利尿激素分泌不适当综合征或反复呕吐引起的低钠血症引起的意识错乱、幻觉、惊厥；
- 尿呈暗红色；
- 死亡：常见原因是心脏骤停和长时间机械通气引起的肺炎。

急性卟啉病的诊断需要对任何不明原因的急性腹痛、精神错乱和神经病变的患者保持高度的怀疑。如果误诊而不及时治疗，急性发作可能是致命的。一旦怀疑是急性卟啉病，应检查尿液以检测是否有高水平的卟啉原（porphobilinogen，PBG）和（或）ALA。PBG 水平可能高达正常水平的 10 倍。ALA 的测定对诊断并不重要，但有助于 AIP 与 ALAD 卟啉病的鉴别。粪便中卟啉水平可以帮助区分 HC 和 VP 与其他类型的急性卟啉病。此外，红细胞 PBG 脱氨酶活性也可能降低；然而，5% 的卟啉病患者的红细胞酶的表达可能正常。DNA 检测也可以检测特定的基因突变并确定卟啉病的类型。酶活性测定和 DNA 检测对急性发作的诊断没有必要，但对不确定病例的诊断和新发现病例的家庭成员筛查有帮助。

可以进行若干研究以帮助诊断相关的并发症（例如，用于检测心律失常的心电图，脑磁共振成像显示可逆的脑白质密度，类似于盲人后部可逆脑病）。

风险评估

美国只有不到 20 万例卟啉病。世界范围内，卟啉病的患病率约为（0.5 ～ 10）/10 万人，其中 30 ～ 40 岁女性占多数。然而，ALAD 卟啉病非常罕见，很少有报道病例。在 AIP 中，已经发现了超过 400 个 PGB 脱氨酶基因突变，但只有 10% ～ 20% 的携带者出现临床表现。

现已确定一些危险因素可以导致卟啉病急性发作。药物（如巴比妥类、灰黄霉素和磺胺类）、激素（雌激素和孕酮）、吸烟和饮酒诱导含血红素的肝酶细胞色素 P-450，增加有缺陷的血红素合成途径，导致卟啉的累积。此外，禁食和发烧可能会诱导血红素加氧酶（将血红素降解为胆绿素的酶），导致血红素储存的耗尽，进而增加 ALAS 活性。心理压力是引发急性发作的另一个危险因素（框 19.1）。

启示

已知的卟啉病病例应进行彻底的术前评估，并记录其神经系统状况。术前麻醉计划应旨在避免诱发急性发作的因素。在全身麻醉期间，不建议使用巴比妥酸盐、依托咪酯和氯胺酮，但可以安全地使用丙泊酚、咪达唑仑、琥珀胆碱，所有非去极化肌松药和阿片类药物。所有吸入麻醉药也被认为可以安全用药麻醉维持。

麻醉类型的选择也很重要。区域麻醉通常不是禁忌证，但在急性发作时最好避免，以防止感觉运动神经病变恶化。利多卡因、布比卡因、丁卡因、普鲁卡因和甲哌卡因被认为是安全的局麻药。表 19.1 列出了安全 / 不安全药物清单。美国卟啉基金会网站（http://www.porphyriafoundes.com/）和欧洲卟啉网络网站（http://porphyria.eu/）提供了更全面的药物清单。

管理

卟啉病患者的治疗是基于避免急性危象的触发因素。对于发生急性发作的患者，建议采取以下措施：

- 去除诱发因素。
- 镇痛药用于疼痛控制：对乙酰氨基酚或阿片类药物（如吗啡）。有些患者可能会发展成慢性疼痛，需要长期的疼痛管理。

框 19.1 可能诱发急性卟啉病的条件

肝酶细胞色素 P-450 的诱导：
- 药物（巴比妥酸盐、灰黄霉素和磺胺类药物）
- 荷尔蒙（雌激素及黄体酮）
- 吸烟
- 酒精

血红素加氧酶的诱导：
- 禁食
- 发烧

心理压力

表 19.1 可能诱发急性卟啉病的麻醉相关药物

使用 / 安全[a]	药物
请勿使用（不安全）	静脉麻醉药：巴比妥酸盐，依托咪酯，氯胺酮 吸入麻醉药：恩氟烷 支持性药物：喷他佐辛，肼屈嗪，钙通道阻滞剂，氯氮卓，酮咯酸，磺胺类
使用（安全）	静脉麻醉药：丙泊酚 吸入麻醉药：异氟烷，七氟烷，地氟烷，氟烷和氧化亚氮 苯二氮䓬类药物：地西泮，咪达唑仑 镇痛药或拮抗药：阿片类药物，阿司匹林，对乙酰氨基酚、纳洛酮 肌肉松弛药和逆转剂：琥珀胆碱，非去极化肌松药，格隆溴铵，新斯的明 局部麻醉药：利多卡因，布比卡因，丁卡因，丙胺卡因和甲哌卡因 其他支持药物：西咪替丁，雷尼替丁，昂丹司琼，硝普钠，甲氧氯普胺，可乐定，血管紧张素转换酶抑制剂，β 受体阻滞剂，氟哌利多，吩噻嗪类，阿托品，皮质类固醇，去氧肾上腺素，右美托咪定，麻黄碱

[a] 来自美国卟啉病基金会的数据（http://www. porphyriafoundation. com/，Spring 2011）和欧洲卟啉病网络的安全药物清单（http://pherolia.eu/，2015 年 4 月修订）

- 增加热量摄入，患者口服摄入或静脉输注（葡萄糖 300 ～ 500 克 / 天）。
- 对症治疗：
  - 心动过速与高血压：普萘洛尔（心得安）；
  - 恶心呕吐：氯丙嗪或丙氯丙嗪；
  - 便秘：乳果糖；
  - 癫痫发作：轻症患者用限制液体治疗低钠血症，重症患者用高渗盐水（3%），加巴喷丁长期控制。
- 血色素或精氨酸血红素：如果上述一般措施在 2 ～ 3 天内不能控制急性发作或出现严重情况（如惊厥），可静脉输注血色素或精氨酸血红素，以补充血红素储备，抑制 ALAS 酶活性。血色素的副作用包括血栓性静脉炎和凝血功能障碍。建议用血色素与白蛋白一起输注，从大静脉中输注，3 ～ 4 mg/kg，持续 30 min，每天一次，连续 4 天。精氨酸血红素是另一种制剂，但只在美国以外的地区有售。

预防

应尽量避免在围术期引发急性发作：

- 避免长时间禁食，静脉注射葡萄糖（300～500 克 / 天）。
- 术前镇静是避免心理压力的重要手段。
- 确定并避免在围术期使用不安全药物（例如，避免双氯芬酸作为镇痛剂药和甲氧氯普胺作为止吐药）。
- 应密切监测卟啉病患者是否出现延迟的急性发作，不应考虑当天手术。应每天进行详细的神经系统检查，以便早期发现神经病变。还应检查电解质，以避免低钠血症诱发抽搐。
- 避免感染和发热。对新诊断为卟啉病患者的家庭成员进行潜在卟啉病筛查，并对携带该病的人进行相关宣教。

（程　芳　译　汪　惠　校）

延伸阅读

Armen TA, Sai-Sudhakar CB, Blais D, et al.: Anesthetic management for combined double-valve and coronary artery bypass in a patient with acute intermittent porphyria, *J Cardiothorac Vasc Anesth* 23:364–368, 2009.

Besur S, Schmeltzer P, Bonkovsky HL: Acute porphyrias, *J Emerg Med* 49:305–312, 2015.

Egger NG, Lee C, Anderson KE: Disorders of heme biosynthesis. In Fernandes J, Saudubray JM, van den Berghe G, et al.: *Inborn metabolic disorders: diagnosis and treatment*, Heidelberg, 2006, Springer Medizin, pp 451–464.

Findley H, Philips A, Cole D, Nair A: Porphyrias: implications for anaesthesia, critical care, and pain medicine, *CEACCP* 12:128–133, 2012.

Herrick AL, McColl KE: Acute intermittent porphyria, *Best Pract Res Clin Gastroenterol* 19:235–249, 2005.

Hift RJ, Thunell S, Brun A: Drugs in porphyria: from observation to a modern algorithm-based system for the prediction of porphyrogenicity, *Pharmacol Ther* 132:158–169, 2011.

James MFM, Hift RJ: Porphyrias. *Br J Anaesth* 85:143–153, 2000.

Jensen NF, Fiddler DS, Striepe V: Anesthetic considerations in porphyrias, *Anesth Analg* 80:591–599, 1995.

Puy H, Gouya L, Deybach JC: Porphyrias. *Lancet* 375:924–937, 2010.

Sassa S: Modern diagnosis and management of the porphyrias, *Br J Haematol* 135:281–292, 2006.

Simon NG, Herkes GK: The neurologic manifestations of the acute porphyrias, *J Clin Neurosci* 18:1147–1153, 2011.

Tracy JA, Dyck PJB: Porphyria and its neurologic manifestations. In José B, José MF, editors: *Handbook of clinical neurology*. Philadelphia, Elsevier, 2014, pp 839–849.

麻醉前评估：假阳性检查 第20章

Jeffrey W. Lee，*Scott R. Springman*

病例概要

患者，男性，25岁，是一名运动员，拟行膝前十字韧带修复术。患者近期无用药史，其个人和家族史中无凝血异常、出血或易挫伤淤血。患者行凝血酶原时间和部分凝血活酶时间（partial thromboplastin time，PTT）在内的多项检测，其PTT结果超过正常值。患者手术被推迟，并进行更完善的血液学检查。最终报告显示，该患者为“正常变异，无凝血缺陷”。

问题分析

定义

只有当达到临床医师（和患者）能够理解一项检查的阳性或阴性结果的程度，该检查才有价值。几乎没有任何检查能正确识别出所有患者是否患病。只有当临床医师明确了解检查的特点，以及应用于特定患者群体的统计预测值时，才能决定如何正确处理“阳性”或“阴性”检查结果。这种“医疗决策分析”直接影响到患者的临床治疗。

部分检查提供了阳性或阴性的二元定性结果。然而，大多数检查结果都是定量的，围绕某一平均值定义了一系列“正常”值。因此，人群中总会有人出现“异常”的检测结果，但其实并未患病。这意味着，检查结果可能因人口的自然变异性而具有一定的误导性。

检查可能由于不准确（inaccuracy）、不精确（imprecision）或操作不当（incorrect performance）而导致错误的结果。**准确性**是指该检查结果的平均值与真实值（遵循金标准得出的结果）的差异。**精确性**是指执行检查的仪器或人员所得到结果的可重复性。**操作不当**的检查可使任何检查结果无效。

准确性

试验的准确性可从以下方面描述。检查的**敏感度**是指患病的个体被准确识别并判定为阳性的比例。检查的**特异度**是指没有疾病的个体被准确识别并判定为阴性的比例。假阳性结果更可能出现在敏感度高、特异度低或两者兼有的检查中。敏感度和特异度是检查所固有的特征，不会随疾病在人群中的患病率（频率）而改变。换言之，检查的敏感度和特异度并不影响患者罹患某一疾病的概率。

预测值

相比之下，检测的**预测值**取决于疾病在人群中的流行程度。检查结果的阳性预测值，是指在检查为阳性的全部患者中，真正罹患某病的例数（真阳性）所占的比例。通常情况下，检查的预测值表示为某一情形存在的概率（probability）或几率（odds）。

似然比（likelihood ratios）表示给定检查结果后出现概率发生的程度（表20.1）。此时，需引出一个重要的概念即贝叶斯定理，它“在基于某种属性（例如异常检查结果）存在时，某个体（如患者）是否属于某一特定群体（如临床分级）的概率，与具有该属性的已知成员的概率及从该群体中随机选取某一个体的概率的关系联系起来。”它允许随着新信息（如检查结果）的出现而计算出疾病的概率变化。“后验”概率发现的疾病可用Fagan列线图估计，如图20.1所示。以下网址可查阅网络交互式Fagan列

表 20.1 试验准确性和预测值

	基于金标准检查的目标疾病		
诊断结果	有疾病	无疾病	出现该结果的患者数量
阳性	a	b	a+b
阴性	c	d	c+d
总计	a+c	b+d	

1. a/（a+c）= 敏感度。患病且检查阳性的患者人数除以患病的患者总人数。敏感度高的检查很少错失真正患有此疾病的患者。
2. d/（b+d）= 特异度。不患病且检查阴性的患者人数除以不患病的患者总人数。特异度高的检查很少将不患病的患者诊断为患病。
3. a/（a+b）= 阳性预测值，或在阳性检查结果患者中诊断为目标疾病的后测概率。
4. d/（c+d）= 阴性预测值，或在阴性检查结果患者中没有诊断为目标疾病的后测概率。
5. c/（c+d）= 阴性检查结果的患者诊断为目标疾病的后测概率。
6.（a+c）/（a+b+c+d）= 目标疾病的患病率或预测率。
7. 敏感度 /（1- 特异度）= 阳性检查结果的似然比（有目标疾病的）=［a/（a+c）］/［b/（b+d）］。
8.（1- 敏感度）/ 特异度 = 阴性试验结果的似然比（有目标疾病的）=［c/（a+c）］/［d/（b+d）］。
9. 目标疾病的后测概率（用概率表示）= 目标疾病的预测概率（用概率表示）× 试验结果的似然比。
10. 几率 = 概率 /［1- 概率］。
11. a= 真阳性检查（TP），b= 假阳性检查（FP），c= 假阴性检查（FN），d = 真正态检查（TN）。

Adapted from Sackett DL：A primer on the precision and accuracy of the clinical examination. *JAMA* 267（19）：2638-2644，1992.

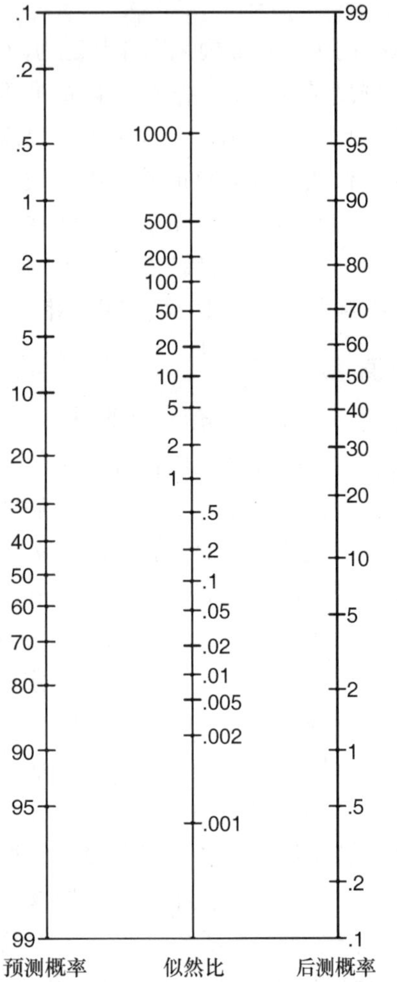

图 20.1 通过似然比从预测概率画线图，确定后测概率
［Adapted from Fagan TJ：Nomogram for Bayes theorem（letter）. *N Engl J Med* 293（5）：257，1975.］

线图 http://araw.mede.uic.edu/cgi-bin/testcalc.pl。此外，还有针对智能手机和平板电脑的移动应用程序、计算机软件用于计算 Bayesian 分析。Fagan 列线图“两步法”通过增加诊断敏感度和特异度，简化了估计值。其方法可在 http://www.adelaide.edu.au/vetsci/research/pub_pop/2step-nomog/ 上查阅。

识别

如果未正确实施检查，即便检查结果阳性实际上也可能是错误的。换言之，假设正确实施某检查，并非金标准的检查所得到的结果也可能错误提示该个体患病。最后，由于人群的变异性，即使金标准的检查所得到的阳性结果（超出“正常”范围），也可能提示该个体为临床正常。

风险评估

如果我们假设正确地实施检查，且其精确度高，则该检查的准确性和疾病的流行率是决定该检查结果是否“正确”的主要因素。接受多次检查的患者，可能至少有一次结果为假阳性，尤其当受检查患者的人群患病率较低时。当无症状患者接受大量术前筛查检查时，这种情况经常发生。

启示

在术前，检查假阳性可能导致对患者的诊断及治疗产生困惑。检查假阳性可能导致手术延迟或取消。医师通常重复进行检查，希望假阳性结果是由操作不当造成，或选择其他检查来证实诊断。然而，这两种选择均增加不必要的成本并导致时间浪费。此外，如果额外检查为有创的，会增加患者身体受到伤害的风险。然而，如果择期手术没有延误，而检查结果并非假阳性，医师可能面临专业审查或医疗诉讼风险，除非能证明进行手术是合理的。围术期管理中任一不必要的改变，均可能增加患者治疗成本和风险。最后，如果行丙型肝炎或人类免疫缺陷病毒筛检的个体出现假阳性结果，可能会对患者个体及筛检者造成一定的心理压力。

管理

决定认可某检查结果"真实可靠"，必须取决于充分了解该检查的特点和不足，还取决于相关患者群体对检测疾病发生率的了解程度。应对每个检查结果进行核验，以确定是否符合患者的真实情况。若不照此进行且没有确凿结果，则可能需要进一步检查，方可认为结果是真实的。在许多情况下，对于单一的阳性结果，应怀疑其真实性，除非所行检查的特异度高或疾病发生率高，或两者兼有。

预防

显然，将检查假阳性结果可能性降至最低的最佳方法是避免不必要的检查。筛检者过度进行术前检查是常见现象，但应根据患者具体情况谨慎安排。患者年龄、个人和家族史、症状和体征及手术类型，都可能决定了检查的适应证。筛检是否适当，应考虑当前科学研究及地方、全国医学专家的意见等。如需要进行筛检，选择特异度高的检查也可减少假阳性结果的数量。使用 Bayesian 评价工具有助于提高某一检查结果并非在所有人群均相似的临床认识，但这种评价方法十分复杂，且需进行主观的价值判断。使用成本效益和风险效益分析，可能也有助于决定是否应进行某一检查。此外，合理的检查方案应只包括可能改变患者围术期管理的检查。

（王家强　译　薄禄龙　译）

延伸阅读

Apfelbaum JL, Connis RT, Nickinovich DG, et al.: American Society of Anesthesiologists: Practice Advisory for Preanesthesia Evaluation: an updated report by the American Society of Anesthesiologists Task Force on Preanesthesia Evaluation, *Anesthesiology* 116(3):522–538, 2012. 116.

Attia J: Moving beyond sensitivity and specificity: using likelihood ratios to interpret diagnostic tests, *Aust Prescr* 26:111–113, 2003.

Baez A: Bayesian approach to clinical decision making (audio podcast). Available at https://vimeo.com/111380685. Accessed January 1, 2016.

Bayes MJ: Medical diagnostics and nomograms. Stanford University video. Available at http://youtu.be/7VTQ1glcXYg. Accessed January 1, 2016.

Berwick DM: Screening in health fairs. A critical review of benefits, risks, and costs, *JAMA* 254(11):1492–1498, 1985.

Caraguel CG, Vanderstichel R: The two-step Fagan's nomogram: ad hoc interpretation of a diagnostic test result without calculation, *Evid Based Med* 18(4):125–128, 2013.

Chen CL, Lin GA, Bardach NS, et al.: Preoperative medical testing in Medicare patients undergoing cataract surgery, *N Engl J Med* 372(16):1530–1538, 2015.

Grimmes DA, Schulz KF: Refining clinical diagnosis with likelihood ratios, *Lancet* 365:1500–1505, 2005.

Kachalia A, Berg A, Fagerlin A, et al.: Overuse of testing in preoperative evaluation and syncope, *Ann Int Med* 162(2):100–108, 2015.

Kirkham KR, Wijeysundera DN, Pendrith C, et al.: Preoperative laboratory investigations: rates and variability prior to low-risk surgical procedures, *Anesthesiology* 124(4):804–814, 2016.

Pasternak LR: Preoperative laboratory testing: general issues and considerations, *Anesthesiol Clin North Am* 22:13–25, 2004.

Rusk MH. Avoiding unnecessary preoperative testing, *Med Clin North Am* 100(5):1003–1008, 2016.

Sackett DL: A primer on the precision and accuracy of the clinical examination, *JAMA* 267:2638–2644, 1992.

第 21 章 检查结果不充分或缺失

Jeffrey W. Lee，*Scott R. Springman*

病例概要 1

患者，男性，64 岁，运动耐量较低，既往有高血压、肥胖，不定时间发作腹上区不适入院，拟行择期开腹结肠部分切除术。术前未检查心电图。患者后来在围术期发生继发于未确诊的冠状动脉疾病导致的心肌梗死。

病例概要 2

患者，女性，73 岁，目前正在服用多种利尿药物，拟行择期髋关节置换术。该患者在外院进行了生化及电解质检查，并将结果传真到外科医师的办公室。手术当天传真无法查阅，外科医师讨论认为有必要进行复查，最终检测到血浆钠含量为 124 mEq/L，手术被推迟。

问题分析

定义

通过了解检查结果以及漏检所带来的影响，有助于有效地选择术前检查。以下为 4 个重要的不利影响：

1. 医务人员或患者对检测重要性的误解；
2. 针对检查结果未处理或处理方式错误，导致的不良医疗事件；
3. 增加了检查、复查、后续检查或操作的医疗成本；
4. 因上述原因引起的诉讼。

仅通过术前检查的结果并不能保证良好的预后。检测的准确性和有效性取决于其本身的敏感性、特异性及疾病发生率。此外，将特定患者患病概率考虑在内，可增加测试的效用。

识别

未被推广、未被评估分析或不易进行的检查不建议应用于临床诊疗。确定某项特定的检查是否有明确的适应证较为困难。事后的认知可能不满足术前的实际需要。只有设计良好的临床研究和逻辑分析才能为临床医师提供循证医学的指导。

风险评估

如果由于疏忽、询问病史和体格检查不充分、指南依据不足或为减少医疗成本而未进行必要的检查，患者将面临不良结果带来的风险。即便完成了相关检查，但检查的结果不能查阅、丢失或者是在麻醉实施前医师没有再次回顾检查结果，也会造成医疗过程的失败。根据患者的病史和身体状况，缺乏恰当的术前检查可能会使患者面临更高的不良结局的风险。然而，健康患者接受常规手术时不需要复杂术前检查，甚至根本不需要进行术前检查。

启示

如果没有按要求做术前检查，患者的预后可能会受影响。例如患者的血钙水平略有升高或轻微贫血，对于大多数手术来说，不会出现不良后果。

然而，如果患者患有严重的、未被发现的冠状动脉疾病，围术期发生心肌梗死，则需要更多的医疗护理、更长的住院时间、更高额的住院费用，以及可能导致长期残疾或死亡。此外，医务人员的情绪、专业、经济和医疗法律风险也将增加。

术前发现的异常检查结果如何指导基本或特殊治疗以改善患者健康，虽然并不在文的讨论范畴，但却很重要。

管理

如果在择期手术麻醉开始前发现检查缺失，那么麻醉科医师和外科医师必须明确是否有院内外规定必须进行这项检查。如果是必需的检查，应补齐，或者医师必须在医疗记录中注明为什么他们愿意在没有检查结果的情况下进行麻醉或手术。对于突发意外或急诊手术，医师应始终权衡补做检查的预期收益和推迟手术的风险。

如果麻醉或手术开始后发现检查缺失，医务人员必须确定此时补做检查，其结果是否有差别，或者是否应该终止手术（幸运的是，这种情况很少发生）。如果缺失的检查仅在术后治疗中需要，并且检查的目的与术前检查相同，可以在麻醉的过程中进行检查。然而，如果一项术前检查结果对手术或麻醉方案有重大影响，则不能等到手术麻醉过程后补做。例如在椎管内麻醉前，发现凝血酶原时间延长的情况。

如果在手术后发现某项检查缺失，是否需要补做检查呢？如果这项检查结果会改变术后或长期的医疗管理，那么补做检查可能是明智之选。

预防

遵循价值的医疗

如果检查缺失导致不良结果，则应重新审视体系制度，以防止再次发生。在确定因果关系时应谨慎行事。不良的结局不一定意味着需要更多的预防性检查。我们必须考虑检查是否真的会对患者结局产生影响。此外，应权衡短期和长期收益与检查潜在的有害影响。这与价值导向的麻醉服务理念是一致的。可能需要复杂的成本效益分析，时间在医疗方面有实际价值，从长远来看，一项昂贵的检查较成本低但耗时更长的检查，可能总的成本更低。

循证医疗

理想情况下，所有的检查都应该按照循证医学的原则进行。关于术前评估的文章很多，但很少有文章引用足够严谨的证据为所有的患者提供确切的答案。最近，美国麻醉科医师协会工作组的一份最新报告再次发现，除了主要基于仔细询问病史和体格检查的医疗实践之外，尚无足够的科学研究结果来支持术前检测的具体方案。

术前重点检查

充分了解病史和体格检查是为了明确术前检查的重点。然而，许多症状或体征可能敏感性高，但并不是特异性高的指标。观察者之间的变异度通常很高。此外，病史的价值还取决于既往病历的充分程度以及患者提供病史的可靠性和沟通技巧。充分的病史或合理的检查也不一定能预测某些疾病的不良结果，特别是出血。而有一些检查，如低钠血症，则可能与较差的结局相关。

美国麻醉科医师协会术前评估指南声明如下：

术前检查作为麻醉前评估的一个组成部分，可用于各种目的（包括但不限于）：①发现或识别可能影响围术期麻醉的疾病或功能障碍；②对已知的可能影响围术期麻醉的疾病、功能障碍、药物或者替代治疗方法进行确认或者评估；③制定围术期麻醉的具体方案和替代方案。

选择性和非选择性检查

大多数术前检查方案可分为非选择性检查和选择性检查两个部分。前者要求即使没有症状，也要对每位患者进行检查或筛查。过去这种方法很常用，但现在不推荐使用。选择性检查要求使用特定的标准来确定检查的必要性。

- **患者因素**。包括但不限于：症状、年龄、既往病史、性别和体格检查。其他因素，如获得可靠病史或进行仔细检查的能力，也应予以考虑。
- **手术类型**。手术本身会导致患者的解剖或生理紊乱，因此需要获得其基础值作为参考标准。

然而，一些手术的风险很低，很少会发生心脏或其他（非手术）并发症。比如眼科手术，只要患者病情稳定，大多数术前检查没有意义。一些人建议取消大多数门诊手术的术前检查。随着门诊患者的并存疾病越来越多，门诊手术越来越复杂，某些类型的门诊手术取消术前检查可能并不合适。

那些对患者生理功能影响大的更复杂的手术需要检查作为基准来追踪围术期的改变。需要谨慎地安排检查，并仔细根据检查结果分析原因。

实践指南

医学机构对**临床实践指南**的定义如下："临床实践指南为一项申明，通过对证据的系统性回顾以及对替代治疗方案的利弊进行评估而获得治疗推荐，目的在于优化患者的治疗。"理想情况下，指南应该以高质量的研究为基础，并遵循与美国心脏病学会（American College of Cardiology）方法类似的原则。由于缺乏严格的结局性研究，标准往往以地方和国家的专家意见和经验为基础。原则或指南需要不断更新，以增加其可信度；地方共识亦有绝对的必要。指南可能有经验性成分在内，也可能来自于复杂且广泛的共识。经典指南包括2016年英国国立健康与临床优化研究所（NICE）指南和美国国立指南库围术期指南。美国心脏病学会/美国心脏协会2014年更新的指南提到可按病史的严重程度和体格检查为标准，判断是否有心脏检查的必要性。以后会越来越多地使用筛选性生化标志物，如B型利尿钠肽（B-type natriuretic peptide，BNP）或高敏肌钙蛋白测定来对围术期心脏风险进行分级。

许多指南只是简单地推荐"根据病史和体检的需要"进行检查。然而，这种非指导性的指南也许会导致检查超过或者不满足实际需要特别是如果非麻醉科医师负责安排检查。指南也许会减少不适当的检查，一项调查发现临床医师经常安排超越指南建议的检查来消除患者或自己的疑虑。

重要的是，我们有充分的理由来省去无适应证的检查。即使检查不需要任何花费，但进一步的检查、不恰当地改变病程管理、给麻醉科医师和外科医师一种虚假的安全感，甚至会转移对更重要问题的关注，这些都会对患者造成伤害。做一些术前本无计划的检查，毫无医学意义，并具有法律风险。

2012年美国麻醉科医师协会术前评估指南推荐根据患者和手术因素进行检查，而不是进行无症状的筛查。引用前文提到的关于病例研究的指南："有报道显示，在无症状或非选择性患者中，约有0.06%～21.2%的患者凝血功能有异常（包括出血时间、凝血酶原时间、部分凝血酶原时间或血小板计数），其中只有0.0～4.0%的患者因发现异常需要取消或改变治疗方案（B2类证据）。"虽然不能确定在已发表的凝血检查研究中，治疗过程中检查报告的变化对治疗结局的影响多频繁，但在没有特定适应证时进行凝血检查并不常见。

近期，为减少不必要的医疗干预做出的努力包括有许多专业协会参与"明智选择"倡议。美国麻醉科医师协会的两项相关声明列于框21.1中。

简单地说，实践指南是很好的参考起点。在决策过程中必须将患者的并存疾病、自述病史、既往病历信息以及手术的类型和范围纳入考虑因素。

麻醉前评估门诊，术前计算机评估系统，围术期外科之家

麻醉前评估门诊可以为术前检查和术前准备提供系统、合理、经济有效、流程化的方法。随着时间的推移，许多术前门诊已经不需要每个患者都来诊所。结构良好的纸质或计算机化的术前评估系统以及电话访视等，都是有用的工具，可增强患者的数据采集、减少不必要的或错过的术前访视。此外，采用集成决策支持的电子病历可大大提高术前评估及检查的质量和可行性。在计算机支持下规范化标准更加统一。这些标准的价值几乎可与人的逻辑相媲美。在实行术前门诊评估和有序的检查后，麻醉科医师浏览患者的评估时会更及时、方便、完整和有效。

随着大型医疗数据库在分析患者预后和风险评估的应用，术前检查的预测性分析将会更加有用。数据分析在依靠群体数据建模中效果很好，但却不能很好地预测单个患者的风险。这也是多数人认为在普通（和围术期）医疗服务中指南和计算机分析

框 21.1　美国麻醉科医师协会"明智选择"倡议

1. 无严重系统性疾病（ASA Ⅰ或Ⅱ）的低危手术患者，在预计失血（或液体交换）较少时，可不做术前基础检查，特别是全血细胞计数、基本或全面的生化检查，或凝血试验。
2. 对于已知心脏疾病（如冠状动脉疾病、瓣膜疾病）病情稳定且无症状的患者，在进行低中危的非心脏手术时，不需进行基础诊断性心脏检查（经胸/食管超声心动图）或心脏应激测试。

Adapted from American Society of Anesthesiologists：Five things physicians and patients should question. Choosing Wisely Initiative. October 2013. Retrieved from http://www.choosingwisely.org/societies/american-society-of-anesthesiologists/. Accessed May 9，2016.

并不能代替医师的原因之一。

优化术前评估过程的关键步骤在于：回顾现有的检查指南，并就检查的适应证、检查的时机、谁安排检查以及谁负责审阅检查结果取得地区性共识。麻醉科医师作为围术期手术之家的一部分，参与围术期治疗，并对术前检查和术前准备产生实质性的影响。

最后，1954 年 Asher 所写仍然正确。临床医师应该经常问自己这些问题：

1. 为什么要做这个检查？
2. 要从结果中寻找什么？
3. 如果发现问题，会影响我的诊断吗？
4. 这将如何影响我对该病例的处理？
5. 最终会使我的患者受益吗？

（赵晗燚 译 李 博 校）

延伸阅读

Apfelbaum JL, Connis RT, Nickinovich DG, et al.: Practice advisory for preanesthesia evaluation: an updated report by the American Society of Anesthesiologists Task Force on Preanesthesia Evaluation, *Anesthesiology* 116(3):522–538, 2012. 116.

Asher R: Straight and crooked thinking in medicine, *Br Med J* 2:460–462, 1954.

Bader AM, Sweitzer B, Kumar A: Nuts and bolts of preoperative clinics: the view from three institutions, *Cleve Clin J Med* 76(Suppl 4):S104–S111, 2009.

Card R, Sawyer M, Degnan B, et al.: *Perioperative protocol.* Bloomington, MN. Retrieved from http://www.guideline.gov/content.aspx?id = 48408, 2014. Accessed January 2, 2016.

Chen CL, Lin GA, Bardach NS, et al.: Preoperative medical testing in Medicare patients undergoing cataract surgery, *N Engl J Med* 372(16):1530–1538, 2015.

Chung F, Yuan H, Yin L, et al.: Elimination of preoperative testing in ambulatory surgery, *Anesth Analg* 108(2):467–475, 2009.

Dexter F, Wachtel RE: Strategies for net cost reductions with the expanded role and expertise of anesthesiologists in the perioperative surgical home, *Anesth Analg* 118(5):1062–1071, 2014.

Dhesi JK, Swart M: Specialist pre-operative assessment clinics, *Anaesthesia* 71:3–8, 2016.

Fleisher LA, Fleischmann KE, Auerbach AD, et al.: ACC/AHA guideline on perioperative cardiovascular evaluation and management of patients undergoing noncardiac surgery: executive summary: a report of the American College of Cardiology/American Heart Association Task Force on Practice Guidelines, *Circulation* 130(24):2215–2245, 2014.

Fritsch G, Flamm M, Hepner DL, et al.: Abnormal pre-operative tests, pathologic findings of medical history, and their predictive value for perioperative complications, *Acta Anaesthesiol Scand* 56(3):339–350, 2012.

Gabriel P, Mazoit X, Ecoffey C: Relationship between clinical history, coagulation tests, and perioperative bleeding during tonsillectomies in pediatrics, *J Clin Anesth* 12(4):288–291, 2000.

Houry S, Georgeac C, Hay JM, et al.: A prospective multicenter evaluation of preoperative hemostatic screening tests, *Am J Surg* 170(1):19–23, 1995.

Institute of Medicine Committee on Standards for Developing Trustworthy Clinical Practice Guidelines. In Graham, editor: *Clinical practice guidelines we can trust,* Washington, DC, 2011, National Academies Press.

Jacobs AK, Anderson JL, Halperin JL: The evolution and future of ACC/AHA Clinical Practice Guidelines: a 30-year journey. A report of the American College of Cardiology/American Heart Association Task Force on Practice Guidelines, *Circulation* 130(14):1208–1217, 2014.

Kachalia A, Berg A, Fagerlin A, et al.: Overuse of testing in preoperative evaluation and syncope: a survey of hospitalists, *Ann Int Med* 162(2):100–108, 2015.

Katz RI, Dexter F, Rosenfeld K, et al.: Survey study of anesthesiologists' and surgeons' ordering of unnecessary preoperative laboratory tests, *Anesth Analg* 112(1):207–212, 2011.

Leung AA, McAlister FA, Rogers Jr SO, et al.: Preoperative hyponatremia and perioperative complications, *Arch Intern Med* 172(19):1474–1481, 2012.

McKinney B, Harvey E: Preoperative investigation of the surgical patient, *Surgery (Oxford)* 29(3):115–117, 2011.

NHS National Institute for Health and Care Excellence (NICE): *Routine preoperative tests for elective surgery,* 2016. Retrieved from https://www.nice.org.uk/guidance/ng45 . Accessed March 5, 2017.

Pasternak LR: Preoperative testing: moving from individual testing to risk management, *Anesth Analg* 108(2):393–394, 2009.

Sniderman AD, D'Agostino Sr RB, Pencina MJ: The role of physicians in the era of predictive analytics, *JAMA* 314(1):25–26, 2015.

Yen C, Tsai M, Macario A: Preoperative evaluation clinics, *Curr Opin Anaesthesiol* 23(2):167–172, 2010.

第22章 术前心脏干预

Lee A. Fleisher

病例概要

患者，男性，65岁，因非梗阻性恶性肿瘤入院接受结肠切除术。患者4个月前因心肌梗死置入了药物洗脱支架，自置入支架后无任何症状。患者目前服用氯吡格雷和阿司匹林，同时阿替洛尔治疗高血压。手术定于7天后。

药物洗脱支架患者的麻醉管理是麻醉科医师、外科医师和心脏病专家面临的主要挑战。自从采用经皮冠状动脉介入放置冠脉支架后，文献中出现了一系列支架血栓形成的病例报告。术前已置入冠状动脉支架患者的关键问题是手术最佳时机和抗血小板药物的管理。具体来说，考虑到支架血栓形成的风险与围术期出血增加的风险，是否应继续使用或停用这些药物？众所周知，冠状动脉支架的急性血栓会导致心肌梗死和潜在的死亡风险。

问题分析

当已放置药物洗脱支架的患者进行手术时，术前的关键决定是应该何时进行手术（即，在放置支架后延迟多长时间）和抗血小板治疗的管理。2016年，美国心脏病学会/美国心脏协会临床实践指南工作组（the American College of Cardiology/American Heart Association Task Force on Clinical Practice Guidelines）发布了关于冠状动脉疾病患者双重抗血小板治疗持续时间的“重点更新”。由于还没有包括桥接疗法在内的最佳围术期策略的随机试验，因此这些建议是基于非手术环境的随机试验和外科患者的队列研究。第二个因素是基于药物洗脱支架升级产生的抗血小板药物管理的变化。更新一代支架需要抗血小板治疗时间更短，因为其血栓形成倾向更低。关键问题是根据支架置入时间、再内皮化及不同抗血小板药物的应用等，来平衡在双重抗血小板治疗下手术出血的风险对血栓及发生心肌梗死的风险。介入心脏病专家还会将支架位置的解剖纳入考虑以决定最佳治疗方案。

定义

对一个有冠状动脉支架置入史的非心脏手术患者，关键要确定①冠脉支架的指征，②冠脉支架的类型（第一代或第二代），③目前的抗血小板治疗，④手术的紧迫性。

识别

虽然冠状动脉支架患者的术前准备工作是主要关注点，但术中识别和治疗支架内血栓形成也很重要。术中或术后冠状动脉支架内血栓形成与围术期其他心肌梗死表现相似，但更可能表现为ST段抬高而不是压低。

支架内血栓形成受累心肌的范围可能很大，因此可能表现为血流动力学变化并可能导致心力衰竭。

管理

证据

一些报告表明，与那些有冠状动脉疾病和非近期支架置入患者相比，药物洗脱支架在较长时间内（最长12个月）可能存在额外风险，特别是如果中断使用抗血小板药物。Schouten小组回顾性评估了192例因不稳定冠状动脉疾病成功进行经皮冠状动脉介入治疗（percutaneous coronary intervention，PCI）后2年内接受非心脏手术的患者。药物洗脱支架占放置支架的52%。在192例患者中，30例患者在建议可中断对特定支架的双重抗血小板治疗期限（金属裸支架 30 天，西罗莫司洗脱支架 6 个月）前接受了手术。对于在必需使用氯吡格雷时间之前（早期手术组）就停止抗血小板治疗的患者，死亡或非致死性心肌梗死（myocardial infarction，MI）的发生率为 30.7%，而持续抗血小板治疗的患者为 0%。然而，支架血栓形成和心血管事件升高的风险似乎随着时间的推移而降低。在药物洗脱支架和缺血性事件评估（the Evaluation of Drug-Eluting Stents and Ischemic Events，EVENT）登记的 4637 例连续患者中，4.4% 的患者在 1 年内接受了非心脏大手术。他们报告手术后 1 周内心血管事件发生率相对于支架置入术后其他任何 1 周增加了 27 倍，但绝对发生率仅为 1.9%。

Wijeysundera 及其同事对加拿大安大略市接受非心脏手术的 8116 例患者进行了评估，发现 34% 的患者在手术前 2 年内置入了冠状动脉支架。药物洗脱支架占放置支架的三分之一。术前 45 天内置入金属裸支架的患者心血管事件发生率为 6.7%，术前 45 ～ 180 天置入的发生率降至 2.6%。置入药物洗脱支架的患者在前 45 天手术有 20.2% 的心血管事件发生率，而当支架置入超过术前 180 天时，心血管事件发生率与无支架患者相似。Bangalore 及同事研究了马萨诸塞州 8415 例患者术前放置药物洗脱支架（drug-eluting stent，DES）与金属裸支架（bare-metal stent，BMS）相比的影响。在这一队列研究中，PCI 术后前 30 天的死亡、MI 和出血事件率为 8.6%，冠状动脉血管重建术后 90 天以上进行手术则降至 5.2%。采用倾向匹配（propensity matching）比较 BMS 和 DES 人群，BMS 队列中的死亡和 MI 率较高。在一项整个苏格兰的回顾性队列分析中，支架置入后 6 周内围术期死亡和缺血性心脏事件比 6 周后更常见，分别为 42.4% 和 12.8%。该队列中 45% 的血管重建是为了治疗急性冠状动脉综合征，增加了该队列的基线风险。6 周内因急性冠状动脉综合征进行血管重建患者的事件发生率更高，达到 65%。与其他报告相对照，BMS 组和 DES 组之间没有显著的时间差异。最近的大型观察性研究的数据表明，无论支架类型（BMS 或 DES）如何，支架血栓形成风险增加的时间范围约为 6 个月。来自退伍军人健康管理局医院患者的一项大型队列研究中，支架置入术后 6 个月手术风险增加最明显的是那些 PCI 指征为 MI 的患者。在使用佐他莫司洗脱支架治疗的稳定型冠状动脉疾病或低风险急性冠状动脉综合征的非手术患者中，3 个月的双重抗血小板治疗与 12 个月治疗相比，心脏转归没有差异。相比之下，与单用阿司匹林治疗相比，放置药物支架后超过 1 年的双重抗血小板治疗显著降低了支架血栓形成和主要心血管及脑血管不良事件的风险，但与出血风险增加有关。

围术期处理指南

截至 2016 年的建议见表 22.1。支架置入 6 个月后可以安全实施手术，如果延迟手术的风险大于支架血栓形成的风险，可以考虑在支架置入后 3 个月进行。理想情况下，双重抗血小板治疗应持续至少 6 个月，然后继续应用阿司匹林。非心脏手术的时机如图 22.1 所示。外科医师、麻醉科医师和心脏病专家之间的积极讨论是最佳策略，但并非总是可行。

表 22.1 围术期管理的推荐—PCI 和 DAPT 治疗患者择期非心脏手术的时机

推荐级别	推荐内容
Ⅰ	择期非心脏手术应延迟到 BMS 置入 30 天后，最好在 DES 置入 6 个月后
Ⅰ	冠状动脉支架置入术后接受 DAPT 治疗的患者如必须接受外科手术且要求中断 $P2Y_{12}$ 抑制剂治疗，推荐尽可能继续服用阿司匹林，并在手术后尽快重新开始 $P2Y_{12}$ 血小板受体抑制剂
Ⅱ a	当目前服用 $P2Y_{12}$ 抑制剂的患者需要进行非心脏手术时，应由参与治疗的医生共同对手术相关风险和中断或持续抗血小板治疗做出决定
Ⅱ b	如果进一步延迟手术的风险大于支架血栓形成的预期风险，对于患者置入 DES 后需要停用 $P2Y_{12}$ 抑制剂治疗的择期非心脏手术可在 3 个月后考虑
Ⅲ	在 BMS 置入后 30 天内或在 DES 置入后 3 个月内，不应实施围术期需中断 DAPT 的择期非心脏手术

BMS，金属裸支架；DAPT，双重抗血小板治疗；DES，药物洗脱支架；PCI，经皮冠状动脉介入治疗

Adapted from Levine GN，Bates ER，Bittl JA，et al：2016 ACC/AHA guideline focused update on duration of dual antiplatelet therapy in patients with coronary artery disease：a report of the American College of Cardiology/American Heart Association Task Force on Clinical Practice Guidelines. *J Am Coll Cardiol* 68（10）：1082-1115，2016.

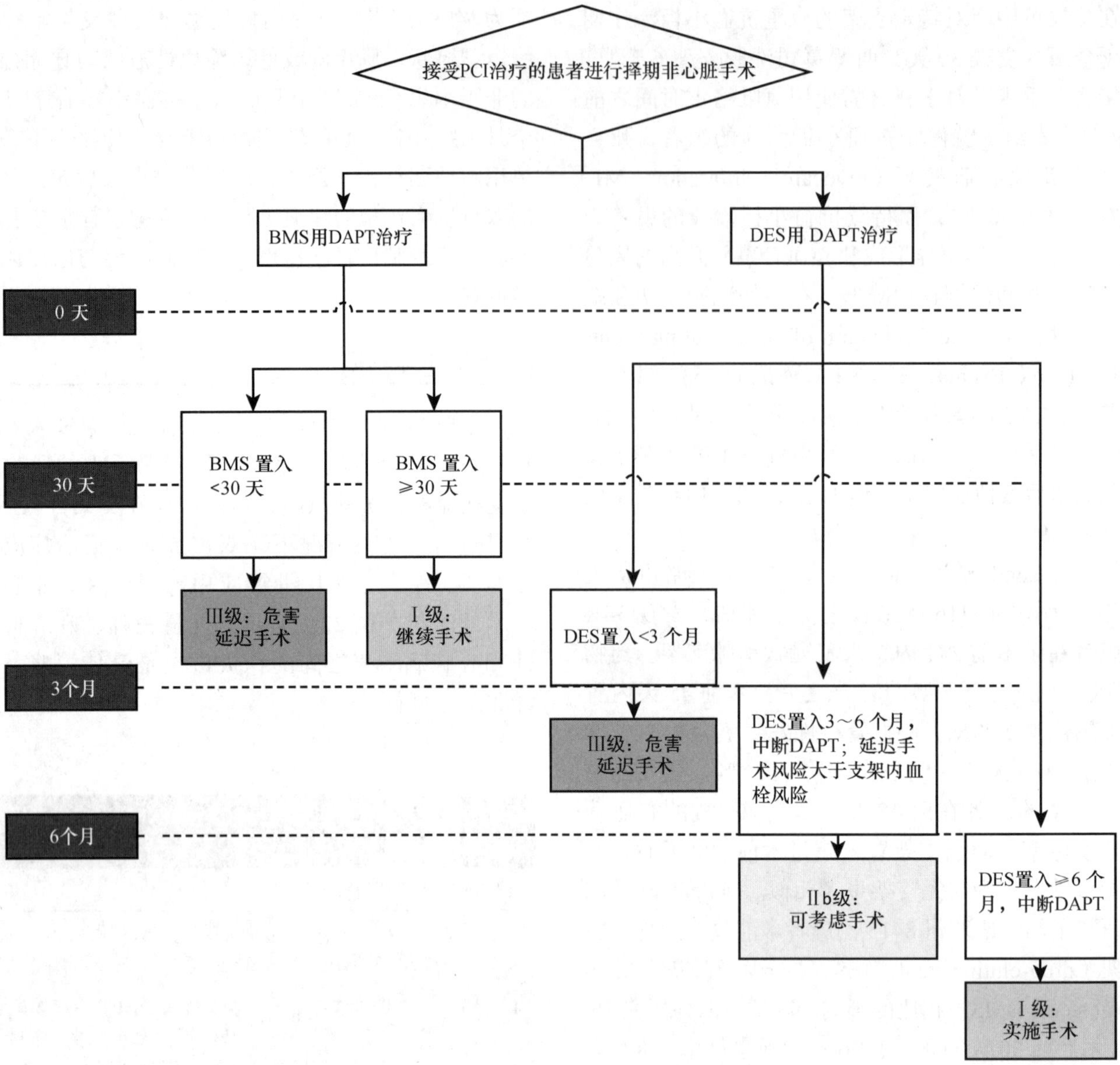

图 22.1 冠状动脉支架患者择期非心脏手术时机的判断原则。灰色底纹对应于推荐类别。BMS，金属裸支架；DAPT，双重抗血小板治疗；DES，药物洗脱支架；PCI，经皮冠状动脉介入治疗（From Levine GN，Bates ER，Bittl JA，et al：2016 ACC/AHA guideline focused update on duration of dual antiplatelet therapy in patients with coronary artery disease：a report of the American College of Cardiology/American Heart Association Task Force on Clinical Practice Guidelines. *J Am Coll Cardiol* 68［10］：1082-1115，2016.）

支架内血栓形成的处理

支架内血栓形成的最佳治疗包括与所有含抗血栓剂治疗相关的出血风险。如果推测诊断为支架内血栓，应立即将患者送往导管室进行血管造影，并尝试打通已形成血栓的支架。

预防

建议静脉注射一种短效糖蛋白Ⅱb/Ⅲa抑制剂作为双重抗血小板治疗患者手术的桥接。在一项对515 例患者进行的回顾性队列研究中，对有冠状动脉支架的手术患者行低分子肝素桥接在 30 天导致更差的缺血结局和显著的出血风险。在另一项小型回顾性连续队列研究中，使用替罗非班的围术期桥接治疗与 30 天主要不良心脏事件（major adverse cardiac event，MACE）发生率降低相关，尤其是在支架置入后 60 天内进行手术时。目前，不推荐使用肝素桥接治疗，因为风险增加且缺乏疗效。关于短效糖蛋白Ⅱb/Ⅲa 抑制剂，数据尚不足以提出建议。

本文作者的推荐是，糖蛋白Ⅱb/Ⅲa 抑制剂仅 5 天即应中断，因为在 7 ～ 10 天左右有反弹性高凝倾向的风险。如果没有重新启动双重抗血小板治疗的计划，根据专家意见，手术应延迟约 2 周。

（黄 成 译 侯 炯 校）

延伸阅读

Bangalore S, Silbaugh TS, Normand SL, et al.: Drug-eluting stents versus bare metal stents prior to noncardiac surgery, *Catheter Cardiovasc Interv* 85:533–541, 2015.

Berger PB, Kleiman NS, Pencina MJ, et al.: Frequency of major noncardiac surgery and subsequent adverse events in the year after drug-eluting stent placement results from the EVENT (Evaluation of Drug-Eluting Stents and Ischemic Events) Registry, *JACC Cardiovasc Interv* 3: 920–927, 2010.

De Servi S, Morici N, Boschetti E, et al.: Bridge therapy or standard treatment for urgent surgery after coronary stent implantation: analysis of 314 patients, *Vascul Pharmacol* 80:85–90, 2016.

Feres F, Costa RA, Abizaid A, et al.: Three vs twelve months of dual antiplatelet therapy after zotarolimus-eluting stents: the OPTIMIZE randomized trial, *JAMA* 310:2510–2522, 2013.

Hawn MT, Graham LA, Richman JR, et al.: The incidence and timing of noncardiac surgery after cardiac stent implantation, *J Am Coll Surg* 214:658–666, 2012. discussion 666-667.

Hawn MT, Graham LA, Richman JS, et al.: Risk of major adverse cardiac events following noncardiac surgery in patients with coronary stents, *JAMA* 310:1462–1472, 2013.

Kristensen SD, Grove EL, Maeng M: Coronary stents and non-cardiac surgery: to bridge or not to bridge? *Thromb Haemost* 114:211–213, 2015.

Levine GN, Bates ER, Bittl JA, et al.: 2016 ACC/AHA guideline focused update on duration of dual antiplatelet therapy in patients with coronary artery disease: a report of the American College of Cardiology/American Heart Association Task Force on Clinical Practice Guidelines, *J Am Coll Cardiol* 68:1082–1115, 2016.

Mauri L, Kereiakes DJ, Yeh RW, et al.: Twelve or 30 months of dual antiplatelet therapy after drug-eluting stents, *N Engl J Med* 371:2155–2166, 2014.

Schouten O, van Domburg RT, Bax JJ, et al.: Noncardiac surgery after coronary stenting: early surgery and interruption of antiplatelet therapy are associated with an increase in major adverse cardiac events, *J Am Coll Cardiol* 49(1):122–124, 2007.

Wijeysundera DN, Wijeysundera HC, Yun L, et al.: Risk of elective major noncardiac surgery after coronary stent insertion: a population-based study, *Circulation* 126:1355–1362, 2012.

第23章 结节病

Barry A. Harrison，Martin L. De Ruyter

病例概要

患者，女性，50岁，非洲裔美国人，被诊断为肺结节病Ⅲ期，拟接受开胸手术切除右上肺叶的肺曲霉球。长期以来，患者表现为声音嘶哑、静息性呼吸困难和脚踝肿胀。现接受皮质类固醇治疗和2 L/min的床旁氧疗，主诉有心悸和昏厥。

问题分析

定义

结节病是一种系统性肉芽肿性疾病，尽管140年前就曾有报道，但其病因仍不明确。遗传、环境和（或）传染性抗原的复杂相互作用会引发1型T淋巴细胞反应，其特点是慢性炎症、单核细胞募集和肉芽肿行成。结节病病理表现：由不连续的非干酪样肉芽肿紧密组成。粒细胞类型主要为单核吞噬细胞，如上皮样细胞和多核巨细胞及淋巴细胞成结。中央细胞被成纤维细胞和肥大细胞包围（图23.1）。

识别

临床特征

- 结节病发病年龄多在20～40岁，在美国患病率约为20/100 000。女性的发病率比男性略高，而非洲裔美国人与白种人的比例为15∶1。
- 结节病可呈急性发作，也可亚急性或隐匿性起病。30%～60%的病例是无症状的，常常是通过胸部X线检查异常才偶然发现。全身症状包括发热、疲劳、厌食、咳嗽、呼吸困难和胸骨后不适。与急性结节病有关的综合征包括结节性红斑、前葡萄膜炎、关节炎、腮腺肿大和面神经麻痹等关。在隐匿起病的患者中，呼吸症状通常是主要表现。
- 目前尚无特异性病原体被确定为致病抗原。然而，暴露在易燃木制品中与发病相关。有趣的是，参与9·11恐怖袭击事件救援工作的消防员中，一种类似肉瘤样肉芽肿性疾病的发病率增加。
- 诊断需要相关的临床特征和组织活检显示为非干酪性肉芽肿。
- 疾病活动的程度、波动性和累及器官的不同，决定了临床表现的多变性，这些因素在肉瘤患者中也常常看到，因而导致结节病确诊时间延长。
- 在结节病确诊前，应排除铍中毒和过敏性肺炎。
- 结节病患者的致死原因通常是由受累的肺、心脏或神经系统病变进展所致。在过去的20年中，结节病的死亡率每年增加3%。

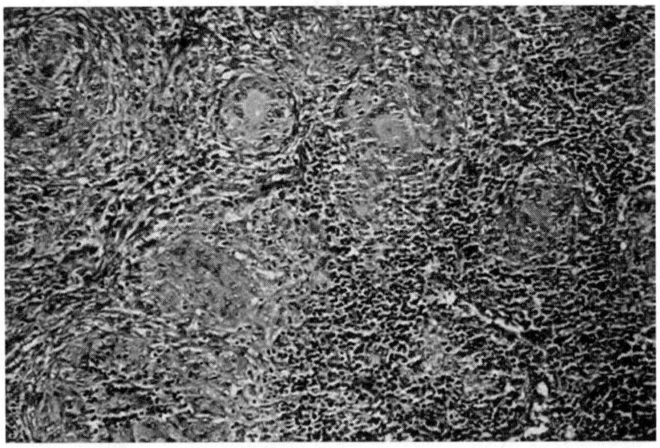

图23.1 肺组织中的结节性肉芽肿（Photomicrograph courtesy of Dr. Thomas A. Gaffey，Department of Pathology，Mayo Clinic and Foundation，Rochester，MN.）

肺部表现

高达95%的结节病患者累及肺部。

上呼吸道。虽然喉结节可能是孤立的症状，但通常与全身表现有关。近5%的结节病患者，喉结节的症状和体征包括吞咽困难、嘶哑、喉咙痛、呼吸困难和喘鸣。

声门上喉部或整个喉部常常发现肉芽肿或结节（图 23.2）。可能会发生气道阻塞，在某些情况下需要行气管造口术。喉返神经受累可导致单侧声带麻痹。

下呼吸道。胸腔内淋巴结肿大可以压迫大气道，导致气管和支气管狭窄、气流受阻和肺不张。

肺实质。90% 的病例累及肺和胸腔内淋巴结。大约 50% 的患者发生永久性肺异常，5% ～ 15% 的患者发生肺纤维化。肺结节病可以引起慢性低氧性呼吸衰竭和肺源性心脏病。

胸部 X 线和实验室检查。90% 的结节病患者在某一时间段的胸部 X 线检查是正常的。与呼吸困难发生频率增加相关的胸部 X 线经典表现有 3 种，随着病程进展，发生呼吸困难的频率会相应增加（表 23.1）。血清血管紧张素转换酶（angiotensin-converting enzyme，sACE）浓度的增加，这是一种由肉芽肿所分泌的酶，有助于临床诊断。但在其他慢性炎症状态 sACE 血清浓度也会增加。最近的研究结果表明，sACE 水平与疾病活动程度或治疗反应并不总是一致。

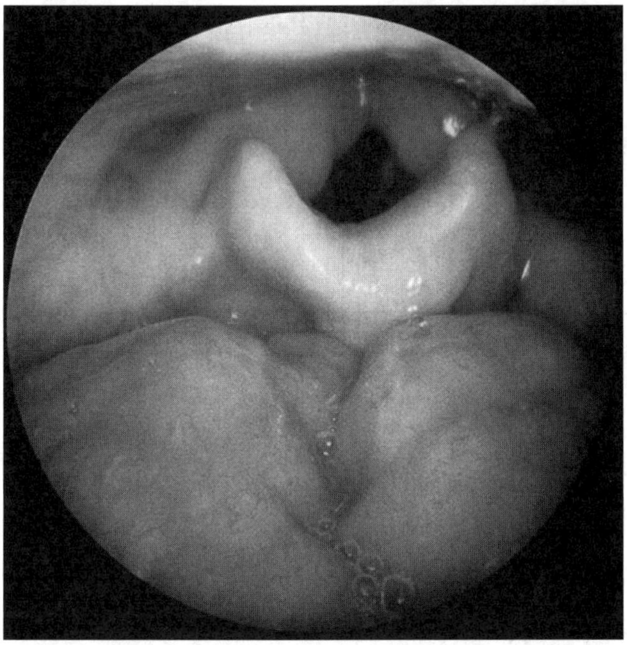

图 23.2 声门上区肉芽肿（From Neel HB，McDonald TJ：Laryngeal sarcoidosis. *Ann Otol Rhinol Laryngol* 91：361，1982.）

表 23.1 结节病的三种典型胸部 X 线表现

胸部 X 线	放射学检查结果	ACE 升高发生率（%）
Ⅰ期	肺门纵隔异常无肺实质异常	67
Ⅱ期	肺门纵隔异常伴肺实质异常	88
Ⅲ期	无结节肿大的弥漫性肺疾病	95

ACE，血管紧张素转换酶

计算机断层扫描（computed tomography，CT）。当仅靠胸部 X 线检查不能确诊时，高分辨率计算机断层摄影（high-resolution computed tomography，HRCT）可有助于将诊断率提高至 75%。HRCT 可用于诊断小而边界清晰的结节及支气管周围的间质增厚，而常规 CT 对弥漫性实质结节病的诊断价值更高（图 23.3）。

经支气管活检。经支气管活检诊断率为 90%。即使在胸部 X 线片上还不能发现到间质浸润，该方法的阳性率也非常高。

支气管肺泡灌洗。灌洗可能有帮助，特别是需要分析淋巴细胞群时；淋巴细胞增多率大于 15% 的冲洗液对诊断的敏感性为 90%。CD4/CD8 比值大于 3.5 时特异性为 94%。

心脏表现

临床上约有 5% 的结节病患者会出现明显的心脏受累，通常没有其他疾病的证据。心脏受累可表现为心律失常（室性多于室上性）、传导障碍、心肌病、心包炎、室壁运动异常或心脏停搏。心电图、超声心动图，以及在经过筛选的患者中行心导管检查结合心肌活检有助于评估患者的心脏受累情况。在无全身表现的情况下，心肌结节病可能很难诊断。由于取样偏差，心肌活检可能为假阴性。肺源性心脏病可由肺实质疾病引起。猝死与心脏结节有关；然而，随着抗心律失常药物、心脏起搏器和自动植入式除颤器的发展，伴发心肌肉瘤的充血性心力衰竭已成为心脏结节病死亡的最常见原因。

肺动脉高压表现

结节病患者合并肺动脉高压的发生率为 5% ～ 15%。最常见的合并情况是毛细血管前高血压。病因包括肺纤维化、肺血管床闭塞、腺病压迫肺血管、肉芽肿性动脉炎、肺静脉闭塞性疾病、缺氧性肺血管收缩。结节性左心室功能障碍也是结节性肺动脉高压的原因之一，与结节相关肺动脉高压的其他病因相比，该亚型有更好的预后。由于结节性肺动脉高压存在多重病因，它被世界卫生组织分

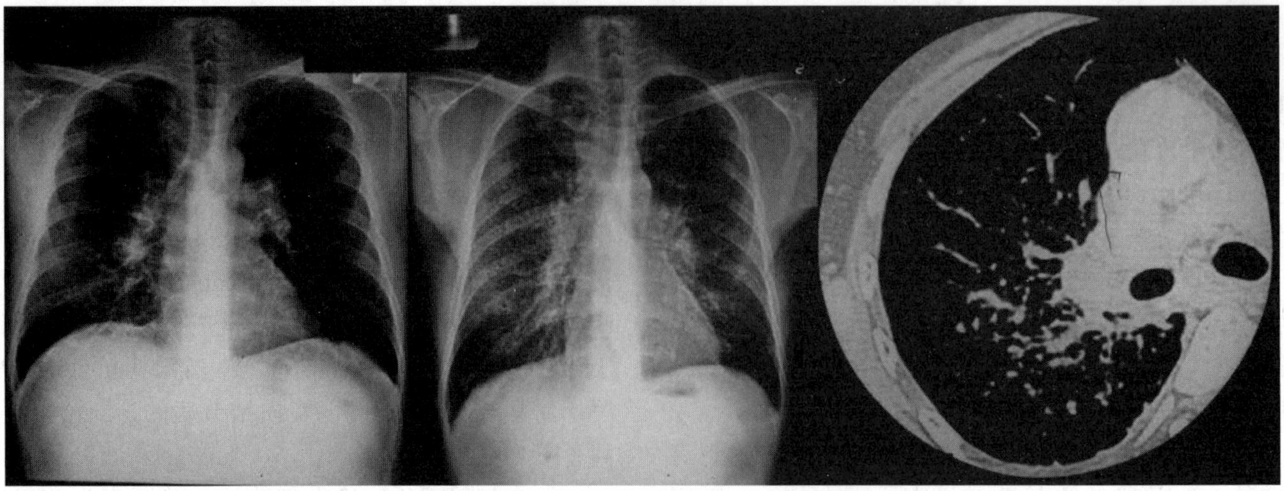

图 23.3 左侧、双侧肺门淋巴结肿大（Ⅰ期）。中间、双侧肺门淋巴结肿大和间质浸润（Ⅱ期）。右侧、高分辨率胸部 CT 扫描显示广泛的结节性间质进程（Radiograph courtesy of Department of Radiology，Mayo Clinic and Foundation，Rochester，MN.）

为五类。

多系统表现

在结节病患者中，超过 40% 的患者心肺系统以外存在疾病。因此，对麻醉科医师而言，这种疾病具有重要的意义（表 23.2）。

风险评估

根据结节病累及器官系统的范围及严重程度进行风险评估。

肺功能测定

肺量计、肺容积和肺二氧化碳弥散量（diffusing capacity of carbon monoxide，$DLCO_2$）是评价肺结节病患者肺功能的初步指标。随着肺的弹性阻力增加，结节病患者可以通过浅快呼吸来减少呼吸做功。最常见的表现是肺容积和 $DLCO_2$ 减少（图 23.4）。呼气流速也可能降低，提示气流阻塞和肺顺应性降低。运动时常会发生动脉低氧血症；但在静息时出现低氧血症则提示病情严重。虽然肺结节病病理改变是由纤维化和肉芽肿形成引起的，肺功能检测可以反

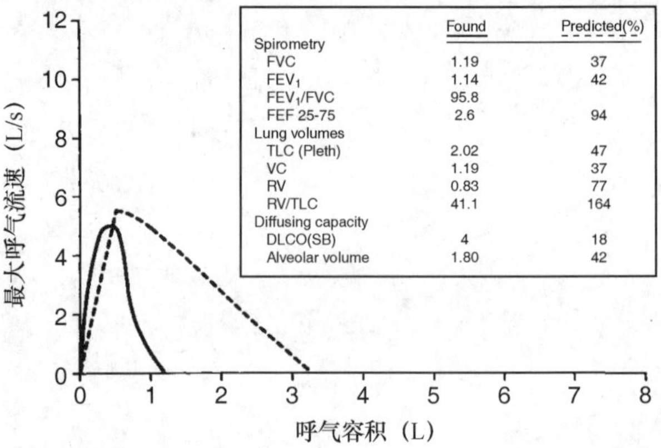

图 23.4 肺结节病的呼气流量环、肺容积和弥散能力（Data from Pulmonary Function Laboratory，Mayo Clinic and Foundation，Rochester，MN.）

表 23.2 结节病的多系统表现

器官系统（受累率）	表现	对麻醉的影响
神经系统（5%）	周围神经病、中枢神经系统症状：脑膜炎、脑炎、癫痫、颅神经异常	注意肌肉松弛药
肌肉骨骼（5%）	周围关节炎：踝关节、膝盖、手腕、手；颞下颌关节强直	检查气道
肾（1% ～ 2%）	高钙尿症伴或不伴高钙血症、肾钙沉着症、肾结石	药物排泄改变
肝脏（20% ～ 30%）	肝大、肝功能异常	药物代谢改变
血液系统（15%）	贫血、血小板减少、中性粒细胞减少、嗜酸性粒细胞减少、脾大	检查全血细胞计数
眼（25%）	葡萄膜炎、结膜结节、巩膜角结膜炎	标准眼预防措施
皮肤（25%）	结节性红斑、色斑、皮下结节	病损可能会有触痛和疼痛
内分泌	垂体后叶：尿崩症、高钙血症	监测血清 Ca^{2+}、Na 和尿量

映疾病的范围，而不一定能反映疾病的活动性。但是，肺功能的动态检查可以为患者的治疗反应提供客观数据。

心肺运动试验，如 6 分钟步行试验，已被用于对肺功能检查和超声心动图检查正常的肺结节病患者的功能状态评估。

心脏评估

心电图、24 小时动态心电图监测、超声心动图及心导管下行心肌穿刺活检可有助于心脏结节病的诊断。铊 -201 心肌显像可显示与肉芽肿或纤维瘢痕相一致的节段性缺损。磁共振成像技术也被用于识别受结节病影响的心肌区域，并引导心肌穿刺活检。

肺动脉高压与右心功能不全

肺动脉高压往往被忽视而没有得到诊断。不明原因呼吸困难、6 分钟步行试验成绩不佳（不到 150 m）以及相关的去氧饱和状态，都表明有指征进行超声心动图检查。超声心动图肺动脉收缩压大于 30 mmHg 与心导管直接测量肺动脉收缩压有显著相关性。三尖瓣反流和三尖瓣环平面收缩期偏移是右心室功能不全的指标。

启示

结节病患者进行活检操作和诊断检查时可能需要麻醉。这些操作包括纤维支气管镜和经支气管活检、斜角结节活检、纵隔镜下肝门淋巴结活检、电视胸腔镜或开胸术行肺活检。许多结节病患者由于治疗的并发症需要麻醉，例如，继发于皮质类固醇治疗的十二指肠溃疡穿孔。结节病患者也常常因为其他并存疾病需要在麻醉下治疗。在病例概要中，患者的肺内有一个由结节病引起的肺组织囊性破坏所致的肺曲霉菌球。肺结节进行性生长会并发慢性缺氧性呼吸衰竭、右心功能衰竭、心脏结节的持续进展等会给麻醉带来难题并增加风险。

管理

大约有 30 ～ 50% 的病例在 3 年内自发恢复，在接下来的 5 ～ 10 年中，30% 的患者出现病情缓解，其余的 20% 保持稳定。因此，并不是所有的结节病患者都需要特殊的治疗，尤其是 I 期 X 线分型的患者。需要系统性治疗的结节病患者比例在 20% ～ 80%。

药物治疗

糖皮质激素

结节病的治疗指征是进行性发展的有症状的疾病。明确的症状如继发于结节病的心脏、神经系统结节病和高钙血症。肺结节病引起的呼吸综合征伴肺功能持续下降也需要治疗。

一项对结节病使用糖皮质激素的系统性循证回顾分析发现，糖皮质激素可以改善 X 线表现（第Ⅱ期和第Ⅲ期 X 线分型）和肺功能检查结果。然而，尚无数据支持糖皮质激素能够显著影响疾病的远期进展。通常，临床医师在重新评估患者的治疗方案之前，会进行为期 3 个月的糖皮质激素试验。吸入性糖皮质激素也被尝试过，然而，迄今为止还没有进行足够的临床试验来确定其疗效。

抗代谢药物——减少糖皮质激素使用

抗代谢物用于控制结节病的进展，特别是糖皮质激素治疗失败或临床医师需要减少患者的糖皮质激素使用量。甲氨蝶呤、硫唑嘌呤、来氟米特、霉酚酸酯均已应用结节病治疗；最常用的药物是甲氨蝶呤。它可能需要使用 6 个月才能正确评估患者的反应。遗憾的是，这些药物都存在严重的毒性，这可能限制了它们的使用。

抗肿瘤坏死因子 -α 生物制剂

经过糖皮质激素或抗代谢治疗，如果器官和（或）生命受到结节样疾病进展的威胁，可以考虑使用抗肿瘤坏死因子 -α（anti-TNF-α）治疗。两种已显示有效的药物是英夫利昔单抗和阿达木单抗。其他 anti-TNF-α 的药物（依那西普和戈利木单抗）尚未证实具有抗结节病的疗效。

肺动脉高压

前列环素、内皮受体拮抗剂、磷酸二酯酶抑制剂以及联合应用已有个案报道、系列和少量前瞻性应用研究。这些研究的结论表明虽然血流动力学得到了改善；但 6 分钟步行试验和血氧饱和度可能没有改善。这种现象的一个解释是，肺血管扩张药的治疗时间有限，或者肺结节严重，限制了对肺血管扩张药的反应。

慢性低氧血症、呼吸衰竭和肺心病

长期进展性的肺结节病可引起慢性低氧性呼吸衰竭和肺心病。**肺心病**是指由影响肺部结构和（或）功能的疾病引起的肺动脉高压，肺动脉高压继而导致右心室扩大［肥厚和（或）扩张］，并可能随着时间的推移导致右心衰竭。这两种情况的治疗首先且重要的方法是持续吸氧，使动脉血氧饱和度提高到90%以上。如果出现右心衰竭，应开始利尿，通常为呋塞米。过多的容量丢失较为危险，因为它可能会减少右心室前负荷。洋地黄的使用是有争议的，因为在低氧血症、碱中毒引起的低钾血症和肺心病状态下，即使洋地黄血清浓度很低，毒性也很大。

肺和心脏移植

对积极的内科治疗没有反应的终末期肺结节病患者可以行肺移植治疗，肺动脉高压是决定是否需要肺移植的重要因素。双肺移植优于单肺移植。肺移植手术因为粘连、肺曲霉菌球和既往的肺手术史而非常复杂。大多数患者的移植肺内会复发结节性肉芽肿，但很少引起临床症状。单肺／双肺移植患者的2年生存率为70%。内科治疗不能控制的终末期结节性心脏病患者也已采用心脏移植。

麻醉

术前

由于结节病是一种多系统疾病，在术前评估时，必须对所有系统进行评估，以确定是否可能被结节累及。必须优先对肺和心脏系统进行评估，重点在于呼吸系统、运动能力、氧含量、持续时间以及并发感染等，都需要进行评估，特别是如果最近病情发生了恶化更要关注。同样的重点是心脏系统，特别是恶性心律失常或左、右心室功能恶化。气管插管前必须特别关注上呼吸道受结节病累及后的症状和体征。必须评估糖皮质激素的使用及继发肾上腺皮质功能不全的可能性，并在术前酌情适当使用糖皮质激素。

术中

监护麻醉

如果慢性低氧性呼吸衰竭和右心衰竭同时存在，必须避免出现缺氧、高碳酸血症和酸中毒，这也通常被认为是一种“安全”的选择，因为缺氧、高碳酸血症和酸中毒都会增加肺动脉压，会进一步加重右心衰竭。必须维持氧饱和度大于92%，动脉血二氧化碳在35～45 mmHg之间。由于晚期肺部疾病会增加死腔量，导致呼气末二氧化碳不能准确地反映动脉血二氧化碳。

全身麻醉

麻醉的目的是维持动脉血氧饱和度大于92%，动脉血二氧化碳35～45 mmHg，pH 7.35～7.45，在最大限度地降低肺动脉压的同时保持全身动脉压，优化输液治疗（避免加重右心衰竭）。为了达到这些目的，应考虑监测中心静脉压和肺动脉压。有创动脉压监测很重要，强烈建议进行中心静脉压和肺动脉压监测。肺动脉导管或经食管超声心动图可达到这些目的。这两种监测将有助于输液治疗的评估管理和管理。需要避免使用的麻醉药是氯胺酮，因为它会增加肺动脉压。

机械通气是合理麻醉管理的重点。晚期肺结节病患者机械通气的目的是避免进一步的肺损伤。若患者正在接受胸外科手术，这一点尤为重要。在机械通气时，吸气平台压力应控制在30 cmH_2O以下，尤其是在肺纤维化的情况下。这可以通过将机械通气潮气量设定在4～8 ml/kg（患者的理想体重）并观察压力来实现。或者，呼吸机可以设置为压力控制通气模式，压力设定在30 cmH_2O。在这两种情况下，记录潮气量和测量呼气末二氧化碳很重要，应该调整参数以确保足够的通气。在肺纤维化患者中，呼气末正压可能需要增加到大于10 cmH_2O的水平，才能提供足够的氧合。为了达到这些机械通气的目的，经常需要使用神经肌肉阻断剂。

区域麻醉

区域麻醉的使用具有潜在的优势，尤其是当手术部位在脐以下时。脐以上的手术使用高位椎管内阻滞可能会干扰肋间肌肉功能和加重呼吸衰竭。在晚期肺结节病患者中，辅助肌功能是通气功能的重要组成部分。由于交感神经阻滞引起的低血压，过多输液可能会加重右心衰竭。使用升压药物维持血压，以确保右心灌注。

术后护理

对于结节病性肺动脉高压、慢性低氧性呼吸衰竭和右心衰竭，应慎重考虑术后镇痛。全身应用阿片类药物可抑制通气，诱发低氧血症。因此，应考虑使用局部麻醉药、阿片类药物或两者合用的椎管内麻醉技术。许多人主张通过周围神经阻滞和持续导管输注局部麻醉药来优化镇痛，减少阿片类药物的用量，从而减少呼吸系统的副作用。推荐滴定吸入氧浓度，以维持血氧饱和度大于 92%，目的是尽量减少肺动脉高压（如果有）的有害影响。长期服用糖皮质激素的患者在术后需要继续使用和逐渐减量，但也存在消化性溃疡的风险，需要预防消化道出血。

（王　春　译　许　华　校）

延伸阅读

Baughman RP, Engel PJ, Nathan S: Pulmonary hypertension in sarcoidosis, *Clin Chest Med* 36:703–714, 2015.

Baughman RP, Grutters JC: New treatment strategies for pulmonary sarcoidosis: antimetabolites, biologic drugs, and other approaches, *Lancet Resp Med* 3:813–823, 2015.

Clark D, Mitchell AW, Dick R, et al.: The radiology of sarcoidosis (review), *Sarcoidosis* 11:90–99, 1994.

Dubret SW, Sharma R, Underwood R, et al.: Cardiac sarcoidosis: diagnosis and management, *Postgrad Med* 91:384–394, 2015.

Harjola VP, Mebazza A, Celutkiene J, et al.: Contemporary management of acute right ventricular failure: a statement from the Heart Failure Association and the Working Group on Pulmonary Circulation and Right Ventricular Function of the European Society of Cardiology, *Eur J Heart Fail* 18:226–241, 2016.

Paramothayan S: Corticosteroid therapy in pulmonary sarcoidosis: a systematic review, *JAMA* 287:1301–1307, 2002.

Valeyre D, Bernaudin JF, Jeny F, et al.: Pulmonary sarcoidosis, *Clin Chest Med* 36:631–641, 2015.

Wills MH, Harris MM: An unusual airway complication with sarcoidosis, *Anesthesiology* 66:554–555, 1987.

第24章 脓毒症、全身炎症反应综合征和多器官功能障碍综合征

Jesse M. Raiten，*Jacob T. Gutsche*

病例概要

患者，男性，35 岁，腹部遭受枪击伤，随后被紧急送往手术室，术中发现结肠穿孔且腹腔有粪水和脓液。患者接受了部分结肠切除和结肠造口术，手术过程中患者心率逐渐变快且出现低血压，需要大量的液体复苏，并启用升压药物以及有创血流动力学监测。手术结束后，患者转运至重症监护室进一步治疗。

问题分析

定义和识别

全身炎症反应综合征（systemic inflammatory response syndrome，SIRS）、脓毒症以及多器官功能障碍综合征（multiple organ dysfunction syndrome，MODS）可发生于患者整个围术期，其可通过特异的症状和体征来定义（框 24.1 和框 24.2）。随着对合并复杂内外科疾病患者所提供的医疗服务质量的改进和治疗水平的提高，加上期待利于对合并多种内科疾病的患者进行分类和比较的方法的出现，SIRS、脓毒症以及 MODS 的概念应运而生并发展演变至今。

SIRS 标准过于广泛，某些术前焦虑患者和几乎所有术后患者可能会达到其标准。因此，它的发生可能无法在围术期引起临床医师的高度关注。但是，SIRS 标准通常预示着更为棘手的脓毒症病情的发生以及由其所带来的相当高的病死率。由于 SIRS 和脓毒症之间的差异仅仅取决于是否存在感染，许多手术患者符合脓毒症的标准。手术固有的促炎特征可使患者进一步发展为脓毒性休克。

MODS 是一个以多器官系统进行性衰竭为特征的动态过程，可能由脓毒症、创伤或其他病理进程引起。MODS 通常在重症监护室（intensive care unit，ICU）的患者中观察到，并且可能在需手术干预的 ICU 患者的围术期遇到。

框 24.1　全身炎症反应综合征的诊断标准

发热或低体温（中心温度 >38℃或 <36℃）
白细胞计数 >12 000 或 <4000，或者中性杆状核粒细胞比例 >10%
心率 >90 次 / 分或者 > 正常年龄基础值的 2 个标准差
呼吸急促（呼吸频率 >20 次 / 分）

框 24.2　脓毒症和脓毒性休克的共识定义

脓毒症：出现感染的 SIRS
严重脓毒症：合并至少一个器官功能障碍的脓毒症
脓毒性休克：容量复苏后仍存在持续低血压的脓毒症

译者注：sepsis 3.0 新定义：
脓毒症：机体对感染反应失调而导致危及生命的器官功能障碍
脓毒性休克：脓毒症合并出现严重的循环障碍和细胞代谢紊乱，其死亡风险较单纯脓毒症显著升高

SIRS，全身炎症反应综合征

风险评估和启示

虽然定义 SIRS 的生理指标很常见且可能代表升高的应激反应，但脓毒症却是一种极度的病理状态。手术和急性病对代谢和免疫功能都有严重的影响，可能会增加患者发生脓毒症和 MODS 的风险。脓毒症患者机体摄取和利用氧的能力受损，乳酸生成增加。内分泌异常紊乱，包括血管加压素产生减少和对其他激素（包括胰岛素和儿茶酚胺）的抵抗。

每年有数百万患者出现手术部位感染，脓毒症患者中 30% 是手术患者。围术期脓毒症的危险因素包括高龄人群、男性和非裔美国人。早期识别脓毒症和 MODS 高危患者有助于早期干预和合理分诊患者到重症监护室。脓毒症患者早期和积极治疗已被证明可以降低病残率并提高生存率。麻醉科医师在启动治疗 SIRS 和脓毒症患者时独特和有利的地位，包括确保开放中心静脉通路和实施有创监测，提供容量复苏和给予抗生素治疗。对于 MODS 患者，超声心动图等诊断性干预可在手术室或 ICU 进行，在麻醉科医师的监测下可启动或者继续支持性治疗。

治疗和预防

对于 SIRS、脓毒症和 MODS 尚无简单的治疗方法。SIRS、脓毒症和 MODS 的生理过程复杂，需要多种方法治疗和限制其发展。目前尚无特定的治疗目标，主要基于**控制感染源、支持治疗以及预防进一步并发症**。拯救脓毒症运动是一个致力于研究脓毒症和脓毒性休克患者治疗进展的国际组织，脓毒症新疗法仍是研究的重点领域。

感染源控制

SIRS 的炎性进程可以由各种对机体的伤害引起——感染、创伤、代谢异常或疾病进程。患者的病史、体格检查、实验室或诊断检查有助于确定持续炎症反应的原因。感染源控制是治疗的关键，早期识别和治疗原发疾病可阻止炎症进展和（或）脓毒症或 MODS 的发展。在某些情况下，如感染的外科手术清创，因患者机体对手术产生额外的应激反应，实现感染源控制可能会暂时加重患者的临床病情。

支持治疗

支持治疗可以分为以下不同的类型。

1. 容量和血制品治疗

SIRS 和脓毒症的特点是全身性毛细血管渗漏，且容量复苏是治疗的基础。Rivers 和其同事开展的“早期目标导向治疗严重脓毒症或脓毒性休克”基准研究旨在实现中心静脉压为 8 ～ 12 mmHg，作为优化患者中心静脉血氧饱和度和血流动力学的一部分。拯救脓毒症运动建议给予低血压或乳酸升高的患者 30 ml/kg 的晶体液。可以通过血流动力学的改善、监测脉压变异度、代谢指标如乳酸水平的趋势来评估患者的容量反应性。血压的恢复通常定义为平均动脉压至 60 ～ 65 mmHg。

尽管给予晶体液与胶体液的研究难以比较，因为患者构成复杂，使用液体持续时间不同，存在偏倚风险等，但与其他液体复苏相比，平衡液或白蛋白复苏可能会降低患者死亡率。红细胞输注指征已在许多患者群体中得到广泛研究，并且大多数研究表明，无活动性出血的危重患者血红蛋白 7.0 g/dl 即已足够。拯救脓毒症运动建议血红蛋白 7.0 g/dl 作为输注红细胞的触发值，如果成人患者无活动性心肌缺血、严重低氧血症或活动性出血，其血红蛋白目标值为 7.0 ～ 9.0 g/dl。

2. 血管收缩药和正性肌力药

脓毒症或脓毒性休克的患者中，液体复苏可能不足以恢复器官的灌注。脓毒症患者的低血压通常由多种因素所致——低血容量、血管扩张和心肌功能障碍。虽然脓毒症诱发的心肌功能障碍可高达 40%，但血管扩张是脓毒症生理学的标志，通常需要使用血管收缩药维持血压。多巴胺过去曾被用于低血压和脓毒症患者，但目前建议去甲肾上腺素作为脓毒症患者低血压的一线药物。去甲肾上腺素可作用于 α- 和 β- 受体，减少血管舒张和增强心脏收缩。

拯救脓毒症指南建议肾上腺素作为第二种药物。脓毒性休克患者体内内源性加压素水平因患者的需求增加而相对减少，即“加压素相对缺乏”，如有必要，应在使用去甲肾上腺素的基础上，加用低剂量加压素。心肌收缩力严重降低的情况下，可以使用正性肌力药物如多巴酚丁胺，尽管其 β- 受体活性可能会加重血管扩张。

3. 机械通气

脓毒症引起的呼吸衰竭很常见。呼吸肌代谢需求增加，加上能量供应和产生受限，导致供需失衡，易出现呼吸衰竭并需要机械通气。急性肺损伤和急性呼吸窘迫综合征（acute respiratory distress syndrome，ARDS）常见于脓毒症患者，呼吸衰竭往往是 MODS 的一部分。脓毒症引起呼吸衰竭患者的呼吸支持与 ARDS 患者的指南相一致。拯救脓毒症运动推荐临床医师使用 6 ml/kg（预测体重）的潮气量且平台压小于 30 cmH_2O。这种肺保护性通气策略已被证明可以改善患者预后。顽固性低氧血症的患者推崇使用呼气末正压（positive end-expiratory pressure，PEEP）和肺复张手法维持肺泡复张。床头应保持在 30° ～ 45° 之间（该策略可能在手术中无法实现）以便降低肺误吸的风险。

4. 抗生素

当确认存在活动性感染时，SIRS 通常进展为脓毒症。早期应用抗生素是治疗脓毒症的基石。抗生素使用延迟导致死亡风险增加，拯救脓毒症指南推荐严重脓毒症或脓毒性休克诊断后 1 h 内开始使用抗生素。尽管抗生素通常在手术开始时使用，但 SIRS 或脓毒症患者应仔细考虑抗生素的选择。详细的病史和体格检查可以推测感染来源，从而指导选择合理的抗生素。在许多情况下，患者在手术之前已经接受了合理的抗生素治疗。

5. 内分泌支持

脓毒症患者内分泌的特征可能是皮质醇产生不足和肾上腺皮质功能相对不全。以往通过 ACTH 刺激试验评估肾上腺反应，但目前不再推荐。大量研究探讨了脓毒症和脓毒性休克患者类固醇激素的使用，结果各异。根据现有数据，大多数研究认为无休克的脓毒症患者不应接受类固醇激素治疗。顽固性脓毒性休克患者（对液体复苏和血管收缩药无反应）有使用应激类固醇激素的指征。通常分次给予氢化可的松，每天共 200 ～ 300 mg。类固醇激素持续时间和后续治疗是否需要减量尚无达成共识。

如上所述，脓毒症期间垂体产生加压素相对缺乏。血管加压素主要调节内脏血管张力，是脓毒症相关血管扩张时内脏血管床内升高的主要物质。输注血管加压素（0.01 ～ 0.04 U/min）恢复正常血压，可能有助于患者脱离其他血管活性物质。

6. 肾替代治疗和酸碱支持

酸血症在脓毒症和 MODS 患者中比较常见，其由多种病因共同导致。脓毒症引起的肾衰竭可导致酸中毒，器官低灌注可能引起乳酸酸中毒，只有潜在的病情得到纠正才会改善。脓毒症和 MODS 患者因各种原因需要肾替代治疗（renal replacement therapy，RRT），包括酸中毒、电解质异常、容量超负荷和尿毒症。持续 RRT 和间歇性血透均为合理的治疗措施，但血流动力学不稳定的患者可以更好地耐受持续 RRT。碳酸氢钠可用来暂时性纠正酸中毒，除非是对升压药无反应的严重酸血症，一般并不推荐使用。

7. 血糖控制

来自 SIRS 和脓毒症的全身炎症和应激反应会导致高糖血症。尽管普遍认为脓毒症患者应该治疗高糖血症，但血糖控制目标尚无一致性较好的标准。严格的血糖控制（80 ～ 100 mg/dl）导致低血糖的风险增加，且许多医疗从业人员和治疗方案以血糖低于 150 mg/dl 为目标。拯救脓毒症运动建议目标血糖低于 180 mg/dl。由于患者代谢状态变化迅速，需要对患者进行频繁的血糖监测，持续输注胰岛素可利于剂量的调整。

进一步预防并发症

源自脓毒症和 MODS 的各种并发症几乎遍及每个器官系统（表 24.1）。“预防远胜于治疗”这句经典教义非常适用于对 SIRS 和脓毒症患者的处理。早期感染源控制、积极的液体复苏、启动抗生素治疗和血流动力学支持可以降低发病率和死亡率。当早期干预和感染源控制涉及手术干预时，麻醉科医师在治疗 SIRS、脓毒症或 MODS 患者中具有举足轻重的作用和地位。

表 24.1 器官功能障碍的标准

器官系统	严重程度	
	中度	重度
肺	低氧或高二氧化碳，需要≥ 3 ～ 5 天的辅助通气	ARDS，需要 PEEP ≥ 10 cmH_2O 且 FiO_2 ≥ 0.5
肝	胆红素≥ 2 ～ 3 mg/dl；凝血酶原时间和其他的肝功能检查≥ 2 倍正常值	黄疸且胆红素≥ 8 ～ 10 mg/dl
肾	少尿（<500 ml/d）或者肌酐升高（≥ 2 ～ 3 mg/dl）	需要透析
胃肠道	不耐受胃管饲养≥ 5 天	需要输血的应激性溃疡；无结石的胆囊炎
血液系统	部分凝血活酶时间≥正常值的 125%，血小板计数 <50 000 ～ 80 000	弥散性血管内凝血
中枢神经系统	意识错乱	昏迷
外周神经系统	中度感觉神经病变	运动和感觉缺失
心血管系统	射血分数降低，持续的毛细血管渗漏	血管收缩药无反应的低动力状态

（卢文斌 译 卞金俊 校）

延伸阅读

NHLBI ARDS Network. http://www.ardsnet.org.

Rochwerg B, Alhazzani W, Sindi A: Fluid resuscitation in sepsis: a systematic review and network meta-analysis, *Ann Intern Med* 161:347–355, 2014.

Russell JA, Walley KR, Singer J, et al.: Vasopressin versus norepinephrine infusion in patients with septic shock, *N Engl J Med* 358:877–887, 2008.

Sprung CL, Annane D, Keh D, et al.: Hydrocortisone therapy for patients with septic shock, *N Engl J Med* 358:111–124, 2008.

Surviving Sepsis Campaign. http://www.survivingsepsis.org.

Vogel TR, Dombrovskiy VY, Lowry SF: Trends in postoperative sepsis: are we improving outcomes? *Surg Infect (Larchmt)* 10:71–78, 2009.

第25章 类固醇

Nancy B. Greilich，Philip E. Greilich

病例概要

患者，男性，55岁，因结肠憩室穿孔引发急腹症，被紧急送往手术室，既往有严重慢性阻塞性气道疾病和类固醇依赖史，过去的1年内每日服用10 mg泼尼松治疗。患者术中血流动力学不稳定，需要大量液体复苏并使用升血压药物。术后，患者带气管导管转入重症加强治疗病房，血流动力学依旧不稳定。

问题分析

定义

类固醇是治疗各种需要抑制免疫反应的一类疾病的主要药物。这些疾病包括皮肤病、肺部疾病和自身免疫性疾病，以及预防器官移植后的排斥反应。它也可用于那些因垂体或肾上腺疾病导致皮质醇分泌不足患者的替代治疗。围术期急性肾上腺功能不全的发生率约为0.01%～0.1%。在这种情况下，最可能引发艾迪生病危象的因素是皮质醇水平不足，无法满足创伤、感染和手术应激对糖皮质激素的需求。血浆皮质醇浓度在术后4～5 h达到峰值，并可能在术后48～72 h持续升高，尤其是在重大手术后。在正常应激反应最初的24 h内，小手术后皮质醇生成量少于50 mg，而大手术在同一时期产生75～100 mg的皮质醇。在最大的应激下（如脓毒性休克或严重创伤），肾上腺每天可产生高达300～500 mg的皮质醇。

根据下丘脑-垂体-肾上腺（hypothalamicpituitary-adrenal，HPA）轴的解剖损伤程度，肾上腺功能不全分为原发性、继发性或三发性。原发性肾上腺功能不全，是肾上腺本身异常。超过90%的肾上腺在糖皮质激素和盐皮质激素缺乏出现明显症状之前肯定已经受损。在美国，原发性肾上腺功能不全最常见的原因是自身免疫性疾病。而继发性肾上腺功能不全表现为垂体异常。这些患者表现出糖皮质激素缺乏的症状，但由于血管紧张素Ⅱ对醛固酮分泌的额外影响，患者通常具有完整的盐皮质激素功能。三发性肾上腺功能不全是围术期最常见的类型，这是由长期使用外源性类固醇抑制HPA轴反应所致，是继发于糖皮质激素给药及其对下丘脑的负反馈作用所引起的血浆皮质醇水平的升高的结果。促肾上腺皮质激素释放激素的减少降低了垂体促肾上腺皮质激素（adrenocorticotropic hormone，ACTH）的分泌，从而减少了内源性肾上腺糖皮质激素的生成（也较小幅度地减少了盐皮质激素的生成）。HPA轴功能的恢复在临床上和生物化学上都是可变的。

除了HPA轴功能损伤的潜在风险，长期使用类固醇还可能在围术期产生许多其他临床问题。皮肤变脆引起静脉注射困难和皮肤破裂的问题。感染风险增加，使得无菌技术尤为重要。最后，患者可能会出现未发现的隐匿性胃肠道出血或溃疡性疾病。

识别

艾迪生病危象的临床表现呈多变性，可从轻微的、非特异性的全身症状到对升压药治疗无反应的严重休克。在围术期，临床医师在治疗长期服用或者近期停用类固醇治疗的患者时，应保持高度警惕。肾上腺功能不全的轻微症状包括恶心、呕吐、厌食、疲劳和腹痛。盐皮质激素缺乏很少伴有艾迪生病危象，但当它发生时，它可能表现为低钠血症、高钾血症和代谢性酸中毒。严重的肾上腺功能不全，体位性低血压较常见。由于血管舒缩对儿茶酚胺的敏感性受糖皮质激素影响较明显，因此这种低血压可能对液体和升压药治疗无效。这种临床表现在接受每日常规剂量类固醇的患者中极少出现，尤其是在他们未经历高强度的生理应激反应时。

风险评估

以下是围术期发生肾上腺功能不全的重要危险因素：

- 每日类固醇的剂量（泼尼松 >20 mg/d 或等效剂量）；
- 类固醇治疗的持续时间（>3 周）；
- 基于血清试验的 HPA 轴抑制（皮质醇水平、ACTH 刺激试验）；
- 高强度的生理应激（手术、创伤、烧伤、感染）；
- 需要类固醇替代治疗的原发性或继发性肾上腺功能不全。

研究表明，类固醇的每日总剂量决定了 HPA 轴对应激的反应。LaRochelle 及其同事证明，当每日泼尼松总剂量≤ 5 mg 时，对 ACTH 刺激试验有正常反应。当剂量 >5 mg/d 时，对 ACTH 试验的反应会有很大差异。另一些人认为，如果泼尼松的给药时间限制在 3 周以内，且停药时间超过 14 天，那么即使剂量达到 20 mg/d，HPA 轴可能也不受抑制。对于接受较高剂量类固醇治疗（泼尼松 >20 mg）和（或）持续时间较长（>3 周）的患者，在停止治疗后，HPA 轴应被视为受损时间长达 6 个月。在有疑问时，建议采用两级方法确认。如果时间允许，可以在患者停止服用类固醇 24 h 后测试早晨的皮质醇。如果皮质醇水平低于 5 μg/dl，则 HPA 轴受损，且需要基于预期的手术应激程度补充类固醇。早晨皮质醇大于 10 μg/dl 意味着 HPA 轴完整，患者除了长期使用的每日剂量外，不需要额外补充。5 ～ 10 μg/dl 之间的结果不能确定 HPA 轴功能是否完整，如果可以则需要进行 ACTH 刺激试验，以确定 HPA 轴是否恢复正常。

对于伴有严重创伤、烧伤或脓毒症的手术患者，随机血清皮质醇水平测定可用于确定对大手术和危重疾病的生理反应是否足够。Marik 和 Zaloga 的一篇综述支持在这些危重患者中以 25 μg/dl 的血清皮质醇水平作为治疗的临界值，可以适当地补充类固醇。当在 ICU 发现随机血清皮质醇水平低时，特别是在脓毒症患者中，通常会使用应激剂量的类固醇。

启示

类固醇补充不足引起的艾迪生病危象十分罕见，但麻醉科医师对肾上腺功能不全的细微迹象保持警惕对于避免并发症的发生十分重要。每日累积剂量、长期类固醇治疗的持续时间和手术性质是预测 HPA 轴完整性和反应性的重要因素。术前库欣样表现提示类固醇使用过度，应警惕 HPA 轴抑制的可能。近期接受依托咪酯作为诱导剂也使患者面临更高的 HPA 轴抑制风险，当术后低血压对常规治疗无反应时应考虑这一点。由于依托咪酯可以抑制类固醇合成，因此麻醉科医师应考虑在 HPA 轴异常风险较高的患者中避免使用此药。局部使用和吸入类固醇通常很少有肾上腺功能不全的风险，但长期大剂量使用类固醇需要特别注意（例如，局部注射强效药物 >2 g/d），在手术后 3 个月内进行 3 次或 3 次以上的关节内或硬膜外类固醇注射也需要引起关注。

伴有脓毒性休克、严重创伤或烧伤的外科患者是一个特殊的群体。Annane 对脓毒性休克患者的研究表明，超生理剂量的类固醇治疗可改善临床疗效。考虑到高剂量类固醇的潜在风险（高血糖、高血压、液体潴留、感染风险增加），使用剂量应基于随机测量的皮质醇水平。最后，原发性或继发性肾上腺功能不全的患者也有较高的围术期加重的风险，因为他们在生理应激时不能增加皮质醇分泌。因此，除了接受长期治疗外，他们还应接受补充剂量治疗。

管理

最近的 Cochrane 系统评价认为，没有足够的证据支持围术期对潜在肾上腺功能抑制进行经验性治疗。然而，它确实支持长期服用类固醇的患者继续每日的剂量。内分泌专家则更进一步地建议选择性地在高风险患者（大手术、脓毒性休克）中使用补充剂量的类固醇。应避免为所有患者提供统一标准剂量。相反，围术期补充类固醇的剂量应基于患者类固醇的使用史以及预期的手术应激程度（详见表 25.1 和 25.2）。

对于那些积极接受治疗的患者，在手术前继续使用规定的晨间剂量是第一步。补充剂量应基于每日总剂量、治疗持续时间、围术期应激的严重程度，以及同时使用地塞米松的止吐剂量（4 ～ 8 mg）。尽

表 25.1　补充类固醇给药（“应激剂量”）指南

每日剂量的强的松	治疗时程	手术应激程度	围术期的处理 [a]
<5 mg	任何时间	不适用	正常 HPA 轴；如果仍服用类固醇，则给予每日剂量
5 ～ 20 mg	<3 周		
5 ～ 20 mg	>3 周，但在 14 天内停止		
5 ～ 20 mg	>3 周，但 14 天内没有停止	如果未测试 HPA 轴，则建议更高（>20 mg/d）的长期类固醇剂量	如果 HPA 轴的状态未知，考虑轴测试；否则，根据手术应激程度进行基础补充 如果使用类固醇，则每天服用一次
>20 mg	任何时间	小手术（如疝气修补）	只给每日剂量
		中手术（如关节置换）	每日剂量加 50 mg 静脉注射前，然后 75 mg 静脉注射氢化可的松超过 24 h，然后恢复每日剂量
		大手术（如 Whipple 术）	每日剂量加 100 mg 氢化可的松静脉注射术前，然后 150 mg 超过 24 h。减量 50%，直到达到每日剂量

HPA，下丘脑–垂体–肾上腺

[a] 同时应用止吐剂量（4 ～ 8 mg）的地塞米松可以减少或消除手术当天额外使用氢化可的松的需要，等效剂量见表 25.2

表 25.2　类固醇比较：糖皮质激素和盐皮质激素的相对效力和作用持续时间

类固醇	糖皮质激素效力	盐皮质激素效力	作用持续时间（h）
氢化可的松 [a]	1	1	8 ～ 10
强的松	4	0.8	18 ～ 36
泼尼松龙	4	0.8	12 ～ 36
甲泼尼龙	5	0.5	18 ～ 36
地塞米松	25 ～ 30	0	36 ～ 54
氟氢可的松	10	120	18 ～ 36

[a] 与皮质醇相同

管一些数据表明至少 2 个月才能恢复正常的皮质醇分泌，但谨慎起见，应认为 HPA 轴功能可能会受损长达 6 个月。尽管 ACTH 刺激测试可有助于确定 HPA 轴的完整性，但是对所有患者都进行测试是不切实际的，也没有必要。那些每天服用少于 5 mg 泼尼松或其等效物的患者可以假设 HPA 轴完整，不需要补充剂量的类固醇；然而，为治疗他们的基础疾病继续长期每日剂量非常重要。

对于小手术（例如局部麻醉、腹股沟疝修补术、腹腔镜手术），在手术当天早晨提供正常的每日类固醇剂量即应足够。如果不能恢复口服治疗，可在术后提供等效剂量给药。对于中度应激的手术（例如全关节、部分结肠切除术），除了手术当天早晨的常规剂量外，还应在静脉使用 75 ～ 125 mg/d 的氢化可的松作为补充剂量。补充的氢化可的松可以连续输注或每 8 h 分次给予。如果没有脓毒性休克的体征和症状，应在 24 h 内停止补充类固醇，并立即恢复长期口服类固醇的剂量。手术应激较大的情况下（如冠状动脉旁路移植术、Whipple 术、食管切除术），除了手术当天早晨的常规剂量外，还应静脉给予 150 ～ 250 mg 的氢化可的松补充剂量。术后 24 h 持续注射或每 8 h 重复给药，然后每天减少 50%，直到达到术前等效的给药剂量为止。如果患者病情危重和（或）有对液体和升压药治疗无反应的脓毒性休克症状，则应继续或增加氢化可的松的补充剂量（每 8 h 静脉注射 100 mg 或 10 mg/h）。理想情况下，治疗前应随机抽取血清皮质醇，以记录是否存在肾上腺功能不全（皮质醇 <25 μg/dl）。

值得注意的是，目前的临床麻醉实践中常使用地塞米松作为止吐剂，因而可能需要调整补充类固醇的剂量。自 20 世纪 90 年代中期以来，地塞米松已被频繁用于术后恶心和呕吐风险较高的患者（经常与其他增效药物联合使用）。4 ～ 8 mg 地塞米松相当于 100 ～ 200 mg 的糖皮质激素效力。如果在手术中给予这种程度的类固醇补充，对于大多数外科手术来说，在最初的 24 h 内应可以消除肾上腺功能不全的风险。

预防

以下方法可用于预防急性肾上腺功能不全和糖皮质激素过量（超生理量）的副作用：

- 识别有发生肾上腺功能不全风险的患者；
- 对有肾上腺功能不全风险的患者进行 HPA 轴测试；
- 如果检测不可行，应警惕急性肾上腺功能不全的细微迹象，并在治疗时使用较低的阈值；
- 根据类固醇使用史和手术应激程度决定围术期的给药剂量；
- 考虑在脓毒性休克患者中使用大剂量类固醇，因为有证据表明此类患者类固醇治疗组的预后有所改善；
- 在手术当天如果同时给予地塞米松作为预防性止吐药，则减少或取消补充氢化可的松的剂量。

致谢

感谢 Bhiken Naik 和 Lisa Tannikary 医生对本章上一版的贡献。

（黄 成 译 石亚平 校）

延伸阅读

Annane D, Sebille V, Charpentier C, et al.: Effect of treatment with low doses of hydrocortisone and fludrocortisone on mortality in patients with septic shock, *JAMA* 288:862–871, 2002.

Axelrod L: Perioperative management of patients treated with glucocorticoids, *Endocrinol Metab Clin North Am* 32(2):367–383, 2003.

Hamrahian AH, Roman S, Milan S: The surgical patient taking glucocorticoids. In Nieman LK, Carty SE, editors: UpToDate, Waltham, MA. Accessed October 15, 2016.

LaRochelle Jr GE, LaRochelle AG, Ratner RE, et al.: Recovery of the hypothalamic-pituitary-adrenal (HPA) axis in patients with rheumatic diseases receiving low-dose prednisone, *Am J Med* 95:258–264, 1993.

Marik PE, Zaloga GP: Adrenal insufficiency in the critically ill, *Chest* 122:1784–1796, 2002.

Schiff R, Welsh GA: Perioperative evaluation and management of the patient with endocrine dysfunction, *Med Clin North Am* 87(1):175–192, 2003.

Udelsman R, Ramp J, Gallucci WT, et al.: Adaptation during surgical stress. A reevaluation of the role of glucocorticoids, *J Clin Invest* 77:1377–1381, 1986.

Yong SL, Coulthard P, Wrzosek A: Supplemental perioperative steroids for surgical patients with adrenal insufficiency, *Cochrane Database Syst Rev* 12, 2012. CD005367.

第26章 耶和华见证会患者

Gail A. Van Norman

病例概要

患者，R女士，45岁，因第4次怀孕收治入院。第二天，她生下了女儿，但出现了与侵入性胎盘有关的出血并发症。由于她的宗教信仰，R女士拒绝输血。尽管如此，当R女士失血达到了总血容量大约80%时，医师首先寻求法律咨询，然后在耽搁一段时间后给她输注了2个单位的血——手术室里唯一可用的血液。R女士在女儿出生大约2.5 h后去世。她的家人以医疗事故为由起诉医师，纽约最高法院陪审团判决赔偿原告125万美元。

问题分析

定义

耶和华见证会关于输血的教义是基于教派对圣经中禁止吸血的经文的解释：

> 创世记9:3—凡活着的动物，都可作你们的食物；这一切我都赐给你们，如同菜蔬一样；惟独肉带着血，那就是它的生命，你们不可吃。
>
> 利未记17:10-16—若吃什么血，我必向那吃血的人变脸，把他从民中剪除……你们都不可吃血；寄居在你们中间的外人也不可吃血……因为一切活物的血就是他的生命。凡吃了血的，必被剪除。
>
> 使徒行传15:28-29—就是禁戒祭偶像的物，和血，并勒死的牲畜和奸淫。这几件你们若能自己禁戒不犯，就好了。愿你们平安。

基于20世纪这段经文的解释，许多耶和华见证会教徒在任何情况下都拒绝输血，即使这种输血可以挽救生命。这可能会给一些麻醉科医师和外科医师带来严重的伦理道德困惑，他们更关注患者当前的身体健康，而不是将来。

伦理意义

在西方医学伦理学中，尊重患者自主性是支配医师行为的主导因素。在20世纪以前，医师依靠家长式的伦理框架，由医师而不是患者来决定什么是患者的“最佳利益”，而最佳利益的确定通常取决于有利于维护生命的决定。然而，在整个20世纪，文化变迁和法律判例将决策的重心从医师转移到了患者身上。伦理医疗的重点并不是“维护生命”，而是生活质量的维护。因此，患者对医疗行为的认可，特别是**知情同意**，成为医学实践中伦理和法律价值的基石。

尊重患者自主意愿也符合医学伦理学的第二条原则，即仁慈或“行善”。通过尊重耶和华见证会患者的意愿，医师表现出对他们的精神信仰以及他们对死后美好精神生活目标优先考虑的尊重。此外，医师应避免参与损害患者的精神信仰。

如果尊重患者的信念会导致医师违背他/她自己的道德准则，医师能成为“良心反对者”吗？医师可以而且确实有时会争辩说，如果可以的话，不进行有效的救命治疗会违背他们个人的道德信仰，拒绝输血（以及其他常见的救命治疗，例如心肺复苏）违反了医师的道德“权利”。然而，医师和他们的患者之间有一种特殊的“社会契约”，这种契约赋予医师重大的社会特权，以回报他们把患者的自主利益置于自己的利益之上，把患者的道德权利置于自己的权利之上。

医师通常都清楚对患者的这些义务，并且可选择不进行医疗行为或避免医疗行为会违反自己道德准则的专业领域。此外，他们通常能够避免可能违反个人道德的特定患者关系。但是，允许个别医师的伦理道德能常规取代医学伦理学的一般原则，这将对整个医学行业内医学哲学的完整性构成挑战。例如，医师在没有知情同意的情况下不允许进行治疗，因为他或她不认为这是一个重要的原则。社会把同意和拒绝的权利放在首位，医师在社会中发挥促进作用。许多麻醉实践的政策都认识到，可以预见会碰到强烈坚持个人道德信仰的情况，可以通过预案和计划避免冲突。在允许对患者进行适当治疗的时间段内，医师可以根据自己的情况做出选择，从伦理上讲，医师可以放弃对患者的治疗，转而选择另一位在道德上没有异议的医师。因此，允许一些医师从例如堕胎手术中“选择退出”的行为。不幸的是，时间并不总是提供这样的选择，医师有义务提供在伦理医疗中需要广泛道德要求的医疗服务，而不是将他们的个人道德信仰强加于患者。

法律层面的考虑

联邦法律和法律判例支持可自主决定的患者有拒绝接受挽救生命输血的权利，尽管也有一些例外。1914 年，具有里程碑意义的“施伦德诉纽约医院协会案”（*Schloendor v. Society of New York Hospital*）裁定，“每个成年且心智健全的人，都有权决定自己的身体该如何处置。”这些权利基于宪法对隐私和不干涉的保障。

Karen Ann Quinlan 和 *Nancy Cruzan* 的案例涉及昏迷患者，他们的代理决策者希望停止维持生命的治疗。新泽西州最高法院和美国最高法院分别认为，基于宪法第 14 条修正案所依据的权利允许患者拒绝接受此类治疗。美国国会于 1990 年通过了《患者自决权法案》，并在联邦法律中确立了患者拒绝任何医学治疗（见第 7 章 7.1 节），包括维持生命治疗的权利。最近的案例涉及一名长期处于植物人状态的妇女，*Terri Schiavo*，她的丈夫想停止管饲，此案例证明了这项宪法权利的持久性。

识别

临床病情发展迅速，需要快速决策。在出现这种情况之前医师应该熟悉基本情况并做出适当的反应。

有决定权的成年患者

如果有决定权的成年患者被告知相关风险，并拒绝接受某种医疗行为，即使生命受到威胁，伦理原则和法律判例都支持其他们决定。

没有决定权的成年患者

尊重患者的自主声明，有决定权的患者可能会宣布未来在他们没有决定权和（或）无法表达自己的意愿时可能出现的医疗问题他们所做的决定。生前遗嘱、不抢救的决定、拒绝输血和器官捐献这些预立指示，在伦理和法律上被视为患者自己的意愿。在许多情况下，代理决策者可以为没有决定权的患者做出决定，许多州已经建立了法律等级制度，规定谁可以代表患者做出并表达此类决定（表 26.1）。

怀孕的患者

伦理原则确立了孕妇决定权的伦理和法律权威，特别是在怀孕早期影响胎儿生命的决定，甚至包括堕胎，都普遍受到尊重。随着孕期的进展和胎儿独立存活的可能性越来越大，母亲决定权的比重可能会降低，母亲的医疗行为决定是否一定会凌驾于胎儿利益之上的问题，法院的判决存在争议。当孕期和分娩期间发生母胎冲突时，母亲的妊娠期越长，她就越有可能在法律上被迫遵从胎儿的利益。然而，正如 *Darlene Brown* 案例的结果所表明的那样，这并不是一个确定的事实。*Brown* 在怀孕 34 周时接受了手术。她表示，作为耶和华见证会信徒，她将拒绝输血。当出现意外的严重失血时，她的医师寻求并获得了法院要求输血的裁决，理由是除了她自身的风险外，不输血还会给她未出生的胎儿带来风险。后来她生下了一名健康的男婴。*Brown* 随后向伊利诺斯州法院提出上诉，要求就先前的裁决做出声明，

框 26.1 代理决策的示例层次结构[*]

- 医疗行为决定的长期授权书
- 有权做出医疗行为决定的监督员或监护人
- 配偶或同居伴侣
- 成年子女或如果意见一致成年子女作为一个群体
- 有监护权父母或如果意见一致的父母
- 如果意见一致的成年兄弟姐妹
- 如果意见一致的成年孙子女
- 其他与患者血缘关系最密切的成年亲属

[*] 各州层次结构可能有所不同

以便为未来的政府官员提供指导，确定医师是否有权推翻她拒绝输血的自主意愿。法庭做出对她有利的判决，声明如下：

> ［怀孕］女性的自由在某种意义上受到威胁，这是人类状况所特有的，对法律亦是殊例……．［女性的］苦难太过私密和个人化，国家不能坚持自己对女性角色的看法，无论这种看法在我们的历史和文化进程中多么占主导地位。女性的命运必须在很大程度上取决于她自己对自己精神需求和社会地位的看法。

未成年患者

由于认知和情感上的不成熟，未成年患者直到18岁才被认为有自主决定能力。在那个时候，除非情况表明患者是没有决定权的，否则认为患者有能力做出医疗决定。在某些情况下，未成年人可以在法律上质疑这一规则，并因其独立的认知和情感能力而被授予做出医疗决定的权利。此外，许多州承认法律赋予未成年人在未经父母知情或同意的情况下做出医疗决定和寻求医疗行为权利的特殊情况。通常这种情况包括生殖健康、成瘾治疗和精神健康障碍治疗等问题。各州的法律不尽相同，医疗人员应该熟悉当地法规。关于未成年人权利的更多信息见第15章。

在大多数“正常”情况下，儿童的医疗决策是由代理决策者根据符合儿童“最佳利益”的原则做出的，而不是基于儿童的意愿。这种决定通常是由父母做出的，因为在大多数情况下，没有理由去质疑是否有人比父母更有资格去做这些决定。然而，当父母决定拒绝为未成年儿童提供救命治疗时，例如为耶和华见证会信徒的孩子做出输血的决定时，伦理原则建议至少应该从“最佳利益”的角度重新审查这一决定。在这种情况下，法院更有可能干预和撤销父母的决定。

紧急情况下

有决定权的患者在紧急情况下不会自动失去他们的宪法权利，如果他们拒绝医疗干预，这些意愿应该在道德和法律上得到尊重。然而，医疗紧急情况下到处都是可能损害患者做出决定能力的情况——头部受伤、中毒、休克等等。患者预立指示的文件，比如生前遗嘱和输血决定，在他们可能无法表达意愿的情况下能准确地决定。在这种情况下应遵守预立指示。在患者没有能力做决定和患者的愿望不明的情况下，医师可能必须实施认为对患者最有利的治疗。

知情同意和耶和华见证会患者

当患者拒绝输血时，确保患者充分了解该决定的风险和益处尤其重要。充分了解风险不仅包括死亡风险，还包括如果在严重失血期间不输血可能发生的其他健康后果的风险。这些问题包括卒中、严重的心脏不良事件、肾衰竭和其他相关后果。如果患者已怀孕，还应包括潜在的胎儿流产或损伤。对于耶和华见证会患者，还应审查其他信息。在实体器官移植的情况下，应告知患者在实体器官中存在一些血细胞。应讨论血液保存技术，包括血液稀释。应描述血液回收技术，如细胞保存技术，并应要求患者指出他们能够接受的血液成分。

强制

耶和华见证教会社区的成员和家庭成员陪同需要治疗的耶和华见证会患者是很常见的，这既是为了支持他们所爱的人，也是为了强化不输血的信条。虽然罕见，但一些医疗服务人员曾经历过这样的情况：耶和华见证会患者私下做出的决定不同于其在家人和社区面前做出的决定。这些合作行为提醒我们，所有患者都应该有机会在一个没有潜在强制的环境中表达他们对医疗行为的意愿。将家庭成员和教会成员送到手术等候区，就可以做到这一点。私下讨论的目的不应该是说服患者强制接受输血，而应该是确保了解患者的真实意愿。患者私下做出的关于输血的任何决定都应严格保密。

管理

我们的病例情节的细节取自一个实际的诉讼，该诉讼证明了拒绝输血两难困境中的一些微妙之处，实际上几乎与任何表示患者拒绝救命治疗的预立指示相关。

在该病例中，输血方面没有母婴冲突。如果母亲需要输血才能存活足够长的时间进行分娩，或者如果母亲需要输血主要是为了挽救胎儿的生命，母亲的拒绝会造成伦理和法律上的两难困境，因为这会使母亲的自主权利与另一个潜在的人即胎儿的利益相冲突。如何从伦理和法律上解决这一问题取决于许多因素：例如，对母亲的伤害（输血）将有利于孩子的可能性。如果可能性很小，那么主张母亲的权利应该受到侵犯的观点就更有争议了。另一方面，如果这种可能性很大，那么就会出现其他伦理问题，即生命的内在价值是否应该超越对自主权的尊重。一般来说，法院不把胎儿视为“未成年人”，也像病例中出生的婴儿很少去干预。在本病例中，孩子已经出生，只有母亲的生命正处于危险之中。

尊重患者自主权的伦理原则要求应该尊重母亲的拒绝。母亲是否应该被迫接受输血，以免孩子失去母亲，法院在裁决中指出，我们通常不要求父母仅仅是因为有孩子就不去参与只对自己有害或其他危及生命的活动（如跳伞、潜水、攀岩）。

在本病例中，医师决定违反这一伦理原则，而对善良原则进行争论（忽略了患者的善良概念与他们的不同）。在美国，无论在道德上还是在法律上，这种对善良的定义一般不会取代对自主的尊重。更严重的问题是，一旦医师做出这个决定，他们就不能按照医疗标准行事。输血太少，太迟——部分原因是医师在行动前等待律师为他们开脱潜在的法律责任。换句话说，医师的做法是保护自己未来不受伤害，而不是防止对患者造成伤害。由于他们的方法，输血几乎没有机会成功拯救患者，尽管它实际上肯定会造成严重的精神伤害。

目前还不清楚，在本病例中，医师是否有机会为拒绝输血的患者可能出现危及生命的失血提前做好准备。一旦确定拒绝输血的患者有发生严重出血的危险，应考虑使用特殊技术来限制失血，如血液稀释和术中血液回收。如果计划行择期手术，应在计划手术前考虑提高血细胞比容的治疗，如促红细胞生成素和补充铁剂治疗。不幸的是，一些未预料会严重失血的手术可能会在术中出现突发性失血。

当医师决定违背患者的自主意愿时，如果他们的做法不符合最低的医疗行为标准，就很难判断他们这样做是正当的。在这种情况下，患者受到双重伤害：不仅患者的自主权被忽视，而且患者还承受了不合格医疗行为的后果。虽然本章的意图不是要表明违反有决定权的患者意愿是有正当理由的，但很明显，这种违反道德的行为需要有良好的医疗技术行为做基础。

只要有可能，如果医师觉得他们的个人道德不允许他们遵循基本的医学伦理原则，如尊重患者的自主权，他们应该退出对患者的治疗，而选择一个没有冲突的医师。这些原则在 1993 年由美国麻醉科医师协会首次出版的《拒绝复苏或其他限制患者治疗要求的麻醉治疗伦理指南》（框 26.2）中得到了阐述。

预防

耶和华见证会患者，实际上是**所有**患者，在法律和道德上都有权利拒绝接受医疗治疗，即使治疗可以挽救生命。对接受手术和麻醉的耶和华见证会患者进行适当的伦理管理涉及每个医师、临床操作者和医疗机构的责任。

每个医师都有责任根据患者的自主意愿为其提供医疗服务。只有在关于风险和利益适当信息的条件下才能自主选择，医师应该与患者就这些问题进行诚恳、非强制性的对话，包括术中血液稀释技术和血液回收技术。对于拒绝输血的患者，在考虑进

框 26.2 美国麻醉科医师协会的《拒绝复苏或其他限制患者治疗要求的麻醉治疗伦理指南》摘要

自动暂停 DNR 或其他限制治疗的政策不能充分表达患者的自决权。应当审查和修订这些政策。

限制复苏操作的声明应与患者或指定的代理人一起审查，必要时应加以修改，以反映患者的意愿。

澄清 / 修改患者的预立指示应该记录在患者的医疗记录中。

术后治疗计划应包括恢复患者预立指示的计划。

讨论和文件应包括是否有针对特定并发症拒绝复苏的例外情况。

应征得患者的主治医师、外科医师 / 操作者和麻醉科医师的同意。

如果发生冲突：

- 当麻醉科医师发现患者或外科医师 / 操作者关于干预限度的决定与麻醉科医师自己的道德观念不一致时，他或她应该以一种非评判的方式退出，提供及时治疗。
- 如果患者或外科医师 / 操作者对干预限度的决定与可接受的治疗标准、伦理行为或制度政策不一致时，麻醉科医师应表达这种担忧，并将其提交给适当的机构。

DNR，拒绝复苏

行可能会大量失血的择期手术时，应考虑提前对患者做好医疗准备，甚至推迟手术，以便进行促红细胞生成素治疗或其他措施。

那些自认为在道德上无法遵守患者关于血液管理要求的医师，应该避免可能出现这种决定的情况，并将患者推荐给与患者的决定没有冲突的医师。

执业团体应该准备好接受一些成员可能在道德上反对某些医疗行为，并制定政策和实践来解决该问题，包括何时以及如何将患者治疗转移给另一个医师。

有自主权的患者拒绝接受挽救生命的治疗时，机构政策应明确规定适当的处理程序。应当明确规定孕妇拒绝输血、父母拒绝输血等特殊情况。

（陈丽茹 译 范晓华 校）

延伸阅读

American Society of Anesthesiologists: *Committee on Ethics: Ethical guidelines for the anesthesia care of patients with do-not-resuscitate orders or other directives that limit treatment.* Last amended October 15, 2013. Park Ridge, IL, 2003, ASA. Available at http://www.asahq.org. Accessed November 12, 2015.

Associated Press: Lawsuit is won on transfusion after childbirth, *The New York Times*, March 1, 1984. Available at http://www.nytimes.com/1984/03/01/nyregion/lawsuit-is-won-on-transfusion-after-childbirth.html. Accessed November 12, 2015.

Cruzan v. Director, Missouri Department of Health, 497 U.S. 261 (1990).

Fosmire v. Nicoleau 551 N.Y.S.2d 876 N.Y., 1990, Jan 18, 1990.

In re Brown 689 N.E. 2d 397 Ill. App. 1 Dist., 1997, Dec 31, 1997.

In re Quinlan (70 N.J. 10, 355 A.2d 647 [NJ 1976]).

In re Schiavo, 90–2908GD-003 (Fla Cir Ct, Pinellas Co, February 11, 2000).

Morgenweck CJ, Jackson S: Physician conscientious objection in anesthesiology practice. In Van Norman GA, Jackson S, Rosenbaum SH, et al.: *Clinical ethics in anesthesiology: a case-based textbook*, Cambridge, 2011, Cambridge University Press, pp 257–260.

Schloendorff v. Society of New York Hospital, 211 N.Y. 125, 105 N.E. 92 (1914).

The Holy Bible, revised standard version.

Weisleder P: The right of minors to confidentiality and informed consent, *J Child Neurol* 19:145–148, 2004.

West JM: Ethical issues in the care of Jehovah's Witnesses, *Curr Opin Anesth* 27:170–176, 2014.

不稳定颈椎：寰枢椎半脱位

第 27 章

Suneeta Gollapudy，*Lois A. Connolly*

病例概要

患者，男性，79 岁，因醉酒从楼梯上摔下，导致 C1 和齿突骨折。受伤 2 天后，在楼梯底部被发现。患者除了酗酒史，还合并高血压病史、吸烟史，每日抽 1 ～ 2 包香烟。患者有不适当的语言反应，且时间、地点或人物定向错乱，但无明显的神经障碍。

问题分析

定义

颈椎稳定性是颈椎在生理负重时能够保持椎骨之间的连接，保证包绕的脊髓不受到损伤。颈椎不稳定是指当生理性负重使部分颈椎移位，并压迫颈部脊髓。颈部的肌肉、韧带、椎间盘、关节结构在颈椎的稳定性上都各自发挥作用。颈椎上部的稳定性会因创伤、先天性疾病和炎性疾病受到影响，以上的所有因素也会导致寰枢椎不稳定（框 27.1）。

框 27.1　与寰枢关节半脱位有关的疾病

- 先天性疾病
  - 唐氏综合征
  - 齿状突异常
  - 黏多糖贮积症
- 后天性疾病
  - 类风湿关节炎
  - 幼年型类风湿关节炎
  - 强直性脊柱炎
  - 银屑病关节炎
  - 肠病性关节炎
    - 克罗恩病
    - 溃疡性结肠炎
- 莱特尔综合征
- 外伤
  - 齿突骨折
  - 韧带损伤

创伤性颈椎不稳定

由于颈椎的柔韧度和头部的重量，颈椎更容易受到损伤。当韧带、肌肉和关节结构无法消除冲击带来的能量，颈椎就会受损。这种能量的传递会导致脊髓中央灰质的微量出血和周围白质中神经传递中断。最初的损害后，生物化学的级联反应使神经轴细胞膜变得不稳定，引起小血管痉挛，造成二次损害。同时，颈部脊髓的初次损害会导致自主神经张力改变、自主调节能力丧失、心血管功能抑制以及低血压。

创伤性寰枢关节脱位（大于 18 岁的成年人寰齿间距 >3 mm，儿童寰齿间距 >5 mm）经常发生在颈部受外力移位，如在足球、橄榄球争球时承受的外力，也和头部外伤相关。如寰枢关节脱位或Ⅱ型齿突骨折发生（骨折发生在齿突基底部，在横向韧带和 C2 椎体之间），通常合并韧带损伤。横向韧带功能正常时，齿状体和寰椎前弓之间通常可以前后移动不超过 3 mm。如果韧带损伤，齿突移位会减少脊髓的空间（图 27.1）。在正常脊椎情况下，脊髓的空间大约是 20 mm。当空间超过 18 mm 时，脊髓不会出现受压，当空间小于 14 mm 时，脊髓就会受压。

先天性颈椎不稳定

先天性或染色体异常疾病可导致颈椎不稳定，主要是由于齿突发育不全或横向韧带松弛造成的寰枢椎不稳定。由于齿突发育不全，齿突在伸展过程

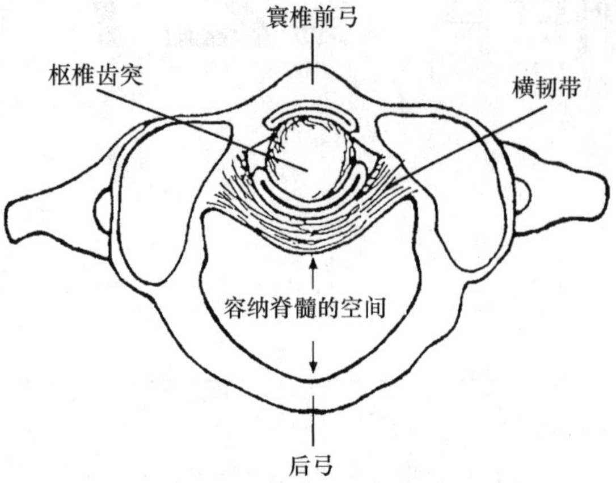

图 27.1 寰枢椎关节——从上方观察（From Crosby ET, Lui A: The adult cervical spine: implications for airway management. *Can J Anaesth* 37［1］: 77-93, 1990.）

中的稳定作用丧失，齿突的半脱位发生在前轴，减少了脊髓的空间。21 三体综合征患者中 14% ～ 22% 合并横韧带松弛。其他关节的过分松动也和寰枢椎不稳定相关。其他先天性伴有骨骼异常的疾病也是颈椎不稳定的高风险因素，例如 Goldenhar 综合征、脊椎骨骺发育不良、Morquio 综合征（黏多糖贮积症Ⅳ型）。

炎性颈椎不稳定

炎性关节病也会侵犯颈椎，例如类风湿关节炎（rheumatoid arthritis，RA）、强直性脊柱炎。RA 的病理生理包括关节翳形成，继而出现软骨和骨的破坏，韧带的松弛和不稳定。约 25% RA 患者中会出现寰枢关节半脱位。男性、病程长、有皮下结节或血清反应阳性、接受类固醇治疗的患者中更为常见。RA 患者也可发生齿突垂直半脱位。

流行病学

- 1.5% ～ 7.7% 的严重创伤患者发生颈椎损伤。
- C4 ～ C6 水平最易发生损伤。
- 最易受伤的年龄是 19 岁。近 1/4 受伤患者年龄在 17 ～ 22 岁（24.3%），近一半的受伤患者年龄在 16 ～ 30 岁（48.9%），10.7% 受伤患者发生在 60 岁以后。受伤患者的平均年龄从 19 世纪 70 年代的 29 岁上升到现在的 42 岁。约 80% 新发的脊髓损伤（spinal cord injury，SCI）患者为男性。
- 导致颈椎损伤的常见原因有机动车事故（motor vehicle accident，MVA；42% ～ 56%），坠落（19% ～ 30%），以及与枪击或运动相关的活动（6% ～ 7%）
- MVA 和运动相关的活动是年轻人颈椎损伤的常见原因，坠落是老年人颈椎损伤的常见原因。
- 年幼的儿童由于体重较轻，相较于成人有更多的软骨，不容易发生颈椎损伤。随着年龄的增长，损伤也会随之增加。
- 小于 2 岁的儿童中的颈椎损伤最常见 C1 ～ C2 节段，因为在这个节段的关节面较平，韧带也较松弛。
- 呼吸系统疾病是导致死亡的主要原因（67.4% 的死亡病例是由于肺炎）。导致死亡的第二位的原因是感染和寄生虫病。这些患者通常为菌血症（89.2%），且通常会出现褥疮、尿道感染和呼吸系统感染。
- SCI 患者 10 年、20 年、30 年、40 年的总生存率分别为 81.71%、68.05%、52.99% 和 37.44%。

识别

病史和体格检查

识别颈椎损伤从病史开始。高风险的因素（例如，MVA、坠落、病程长的 RA）和已知的染色体异常疾病，这些均可提示临床医师关注颈椎不稳定的临床表现。例如，患有 RA 患者可能会主诉弯曲颈部时发出的咔哒声以及颈部疼痛和僵硬。创伤的患者会主诉颈部疼痛和压痛。无颈部疼痛和神经损伤的警醒患者，不需要在气道操作时进一步评估颈椎情况、制动和特殊的防范措施。若患者不完全警醒，但主诉颈部疼痛，有神经损伤或有其他疼痛的损伤，应采取保护颈椎的预防措施。

由于椎管是脊椎中最宽的区域，可能发生脊椎损伤，脊髓并无损伤。46% 脊椎受损的患者中存在神经损伤，在 C5 ～ C7 损伤的患者中，发生率更高。全面详细的神经系统检查可以鉴别和区分脊髓受累的节段水平。

急性发作的自主神经功能不稳定，称之为**脊髓休克**。脊髓休克后，失去对交感神经的支配，导致全身的血流动力学不稳定，其特征为心动过缓，外周动、静脉血管舒张，低血压和心律失常。

由于失去对肋间神经的支配，或由于高位颈部损伤，失去对膈神经的支配，可能会急性出现呼吸功能受损。正常人中，胸腔扩张占静止时潮气量的 60%。即使膈神经功能完好，肺泡通气和咳嗽的力气也会受到失去肋间肌神经功能而降低。急性颈髓损伤可能会发生缺氧、肺不张和呼吸衰竭。如果并发吸入性肺炎，情况可能更加复杂。此外，由于 SCI，交感神经大量放电，也可导致神经性肺水肿。

颈椎损伤可能伴发椎动脉损伤。如果未得到诊断和治疗，发生脑缺血导致的死亡率高达 30%。椎动脉最易在 C6 进入横突孔的部位损伤。第二个常见部位是 C1 ～ C2。即使诊断明确和进行抗凝治疗，仍有 5.8% 的患者会出现临床症状，2.9% 的患者死于脑缺血。

影像学评估

国家急诊影像学应用研究（National Emergency X-radiography Use Study，NEXUS）低风险（Low Risk，NLR）标准和加拿大 C- 脊柱规则（Canadian C-Spine Rule，CCR）的项目旨在不需要让患者进行影像学检查就可以排除颈椎重大损伤。只有患者符合这 5 个特征，才有指征行颈椎（cervical spine，CS）影像学检查。

1. 患者警醒；
2. 无醉酒；
3. 无颈后压痛；
4. 无神经系统变化；
5. 无转移注意力的其他部位的损伤，如挤压伤、烧伤、大面积撕脱伤或严重的骨折。

CCR 在检测损伤方面的灵敏度为 99.4%（NLR 为 90.7%），并提出 3 个问题：

1. 患者是否有损伤的高风险因素（年龄 > 65 岁，是否为高危的受伤，如 MVA、坠落、自行车事故）?
2. 患者是否有安全评估颈椎运动范围的低风险因素？低风险因素包括简单的追尾碰撞、能坐直、能行走、迟发的颈部疼痛或无颈部压痛。
3. 患者是否能够自主向右和向左 45°转动颈部?

如果患者有低风险因素，同时能自主转动颈部且无任何高风险因素，医师可以安全地排除颈椎问题，不需要影像学检查。

X 线平片通常包含 3 个角度：前后位、侧位和齿突位。由于 X 线平片的假阴性率比计算机断层扫描（computed tomography，CT）高，X 线平片已经基本被 CT 取代。急诊医师通常依靠 CT 来评估患者的损伤情况。CT 最适合检测骨骼异常。对于哪种方法最合适用来排除精神状态改变患者的颈椎损伤情况仍存在争议。2009 年东部创伤外科学会创伤后颈椎损伤识别实践管理指南指出，自 1998 年第一版颈椎损伤指南发布以来，临床实践发生了重大变化。如今，CT 已代替 X 线平片成为影像学检查的主要筛查工具。在反应迟钝的患者中，床旁屈 / 伸动态透视不会增加有用的信息，不足以诊断并可能具有风险。对于颈椎 CT 阴性且反应迟钝患者，可以通过磁共振成像（magnetic resonance imaging，MRI）以进一步检查韧带损伤。如果 MRI 为阴性，则可以取消颈椎制动。存在争议的是 CT 扫描阴性的患者发生韧带损伤的发生率非常低。在 2005 年，Hogan 团队研究了 366 例 CS 损伤且 CT 检查阴性的患者。96.7% 患者 MRI 检查阴性，1.1% 患者检出韧带损伤。脊髓损伤最常与如骨折、韧带损伤或半脱位等影像学检查结果有关。但是，约有 3.3% 的成人无放射影像学异常的脊髓损伤（spinal cord injury without radiographic abnormality，SCIWORA），却在 MRI 上检测到 SCI。因此，目前在患者 CT 检查阴性后，是否需要 MRI 检查尚无明确推荐。对反应迟钝的患者进行额外的 MRI 筛查价格昂贵，且具有显著的风险。此外，当使用颈托超过 72 h 后，可能会发生颈托相关并发症，如颈托相关的皮疹，皮肤破裂和压力相关的伤害，颅内压增高，使用呼吸机天数和重症监护室时间延长，谵妄发生率升高，中心静脉通路穿刺困难，耽误气管切开术。这些问题须与潜在漏诊 CS 损伤的风险进行权衡。

潜在颈椎损伤患者的诊断参见颈椎损伤的评估流程（图 27.2）。

对合并慢性病相关的潜在寰枢关节半脱位 (如 RA、唐氏综合征)，可通过自然、弯曲和延伸位获取颈椎矢状面影像 (图 27.3)。应寻找前后或垂直半脱位的证据，测量脊髓可用空间大小。对 RA 患者，可通过前后位影像确定是否出现喉偏移。

风险评估

对已知不稳定 CS 的患者进行术前评估应包括以下内容：

- 通过影像学评估颈椎情况；
- 判断呼吸情况（血气分析或肺量计）；
- 检查是否有脊髓休克的证据（血压、心率、心律失常、心电图改变、是否需要升压药）；

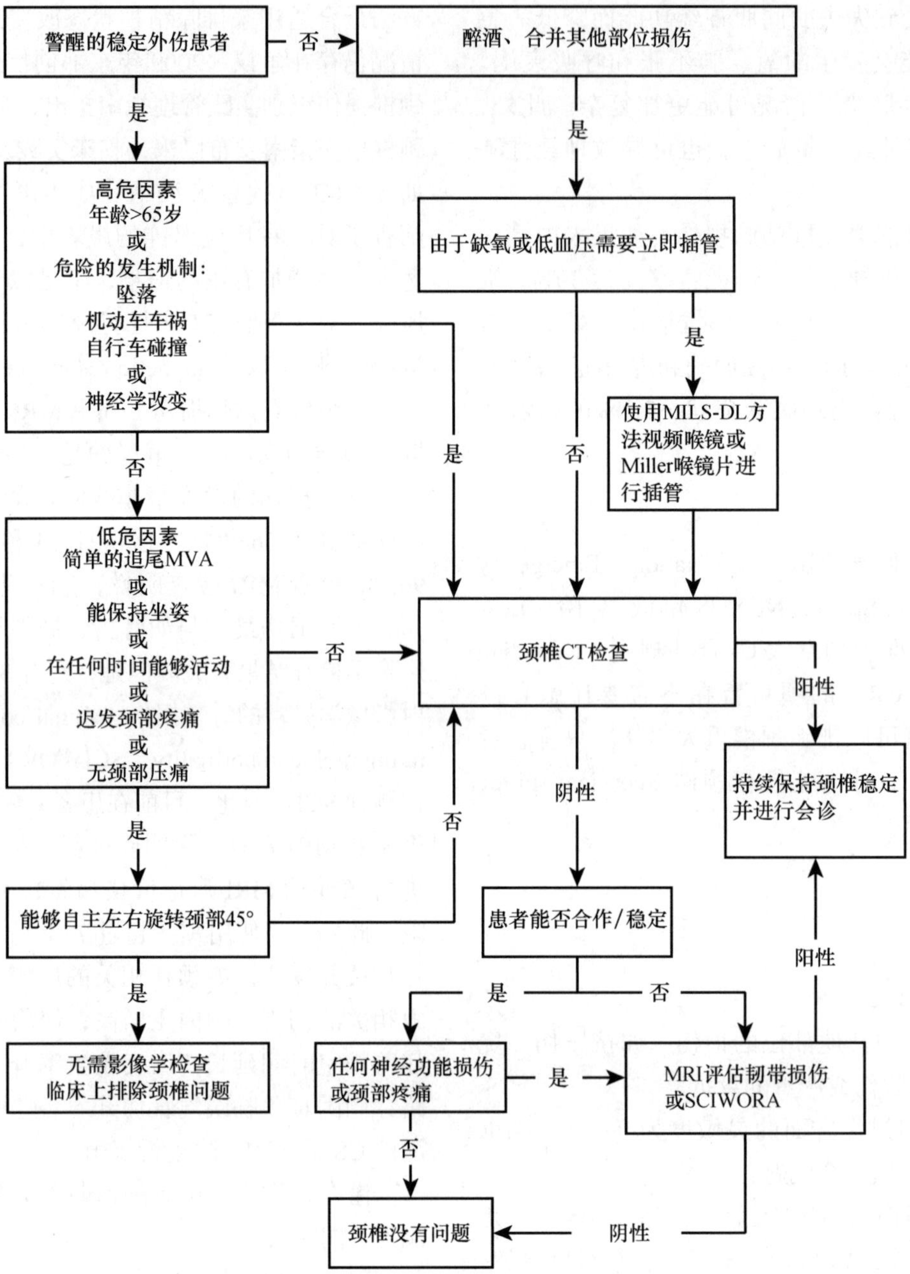

图 27.2 颈椎损伤的评估流程。CT，计算机断层扫描；DL，直接喉镜；MILS，保持中线固定手法；MRI，磁共振成像；MVA，机动车事故；SCIWORA，无放射影像学异常的脊髓损伤

- 评估损伤对中枢神经系统的影响（神经学评估，是否有闭合性颅脑外伤的证据）；
- 检查相关损伤（胸部 X 线片或 CT 和心电图以排除胸部损伤）；
- 确定血红蛋白、电解质水平、凝血功能和肌酐；
- 评估体温。

启示

如上所述，多个器官会受急性脊髓损伤的影响。发生脊髓休克的患者需要有创动脉监测、中心静脉通路和滴定升压药以确保足够的灌注压。如果存在神经源性肺水肿，需要进一步行肺动脉导管或经胸/经食管超声心动图监测。急性脊髓损伤以往使用大剂量甲泼尼龙治疗。根据国家急性脊髓损伤研究（National Acute Spinal Cord Injury Study，NASCIS）Ⅱ，在损伤的最初 8 h 内输注 30 mg/kg 甲泼尼龙，以 5.4 mg/（kg·h）持续输注 24 h。NASCIS Ⅲ 则评估了以 5.4 mg/（kg·h）持续输注 48 h 甲泼尼龙，并未发现任何益处。美国神经外科医师协会（American Association of Neurological Surgeons，AANS）和神

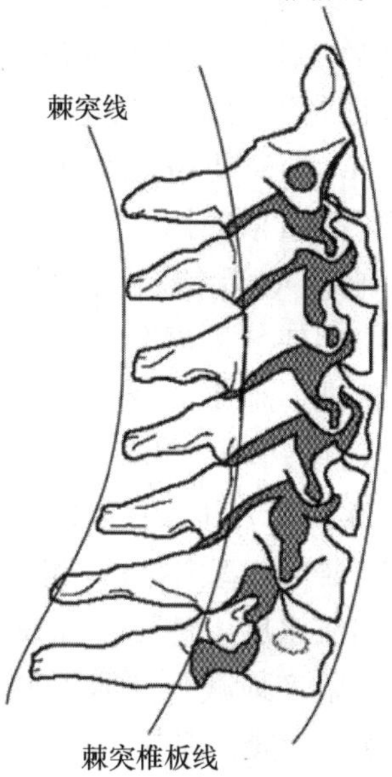

图 27.3 颈椎矢状面

经外科医师学会（Congress of Neurological Surgeons，CNS）的最新指南现已将使用甲泼尼龙重新分类在选择项，而不再是必须项。基于这种降级，鉴于观察到的甲泼尼龙缺乏疗效以及并发症增加，如伤口感染率和胃肠道出血的风险增加等，大多数 I 级创伤中心完全放弃了使用。最初的制动可通过骨骼牵引，在指导下进行复位和重新对齐。颈椎固定至关重要，在气道操作期间也必须保持。

管理

术中关注点

主要术中关注点如下：

- 监护；
- 气道管理；
- 体位；
- 心肺管理；
- 麻醉药物的使用（琥珀胆碱）；
- 液体管理，含葡萄糖液体使用；
- 术后视力丧失。

术中管理需要气管插管。气道干预的紧迫性可能是规划气道管理方案的最重要因素。其他因素包括患者的合作程度、气道评估以及颈部运动导致的脊髓损伤的风险。在颈椎不稳定的情况下进行气管插管增加了脊髓损伤的风险。顾虑在于，常规直接喉镜的力度可能导致不稳定颈椎节段发生异常大（病理）的活动并导致颈髓压迫和损伤。尽管 C3 以下运动最小，直接喉镜检查仍需要寰枢椎伸展和 C3 ～ C5 的轻度下旋。C1 ～ C2 损伤最容易引起神经损伤。手法中线牵引减少了插管期间的寰枕伸展，已发表的系列研究详细介绍了使用直接喉镜检查与中线牵引的方法，且无神经学加重的证据。

与使用弯曲（如 Macintosh）喉镜片相比，使用 Miller 型喉镜片颈椎移动较小（即轴向分散）。插管前，如提颏抬颌手法，引起的移动最大，并缩小脊髓的空间。在进行这些操作时必须非常小心。插管操作者的视野可能因患者需要固定而受到影响，因此插管失败风险也增加。但当需要快速控制气道时（如呼吸衰竭、血流动力学不稳定、颅内压增高的患者），在手法保持中线固定下直接喉镜插管最为有用。新型的视频喉镜已取代直接喉镜开始流行。Glidescope、Airtraq 和 CMAC 已经在临床使用。Glidescope 与手法中线固定（manual inline stabilization，MILS）下使用直接喉镜相比，C2 ～ C5 的运动减少 50%。光棒也是直接喉镜的另一种替代工具，颈椎运动比使用直接喉镜少 57%（表 27.1）。

控制颈椎不稳定患者的气道，清醒气管插管可能是最理想的方式，但如果需要快速插管，清醒插管可能并不合适。使用纤支镜可以在直视下插管，但如果患者咽部出血或不合作，插管可能会很困难。其他清醒下插管的技术也可采用，包括经鼻盲探插管或导丝引导下逆行插管。

由于喉罩对颈椎施加的压力较大，通常不建议使用喉罩，但它已成为插管失败或困难插管流程的一部分。使用喉罩可能会使颈椎后移（C2 ～ C6）和后纵韧带破裂。如果通过其他方式气管插管不成功，可考虑行环甲膜切开术或气管切开术。应考虑置入加强型气管导管，因其可降低摆放患者体位时导管打折的风险。

对有意识的患者实施气管插管后，搬动体位时仍需要持续保持颈椎稳定性。通常在患者处于清醒状态下摆体位，这样可以立即识别任何神经系统恶化。

由于相关损伤引发出血或由于自主神经不稳定引起神经源性休克，全身性低血压较为常见。AANS 发布了 SCI 患者血流动力学目标的推荐。应避免低血压（收缩压 <90 mm Hg），建议在急性脊髓损伤后 7 天内，维持平均动脉压（mean arterial pressure，

表 27.1 气道管理技术及其对颈椎的影响

手法保持中线稳定	消除偏移和减少角度，但增加半脱位风险
面罩通气	明显的前后移位，最大的头颈部的屈曲和伸展
口 / 鼻咽通气道	在受伤节段上扩大椎间盘≈ 2 mm 的空间
提颏 / 托下颌	在受伤节段上扩大椎间盘 >5 mm 的空间
压迫环状软骨	单手压迫环状软骨导致颈部垂直位移≈ 5mm 但没有脊柱运动
喉镜	在枕骨和 C1 ～ C2 关节伸展，C2 ～ C5 最小限度地移位，嗅花位：位于胸部的下颈部屈曲，在上颈部头部伸展；在受伤节段上扩大椎间盘 3 ～ 4 mm 的空间
Glidescope	与使用弯喉镜片相比，C2 ～ C5 的整体脊柱运动减少了 50%
光棒	所有节段的运动减少 57%
喉罩	可能会产生上颈椎后移；插入过程中：C5 和上段屈曲 <2°；插管期间：C4 和上段屈曲 <3°；C3 以上几乎无运动

MAP）在 85 ～ 90 mmHg 以改善脊髓灌注。如果平均动脉压低于 85 mmHg，先静脉输注晶体液。如果血细胞比容低（血液）或作为扩容使用（白蛋白），则给予胶体液。如果患者的体液容量状态正常，但 MAP 仍然低于阈值，AANS 建议使用血管活性药物，在使用 α- 激动剂（去氧肾上腺素）之前，通常使用 β_a- 激动剂（多巴胺），以提高 MAP。

创伤性颈椎损伤后常见呼吸功能不全和肺功能障碍。严重受伤的患者可能出现肺活量显著减少，并且更容易发生低氧血症，这可能会加重脊髓缺血。因此，仔细监测并经常进行动脉血气分析非常重要。在手术结束时，要对拔管进行严格的临床评估。

除了保证气道和正确的患者体位外，麻醉药物的选择也至关重要。在受伤后的第一个 24 h 内，琥珀胆碱可能引起高钾血症。在去神经支配的肌肉中，运动终板增殖，琥珀胆碱会产生放大的去极化反应，并释放大量的钾。钾的急剧上升可导致心律失常、心脏停搏和死亡。

麻醉药物的选择根据药物能否保护脊髓灌注和自主调节功能，以及药物是否具有神经保护作用。如果术中进行躯体感觉诱发电位监测，麻醉药物可能会影响诱发电位的潜伏期或幅度。低血压和低体温也可能影响躯体感觉诱发电位监测。以静脉麻醉药物、阿片类药物和非去极化肌松药为基础，加用最少量的强效吸入麻醉药物的麻醉方案似乎最具优势。如果同时监测运动诱发电位（motor evoked potential，MEP），则应使用全凭静脉麻醉。已经证实吸入麻醉药以剂量依赖性方式降低皮质振幅，且氧化亚氮比其他吸入麻醉药物更能降低皮质振幅。丙泊酚已被证明即使剂量逐渐增加也能维持皮质波形的振幅和潜伏期。临床剂量的右美托咪定作为全凭静脉麻醉的辅助药物，几乎不会改变诱发电位（evoked potential，EP），因此可以安全使用。

液体管理应维持血管内容量，以确保充分灌注，同时应当避免间质水肿。使用目标导向的液体管理方案有助于最大限度地减少液体正平衡。避免使用低渗和含葡萄糖的溶液，因其可能会加剧脊髓水肿。已经证实，神经学结局恶化与短暂的脊髓缺血和血浆葡萄糖浓度的升高相关。

颈椎手术后的术后视力丧失较少见，但应与俯卧位手术的患者进行讨论。风险因素包括手术时间、失血量、非胶体的使用、贫血和长时间低血压。

术后关注点

气管拔管取决于神经受损伤的水平以及有无头胸部相关损伤。脱机标准包括最大吸气压力为 -20 cm H_2O，肺活量为 1000 ml，PaO_2/FiO_2 大于 250，此标准可能不适合四肢瘫痪患者。在手术结束后是否拔管须由外科医师和麻醉科医师共同决定。理论上，颈椎前路软组织创伤和俯卧患者的体位可能会导致上呼吸道水肿和潜在呼吸窘迫可能。Epstein 及其同事探索了一种方案，接受颈椎前路和后路手术的患者术后带管过夜，在术后第 1 天，经过纤支镜评估气道水肿情况后，进行拔管。Kwon 及其同事认为，气道水肿是导致气道受损和术后发生呼吸困难的最终病理途径。他们也采取保留气管导管过夜来预防任何不良的呼吸道紧急情况。通过气囊漏气试验评估拔管的条件，针对这些患者的气道管理提供了安全且有效的术后方案。他们认为长时间的手术、大量晶体液和输血以及失血与延迟拔管相关。气囊漏气试验是先抽掉气管导管套囊的气体，用手指堵住气管导管，观察清醒的患者能否使导管周围的气体流动。如果空气在吸气和呼气时都流动，则可认为气道通畅。如果手术入路包括前颈部，进行气囊漏气试验有助于排除水肿或颈部血肿引起的气道压迫。在颈部手术期间，喉返神经和迷走神经分支都可能受损（右侧比左侧更常见），可能导致拔管后声带麻痹和喘鸣，以及吞咽困难。

预防

预防颈椎不稳定患者出现神经功能恶化需要注意以下方面：

- 在气道操作和体位变化期间识别颈椎损伤和保持颈椎稳定；
- 通过优化 MAP 维持脊髓灌注；
- 注意液体管理，尽量减少脊髓水肿；
- 及时治疗呼吸系统损伤，防止缺氧及其带来的进一步神经系统恶化；
- 神经保护。

改善脊髓损伤患者神经系统结局的探索已转向针对如缺血、轴索变性和炎症等的继发性损伤机制。尽管许多临床试验评估了可能的神经保护疗法的有效性，但没有任何一种方法在保留或改善脊髓功能方面表现出决定性的优势。被评价过的神经保护剂包括甲泼尼龙、神经节苷脂 GM-1、加环利定（天冬氨酸受体拮抗剂）、替拉扎特（自由基清除剂）和纳洛酮。这些药物的保护效果从未被证实，并且许多治疗方案具有严重的副作用。此外，也没有证据表明低体温有效。

总之，不稳定的颈椎需要及时识别、评估神经系统损伤，并对全身的影响进行评估及治疗，以及细致的气道管理，以确保颈椎损伤获得最佳治疗结局。

（郭品豪 译 余喜亚 校）

延伸阅读

Austin N, Krishnamoorthy V, Dagal A: Airway management in cervical spine injury, *Int J Crit Illn Inj Sci* 4:50–56, 2014.

Blood pressure management after acute spinal cord injury: *Neurosurgery* 50:S58–S62, 2002.

Boisseau N, Madany M, Staccini P, et al.: Comparison of the effects of sevoflurane and propofol on cortical somatosensory evoked potentials, *Br J Anaesth* 88:785–789, 2002.

Chaudhary SB, Hullinger H, Vives MJ: Management of acute spinal fractures in ankylosing spondylitis, *ISRN Rheumatol* 150484:2011, 2011.

Como JJ, Diaz JJ, Dunham CM, et al.: Practice management guidelines for identification of cervical spine injuries following trauma: update from the eastern association for the surgery of trauma practice management guidelines committee, *J Trauma* 67:651–659, 2009.

Consortium for Spinal Cord Medicine: Early acute management in adults with spinal cord injury: a clinical practice guideline for health care professionals, *J Spinal Cord Med* 31:403, 2008.

Dooney N, Dagal A: Anesthetic considerations in acute spinal cord trauma, *Int J Crit Illn Inj Sci* 1:36–43, 2011.

Emery SE, Akhavan S, Miller P, et al.: Steroids and risk factors for airway compromise in multilevel cervical corpectomy patients: a prospective, randomized, double-blind study, *Spine (Phila Pa 1976)* 34:229–232, 2009.

Epstein NE, Hollingsworth R, Nardi D, et al.: Can airway complications following multilevel anterior cervical surgery be avoided? *J Neurosurg* 94:185–188, 2001.

Hindman BJ, Santoni BG, Puttlitz CM, et al.: Intubation biomechanics: laryngoscope force and cervical spine motion during intubation with Macintosh and Airtraq laryngoscopes, *Anesthesiology* 121:260–271, 2014.

Hogan GJ, Mirvis SE, Shanmuganathan K, et al.: Exclusion of unstable cervical spine injury in obtunded patients with blunt trauma: is MR imaging needed when multi-detector row CT findings are normal? *Radiology* 237(1):106–113, 2005.

Jung JY: Airway management of patients with traumatic brain injury/C-spine injury, *Korean J Anesthesiol* 68:213–219, 2015.

Kasodekar VB, Chen JL: Monocular blindness: a complication of intraoperative positioning in posterior cervical spine surgery, *Singapore Med J* 47:631–633, 2006.

Kill C, Risse J, Wallot P, et al.: Videolaryngoscopy with glidescope reduces cervical spine movement in patients with unsecured cervical spine, *J Emerg Med* 44:750–756, 2013.

Kwon B, Yoo JU, Furey CG, et al.: Risk factors for delayed extubation after single-stage, multi-level anterior cervical decompression and posterior fusion, *J Spinal Disord Tech* 19:389–393, 2006.

Lauweryns P: Role of conservative treatment of cervical spine injuries, *Eur Spine J* 19:23–26, 2010.

Lee LA: Perioperative visual loss and anesthetic management, *Curr Opin Anaesthesiol* 26:375–381, 2013.

Mueller CA, Peters I, Podlogar M, et al.: Vertebral artery injuries following cervical spine trauma: a prospective observational study, *Eur Spine J* 20:2202–2209, 2011.

National Spinal Cord Injury Statistical Center: 2014 Annual statistical report for the spinal cord injury model systems public version. University of Alabama at Birmingham, Birmingham, AL. Available at https://www.nscisc.uab.edu/reports.aspx. Accessed May 10, 2016.

Pimentel L, Diegelmann L: Evaluation and management of acute cervical spine trauma, *Emerg Med Clin North Am* 28:719–738, 201https://www.nscisc.u

Postab.edu/reports.aspxss Study Group: Risk factors associated with ischemic optic neuropathy after spinal fusion surgery, *Anesthesiology* 116:15–24, 2012.

Readdy WJ, Whetstone WD, Ferguson AR, et al.: Complications and outcomes of vasopressor usage in acute traumatic central cord syndrome, *J Neurosurg Spine* 1–7, 2015. [epub ahead of print].

Rozet I, Metzner J, Brown M, et al.: Dexmedetomidine does not affect evoked potentials during spine surgery, *Anesth Analg* 121:492–501, 2015.

Ryken TC, Hurlbert RJ, Hadley MN, et al.: The acute cardiopulmonary management of patients with cervical spinal cord injuries, *Neurosurgery* 72(Suppl 2):84–92, 2013.

Selvarajah S, Hammond ER, Haider AH, et al.: The burden of acute traumatic spinal cord injury among adults in the united states: an update, *J Neurotrauma* 31:228–238, 2014.

Stier GR, Gabriel CL, Cole DJ: Neurosurgical diseases and trauma of the spine and spinal cord: anesthetic considerations. In Cottrell JE, Young WL, editors: *Cottrell and Young's neuroanesthesia*, 5th ed., Philadelphia, 2010, Elsevier, pp 343–389.

Turkstra TP, Craen RA, Pelz DM, et al.: Cervical spine motion: a fluoroscopic comparison during intubation with lighted stylet, GlideScope, and Macintosh laryngoscope, *Anesth Analg* 101:910–915, 2005.

Wong DM, Prabhu A, Chakraborty S, et al.: Cervical spine motion during flexible bronchoscopy compared with the Lo-Pro GlideScope, *Br J Anaesth* 102:424–430, 2009.

Wuermser LA, Ho CH, Chiodo AE, et al.: Spinal cord injury medicine. 2. Acute care management of traumatic and nontraumatic injury, *Arch Phys Med Rehabil* 88:S55–S61, 2007.

Yang SY, Boniello AJ, Poorman CE, et al.: A review of the diagnosis and treatment of atlantoaxial dislocations, *Global Spine J* 4:197–210, 2014.

第28章 上呼吸道感染

Harshad Gurnaney，Arjunan Ganesh

病例概要

患儿，女性，4 岁，最近有上呼吸道感染（upper respiratory tract infection，URI）病史，症状为清涕和偶尔干咳，3 天前有低烧病史，拟全麻下行扁桃体切除术及腺样体切除术。她有频繁上呼吸道感染的病史，在过去的 3 个月中发作 4 次。患儿在七氟烷麻醉时发生喉痉挛。

问题分析

定义

患有活动性 URI 的儿童，其择期手术麻醉的结局存在相互矛盾的信息。一些研究表明，URI 的儿童在围术期发生呼吸并发症的风险增加。其他研究则认为这类患儿并没有增加患病风险（表 28.1）。任何对照研究都没有显示死亡率增加。临床医师在得出麻醉风险效益比结论时需要了解的研究设计的局限性包括：病例对照研究的回顾性数据收集，研究间缺乏明确的 URI 定义标准，年龄、手术类型、麻醉方法的多样性，不同研究对不良事件的定义和报告不一致，以及每个麻醉科医师取消手术的选择偏差。回顾性数据表明，近期 URI（在 2 ~ 6 周内）的儿童与无 URI 或有活动性 URI 的儿童相比，发生肺部并发症的风险更高。这些潜在并发症的临床重要性将进一步影响取消或继续手术。例如，喉痉挛发生率的增加是否会导致呼吸系统并发症发生率的增加，或者麻醉科医师能否在不造成伤害的情况下识别和治疗这种并发症？最近的一项前瞻性研究表明，虽然急性和近期 URI 的儿童发生呼吸道并发症的风险较大，但大多数儿童可以进行择期手术，且不增加不良麻醉后果。然而，这项研究是非随机的，继续手术的决定是由负责患者的主治麻醉科医师决定的。取消手术的常见原因是严重的 URI、存在下呼吸道感染和细菌感染。一项前瞻性队列研究发现，在接受择期手术的喉罩全麻的儿科患者中，近期 URI 的存在与围术期呼吸并发症发生的概率增加有关（OR 1.8；CI：1.3 ~ 2.6）。

识别

诊断 URI 的儿童至少应有以下的体征和症状中

表 28.1　患儿上呼吸道感染全身麻醉后呼吸道并发症的发生率

	频率（%）（上呼吸道感染症状）					
观察指标	活动性	最近	无	数量	气管插管	研究设计
气道阻塞[*]	1.6	5.3	1.6	3585	大多数	R
喉痉挛	1.3	2.4	1.2	489	没有	P
支气管痉挛	13.3		0.6	402	一半	P
咽喉炎	3.8		0.7	22159	一些	P
低氧血症	32	25	10	130	没有	P
低氧血症	40		16	402	一半	P
低氧血症	20		0	50	大多数	P

[*] 包括喉痉挛和支气管痉挛。

P，前瞻性；R，回顾性

的两个：①喉咙痛或发痒，②打喷嚏，③流鼻涕，④鼻塞，⑤不适，⑥干咳，⑦发热低于 38.5℃，⑧喉炎。第 1 项和第 5 项、第 2 项和第 3 项、第 3 项和第 6 项以及第 4 项和第 6 项的组合要求至少存在一个额外的症状来满足 URI 的诊断。有高热和全身症状及（或）下呼吸道受累症状的患者不止存在简单的上呼吸道感染，从某种意义上来说他们的疾病不仅仅局限于上呼吸道。

风险评估

儿童每年发生 5 ~ 8 次 URI（在儿童日托中心和父母吸烟的儿童中发病率更高）。在所有的小儿外科手术申请者中，6% 的麻醉和手术患者存在活动性上呼吸道感染。症状消失后，肺部变化可持续 4 ~ 7 周。上呼吸道感染的阶段（开始、活跃、消散等）可能会影响风险。此外，在评估风险时应考虑手术类型、儿童年龄、麻醉计划（插管）和并存内科疾病。

启示

继发于分泌物和（或）气道应激的潜在呼吸并发症包括喉痉挛（喉痉挛的其他危险因素包括低龄、气道手术、麻醉科医师经验不足）；支气管痉挛（仅插管患者）；拔管后喘鸣；围术期动脉血氧饱和度降低。

与这些并发症相关的费用包括日间手术住院时间延长、门诊患者意外住院、未预期的重症监护病房入住以及这些并发症继发的潜在医疗法律问题。与取消手术相关的费用包括：额外的术前预约和重复检查（必要时），因临时通知取消而导致的手术室使用效率下降造成的收入损失，给患者和家庭带来的不便，以及可能给家庭带来的收入损失。

管理

注意潜在的并发症。所有的患者都不一样，在决定是否继续治疗时，医师应考虑儿童的年龄；URI 发生的频率（除了患者本身，还需要与年龄匹配的对照组相比）；手术的类型及紧急程度，以及手术是否可舒缓或减少慢性鼻塞或复发性耳部感染的次数；儿童的其他健康问题；麻醉科医师的技术和经验；父母对最近 / 当前 URI 麻醉用药风险的理解；以及其他问题（例如，外科医师是否可以手术，特定或自体血液即将到期）。

如果决定继续手术，应详细记录外科医师和家属讨论的风险，且家属接受增加的风险，并愿意继续手术。然后制订一个麻醉方案，该方案需要考虑以下内容：①术前服用抗胆碱能药物（阿托品、异丙托溴铵雾化）；②支气管扩张剂治疗支气管痉挛；③使用较小的气管导管、喉罩或者面罩麻醉；④术后监测动脉血氧饱和度并适当补充氧气。

预防

许多学龄前和学龄早期儿童在任何给定的时间内都有 URI 或者正在从 URI 中恢复。所有 URI 患儿的手术不可能推迟到症状消除后 4 ~ 6 周。这种策略会导致许多儿童可以进行手术干预的治疗时间窗狭小或根本无法手术。良好的临床判断、患者家属和外科医师的讨论、书面的知情同意以及麻醉科医师的经验，在决定处理每一个病例时都至关重要。

（陈丽茹　译　赵珍珍　校）

延伸阅读

Cote CJ: The upper respiratory tract infection (URI) dilemma: fear of a complication or litigation? *Anesthesiology* 95:283–285, 2001.

Cohen MM, Cameron CB: Should you cancel the operation when a child has an upper respiratory tract infection? *Anesth Analg* 72:282–288, 1991.

Rolf N, Coté CJ: Frequency and severity of desaturation events during general anesthesia in children with and without upper respiratory infections, *J Clin Anesth* 4:200–203, 1992.

Schreiner MS, O'Hara IB, Markakis DA, et al.: Do children who experience laryngospasm have in increased risk of upper respiratory tract infection? *Anesthesiology* 85:475–489, 1996.

Tait AR, Knight PR: The effects of general anesthesia on upper respiratory tract infection in children, *Anesthesiology* 67:930–935, 1987.

Tait AR, Knight PR: Intraoperative respiratory complications in patients with upper respiratory tract infection, *Can J Anaesth* 34:300–303, 1987.

Tait AR, Malviya S, Voepel-Lewis T, et al.: Risk factors for perioperative adverse respiratory events in children with upper respiratory tract infections, *Anesthesiology* 95:299–306, 2001.

von Ungern-Sternberg BS, Boda K, Habre W, et al.: Laryngeal mask airway is associated with an increased incidence of adverse respiratory events in children with recent upper respiratory tract infections, *Anesthesiology* 107(5):714–719, 2007.

第二部分

手术相关并发症

第29章 腹主动脉瘤修复术

Christopher J. O'Connor，Anthony de la Cruz

病例概要

患者，男性，74岁，全身麻醉下行肾下型吻合口旁腹主动脉瘤腔内修复术（endovascular aneurysm repair，EVAR）。患者既往有慢性稳定性心绞痛、高血压和陈旧性心肌梗死。术前的双嘧达莫试验显示患者有较大面积的固定的心肌缺损，但无可逆性疾病的证据。患者4个月前行开腹腹主动脉瘤（abdominal aortic aneurysm，AAA）修复手术，术后因急性肾损伤（acute kidney injury，AKI）在ICU治疗1周。在撑开血管内移植物时，有轻微的血压升高，但在球囊释放后迅速好转。术中共输入2 L勃脉力（Plasmalyte）。患者术后成功拔管并转运至ICU。

问题分析

定义

EVAR正在成为治疗原发性和再次手术的AAA的常用方法（图29.1）。EVAR与开放式AAA修复术在麻醉管理上有很大不同。了解每种手术方式的特点有助于我们制订合适的麻醉计划，包括选择合适的监测项目，麻醉方式以及围术期可能出现的并发症。

AAA的开放手术修复（open surgical repair，OSR）涉及肾下主动脉的阻断。导致主动脉血流阻断的外科分离、主动脉本身的血流阻断、主动脉夹闭开放后引起的病理生理改变，导致术中不同程度的血流动力学变化。大面积的开放手术期间的低血压相对常见，尽管它通常短暂且耐受性良好。在已知或之前未确诊的冠状动脉疾病（coronary artery disease，CAD）患者中有时会发生心肌缺血，并且可能伴有肺毛细血管楔压升高，心排血量减少，经食管超声心动图（transesophageal echocardiogram，TEE）可以看到室壁运动异常。在主动脉血流阻断期间，可能发生高血压和左心室（left ventricular，LV）功能障碍。表29.1比较了不同水平主动脉血流阻断引起的血流动力学变化。主动脉夹闭开放后出现低血压是常见的并可预知的并发症。

识别

根据患者的并存疾病制订合适的术中监测计划有助于识别这些血流动力学事件。对于OSR，通常采用直接动脉压和中心静脉压监测，而严重CAD或左心室功能障碍患者需置入肺动脉导管和TEE监测，以进一步评估前负荷、心室功能和作为心肌缺血的指标。通过肺毛细血管楔压、肺动脉舒张末压或TEE显示LV舒张末期容积的显著降低可诊断低血容量。心肌缺血通常表现为ST段改变并伴有TEE上新的区域性室壁运动异常。

清晰了解手术不同时期和夹闭肾上型主动脉相关的病理生理学变化，可有助于预测术中可能发生的血流动力学变化。手术暴露动脉瘤期间的低血压可能是由肠道膨出及肠系膜牵拉引起的前列环素释放导致，导致严重的血管舒张、心动过速和面部潮红。虽然这种所谓的**肠系膜牵引综合征**是一种短暂事件，但它通常需要用升压药如去氧肾上腺素治疗。同时使用硬膜外麻醉可能通过降低体循环阻力（systemic vascular resistance，SVR）和LV前负荷而导致低血压。

轻度高血压（hypertension，HTN）在肾下夹闭主动脉期间相对常见，通常认为是由主动脉阻力的突然增加和后负荷的增加引起。相反，如果主动脉夹闭位置在主动脉腹腔干上方，则HTN更为明显，

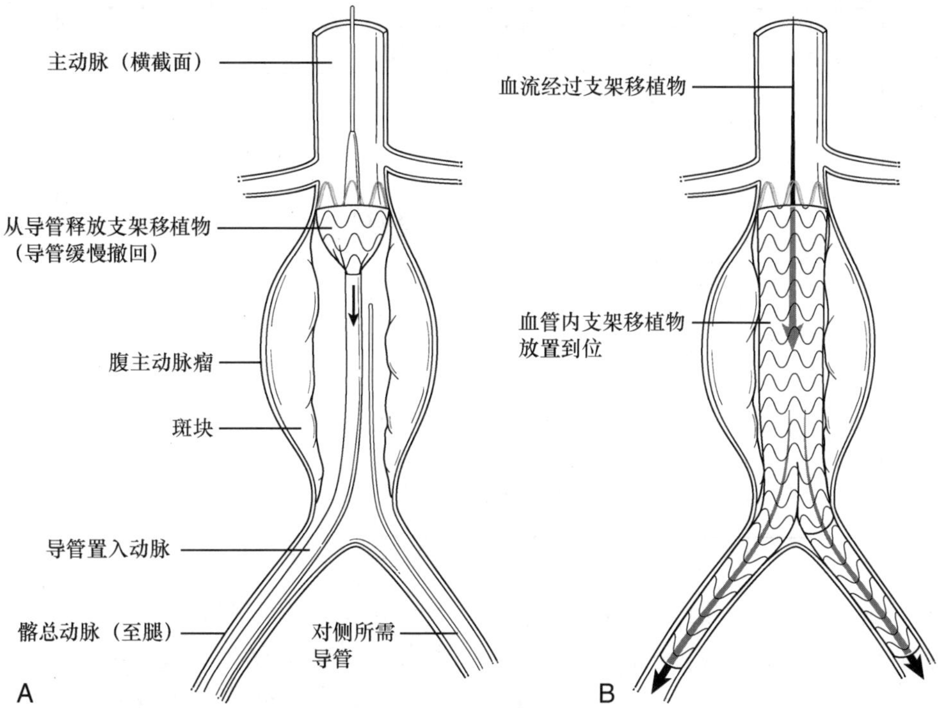

图 29.1 主动脉瘤内支架移植物置入。A. 将导管插入腹股沟（大腿上部）的动脉。导管经过腹主动脉，支架从导管中释放。**B.** 支架移植物允许血液流经动脉瘤（Redrawn from National Heart, Lung, and Blood Institute, National Institutes of Health（NIH）, Department of Health and Human Services [DHHS]：How is an aneurysm treated? 2011. Available at https：//www.nhlbi.nih.gov/health/health-topics/topics/arm/treatment. Accessed January 26，2016.）

表 29.1 肾上型和肾下型腹主动脉瘤手术主动脉血流阻断开始时心血管参数的变化百分比

	主动脉血流阻断水平		
变量	腹腔干上	腹腔干下–肾上	肾下
平均动脉压	+54	+5*	+2*
肺毛细血管楔压	+38	+10*	0*
舒张末期面积	+28	+2*	+9*
收缩末期面积	+69	+10*	+11*
射血分数	-38	-10*	-8*
室壁运动异常患者	+92	+33	0
新发心肌梗死	+8	0	0

* 与行腹腔干上主动脉血流阻断组相比，有统计学差异（$P<0.05$）

From Roizen MF, Beaupre PN, Alpert RA, et al：Monitoring with two-dimensional trans esophageal echocardiography：comparison of myocardial function in patients undergoing supraceliac, suprarenal-infraceliac, or infrarenal aortic occlusion. *J Vasc Surg* 1：300-305, 1984.

这可能是由于血流从内脏血管床转移到体循环导致静脉回流和心排血量增加。然而，尽管发生 HTN，腹腔干下阻断并不会产生血容量再分布。

然而，重要的是，在主动脉血流阻断期间未发生 HTN 或低血压时应该立即启动对 LV 功能、血容量和手术失血的即时评估。血容量不足的低血压通常是由于在主动脉血流阻断之前和阻断期间未发现的失血和第三间隙液体丢失引起。此外，如果出现心肌缺血，LV 功能障碍可能进一步减少心排血量，从而加剧血容量不足和血管舒张的不良影响。

主动脉夹闭开放后的低血压是一种可预知的常见事件，其原因在于 SVR 的减少和中心血容量不足。在阻断期间，下肢发生缺血性血管舒张，并且随着这些血管床的再灌注，缺血代谢物和体液因子被释放到体循环中，导致 SVR 降低。此外，这些扩张的静脉和动脉血管中的血液淤积导致静脉回流减少和中心血容量不足。发生低血压的程度取决于主动脉血流阻断的水平和持续时间、钳夹移除的速度、主动脉开放前的血管内容量状态以及麻醉药和血管扩张药的持续影响。在开放主动脉之前，适当补充液体以替代血液丢失以及缓慢释放主动脉钳可以在很大程度上避免严重的低血压。由阻断钳释放引起低血压的病理生理学如图 29.2 所示。

与 OSR 相比，EVAR 很少会出现术中明显的血流动力学变化。使用经皮血管通路装置代替开腹手术，仅短时间阻断主动脉腔，这是 EVAR 相对于

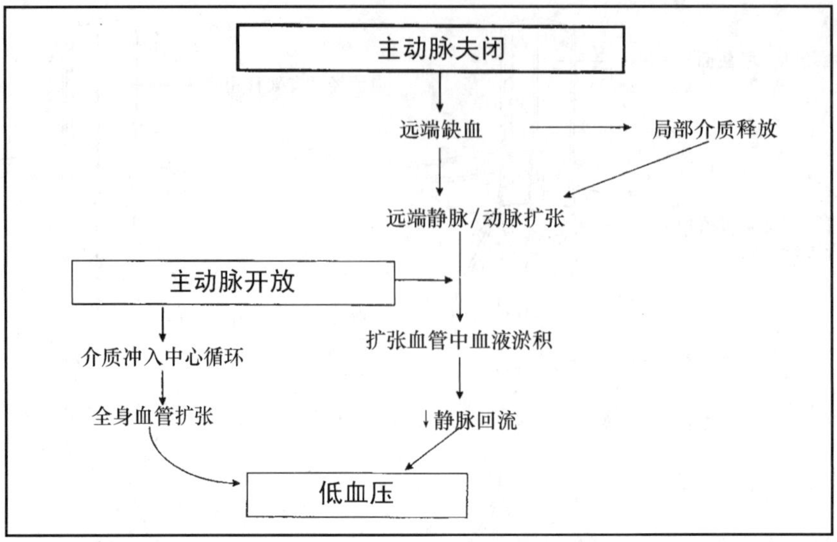

图 29.2 主动脉开放后低血压的原因

OSR 的显著优势。在 EVAR 球囊阻断主动脉期间，很少发生血流动力学紊乱及后遗症。因此，与 OSR 相比，EVAR 通常不需要高级别的监测和静脉通路选择，只需单根大口径静脉通路和动脉导管即可。此外，经典的麻醉方式是使用小剂量短效阿片类药物如芬太尼（或输注瑞芬太尼）浅麻醉和吸入全身麻醉。如果进行全身麻醉，则术后常规拔管。

在麻醉性监护（monitored anesthesia care，MAC）下进行局部/区域（L/R）麻醉代替全身麻醉进行 EVAR 手术时，应考虑以下因素：

- 已证实在 L/R 麻醉下行 EVAR 的成功率为 75%；
- 与全身麻醉相比，L/R 麻醉下 EVAR 的围术期心肺并发症较少；
- 与全身麻醉相比，区域麻醉与输血减少有关；
- 与全身麻醉相比，L/R 麻醉与较短的手术时间和较短的 ICU 时间、住院时间和总体成本下降有关；
- 外科医师可能更倾向于在主动脉支架展开时使患者屏住呼吸，这可能会限制 MAC 下 L/R 麻醉的应用。

风险评估

EVAR 术中即可能发生并发症，如切口部位血肿、下肢缺血、动脉闭塞、股动脉假性动脉瘤、血管破裂（如髂动脉）和支架移位。然而，EVAR 总体的手术即刻预后远优于 OSR。EVAR 组的病残率和死亡率显著低于 OSR 组。尽管在 EVAR 期间使用静脉造影剂，但与 OSR 相比，AKI 的发生率仍然较低。此外，EVAR 与 OSR 相比，失血量减少，输血减少，ICU 和住院时间也通常较短。然而，远期结局差异仍存在争议，最近的研究才显示 1 年后 EVAR 的全因死亡率和主要病残率较 OSR 低。总之，EVAR 的 30 天死亡率风险较小，但两种方法的 4 年内的总死亡率并无差异（表 29.2）。

启示

腔内介入治疗 AAA 是目前的趋势。然而，由于解剖学原因，并非所有患者都适合 EVAR。进一步的研究可能会在某些患者人群中重新探索开放手术技术，因此，开放手术修复 AAA 的麻醉管理仍然重要，破裂 AAA 的紧急修复也是如此。

当发生低血压时，首要诊断措施是积极评估血管内容量和失血程度，因为低血容量是最可能的原因。应用心电图 ST 段分析、TEE 或两者结合来评估是否存在心肌缺血。静脉注射硝酸甘油可用来提高冠状动

表 29.2 腹主动脉瘤腔内修复与开放手术并发症发生率比较

并发症	腔内修复（EVAR）	开放手术	优势比（EVAR）
30 年死亡率（%）	1.4	4.2	0.33
4 年死亡率（%）	37.3	37.8	无差异
致命脑卒中（%）	0.02	0.03	无差异
心脏死亡（%）	0.08	0.07	无差异
肺部并发症（%）	0.03	0.08	0.36
肾并发症（%）	0.02	0.01	无差异

From Paravastu SC，Jayarajasingam R，Cottam R，et al：Endovascular repair of abdominal aortic aneurysm. Cochrane Database *Syst Rev* 1：CD004178，2014.

脉灌注压，当伴有心动过速时，应用 β 受体阻滞剂来治疗。在整个围术期应用 β 受体阻滞对于因 CAD 导致术后心脏病发病风险的患者至关重要。

低血压的处理取决于它与主动脉血流阻断的关系：

- **主动脉血流阻断前低血压**：考虑硬膜外麻醉、肠系膜牵拉或术前低血容量的影响。
- **主动脉血流阻断时低血压**：考虑严重的低血容量。在主动脉夹闭开放前应用血液和晶体液进行积极的容量复苏，使中心静脉压或肺毛细血管楔压增加至比基线水平高 10% ～ 20%。
- **主动脉夹闭开放后低血压**：应酌情暂时停用所有麻醉剂和血管扩张剂。应备好血管收缩剂如去甲肾上腺素、血管加压素或去氧肾上腺素等治疗伴发的血管舒张和前负荷降低。如果出血严重，应备好血液制品，强烈建议术中使用血液回收系统。

（李之娥　译　李斌本　校）

延伸阅读

Edwards MS, Andrews JS, Edwards AF, et al.: Results of endovascular aortic aneurysm repair with general, regional, and local/monitored anesthesia care in the American College of Surgeons National Surgical Quality Improvement Program Database, *J Vasc Surg* 54(5):1273–1282, 2011.

Elkouri S, Gloviezki P, McKusick MA, et al.: Perioperative complications and early outcome after endovascular and open surgical repair of abdominal aortic aneurysms, *J Vasc Surg* 39:497–505, 2004.

Fleisher LA, Fleischmann KE, Auerbach AD, et al.: 2014 ACC/AHA guideline on perioperative cardiovascular evaluation and management of patients undergoing noncardiac surgery: a report of the American College of Cardiology/American Heart Association Task force on practice guidelines, *J Am Coll Cardiol* 64(22):e77–137, 2014.

Gelman S: The pathophysiology of aortic cross-clamping and unclamping, *Anesthesiology* 82:1026–1060, 1995.

Johnston WE, Balestrieri FJ, Plonk G, et al.: The influence of periaortic collateral vessels on the intraoperative hemodynamic effects of acute aortic occlusion in patients with aorto-occlusive disease or abdominal aortic aneurysm, *Anesthesiology* 66:386–389, 1987.

Karthiksalingam A, Thrumurthy S, Young E, et al.: Locoregional anesthesia for endovascular aneurysm repair, *J Vasc Surg* 56(2):510–519, 2012.

Lederle FA, Freischlag JA, Kyriakides TC, et al.: Outcomes following endovascular vs open repair of abdominal aortic aneurysm a randomized trial, *JAMA* 302(14), 2009. 1535–1532.

Paravastu SC, Jayarajasingam R, Cottam R, et al.: Endovascular repair of abdominal aortic aneurysm, *Cochrane Database Syst Rev* 1:CD004178, 2014.

Prinssen M, Verhoeven EL, Buth J, et al.: A randomized trial comparing conventional and endovascular repair of abdominal aortic aneurysms, *N Engl J Med* 351(16):1607–1618, 2004.

Ruppert V, Leurs L, Steckmeier B, et al.: Influence of anesthesia type on outcome after endovascular aortic aneurysm repair: an analysis based on EUROSTAR data, *J Vasc Surg* 44(1):16–21, 2006.

Wald R, Waikar SS, Liangos O, et al.: Acute renal failure after endovascular vs open repair of abdominal aortic aneurysm, *J Vasc Surg* 43(3):460–466, 2006.

第30章 腺样体扁桃体切除术

Lynne R. Ferrari

病例概要

肥胖患儿，男性，3 岁（体重指数 30），患有阻塞性睡眠呼吸暂停（呼吸暂停低通气指数 10），拟行扁桃体切除术和腺样体切除术。在麻醉恢复室，他的呼吸频率为 10 次 / 分伴严重的呼吸暂停，心率为 140 次 / 分。口咽部见少量血，且听诊双侧有啰音。脉搏氧饱和度为 86%。

问题分析

定义

在美国，扁桃体切除术伴或不伴腺样体切除术，是最常实施的外科手术之一，每年完成 700 000 多例。很多患者都伴有内科并存疾病需在术前调理，要充分理解围术期并发症的可能性。绝大多数儿童都能在术后恢复得很好，但并发症也可能会非常严重，有时可威胁生命。扁桃体切除术患者术后死亡风险是 1∶10 000。合理筛选患者、重视麻醉风险和技术可降低死亡风险，减少与下列因素相关并发症的发生：

- 出血；
- 低龄；
- 术后肺水肿；
- 术后疼痛；
- 阻塞性睡眠呼吸暂停。

识别

失血

患者术后大出血的概率为 0.1% ～ 8.1%。75% 的出血病例发生于手术 6 h 内，多为外科技术所致；剩下的 25% 在术后第 8 天有可能发生，与术后血痂脱落有关。多数出血情况可通过痰中血迹或呕吐物中“咖啡渣”样物质来发现。

低龄

过去所有接受扁桃体切除术的儿童患者术后都需要收治入院以控制呕吐、脱水、出血、疼痛和窒息等症状。然而成本控制的出现和日间手术的趋势改变了这种状况。近期指南建议只有 3 岁或更小的儿童才需要在术后常规收治入院，此外，伴有严重阻塞性睡眠呼吸暂停综合征（obstructive sleep apnea syndrome，OSAS）（呼吸暂停低通气指数为 10 或每小时更多阻塞性事件）或氧饱和度最低值低于 80%（或两种状况都存在）的儿童也需要常规办理住院。

肺水肿

肺水肿可表现为气管导管内泡沫样粉色液体、氧饱和度降低、哮鸣音、呼吸困难或拔除气管导管后呼吸频率增加。阻塞后肺水肿的鉴别诊断包括胃内容物误吸、呼吸窘迫综合征、充血性心力衰竭、容量负荷过重和过敏反应。胸部 X 线片表现出弥漫性间质性肺浸润影，通常为双侧，结合相关临床病史，即可明确诊断。

术后疼痛

腺样体切除术后的疼痛轻微，但扁桃体切除术后疼痛常很剧烈。胃中的刺激性血液、水肿引起咽反射的干扰以及化学感受器触发区受体的激活等因素综合影响造成术后呕吐现象常见，在未接受预防性止吐剂治疗的扁桃体切除患者中发生率可高达 70%。

阻塞性睡眠呼吸暂停

在约 3% ～ 12% 的儿童中，肥大的扁桃体会在睡眠中阻塞上呼吸道而导致 OSAS。5 岁以下儿童的发病率最高。多导睡眠图是自然睡眠过程中呼吸活动的图像记录，是 OSAS 的最终确诊手段；然而要给所有疑似 OSAS 和睡眠呼吸失调的儿童进行测试并不可行。因此许多作者尝试设计一个儿童术前问卷调查来辅助 OSAS 的诊断，如同在成年人中得到验证的 STOP-BANG 问卷。睡眠监测阳性是扁桃体切除术的适应证，尤其伴有相关系统异常时。OSAS 的临床表现因人而异，有些患者所受限制很大，而其他则所受影响很小（框 30.1）。

风险评估

失血

扁桃体窝、鼻咽部或二者皆有出血的占比分别为 67%、27% 和 6%。

低龄

年龄小于 3 岁是腺样体切除术后呼吸系统并发症的最重要危险因素。**呼吸系统并发症**的定义是血氧饱和度低于 90% 且伴有阻塞性呼吸类型或需干预的急性呼吸窘迫症状。

肺水肿

增加无论哪一侧心室静脉回流和前负荷，或降低肺淋巴系统清除大量液体的能力的因素，都会增加阻塞性肺水肿的风险。术后喉痉挛以及声门紧闭时呼吸会导致负跨肺压，从而引起静水压梯度增加，进而产生肺水肿。

术后疼痛和呕吐

术后疼痛程度的显著差异与扁桃体切除的外科技术有关。与接受锐器切开手术的患者相比，在接受电灼和激光切除扁桃体的患者中可观察到镇痛药物需求增加、耳痛和易怒等现象。有证据表明扁桃体部分切除术（Tonsillotomy 或 Partial tonsillectomy）术后出血和疼痛的发生率更低，正越来越多地被用作扁桃体切除术的一种替代疗法。呕吐是多因素的，部分原因可能是下咽部迷走神经的刺激，以及全身 5- 羟色胺的释放。

框 30.1　阻塞性睡眠呼吸暂停的临床表现

- 低龄（<6 岁）
- 睡觉时打鼾
- 生长迟缓
- 反复呼吸道感染
- 头面部畸形
- 心律失常
- 睡眠呼吸暂停
- 清醒时嗜睡
- 发育延迟
- 肥胖
- 行为障碍
- 肺心病

阻塞性睡眠呼吸暂停

扁桃体肥大的程度与 OSAS 患者上气道梗阻的严重程度无关。扁桃体轻度肿大的儿童可能有严重的 OSAS 症状，而扁桃体重度肿大的儿童可能完全没有 OSAS 表现。发生 OSAS 的风险随着鼻咽气道的改变和肥胖而增加。因 OSAS 患儿鼻咽气道孔径较窄，所以舌后坠会引起下咽梗阻。多达 60% 的 OSAS 患儿为肥胖儿童，有人建议有必要为肥胖儿童制定一份特殊的 OSAS 筛查问卷。颈部脂肪浸润与咽肌的松弛可加重梗阻，因为此时吸气负压产生气道塌陷的收缩力超过了咽肌收缩的扩张力。这些儿童发生呼吸相关不良事件的风险增加，他们也对阿片类药物的呼吸抑制作用也更敏感。

启示

失血

扁桃体切除术后出血可通过局部用药促进凝血来控制。然而，大多数病例需要手术探查和治疗。患者可能会吞下大量的血液，导致患者本人、父母或外科医师都没有重视。因此，所有扁桃体切除术后出现扁桃体出血的患者都被认为是饱胃状态，必须采取适当的麻醉措施。由于吞下的血液量通常被低估，因此需要检查体位性低血压以衡量血管内容量是否充足。

低龄

3 岁以下的儿童口服摄入不足以及随后在手术后立即脱水的风险增加。他们术后发生呼吸系统并发症的风险也会增加。

肺水肿

扁桃体切除后气道阻塞解除时可发生肺水肿。有研究表明，气道阻塞引起的负压升高会增加静脉回流和肺血容量（图 30.1）。吸气时胸膜内负压峰值通常为 2.5 ～ 10 cmH_2O，随着气道阻塞可增加至

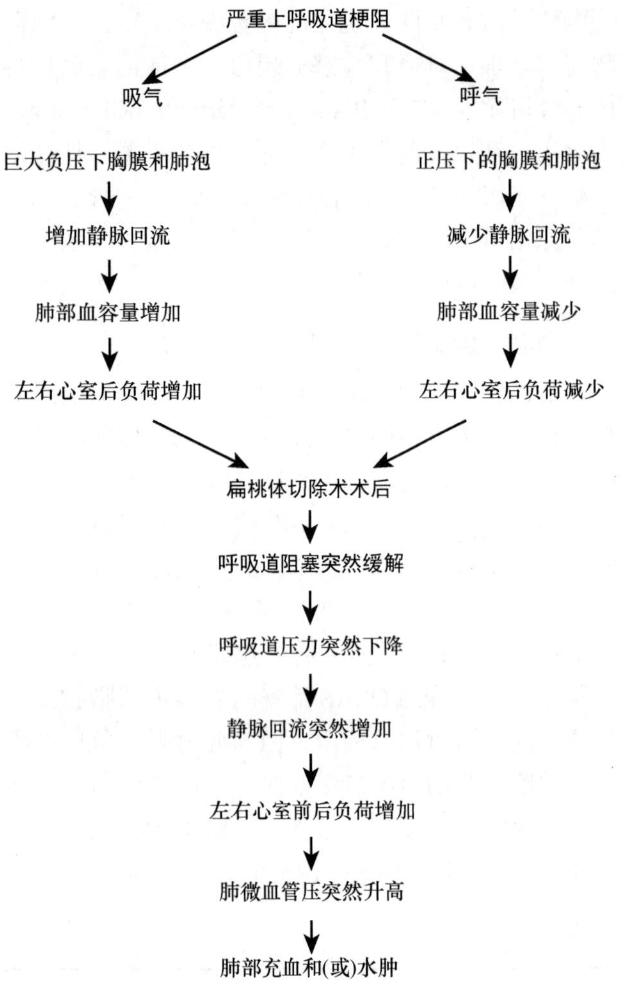

图 30.1 上呼吸道梗阻治疗后导致肺水肿的生理改变（Adapted from Galvis AG，Stool SE，Bluestone CD：Pulmonary edema following relief of acute upper airway obstruction. *Ann Otol Rhinol Laryngol* 89 [2 Pt 1]：124-128，1980.）

30 cmH_2O。这种程度的负性跨肺压力梯度会破坏肺毛细血管壁的完整性。同时，增加肺动脉血流和静水压力有助于液体进入肺泡腔。为了抵消这一点，呼气时产生正的胸膜内和肺泡压力（类似于打鼾或 Valsalva 动作），减少了肺静脉回流和血容量。扁桃体切除术后气道阻塞的缓解降低了气道压力，但也增加了静脉回流和肺静水压力。这会导致肺充血，最终导致肺水肿。需注意的是呼气时打鼾限制肺静脉回流的平衡作用可随着气道阻塞的减轻而消失。

术后疼痛和呕吐

扁桃体切除术后，疼痛控制不佳、血液吞咽和口腔摄入过少会导致恶心呕吐。1% 的患者会有脱水症状，脱水症状可通过静脉补液恢复血管内容量来预防。脱水的患者需要收治入院以接受静脉补液。

阻塞性睡眠呼吸暂停

中枢神经功能障碍导致许多 OSAS 患儿心肺功能恶化。持续性高碳酸血症、低氧血症和右心室功能障碍可造成心律失常和肺心病。部分患儿可出现肺动脉压持续升高，可能是因为 OSAS 使血管反应性增强。

管理

失血

出血通常采用咽部加压包、局部药物或两者结合的方式来控制。如果这些方法失败，患者要被送回手术室进行探查和手术止血。静脉注射和吸入麻醉的方法都是合适的，但患者应在手术结束时反应良好，并在清醒时拔管。提倡采用快速序贯诱导，并压迫环状软骨和探条引导气管插管。最后，控制出血的外科手术通常很简单，因此应该做好相应的麻醉计划。

低龄

3 岁以上的健康儿童观察 4 h 后，在没有发现扁桃体切除术后并发症证据的情况下，即可出院回家。

肺水肿

以支持治疗为主，保持患者呼吸道顺畅，必要时吸氧和使用利尿剂。在严重的情况下，可能需要进行气管插管和给予带呼气末正压的机械通气。肺水肿的消除一般很快，通常在术后几小时以内。很多病例在术后 24 h 内无需处理即可自行缓解。

术后疼痛

术中给予皮质类固醇可减少水肿产生和之后的患者不适。用局部麻醉剂和肾上腺素浸润扁桃体周围组织可以减少术中失血，并能缓解即时和长期的术后疼痛。长期的术后疼痛缓解可能是因为神经阻滞防止了伤害性冲动在术中和术后传入中枢神经系统，从而抑制了促进疼痛感知的持续过度兴奋状态。但是局部麻醉和肾上腺素浸润并非没有风险，血管内注射（尤其是动脉内）可能是致命的。小剂量重复注射镇痛药物有助于缓解疼痛。由于一些儿童的遗传基因中有可以将可待因转换为致命剂量的吗啡的能力，因此禁止使用口服可待因来处理扁桃体切除术后的疼痛。高达 16% 的术后病残率和死亡率与阿片类药物的使用有关。最近有关非甾体类药物的研究表明，它们对血小板功能的影响并未导致术后出血的增加。除酮咯酸外，其他非甾体类药物均可用于术后疼痛的控制。扁桃体切除术后可应用止吐药物包括昂丹司琼和类固醇等，利用经口胃管进行胃减压（腺样体切除术后禁用鼻胃管），以及充分镇痛等措施来控制术后呕吐。

阻塞性睡眠呼吸暂停

应保证 OSAS 患者在扁桃体切除术后拔管前具有自主呼吸和保护其气道的能力。应非常小心地滴定镇静药和镇痛药的剂量，以平衡镇痛需求和呼吸抑制的风险。尽管扁桃体切除术可缓解气道阻塞，但术后残留的中枢神经系统功能障碍、高碳酸血症和低氧血症仍可能持续存在。因此，患有 OSAS 的儿童应在术后住院接受呼吸暂停的监测（框 30.2）。大多数 OSAS 患者的二氧化碳分压（Pco_2）水平正常并于麻醉后即拔管；但是，患有严重 OSAS 的患者（即肺心病，静息 Pco_2 大于 50 mmHg）应保留插管并进行机械通气直至 Pco_2 正常化，随后拔管并仔细观察。

框 30.2　腺样体扁桃体切除术后患者入院标准

如果患者符合美国耳鼻咽喉头颈外科–儿科耳鼻喉科委员会的以下任何标准，则必须入院：

患者或家庭中有或没有已知出血性疾病的凝血值异常。

由扁桃体或腺样体肥大引起的阻塞性睡眠障碍或呼吸暂停的证据。

使患者术后心肺、代谢或一般医疗风险增加的系统性疾病。

存在头面部或其他气道异常，包括但不限于以下内容：

- 特雷彻·柯林斯综合征
- 克鲁宗综合征
- 戈尔登哈尔综合征
- 皮埃尔·罗班异常
- CHARGE 联合缺陷*
- 软骨发育不全
- 唐氏综合征

孤立性气道异常

- 鼻后孔闭锁
- 喉气管狭窄

针对急性扁桃体周围脓肿实施的手术。

主治医师判断路程时间较长、天气或家庭社会状况等因素导致患者无法接受密切观察、配合或快速返回医院时。

*CHARGE 联合缺陷包括色素瘤畸形序列（从孤立的虹膜眼组织到临床无眼畸形）、心脏缺陷（如法洛四联症、房间隔或室间隔缺损、动脉导管未闭）、胆管闭锁、生长发育迟缓或中枢神经系统异常、生殖器异常或性腺功能减退（男性）、耳部异常或耳聋。

预防

失血

术中常规静注地塞米松 0.5 mg/kg 预防呕吐可降低扁桃体切除术后出血的风险。轻度出血可以局部应用硝酸银治疗；但是，有些患儿需要手术探查以达到止血的效果。可在麻醉诱导前进行倾斜试验以评估出血引起的直立性变化，建立静脉通路，开始容量替代治疗，测量血细胞比容，并且送出血液样品用于血型测定和交叉配型。应保证各种喉镜片、镜柄和气管导管随时可用，并且至少应有两个抽吸装置，以防探查气道气管插管时吸引管因血栓阻塞。

低龄

在低龄儿童中扁桃体切除术后的并发症发生率已得到充分证实；因此，美国耳鼻喉科学会指南建议 3 岁以下儿童或符合其他标准的儿童需住院过夜（见框 30.2）。

肺水肿

尚无可靠的方法来预测哪些患者会在手术后出现阻塞性肺水肿。麻醉期间持续的中等气道正压可以为循环适应提供时间。这类似于会厌炎或喉痉挛所致急性上气道阻塞的处理方法。阻塞性肺水肿在患有长期气道阻塞的儿童中并不常见，但不幸的是，在某些儿童中扁桃体切除后仍不可避免。

术后疼痛和呕吐

止吐药、经口胃减压、充分的疼痛缓解和麻醉后平稳苏醒有助于降低扁桃体切除术后呕吐的频率。

阻塞性睡眠呼吸暂停

应用高频速离技术或通过手术切除扁桃体和腺样体可以逆转大多数 OSAS 患者的进行性心血管改变。儿童中 OSAS 的发病通常是无法预防的。美国耳鼻喉科头颈外科协会建议 3 岁以下儿童或呼吸暂停低通气指数大于 10 的儿童入住加强医疗病房，美国儿科学会则建议呼吸暂停低通气指数大于 24 的儿童入住加强医疗病房。他们已经多次尝试设计术前问卷，以筛选术后有 OSAS 风险的儿童。

（王云鹏　译　王嘉锋　校）

延伸阅读

Alonso-Alvarez ML, Cordero-Guevara JA, Teran-Santos J, et al.: Obstructive sleep apnea in obese community-dwelling children: the NANOS study, *Sleep* 37(5):943–949, 2014.

Amoils M, Chang KW, Saynina O, et al.: Postoperative complications in pediatric tonsillectomy and adenoidectomy in ambulatory vs inpatient settings, *JAMA Otolaryngol Head Neck Surg* 142(4):344–350, 2016.

Baugh RF, Archer SM, Mitchell RB, et al.: Clinical practice guideline: tonsillectomy in children, *Otolaryngol Head Neck Surg* 144(Suppl 1):S1–30, 2011.

Blum RH, McGowan Jr FX: Chronic upper airway obstruction and cardiac dysfunction: anatomy, pathophysiology and anesthetic implications, *Paediatr Anaesth* 14:75–83, 2004.

Brown KA, Brouillette RT: The elephant in the room: lethal apnea at home after adenotonsillectomy, *Anesth Analg* 118(6):1157–1159, 2014.

Brown OE, Cunningham MJ: Tonsillectomy and adenoidectomy inpatient guidelines, *Am Acad Otololaryngol Head Neck Surg Bull* 15:13, 1996.

Cote CJ, Posner KL, Domino KB: Death or neurologic injury after tonsillectomy in children with a focus on obstructive sleep apnea: Houston, we have a problem!, *Anesth Analg* 118(6):1276–1283, 2014.

Feinberg A, Shabino C: Acute pulmonary edema complicating tonsillectomy and adenoidectomy, *Pediatrics* 75:112–114, 1985.

Galvis A, Stool S, Bluestone C: Pulmonary edema following relief of acute upper airway obstruction, *Ann Otol Rhinol Laryngol* 89:124–128, 1980.

Goldman JL, Baugh RF, Davies L, et al.: Mortality and major morbidity after tonsillectomy: etiologic factors and strategies for prevention, *Laryngoscope* 123(10):2544–2553, 2013.

Kelly LE, Sommer DD, Ramakrishna J, et al.: Morphine or ibuprofen for post-tonsillectomy analgesia: a randomized trial, *Pediatrics* 135(2):307–313, 2015.

Patino M, Sadhasivam S, Mahmoud M: Obstructive sleep apnoea in children: perioperative considerations, *Br J Anaesth* 111(Suppl 1):i83–95, 2013.

Raman VT, Splaingard M, Tumin D, et al.: Utility of screening questionnaire, obesity, neck circumference, and sleep polysomnography to predict sleep-disordered breathing in children and adolescents, *Paediatr Anaesth* 26(6):655–664, 2016.

Roland PS, Rosenfeld RM, Brooks LJ, et al.: Clinical practice guideline: polysomnography for sleep-disordered breathing prior to tonsillectomy in children, *Otolaryngol Head Neck Surg* 145(Suppl 1):S1–15, 2011.

Subramanyam R, Chidambaran V, Ding L, et al.: Anesthesia- and opioids-related malpractice claims following tonsillectomy in USA: LexisNexis claims database 1984-2012, *Paediatr Anaesth* 24(4):412–420, 2014.

Tait AR, Bickham R, O'Brien LM, et al.: The STBUR questionnaire for identifying children at risk for sleep-disordered breathing and postoperative opioid-related adverse events, *Paediatr Anaesth* 26(7):759–766, 2016.

电休克治疗的麻醉

第 31 章

Ross MacPherson

病例概要

患者，男性，65 岁，患有严重抑郁症，拟实施第一个疗程的电休克治疗（electro-convulsive therapy，ECT）。开始治疗前的内科评估提示，除了有高血压（多次测量在 180/95 mmHg 左右）外，其他方面均正常。目前他正在服用反苯环丙胺、锂剂和丙戊酸钠控制精神疾病。使用硫喷妥钠和琥珀胆碱实施麻醉，并进行一段时间的过度通气后，对患者实施了刺激。患者有一次明显的运动性癫痫发作，表现为所有肢体的强直性-阵挛运动，发作时伴心率明显增加。随着癫痫发作的结束，心率也随之迅速下降。进入麻醉后复苏室，血压持续升高 15 min，后缓慢恢复到 ECT 前的水平。麻醉苏醒后，患者出现意识错乱和挣扎现象。予小剂量咪达唑仑帮助患者安静。最终，他清醒后对时间和地点有定向力，对近期事件无记忆。

当他准备下一次治疗的时候，患者主诉有严重的广泛的肌肉疼痛。

问题分析

这个病例显示了 ECT 麻醉的主要并发症：药物治疗、肌肉松弛不够充分、血流动力学改变、苏醒期躁动以及琥珀胆碱诱发的肌肉酸痛。

尽管 ECT 麻醉通常是一个相当简单的过程，但仍可能出现与操作相关的严重并发症（表 31.1 和 31.2），通过仔细地管理可将这些并发症的风险降至最低。最初的治疗阶段被称为“滴定”阶段，在此期间，通常会施加一系列刺激，旨在确定个体患者引发癫痫的阈值。此阶段通常比标准治疗期稍长，整体的不良反应的发生率通常稍高。麻醉科医师在滴定阶段需要特别警惕。在长时间的系列治疗中，由于电极位置的改变或需要重新确定刺激的水平时，患者可能会需要多次这样的滴定过程。

表 31.1　ECT 治疗中的并发症

并发症	治疗选择
对治疗反应不佳或短时程发作	使用最低剂量的诱导药物，必要时加入瑞芬太尼以降低清醒程度。确保具有抗惊厥活性的药物已经停止使用
肌肉松弛不够充分	增加珀酰胆碱的剂量。注射后等待 90 s，使用肌腱锤检查肌腱反射
长时程癫痫发作	用小剂量的诱导药物终止。通常反应迅速
治疗过程中脉率和血压的变化	变化通常为一过性的，但干预措施并未显示出特别益处
治疗期间缺氧	在治疗前确保氧合充分并过度通气。在治疗期间尽量减少肌肉活动（因为会增加氧耗）

表 31.2　治疗后的并发症

并发症	治疗
长时程高血压	通常无需处理；或使用硝酸甘油、肼屈嗪（肼苯哒嗪）或美托洛尔
ECT 后躁动	合理抑制；咪达唑仑或丙泊酚静脉滴注
肌痛	无有效治疗；往往在首次治疗后得到缓解
恶心	标准止吐药物

管理

患者选择

在过去的几年里许多出版物都发表了全面详细实施 ECT 的禁忌证。对于有脑动脉瘤和脑占位性病变等疾病的患者，对其实施 ECT 可引起血压上升和脑血流量增加，因而是一种高风险的治疗手段。然而，尽管风险增加，但 ECT 已成功地应用于此类患者及有其他疾病的患者，如腹主动脉瘤或主动脉狭窄患者。

对于既往有心脏疾病的患者，尚无风险增加的证据，通常不需要干预。心脏起搏器患者可以安全地接受 ECT 治疗，无需任何特殊的干预。

为了帮助指导 ECT 前的患者评估，最近发表的一些综述提供了有用的信息，尽管大多数这样的建议都是基于临床逻辑而非临床试验数据。

麻醉实施

在给予适当剂量的诱导药物和肌肉松弛药后，患者需要充分通气。ECT 时过度通气是一个有用的策略，因为它不仅能确保肺的最佳给氧去氮，也被证明能改善癫痫发作。

实施 ECT 前充分氧合通常能确保操作过程顺利进行，不会出现氧饱和度骤然下降，患者通常会维持 2 min 的呼吸暂停状态。然而，患有病态肥胖的患者，或有特别剧烈的运动性痉挛的患者，在手术过程中可能会出现脱氧饱和现象。这在一定程度上是有问题的，因为在癫痫发作期间试图提供有效的通气可能很困难。如果出现这种情形，除了等待癫痫发作结束，并大力通气以恢复氧和外，我们别无选择。

ECT 期间的心血管变化已得到很好地阐述。在实施刺激之后即刻可能会有一个严重的心动过缓阶段，甚至是短暂的心搏骤停期，与单侧治疗或双颞叶治疗相比，双额叶治疗更为常见。随后将会出现心动过速和副交感神经放电期及心动过缓。如果对血压进行了监测，则该参数也会随之升高。在恢复期，心率和血压将再次上升。使用丙泊酚而非巴比妥类在一定程度上可以减轻心血管反应。所有这些心脏反应都会遵循常规模式，通常为一过性，且很少需要干预，大多数权威均不推荐使用任何形式的预防措施。

使用琥珀胆碱引起的肌痛比较常见，且与药物剂量或肌震颤的程度无关。通常很少需要干预。可以让患者安心，在第一次或第二次治疗后，肌痛将会减轻。尽管多年来提出了一系列的干预措施，但在改善这一问题方面似乎仍无能为力。

苏醒室问题

心血管挑战

实施 ECT 后常出现高血压，在操作之后收缩压会立即升高 20% 或更多。但由于测量读数很快会下降至 ECT 前水平，因而很少需要快速的干预。如果高血压确实持续存在，起效迅速且持续时间短的药物，如硝酸甘油或艾司洛尔，可作为有效的一线用药。对于接受抗高血压药物治疗的患者，确定这些药物是否已经服用非常重要。如上文所述，如果患者既往有高血压，通常需要一些干预措施。

缺氧事件

治疗之后，一旦自主呼吸恢复，只要气道保持通畅，患者通常在 5 ～ 7 min 内恢复意识，但上呼吸道梗阻仍可能发生。虽无必要常规使用 Guedel 口咽通气道，但推荐在治疗后将患者置于侧卧位。苏醒室工作人员需要警惕上呼吸道梗阻和缺氧的发生。

苏醒期躁动

大多数患者经 ECT 治疗后会正常苏醒，偶尔也会伴有不同程度的癫痫发作后精神错乱不清，只需要稍作再定向干预即可。

然而，患者偶尔会苏醒时精神极其错乱，且可能行为粗暴，对患者自身和其他人均带来危险。这可能会构成真正的紧急情况。试图预测哪些患者会出现这样的事件并不容易，虽然一些研究表明，这种情况在年轻的患者、单侧 ECT 治疗的患者、接受锂剂治疗的患者以及接受第一次（滴定）治疗后的患者中更为常见。在这种情况下，没有任何办法可以代替牢固固定的静脉置管内的药物治疗。

咪达唑仑是治疗这类患者的常用选择药物，尽管有人建议在治疗结束时使用小剂量的丙泊酚；然而，这种情况的发生率很低，因此（如果需要的话）使用合适剂量的咪达唑仑治疗个别患者似乎更为合理。

预防

大多数患者进行 ECT 时很少会出现并发症，因此减少 ECT 并发症的预防策略亦很少。在大多数患者中，当出现并发症时必须予以处理。但在某些情形下，预防性措施可以改善治疗结局。

既往高血压病史

如果确定存在未控制或控制不佳的高血压时，在可能的情况下应在开始治疗之前进行治疗，因为它会影响围术期血流动力学的变化。在 ECT 开始前进行适当控制，术后治疗过程将更顺利。

药物治疗

术前用药应继续服用。重要的是，停用单胺氧化酶抑制剂尚无实质性理由。虽然理论上存在停用的原因，但这种干预可能会对患者产生严重的不良影响，至少有一项试验表明，服用这些药物的患者其发生麻醉不良反应的风险并不高于一般人群。

然而，有些药物确实需要特别注意。首先，抗癫痫药物越来越多地作为“情绪稳定剂”用于一些拟行 ECT 的患者。如果有可能，这些药物应该在开始治疗前停止使用，但这种做法通常并不切实际。虽有一种常见的替代方法，即停服该类制剂的晚间剂量，但不太可能产生明显的益处，因为这类药物多数是中效半衰期的制剂。

苯二氮䓬类药物的情况与此相似，特别是具有显著抗惊厥作用的长半衰期药物。同样，如果可能的话，这类药物需要在 ECT 之前逐渐减量，最好是停止使用。不推荐常规使用氟吗西尼作为停止药物的替代药物。

碳酸锂的相关情况尚不清楚。有人建议在治疗期间可以持续服用，而另一些人则建议停用。碳酸锂的应用被认为与 ECT 治疗后躁动的风险增加相关，这是发生在苏醒室的严重问题。虽然理论上存在药物相互作用，即锂剂可能延长琥珀胆碱的活性，但在临床上这似乎并不是问题。

肌肉松弛

显然，骨骼肌充分松弛对于减少 ECT 治疗期间患者的损伤风险至关重要。在癫痫诱发期间用麻醉来降低患者伤害的风险极难实现。在所有患者中，试图达到骨骼肌的完全松弛并不容易，特别是在肌肉发达的年轻患者中。一般来说，以大剂量琥珀胆碱开始是最安全的方案，剂量范围为 75 ～ 100 mg，并根据需要调整用量。在某些情况下，剂量甚至需要超过 100 mg。琥珀胆碱给药后，完全肌松时间通常为 90 s 左右。一些作者建议，在肌束震颤（如果出现）停止后等待 15 s 也具有一定的指导用途。

由于牙齿损伤的风险一直存在，因此必须提供详细的牙科病史，并关注牙帽和牙冠的情况。如果偶有患者存在特殊问题，特别是松动的牙齿或牙冠，可能需要在 ECT 开始前进行治疗。

牙垫常用来减少牙齿损坏的风险，并且应该由麻醉科医师亲自置入。牙垫有多种不同的类型可供选择，但无论使用何种形式，它都需要被很好地放入与磨牙相邻的口腔中。

预防血流动力学变化

除了对既往存在的高血压进行治疗外，几乎没有什么措施可以改善与 ECT 治疗有关的血流动力学变化。尽管一些权威建议常规使用抗胆碱能、β 受体阻滞剂或其他抗高血压药物作为降低血压和减慢心率的一种方法，但尚缺乏确凿的证据证明这种干预措施有任何益处。现在许多权威机构倾向于对特定的患者在其有需要时进行治疗，而不是对所有患者都进行超前干预。

（蒲君涔　译　代元强　校）

延伸阅读

Cristancho MA, Alici Y, Augoustidies JG, O’Reardon JP: Uncommon but serious complications associated with electroconvulsive therapy: recognition and management for the clinician, *Curr Psychiatry Rep* 10:474–480, 2008.

Dolenc TJ, Rasmussen KG: The safety of electroconvulsive therapy and lithium in combination: a case series and review of the literature, *J ECT* 21(3):165–170, 2005.

Kellner CH, Bryson EO: Electroconvulsive therapy anesthesia technique: minimalist versus maximally managed, *J ECT* 29(3):153–154, 2013.

MacPherson RD: Which anesthetic agents for ambulatory electroconvulsive therapy? *Curr Opin Anaesthesiol* 28(6):656–661, 2015.

Sundsted KK, Burton MC, Shah R, et al.: Preanesthesia medical evaluation for electroconvulsive therapy: a review of the literature, *J ECT* 30(1):35–42, 2014.

Tess AV, Smetana GW: Medical evaluation of patients undergoing electroconvulsive therapy, *N Engl J Med* 360(14):1437–1444, 2009.

Tzabazis A, Schmitt HJ, Ihmsen H, et al.: Postictal agitation after electroconvulsive therapy incidence severity and propofol as a treatment option, *J ECT* 29:189–195, 2013.

Van den Broek WW, Groenland TH, Mulder PG, et al.: Beta blockers and electroconvulsive therapy: a review, *Curr Drug Ther* 2:121–126, 2007.

第32章 胎儿手术的麻醉并发症：宫外产时治疗手术

Jagroop Mavi，*Joseph Previte*

病例概要

患者，女性，28 岁，孕 36+2 周，G2P1，产前胎儿被诊断出左肺巨大囊性肿块。宫外产时治疗计划为分娩前建立气道，有可能将胎儿转为体外膜氧合。

问题分析

定义

胎儿手术包括多种不同类型，可分为三大类：①微创手术（胎儿镜手术），②妊娠中期胎儿开放式手术，③宫外产时治疗（ex utero intrapartum therapy，EXIT）。胎儿镜检查或微创手术（表 32.1）涉及内窥镜下处理胎盘或脐带，只需要局部或区域麻醉。开放式胎儿手术（表 32.2）需要子宫完全松弛，通常需要术中高浓度的吸入麻醉药以及区域麻醉控制术后疼痛。胎儿镜手术和开放式胎儿手术均在妊娠中期进行，以利于术后胎儿生长发育。

相反，EXIT 手术是用于那些出生前影像学提示出生后保守治疗可能不能提高生存率的新生儿。该手术通常基于母体和胎儿的情况，尽可能推迟到妊娠晚期进行。EXIT 中实施的特殊干预因适应证而异（表 32.3），可能涉及气道保护，胸腔内肿块切除，在一定条件下颈部肿块切除，胸脐连体双胞胎等特殊情况，或建立体外膜氧合（extracorporeal membrane oxygenation，ECMO）插管。由于在通气的最初几分钟很难评估是否真的需要行 ECMO，尤其是此时胎儿仍然得到胎盘支持，故 EXIT 转为 ECMO 存在争议。在该病例概要中，保守治疗后常规分娩，肺部巨大肿块如果导致供氧和通气困难甚至无法供氧和通气，则使胎儿面临围产期窒息的风险。EXIT 通过直接喉镜、硬质或纤维支气管镜气管插管，以及必要时置入 ECMO 导管来提供气道保护，

表 32.1　微创胎儿镜手术的适应证

疾病	手术操作
双胎输血综合征	胎盘血管的激光凝固
双胎反向动脉灌注	脐带凝固
羊膜带综合征	羊膜带松解

表 32.2　妊娠中期胎儿开放手术的适应证

疾病	手术操作
脊髓膜膨出症	神经管缺损修复术
骶尾部畸胎瘤	畸胎瘤切除术
胸腔肿块	肿块切除术
肺头比低的先天性膈疝	气管堵塞术

表 32.3　宫外产时治疗（EXIT）的适应证

疾病	手术操作
严重的主动脉瓣狭窄或左肺发育不全	ECMO 置管
先天性膈疝	宫内气管夹或球囊移除 ECMO 置管
先天性上气道阻塞综合征	气管造口
巨大颈部肿块	肿块切除
胸腔肿块所致严重肺发育不良或 CPAM	肿块切除 ECMO 置管
预计困难插管	建立外科气道

CPAM，先天性肺气道畸形；ECMO，体外膜氧合

可延长子宫胎盘对胎儿的支持。通过最大限度地松弛子宫和维持子宫胎盘血流的技术，目前可使胎儿分娩和脱离胎盘循环前维持胎盘支持长达 180 min。

识别

产前检查对产前诊断胎儿异常至关重要，超声和磁共振成像的进步能够更好地判断胎儿结构异常及其对胎儿或新生儿的潜在影响。大多数胎儿疾病最初通过超声检查发现异常，从而提示进一步检查。最佳成像技术包括高分辨率胎儿超声检查、三维胎儿超声检查、快速胎儿磁共振检查和胎儿超声心动图检查。全面深入的超声检查用于评估胎儿体重和整体健康状况。评估胎儿体重对于准备胎儿确切剂量的镇痛药、肌肉松弛药以及复苏药物至关重要。羊膜穿刺术可提供羊水用于分析，包括核型分析。胎儿超声心动图可识别心脏结构上或功能上的缺陷。连续影像学检查对监测肿块的生长、治疗药物的反应和胎儿水肿的发展至关重要。胎儿水肿是一种威胁生命的状况，可引起两个或多个器官系统水肿，进而导致免疫紊乱、心肺功能障碍以及严重的胎儿贫血或发育缺陷。术前胎盘的位置需仔细评估，因为异常胎盘，如前置胎盘或绒毛膜下出血可能会增加术中发生并发症的风险。

虽然确定胎儿能否从 EXIT 手术中受益的具体标准因适应证不同而有所不同，但很多情况有着相似的表现。例如，颈部肿块会阻止胎儿吞咽羊水，导致羊水过多。肺内羊水聚积导致肺部变大且回声增强。多种原因所致的慢性胎儿疾病可导致胎儿水肿、进行性腹水、胸腔及心包积液，而未干预的全身性水肿最终会导致胎儿死亡。

风险评估

胎儿风险

胎儿无论在 EXIT 手术期间和之后都存在发生不良事件的风险。手术期间，由于胎儿皮肤容易蒸发水分和热量损失，导致暴露的胎儿难以维持正常体温。由于早产儿器官功能不成熟、髓鞘形成不全以及药物消除延长，导致麻醉药物的作用和持续时间增加。

由于胎儿心脏收缩力下降，胎儿可能无法代偿血流动力学的变化。胎儿对心率变化（如切皮时的心动过速，子宫胎盘灌注不足或脐带受压导致的心动过缓等）的耐受时间很短。产妇缺氧、体循环阻力增加或麻醉药的负性肌力作用可能进一步损害胎儿心脏功能。手术操作静脉回流受阻导致心脏前负荷降低，或失血则可导致胎儿低血压、心动过缓、休克甚至心脏停搏。应随时备好温热的胎儿血制品，以治疗低血容量所导致的胎儿心脏功能不全。

在 EXIT 手术期间，胎儿在与脐带分离之前仍保持在无菌区域，使得监测生理异常的监测选项受限。血流动力学数据从无菌胎儿脉搏血饱和度仪（正常胎儿血氧饱和度为 60% ～ 70%）和间断性胎儿超声心动图获得。胎儿超声心动图有助于识别一些早期问题，如灌注不足、心动过缓、心肌收缩力下降，肺动脉导管缩窄和房室瓣膜功能不全。理想情况下，外科医师可放置一个胎儿静脉导管，麻醉科医师可经静脉导管给予正性肌力药物、血液和液体。如果胎儿没有静脉通路，复苏仅限于外科医师肌内注射以及麻醉科医师对产妇进行干预。外科医师通常在胎儿肩部暴露后立即肌肉注射阿托品、芬太尼和非去极化肌肉松弛药的混合物。产妇血压的维持和分娩时充足的氧供对胎儿健康至关重要，确保子宫完全松弛和脐带血流通畅也同样至关重要。

胎儿最大风险是胎儿死亡或潜在疾病进程导致的严重残疾。胎儿必须要在无干预的情况下存在预后不良，才考虑 EXIT 手术。如果进行干预，除了存在已经提到的风险之外，还存在疾病过程及其治疗相关的特殊风险。分娩后有时需要一个由外科医师、麻醉科医师和护士组成的独立团队在相邻手术室继续对新生儿进行持续治疗。最后，基于 EXIT 手术的时限性，早产可能会使婴儿的情况进一步复杂。从胎儿的角度来看，EXIT 手术对酸碱状态通常具有良好的耐受性，这表明尽管长时间使用高浓度的吸入麻醉药，子宫胎盘仍然具有良好的灌注。

产妇风险

EXIT 期间，产妇也面临重大风险。同所有其他产妇一样，EXIT 产妇同样经历妊娠期生理变化并且面临全身麻醉的相关风险（表 32.4）。气道水肿可能使插管困难，而胃反流和妊娠子宫增加产妇发生吸入性肺炎的风险。妊娠高凝状态合并手术时间延长使产妇面临发生静脉血栓栓塞事件的风险，因此，除非患者能完全自由活动外都需要使用充气

表 32.4 孕妇生理的改变

器官系统	孕妇改变	麻醉风险
神经系统	MAC 降低	对麻醉药更敏感
	硬膜外神经丛丰富	对椎管内麻醉更敏感
呼吸系统	上呼吸道水肿	潜在面罩通气和插管困难
	功能残气量降低和分钟通气量增加	呼吸暂停导致氧饱和度降低速度更快
循环系统	下腔静脉位于子宫后方	仰卧位下腔静脉受压迫
	血容量增加大于血细胞比容增加	孕期相对贫血；血压改变较小或无改变
	心排血量增加，外周血管阻力降低	对麻醉药更敏感
胃肠道及肝	食管下段括约肌张力降低，腹内压增加	误吸风险增加
	血浆蛋白和白蛋白下降	肺水肿风险增加
	血浆胆碱酯酶下降	延长琥珀胆碱作用

MAC，最低肺泡有效浓度

加压靴。产妇在分娩或腹腔内手术时也存在发生羊水栓塞和术后伤口感染的风险。EXIT 手术特有的其他风险包括：

- **未来的生产必须采取剖宫产分娩**：EXIT 的切口通常比标准剖宫产切口大且子宫切开的位置不同，这增加了患者再次分娩时和经阴道分娩时子宫破裂的风险。
- **有创监测的风险**：胎儿安危取决于子宫胎盘的灌注，而子宫胎盘的灌注取决于产妇血压，因此 EXIT 和妊娠中期开放手术期间需要持续监测产妇血压。
- **失血及输血的风险增加**：EXIT 期间，子宫需完全松弛来维持子宫胎盘的灌注，加重第三产程后子宫收缩无力进而导致循环不稳定的风险。即使是子宫收缩迅速恢复，EXIT 手术输血制品的可能性仍比常规剖宫产更大。如果病情需要，应备好血液制品随时可供使用。

EXIT 恢复期的产妇患者有类似于剖宫产患者潜在的术后并发症，包括伤口裂开、感染、出血和尿潴留。

启示

只有在胎儿治疗委员会进行全面评估并认真权衡产妇和胎儿的风险和益处后，才能进行胎儿手术。因为胎儿手术涉及诸多风险，只有当胎儿“生病”而产妇“健康”时，才适合手术。一旦认为胎儿适合进行干预，应当举行包括母亲、特定的家庭成员或朋友以及相关医师参加的团队会议。小儿外科医师、产科医师、新生儿科医师、麻醉科医师以及其他相关医学专家对风险和获益进行完整的阐释。一旦产妇同意，该手术的复杂性要求人员和手术室资源的密切协调。

管理

剖宫产分娩在区域麻醉或全身麻醉下进行，胎儿无需麻醉，而 EXIT 手术通常需要胎儿和产妇都实施全身麻醉。EXIT 手术的麻醉管理目标包括以下内容：

- 产妇麻醉；
- 胎儿麻醉；
- 完全的子宫松弛以便手术和暴露；
- 无宫缩；
- 血流动力学稳定状态下保留胎盘灌注和气体交换；
- 脐带断开前维持子宫胎盘灌注。

产妇实施全身气管内麻醉在某种程度上实现了以上目标。术中需要辅助其他药物作为补充以实现以上目标。

诱导前

对于任何需要麻醉的孕妇而言，误吸预防措施包括诱导前 8 h 禁食、静脉注射甲氧氯普胺和口服双辛酸钠。如果术后产妇计划实施硬膜外镇痛，术前放置导管并且使用试验剂量以确认导管位置。将子宫向左侧推移可防止下腔静脉压迫和增加静脉回流并保持足够的产妇心排血量。

术前必须确定单纯硬膜外麻醉是否能够适合应用于该手术作，并且切皮之前确认局麻药的剂量和麻醉平面达到 T4 ～ T6 水平。

诱导

在充分预充氧后，进行快速序贯诱导并且用带套囊的气管导管确保气道安全。由于孕妇口咽部发生改变，经常选择较小型号的气管导管。紧急气道设备应该一直处于随时备用状态。插管后，另外开放静脉通路以及动脉置管和插导尿管。手术切皮前，使用非去极化神经肌肉阻滞药物实现肌肉松弛。

手术开始

手术准备之前使用超声检查确认胎儿情况良好及确定胎盘的位置。子宫切开之前，至少使用 2 倍最低肺泡吸入麻醉药浓度（minimum alveolar anesthetic concentrations，MAC）诱导子宫完全松弛，必要时，使用硝酸甘油（分次给予 100 ～ 200 μg）作为辅助用药，然后以 0.5 ～ 1 μg/（kg·min）速度维持。据报道，使用硝酸甘油的好处包括其效能强、易滴定以及作用时间短。通常外科医师通过术中触诊确定子宫张力。随着吸入麻醉药浓度增加，停止使用氧化亚氮，使用 100% O_2 最大限度地提高氧供。尚无研究比较何种卤族吸入麻醉药能提供的子宫松弛程度最大；因此目前临床中通常使用七氟烷、地氟烷和异氟烷。

高剂量的吸入麻醉药会降低产妇体循环阻力和心排血量。可使用麻黄碱和去氧肾上腺素滴定以维持产妇收缩压波动在基础值的 20% 以内。产妇血压降低对胎儿产生不良影响，因为子宫胎盘灌注与产妇血压直接相关。去氧肾上腺素已被证实可较有效地提高产妇血压，进而提高子宫胎盘灌注。一些机构已经发现，在不需要子宫松弛的时期内，全凭静脉麻醉技术有助于保持血流动力学平稳。

一旦确认手术部位后，行 U 形子宫切开术并使用子宫吻合器止血以便尽量减少产妇出血。通过超声定位胎盘并且距离胎盘边缘 5 cm 处切开子宫以减少胎盘早剥的风险。子宫温水灌洗预防胎儿低体温和维持子宫容积。通过关注子宫完全松弛、维持产妇正常血压、氧合以及避免扭曲或压迫脐带以便确保维持子宫胎盘血流量充足。

为监测胎儿，将无菌脉搏血氧饱和度仪探头放在肢体末端并用箔片覆盖减少环境光线的干扰。通过静脉内或肌内给予由非去极化肌肉松弛药、麻醉镇痛镇静药物以及有或无阿托品组成的“鸡尾酒混合剂”为胎儿追加麻醉。在颈部肿块的病例中，将胎儿头部和躯干作为手术区域以便进行直接喉镜检查和可能需要的气管切开术。间段的无菌胎儿超声心动图可以监测心脏功能、导管通畅和容量状态。

EXIT 后治疗

一旦 EXIT 手术完成，可以通过 Seldinger 技术放置脐带、动脉和静脉导管，此时脐带仍然充满了来自子宫胎盘的血流。脐带断离之前，需要确保足够的胸廓起伏，并确认血氧饱和度适当上升。子宫内胎儿血氧饱和度通常是 55% ～ 65%。100% 纯氧通气应使血氧饱和度增加到 95% ～ 100%。当脐带断离时，记录分娩时间，并从无菌区域中取出婴儿进行评估和复苏。分娩后应立即行简短的体格检查，快速确定双肺呼吸音和血流动力学稳定。如果存在其他即刻手术的指征，则通常将婴儿带至紧邻的手术间，由等候的麻醉科医师、外科医师和护士组成的第二团队术间实施手术。

胎盘娩出后，降低吸入麻醉药浓度，催产素 20 单位稀释于 1000 ml 的乳酸钠林格液静脉滴注以恢复子宫张力。如果产妇血流动力学稳定，可采用硬膜外给药镇痛。产妇出现顽固性子宫无力可肌内注射甲麦角新碱 0.2 mg 和（或）卡前列素氨丁三醇 250 μg。当子宫切口和腹部切口缝合完毕，可根据产妇生命体征和估计失血量来进行容量复苏。手术结束时，需要逆转肌肉松弛，当产妇完全清醒时拔管，然后转移于恢复室。

预防

虽然不可能预防所有不良后果，但合理的麻醉准备可有助于减少相关的风险。EXIT 手术中，麻醉准备必须考虑两个患者的因素——产妇和胎儿。而后，进行简洁沟通，包括 EXIT 计划期间专科医师和护理人员之间的术前汇报，可以识别潜在的风险和问题，并尽量做到为两位患者提供最佳治疗。

致谢

感谢 Marnie Robinson 博士对本章上一版的贡献。

（卢文斌 译 沈 镀 校）

延伸阅读

Adzick NS, Harrison MR: Fetal surgical therapy, *Lancet* 343:897–902, 1994.

Dahlgren G, Tornberg DC, Pregner K, et al.: Four cases of the ex utero intrapartum treatment (EXIT) procedure: anesthetic implications, *Int J Obstet Anesth* 13:178–182, 2004.

Gaiser RR, Cheek TG, Kurth CD: Anesthetic management of cesarean delivery complicated by ex utero intrapartum treatment of the fetus, *Anesth Analg* 84:1150–1153, 1997.

Harrison MR, Keller RL, Hawgood SB, et al.: A randomized trial of fetal endoscopic tracheal occlusion for severe fetal congenital diaphragmatic hernia, *N Engl J Med* 349:1916–1924, 2003.

Hirose S, Farmer DL, Lee H, et al.: The ex utero intrapartum treatment procedure: looking back at the EXIT, *J Pediatr Surg* 39:375–380, 2004.

Liechty KW: Ex-utero intrapartum therapy, *Semin Fetal Neonatal Med* 15:34–39, 2010.

Liechty KW, Crombleholme TM, Timothy M, et al.: Intrapartum airway management for giant fetal neck masses: the EXIT procedure, *Obstet Gynecol* 177:870–874, 1997.

Lim BF, Crombleholme TM, Hedrick JL, et al.: Congenital high airway obstruction syndrome: natural history and management, *J Pediatr Surg* 38:940–945, 2003.

Marwan A, Crombleholme T: The EXIT procedure: principles, pitfalls, and progress, *Semin Pediatr Surg* 15:107–115, 2006.

Moldenhauer JS: Ex utero intrapartum therapy, *Semin Pediatr Surg* 22:44–49, 2013.

Myers LB, Cohen D, Galinkin J, et al.: Anaesthesia for fetal surgery, *Paediatr Anaesth* 12:569–578, 2002.

Noah MM, Norton ME, Sandberg P, et al.: Short-term maternal outcomes that are associated with the EXIT procedure, as compared with cesarean delivery, *Am J Obstet Gynecol* 186:1299–1303, 2002.

Oluyinka O, Olutoye O: EXIT procedure for fetal neck masses, *Curr Opin Pediatr* 24:386–393, 2012.

Rychik J, Tian Z, Cohen MS, et al.: Acute cardiovascular effects of fetal surgery in the human, *Circulation* 110:1549–1556, 2004.

产前出血

第33章

Elizabeth M.S. Lange，*Paloma Toledo*

病例概要

患者，女性，30岁，G3P2，孕28周时出现阴道出血，既往有子宫肌瘤切除以及2次剖宫产史。此次为该患者首次在孕期出血，估计出血量为200 ml，目前患者循环状况稳定，血细胞比容30%。超声检查结果提示为侵入性胎盘。

问题分析

定义

产前出血的定义为分娩前出现的阴道出血。3%～5%的妊娠因产前出血而变得复杂，这仍然是全世界孕产妇在围产期病残和死亡的主要原因。

许多综述观点显示，通过改善医疗措施可以避免出血相关的死亡情况发生。改善医疗措施的建议包括：①识别出血高风险孕产妇；②改善对出血的认识；③及时治疗出血。对孕期出血的识别具有挑战性，因为与非孕期相比，孕期的生理状况允许孕妇在出现血容量不足的体征或症状前有相对更多的失血。而且，临床医师很难估计失血量。目前，已经提出了多学科协作来使出血孕产妇的处理方法和管理方案标准化。

流产、异位妊娠、前置胎盘、胎盘早剥、子宫破裂和血管前置是导致产前出血的最常见原因。产前出血的病因可能随孕龄的变化而变化。妊娠早期（妊娠20周前）出血可能是胚胎植入异常（如前置胎盘、侵入性胎盘、胎盘早剥或血管前置）、流产、异位妊娠、妊娠滋养细胞疾病、功能性子宫出血和生殖道良恶性肿瘤。妊娠早期并发出血的孕妇中，进展超过孕期20周的病例通常不到50%；10%～15%是异位妊娠，0.2%是葡萄胎，超过30%导致流产。妊娠20周以上出血的最常见原因是胎盘早剥和前置胎盘。

胎盘早剥

胎盘早剥的定义为：胎儿出生前，正常位置的胎盘从胎盘蜕膜基底附着部位的剥离。这种剥离被认为是胎盘动脉或静脉破裂的结果。胎盘早剥在所有妊娠中发生率为0.5%～1.8%，约40%的病例发生在妊娠第37周之后，40%的病例发生在妊娠第34周和第37周之间，不到20%的病例发生在妊娠第32周之前。在20%～35%的病例中，出血可能是隐匿性（即未见明显阴道出血）；因此，对产妇低血容量的体征和症状的关注非常重要。

前置胎盘

前置胎盘是指胎盘附着于子宫下段。其分型主要依据宫颈口被侵犯或覆盖的程度（图33.1）。由于子宫下段在妊娠期间逐渐伸长，在宫颈口的前置胎盘的入侵程度减少（因而出血风险也降低）。前置胎盘在妊娠晚期的发病率高达1%。

侵入性胎盘

有时，胎盘可以在没有蜕膜的情况下黏附到植入部位，这是一种通过蜕膜层产生的生理裂解线的异常。胎盘还可以侵入子宫肌层（植入性胎盘）或延伸穿过子宫肌层并黏附到周围结构（穿透性胎盘）。

血管前置

虽然脐带通常附着在胎盘上，但在约1%的单胎妊娠和约9%双胎妊娠中，脐带会附着于绒毛膜羊膜。这种非典型或帆状附着使脐带血管在羊膜和绒毛膜之间穿过到达胎盘时受到创伤或压迫。当帆状脐带血管出现在胎儿前方时存在血管前置，使胎儿胎膜破裂的风险更大，经常导致胎儿放血（exsanguination）和死亡。

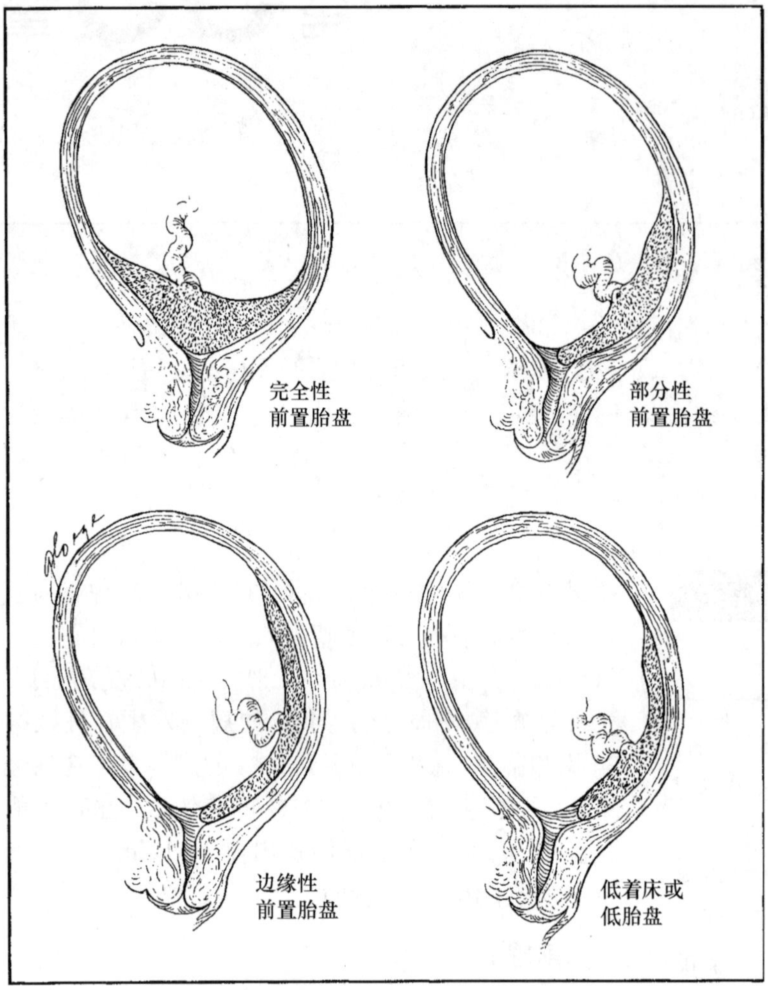

图 33.1 胎盘前置的类型（From Ricci JM：Antepartum hemorrhage. In Hacker NF，Moore JG，editors：*Essentials of obstetrics and gynecology*，2nd ed. Philadelphia，WB Saunders，1992，p 156.）

子宫破裂

子宫破裂被定义为子宫壁的缺陷，与胎儿窘迫或产妇出血相关，一旦发生需行剖宫产术或产后剖腹探查术。妊娠期子宫破裂的发生率不到1%，多发生在有子宫外伤的患者中。子宫瘢痕裂开无需进行手术，尽管这比真正的子宫破裂更常见，但大多数病例无症状且不太可能导致母体或胎儿死亡。然而，子宫瘢痕裂开可导致显著的发病率，尤其是当它导致胎盘向外侧延伸侵犯子宫主要血管或有异常胎盘形成（侵入性胎盘、植入性胎盘或穿透性胎盘）。如果引产、剖宫产则瘢痕破裂的可能性更大。

流产

流产（即自然流产）的定义是在孕 20 周前确认怀孕失败。流产可分为先兆流产、难免流产、完全流产、不完全流产、流产感染、反复流产或稽留流产。在所有临床诊断的妊娠中，有 15% ～ 20% 的妊娠会导致流产，但根据流产的定义，实际发生率可能更高。典型表现包括阴道点滴出血或轻度出血。当怀孕前 12 周阴道出血与正常月经失血一样严重时，妊娠很少成功。当发生宫内胎儿死亡时，尤其是在妊娠期，可以观察到大量的失血。

异位妊娠

约 2% 的妊娠中受精卵未在子宫内正常着床，且发生率似乎在增加。虽然异位妊娠通常表现为盆腔疼痛伴腹腔出血，但也可能被误诊为其他疾病，包括阑尾炎、卵巢囊肿扭转、子宫内膜异位症和盆腔炎症。已有关于异位妊娠导致的重大失血与猝死的相关报道。出血的风险和结果与着床部位（如输卵管峡部或间质部、卵巢、子宫颈、腹部）和诊断时间有关。异位妊娠可自行解决，可通过药物治疗，或需要腹腔镜或开腹手术。一般在出现相关腹膜征象、血流动力学不稳定或保守治疗失败的情况下，建议手术治疗。

未分类出血

未分类出血几乎占产前出血的一半（血管前置有时也归为此类）。它通常发生在妊娠晚期，其原因要么未知，要么知之甚晚。这种类型的出血虽然通常是轻微的，并可自行消退，但仍有极高的围产期死亡率（3.5% ～ 15.7%）。这可能是由于胎盘功能障碍和未分类出血患者早产率较高所致。

识别

妊娠期出血可被妊娠期正常的生理变化所掩盖。早在妊娠 6 ～ 8 周时，孕妇血容量就有逐渐增加的趋势，在妊娠 32 周时血容量达到峰值（4700 ～ 5200 ml）。该容量比非妊娠妇女增加了 45%，孕妇血容量会因多胎妊娠进一步增加，且似乎与胎儿体重有关。胎盘绒毛膜生长催乳素、孕酮、促红细胞生成素和催乳素共同作用，可使妊娠期红细胞容量增加 250 ～ 450 ml，比妊娠前期增加 20% ～ 30%。血容量与红细胞容量不成比例地增加导致了相对的血液稀释和妊娠中晚期可见的血细胞比容的最大限度地下降。由此导致的血液黏度降低被认为可以改善绒毛间灌注，降低血栓栓塞事件的风险。它还可以减少分娩过程中红细胞的损失。血细胞比容和血容量的变化有助于提高产妇的心排血量。心率从妊娠第 5 周开始增加，到 32 周时达到 15 ～ 20 次 / 分钟的最大增幅。这是对相对贫血、迷走神经控制减弱和交感神经张力增强的反应。每搏输出量的增加是早期心排血量增加的主要原因，与妊娠前期心肌重量的增加以及妊娠中期和妊娠晚期舒张末期体积的增加有关。总的来说，怀孕期间心排血量增加了 30% ～ 50%。一半的增长发生在怀孕的前 8 周，最大的增长出现在产后。正常妊娠期间出现的贫血、心动过速和血压下降与出血时出现的生理紊乱相似。

这些生理上的改变使孕妇能够承受 1000 ～ 1500 ml 的失血而不引起血流动力学的重大变化。然而，由于每分钟有近 20% 的心排血量（600 ～ 700 ml 血液）流经胎盘绒毛间隙，产科出血可迅速导致严重休克症状（表 33.1）。此外，由于产前出血可能导致严重失血，应回顾出血常见原因的特点，以协助早期诊断和治疗（表 33.2）。

表 33.1 产科出血的评估

休克严重程度	表现	失血量（%）
无	无	15 ～ 20
轻度	心动过速（<100 bpm） 轻度低血压 周围血管收缩	20 ～ 25
中度	心动过速（100 ～ 120 bpm） 低血压（80 ～ 100 mmHg） 烦躁不安，少尿	25 ～ 35
重度	心动过速（>120 bpm） 低血压（SBP<60 mmHg） 意识障碍，无尿	>35

bpm，次 / 分钟；SBP，收缩压

表 33.2 产前出血的早期和晚期诊断特征

诊断	特征
妊娠早期（<20 周）	
流产	末次月经后，阴道出血（伴或不伴疼痛）>8 周；子宫检查轻度压痛；无附件肿物
异位妊娠	可能无阴道出血；末次月经后，疼痛 <8 周；子宫检查有单侧压痛；可能存在休克；子宫大小可能正常
妊娠晚期（≥ 20 周）	
前置胎盘	无痛性阴道出血（≤ 10% 有胎盘早剥引起的疼痛）；胎儿畸形（35%）；难以触及胎儿位置
胎盘早剥	有痛觉的阴道出血；子宫易激惹或抽搐；凝血功能障碍；胎儿窘迫或死亡
子宫破裂	阴道出血（伴或不伴疼痛）；低血压；分娩终止；胎儿窘迫
前置血管	无痛性阴道出血；引流血液中存在胎儿血红蛋白
未分类的出血	无痛性阴道出血；轻微出血（通常会自行消散）；通常发生在妊娠 37 周后

风险评估

出血的风险受到许多因素的影响，包括是否存在产科异常状况、医疗条件或胎儿畸形（表 33.3）。早期发现出血的危险因素对调动医疗资源非常重要。输血前血液测试（即根据出血量、持续出血量及输血需求进行血型筛查与交叉配型）。对于正在出血或有潜在大出血可能的患者，也应启动所在机构的相关预案。

启示

除了产后出血的风险外，产前出血可能还有重

表 33.3 产前出血相关的危险因素	
诊断	特征
妊娠早期（<20 周）	
流产	早期流产；产妇年龄的增加；基因畸变；子宫畸形；内分泌异常；感染；血栓形成；免疫反应异常；烟草、酒精、药物
异位妊娠	子宫内膜异位症；不孕症；感染；既往输卵管绝育或再造术；子宫内避孕器
妊娠晚期（≥ 20 周）	
前置胎盘	分娩次数或产妇年龄的增加；既往有过胎盘前置或剖宫产史
胎盘早剥	创伤；胎膜破裂；接触过可卡因、美沙酮、烟草；子痫前期；子宫肌瘤
子宫破裂	既往有子宫手术史；创伤；既往有宫内操作史，包括胎盘取出、刮除、倒转术、钳检；多胎；子宫发育异常；穿透性胎盘；肿瘤；胎儿问题（如胎儿巨大、胎位不正、畸形）；引产或增产
前置血管	多胎妊娠；低位胎盘；体外受精后怀孕；帆状胎盘；双胎盘和副胎盘

要的后遗症，包括凝血病、急性肾衰竭、垂体坏死、休克以及孕产妇和胎儿死亡。围产期的病残率和死亡率主要与胎盘灌注不良或早产相关。

凝血病最初是由持续的血液成分丢失和快速容量置换引起的血液稀释，可伴有弥散性血管内凝血（disseminated intravascular coagulation，DIC）。尽管 DIC 一直是所有产前出血病例的关注焦点，但最常见的病种是胎盘早剥（高达 20%）。DIC 的实验室诊断特征包括：凝血酶原时间延长、部分凝血活酶时间延长、血纤维蛋白原过少、血小板减少和纤维蛋白降解产物升高。虽然 DIC 的治疗存在争议，但凝血相关因素（特别是纤维蛋白原）的恢复是关键。体重 70 kg 的成年人，需 4 g 的纤维蛋白原使纤维蛋白原水平增加 1000 mg/L。纤维蛋白原在冷沉淀中的浓度是新鲜冰冻血浆的 3 ～ 10 倍。妊娠期纤维蛋白原水平可升高至 4000 mg/L 或更高。在持续出血情况较为严重时，纤维蛋白原水平低于 2000 mg/L 是输血的一个指标。

严重产前出血患者中，约 10% 存在急性肾衰竭（伴或不伴 DIC）。急性肾衰竭与低血压、肾缺血、纤维蛋白沉积、微血管凝块和肌红蛋白尿有关。急性肾衰竭最常与胎盘早剥同时出现，可通过积极输血和容量复苏加以预防。

缺血性脑垂体坏死（Sheehan 综合征）可伴有严重出血，甚至分娩时无明显失血。垂体增大、蝶鞍小、DIC 或自身免疫也可导致 Sheehan 综合征，最常见的表现为轻度垂体功能障碍，如不能分泌乳汁或月经恢复。急性低钠血症和低血糖也可能伴随 Sheehan 综合征。

治疗

血流动力学管理

虽然只有不到 1% 的产妇需要输血，并且健康且能够耐受无明显症状的贫血，但医务人员需要意识到大量出血可能很快发生并需要做好复苏的准备。对失血的低估和容量复苏不足在产前出血患者中很常见，并可能影响相关的孕产妇死亡率。一份报告中指出，在 79% 产前出血相关的孕产妇死亡中，监护不力被认为是促发因素。

大多数机构都制订了产科出血管理方案。孕产妇安全国家伙伴关系组织最近发表了一份关于产科出血的共识，强调应对措施的重要性，在每个产科单位制定了分阶段进行的产科出血应急管理计划和清单。管理方案中应酌情考虑调动相关资源，包括血库和其他相关学科（例如介入放射学）。同时应根据分娩的风险和胎儿的胎龄请新生儿相关学科的介入。

容量治疗是维持组织灌注和氧合的重要手段。如有需要，应及早应用胶体液和血液制品，同时应请求协助，开放第二路大静脉输液通道，并使用加压输液设备。血流动力学监测与有创血压监测或经胸超声心动图可帮助评估容量状态和是否需要强心药或血管升压药。在更严重的出血病例中，中心静脉导管或经食管超声心动图可能是必要的。

有很多关于最佳输血策略的研究，然而到目前为止，还没有对产科出血患者进行的随机对照试验报道。美国血库协会建议通过症状而非血红蛋白水平来决定输血的必要性。目前，除了辅助治疗措施外，辅助性药物在产科出血中的应用也越来越受到关注，包括促红细胞生成素、预存式自体血回输、术中自体血回输、急性等容性血液稀释和抗纤维蛋白溶解治疗。这些疗法的有效性需进一步研究来确定。

麻醉管理

发生出血的产妇应在优化血流动力学状态的同时做好手术准备。术前对失血状况进行全面控制是不现实的，因为出血会一直持续到病因消除。虽然可以考虑局部麻醉，但气管内插管的全身麻醉可能更有利于其他紧迫的临床场景。这些情况包括：

- 血流动力学不稳定的患者；
- 因分娩加重的持续出血以及容量复苏；
- 未建立气道保护可能导致的意识丧失；
- 凝血功能障碍。

全身麻醉可能导致患者血流动力学的不利影响，休克患者在诱导前应准备好升压药。低血压通常从诱导时就会出现，对于已经表现出血流动力学不稳定的患者，低血压的处理是非常具有挑战性的。在进行子宫左倾、充分去氮给氧、快速诱导和气管插管后，应尽量减少吸入麻醉药的使用剂量，因为它们会促进子宫肌肉松弛。相反，氧气和氧化亚氮、苯二氮䓬类药物和短效麻醉药物的使用剂量应控制在可耐受的范围内。应经常检查尿量，并评估是否需要开放额外的静脉通道或进行必要的有创监测。胎儿和胎盘取出后，应根据需要给予子宫收缩剂（缩宫素、甲基麦角新碱、15-甲基前列腺素 F2α）。然而，潜在的子宫内膜病变可能不允许恢复正常的子宫张力或难以停止出血。这种情况下，可能需要行妊娠子宫切除术。如果在分娩时孕妇配合且硬膜外导管在位通畅，则可以选择使用硬膜外麻醉进行子宫切除术，否则应选择全身麻醉。

预防

预防与严重产前出血相关的并发症需要根据患者的病史和症状、超声或磁共振成像，给予保持高度的警惕并加快团队反应的速度。影像学检查，特别是彩色多普勒超声的血流增强显影，极大程度地提高了对前置胎盘、侵入性胎盘子宫壁（侵入性胎盘、植入性胎盘、穿透性胎盘）、血管前置的诊断水平，改善了母婴最终的结局。即便如此，这些影像学方法的诊断敏感性和特异性仍存在一定局限性，而且在某些方面的可行性有限。因此，可能需要双重检查。这包括在手术室行阴道穹窿指诊，为紧急剖宫产做好准备。目前，这种方法仅适用于活动性出血、胎儿健康状况已知以及影像学检查不明确的患者。或者，介入放射科医师可以在高危产妇的子宫动脉内放置气囊栓塞导管，以便在必要时迅速控制出血。

（常永青 译 杨 涛 校）

延伸阅读

Anderson FW, Hogan JG, Ansbacher R: Sudden death: ectopic pregnancy mortality, *Obstet Gynecol* 103:1218–1223, 2004.

Berg CJ, Harper MA, Atkinson SM, et al.: Preventability of pregnancy-related deaths: results of a state-wide review, *Obstet Gynecol* 106:1228–1234, 2005.

Bick RL: Syndromes of disseminated intravascular coagulation in obstetrics, pregnancy, and gynecology: objective criteria for diagnosis and management, *Hematol Oncol Clin North Am* 14:999–1044, 2000.

Bick RL: Disseminated intravascular coagulation: a review of etiology, pathophysiology, diagnosis, and management: guidelines for care, *Clin Appl Thromb Hemost* 8:1–31, 2002.

Callaghan WM, Kuklina EV, Berg CJ: Trends in postpartum hemorrhage: United States, 1994–2006, *Am J Obstet Gynecol* 202(353):e1–e6, 2010.

Carretti N, La Marca A: Maternal serum levels of human chorionic somatotropin correlates with transferrin and erythropoietin in pregnancy, *Gynecol Obstet Invest* 53:28–31, 2002.

Centre for Maternal and Child Enquiries (CMACE): Saving Mothers' Lives: reviewing maternal deaths to make motherhood safer: 2006–08. The Eighth Report on Confidential Enquiries into Maternal Deaths in the United Kingdom, *BJOG* 118(Suppl 1):1–203, 2011.

Chan CC, To WW: Antepartum hemorrhage of unknown origin—what is its clinical significance? *Acta Obstet Gynecol Scand* 78:186–190, 1999.

Chestnut DH, Dewan DM, Redick LF, et al.: Anesthetic management for obstetric hysterectomy: a multi-institutional study, *Anesthesiology* 70:607–610, 1989.

Coste J, Bouyer J, Ughetto S, et al.: Ectopic pregnancy is again on the increase: recent trends in the incidence of ectopic pregnancies in France (1992–2002), *Hum Reprod* 9:2014–2018, 2004.

Duvekot JJ, Cheriex EC, Pieters FA, et al.: Maternal volume homeostasis in early pregnancy in relation to fetal growth restriction, *Obstet Gynecol* 85:361–367, 1995.

Faiz AS, Ananth CV: Etiology and risk factors for placenta previa: an overview and meta-analysis of observational studies, *J Matern Fetal Neonatal Med* 13:175–190, 2003.

Gilson GJ, Samaan S, Crawford MH, et al.: Changes in hemodynamics, ventricular remodeling, and ventricular contractility during normal pregnancy: a longitudinal study, *Obstet Gynecol* 89:957–962, 1997.

Gonik B: Intensive care monitoring of the critically ill pregnant patient. In Creasy RK, Resnik R, editors: *Maternal-fetal medicine*, Philadelphia, 1994, WB Saunders, pp 865–890.

Guise JM, McDonagh MS, Osterweil P, et al.: Systematic review of the incidence and consequences of uterine rupture in women with previous caesarean section, *BMJ* 329:19–25, 2004.

Hansch E, Chitkara U, McAlpine J, et al.: Pelvic arterial embolization for control of obstetric hemorrhage: a five-year experience, *Am J Obstet Gynecol* 180:1454–1460, 1999.

Hunter S, Robson SC: Adaptation of the maternal heart in pregnancy, *Br Heart J* 68:540–543, 1992.

Kacmar RM, Scavone BM, Mhyre JM, et al.: The use of postpartum hemorrhage protocols in United States academic obstetric anesthesia units, *Anesth Analg* 119:906–910, 2014.

Kelestimur F: Sheehan's syndrome, *Pituitary* 6:181–188, 2003.

Koonin LM, MacKay AP, Berg CJ, et al.: Pregnancy-related mortality surveillance—United States, 1987–1990, *MMWR CDC Surveill Summ* 46:17–36, 1997.

Lund CJ, Donovan JC: Blood volume during pregnancy: significance of

plasma and red cell volumes, *Am J Obstet Gynecol* 98:394–403, 1967.
Main EK, Goffman D, Scamove BM, et al.: National Partnership for Maternal Safety: consensus bundle on obstetric hemorrhage, *Obstet Gynecol* 126:155–162, 2015.
Mercier FJ, Van de Velde M: Major obstetric hemorrhage, *Anesthesiol Clin* 26:53–66, 2008.
Oppenheimer LW, Farine D: A new classification of placenta previa: measuring progress in obstetrics, *Am J Obstet Gynecol* 201:227–229, 2009.
Oyelese Y, Smulian JC: Placenta previa, placenta accreta, and vasa previa, *Obstet Gynecol* 107:927–941, 2006.
Paterson ME: The aetiology and outcome of abruptio placentae, *Acta Obstet Gynecol Scand* 58:31–35, 1979.
Porreco RP, Clark SL, Belfort MA, et al.: The changing specter of uterine rupture, *Am J Obstet Gynecol* 200(269):e1–e4, 2009.
Practice Guidelines for Obstetric Anesthesia: An updated report by the American Society of Anesthesiologists Task Force on Obstetric Anesthesia and the Society for Obstetric Anesthesia and Perinatology, *Anesthesiology* 124:270–300, 2016.
Pritchard JA, Brekken AL: Clinical and laboratory studies on severe abruptio placentae, *Am J Obstet Gynecol* 97:681–700, 1967.
Rao KP, Belogolovkin V, Yankowitz J, Spinnato JA: Abnormal placentation: evidence-based diagnosis and management of placenta previa, placenta accreta, and vasa previa, *Obstet Gynecol Surv* 67:503–519, 2012.
Rosevear S: Bleeding in early pregnancy. In James DK, Steer PJ, Weiner CP, Gonik B, editors: *High risk pregnancy management options*, London, 1999, WB Saunders.
Thachil J, Toh CH: Disseminated intravascular coagulation in obstetric disorders and its acute haematological management, *Blood Rev* 23:167–176, 2009.
Toledo P, McCarthy RJ, Hewlett BJ, et al.: Accuracy of blood loss estimation after vaginal delivery, *Anesth Analg* 105:1736–1740, 2007.
Why Mothers Die 1997–1999: *Confidential enquiries into maternal deaths in the United Kingdom*, London, 2001, Department of Health, HMSO, pp 36–37.
Williams MA, Mittendorf R, Lieberman E, Monson RR: Adverse infant outcomes associated with first-trimester vaginal bleeding, *Obstet Gynecol* 78:14–18, 1991.

前纵隔肿物

第 34 章

Devon Aganga，*Randall P. Flick*

病例概要

患者，女性，8 岁，既往体健，因呼吸困难、喘息和喘鸣入院。她的症状在 2 周内逐渐加重，并伴有夜间发热和运动耐量降低。胸部 X 线显示纵隔扩大和胸骨后肿块（图 34.1）。胸部计算机断层扫描（CT）证实存在前纵隔肿物（图 34.2）。拟对其肿块进行活检。

问题分析

引言

接受前纵隔肿物组织活检或手术切除的儿童和成人的麻醉管理是我们目前在麻醉方面所遇到的最大挑战之一。这是因为，这些患者在麻醉诱导和麻醉维持期间的任何时刻都可能遭受危及生命的气道外源性受压、心排血量受阻或静脉回流受阻。看似无症状的患者也可能在麻醉期间发生上述灾难性事件之一。尽管对前纵隔肿物患者的病理生理学和管理有了更好的了解，但麻醉过程中从轻度气道阻塞到完全心肺衰竭的围术期并发症发生率估计仍在 9% ～ 20%。为这些患者实施麻醉最安全的方法是什么？我们如何在术前确定哪些患者的风险最大？有没有办法在优化组织诊断的同时降低患者的风险？这些是患有前纵隔肿物的患者所面临的一些挑战。

定义

纵隔定义为胸腔胸膜内侧面的一部分，位于膈肌上方和胸腔入口下方。前方为胸骨，后方为胸椎。第四胸椎和胸骨角连线将纵隔腔分为下纵隔和上纵隔。下纵隔被心包进一步分为前纵隔、中纵隔和后纵隔。前纵隔位于胸骨和心包之间。中纵隔包括心包及其内容物，后纵隔包括心包和胸椎之间的空间。没有筋膜平面将这些区域分开，因此起源于一个纵隔区域的肿块可能会侵袭至另一个区域。纵隔肿块可影响许多胸腔内结构。最严重的是压迫心脏或各纵隔区域内主要血管肿块。通常情况下出现于前纵隔，较少涉及中纵隔和后纵隔。基于纵隔肿块的位置，无论其为良性还是恶性，都具有特征性。它为临床医师提供了肿块起源的线索，并确定了它对周围纵隔和其他胸廓结构的影响。前纵隔肿物的鉴别诊断包括 T 字开头的恶性肿瘤：**恶性淋巴瘤（terrible lymphoma）、胸腺瘤（thymoma）、畸胎瘤（teratoma）和甲状腺肿瘤（thyroid tumor）**。儿童中报道的最常见的是恶性淋巴瘤，占前纵隔肿物的 45%。据报道，在成人中胸腺瘤和淋巴瘤占前纵隔肿物的 50% 以上。前纵隔肿物的其他潜在病理类型包括转移瘤、胸内甲状腺肿、神经母细胞瘤、胸腺囊肿、支气管囊肿和心包囊肿。

识别

前纵隔肿物的成人患者存在多种体征和症状。然而，大多数是无症状或有轻至中度症状，包括咳嗽、劳力性呼吸困难、胸痛、乏力和声带麻痹。少数成年患者的严重症状包括端坐呼吸、喘鸣、发绀、颈静脉怒张或上腔静脉综合征。儿童可能会表现为看似良性呼吸系统疾病的健康状况，如持续性感冒、喘息、咳嗽或喘鸣，但胸部 X 线可使医师发现更为危险的病因。无论临床表现如何，组织活检对于建立准确的诊断以指导最终治疗至关重要。这对于根据组织诊断确立的化疗方案显著不同的儿童尤为如此。

风险评估

对患有前纵隔肿物的患者进行彻底的术前评估

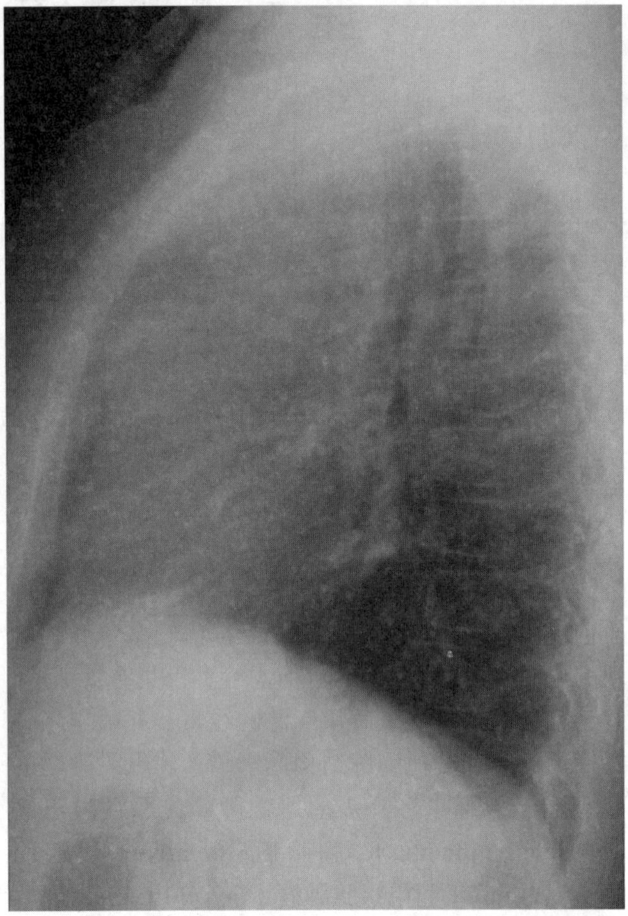

图 34.1 一名 8 岁女孩的侧位胸片，后被确定患有淋巴瘤。前纵隔可见一个大肿块。在活检之前即开始治疗

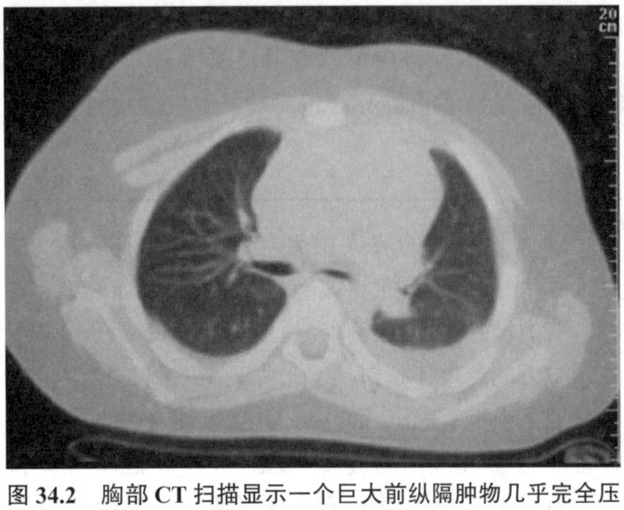

图 34.2 胸部 CT 扫描显示一个巨大前纵隔肿物几乎完全压闭远端气管和主支气管。经测量肿块大小约为 7 cm × 7 cm，不仅侵袭气管，还侵袭大血管和心包

对于保证麻醉安全至关重要。举例来讲，典型的实验室评估包括全血细胞计数、血涂片、电解质、尿酸、乳酸脱氢酶和流式细胞术。患者也可能接受各种诊断性操作，包括腰椎穿刺、骨髓穿刺、CT、经胸超声心动图和肺功能检查。此类患者在接受包括颈部淋巴结活检、Chamberlain 术（纵隔淋巴结活检）、骨髓活检、化疗用中央静脉导管置入以及肿瘤切除术（不太常见）时，均应引起麻醉科医师的高度关注。对于患有前纵隔肿物患者的麻醉注意事项取决于个体解剖结构、症状、患者年龄和拟进行的手术。尽管存在保证麻醉安全的一般原则，但的确需要对每个患者进行个体化管理。所有患者均应进行有针对性的询问病史和体格检查，胸部 X 线检查和 CT 扫描作为术前评估的一部分。端坐呼吸，仰卧位时出现咳嗽、喘鸣、喘息、面部肿胀或上半身水肿等，提示麻醉科医师应注意围术期风险增加的可能。应注意的是，没有临床症状并不排除出现危及生命的并发症的可能性。尤为重要的是，麻醉科医师应确定症状是否存在体位因素并明确患者症状最轻的体位。

CT 扫描将显示肿块的范围、是否存在气道受压及程度，以及对其他周围结构的侵袭和（或）压迫。磁共振成像未必可常规获得，幼儿需要镇静或全身麻醉才能获得图像。超声心动图可用于评估前纵隔肿物心血管受累患者的心脏功能；肿瘤是否浸润心包和心肌组织；是否压迫上腔静脉、肺动脉、右心房和右心室；是否存在心包积液，并评估心脏压塞时的生理功能。一些作者提倡在儿童和成人前纵隔肿物的检查中进行直立和仰卧位的肺功能检查（pulmonary function test，PFT）。纤维支气管镜检是动态评估气道阻塞的另一个有用工具。

最大呼气流速已被用于评估动态气道塌陷。流速-容量环的形状可提供气道阻塞部位（胸内或胸外）的线索，并提示阻塞是固定的还是可变的。曾有文献中提到，仰卧位最大呼气流速小于预测值的 50% 或 PFT 伴限制性和阻塞性混合通气功能障碍与术前呼吸并发症发生率的增加有关。最近的文献质疑了 PFT 的必要性，并认为 PFT 在前纵隔肿物患者的术前评估中用处极少。一项此类研究发现，流速-容量环与存在症状或 CT 扫描中所见气道受压程度的相关性均较差。

将临床症状和体征与诊断性检查结果相结合，可帮助识别出术前并发症风险较高的患者。在全身麻醉下心肺功能受损的预测指标包括以下几点：

- 存在严重的术前症状，尤其是端坐呼吸；
- 上腔静脉阻塞的患者；
- 存在肺动脉流出道梗阻的证据；
- 心室功能障碍；

- 存在心包积液 / 心脏压塞的生理；
- CT 显示横截面减少 50% 以上的气管受压，和（或）隆突或支气管受压；
- 仰卧位最大呼气流速小于预测值的 50%；
- 肺功能检查提示存在阻塞性和限制性混合通气功能障碍。

对于存在上述情况的患者，应仔细考虑能否安全地施行全身麻醉。应该充分考虑在局部麻醉辅助或不辅助镇静下进行组织活检的可能性。对于那些认为风险很高的患者，应考虑在手术前给予皮质类固醇治疗和（或）放射治疗。治疗可引起广泛的肿瘤溶解并缓解气道阻塞和心血管症状，从而降低患者的麻醉风险。对于此类治疗的担忧之处在于类固醇和辐射可能会影响后期组织诊断结果。然而，据一项研究报道，接受短期类固醇治疗不超过 5 天的患者组织诊断成功率高达 95%。

管理

对于治疗前纵隔肿物患者来说，最理想的方法是由肿瘤学、麻醉学、放射肿瘤学、放射学和外科专科的专家组成的多学科联合治疗。在回顾患者的临床资料和影像以及评估患者的术前风险后，需要决定做出组织诊断的最佳方案。麻醉的选择可归结为以下几点：

- 全身麻醉 [吸入和（或）静脉]；
- 仅采用局部麻醉；
- 施行镇静辅助的局部麻醉。

较大和较合作的儿童如考虑为心肺高危人群，可在局麻或局麻辅助镇静下对其肿块进行活检。据报道，细针穿刺活检足以对 80% 以上的病例做出准确的诊断。对于幼儿，即使是颈部淋巴结和骨髓等外周部位活检，如未实施全身麻醉很难提供理想的手术条件（无体动）。

了解作用于前纵隔肿瘤的压力平衡是关键。实质上，在仰卧位时，重力下拉纵隔肿瘤的效应被胸腔和肺部的回弹所产生的胸腔内负压所抵消。胸腔内负压是结构性（肋间肌和其他呼吸肌）和生理性（呼吸）力的总和。仰卧位时，膈肌更加向头侧偏移，胸膜腔内压较低，重力效应导致肿物对其背侧的结构即气道、右心和大血管施加更大的压力。因此，任何降低胸膜腔内压的操作都可能进一步加重前纵隔肿块的生理效应。这种操作包括全身麻醉的实施和自主通气的停止。麻醉药物和神经肌肉阻滞药物都会导致肌张力降低，这将使纵隔肿块的力量平衡向重力的方向偏移。

全身麻醉期间，在整个麻醉过程中或在气道得到明确保障之前维持自主呼吸是最安全的方法。可通过气道局部麻醉和纤支镜插管建立气道，或通过吸入诱导或滴定式输注静脉麻醉药物来实现。有几份病例报告了使用氯胺酮、丙泊酚、瑞芬太尼和右美托咪定的各种组合输注以达到这一目的。在小儿麻醉文献中也曾报道了在全身麻醉中使用面罩诱导并通过面罩通气维持自主呼吸。在麻醉诱导前建立静脉通路可能是最安全的。临床上有症状或影像诊断为高风险的儿童最好避免术前用药。上腔静脉综合征患者最好在下肢建立静脉通路。

保持床头抬高将减少膈肌向头侧的偏移。患者可以取坐位或侧卧位，以帮助维持气道的张力和减少心血管压迫。麻醉开始前的多学科团队应制订应急计划以管理手术期间的任何心肺功能衰竭。手术团队、麻醉团队和手术室工作人员均应该熟悉这个计划。如果发生气道阻塞，取俯卧位、头高脚低位或侧卧位（或采取患者术前描述的最舒适体位）可能改善患者病情。可通过将气管内导管向前推进至超过梗阻部位来减轻气道阻塞。在严重气道梗阻的情况下，或阻塞位置在远端，插入硬支气管镜可能改善这种情况。因此，在整个手术过程中应配备硬支镜和操作经验丰富的人员。出现危及生命的心血管压迫或气道阻塞且插入硬支气管镜无法缓解时，可能需要外科医师提起胸骨（将手指放在胸骨切迹和剑突下并提起）或紧急行胸骨切开术以抬起肿块。一些作者讨论了在心血管衰竭的情况下实施心肺转流术（体外循环）或体外膜氧合（extracorporeal membrane oxygenation，ECMO）的可行性，表达了对小儿和成人纵隔肿瘤患者实施 ECMO 的支持，并报道了可对清醒成人实施 ECMO 的机构。然而，最近的研究对 ECMO 或体外循环用于“待命”的有效性提出了质疑，例如，在心肺功能衰竭的情况下，当 ECMO 成功实施时，患者很可能已经遭受了严重缺氧缺血性神经损伤。

高风险的患者术后应在重症监护室进行监护。拔管应在患者完全清醒并处于头高位时进行。有明显气道阻塞的患者在术后可能出现呼吸困难。此时的治疗应重新定位，如果患者有呼吸衰竭的风险，应再次插管。

预防

对于有症状的纵隔肿块患者，避免全身麻醉或深度镇静是预防急性气道压迫的最佳方法。相反，活检应尽可能在局部麻醉下进行。或者，在实施全身麻醉行组织活检之前，给予放疗或皮质类固醇治疗可以减小肿块的大小。虽然仍有争议，但即使在放射治疗或短暂的类固醇治疗后，进行分子诊断的能力似乎也有了很大的提高。对于必须全身麻醉的患者，麻醉科医师必须保持高度警惕和谨慎。

（成雨彤 译 孟 岩 审校）

延伸阅读

Anghelescu DL, Burgoyne LL, et al.: Clinical and diagnostic imaging findings predict anesthetic complications in children presenting with malignant mediastinal masses, *Paediatr Anaesth* 17:1090–1098, 2007.

Bechard P, Letourneau L, Lacasse Y, et al.: Perioperative cardiorespiratory complications in adults with mediastinal mass: incidence and risk factors, *Anesthesiology* 100:826–834, 2004.

Blank RS, de Souza DG: Anesthetic management of patients with an anterior mediastinal mass: continuing professional development, *Can J Anesth* 58:853–867, 2011.

D'Cruz IA, Feghali N, Gross CM: Echocardiographic manifestations of mediastinal masses compressing or encroaching on the heart, *Echocardiography* 11:523–533, 1994.

Erdos G, Tzanova I: Preoperative anaesthetic management of mediastinal mass in adults, *Eur J Anaesth* 26:627–632, 2009.

Ferrari LR, Bedford RF: General anesthesia prior to treatment of anterior mediastinal masses in pediatric cancer patients, *Anesthesiology* 72:991–995, 1990.

Hack HA, Wright NB, Wynn RF: The anaesthetic management of children with anterior mediastinal masses, *Anaesthesia* 63:837–846, 2008.

Lerman J: Anterior mediastinal masses in children, *Semin Anesth Perioperat Med P* 26:133–140, 2007.

Pearson JK, Tan GM: Pediatric anterior mediastinal mass: a review article, *Semin Cardiothorac Vasc Anesth* 19:248–254, 2015.

Prakash YS, Abel MD, Hubmayr RD: Mediastinal mass and tracheal obstruction during general anesthesia, *Mayo Clin Proc* 63:1004–1011, 1988.

Pullerits J, Holzman R: Anaesthesia for patients with mediastinal masses, *Can J Anaesth* 36:681–688, 1989.

Rath L, Gullahorn G, Connolly N, et al.: Anterior mediastinal mass biopsy and resection: anesthetic techniques and preoperative concerns, *Semin Cardiothorac Vasc Anesth* 16:235–242, 2012.

Robie DK, Mustafa HG, Pokorny J: Mediastinal tumors—airway obstruction and management, *Semin Pediatr Surg* 3:259–266, 1994.

Shamberger RC, Holzman RS, Griscom NT, et al.: Prospective evaluation by computed tomography and pulmonary function tests of children with mediastinal masses, *Surgery* 118:468–471, 1995.

Sinner WN: Directed fine needle biopsy of anterior and middle mediastinal masses, *Oncology* 42:92–96, 1985.

Slinger P, Karsli C: Management of the patient with a large anterior mediastinal mass: recurring myths, *Curr Opin Anaesthesiol* 20:1–3, 2007.

Vader Els NJ, Sohage F, Bach AM, et al.: Abnormal flow volume loops in patients with intrathoracic Hodgkin's disease, *Chest* 117:1256–1261, 2000.

抗凝药和周围神经阻滞 第35章

Christina M. Spofford

病例概要

患者，男性，70岁，既往有心脏瓣膜病史、周围血管疾病及糖尿病病史，拟行膝下截肢手术。该患者5年前行主动脉瓣置换术，现每天服用华法林进行抗凝治疗。手术前5天，基层医师让患者停用华法林，并让他开始使用低分子肝素进行抗凝桥接治疗。患者在术前24 h最后一次接受低分子肝素注射。骨科医师打算在术后12 h再次恢复使用低分子肝素抗凝。在麻醉前访视时，患者要求周围神经阻滞置管以期长时间的术后镇痛。

问题分析

定义

周围神经阻滞（peripheral nerve block，PNB）在围术期麻醉和镇痛中的应用越来越多。PNB应用增加的原因在于其潜在的益处（框35.1），还包括其可避免与全身麻醉和（或）椎管内麻醉相关的并发症。这些并发症包括术后恶心和呕吐、胃肠外应用阿片类药物引起的呼吸抑制、交感神经阻滞引起的血流动力学不稳定以及门诊手术患者延迟出院。

然而，应用PNB也有其独特的担忧和并发症。特别是，随着临床实践的改变（如积极的围术期抗凝、新型局部技术和新型抗凝药物），出血并发症也越来越频繁。尽管出血性并发症非常罕见，但却是PNB最为严重的并发症，并且在各种PNB中均有报道。

框35.1　周围神经阻滞的潜在益处

- 更佳的术后镇痛
- 提高康复效果（由于镇痛）
- 术后恶心和呕吐发生率低
- 更快速的苏醒和康复
- 早期活动（单侧神经阻滞）
- 加快门诊患者出院
- 改善受累及肢端的血供
- 可置入连续镇痛导管

识别

一般来说，PNB后的局部淤血和压痛比较常见，其报道的发生率为8%～23%。真正的出血并发症似乎较为少见。例如，臂丛神经阻滞后血肿形成的发生率为0.2%～3%。大多数血肿很小，不易识别，临床意义也比较小。然而，文献报道了更严重的出血并发症，以及血肿形成后造成严重的神经功能损害。出血并发症的识别依赖于围术期临床医师敏锐的警惕性，这对于围术期接受抗凝治疗的患者尤为重要。严重低血压、局部疼痛或压痛、严重淤血、不明原因的贫血或出现神经功能缺损均可能预示有潜在的出血或压迫性血肿。可能需要影像学检查以证实和判断损伤的位置和范围。

风险评估

接受抗凝药物治疗的患者进行PNB，其出血并发症的发生率或严重程度目前尚无文献报道。PNB后造成的血管直接损伤仅限于病例报道。这些并发症在凝血功能正常和接受抗凝治疗的患者中均有发生。出血造成神经损伤通常是短暂性的，且具有自限性。因此，与椎管内出血相比，顺应性较好的周围神经部位出血似乎不太可能出现不可逆的永久性神经损伤。

PNB后的严重出血并发症大多发生在腰后丛（即腰大肌间隙；见第175章）或腰交感神经阻滞。在所有病例中，患者在进行PNB之前、期间或之后都接受抗凝药物治疗。不可逆的血小板聚集抑制剂（如噻氯匹定、氯吡格雷）也与PNB患者的出血并发症密切相关。抗凝患者进行PNB后最严重的并发症是需要输血的严重出血，而并非永久性神经损伤。如果PNB在隐蔽的非顺应性部位（如腰大肌间隙）实施，则最有可能发生严重出血和相应的损伤。此外，这种隐匿性出血可能在数小时至数天都不会被察觉。

启示

预防静脉血栓的围术期抗凝可导致显著的病残率、死亡率以及资源浪费。了解血栓栓塞的临床危险因素（框35.2）是合理应用围术期抗凝治疗或预防的基础。较高比例的住院患者通常存在一种或多种危险因素。因此，许多接受择期或急诊手术的患者正在或即将接受改变正常凝血状态的药物治疗。所有临床医师在实施区域麻醉时应该意识到这一点。

治疗

接受抗凝药物治疗的患者实施PNB后发生出血

框35.2 静脉血栓栓塞的临床风险因素

高龄
长期制动（麻痹）
卒中或瘫痪病史
静脉血栓病史
肿瘤（活动性或隐匿性）或肿瘤治疗
大手术
　腹部手术
　骨盆手术
　下肢手术
创伤，尤其下肢损伤
肥胖
静脉曲张和其他血流受阻（肿瘤、动脉畸形）
心功能障碍
留置中心静脉导管
炎症性肠病
肾病综合征
妊娠，产后期间，应用雌激素，雌激素受体调节剂
红细胞生成刺激剂
阵发性睡眠性血红蛋白尿
血栓生成倾向（获得性或者先天性）

Adapted from Geerts WH，Bergqvist D，Pineo GF，et al：Prevention of venous thromboembolism：American College of Chest Physicians evidence-based clinical practice guidelines（8th edition）. *Chest* 133（6 Suppl）：381S-453S，2008.

并发症的风险最大。因此，临床医师必须保持敏锐的警惕性。如果怀疑该出血并发症，应立即进行临床评估，包括以下内容：

- 重点回顾患者围术期病史：
  - 既往史；
  - 术前凝血状态；
  - 术前和围术期用药（例如改变凝血状态的药物、草药）；
  - 手术情况包括术中和术后失血；
  - 术后即刻情况。
- 考虑患者主诉：
  - 疼痛（位置、持续时间、性质）；
  - 神经功能缺损（感觉或运动、发作、持续时间、波动）；
  - 直立位症状；
  - 疲劳、晕厥、头晕、体位性低血压。
- 体格检查（包括详细的神经学评估）。
- 实验室检查（全血计数、术前凝血状况、电解质）。
- 用于确诊的影像学检查（计算机断层扫描成像、磁共振成像、超声）。

如果①血肿继续扩大，②神经症状恶化，③血肿消退后神经功能障碍仍未改善，或④气道、血管或淋巴管发生阻塞，则需要通过手术减压清除血肿。如果没有出现以上情况，则继续观察和保守治疗。所以，及时评估和适度干预能够有效预防出血和不可逆神经损伤。

预防

出血进入不可压缩的部位就可以发展成椎管内血肿，这才是区域麻醉最严重的出血并发症。为了减少这种风险，美国区域麻醉和疼痛医学学会为抗凝患者提出了基于循证医学的椎管内麻醉和镇痛指南（表35.1）。由于抗凝患者在接受PNB时发生此类并发症的风险没有明确定义，这些指南中接受区域麻醉的患者可能应用同一种方法。然而，这可能过于谨慎。相反，更谨慎的情况可能是考虑PNB穿刺部位的可压缩性、神经部位的超声图像、血管结构以及利弊权衡。如果实施PNB在血肿可能压迫气道的区域（颈深丛、肌间沟或锁骨上臂丛神经阻滞）或在不可压缩部位（如腰丛阻滞的腰大肌间隙），那么患者可能数小时至数天内都不会有明显症状。无

表 35.1 美国区域麻醉和疼痛医学学会对预防血栓患者接受椎管内麻醉推荐指南

抗凝药	推荐
抗血小板	NSAIDs 无禁忌 噻氯匹定停用 14 天 氯吡格雷停用 7 天 糖蛋白Ⅱ b/ Ⅲ a 抑制剂停用 8 ～ 48 h
皮下注射肝素	每天少于 10 000 单位无禁忌 若阻滞技术困难则延迟术后应用华法林
静脉注射肝素	椎管内阻滞 1 h 后肝素化 肝素化 2 ～ 4 h 后拔出阻滞导管 若置入创伤针则不强制延迟
低分子量肝素	术前剂量： • 常规剂量低分子肝素应用 10 ～ 12 h 后或者高剂量应用 24 h 后，再置入穿刺针 术后一天两次剂量： • 手术 24 h 后应用低分子肝素 • 首次应用低分子肝素前拔除椎管内阻滞导管 术后一天一次剂量： • 手术 6 ～ 8 h 后应用低分子肝素 • 首次应用 24 h 后立即给予第二次术后剂量 • 留置导管无禁忌 • 低分子肝素应用 10 ～ 12 h 后可拔除导管，拔除导管 2 h 后可再次应用低分子肝素
华法林	椎管内阻滞前维持正常 INR INR ≤ 1.5 h 时拔除导管（开始治疗）
磺达肝素	单次注射可应用无创伤针 避免留置导管
直接凝血酶抑制剂	暂时没有证据推荐 避免椎管内阻滞和留置导管
溶栓	绝对禁忌
草药治疗	没有证据支持椎管内阻滞前停用药物 警惕药物潜在的相互作用

INR，国际标准化比值；NSAIDs，非甾体抗炎药

Data from Horlocker TT，Wedel DJ，Rowlingson JC，et al：Regional anesthesia in the patient receiving antithrombotic or thrombolytic therapy：American Society of Regional Anesthesia and Pain Medicine Evidence-Based Guidelines（third edition）. *Reg Anesth Pain Med* 35（1）：64-101，2010.

论如何，对于接受影响止血药物的患者而言，临床医师之间的良好沟通可以有效地降低严重出血并发症的风险。

（林省伟　译　卞金俊　校）

延伸阅读

Aida S, Takahashi H, Shimoji K: Renal subcapsular hematoma after lumbar plexus block, *Anesthesiology* 84:452–455, 1996.

Ben-David B, Stahl S: Axillary block complicated by hematoma and radial nerve injury, *Reg Anesth Pain Med* 24:264–266, 1999.

Benzon HT, Avram MJ, Green D, Bonow RO: New oral anticoagulants and regional anaesthesia, *Br J Anaesth* 111(Suppl 1):i96–i113, 2013.

Bergman BD, Hebl JR, Kent J, Horlocker TT: Neurologic complications of 405 consecutive continuous axillary catheters, *Anesth Analg* 96:247–252, 2003.

Clergue F, Auroy Y, Perquignot F, et al.: French survey of anesthesia in 1996, *Anesthesiology* 91:1509–1520, 1999.

Ekatodramis G, Macaire P, Borgeat A: Prolonged Horner syndrome due to neck hematoma after continuous interscalene block, *Anesthesiology* 95:801–803, 2001.

Fransson SG, Nylander E: Vascular injury following cardiac catheterization, coronary angiography, and coronary angioplasty, *Eur Heart J* 15:232–235, 1994.

Geerts WH, Bergqvist D, Pineo GF, et al.: Prevention of venous thromboembolism: American College of Chest Physicians evidence-based clinical practice guidelines (8th edition), *Chest* 133:381S–453S, 2008.

Hadzic A, Vloka JD, Kuroda MM, et al.: The practice of peripheral nerve blocks in the United States: a national survey, *Reg Anesth Pain Med* 23:241–246, 1998.

Horlocker TT: Peripheral nerve blocks: Regional anesthesia for the new mil-

lennium, *Reg Anesth Pain Med* 23:237–240, 1998.
Horlocker TT, Wedel DJ, Rowlingson JC, et al.: Regional anesthesia in the patient receiving antithrombotic or thrombolytic therapy: American Society of Regional Anesthesia and Pain Medicine evidence-based guidelines (third edition), *Reg Anesth Pain Med* 35:64–101, 2010.
Idestrup C, Sawhney M, Nix C, Kiss A: The incidence of hematoma formation in patients with continuous femoral catheters following total knee arthroplasty while receiving rivaroxaban as thromboprophylaxis: an observational study, *Reg Anesth Pain Med* 39:414–417, 2014.
Gogarten W, Vandermeulen E, van Aken H, et al.: Regional anaesthesia and antithrombotic agents: recommendations of the European Society of Anaesthesiology, *Eur J Anaesthesiol* 27:999–1015, 2010.
Johr M: A complication of continuous blockade of the femoral nerve [German], *Reg Anaesthesie* 10:37–38, 1987.
Klein SM, D'Ercole F, Greengrass RA, Warner DS: Enoxaparin associated with psoas hematoma and lumbar plexopathy after lumbar plexus block, *Anesthesiology* 87:1576–1579, 1997.
Maier C, Gleim M, Weiss T, et al.: Severe bleeding following lumbar sympathetic blockade in two patients under medication with irreversible platelet aggregation inhibitors, *Anesthesiology* 97:740–743, 2002.
Neal JM, Hebl JR, Gerancher JC, Hogan QH: Brachial plexus anesthesia: Essentials of our current understanding, *Reg Anesth Pain Med* 27:402–428, 2002.
Nielsen CH: Bleeding after intercostal nerve block in a patient anticoagulated with heparin, *Anesthesiology* 71:162–164, 1989.
Sada T, Kobayashi T, Murakami S: Continuous axillary brachial plexus block, *Can Anaesth Soc J* 30:201–205, 1983.
Thomas PW, Sanders DJ, Berrisford RG: Pulmonary haemorrhage after percutaneous paravertebral block, *Br J Anaesth* 83:668–669, 1999.
Vaisman J: Pelvic hematoma after an ilioinguinal nerve block for orchialgia, *Anesth Analg* 92:1048–1049, 2001.
Weller RS, Gerancher JC, Crews JC, Wade KL: Extensive retroperitoneal hematoma without neurologic deficit in two patients who underwent lumbar plexus block and were later anticoagulated, *Anesthesiology* 98:581–585, 2003.

心脏手术的抗凝启动与逆转

第 36 章

Peter Tassani-Prell

病例概要

患者，女性，81 岁，因主动脉瓣狭窄（瓣口面积 0.4 cm^2，平均跨瓣压差 50 mmHg），静息状态下呼吸困难，拟行主动脉瓣置换术。既往因近期肺栓塞，接受静脉肝素治疗。手术时，抗凝血酶Ⅲ（antithrombin Ⅲ，AT-Ⅲ）水平低，活化部分凝血活酶时间升高。肝素化后（375 U/kg），活化凝血时间（activated clotting time，ACT）增高至 325 s。另外给予 125 U/kg 肝素和 2000 U AT-Ⅲ浓缩液。在 ACT 增高至 866 s 后，开始心肺转流术（cardiopulmonary bypass，CPB），无其他并发症。

问题分析

定义

普通肝素是硫酸化寡糖的非均相混合物，分子量在 5000 ～ 50 000 道尔顿。肝素的抗凝活性通过与 AT-Ⅲ结合而启动，这导致其构象改变，从而促进了凝血酶和凝血因子Ⅹa 和Ⅸa 的失活。在 AT-Ⅲ活性低的情况下，肝素的临床效应也相应降低。

识别、风险评估和启示

临床单剂量肝素抗凝反应存在着较大的个体差异。这需要通过床旁或实验室凝血检测进行评估。由于在 CPB 开始前确保充分抗凝极其重要，所以首选床旁检测。临床上有多种方法可用于评估肝素诱导的抗凝。

活化部分凝血活酶时间对血浆低肝素浓度（0.1 ～ 1.0 U/ml）敏感。然而，随着 CPB 所需的肝素剂量持续升高，其数值超过了该检测的阈值。

ACT 可以有效地评估 CPB 时所需的大剂量肝素（200 ～ 400 U/kg）的临床抗凝效果。在 1975 年的一项回顾性研究中，Bull 等发现 50 例患者的 ACT 达到 300 s 即足够。作者增加了 60% 的安全界限（180 s），使 ACT 达到 480 s。40 年后，全世界公认，在常规 CPB 期间，ACT 在 480 s 以上是安全的。即便如此，ACT 值可能会产生误导，因为它们可以被肝素以外的因素延长，如低温、血液稀释和血小板减少。此外，有临床研究表明，在轻度低温的 CPB 期间，ACT 值与患者血浆肝素浓度相关性较差。然而，使用肝素浓度替代 ACT 检测作为金标准并无优势，同时更加复杂且昂贵。在抑肽酶存在的条件下，使用硅藻土活化的 ACT 试管可出现虚假高值，但随着此药物（抑肽酶）从市场撤出，便可排除此误差。

在初始和追加肝素后，肝素抵抗会导致 ACT 值意想不到的小幅增加。大约 2000 例患者中会有 1 例存在 AT-Ⅲ杂合子缺陷（40% ～ 70% 活性），因此易发生深静脉血栓和肺栓塞。在肝素治疗期间，AT-Ⅲ水平的显著降低也可继发于 AT-Ⅲ大量消耗。肝素抵抗的其他原因包括左心室血栓、使用口服避孕药和血小板增多症。这些原因可使肝素与血浆蛋白和内皮结合增加，从而引起血浆肝素浓度降低。

肝素可通过免疫介导和非免疫介导机制引起血小板减少。肝素的使用可诱导两种类型血小板减少症（heparin-induced thrombocytopenia，HIT）。Ⅰ型为非免疫介导型，Ⅱ型为免疫介导型。为便于标准化，**非肝素免疫相关的血小板减少症**特指Ⅰ型 HIT，这是一种良性疾病，其不存在肝素依赖性抗体。**肝素诱导的血小板减少症**特指Ⅱ型 HIT，其可检测到肝素依赖性抗体，并导致血小板减少症。

治疗

此处讨论了心脏手术 CPB 抗凝治疗的不同方面：使用肝素抗凝和鱼精蛋白中和的常规管理、AT-Ⅲ缺陷的管理（如病例概要所示）和 HIT。

CPB 开始前，肝素剂量基于患者体重（300～400 U/kg）。确保 CPB 开始前 ACT 至少达到 480 s。CPB 开始前确定 ACT，以此判断是否存在肝素剂量不足或 AT-Ⅲ缺乏。临床上还建议在确保静脉管路通畅且回抽见血后，再通过中心静脉管路给予肝素注射液。随后，在 CPB 期间，可凭经验给予肝素（例如，5000～10 000 U/h、每小时初始剂量的三分之一）。临床上，强烈建议在 CPB 过程中每 30 min 检测一次 ACT，如果 ACT 小于 480 s，应追加肝素（详见前面讨论）。低温和血液稀释可延长 ACT，且与肝素浓度无关。根据 ACT 来追加肝素的方法可导致凝血酶活性抑制不足和亚临床血栓形成、纤维蛋白溶解、凝血因子和血小板耗竭。CPB 期间维持患者特异性肝素浓度可使肝素剂量更准确，凝血酶抑制更完全，并减少术后出血和血液制品的使用。

对于疑似肝素抵抗的患者，首先必须确认肝素确实进入了静脉，随后再给予另一瓶或另一批次的肝素，以排除同一批次中特异性肝素活性降低。如果大剂量肝素治疗后，ACT 仍低于预期，则应给予 AT-Ⅲ浓缩液，初始剂量至少为 2000 U。由于存在 AT-Ⅲ缺陷（CPB 期间血栓形成）的危险，大多数中心在进行需要 CPB 的手术前，确保患者体内有足够的 AT-Ⅲ水平。

非肝素免疫相关血小板减少症（Ⅰ型 HIT）意味着体内缺乏肝素依赖性抗体，其病因可能是肝素直接激活了非免疫性血小板。Ⅰ型 HIT 通常与大剂量肝素相关。相反，任何剂量肝素均可引起Ⅱ型 HIT。此外，在接受静脉肝素治疗的 30% 患者中，Ⅰ型 HIT 在临床治疗过程中发生较早（通常在 4 天内），即使持续给予肝素，被诱导的血小板功能异常也通常为轻度且可逆的。Ⅰ型 HIT 具有自限性，通常不会引起严重并发症（如血栓形成）。尽管血小板计数低，仍需继续肝素治疗。Ⅰ型 HIT 的临床意义在于必须将其与更严重的Ⅱ型 HIT 区分开来。

Ⅱ型 HIT[或肝素诱导的血小板减少伴血栓形成（heparin-induced thrombocytopenia with thrombosis，HITT）综合征] 是一种免疫介导的肝素反应，通常诊断不出来，可能导致静脉和动脉血栓形成。Ⅱ型 HIT 有 3 种不同的情况：①潜伏（抗体存在但无血小板减少），② HIT（抗体存在同时血小板减少）和③ HITT（抗体存在同时血小板减少和血栓形成）。

Ⅱ型 HIT 可能比Ⅰ型 HIT 更危险，因为它可能与血栓栓塞并发症相关（Ⅰ型中不存在）。给予肝素的患者中约 0.5%～3% 发展为Ⅱ型 HIT 和中度血小板减少。在某些情况下，这会导致静脉或动脉血栓形成，且会引起灾难性的临床后遗症，包括截肢，甚至死亡。这种严重药物不良反应的基础是产生与肝素和血小板因子 4 抗原复合物反应的免疫球蛋白 G 抗体。Ⅱ型 HIT 的诊断依据为“4 个 T”：血小板减少、血小板计数下降时机、血栓形成或其他后遗症和导致血小板减少的其他原因（表 36.1）。此依据不仅使用了实验室诊断，而且纳入了患者临床表现。在多达 20% 的患者中，可检测到肝素-血小板因子 4 抗原复合物的抗体。依据 4 个 T 并不能单独诊断 HIT。肝素诱导的血小板聚集试验（heparin-induced platelet aggregation test，HIPA）是诊断 HIT 的金标准。

对于接受 CPB 的Ⅱ型 HIT 患者，治疗通常包括使用替代抗凝剂或联合使用血小板功能抑制剂与肝素。作者推荐以下替代方案：

- **比伐芦定**，一种直接凝血酶抑制剂，来源于水蛭素的肽片段水蛭素的类似物。一些临床研究推荐，使用比伐芦定优于其他非肝素抗凝药物。
- **替罗非班**。在有 HIT 病史的患者中，最近的一种方法是使用针对糖蛋白Ⅱb/Ⅲa（GP Ⅱb/Ⅲa）的单克隆抗体选择性阻断血小板聚集，或使用特异性 GP Ⅱb/Ⅲa 抑制剂（例如替罗非班）。当 80% GP Ⅱb/Ⅲa 受体阻断和抑制血小板聚集（<20%）时，临床上可常规使用普通肝素和 CPB。CPB 后，常规使用鱼精蛋白中和普通肝素。
- **血浆置换**。一些病例报告和小型系列研究报告显示，在手术 CPB 前使用血浆置换，然后使用常规肝素-鱼精蛋白管理。

作者赞成在 CPB 期间使用替罗非班和单剂量肝素，并且按时使用鱼精蛋白拮抗。术后不应再使用

表 36.1 HIT 预测试评分系统：4 个 T

4 个 T	2 分	1 分	0 分
血小板减少症（Thrombocytopenia）	血小板计数下降 >50%，并且最低血小板值≥ 20[a]	血小板计数下降 30% ～ 50% 或血小板最低值 10 ～ 19	血小板计数下降 <30% 或血小板最低值 <10
血小板计数下降时机（Timing of platelet count fall）	5 ～ 10 天内明确发病或血小板下降≤ 1 天（发病前 30 天内使用过肝素）[b]	5 ～ 10 天的下降，但不明确（例如，血小板计数缺失）；10 天后发病[c]；或下降≤ 1 天（发病前 30 ～ 100 天内使用过肝素）	血小板计数下降 <4 天，无近期肝素暴露
血栓形成或其他后遗症（Thrombosis or other sequelae）	新发血栓形成（并发症）；皮肤坏死[d]；静脉推注普通肝素（UFH）后急性全身反应	进行性或复发性血栓形成[e]；非坏死性（红斑性）皮损[d]；疑似血栓形成（未证实）[f]	无
血小板减少的其他原因（Other causes for thrombocytopenia）	不明显	可能的[g]	明确有[g]

[a] Greifswald，Germany（GW）：血小板计数下降 >50% 或最低值 20 ～ 100；Hamilton，Canada（非 GW）：手术直接导致的血小板计数下降 >50% 为 1 分，而非 2 分。
[b] GW：5 ～ 14 天发病（而不是 5 ～ 10 天）；血小板在 1 天内下降（100 天内肝素暴露）。
[c] GW：14 天后发病。
[d] 肝素注射部位的皮肤损伤。
[e] 进展是指客观记录的血栓大小增加（通常是超声检查显示深静脉血栓形成的扩展）；复发是指既往受累区域新形成的血栓栓子（通常是既往肺栓塞患者的新灌注缺损）。
[f] 在 GW 中未将疑似血栓形成（未证实）作为标准。
[g] 由研究者决定是否可能存在另一种血小板减少的明显原因或是否存在其他原因。
From Lo GK：Evaluation of pretest clinical score（4 T's）for the diagnosis of heparin-induced thrombocytopenia in two clinical settings. *J Thromb Haemost* 4（4）：759-765，2006.

肝素，因为可能会产生抗体。临床上，我们在给予肝素前约 15 min，使用 10 μg/kg 负荷量的替罗非班，随后以 0.15 μg/（kg·min）持续泵注替罗非班，直至预计 CPB 结束前 1 h 停药。

在有 HIT 病史但未检测到抗体的患者中，肝素是目前 CPB 大剂量抗凝治疗的最安全方法。但在手术前后应使用替代抗凝剂。

大约 2 ～ 12 个月后，大多数有Ⅱ型 HIT 病史的患者不再有肝素诱导血小板聚集的实验室证据。如果这样，则可以接受使用肝素。但是，在术后阶段应谨慎再次使用肝素（如肝素冲洗、心导管检查）。

鱼精蛋白，一种从鲑鱼精子衍生的蛋白质，通常用于 CPB 后肝素的拮抗。但何为合适的剂量仍存争议。多数心脏麻醉科医师选择每 100 U 之前注射的肝素给予鱼精蛋白 1.0 ～ 1.3 mg。商品化系统可用于全血及循环肝素的测定，可精确滴定所需鱼精蛋白的量；然而，尽管理论上具有优势，但临床使用鱼精蛋白的量还是常规根据肝素用量来计算。在肝素拮抗后约 30 min 可追加鱼精蛋白。鱼精蛋白具有大量带正电荷的精氨酸残基，其与带负电荷的肝素形成稳定的复合物，并通过网状内皮系统消除。

鱼精蛋白具有显著的临床并发症，主要包括 3 种类型的不良反应：

- Ⅰ型最常见，包括鱼精蛋白给药速度过快引起的低血压，其可能与组胺释放有关。低血压可能与体循环阻力显著降低有关。
- Ⅱ型为过敏反应，可由免疫球蛋白介导。既往有海鲜过敏史的患者发生率较高。随后组胺和白三烯的释放导致全身和肺毛细血管渗漏。
- Ⅲ型与肝素－鱼精蛋白复合物的形成有关。肺巨噬细胞激活补体和白细胞聚集，引起自由基的释放和花生四烯酸途径的激活，从而导致血栓素的形成。这些可以引起强烈的肺血管收缩、肺动脉高压和左心房压力降低。最终结局是右心腔扩张和心力衰竭。幸运的是Ⅲ型反应非常罕见。

预防

肝素抵抗可能会使手术延迟并打乱手术室计划安排。因此，一些临床医生建议对所有需要 CPB 的患者，常规进行术前 AT-Ⅲ水平的筛查。测定肝素剂量－反应曲线还可以提醒临床医生 CPB 前的肝素抵抗，因此可提前计划好后续肝素剂量。如果可能，对Ⅱ型 HIT 患者推迟手术，直到不再出现抗体滴度。比伐芦定之类的新药可能是此类患者肝素的有效替代药物。

为消除鱼精蛋白反应，临床上可使用抗组胺药。此外，最好在大量稀释后通过外周静脉缓慢给予鱼精蛋白。一些外科医师将鱼精蛋白直接注入主动脉根部，以使其在初始分布期间绕过肺部。尽管肝素被覆的 CPB 回路的应用可降低的静脉肝素用量，但该技术效果尚未得到证实。

（范丰启 译 吉 栋 校）

延伸阅读

Anderson EF: Heparin resistance prior to cardiopulmonary bypass, *Anesthesiology* 64:504–507, 1986.

Bull BS: Heparin therapy during extracorporeal circulation. II. The use of a dose-response curve to individualize heparin and protamine dosage, *J Thorac Cardiovasc Surg* 69:685–689, 1975.

Despotis GJ: Antithrombin III during cardiac surgery: effect on response of activated clotting time to heparin and relationship to markers of hemostatic activation, *Anesth Analg* 85:498–506, 1997.

Ganzel C: Platelet factor 4/heparin-particle gel immunoassay (PaGIA) is a weak method for heparin-induced thrombocytopenia (HIT) evaluation of post cardio-pulmonary bypass surgery patients, *J Thromb Thrombolysis* 38:314–320, 2014.

Greinacher A: The use of direct thrombin inhibitors in cardiovascular surgery in patients with heparin-induced thrombocytopenia, *Semin Thromb Hemost* 30:315–327, 2004.

Grubb KJ: Bivalirudin: alternative anticoagulation during cardiopulmonary bypass in patients with heparin-induced thrombocytopenia, *Recent Pat Cardiovasc Drug Discov* 5:20–24, 2010.

Jaben EA: Use of plasma exchange in patients with heparin-induced thrombocytopenia: a report of two cases and a review of the literature, *J Clin Apher* 26:219–224, 2011.

Linkin LA: Treatment and prevention of heparin-induced thrombocytopenia: antithrombotic therapy and prevention of thrombosis, 9th ed: American College of Chest Physicians Evidence-Based Clinical Practice Guidelines, *Chest* 141(Suppl):e495S–e530, 2012.

Lo GK: Evaluation of pretest clinical score (4 T's) for the diagnosis of heparin-induced thrombocytopenia in two clinical settings, *J Thromb Haemost* 4:759–765, 2006.

Pravinkumar E, Webster NR: HIT/HITT and alternative anticoagulation: current concepts, *Br J Anaesth* 90:676–685, 2003.

Walenga JM, Jeske WP, Prechel MM: Newer insights on the mechanism of heparin-induced thrombocytopenia, *Semin Thromb Hemost* 30(Suppl 1):57–67, 2004.

动静脉畸形：正常灌注压力突破

第 37 章

Jason A. Ellis，*Shailendra Joshi*

病例概要

健康男性，41 岁，向他的初诊医师介绍他有 3 个月的右侧颞枕头痛病史。他最初采用口服镇痛药保守治疗，后接受枕部神经阻滞，无明显改善。最终在磁共振成像（magnetic resonance imaging，MRI）下证实位于右颞叶存在 2 cm × 3 cm 动静脉畸形（arteriovenous malformation，AVM）（图 37.1）。经过神经外科会诊，行导管脑血管造影后，证实存在 Spetzler-Martin 分级为三级的动静脉畸形（表 37.1）。AVM 由大脑中动脉和大脑后动脉分支供血，并由侧裂浅表静脉和横窦-乙状窦交汇处的 Labbé 静脉引流。

与患者讨论了治疗方案，包括放射外科、栓塞、手术切除和保守治疗。他被告知，延迟 2 ～ 3 年期间的治疗效果，放射外科治疗不会降低出血风险。此外，虽然放射外科治疗后的治愈率良好（70% ～ 80%），但并不能保证治愈。况且单纯栓塞不能治愈 AVM，但将是手术切除前一个很好的辅助治疗。他还被告知，一旦 AVM 治愈，改善头痛症状的预后良好。最终患者决定在手术前行分期栓塞，然后开颅手术切除 AVM。

患者择期被送至神经腔内血管治疗手术室，动脉穿刺置管后，监测其动脉基础血压为 130/70 mmHg。全身麻醉诱导并行气管插管。对股动脉进行穿刺置管，并使用氰基丙烯酸正丁酯（N-butyl cyanoacrylate，NBCA）胶开始栓塞 AVM。在手术治疗顺利接近尾声时，发现在 AVM 附近存在显著的造影剂外溢（见图 37.1）。患者收缩压突然升高到 170 mmHg。Dyna CT 旋转血管造影证实存在大出血，肿块影响附近的 AVM。患者立即被送往手术室接受颅骨切除、颅内血肿清除术和 AVM 切除。术后经导管脑血管造影显示无残余动静脉分流。

患者被送往神经科重症监护治疗病房，在那里他慢慢苏醒，并使用尼卡地平泵注将收缩压维持在 90 ～ 120 mmHg。第二天早晨拔除气管导管，并发现他轻度左侧偏瘫和上象限斜视。患者最终被送往急症康复中心，并已完全康复。

问题分析

正常灌注压突破（normal perfusion pressure breakthrough，NPPB）理论最初是由 Spetzler 和同事于 1978 年提出的，用来解释术后 AVM 患者的脑水肿和出血，尽管该理论最初只适用于在 AVM 切除后的患者，但也可应用于在单次手术中进行过广泛的 AVM 栓塞的患者。在急性期，栓塞过程中大动静脉分流突然闭塞与手术切除有相似之处。提出 NPPB 的病理生理学如下：通过动静脉瘘的高血流在邻近

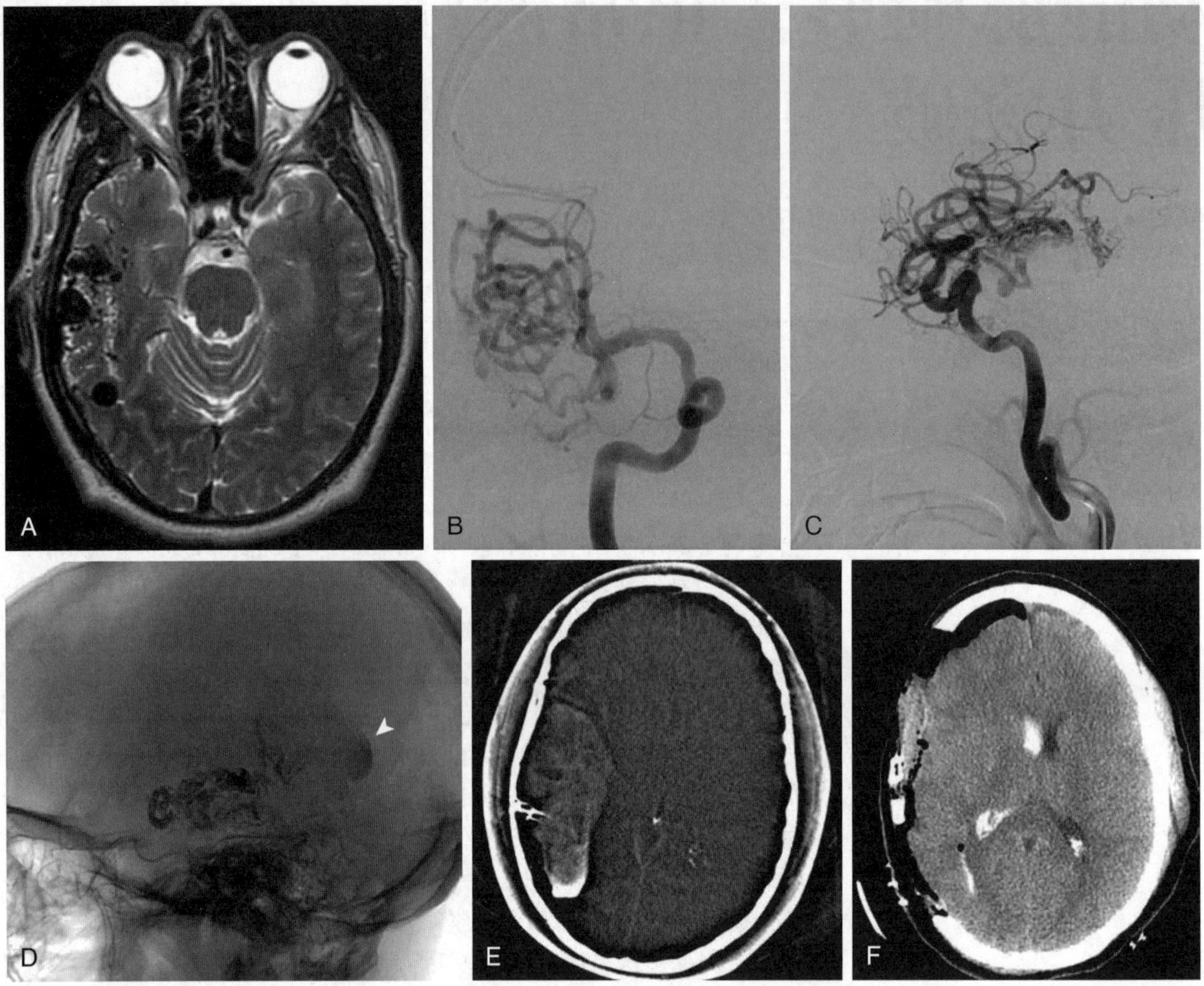

图 37.1 AVM 栓塞后出血。轴向 T2 MRI 显示了右颞叶内出现与 AVM（A）的存在相一致的明显的血流空洞。颈内动脉造影在前后位（B）和外侧（C）投射显示大脑中动脉分支供血的 AVM 病灶的复杂动脉网络。内固定物 NBCA 胶清晰可见于栓塞后侧位头颅 X 线（D）。在颞枕区（箭头）铸型胶后方可见淤血。血管造影三维软组织成像技术（DynaCT）旋转透视显示存在大出血，这可能是由于栓塞后即刻出现的 NPPB 现象（E）。术后头颅 CT 平扫显示单侧颅骨切除、脑出血清除和动静脉畸形切除术后减压良好（F）

表 37.1 Spetzler-Martin 分级

	分值
体积	
<3 cm	1
3 ～ 6 cm	2
>6 cm	3
位置	
非语言区	0
语言区	1
静脉引流	
浅静脉	0
深静脉	1

血管区域形成长期的低血压性脑区域。长期的脑区域性低血压导致接受最大限度的血管扩张和血管麻痹，破坏血管有效收缩能力甚至扩张的能力。低阻力 AVM 分流的切除术可恢复先前低血压脑区的灌注。然而，由于这些血管床不能有效地收缩，脑灌注压力恢复正常就会导致脑充血（“过度灌注”）伴随出现脑水肿形成和脑出血。颈动脉内膜切除术后可观察到的典型的脑灌注亢进综合征与 NPPB 可能具有某种相同的病理生理特征。

有人提出了原因不明的脑出血或水肿的其他机制，包括：①在手术时未被发现的技术性并发症；②由于自主神经活动异常而引起的血管紊乱，导致其支配的脑血管分泌血管活性肽；③毗邻 AVM 的结构缺陷的毛细血管床出血，可能是继发于血管生成因子（如血管内皮生长因子或血管生成素 -2）过度表达；④ AVM 切除后的静脉阻塞。事实上，静脉阻塞是 NPPB 理论最常被引用的替代机制的中心，也就是 Al-Rodhan 和同事在 1993 年提出的闭塞性充血理论（表 37.2）。

治疗

脑水肿和脑出血更常见的病因排除之后，NPPB 可作为一种排除性诊断。如果以前没有按照我们建议的那样在 AVM 切除后立即行导管造影，那么应该考虑残留 AVM 的可能性并通过血管造影予以排除。在可能的情况下，应考虑并纠正术后脑水肿和（或）脑出血的原因，包括缺氧、低钠血症、系统性高血压、凝血功能障碍、血小板功能异常、手术止血不充分和机械操作。治疗脑水肿 / 脑出血需要严格管理液体和控制电解质平衡，谨慎使用渗透和袢利尿剂，并注意脑灌注压。肿胀症状严重时可能需要机械通气、低体温和（或）巴比妥酸盐镇静。如果实施深度镇静，颅内压监测和脑电图（electroencephalography，EEG）是有用的辅助手段。

表 37.2　术后脑水肿和脑出血的原理

	主要特点
正常灌注压突破	• 周围脑组织中动脉 / 小动脉自身调节功能丧失 • 将高血流量分流至慢性扩张的畸形团周围的血管
阻塞性充血	• 周围脑组织中静脉流出阻塞 • 畸形团周围血管内血流淤滞
其他	• 残余动静脉畸形 • 手术创伤 • 止血不充分 • 凝血障碍 • 缺血 / 休克

如果不需要手术减压，在神经科 ICU 中积极的支持治疗对于取得满意的临床效果非常重要（图 37.2）。我们成功地运用了一套旨在维持正常血压、正常血钠、正常二氧化碳分压、正常体温和正常血糖的策略。就血压参数而言，维持初始收缩压目标在 90 ～ 140 mmHg 比较合理。在一些高风险的患者中，轻微的体循环低血压可能会降低充血、水肿和脑出血进展的概率。然而，这样的操作可能会危及大脑中依赖于侧支循环来维持灌注的区域。

持续的症状，如反应迟钝、轻瘫或颅神经功能障碍，可能需要快速输注甘露醇或高渗盐水（一般

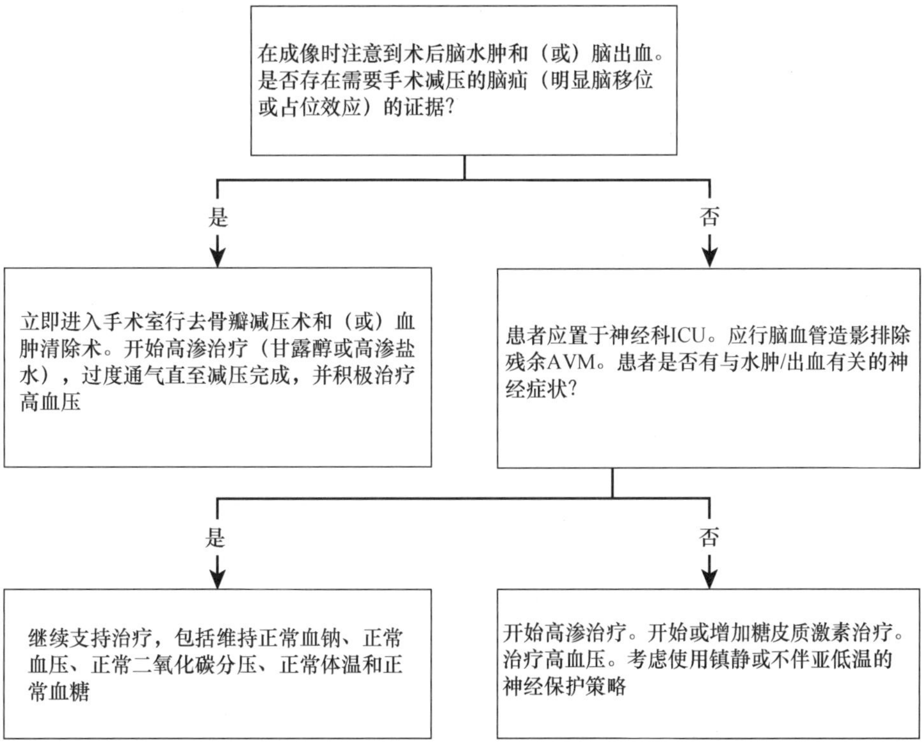

图 37.2　治疗流程

为 2%、3% 或 23%）进行高渗治疗，目标血清钠大于 140 mEq/L。糖皮质激素治疗（每 6 h 4 ～ 10 mg 地塞米松静脉注射）可改善血管源性水肿，但应根据需要输注胰岛素控制血糖。

预防

有人建议手术切除前分期栓塞可降低 NPPB 的发生率。分期栓塞可能使畸形团周围血管逐渐适应增加的灌注压，但机制尚不明确。自从为所有大型 AVM 制定这样的方案以来，我们确实很少观察到这种并发症。在手术过程中和围术期保持正常血压，使收缩压低于 140 mmHg，避免 Valsalva 动作平稳拔管，以及充分的术后镇痛亦为重要的预防策略。

致谢

我们感谢已故的 William L. Young 博士。他不仅贡献了本章的前一版，而且还对脑血管生理学和神经麻醉领域做出了巨大贡献。出于对 Bill 的敬意，我们从第 2 版中保留了本章的相关部分。

（成雨彤　译　代元强　校）

延伸阅读

Al-Rodhan NR, Sundt Jr TM, Piepgras DG, et al.: Occlusive hyperemia: a theory for the hemodynamic complications following resection of intracerebral arteriovenous malformations, *J Neurosurg* 78(2):167–175, 1993.

Ellis JA, Lavine SD: Role of embolization for cerebral arteriovenous malformations, *Methodist Debakey Cardiovasc J* 10(4):234–239, 2014.

Ellis JA, Mejia Munne JC, Lavine SD, et al.: Arteriovenous malformations and headache, *J Clin Neurosci* 23:38–43, 2016.

Gutiérrez-González R, Pérez-Zamarron A, Rodríguez-Boto G: Normal perfusion pressure breakthrough phenomenon: experimental models, *Neurosurg Rev* 37(4):559–567, 2014.

Rangel-Castilla L, Spetzler RF, Nakaji P: Normal perfusion pressure breakthrough theory: a reappraisal after 35 years, *Neurosurg Rev* 38(3):399–404, 2015.

Spetzler RF, Martin NA: A proposed grading system for arteriovenous malformations, *J Neurosurg* 65(4):476–483, 1986.

Spetzler RF, Wilson CB, Weinstein P, et al.: Normal perfusion pressure breakthrough theory, *Clin Neurosurg* 25:651–672, 1978.

Zacharia BE, Bruce S, Appelboom G, et al.: Occlusive hyperemia versus normal perfusion pressure breakthrough after treatment of cranial arteriovenous malformations, *Neurosurg Clin North Am* 23(1):147–151, 2012.

心脏手术术后出血　第38章

Klaus Martin，Peter Tassani-Prell

病例概要

患者，男性，73岁，既往合并主动脉瓣狭窄、冠心病、周围血管疾病、静息时呼吸困难和慢性肾衰竭（肌酐1.6 mg/dl）。患者心肌功能中度减退（左室射血分数为35%）。行主动脉瓣置换术联合冠状动脉搭桥术。心肺转流术（cardiopulmonary bypass，CPB）总时长142 min。术后24 h胸管引流显著增多，达2200 ml。

问题分析

定义

心脏手术术后出血过多基本上分为手术原因和非手术原因两大类。手术出血最常发生于多个部位，如血管吻合口、动静脉插管部位、内乳动脉采集部位、胸骨钢丝或房室切口部位。因此，减少手术出血需要足够的手术技巧。非手术出血是指凝血功能障碍，最近被归因分类为血液稀释、纤溶酶原激活和凝血因子消耗。为制订合适的治疗方案，我们需要了解与心脏手术围术期可能出现的所有情况相关的特定病理生理学知识。

识别

在使用足量鱼精蛋白拮抗肝素化之前，应对大血管吻合口出血的术野进行严格检查。为区分手术和非手术出血，最重要的是手术缝合结扎是否紧密，通过细致的缝合止血避免肉眼可见的出血。如果注射鱼精蛋白后仍有出血而无明显血管渗漏，则应由麻醉科医师寻找并纠正所有的凝血障碍。术后每小时监测纵隔胸管引流量。一个粗略的经验算法是术后首个4 h引流量不超过100～125 ml/h，在此期间任何1 h的引流量不应超过250 ml，或随后24 h引流量不应超过50～75 ml/h。

术后出血导致的心脏压塞或血容量不足，可能引起危及生命的低血压。非手术止血性出血，应在患者从手术室转入ICU之前，尽早通过实验室检查明确其特异性原因。及时发现特异性的止血障碍并确保特效性治疗，不应非特异性地输注多种类型血制品和凝血治疗（霰弹疗法）。

风险评估

术后出血的危险因素包括：

- 患者相关：
    - 高龄；
    - 长期使用类固醇药物；
    - 女性；
    - 慢性肝功能不全；
    - 合并血液疾病或凝血障碍疾病；
    - 术前使用抗凝药物。
- 操作相关：
    - CPB持续时间延长；
    - 再次心脏手术；
    - 多种手术联合（如冠状动脉旁路移植和瓣膜手术）；
    - 术后低体温；
    - 自体血回收应用增多；
    - 意外的手术难度增加；
    - 主动脉内球囊反搏；
    - 采集内乳动脉。

术前对患者相关危险因素进行个体化筛查，对识别患者术后出血风险是否增加至关重要。除病史外，还必须填写一份关于临床非常规止血的标准化问卷，并仔细评估。

影响凝血系统或血小板功能的药物常用于拟行心脏手术的患者。血小板糖蛋白Ⅱb/Ⅲa受体抑制剂，如阿昔单抗、依替巴肽和替罗非班，越来越多地被用作肝素或阿司匹林的辅助用药，应用于急性冠状动脉综合征患者或术前经皮冠状动脉介入治疗患者。它们甚至可作为长效抗凝药物，预防继发性血栓形成。需要紧急心脏手术的患者在转入手术室前，通常可能已在导管室接受抗凝治疗，特别是抗血小板治疗。如有疑问，可根据已行的治疗对特定凝血障碍进行额外的实验室检查。

相反，术前只能部分预测手术相关的风险因素。在手术过程中可能会出现一些有重大影响的问题，如CPB持续时间、主动脉内球囊反搏和自体血回输的应用增加。意外的手术难度增加也不例外。无论何种风险因素，麻醉科医师必须明确该风险的血液学相关原因，以便进行特定的治疗。

启示

心脏外科与其他外科的主要区别是使用体外循环机。体外循环使外科医师有机会将血液循环与心脏分离并维持机体的正常灌注。然而，这一手术需要暂时的医源性抗凝，以避免在体外循环中血液凝固。通常经静脉推注大剂量肝素来完成抗凝。此外，CPB的使用对凝血障碍的发病机制有多重影响，如血小板的短暂活化、血液稀释、低温、肝素和鱼精蛋白。

机械性压力和接触激活

当连接到CPB回路时，患者血液暴露于泵管的人造材料表面。这种接触会导致凝血、纤维蛋白溶解和炎症级联机制的激活。另外，血液通过滚压泵系统泵送。泵送血液时机械会对血液中的所有红细胞造成机械性压力，产生潜在损伤。因此，血小板功能受此影响并造成术后出血，机械性压力也被认为是主要原因。此外，在手术过程中使用心包吸引器也会损伤血细胞，并通过静脉贮血器将凝血激活剂回收进体外循环系统。目前提议使用闭合的贮血器、覆盖涂层的回路以及在自体血回输机中处理后再输注吸引的血液，这些方法可减少对凝血系统的影响。

血液稀释

CPB晶体液预充和心脏停搏液，或多或少会导致患者血液的显著稀释。红细胞、血小板和凝血因子的浓度降低，取决于患者血容量以及预充液和心脏停搏液容量。成人患者CPB组件小型化，使预充量从20世纪90年代的2 L下降至2010年的1 L左右。随着临床血液稀释量的减少，其对凝血系统的影响也明显下降。血液稀释已很少成为术后出血的唯一原因。如果血小板功能正常，凝血因子浓度为25%～30%、血小板计数为50 000～100 000/μl是可以耐受的，不会造成过多出血。由于CPB回路的小型化受技术限制，体型小的患者、儿童和新生儿仍会受到≥200%血液稀释造成的影响，但这取决于人体的容量比。尽管如此，该技术的进展仍然成就了首例无输血心脏手术的诞生。

低体温

术中低温可导致血小板功能受损并降低温度依赖性凝血因子的功能。此外，实验室凝血系统评估统一在37℃下进行。在分析CPB期间获得的低温血样本时，可能会出现误导性结果。CPB期间降至更温和的温度（亚低温）的概念被提出，以减少炎症级联的激活并减轻凝血功能紊乱。

自体血回输系统

由于凝血因子和血小板在常规红细胞回收过程中被清除，来自自体血回输装置的血制品几乎不含上述血浆成分。值得一提的是，直接从术后胸管引流回输纵隔内的血液并不合适，胸液引流瓶不能用于血液保存，输注此类血液可能对患者造成伤害（美国胸外科医师协会心血管麻醉科医师协会指南，2008年）。

肝素和鱼精蛋白

肝素是最常用的抗凝药物，应在患者连接CPB系统开始体外循环之前给药。停机后，给予鱼精蛋白可拮抗其抗凝效果。肝素和鱼精蛋白均有抗凝作用，剂量适当非常重要。肝素-鱼精蛋白复合物本身可以部分抑制血小板功能，可通过血小板功能分析仪测定。尽管最初用鱼精蛋白充分中和，但肝素可在2 h～6 h后出现反弹，导致血小板功能受到抑制。

管理

术后出血的原因复杂多样，其治疗具有很强的挑战。纵隔管引流过多需要急诊再次手术探查，阻止可能的手术相关出血，特别是当血流动力学不稳定时。然而，再次手术探查显著增加患者风险，即围术期病残率和死亡率增加。因此，再次手术探查的指征至关重要。对出血并不严重的患者，是否探查不应仅基于胸管引流量。视具体情况具体分析尤为重要，不同的外科手术有不同的出血风险。例如，除 CPB 插管部位外，仅采用一条心房切口缝合的一期二尖瓣修复术，出血风险远小于主动脉夹层手术或正在进行的抗血小板药物治疗的采集两条内乳动脉的冠状动脉搭桥手术。过去，在没有足够快捷的临床检测手段并在适当的时间监测凝血系统时，医师必须根据临床经验和常备止血药物来治疗患者。指征标准还取决于实验室检验的配合和速度，因此具有很大的不确定性。最近，随着床旁检测（point-of-care，POC）设备技术的改进，医师有机会对凝血系统进行不同方面的床旁快速测试，并随后对特定的影响因素进行目标导向治疗。同时，几种输血和凝血管理流程已经发表。根据当地实际情况和能力，每个机构都必须创建自己的流程。一般而言，这种结构化处理流程在减少术后出血、输血需求和住院费用以及改善患者预后方面似乎有一定的效果。

肝素和鱼精蛋白

如前所述，停机后恢复正常凝血的第一步是用适当剂量的鱼精蛋白完全拮抗肝素化。大多数机构倾向于对鱼精蛋白的使用剂量进行经验性计算。有趣的是，这种计算存在广泛的机构间差异。据我们所知，范围大约为总肝素用量的 70% ～ 125%。

有几种方法可验证肝素是否被充分拮抗。活化凝血时间（activated clotting time，ACT）测量值回到基础值通常被解释为完全肝素中和。但必须记住，ACT 的测量并不像预期的那么准确。即使 ACT 已回到基础值，肝素血浆浓度仍可高达 0.2 U/ml。更为循证的方法是，测量 CPB 结束时的肝素浓度，然后根据估计的血容量计算鱼精蛋白用量。Hepcon HMS 系统是一种测量临床相关肝素浓度的相对简单的装置。通过鱼精蛋白的滴定和凝血时间测定来定量肝素浓度。了解患者身高和体重后，系统会计算血容量和鱼精蛋白用量。可以记录是否完整拮抗肝素或仍有残余。残余肝素化的另一种敏感但仅定性的试验是血栓弹力图（ROTEM）。如果 INTEM 中的血凝块形成时间明显高于 HEPTEM，则可能存在残余肝素化。第三种方法是活化部分凝血活酶时间敏感且可定量，但肝素浓度无法计算。肝素浓度可被直接测量，但在大多数临床实验室，特别是在紧急情况下，这一方法并非万全之策。

血小板

初级凝血是指血小板黏附于损伤的血管内皮，并发生脱颗粒。血小板改变形状，增加其形成稳定止血栓子的能力。受损血管的生理性修复需要有足够数量的有功能的血小板。临床上通常检测血小板计数和功能。当持续出血时，血小板计数应至少维持在 50 000/μl，最好达 100 000/μl，以保持足够的凝血功能进行生理性止血。血小板计数在临床实验室中很容易测定，但不能反映血小板功能。血小板功能的评估可间接通过整体凝血功能分析如血栓弹力图进行测定，或通过更加具体的光透射凝集测定法或全血凝集测定法（多板分析）进行测定。这些设备对于可能需要抗血小板治疗的患者或 CPB 时间长且怀疑血小板受损的患者尤为重要。当血小板计数可接受且血小板功能仅轻度下降时，可尝试给予抗利尿激素的合成类似物醋酸去氨加压素（desmopressin acetate，DDAVP）。DDAVP 被认为可使内皮细胞释放凝血Ⅷ因子和血管性假血友病因子从而增强血小板功能。更有其他研究表明，DDAVP 可能对血小板有直接益处，如增加黏附受体（血小板糖蛋白Ⅰb）的表达。DDAVP 常规使用剂量为 0.3 ～ 0.4 μg/kg，连续给药 30 min 以上。主要不良反应是低血压。

输注浓缩血小板是血小板计数低或血小板功能明显下降唯一的病因治疗方法。多供体采集浓缩血小板和单采血小板哪个作为首选，一直是个持续争论的话题。两种制剂在临床上都有使用，但使用比例有所不同。在剂量适当的情况下，存在着治疗矛盾。一方面，应该使用足够大的剂量，以便尽快完成初期止血；另一方面，血小板在传播感染和细菌污染的风险上最高。另外，这些血液制品在用量上通常有限，而且成本高昂。

凝血因子障碍

最近几项研究表明，术后出血与特异性的凝血功能障碍如低血小板计数、低纤维蛋白原水平或其他因素的减少有关。由于床旁设备的开发，许多临床医师试图进行目标导向治疗，以迅速纠正特异性的凝血功能障碍。这增加了单一凝血因子和单种血液成分的使用量。纤维蛋白原、凝血酶原复合物，甚至活化凝血Ⅶ因子在许多试验中被研究。几项试验显示，纤维蛋白原或其他凝血因子缺陷与术后出血存在显著关联。干预性研究大多证明了输注凝血因子对止血具有益处。因此，临床策略越来越倾向于这种目标导向策略，使得直接输注血浆明显减少。

抗纤维蛋白溶解的预防和治疗

已知，血纤蛋白溶解系统在 CPB 期间因多种生理系统的激活而表达上调。这导致血凝块溶解、凝血因子消耗和血小板功能障碍。许多临床研究表明，预防性应用抗纤维蛋白溶解药物可减少心脏手术患者术后失血量和输血次数，特别是再次手术。直到 2007 年为止，抑肽酶是全世界最常用的抗纤溶药物。在 Mangano 对外公布并提前中止了 BART 试验后，人们对其临床安全性产生严重担忧。制造商立即停止分销，但其在大多数国家仍然被使用。（2011 年加拿大卫生部和 2012 年欧洲药品管理局允许在特定情况和安全预防措施下重新引入该药物。）两种赖氨酸类似物氨甲环酸和氨基己酸，被认为是更安全且同样有效的替代药物。这些药物的使用情况因国家而异，但氨甲环酸似乎在大多数机构中更受青睐。虽然安全剂量和应用范围很广，但建议的方案是在给予肝素后使用氨甲环酸 10 mg/kg 的初始负荷剂量，维持剂量为 1 mg/（kg·h），或者每 2 h 重复给药 5 mg/kg，直至关闭胸腔。由于氨基己酸的有效成分仅为氨甲环酸的十分之一左右，因此等效剂量必须高出 10 倍：负荷剂量 100 mg/kg，维持剂量 10 mg/（kg·h），每 2 h 重复给药 50 mg/kg。

（范丰启 译 薄禄龙 校）

延伸阅读

Boettcher W, Merkle F, Huebler M, et al.: Transfusion-free cardiopulmonary bypass in Jehovah's Witness patients weighing less than 5 kg, *J Extra Corpor Technol* 37:282–285, 2005.

Caputo M, Bryan AJ, Calafiore AM, et al.: Intermittent antegrade hyperkalaemic warm blood cardioplegia supplemented with magnesium prevents myocardial substrate derangement in patients undergoing coronary artery bypass surgery, *Eur J Cardiothorac Surg* 14:596–601, 1998.

Dunning J, Versteegh M, Fabbri A, et al.: Guideline on antiplatelet and anticoagulation management in cardiac surgery, *Eur J Cardiothorac Surg* 34:73–92, 2008.

Fergusson DA, Hebert PC, Mazer CD, et al.: A comparison of aprotinin and lysine analogues in high-risk cardiac surgery, *N Engl J Med* 358:2319–2331, 2008.

Ferraris VA, Brown JR, Despotis GJ, et al.: 2011 update to the Society of Thoracic Surgeons and the Society of Cardiovascular Anesthesiologists blood conservation clinical practice guidelines, *Ann Thorac Surg* 91:944–982, 2011.

Ferraris VA, Ferraris SP, Moliterno DJ, et al.: The Society of Thoracic Surgeons practice guideline series: aspirin and other antiplatelet agents during operative coronary revascularization (executive summary), *Ann Thorac Surg* 79:1454–1461, 2005.

Gertler R, Wiesner G, Tassani-Prell P, et al.: Are the point-of-care diagnostics MULTIPLATE and ROTEM valid in the setting of high concentrations of heparin and its reversal with protamine? *J Cardiothorac Vasc Anesth* 25:981–986, 2011.

Gombotz H: Patient blood management: a patient-orientated approach to blood replacement with the goal of reducing anemia, blood loss and the need for blood transfusion in elective surgery, *Transfus Med Hemother* 39:67–72, 2012.

Gross I, Seifert B, Hofmann A, et al.: Patient blood management in cardiac surgery results in fewer transfusions and better outcome, *Transfusion* 55:1075–1081, 2015.

Gorlinger K, Fries D, Dirkmann D, et al.: Reduction of fresh frozen plasma requirements by perioperative point-of-care coagulation management with early calculated goal-directed therapy, *Transfus Med Hemother* 39:104–113, 2012.

Gorlinger K, Shore-Lesserson L, Dirkmann D, et al.: Management of hemorrhage in cardiothoracic surgery, *J Cardiothorac Vasc Anesth* 27:S20–S34, 2013.

Herbertson M: Recombinant activated factor VII in cardiac surgery, *Blood Coagul Fibrinolysis* 1)(15(Suppl):S31–S32, 2004.

Karkouti K, McCluskey SA, Callum J, et al.: Evaluation of a novel transfusion algorithm employing point-of-care coagulation assays in cardiac surgery: a retrospective cohort study with interrupted time-series analysis, *Anesthesiology* 122:560–570, 2015.

Karkouti K, McCluskey SA, Syed S, et al.: The influence of perioperative coagulation status on postoperative blood loss in complex cardiac surgery: a prospective observational study, *Anesth Analg* 110:1533–1540, 2010.

Levi M, Fries D, Gombotz H, et al.: Prevention and treatment of coagulopathy in patients receiving massive transfusions, *Vox Sang* 101:154–174, 2011.

Mangano DT, Tudor IC, Dietzel C, et al.: The risk associated with aprotinin in cardiac surgery, *N Engl J Med* 354:353–365, 2006.

Mongan PD, Hosking MP: The role of desmopressin acetate in patients undergoing coronary artery bypass surgery: a controlled clinical trial with thromboelastographic risk stratification, *Anesthesiology* 77:38–46, 1992.

Ohata T, Sawa Y, Kadoba K, et al.: Effect of cardiopulmonary bypass under tepid temperature on inflammatory reactions, *Ann Thorac Surg* 64:124–128, 1997.

Remadi JP, Marticho P, Butoi I, et al.: Clinical experience with the mini-extracorporeal circulation system: an evolution or a revolution? *Ann Thorac Surg* 77:2172–2175, 2004.

Richter JA, Meisner H, Tassani P, et al.: Drew-Anderson technique attenuates systemic inflammatory response syndrome and improves respiratory function after coronary artery bypass grafting, *Ann Thorac Surg* 69:77–83, 2000.

Ternström L, Radulovic V, Karlsson M, et al.: Plasma activity of individual coagulation factors, hemodilution and blood loss after cardiac surgery: a prospective observational study, *Thromb Res* 126:e128–e133, 2010.

心肌病

第39章

Mallik G. Reddy，*B. Craig Weldon*

病例概要

患儿，男性，3岁，拟行腹股沟疝修补术。患儿既往无显著疾病史，除3周前经历一次上呼吸道感染，当时的症状是低热、鼻腔稀薄分泌物、轻微咳嗽，上述症状于上周已消失。其体格检查与生命体征基本正常。全麻诱导过程使用了氧化亚氮、氧气和七氟烷，期间患儿心率增加至180次/分，心电图QRS波逐渐宽大，脉搏血氧饱和度曲线变平，无法触及股动脉搏动。遂进行紧急心肺复苏，但未成功。尸检结果显示该患儿存在左心室肥大和心肌炎症，与病毒性心肌炎的诊断依据一致。

问题分析

定义

世界卫生组织（World Health Organization，WHO）将心肌病（cardiomyopathy，CM）定义为与心功能不全相关的心肌疾病，原发性CM按照主要的病理生理进行分类：

- 扩张型心肌病（dilated cardiomyopathy，DCM）；
- 肥厚型心肌病（hypertrophic cardiomyopathy，HCM）；
- 限制性心肌病（restrictive cardiomyopathy，RCM）；
- 致心律失常性右心室发育不良/心肌病（arrythmogenic right ventricular dysplasia/cardiomyopathy，ARVD/CM）；
- 左心室小梁过度形成/致密化不全（left ventricular hypertrabeculation/noncompaction，LVHT/NC）。

继发性CM可能为多种不同病因造成的：

- 缺血；
- 瓣膜；
- 高血压；
- 炎症；
- 代谢；
- 围产期；
- 接触毒性物质；
- 维生素缺乏；
- 某些神经肌肉疾病。

识别

不幸的是，许多CM患儿并无症状或仅有轻微的心力衰竭表现，这使得术前对他们的病情认识非常困难。此类患儿可能存在运动耐量下降、咳嗽、呼吸困难、晕厥、胸痛或营养不良的病史。存在此类症状或有已知与CM相关病症的患儿，应立即详细检查，寻找心力衰竭的迹象，进行心电图检查，必要时应咨询儿科心脏病专家。超声心动图通常对于CM的病理生理类型具有诊断价值。存在心源性猝死（sudden cardiac death，SCD）家族史可能是外表健康的儿童或青少年潜在CM可能的唯一指标。

DCM以左心室腔扩张和收缩功能受损为特征，累及左心室（left ventricle，LV）、右心室（right ventricle，RV）或两者兼有。DCM可能与炎症（病毒或免疫学）、特发性或遗传因素相关。CM的家族特征性与SCD相关。DCM可能是接触毒性物质的结果，或在幼儿中，与可治疗的先天性心脏病（如左冠状动脉异常或严重的主动脉瓣缩窄）有关。据报道，在诊断为CM的儿童中，5年死亡率为35%～70%。超声心动图通常表现为心室扩大、收缩不良、双房增大和房室（atrioventricular，AV）瓣膜反流。

肥厚型心肌病（HCM）可累及左心室、右心室，或两者兼有，且通常是不对称的。心室容量可能正常或减少，并以舒张功能障碍为特征，可保持收缩功能。心电图可正常或提示心室肥厚，超声心动图可进行相关诊断。HCM 通常是一种遗传性或特发性疾病，但也可能与畸形综合征、各种神经肌肉疾病和先天性疾病、代谢功能异常（如Ⅱ型糖原贮积症或 Pompe 综合征）有关。特发性 HCM 患者可能无症状或出现劳力性呼吸困难、胸痛和晕厥。ECG 表现为从心室间隔肥厚到广泛性左心室肥厚的进展型改变。通常此类患者会出现左心室流出道梗阻，这也可能是导致上述症状的原因。然而，也有部分患者的冠状动脉被局限性的心肌肥厚所包裹（即心肌桥），这些患者容易发生劳力性心肌缺血和室性心律失常。这使 HCM 成为引起儿童和青少年运动员 SCD 的最常见原因。

限制性心肌病（RCM）是一种罕见的 CM，其特征是由于心室舒张顺应性降低而导致左或右（或两者兼有）心室充盈。RCM 可能是特发性的，也可能与心内膜纤维化或嗜酸粒细胞增多综合征有关。在疾病的早期阶段，随着时间的推移，可能会有正常或接近正常的收缩功能。左心室舒张期末压升高导致肺血管阻力持续增加，随后出现肺心病和死亡。超声心动图的特征是心室容积减小，心房扩张增大。

致心律失常性右心室心肌病（arrhythmogenic right ventricular cardiomyopathy，ARVCM）的特点是右心室或左心室（或两者兼有）心肌被纤维脂肪替代。ARVCM 是一种常染色体显性遗传和外显不完全的遗传性心脏病。ARVCM 患者常表现为呼吸困难、乏力、肝大和腹水，但 SCD 可能是无症状患者的最初表现。其中有 50% 的患者存在 ECG 异常，可能显示房室传导受损。通过心肌活检可做出明确的诊断，但 ARVCM 是由室性心律失常（最常见的持续性室性心动过速）与左束支传导阻滞相结合而呈现出相关变化。超声心动图可见右心室游离壁的室壁运动异常。超声心动图还可显示心房扩张，并伴有接近正常的心室大小和 AV 瓣膜反流。

左心室小梁过度形成 / 致密化不全（LVHT/NC）是一种罕见的疾病，常与神经肌肉疾病相关，包括肌营养不良、肌病、线粒体疾病等。这些患者常表现出心力衰竭、心律失常和 ECG 异常的症状。超声心动图显示左心室功能降低，但诊断可能需要磁共振成像。疾病的自然病程取决于任何潜在的神经肌肉疾病，以及心肌功能障碍的严重程度。

风险评估

DCM 是儿童 CM 中最常见的一种形式，在男性和女性中具有相似的流行病学分布特征。HCM 通常在青春期前较为少见，但发病率和死亡率在诊断年龄较小的患者中最高。早期死亡通常是由心室纤颤引起的。RCM 在儿童中并不常见，但 RCM 出现通常是心肌炎后或伴有浸润性心肌疾病的终末期发现。ARVCM 并不常见，但在儿童和青少年心源性猝死中所占比例很高。女性的发病率是男性的 3 倍。LVHT/NC 应考虑以下神经肌肉疾病：迪谢贝 / 贝克肌肉营养不良和强直性营养不良、Charco-Marie-Tooth 病、Friedreich 共济失调、Barth 综合征、线粒体病、肌营养不良症、糖原增多症、肌腺苷酸脱氨酶缺乏症和肌萎缩侧索硬化症。

启示

在 DCM 病例中，心排血量是由心动过速和心室腔扩张引起的每搏输出量增加所维持的。然而，这导致心肌壁张力和氧利用率的增加。在 HCM 中，有心室舒张功能不全所致的心肌梗死。大约 25% 的患者有左心室流出道的动态梗阻。左心室收缩期容积、左心室收缩力和跨室壁扩张的压力梯度决定梗阻的严重程度。RCM 使射血分数在此过程的早期得以维持。然而，随着心室肌纤维化的进展，左心室舒张期末压升高，导致肺动脉高压，每搏量和心排血量减少。ARVCM 最初的收缩力是正常的，但室性心律失常的发生与右心功能的恢复缓慢具有一致性。最终，室性心律失常（室性心动过速或心室颤动）对抗心律失常治疗产生抵抗效应。LVHT/NC 表现为不同程度的心功能障碍，并与心室内血栓形成有关。潜在的神经肌肉疾病会使这些患者的麻醉管理更加复杂。

管理

确诊 CM 患儿围术期的处理需要了解正常的心血管生理状况和对脑缺血再灌注损伤与患者 CM 相关的特殊病理生理学。通过对前负荷、收缩力、后负荷和心率的管理以维持心排血量是首要目标。如病例概要所示，麻醉诱导可导致心肌抑制或全身血管张力急剧下降，导致循环突然衰竭，并可能导致恶性心律失常和心脏停搏。

存在心肌病的心室至少需要常规提升前负荷来维持足够的每搏量。然而，静脉容积负荷增加可能会打破一个微妙的平衡，即充分的前负荷与心室扩大以及舒张末期压力增加之间的平衡。后者会减少心内膜灌注，导致每搏量减少而非增加。有创性监测措施有助于评估静脉注射后的血流动力学变化，以及间歇正压通气效果。术前液体受限的患者最易发生间歇正压通气引起的严重低血压。

一旦前负荷得到改善，就应该解决心肌收缩力问题。除 HCM 患者外，CM 患儿也存在心肌收缩功能受损和心肌功能储备受限。麻醉药物的选择与使用应牢记这一点。围术期可能需要使用强心药（如多巴胺、多巴酚丁胺、肾上腺素）或正性肌力-血管扩张药（如米力农）来维持心排血量，增加心肌收缩力，提升每搏量，但同时以增加心肌耗氧量为相应代价。

由于全身或肺血管阻力增加，后负荷增加，使左心室和右心室的收缩受限。根据 Laplace 原理，心肌内壁应力（后负荷的主要决定因素）随心室直径的增加而增加。因此，在相同的动脉压水平下，增大的心室所遇到的后负荷要高于正常大小的心室。

终末期 CM 患儿可能合并肺动脉高压。应尽一切努力避免肺血管阻力增加。这需要通过降低气道平均压力、维持正常呼吸或轻度低碳酸血症、允许性代谢性碱中毒，以及给予外源性肺血管扩张剂（如一氧化氮、前列腺素）来实现的。

最后，每搏量的减少通常会导致交感神经相关的心率增加，以代偿心排血量的减少。维持窦性或房源性节律（如使用游走性心房起搏器），以及心房对心室充分的灌注是至关重要的。伴有非心房、较低起搏器逃逸节律（例如房室交界处或室性异搏心律或心动过速）的窦房结节律缺失会导致舒张期充盈不足和舒张末期容量降低。这会加重任何已有的舒张功能障碍。

特定 CM 子类型的管理目标可在表 39.1 中查看。

表 39.1　心肌病的病理生理特征和麻醉管理目标

亚型	病理生理学	麻醉管理目标
扩张型心肌病（DCM）	心肌收缩力↓ 心排血量↓ CHF	前负荷：正常 心率：正常至↑ 后负荷：正常至↓ 收缩力：↑ 优先选正性肌力-血管扩张药
肥厚型心肌病（HCM）	动态左心室流出道梗阻 正常的收缩性 每搏量↓↓ 心室各向异性↓	前负荷：正常至↑ 心率：↓ 后负荷：正常至↑ （心肌缺血 / 血压↓：建议使用去氧肾上腺素）
限制性心肌病（RCM）	心室各向异性↓ 心肌收缩性逐渐下降 肺动脉高压	前负荷：正常 心率：正常至↑ 后负荷：正常 收缩性：↑ 避免 PVR ↑
房源性右心室发育不良 / 心肌病（ARVD/CM）	右心室纤维脂肪浸润 右心衰竭 围术期致命性室性心律失常	前负荷：正常 心率：窦性心律 手术室内准备起搏器除颤仪电极片 后负荷：避免↑或者减少 收缩性：正常
左心室高小梁形成 / 致密化不全（LVHT/NC）	多变的心肌功能障碍 心律失常 相关神经肌肉功能障碍 可能存在心室内血栓	前负荷：正常至↑ 心率：正常 后负荷：正常至↓ 收缩性：正常 避免使用负性肌力药

CHF，充血性心力衰竭；PVR，肺血管阻力

预防

为了避免CM患儿在麻醉和手术期间心排血量的急剧减少，必须首先识别出这种情况的发生。但如前所述，这通常不可能实现，问题的最初迹象发生于麻醉诱导。预知潜在的CM风险可使接受择期或非紧急手术的患者做好充分的术前准备，并有助于降低围术期病情恶化的风险。与患儿的心脏病学专家、外科医师和家长进行充分的沟通与讨论是必不可少的。

当需要进行比较紧急的手术时，通常难以在患者到达医院前优化其内科病情。因此，心脏病学专家需随时能够到场与麻醉团队一起会诊。总之，术前准备工作需遵循文章中所提及的处理目标。

（段盼盼 译 杨 涛 校）

延伸阅读

Carvahlo JS: Cardiomyopathies. In Anderson RH, Baker EJ, Macartney FJ, editors: *Pediatric cardiology*, Philadelphia, 2002, Lippincott Williams & Wilkins, pp 1595–1643.

Ing RJ, Ames WA, Chambers NA: Paediatric cardiomyopathy and anaesthesia, *Br J Anaesth* 108:4–12, 2012.

Lynch J, Pehora C, Holtby H, et al.: Cardiac arrest upon induction of anesthesia in children with cardiomyopathy: an analysis of incidence and risk factors, *Pediatr Anesth* 21:951–957, 2011.

McKenzie IM: Cardiomyopathies. In Lake CL, Booker PD, editors: *Pediatric cardiac anesthesia*, Philadelphia, 2005, Lippincott Williams & Wilkins, pp 530–535.

Ramamoorthy C, Haberkern C, Sanjay B, et al.: Anesthesia-related cardiac arrest in children with heart disease: data from the pediatric perioperative cardiac arrest (POCA) registry, *Anesth Analg* 110:1376–1382, 2010.

Richardson P, McKenna W, Bristow M, et al.: Report of the 1995 World Health Organization/International Society and Federation of Cardiology task force on the definition and classification of cardiomyopathies, *Circulation* 93:841–842, 1996.

Rosenthal DN, Hammer GB: Cardiomyopathy and heart failure in children: anesthetic implications, *Pediatr Anesth* 21:577–584, 2011.

Tabib A, Loire R, Miras A, et al.: Unsuspected cardiac lesions associated with sudden unexpected perioperative death, *Eur J Anaesthesiol* 17:230–235, 2000.

Venugolapan P, Agarwal AK, Worthing EA: Chronic cardiac failure in children due to dilated cardiomyopathy: diagnostic approach, pathophysiology and management, *Eur J Pediatr* 159:803–810, 2000.

心脏复律

第40章

Johnny J. Kenth，Andrew F. Smith

病例概要

患者，女性，88 岁，既往有高血压、心绞痛、轻度哮喘病史，因腹痛伴恶心呕吐及进食减少 10 天于急诊科（emergency department，ED）就诊。急诊首先就其因胃肠炎导致的急性脱水症状进行了处理。进一步询问病史时发现，患者有严重的缺血性心脏病（ischemic heart disease，IHD）病史，运动耐量受限，此前右冠状动脉区域发生过心肌梗死，曾于急诊行经皮冠状动脉介入治疗。患者体检气道通畅，呼吸费力 30 次 / 分，5 L 氧流量面罩给氧，患者动脉血氧饱和度仅 92%，心率不规则，137 次 / 分，血压为 94/45 mm Hg。实验室结果显示血清钾为 3.1 mEq/L，血尿素氮为 33 mg/dl，肌酐为 310 mmol/L，镁为 0.57 mmol/L，磷酸盐为 0.38 mmol/L。12 导联心电图显示新发心房颤动伴有快速心室率，Ⅱ、Ⅲ、aVF 出现 Q 波且 ST 段压低。经过初始液体复苏后，腹部 CT 发现一小段肠梗阻，决定行急诊手术处理。尽管进行了液体复苏，患者血压仍为 60/35 mmHg，为了协助在实施紧急直流电复律，麻醉科医师对患者诱导全身麻醉，复律使用 150 J 能量，在第三次电击后成功复律至窦性心律。随后对患者建立了有创监测，患者被转运至手术室进行急诊手术治疗。

问题分析

定义

心脏复律可以是电疗或化学疗法，用于在各种情况下恢复窦性心律。直流电心脏复律主要在 3 种情况下使用：第一，出现快速型心律失常且血流动力学不稳定的患者选用的方法；第二，当药物治疗无效，使用禁忌或不能耐受时；第三，在有时间选择余地的情况下使用药物治疗无效的心律失常患者。

直流电心脏复律包括将电能同步应用于心动周期的 QRS 阶段。电能透过胸壁，刺激心肌，同时激发心肌细胞，诱导心室节律性收缩。心室肌细胞同时发生的激活和收缩导致心肌进入有效不应期，减少了折返电路的传导。根据电生理学依据，直流电心脏复律不能成功的原因被归纳为两种理论，第一种是临界数量理论，第二种是上限易损性理论。前者的理论前提基于：心律失常的产生和传导需要有一定数量（临界数量）心肌细胞参与。如果周围的心肌细胞都处于不应期，则心律失常就不能被传出，从而终止心律失常。第二种理论前提则基于：亚治疗性除颤不能使临界数量的心肌细胞全处于不应期，它会使部分心肌细胞处于不应期，而在心动周期的易损期刺激其他心肌细胞，最终形成致心律失常的折返环路。

直流电心脏复律的使用和操作方式与除颤（defibrillation，DF）不同。除颤不与心动周期的特异相同步，它用于紧急情况下，例如无脉性室性心动过速（ventricular tachycardia，VT）或心室颤动（ventricular fibrillation，VF）。直流电心脏复律可用于多种快速性心律失常，无论是起源于心房、房室（atrioventricular，AV）结 [共同形成室上性心动过速（supraventricular tachycardia，SVT）] 还是心室。SVT 包括折返传导，包括房颤和房扑。室性心律失常（室性快速性心律失常）包括 VT 和 VF。

除颤器是一种根据预定和预设量以可控和协调的方式存储电荷并释放预定能量的装置，通常以焦耳（能量的国际单位）测量。电流通过除颤垫或电极释放。电极板片放置的最佳位置包括前侧（前尖部）或前后位。前侧位是指将一个电极片放置于右锁骨下，胸骨右缘第二肋间水平。第二个电极片位于第二肋间水平，位于心尖部上方。在前后位，前电极片位于胸骨左缘，上覆心尖部，后电极片位于肩胛骨之间。现代除颤器使用导电性衬垫，通过降低胸部阻抗来改善电流传递。一些研究表明，除颤电极很可能与心脏复律至窦性心律的成功率增高有关。

直流电心脏复律能否成功的影响因素大致可分为与患者相关的因素和与设备相关的因素。

与患者相关的因素包括：

- 胸部阻抗：能量大小，电极-皮肤接触面，距离，极性，通气相，内在心肌特性和整体导电能力；
- 心律失常类型；
- 心律失常的持续时间；
- 电解质失衡（钾、镁和磷）；
- 毒素和促血栓形成药物（心脏变时性、变兴奋性和变传导性药物）；
- 合并慢性疾病；
- 内有植入式心脏装置。

与设备相关的因素包括：

- 电极：类型、大小和位置；
- 除颤电极板与粘贴除颤电极片；
- 使用的总能量和持续时间；
- 波形：单相与双相。

除颤电极板和电极片之间的重要区别是，对于前者，操作者必须用大约 110 牛顿（25 磅）的力将电极板加压至患者胸壁。对于后者，在除颤期间则不需要操作者保持与患者胸部接触，从而提高了安全性。除颤电极片还提供额外的功能，如进行经皮起搏的能力。

识别

病例中出现的紧急问题包括：

- 高龄；
- 缺血性心脏病病史，急性发作伴快速心室率的心房颤动；
- 严重脱水；
- 电解质异常：低钾血症，低镁血症，低磷血症；
- 严重血流动力学不稳定；
- 吸氧时仍觉气短；
- 急性肾损伤。

病例概要表明患者有不稳定快速心律失常合并脱水和电解质失衡。急性内环境紊乱与心血管并发症的明确病史（缺血性心脏病，陈旧性心肌梗死需要置入冠状动脉支架，舒张功能障碍）的并存导致氧供需失衡。这种不平衡最终导致房颤并伴有快速心室反应，减少舒张期充盈，并进一步拉大氧供需之间的差异。

高级心血管生命支持（advanced cardiovascular life support，ACLS）和高级生命支持（advanced life support，ALS）指南均推荐直流电心脏复律治疗血流动力学不稳定患者的不稳定性快速心律失常。

心脏节律不稳定带来的不良影响包括：

- 心肌功能不全，缺血（胸痛，气短，交感神经兴奋）；
- 心力衰竭 [疲劳，气短，端坐呼吸，外周组织水肿和（或）肺水肿]；
- 终末器官灌注不足 [心脏（缺血，衰竭），肾（尿量减少）]；
- 脑灌注不足（精神状态改变，意识减退，晕厥）。

即使在稳定的患者中，直流电心脏复律也被推荐作为优于药物的治疗方式，因为它们可以防止不良反应和降低致心律失常的影响（见第 161 章）。这对于可能患有结构性心脏病或心肌病变 [如既往心肌梗死、急性缺血和心力衰竭（射血分数低于 35%）] 的患者尤为重要。在这些情况下，药物的副作用可能确实超过了其益处。

心脏复律的主要禁忌证包括缺乏操作经验和技术专长，出现多形心房（异位）心动过速，以及由于心脏自律性增强（即洋地黄中毒）引起的心律失常。怀孕和植入设备的存在不是绝对禁忌证，但是应采取某些预防措施。包括使用最低适用能量，将电复律仪电极片放置在距离植入设备至少 12 cm 的位置，如可能，将植入设备关闭或调为非感知模式。

风险评估

当遇到患者出现心律失常时，最重要的是采用结构化和流程化的途径来治疗不舒服的患者，使用气道（A），呼吸（B），循环（C）和功能障碍（D；ABCD）模式。此外，在进行初步评估时，同步纠正任何危及生命的情况也很重要。使用这种方法可以通过恢复组织和器官再灌注来减轻终末器官损伤。同样重要的是，不稳定患者的紧急心脏复律要重视时间紧迫性，需要迅速采取行动。

在稳定的患者中，心律失常不需要紧急纠正，最新的证据倾向于对速率控制而非对节律的控制。如果需要进行心脏复律，则仅应在抗凝后进行，抗凝治疗可以在有时间选择余地的情况下进行（后面讨论）。

启示

对稳定患者择期进行心脏复律是一种安全且常用的操作方法。相比之下，就患者、设备和位置相关因素而言，紧急病情则带来了多重挑战：

患者相关因素：

- 急诊病例；
- 生理紊乱；
- 既往心肌疾病；
- 合并慢性疾病；
- 氧供需失衡。

设备和位置相关因素：

- 远离具备复律条件的地点；
- 对可用设备不熟悉和设备的局限性；
- 麻醉和复苏药物供应有限；
- 可用的最低监测标准；
- 训练有素的助手。

改进技术和药物的发明以及良好的培训提高了心脏复律的安全性。采用双相波形的心脏复律可显著降低成功的心脏复律所需要的能量。与单向单极波形相比，双相心脏复律和除颤通过变更极性和电轴，在两个（相对的）矢量平面中传递能量。单极单相除颤时需要相当大的能量（360 J），而双相除颤需要 200 J。心脏复律则通过传递电流来刺激心肌，所引发的严重的肌肉收缩可导致疼痛和不适。为了减轻这些疼痛和不适，需要进行麻醉或镇静。稳定的患者在日间手术环境中行择期心脏复律时，由于其血流动力学稳定，同样可满足日常手术的一般要求。尽管心脏复律经历了长时间的检验是安全的，但是，特别是在择期复律的场合中，它仍有几种令人担忧的并发症（可能会致命），包括以下方面：

气道与呼吸：

- 胃内容物的肺误吸，尤其是未禁食或胃潴留的患者；
- 插管失败；
- 球囊活瓣面罩（bag-valve-mask, BVM）通气困难；
- 丧失气道。

心血管系统：

- 心律不能复律至窦性；
- 麻醉药导致的低血压和心肌不稳定；
- 心动过缓，特别是并发心房颤动；
- 进展为室性心律失常；
- 心脏骤停：无脉性室性心动过速，心室颤动，心搏停止，无脉性电活动。

神经系统：

- 静脉血栓栓塞事件：脑血管意外，短暂性脑缺血发作；
- 意识改变，易与全身麻醉相混淆。

肌肉骨骼系统：

- 长骨和椎骨骨折，特别是患有骨关节炎，矿物质缺乏和代谢性骨病的患者（风险增加 1.5 倍）；
- 肌病疼痛。

管理

需要进行心脏复律的患者范围很广泛，从日间手术的择期稳定病例，到不稳定患者（可能在陌生环境中）的紧急情况。镇静可以被概念化为一个连续过程，即从清醒、警觉和有意识的患者，抗焦虑，进展到中度（有意识的）镇静，深度镇静，最后是全身麻醉[参见美国麻醉科医师协会（American Society of Anesthesiologists，ASA）镇静分级，见表 40.1]。实施镇静的医务人员应能将镇静目标维持在某一特定深度，且有能力管理意外出现深度镇静的患者，包括维护患者生理性内环境的干预措施。

用于心脏复律的镇静药，已经从具有众多副作用（包括呼吸暂停、嗜睡、宿醉感和低血压）的长效药物，发展到副作用更少的新型药物。这些超短效药物可以快速起效和失效，减轻宿醉感，同时可达到更深层的镇静作用。需要注意的是，临床医师必须训练有素，具备处理任何潜在并发症的经验，

表 40.1 ASA 镇静分级

	镇静状态类别			
	最小 / 抗焦虑	中度 / 意识镇静	深度镇静	全身麻醉
气道	未受影响	保持，无需干预	可能需要干预	通常需要干预
呼吸	不受影响 / 维持	充足，仅需吸氧	可能不够充分	常不足
自主呼吸		无需使用 IPPV		
心血管功能	不受影响 / 维持	通常不变	通常保持	可能会受损
神经功能 / 反应性	对言语刺激的反应正常	对言语或触觉刺激有目的反应	反复或疼痛刺激后有目的反应	即使有疼痛刺激也无法唤醒

ASA，美国麻醉科医师协会；IPPV，间歇正压通气

包括患者被意外诱导为全身麻醉的处理。

镇静剂的选择取决于持续时间、镇静深度、患者的不适和疼痛。临床医师还应注意不同药物的广泛个体差异及其潜在的不良反应。本章作者进行的 Cochrane 系统回顾认为，没有证据表明一种药物优于另一种药物。作者推荐运用医师经验、使用短效药物，并强调维持血流动力学稳定的重要性。尽管临床经验、国家指南和地方文化和习俗在实践中存在差异，但该综述强调了在不考虑后果的情况下坚持使用任何特定药物的谬误；强调成功地治疗并发症对于成功的结局至关重要（表 40.2）。

尽管有关心脏复律麻醉或镇静的多数研究药物为静脉制剂，但氧化亚氮和（或）挥发性吸入麻醉药亦有使用。氧化亚氮被证实与缺血性心脏病患者的较差预后有关，并且在长期和重复暴露后，其可抑制维生素 B_{12} 和蛋氨酸合成。

不管患者病情如何，无论何时进行心脏复律，都应进行彻底的术前评估，包括病史、体格检查和相关检查的评估。ASA 主张在进行镇静或麻醉时，应强制执行大不列颠和爱尔兰麻醉科医师协会（Association of Anaesthetists of Great Britain and Ireland，AAGBI）制定的最低监测标准。这些包括连续 ECG（最少 3 个导联）、无创血压，SpO_2、能监测 FiO_2 和二氧化碳描记波形。此外，自充气球囊、Mapleson C 呼吸回路、备用氧气瓶和各种搭配的气道装置，包括气管内导管、声门上气道装置（supraglottic airway devices，SAD），以及急救技术（如紧急环甲膜切开术）应该保证随时可以开展。根据 ASA 和英国皇家医学院安全镇静标准，实施镇静的医师应能胜任做到以上几点，包括处理任何潜在的并发症的能力。此外，操作除颤器的医师与实施镇静的医师不能为同一人，后者还应负责监测患者。根据需要，可以使用带有或不带有口咽气道（如 Guedel 气道）或 SAD 的球囊活瓣面罩以保证气道得到安全的管理。在紧急情况下，或可能存在胃内容物误吸的风险时，必须进行气管内插管。

心脏复律的并发症前文已有提及。具体而言，低血压可用静脉快速补充液体进行治疗，如乳酸林格；对于心血管不稳定的患者可能还需要血管收缩和正性肌力药物。急性神经系统后遗症（CVA，TIA）和肌肉骨骼损伤（椎骨骨折）在需要时可以通过一系列的综合治疗进行处理，包括：一般支持措施，特定的影像学检查和专家会诊等。对任何新的体征和症状的出现应保持高度的怀疑，因其可以提醒临床医师谨防这些已被根除的潜在并发症。

针对不稳定性快速心律失常的紧急心脏复律

与择期的心脏复律不同，紧急心脏复律可能存在诸多挑战。这些挑战包括患者因素，如基础疾病进程、血流动力学不稳定和心血管功能不稳定；和麻醉因素、包括麻醉剂的心脏抑制、降低血压和致心律失常作用。远离手术室的麻醉地点、设备不熟悉和不可用的情况，这些都是需要我们在实施紧急心脏复律麻醉时进一步考虑的问题和需要特别注意的风险。

ACLS 和 ALS 指南均推荐了针对不稳定节律的心脏复律的方案。他们主张采用 ABCDE 方法对不稳定的患者进行治疗，同时进行评估和复苏。如上所述，对心脏复律实施安全的麻醉需要 AAGBI 监测的最低标准、训练有素的助手、可用的复苏药物以及适当的设备。此外，除颤器应该经过测试并且确认正常运行。在某些情况下，最好通过将患者转移

表 40.2 心脏复律常用药物、建议剂量和常见优缺点

药物名称	建议剂量	优点	缺点
丙泊酚	单次注射剂量 0.5 ~ 2 mg/kg	起效 / 消退迅速	负性变时、变力、变传导
催眠，丙基苯酚	TCI C_{ET} 1.5 ~ 3 μg/ml	可在肝肾衰竭患者中安全使用 易于滴定镇静 能达到非常深的镇静或全身麻醉水平 止吐作用	↓ HR，↓ SVR，↓ CI 对不稳定患者会出现严重心血管功能不稳定和低血压 ↑ 呼吸暂停发生率增高 注射痛[a] 不自主的肌肉运动（非癫痫发作）[b]
硫喷妥钠硫代巴比妥	2 ~ 5 mg/kg	起效迅速，单个臂脑循环时间[b] 比丙泊酚对降低 SVR 和 CI 的影响较小 RSI 的经典组成部分	宿醉感：清除较慢 较少滴定使用 会导致↓ HR，↓ SVR，↓ CI 有致组胺释放和卟啉症风险 呼吸暂停，不会使喉反射迟钝
咪达唑仑苯二氮草	0.5 ~ 2 mg，最多不超过 10 mg	安全，熟悉，使用已久（如：非麻醉科医师使用） 心血管稳定 保持 MV[c] 不太可能产生更深层的镇静作用	显著的个人差异 较长的终末半衰期 $T_{1/2}$（可达 6 h） 肝 / 肾损伤患者的消退 / 残留作用时间显著延长 代谢物具活性
依托咪酯	50 ~ 100 μ/kg	起效迅速，单个臂脑循环时间维持 SVR 和 CI 心血管稳定的催眠药物 对休克患者特别有用	抑制肾上腺皮质功能令人担忧呼吸暂停 肌阵挛性抽搐[d] 致吐 消退较慢 / 后遗效应
氯胺酮	0.5 ~ 2 mg/kg 静脉注射 2 ~ 4 mg/kg 肌内注射	循环稳定 镇痛特性 保持 MV[c]	幻觉和突发现象 ↑交感张力，↑ MVO_2（缺血性心脏病） 致吐 药物滥用
瑞芬太尼	0.05 ~ 0.20 μg/(kg · min) TCI C_{ET} 1.5 ~ 3 μg/mL	起效 / 消退迅速 对患者病情不敏感 达到更深层次的镇静 与丙泊酚有协同作用 强效止痛作用	中度的↓ HR，↓ SVR，↓ CI，休克状态下降加重 心血管稳定性不如阿芬太尼 ↓ RR，↓ MV；导致胸壁僵硬 药物经济学：仅提供安瓿剂型，导致成本过高 镇痛消退迅速
阿芬太尼	5 ~ 20 μg/kg 0.02 ~ 0.7 μg/(kg · min)	所有阿片类药物中起效最快 因再分布作用消退迅速 比其他阿片类药物心血管系统更稳定 经济	清除率低于瑞芬太尼；对非常短小的手术，临床意义不大 呼吸系统影响如上 稍长的镇痛作用
芬太尼	0.5 ~ 1 μg/kg	心血管稳定 强效镇痛	作用时间远长于所提到的其他阿片类药物；可导致更长的药物残留 呼吸系统影响如上

CI，心脏指数；CV，心血管；C_{ET}，效应位浓度；MV，每分通气量；MVO_2，心肌耗氧量；RR，呼吸频率；RSI，快速序贯诱导；SVR，体循环阻力；TCI，靶控输注

[a] 注射痛可以通过预先注射利多卡因（最多 50 mg）和避免使用小静脉来减轻。超过 100 mg 的利多卡固可通过其作为膜稳定剂的作用，通过抑制钠离子内流，影响心脏复律的阈值。

[b] 药物从注射部位（如手臂）到作用部位（即大脑）所花的时间。

[c] 咪达唑仑和氯胺酮均维持自主呼吸和 MV，显著降低呼吸抑制风险。

[d] 肌阵挛运动（如依托咪酯）可能干扰心电图读数，影响同步心脏复律的感知，由于感知出错，在心脏周期的易损期会发生除颤器放电的危险。

到安全且更熟悉的环境（例如手术室）来稳定患者。然而，不稳定患者的转移可能导致有害的结局，其益处必须大于风险才考虑转移。

在初始评估中必须判断患者的病情是否稳定。临床医师可以询问节律是否是窦性，QRS 波群是宽的还是窄的复合波（大于 120 ms），心室节律是否规则。需要确定特定节律的原因是对不同的心律失常进行复律时需要不同的能量。

心脏复律的具体能量剂量包括以下内容：

- 窄 \ 规则：50 ～ 100 J 双相
- 窄 \ 不规则：120 ～ 200 J 双相或 200 J 单相
- 宽 \ 规则：100 J
- 宽 \ 不规则：200 J 双相或 360 J 单相（非同步）

当滴定心脏复律的能量剂量时，应使用尽可能低的能量，因为累积能量与心肌功能障碍的风险存在正相关。在进行直流电心脏复律后，可能需要药物治疗以预防快速型心律失常的复发或恶化。胺碘酮负荷剂量 150 mg，输注时间为 15 ～ 30 min，然后在 23 h 内维持输注 900 mg。心律失常的药物治疗在第 133 章和第 161 章将会有详细讨论。

儿童，尤其是新生儿和婴儿，心率比成人快，他们正依靠较快的心率来维持心排血量。儿童的快速型心律失常较少见，通常来源为室上性心动过速，可能需要进行直流电复律。这些病例通常很复杂，可能给患儿带来严重的风险和并发症，所以应尽早寻求专家帮助。与成年人一样，他们也必须使用通用的 ABCD 模式（如前所述）。儿童心脏复律的能量水平从 0.5 到 2 J/kg 开始，在无脉性室性心动过速 / 心房颤动中用于除颤的能量为 4 J/kg。室性心动过速在儿童中罕见，尤其在无结构性心脏病、异常传导通路、离子通道疾病、严重的生理异常或中毒的情况下。在血流动力学稳定的患儿中，可以使用负荷剂量的胺碘酮，在 30 min 内以 5 mg/kg 滴注，然后以 15 mg/（kg · d）的速度维持输注。

用于儿童的麻醉药物取决于临床医师的经验和偏好，但也必须考虑儿童的急性生理状况。氯胺酮对患儿有利，因其具有较小的副作用，如心血管稳定，不抑制迷走神经，可用亚催眠剂量进行镇静。氯胺酮对呼吸抑制极小，并具有镇痛作用。与成人相似，如果患儿未禁食或有肺误吸的风险，则必须进行气管内插管。否则可以使用 BVM。由于短暂的心动过缓可能会迅速恶化，应准备好预先计算好剂量的阿托品并能随手可用。

心房颤动的心脏复律

心房颤动患者管理的原则包括以下内容：

- 心率控制；
- 窦性心律的重建与维持；
- 避免血栓栓塞事件，尤其是有其他危险因素的患者。

心脏复律经常应用于稳定和不稳定患者的心房颤动病例中。心房颤动持续时间超过 48 h 是心脏复律的相对禁忌证，因其存在严重的血栓栓塞风险。因此，开始口服抗凝剂需至少 3 ～ 4 周，并行经食管超声心动图检查来排除心房内血栓。新型口服抗凝剂已经出现，并可替代维生素 K 拮抗剂（vitamin-K antagonists，VKA），例如华法林。这些可分为Ⅹa 因子抑制剂和直接凝血酶（Ⅱ因子）抑制剂。尽管这些较新的药物可能比 VKA 具有某些优势，但对这些新药仍不熟悉，且用于评估凝血抑制程度（定量和定性）的特定检测并未普及，不能随时可用。

从随机对照试验的系统回顾来看，复律成功率已高达 90%。成功复律和维持正常窦性心律 [在无结构性心脏病或急性冠状动脉综合征（acute coronary syndrome，ACS）后] 的可能性与持续时间呈正相关。长期慢性心房颤动的复律成功率明显低于近期起病的心房颤动。辅助药物治疗（在心脏复律之前或之后）可有助于窦性心律的维持，并且已经证明在心脏手术后是对患者有益的预防措施。

在心房颤动的情况下，除了心脏复律的一般并发症之外，心动过缓更为普遍且棘手。特别危险的患者包括患有病态窦房结综合征的患者，急性冠脉综合征后（特别是如果右冠状动脉的窦房结分支闭塞），离子通道病或存在病理折返回路。心室颤动是心脏复律的潜在致命并发症，通常由于非同步性电击的错误执行，特别是在心动周期的易损期，出现 R-on-T 现象。这可以通过将电击与主导联上的 R 波同步化来降低风险。心脏复律后可能发生 ST 段抬高等短暂 ST 段改变；这些通常因冠状动脉痉挛而发生并可能消退。如发生持续性不断演变的 ST 段变化、持续的胸痛和心肌坏死的生化证据，如肌钙蛋白升高，临床医师应注意潜在的急性冠脉综合征的存在。

预防

许多有助于降低心脏复律的麻醉风险的预防措施在前文已经提及。在择期或血流动力学参数稳定的患者中，所有患者必须遵循标准化禁食方案。这包括 6 h 的固体食物，包括含有颗粒物质的饮料，以及 2 h 的清饮。预防药物包括甲氧氯普胺、雷尼替丁和柠檬酸钠（30 ml，0.3 M），因为这些有助于降低胃液 pH 和胃液量，可以降低胃内容物肺误吸的风险。在紧急情况下，可能未按规定禁食，该方案仍可有助于降低肺误吸的风险。

在未使用气道设备的择期患者中，可以使用牙垫来防止唇部、舌头和牙龈的损伤。较新型的声门上气道装置，例如 Igel，其外壳内置有咬合防护装置，以及胃吸引口，因此是择期病例的理想选择。在紧急情况下，应对非禁食患者强制进行气管内插管，谨慎滴定药物使对心脏抑制作用最小。在心脏复律之前，如果患者呼吸暂停，应通过 BVM 辅助通气以预防呼吸性酸中毒，因其可降低快速型心律失常的阈值。短效肌松药物可以降低持续骨折或脱位的风险，虽然很少使用。

最后，心脏复律麻醉是一种常见且安全的手术操作。对患者进行全面的术前评估，重点关注不稳定患者的复苏和稳定，将有助于预防潜在的并发症。

致谢

感谢 M. Franckowiak 博士和 N. D. Nader 博士对本章上一版的贡献。

（杨心月 译 卞金俊 校）

延伸阅读

Academy of Medical Royal Colleges: *Safe sedation practice for healthcare procedures: standards and guidance. Report of an Intercollegiate Working Party chaired by the Royal College of Anaesthetists*, UK Academy of Medical Royal Colleges and Faculties, 2013. Available from http://www.aomrc.org.uk/publications/reports-guidance/safe-sedation-practice-1213/. Accessed November 7, 2016.

American Society of Anesthesiologists: *Continuum of depth of sedation: definition of general anesthesia and levels of sedation/analgesia*, 2009. Available from http://www.asahq.org, 2009. Accessed November 7, 2016.

Checketts MR, Alladi R, Ferguson K, et al.: Recommendations for standards of monitoring during anaesthesia and recovery 2015: Association of Anaesthetists of Great Britain and Ireland, *Anaesthesia 1* 71(1):85–93, 2016.

Eng MR: Procedural sedation for adult patients: an overview, *Contin Educ Anaesth Crit Care Pain* 12(4):176–180, 2012.

Fuster V, Rydén LE, Cannom DS, et al.: 2011 ACCF/AHA/HRS focused updates incorporated into the ACC/AHA/ESC 2006 guidelines for the management of patients with atrial fibrillation: a report of the American College of Cardiology Foundation/American Heart Association Task Force on practice guidelines, *Circulation* 123:e269–e367, 2011.

Knight BP: Basic principles and technique of cardioversion and defibrillation. In Page RL, Downey BC, editors: *UpToDate*, Waltham, MA. Available from https://www.uptodate.com/contents/basic-principles-and-technique-of-electrical-cardioversion-and-defibrillation. Accessed November 7, 2016.

Lewis SR, Nicholson A, Reed SS, et al.: Anaesthetic and sedative agents used for electrical cardioversion, *Cochrane Database Syst Rev* 2015(3), CD010824.

Mittal S, Ayati S, Stein KM, et al.: Transthoracic cardioversion of atrial fibrillation: comparison of rectilinear biphasic versus damped sine wave monophasic shocks, *Circulation* 101(11):1282–1287, 2000.

Siaplaouras S, Jung J, Buob A, Heisel A: Incidence and management of early recurrent atrial fibrillation (ERAF) after transthoracic electrical cardioversion, *Europace* 6(1):15–20, 2004.

第41章 颈动脉内膜切除术

Mark D. Stoneham

病例概要

患者，女性，82岁，既往高血压和冠状动脉疾病史，在区域麻醉下行颈动脉内膜切除术（carotid endarterectomy，CEA）。在3天前有短暂的语言障碍和左侧肢体功能丧失。检查显示右侧颈内动脉80%狭窄。术前血压180/95 mmHg。尽管患者一直处于高血压状态，但是手术进展顺利。术后在麻醉恢复室，患者的血压为200/100 mmHg，并出现烦躁和额部头痛。静脉注射拉贝洛尔（50 mg，分次给药）和肼屈嗪（20 mg）快速降压。患者意识水平下降，出现了语言障碍和偏瘫症状，提示缺血性脑卒中。进行头颅CT检查，显示为与脑梗死相一致的影像。不幸的是，患者病情恶化，第2天死亡。

问题分析

定义

CEA的目的是降低颈动脉严重狭窄患者将来发生卒中的风险，但只有在围术期发病率和死亡率较低的情况下才能实现其益处。接受CEA的患者由于存在心血管并存疾病因而其发生并发症的风险增加（表41.1）。动脉压可能难以控制。然而，围术期血流动力学不稳定可直接或间接影响发病率和死亡率。

CEA的独特之处在于，颈动脉窦的压力感受器是动脉压力生理控制机制的主要组成部分之一，它与疾病过程本身有关，并可能受到外科手术、药物治疗、麻醉药物的影响。近期短暂性脑缺血发作（transient ischemic attack，TIA）或卒中患者压力感受器敏感性改变，血流动力学不稳定风险增加。许多CEA患者有原发性高血压，部分患者在出现TIA或卒中后被诊断为高血压，因此短期内才开始进行降压治疗。在患者出现神经性症状的几天内就接受手术，这使得并发症往往更加严重。

因此，CEA期间的血压管理需要在两个极端之间“走钢丝”。一方面，血压必须维持在足够高的水平，以维持脑灌注，特别是在颈动脉夹闭阻断期，此时同侧大脑皮质依赖Willis环周围的侧支循环（Willis环）。另一方面，血压不能太高，以免出现心肌缺血、高灌注综合征或出血性卒中等高血压并发症。这可能很难控制，这就解释了为什么CEA围术期脑卒中和死亡率仍然相对较高。

CEA麻醉的选择对术中及术后血流动力学确实有一定的影响。区域麻醉下CEA患者在颈动脉阻断期间易出现高血压，恢复脑血流后和进入术后阶段发生低血压。相反，在全身麻醉下常见的模式是术中相对低血压和术后相对高血压。

识别

脑灌注风险贯穿整个颈动脉手术。在颈内动脉

框41.1 CEA的术后问题

- 血流动力学不稳定
  - 高血压
  - 低血压
  - 心肌梗死
- 伤口血肿
- 舌咽部水肿伴气道受损
- 颅神经损伤
- 神经功能障碍
- 急性移植物血栓形成（可能需要再次探查）
  - 微小局灶缺陷
  - 分水岭缺血
  - 高灌注综合征导致蛛网膜下腔出血

阻断前，通过狭窄的颈动脉维持同侧大脑皮质的灌注可能依赖于相对较高的血压的维持。在阻断时，同侧大脑皮质的灌注减少，依赖于 Willis 环周围的对侧血流。一旦阻断松开，两侧灌注可能会受到动脉压力波动的影响。脑血管亦受麻醉方式的影响。与区域麻醉相比，全身麻醉对脑自动调节和压力感受器功能的影响更大。动脉二氧化碳水平对脑血管扩张和收缩也有显著影响。

因此，在整个手术过程中，动脉压的严密控制再加上一些评估颈动脉夹闭时脑灌注的方法是至关重要的。选择哪种监测技术可能会受到外科医师是否使用颈动脉分流术的影响（一种绕过颈动脉阻断从而在阻断期维持其同侧灌注的方法）。一些外科医师选择在所有患者身上放置分流管，而另一些则从不使用分流管，而是依靠手术的速度来减少脑缺血时间。而第三类血管外科医师使用术中脑灌注和缺血监测仪来指导他们是否放置分流管。分流并非没有风险，血管壁破裂、动脉粥样斑块脱落伴血栓栓塞、分流管扭结或空气栓塞均可能发生，如果分流管意外脱出，还可发生动脉大出血。

用于评估分流引流必要性的方法：清醒患者的神经学评估（在局部或区域麻醉下，如颈丛阻滞），经颅多普勒超声，脑电图（electroencephalogram，EEG）、体感诱发电位（somatosensory evoked potentials，SEP），测量脑动脉远端残端压（对侧颈动脉回流穿过 Willis 环产生的压力），使用氙直接测定脑血流（表 41.1）。任何检测围术期缺血的技术敏感性均有限，因为大多数发生在术后的脑卒中，很可能是由血栓栓塞现象引起的。

术后患者在麻醉后监护病房（postanesthesia care unit，PACU）接受持续数小时的动脉压监测，并频繁评估神经功能。动脉压管理方案和合理的血管活性药物可用于控制患者在 PACU 的血流动力学稳定性（框 41.2）。

表 41.1　颈动脉内膜切除术中脑缺血的监测

区域麻醉	
清醒患者的中枢神经系统检查	“金标准” 在颈动脉夹闭期间，定期评估对侧握力、语言和大脑活动
全身麻醉	
脑电图（EEG）	EEG 皮质电活动随脑缺血而减少。EEG 监测的缺点包括不能监测脑深部结构变化，由于先前存在或波动的神经功能缺损而出现假阴性结果，以及全身麻醉对 EEG 模式的影响
躯体感觉诱发电位（SEP）	SEP 可以监测大脑的深层结构。SEP 是一种产生于周围的电脉冲，通过一、二级神经元传递到脑干突触的结果。随后，这些冲动被传递到躯体感觉皮质。与 SEP 监测一样，如果麻醉药产生类似脑缺氧的 SEP 变化，可能会出现假阴性
颈内动脉残端压力	目前主要的监测方式。可触及脉搏或平均残端压力大于 60 mmHg 提示有足够的回流以防止缺血
氙 -133 显像	静脉或颈动脉内注射放射性氙或氪。该方法专业且昂贵，而且更多是作为一种研究方法在使用
经颅多普勒超声（TCD）	TCD 测量大脑中动脉的血流速度。它可用于检测颈动脉手术中或术后的急性血栓性闭塞或栓塞，或发现术后出现高灌注综合征的危险患者
近红外光谱（rSO_2）	使用前额传感器对皮质氧饱和度进行无创评估。从狭窄到早期狭窄闭塞 rSO_2 降低 <20% 具有较高的阴性预测值。然而，其假阳性率很高

风险评估

根据定义，所有接受 CEA 的患者均患有动脉疾病，有发生心脑血管并发症的风险。颈动脉疾病的重要危险因素包括高龄、高血压、吸烟和糖尿病史。由于这些患者脑卒中的风险很高，但更有可能死于心肌梗死，因此术前的风险评估、检查和手术时机可能具有挑战性和争议性。

心脏风险评估可包括：运动或多巴酚丁胺负荷试验或心肺运动试验，以确定术前冠状动脉重建的必要性（如冠状动脉旁路移植术或经皮冠状动脉腔内成形术）。然而，冠状动脉重建的益处必须与因延迟或在冠状动脉旁路移植术中应用体外循环的卒中风险相平衡。关于麻醉科医师管理晚期颈动脉和冠状动脉疾病的患者尚无明确的指南，实施有创干预的决定通常基于患者的临床病史、症状的稳定性以及机构规定和个人选择偏好。

启示

在迄今为止完成的最大研究（GALA 试验）中，

框 41.1 CEA 术后血压管理方案

（1）PACU 患者：收缩压 >170 mmHg

一般观点

- 患者是否有尿潴留或疼痛？
- 患者今天是否接受了正常的降压药治疗？
- 当任何血管活性药输注正在运行时，患者应留在 PACU 中，观察至停止输注后 >2 h。

一线药物：拉贝洛尔

100 mg 拉贝洛尔溶于 20 ml 0.9% 氯化钠溶液（即 5 mg/ml）。每 2 min 缓慢推注 10 mg（2 ml），直至 100 mg（20 ml，20 min 以上）。

如果 20 min 后血压仍然升高，换用二线药物治疗。

如果血压下降且没有反弹，继续定期观察血压。

如果血压一开始下降，但又上升，开始输注 50 ～ 100 mg/h，滴定剂量控制血压。

二线药物：肼屈嗪

10 mg 肼屈嗪溶于 10 ml 0.9% 氯化钠溶液（即 1 mg/ml）。

每 5 min 缓慢推注 2 mg（2 ml），直到 10 mg（10 ml，25 min 以上）。

如果 25 min 后血压仍然升高，换用三线药物。

如果血压下降而没有反弹，继续定期观察血压。

如果血压一开始下降，但又上升，则换用三线药物。

三线药物：硝酸甘油（GTN）

50 mg GTN 注入 50 ml 0.9% 氯化钠溶液（即 1 mg/ml）。

以 5 ml/h（5 mg/h）开始输液，增加速度至 12 ml/h（12 mg/h），滴定调节血压。

（2）患者在外科病房：收缩压 >170 mmHg，无头痛或神经学症状

三种情况：

（1）患者平时不进行抗高血压治疗。

（2）患者平时进行抗高血压治疗。

（3）患者不能吞咽药片。

（2.1）患者平时不进行抗高血压治疗

一线药物：硝苯地平缓释剂

10 mg，如果血压无变化，1 h 后再次应用。

不要使用碾碎的硝苯地平胶囊。

如果血压没有下降，则使用二线药物。

二线药物：比索洛尔

5 mg，如果为禁忌证或无效，则使用三线药物。

三线药物：雷米普利

5 mg，如有需要，3 h 重复使用。

联系高血压专科医师进行评估。

（2.2）患者正常进行抗高血压治疗

一线药物：

核实患者是否正常服用降压药。如果没有，执行此方案

二线药物：

联系专科医师进行临床评估。

A=ACEI 类，B=β 受体阻滞剂，C= 钙通道阻滞剂，D = 利尿剂

如果患者在服用 A，加用 C（硝苯地平 10 mg）。

如果患者在服用 C，则加用 A（雷米普利 5 mg）。

如果患者在服用 D，则加用 A（雷米普利 5 mg）。

如果患者在服用 A+C，则加用 D（苄氟噻嗪 2.5 mg）。

如果患者在服用 A+D，则加用 C（硝苯地平 10 mg）。

如果患者在服用 A+C+D，则加用 B（比索洛尔 5 mg）。

（2.3）患者无法吞咽药片

按上述方案通过鼻胃管给药。

（3）患者在外科病房：收缩压 >170 mmHg + 头痛 / 癫痫发作或中枢神经系统症状。

治疗应立即开始并在病房使用无创监测。使用一线、二线和三线方案，如上面（1）所示。

- 抗高血压方案与术后恢复的方案相同。
- 值班外科住院医师必须做以下工作：
  - 联系血管外科医师，告知其与癫痫 / 头痛或中枢神经系统症状发作相关的高血压。
  - 联系 ICU 安排紧急转入进行有创血压监测。
  - 考虑使用类固醇（如地塞米松 IV，8 mg）。

CEA 的总死亡率和卒中率为 4.5%。最权威的中心报告的卒中 / 死亡率在 1% ～ 2%。CEA 术后卒中或死亡的危险因素包括女性、充血性心力衰竭、周围血管疾病、手术医师手术量低以及对侧颈内动脉闭塞。

管理与预防

从门诊、术前评估门诊以及患者入院时的血压来获得患者血压“正常值”是十分重要的。

一般来说，许多麻醉科医师和外科医师的目标是在选择 CEA 之前，将收缩压控制在 160 mmHg 或以下。抗高血压治疗（包括 β 受体阻滞剂但不包括血管紧张素转换酶抑制药和血管紧张素 Ⅱ 受体拮抗剂）应该继续应用到术晨，并在手术后立即恢复应用。然而，β 受体阻滞剂的引入，尤其是美托洛尔使用后立即行手术与低血压患者卒中的风险增加相关。他汀类药物已被证明可以改善 CEA 患者的预后，建议所有患者服用。建议对每位患者继续服用抗高血压和抗血小板药物的风险与效益进行评估。

传统的血管外科麻醉教学建议维持收缩压在术前基线值的 ±20%。然而，对颈动脉夹闭期“分水岭”脑卒中的关注，以及清醒 CEA 患者的一些临床证据表明，血压升高至“正常”值可逆转其发展中的神经功能缺损，这些证据已将 CEA 患者的这些限制修订为正常至高于基线 20% 之间。

在术前、术中和术后期间，需要考虑的事项略有不同。术前控制和维持血压很重要，但要避免颈动脉狭窄远端脑灌注过度减少。术中目标是维持脑灌注压和侧支血流，使其能在麻醉作用可能影响脑压力自动调节时维持正常灌注。压力反射受到手术的直接影响，但颈动脉夹闭或手术本身可能会影响脑血流。与术前自我调节和压力反射受损的情况相比，术后手术部位远端的脑循环较术前增加。

术中管理的主要目标是保护大脑和心脏，但这两个目标可能相互冲突。例如，通过增加血压来增加脑血流量可以增加后负荷或心肌收缩力，从而增加心脏的氧耗。

在全身麻醉下，动脉二氧化碳分压（$PaCO_2$）变化影响脑血流。尽管允许性高碳酸血症会扩张大脑非缺血区域的脑血管，但如果血液从已经最大程度扩张的脑动脉流向缺血区域，则可能是有害的。相反，低碳酸血症可能会使灌注充分的大脑非缺血区域的血管收缩，使血液重新流向缺血区域，从而导致反向窃血现象。因为这两种反应均不可预测，大多数专家建议维持正常的血碳酸浓度。

颈动脉内膜切除术的监测包括全身或区域麻醉的标准监测：体温探头、血压袖带、脉搏血氧仪和呼气末二氧化碳检测。放置动脉内导管进行即时动脉血压监测，以便及早发现和治疗血压变化。由于颈动脉再灌注后心肌缺血发生率较高，应监测心电图导联Ⅱ、V5 ST-T 段变化。

术后需立即评估和监测神经功能变化，包括颈动脉血流多普勒评估和脑成像。某些患者可能需要立即返回手术室再次手术。

（卢凌宇　译　严姝姝　校）

延伸阅读

AbuRahma AF, Srivastava M, Stone PA, et al.: Effect of statins on early and late clinical outcomes of carotid endarterectomy and the rate of post-carotid endarterectomy restenosis, *J Am Coll Surg* 220(4):481–487, 2015.

Ashes C, Judelman S, Wijeysundera DN, et al.: Selective β_1-antagonism with bisoprolol is associated with fewer postoperative strokes than atenolol or metoprolol, *Anesthesiology* 119:777–787, 2013.

Dua A, Romanelli M, Upchurch Jr GR, et al.: Predictors of poor outcome after carotid intervention, *J Vasc Surg* 64:664–670, 2016.

GALA Trial Collaborative Group, Lewis SC, Warlow CP, et al.: General anaesthesia versus local anaesthesia for carotid surgery (GALA): a multicentre, randomised controlled trial, *Lancet* 372:2132–2142, 2008.

Study Group POISE, Devereaux PJ, Yang H, et al.: Effects of extended-release metoprolol succinate in patients undergoing non-cardiac surgery (POISE trial): a randomised controlled trial, *Lancet* 371(9627):1839–1847, 2008.

Stoneham MD, Stamou D, Mason J: Regional anaesthesia for carotid surgery, *Br J Anaesth* 114(3):372–383, 2015.

Stoneham MD, Thompson JP: Arterial pressure management and carotid endarterectomy, *Br J Anaesth* 102(4):442–452, 2009.

Vlisides P, Mashour GA: Perioperative stroke, *Can J Anesth* 63:193–204, 2016.

第42章 长期应用非甾体抗炎药

Arthur Kitt，*Celeste M. Lombardi*

病例概要

患者，男性，60 岁，患有骨关节炎病史，服用萘普生（naproxen）3 年，未发现有任何并发症或副作用。某日突发严重恶心、呕鲜血，被送往急诊室并接受了紧急上消化道（gastrointestinal，GI）内镜检查，结果显示有出血性胃溃疡。

问题分析

定义

非甾体抗炎药（nonsteroidal antiinflammatory drugs，NSAIDs）应用广泛，其通过抑制环氧合酶以及前列腺素的合成发挥作用。前列腺素衍生自花生四烯酸，由作用于细胞膜磷脂的磷脂酶 A_2 形成（图 42.1）。NSAIDs 是世界上最常用的药物之一，通常具有良好的耐受性。然而，像所有药物一样，NSAIDs 并非没有副作用。众所周知，它们会导致以下情况：

- 胃肠道毒性，导致消化性溃疡的形成；
- 不需要的抗血小板作用（非选择性环氧合酶抑制剂）；
- 潜在致血栓形成的风险增加 [选择性环氧合酶 -2（cyclooxygenase-2，COX-2）抑制剂]；
- 肾毒性，可能会引起体液和钾离子失衡，肾功能下降，导致肾病综合征与原发性肾炎、肾乳头坏死以及横纹肌溶解症；
- 部分患者发生过敏和类过敏反应。

识别

胃肠道的影响

除幽门螺杆菌感染以外，应用 NSAIDs 是引起消化性溃疡的第二大重要原因。尽管也可能涉及一氧化氮和降钙素基因相关肽的减少，但溃疡形成的主要机制是抑制胃前列腺素。它可导致上皮黏液、碳酸氢盐分泌减少，降低黏膜对损伤的抵抗力。NSAIDs 还会减少胃黏膜血流量，继之损伤血管内

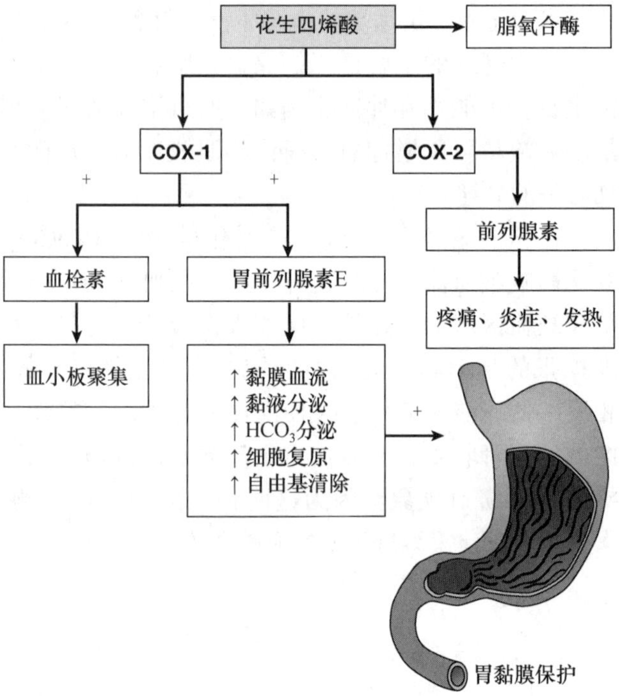

图 42.1　通过环氧合酶（COX-1 和 COX-2）途径由花生四烯酸合成为前列腺素。花生四烯酸是前列腺素的前体，它是由两种 COX 同工酶催化反应中的膜磷脂衍生而来的。COX-1 的基因（“管家”酶）可持续性表达并维持器官稳态，包括胃黏膜的完整性。COX-2 的基因（“炎性”酶）可诱导性表达。通过 COX-1 衍生的血栓素导致血小板聚集或表现出胃黏膜保护作用。相反，通过 COX-2 衍生的前列环素 [如前列环素（PGI_2）] 是疼痛、炎症和发热的介质。PGE，前列腺素 E（Adapted from Wolfe MM：Therapy and prevention of NSAID-related gastrointestinal disorders. In Wolfe MM，editor：*Therapy of digestive disorders*：*a companion to Sleisenger and Fordtran gastrointestinal diseases*. Philadelphia，WB Saunders，2000，pp 96-112.）

皮（NSAIDs 给药的早期影响），同时增强中性粒细胞对血管内皮的黏附。中性粒细胞黏附通过释放氧

衍生的自由基引起内皮损伤。

血栓形成的影响

血栓素 A_2 是血小板中 COX-1 代谢的主要产物（见图 42.1）。它引起血小板聚集、血管收缩和平滑肌增殖。在患有外周血管疾病的患者中，血栓素产生增加与大血管事件的风险增加相关。阿司匹林是血小板环氧合酶（COX-1）的强效抑制剂，其在血小板存活期间能阻止血栓素产生。对于其他 NSAIDs，此过程可持续 24 h 或更短时间。这种效应是阿司匹林降低高危患者心源性死亡、心肌梗死和脑卒中发生率的基础。然而，大剂量或中毒剂量的阿司匹林会抑制维生素 K 依赖性凝血因子，导致凝血酶原时间延长和国际标准化比值增加。

相反，前列环素是血管内皮中 COX-2 代谢的产物。人们据此推测在 COX-2 受到抑制后前列环素的合成也相应被抑制。前列环素可抑制血小板聚集、平滑肌增殖以及引起血管舒张。萘丁美酮（nabumetone），依托度酸（etodolac）和非乙酰化水杨酸盐（相对 COX-2 选择性 NSAIDs）会抑制 COX-2 介导的前列环素合成，并且对血小板聚集几乎没有影响。而其他 NSAIDs 选择性较差，会同时阻断 COX-1 血栓素合成和 COX-2 前列环素产生（表 42.1；图 42.2）。

肾影响

常规应用 NSAIDs 治疗的患者中，高达 5% 的患者会出现一种或多种肾毒性副作用，包括体液和电解质异常、急性肾衰竭和肾病综合征（框 42.1）。这些副作用的作用机制是通过阻断 COX-1 同工酶来抑制前列腺素 I_2、E_2 和 D_2 的产生。这会引起急性肾动脉血管收缩、肾髓质缺血甚至急性肾衰竭，进而减少肾灌注。NSAIDs 也会降低降血压药物的疗效，因为它们大多需要依赖完整的肾前列腺素功能。钙

表 42.1　抑制前列环素和血栓素的生物合成以及血栓形成的风险

药物	前列环素	血栓素	血栓形成风险
小剂量阿司匹林	±	↓↓	↓
常规	↓	↓	尚不清楚
选择性 COX-2 抑制剂	↓	±	尚不清楚

COX，环氧合酶

From Catella-Lawson F，Crofford LJ：Cyclooxygenase inhibition and thrombogenicity. *Am J Med* 110：28-32，2001.

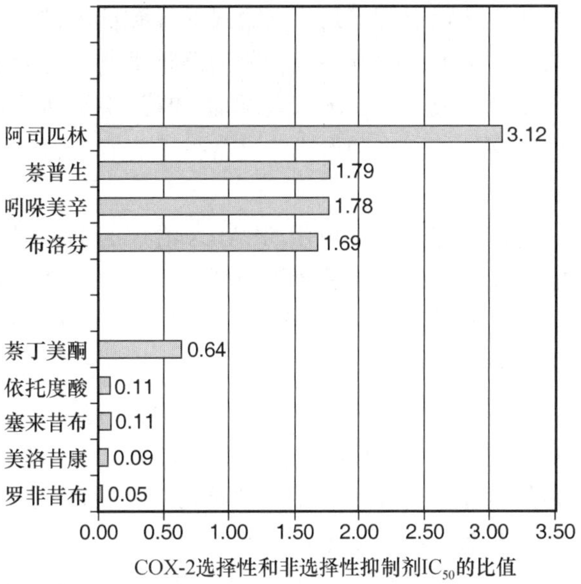

图 42.2　COX-2 抑制剂的选择性。比较选择性和非选择性非甾体类抗炎药物的体内抑制浓度（IC_{50}）比值（COX-2/COX-1）。比值低则表明 COX-2 的选择性较高（Adapted from Feldman M，McMahon AT：Do cyclooxygenase-2 inhibitors provide benefits similar to those of traditional anti-inflammatory drugs，with less gastrointestinal toxicity？ *Ann Intern Med* 132：134-143，2000.）

框 42.1　肾性综合征与传统的非甾体抗炎药治疗相关

- 体液和电解质异常
- 急性肾衰竭
- 血流动力学改变
- 肾病综合征（微小病变型肾小球病，间质性肾炎）
- 急性肾乳头状坏死（通常是由单一药物引起）
- 其他系统性相互作用
- 高钠血症
- 水潴留
- 高钾血症
- 膜性肾小球病
- 慢性肾乳头状坏死（通常是由多种药物引起）
- 慢性心力衰竭
- 高血压（治疗后）

通道阻滞剂和血管紧张素Ⅱ受体拮抗剂除外，因为它们不受肾前列腺素的影响。各种 NSAIDs 对血压有不同的影响，这取决于它们对肾血管舒张性前列腺素抑制的程度。例如，舒林酸（Sulindac）可能是较弱的肾前列腺素抑制剂，因此对高血压患者的血压影响较小。开始接受 NSAIDs 治疗并服用降血压药物的患者需要密切监测血压，特别是 55 岁及以上的患者。

体液和电解质紊乱是常见的 NSAIDs 相关的肾副作用。其发生原因是由于抑制了 Henle 环的升支

粗段和远端肾小管前列腺素合成而导致低渗钠和水潴留。理论上，随着环氧合酶通路被抑制，经脂氧合酶途径形成的白三烯就会增加，导致毛细血管通透性增高，加剧水肿形成。这常见于患有充血性心力衰竭的患者。

高钾血症是长期应用 NSAIDs 治疗的罕见但严重的并发症，这可能是由于前列腺素介导的肾素释放被抑制而导致的，这会引起远端肾小管中醛固酮形成减少和钾分泌减少。

肾病综合征伴间质性肾炎的形成很少见，其机制尚不清楚。从理论上讲，倾向于解释为白三烯形成和前列腺素受抑制增加血管通透性，进而引发肾病性范围蛋白尿和间质性肾炎。

肾乳头坏死也很罕见，且多发生于摄入 NSAIDs 过量的严重脱水患者。前列腺素受抑制和肾乳头内高浓度的 NSAIDs（其本身可能是细胞毒性的）的联合作用导致肾乳头坏死。常规剂量的 NSAIDs 极少发生这种情况。

过敏和类过敏反应

少数患者对阿司匹林和 NSAIDss 有过敏和假性过敏反应。部分是由传统 NSAIDs 类似的药理学特性引起的，即对 COX-1 和 COX-2 的抑制。前列腺素 E_2 的形成被 COX-1 的抑制阻断，导致白三烯形成和肥大细胞释放组胺相对增加。这种假性过敏反应多发生于初次暴露于 NSAIDs，不存在有先前致敏的可能。对于有鼻窦炎和哮喘病史的患者，应用阿司匹林和比对 COX-2 更具特异性的 COX-1 的其他 NSAIDs（见图 42.2）可以诱发流鼻涕、支气管痉挛和喉痉挛。阿司匹林和其他相对具 COX-1 特异性的 NSAIDs 与新型 COX-2 选择性拮抗剂的交叉敏感性并不会发生，这进一步证明 COX-1 抑制是阿司匹林诱发呼吸道症状的主要原因。

一些患者对特定的 NSAIDs 表现出真正的过敏反应，初次暴露会导致免疫球蛋白 E（immunoglobulin E，IgE）抗体的形成。在随后的暴露中，他们会表现出症状，包括荨麻疹、血管神经性水肿和过敏反应。目前还没有针对特定药物半抗原的检测，并且在这类患者的血液中很少发现 IgE 抗体。因此，**过敏反应**这个词已被用于描述这种反应。这些反应是由特定的 NSAIDs 引起的，患者服用其他 NSAIDs 则不会出现。

风险评估和启示

胃肠道损伤

消化不良并不是评估胃肠道黏膜损伤的可靠方法。有 10% ～ 20% 的 NSAIDs 治疗患者主诉消化不良，但 50% 的内镜检查结果显示胃肠道黏膜正常。大多数患者在出现危及生命的上消化道出血之前不会主诉胃肠道症状。发生溃疡的危险因素包括高龄（65 岁以上）、肾或肝损害、溃疡病史、吸烟、饮酒、同时使用口服皮质类固醇或抗凝剂、大剂量和长时间的 NSAIDs 治疗。

随着人们对环氧合酶两种亚型的认识，COX-1 酶被认为是负责胃前列腺素 E_1 形成的酶，并且使用非选择性 NSAIDs 发生胃肠道并发症风险更高。重要的是要了解 NSAIDs 对 COX 亚型的相对选择性，因为这决定了给患者选择哪种药物。例如，依托度酸（etodolac）、美洛昔康（meloxicam）和萘丁美酮（nabumetone）对 COX-2 的亲和力比对 COX-1 的亲和力高（见图 42.2），并且在胃肠道毒性方面更加安全。

塞来昔布长期治疗关节炎安全性研究（The Celecoxib Long-Term Arthritis Safety Study，CLASS）是一项为期 6 个月的随机、双盲、对照试验，比较了塞来昔布（400 mg，每天 2 次）与更传统的 NSAIDs（双氯芬酸 75 mg，每日 2 次；布洛芬 800 mg，每日 3 次）的胃肠道毒性。主要终点是溃疡相关并发症（胃穿孔、胃出口综合征、胃肠道出血），次要终点是症状性溃疡。尽管症状性和复杂性溃疡似乎存在差异，但这在统计学上并不显著。该研究中的两个混杂因素是使用塞来昔布的超治疗剂量，以及有 21% 的患者使用低剂量阿司匹林预防心血管疾病。已知阿司匹林会增加上消化道出血的风险。服用塞来昔布的非阿司匹林使用者的溃疡并发症发生率与一般人群相似，但由于没有安慰剂组，因此很难用塞来昔布评估溃疡的风险。然而，我们能够确定患者对塞来昔布的耐受力比双氯芬酸和布洛芬更高，血细胞比容下降较小，消化不良发生率更低，内镜检查需要较少。

罗非昔布（Vioxx）胃肠道预后研究（Vioxx Gastrointestinal Outcomes Research，VIGOR）是一项为期 12 个月的试验，旨在比较罗非昔布每日 50 mg 与更传统的 NSAIDs 萘普生每日 2 次 500 mg 的胃肠道毒性。主要终点是临床上确诊的胃肠道事件，包括症状性胃十二指肠溃疡、穿孔或梗阻以及上消化道出血。次要终点是复杂的胃肠道事件导致患者病情加重。结果显示，与萘普生相比，罗非昔布的胃肠道事件发生率显著降低，且有统计学意义。甚至在胃肠道事件高危患者中，包括高龄、使用皮质类固醇、有胃肠道穿孔或梗阻的既往病史以及幽门螺杆菌感染者，罗非昔布的胃肠道毒性发生率也显著降低。这是第一项证明使用选择性 COX-2 抑制剂有确切益处的研究。之后，一项多国参与研究的依托考昔和双氯芬酸关节炎长期（Multinational Etoricoxib and Diclofenac Arthritis Long-term，MEDAL）计划，比较了服用依托考昔和双氯芬酸患者的上消化道事件发生率，显示服用依托考昔的患者中无并发症的胃肠道事件发生率较低 [风险比（HR）0.57，95% 置信区间（CI）0.45 ～ 0.74]。对于同时服用阿司匹林和质子泵抑制剂的患者，两者情况相同。无并发症的胃肠道事件包括无并发症出血以及有胃食管溃疡形成的证据。然而，依托考昔组和双氯芬酸组之间的复杂胃肠道事件发生率没有差异。

血栓形成

选择性 COX-2 抑制剂优先阻断前列环素的合成，对血栓素的产生几乎没有影响。因此理论上来说，可能会增加血栓形成风险，尤其是动脉粥样硬化疾病风险较高的老年患者。

一项关于使用塞来昔布预防腺瘤研究（Adenoma Prevention with Celecoxib，APC）发现，与安慰剂相比，每日 2 次服用塞来昔布 200 mg 和 400 mg 均与心血管事件发生率增加相关。安慰剂组 679 名患者中有 7 名（1.0%）患有心肌梗死、卒中或心力衰竭；而每天 2 次接受 200 mg 塞来昔布的 685 名患者和每天 2 次接受 400 mg 塞来昔布的 671 名患者中各有 16 名（2.3%；95%CI 0.9 ～ 5.5）和 23 名（3.4%；95%CI 1.4 ～ 7.8）患有心肌梗死、卒中或心力衰竭。在 MEDAL 研究中，双氯芬酸似乎与每年 1.3% 的心血管事件风险相关，而选择性 COX-2 抑制剂依托考昔与 1.46% 的年度风险相关——尽管无明显统计学差异。2015 年，美国食品和药物管理局（FDA）加强了所有非阿司匹林类 NSAIDss 的标签警告，声称这些药物会增加心脏病发作和卒中的风险。

肾损伤

老年人和患有肾病或肝病、高血压、一定程度的心血管损伤、充血性心力衰竭或血容量不足的患者是因抑制肾前列腺素而发生肾功能不全的高危人群。人们发现肾也会产生 COX-2，因此 COX-2 的非选择性和选择性抑制剂都会导致水肿形成。

塞来昔布对肾功能的损害作用已有评估，尤其指肾病综合征、间质性肾炎、血清肌酐水平升高和肾乳头状坏死。与非选择性 COX 抑制剂相比，塞来昔布的肾损伤作用更小，但尚未经过严格测试。因此，至少就目前而言，对于既往有肾病史的患者应谨慎使用选择性 COX-2 抑制剂，如同传统的 NSAIDs 一样。

变态反应

据报道，患有关节炎的患者在接受数月特定 NSAIDs 治疗后，有少数病例可发生无菌性脑膜炎。这些病例中，无菌性脑膜炎被认为是对 NSAIDs 的免疫反应。并且在这些患有无菌性脑膜炎患者的脑脊液中发现了 IgG 和免疫复合物。尚未见报道阿司匹林会引发这一情况。另有少数报道认为应用除阿司匹林以外的多种 NSAIDs 还会引发咳嗽、发热、肺部浸润和嗜酸性粒细胞增多。这种变态反应肺泡炎或超敏性肺炎也被认为是由免疫反应介导的，因为对这些患者的肺组织活检发现了间质淋巴细胞和嗜酸性粒细胞。这可能是由 IgE 介导的反应或迟发型超敏反应。

管理

胃肠道毒性

每年约有 15 000 人死于 NSAIDs 的胃肠道并发症（包括出血、穿孔和梗阻）。在停用 NSAIDs 后，其诱发的溃疡会缓慢自愈；抗分泌治疗可加速溃疡愈合。尽管 H_2- 拮抗剂价格上更加便宜，但质子泵抑制剂通常是首选药物。它们可使溃疡更快地愈合，并且缓解早期症状。如果患者在用 H_2- 拮抗剂（例如，雷尼替丁 150 mg，每天 2 次）或质子泵抑制剂（例如，奥美拉唑，每天 20 mg）进行溃疡治疗时继续服用 NSAIDs，则溃疡复发率高。手术治疗适用于出现严重胃肠道出血或穿孔的患者。服用抗血小板药物（如氯吡格雷）或抗凝药物的患者应避免使用 NSAIDs，因为这可能会进一步增加出血风险。

变态反应

患者服用阿司匹林 650 mg，每天 2 次，持续 2 周后，就可以达到阿司匹林脱敏。持续监测尿白三烯，脱敏后可见显著降低。这种脱敏可能对需要长期服用阿司匹林的心血管疾病老年患者特别有益。

预防

胃溃疡

米索前列醇是一种前列腺素 E_1 类似物，可降低胃和十二指肠溃疡的风险。H_2- 拮抗剂和质子泵抑制剂分别用于降低十二指肠溃疡和胃溃疡的发生率。对于易发生胃肠道并发症的高风险患者，优先选用选择性 COX-2 拮抗剂。研究还表明，局部应用 NSAIDs，如双氯芬酸，可降低所有年龄段患者的消化性溃疡风险。

血栓形成

心血管事件高危患者，在服用传统的 NSAIDs 和 COX-2 选择性拮抗剂的同时，应服用低剂量阿司匹林。由于传统的 NSAIDs 和阿司匹林抑制 COX-1，可能存在竞争性拮抗作用，可能会增加胃肠道出血的风险。因此，对于服用阿司匹林的患者，H_2- 拮抗剂可能是更好的胃肠道保护选择。奥美拉唑可提高阿司匹林的吸收率。它可以迅速增加水杨酸盐水平，具有潜在的毒性作用。

肾毒性

一般而言，血清肌酐水平在 25 mg/L 或更高的患者，不应常规首选 NSAIDs 治疗。那些接受抗高血压治疗的患者，需要在应用 NSAIDs 治疗期间，密切监测他们的血压。最近的一项研究还表明，与一般人群相比，高血压患者接受 NSAIDs 治疗更可能引起慢性肾疾病。有发生充血性心力衰竭风险的患者，在 NSAIDs 治疗期间也应密切注意监测。

（刘洪君 译 熊源长 校）

延伸阅读

Baraf HS, Gloth FM, Barthel HR, et al.: Safety and efficacy of topical diclofenac sodium gel for knee osteoarthritis in elderly and younger patients: pooled data from three randomized, double blind, parallel-group, placebo-controlled, multicentre trials, *Drugs Aging* 28(1):27–40, 2011.

Boyce EG, Takiya L: Nonsteroidal anti-inflammatory drugs: review of factors guiding formulary selection, *Formulary* 35:142–168, 2000.

Buttgereit F, Burmester GR, Lee LS: Gastrointestinal toxic side effects of nonsteroidal anti-inflammatory drugs and cyclooxygenase-2-specific inhibitors, *Am J Med* 110(Suppl 3A):13S–19S, 2001.

Cannon CP, Curtis SP, Bolognese JA, et al.: Clinical trial design and patient demographics of the Multinational Etoricoxib and Diclofenac Arthritis Long-term (MEDAL) study program: cardiovascular outcomes with etoricoxib versus diclofenac in patients with osteoarthritis and rheumatoid arthritis, *Am Heart J* 152(2):237–245, 2006.

Catella-Lawson F, Crofford LJ: Cyclooxgenase inhibition and thrombogenicity, *Am J Med* 110(Suppl 3A):28S–32S, 2001.

Frishman WH: Effects of nonsteroidal anti-inflammatory drug therapy on blood pressure and peripheral edema, *Am J Card* 89:18D–25D, 2002.

Hsu CC, Wang H, Hsu YH, et al.: Use of nonsteroidal anti-inflammatory drugs and risk of chronic kidney disease in subjects with hypertension: nationwide longitudinal cohort study, *Hypertension* 66(3):524–533, 2015.

Laine L, Curtis SP, Cryer B, et al.: Assessment of upper gastrointestinal safety of etoricoxib and diclofenac in patients with osteoarthritis and rheumatoid arthritis in the multinational etoricoxib and diclofenac arthritis long-term (MEDAL) programme: a randomised comparison, *Lancet* 369(9560):465–473, 2007.

Oviedo JA, Wolfe MM: Gastroprotection by coxibs: what do the Celecoxib Long-Term Arthritis Safety Study and the Vioxx Gastrointestinal Outcomes Research Trial tell us? *Rheum Dis Clin North Am* 29:769–788, 2003.

Pirlamarla P, Bond RM: FDA labeling of NSAIDs: review of nonsteroidal anti-inflammatory drugs in cardiovascular disease, *Trends Cardiovasc Med*, 2016 Apr 29. [epub ahead of print].

Shiotani A, Graham DY: Pathogenesis and therapy of gastric and duodenal ulcer disease, *Med Clin North Am* 86:1447–1466, 2002.

Stevenson DD: Anaphylactic and anaphylactoid reactions to aspirin and other nonsteroidal anti-inflammatory drugs, *Immunol Allergy Clin North Am* 21:745–768, 2001.

Stevenson DD: Aspirin and NSAID sensitivity, *Immunol Allergy Clin North Am* 24:491–503, 2004.

Whelton A: Renal aspects of treatment with conventional nonsteroidal anti-inflammatory drugs versus cyclooxygenase-2-specific inhibitors, *Am J Med* 110(Suppl 3A):33S–42S, 2001.

全肺切除术后并发症 第43章

Harleena Gulati，*Eric Jacobsohn*

病例概要

患者，男性，72 岁，因患非小细胞肺癌拟行右侧肺部切除术。患者长期吸烟，既往有高血压和糖尿病，同时有非 Q 波心肌梗死的病史，并在冠状动脉左前降支放置支架一枚。患者曾在 1 年前进行了核医学应激测试，结果提示心肌缺血为阴性。患者使用的药物包括：阿司匹林、辛伐他汀和美托洛尔。

患者手术过程并不复杂，包括全身麻醉–胸段硬膜外联合麻醉和标准的后外侧胸部切口，术中失血量极少，术中和术后接受限制性补液，术后第 1 天拔除胸管，术后第 3 天患者呼吸困难加重，胸部 X 线片显示左肺弥漫状浸润影伴肺水肿，由于患者进行性呼吸窘迫，对其行气管插管，并开始机械通气，在 100% 氧气，10 cmH_2O 呼气末正压和最佳呼吸机的设置下，患者的血氧饱和度保持在 90% ～ 94% 之间。经慎重评估后行肺动脉置管，并通过胸部 X 线片确定位置正确，测得心排血量和肺动脉楔压低，中度肺动脉高压和跨肺压、右心房压力升高，经食管超声心动图显示轻度右心室和右心房扩张，没有明显的心内分流。诊断性支气管肺泡灌洗发现炎性细胞或微生物为阴性（培养物为阴性），诊断为全肺切除术后肺水肿并发右心室功能障碍。对患者采用了支持性疗法，包括利尿、肺保护通气支持、小剂量多巴酚丁胺、糖皮质激素和吸入前列环素（用于增加肺动脉压和难治性低氧血症）。在术后第 5 天，出现血流动力学不稳定的心房颤动，行电复律处理并开始输注胺碘酮。患者的肌钙蛋白水平增加至 1.1 ng/ml。患者机体完全肝素化，并予 β 受体阻滞剂强化治疗。经过 14 天的支持性治疗：包括早期气管切开，患者成功脱离机械通气，并转出 ICU，血管造影显示稳定的冠状动脉疾病。

问题分析

定义和识别

全肺切除术是非小细胞肺癌有效的外科治疗方法之一。它最常用于涉及肺门的支气管肺癌，是联合化疗和放疗的多模式治疗方法的一部分。但很少用于炎性肺疾病、创伤性肺损伤、先天性肺疾病、不可逆性肺不张的患者。如果考虑用肺叶切除术处理中心位置的病变，则保留实质的袖式肺叶切除术可能有一些益处。虽然从技术上讲，这是一项更为复杂的手术，但也有一些优点，如保留肺功能，避免全肺切除术后并发症，提高患者的生活质量。

胸膜外全肺切除术（extrapleural pneumonectomy，EPP）通常用于局部控制恶性胸膜间皮瘤。除了肺单侧切除术，EPP 手术还需要切除肺、胸膜、心包和膈肌。

全肺切除术是一种导致解剖学和心肺生理学变化的大手术。全肺切除术后并发症包括肺、心血管或其他并发症相对较常见，但可能比较严重甚至会危及生命。框 43.1 中对这些并发症进行了小结。

框 43.1 全肺切除术后并发症

肺
- 低氧血症
- 术后呼吸衰竭
- 肺炎
- 急性肺损伤
- 慢性肺功能减退或缺乏
- 全肺切除术后肺水肿
- 全肺切除术后综合征
- 支气管胸膜瘘
- 肺栓塞
- 脓胸
- 食管胸膜瘘
- 血胸
- 乳糜胸
- 对侧气胸
- 纵隔气肿
- 纵隔感染（纵隔炎症）
- 声带麻痹
- 肺不张

心血管
- 室上性快速性心律失常
- 持续室性心动过速 / 颤动
- 非持续室性心动过速
- 心动过缓
- 心肌梗死
- 心内分流
- 心脏压塞或疝
- 心包积气

其他
- 全肺切除术后瘫痪
- 全肺切除术后脊柱侧弯
- 肺动脉导管数据解读困难
- 伤口感染
- 深静脉血栓形成
- 肾衰竭

风险评估

通过选择合适的患者可以将术后并发症降至最少。需要对患者的呼吸力学 [1 秒用力呼气容积（forced expiratory volume over 1 second，FEV_1）]、心肺储备 [最大摄氧量（maximum oxygen uptake，VO_2 max）] 和肺实质功能 [肺一氧化碳弥散功能（diffusing capacity of the lung for carbon monoxide，DLCO）和动脉血气分析] 进行全面评估（图 43.1）。预测术后 DLCO 是预测术后呼吸系统死亡率增加的最有力指标。对患者任何共存的疾病或病情进行评估和调节治疗亦很重要，包括肥胖、吸烟、可逆性肺部疾病和冠状动脉疾病。

日常肺功能检查 ⇒ FEV_1>60% 或 DLCO >60% ⇒ 进行手术
⇓
FEV_1<60% 或 DLCO <60% ⇒ 进行肺部扫描
⇓
PPO FEV_1 >40% 或 PPO DLCO >40% ⇒ 进行手术
⇓
PPO FEV_1 <40% 或 PPO DLCO <40%
⇓
行VO_2 max运动测试 >15 ml/kg/min ⇒ 进行手术
⇓
VO_2 max <15 ml/kg/min ⇒ 在术前使用其他治疗方法

图 43.1 肺切除患者术前肺评估流程。DLCO，肺 CO 弥散能力；FEV_1，1 秒用力呼气容积；PFT，肺功能测试；PPO，术后预测；VO_2 max：最大摄氧量

死亡率

与左侧全肺切除术相比，右侧全肺切除术与较高的死亡率有关（10% ～ 12% vs. 1% ～ 3.5%）。全肺切除术的适应证可能影响预后；例如，肺癌全肺切除术的死亡率为 3% ～ 4%，而良性疾病的死亡率可能高达 26%。急诊全肺切除术在创伤或大量咯血的情况下，死亡率大于 30%。此外，胸外科医师行全肺切除术的死亡率低于普通外科医师。术前患者相关肺部疾病、冠心病史、充血性心力衰竭史、高血压、心房颤动，脑血管意外，吸烟、手术前 6 个月内体重减轻 10% 或以上，都可增加死亡风险。

全肺切除术术后心肺功能

多项研究观察了全肺切除术后肺和心功能的变化。研究结果小结于框 43.2 中。

全肺切除术后肺功能呈可预测性地下降，但是下降的程度往往小于根据除切除肺叶比例的预测。FEV_1、DLCO 和用力肺活量（forced vital capacity，FVC）通常下降不到 50%。FEV_1 继续以每年 3% ～ 4% 的速度下降。肺动脉氧饱和度、PO_2、PCO_2 在肺相对健康的患者中没有变化。有足够剩余肺功能的患者已被证明能够耐受进一步的大手术。

全肺切除术后心血管功能发生改变，但根据不同的研究其结果不一致。有研究表明，术后右心室射血分数随右心室舒张末期容积增加而降低；但也有不同的研究结果。

管理与预防

全肺切除术后发生的并发症可累及肺、心或与

框 43.2 全肺切除核心肺功能的变化

肺

肺容量下降（<50%）

FEV_1、FVC 下降（<50%）

FEV_1 下降 3 ～ 4 ml/ 年

DLCO 降低（<50%）

肺顺应性降低

呼吸道阻力增加

无效腔增加或减少

Po_2 和 Pco_2 几乎没有变化

心血管

右心室射血分数降低

右心室舒张末期容积增加

肺动脉收缩压瞬时升高

右心房压力增加

DLCO，肺一氧化碳弥散能力；FEV_1，1 秒用力呼气容积；FVC，用力肺活量

心肺系统均无关。

肺部并发症

术后呼吸衰竭

合适的患者选择以及心肺可逆性疾病的判别和治疗，可大大减少术后呼吸衰竭的发生。以下因素也可减少全肺切除术相关围术期呼吸并发症的发生率：

- 手术由一名有资质的胸外科医师在具有较大肺部手术数量的医疗中心实施；
- 合理的围术期肺部康复训练、支气管扩张剂、类固醇和抗生素的使用；
- 手术前戒烟；
- 有效的术后物理治疗和诱发性肺活量测定；
- 良好的术后疼痛控制（如胸段硬膜外镇痛）。

慢性肺功能不全

通过合适的患者选择和肺功能的术前评估，这种情况在很大程度上是可以预防的。

全肺切除术后肺水肿

在接受肺单侧切除术的患者中，肺水肿并发症的发生率高达 5%，而右侧肺叶手术的发生率更高。死亡率超过 50%。全肺切除术后肺水肿导致低氧性呼吸衰竭，胸部 X 线片显示弥漫性浸润，类似于急性呼吸窘迫综合征。通常发生在手术后 72 h 内。其发病机制是多因素的，尚不完全清楚，包括：

- 输注过多液体或者使用新鲜冰冻血浆；
- 单肺通气时的过度肺膨胀损伤；
- 并发肺动脉高压；
- 手术切除肺门淋巴结导致淋巴引流功能受损；
- 隐匿性肺误吸。

目前尚无治疗或预防全肺切除术后肺水肿的具体措施。可能的有益措施包括：避免高血容量和过度利尿，肺保护性通气支持，如果全肺切除术与难治性低氧血症或肺动脉压力升高相关，则可吸入肺动脉血管舒张剂。类固醇治疗仍有争议。这种病情下患者也可能获益于早期气管造口。

全肺切除术后综合征

此综合征是气管远端及主干支气管受外部压迫所致，由纵隔向肺切除一侧移位及残余肺的过度膨胀所引起。它发生在术后 6 个月左右，多见于儿童时期全肺切除术的患者，并且通常是右侧全肺切除术的并发症。治疗包括纵隔改位和用不可吸收的材料填充胸腔。

肺炎

根据研究人群的不同，术后肺炎的发生率为 2% ～ 40%。它与气管再插管率增高、住院时间延长和死亡率增加（高达 19%）有关。建议预防性使用第一代和第二代头孢菌素。

支气管胸膜瘘

支气管胸膜瘘发生率 1.5% ～ 4.5%；它与 30% ～ 80% 的死亡率相关，并且在右侧全肺切除术后更为常见。通常在术后 1 ～ 2 周出现发热、咳痰、咯血、皮下气肿。其他相关因素包括支气管残端大小、肿瘤切除不全、同时放疗或化疗、伤口愈合不良（如虚弱患者、类固醇治疗）。治疗方法包括抗生素治疗、长期胸腔引流，以及在必要时用肌瓣手术修复任何空气泄漏的死腔。

急性呼吸窘迫综合征（ARDS）

全肺切除术后急性呼吸窘迫综合征的发生率为 1% ～ 3%。

肺栓塞

大多数肺栓塞来自于腿部深静脉血栓。它们很少来自于肺动脉残端或肿瘤本身。对于肺血管储备已经减少的患者，这种并发症可能是致命性的。围

术期深静脉血栓形成的正确预防至关重要。处理包括抗凝，但也可能术后立即需要行紧急血栓切除术。对于不能手术切除的患者，应考虑静脉溶栓。对于那些有明显的深静脉血栓形成和无肺栓塞的患者，可建议放置可回收的下腔静脉过滤器。

其他肺部并发症

其他并发症包括脓胸、乳糜胸和急性血胸、食管胸膜瘘、对侧气胸和声带麻痹。治疗可能需要手术（切开和引流、瘘管闭合、纵隔改位，以及用不可吸收材料填充空胸腔）。对于部分或完全声带麻痹，建议请耳鼻喉科医师会诊。

心脏并发症

心律失常

房性快速性心律失常（见 161 章），尤其是心房扑动或颤动，在胸外科手术后很常见，约 20% 的病例发生。80% 发生在术后 72 h 内。心律失常的危险因素包括：年龄 60 岁以上、右侧全肺切除术、经心包全肺切除术、既往有冠心病和慢性高血压。全肺切除术后房性快速心律失常的一级预防是 β 受体阻滞剂——任何常见的 β 受体为主的阻滞剂或索他洛尔（既是 β 受体阻滞剂，同时还具有Ⅲ类抗心律失常的活性）（见第 161 章）。胺碘酮也可能有效，而且越来越多的证据表明，胺碘酮在全肺切除术或开胸术后预防心房颤动中发挥作用。肺毒性可发生于短期应用胺碘酮的患者，长期应用则更为常见。血流动力学不稳定的心房扑动或颤动需要立即进行直流电复律，并根据现有指南（高级心血管生命支持）进行进一步的治疗和预防（见第 161 章）。

心肌梗死

胸外科手术患者发生围术期心肌梗死（myocardial infarction，MI）的发生率为 1% ～ 5%。围术期预防性应用 β 受体阻滞剂可减少急性 MI 和其他胸外科手术后的心脏事件发生率。接受全肺切除术患者的术前风险分层应遵循美国心脏学会（American Heart Association-American College of Cardiology）的新指南，该指南将全肺切除术归类为一种风险较高的外科手术（已去除中度风险类别）。病例概述中所描述的患者已经血运重建并具有身体活动能力。在计划行全肺切除术的前一年，他的应激试验呈阴性，无需再进一步的术前测试。所有接受长期 β 受体阻滞剂治疗的患者，应该继续这些药物。已知患有冠状动脉疾病或外周血管疾病的患者，以及有 2 个或 2 个以上的冠状动脉疾病的危险因素 [年龄超过 65 岁、治疗或未治疗的高血压、糖尿病、高胆固醇血症，当前或近期 MI（≤ 6 个月）] 的患者，应该接受围术期 β 受体阻滞剂治疗。

对于有冠状动脉疾病或外周血管疾病的患者，在大手术术前常规停用阿司匹林治疗可能是禁忌。然而，是否停止这种治疗应根据患者的个体化病情决定。长期使用阿司匹林治疗的冠状动脉疾病患者突然停药可能会出现导致急性心肌梗死的阿司匹林停药综合征。必须考虑心脑血管疾病的严重程度，以及支架的存在和使用年限等因素。停用阿司匹林的风险必须和继续应用可能增加出血的风险进行权衡。

越来越多的证据表明，他汀类药物在心血管疾病患者围术期可能具有保护作用。这可能与药物的多效性有关。服用他汀类药物的患者在围术期不应中断治疗。

心内分流

全肺切除术后 30% 的人群中可能出现卵圆孔开放。如果右心压力升高，可引起明显的右向左分流和严重的低氧血症。这可能是由于患者选择不当、术前肺动脉压升高、肺栓塞、肺炎、气胸、全肺切除术后肺水肿或肺误吸所致。治疗右心房压升高的潜在原因至关重要。这包括优化右心室功能和降低肺动脉压力（如果升高）。措施包括吸入性肺动脉血管扩张剂，如前列环素或一氧化氮。某些患者可能需要经皮闭合分流术。

心脏疝

通过心包缺损引起的心脏疝可以发生于术后任何时间。除了由于心包缺损造成的疝外，如果不小心将胸管置于吸引器上，心脏或纵隔内容物也可能会疝入胸膜腔。因此，许多外科医师认为在全肺切除术后禁忌常规放置胸管放置，即使短时间放置也是禁忌的。心脏疝表现为突发性低血压和休克、发绀、胸痛以及上腔静脉综合征的症状。需行紧急重新开胸使心脏复位。术中将心包边缘缝合至心肌或在心包缺损处放置假体补片均可预防该并发症的发生。如果是由无意中的胸管抽吸，必须立即停止。

改变患者体位，肺切除侧向上可能对患者也有帮助。

与心肺系统无关的并发症

这里只讨论了与心肺无关的一些比较常见和难处理的并发症。

全肺切除术后脊髓缺血和瘫痪

这是由于术中肋间动脉对脊髓胸腰椎区域的损伤引起的罕见并发症，导致脊柱前动脉综合征。治疗方法有限，且大多未经证实。它们包括维持高的脊髓灌注压力和使用脑脊液引流。

全肺切除术后的脊柱侧凸

据估计，接受过全肺切除术的患者 90% 会发生脊柱侧凸。这种并发症是由于手术后胸腔收缩引起的。相关症状通常较轻，且大多无关紧要。

肺动脉导管数据解读困难

全肺切除术通常不需要肺动脉导管或中心静脉通路。然而，如果在胸外科手术中使用肺动脉导管，需要注意的是，根据导管漂浮到哪侧肺或肺段（如重力依赖区或非重力依赖区）、是否使用单肺通气以及何时进行读数，从导管中获得的数据可能有所不同。根据临床情况，肺动脉导管有可能提供误导的数据。如果在术后期间放置，在新缝合或钉合的肺动脉内漂浮和充气气球时必须谨慎。此外，应考虑在透视或超声心动图指导下漂浮放置肺动脉导管。

其他并发症

全肺切除术后的其他并发症主要累及胃肠道系统，包括运动障碍和胃扭转。内科或外科治疗均为可行的治疗方法；如有必要，当出现这些并发症时，应该立即寻求相应的专科会诊。

（董 朋 译 马 宇 校）

延伸阅读

Attar S, Hankins JR, Turney SZ, et al.: Paraplegia after thoracotomy: report of five cases and review of the literature, *Ann Thorac Surg* 59:1410–1415, 1995.

Bachamn DS: Discontinuing chronic aspirin therapy: another risk factor for stroke? *Ann Neurol* 51:137–138, 2002.

Cerfolio RJ, Bryant AS, Thurber JS, et al.: Intraoperative Solu-Medrol helps prevent postpneumonectomy pulmonary edema, *Ann Thorac Surg* 76:1029–1033, 2003.

Collins G, Jacobsohn E: Complications after pneumonectomy. In Atlee JL, editor: *Complications in anesthesia*, 2nd ed, Philadelphia, 2007, Elsevier, pp 376–379.

Datta D, Lahiri B: Preoperative evaluation of patients undergoing lung resection surgery, *Chest* 123:2096–2103, 2003.

De Wet CJ, Affleck DJ, Jacobsohn E, et al.: Inhaled prostacyclin is safe, effective, and affordable in patients with pulmonary hypertension, right heart dysfunction, and refractory hypoxemia after cardiothoracic surgery, *J Thorac Cardiovasc Surg* 127:1058–1067, 2004.

De Wet CJ, McConnell K, Jacobsohn E: Progress in postoperative ICU management, *Thorac Surg Clin* 15:159–180, 2005.

Eagle KA, Berger PB, Calkins H, et al.: ACC/AHA update for perioperative cardiovascular evaluation for noncardiac surgery, *Circulation* 105:1257–1267, 2002.

Fleisher LA, Fleischmann KE, Auerbach AD, et al.: 2014 ACC/AHA guideline on perioperative cardiovascular evaluation and management of patients undergoing noncardiac surgery: executive summary: a report of the American College of Cardiology/American Heart Association Task Force on Practice Guidelines, *Circulation* 130(24):2215–2245, 2014.

Guggino G, Doddoli C, Barlesi F, et al.: Completion pneumonectomy in cancer patients: experience with 55 cases, *Eur J Cardiothorac Surg* 25:449–455, 2004.

Handschin AE, Lardinois D, Schneiter D, et al.: Acute amiodarone-induced pulmonary toxicity following lung resection, *Respiration* 70:310–312, 2003.

Hoff WS, Hoey BA, Wainwright GA, et al.: Early experience with retrievable inferior vena cava filters in high-risk trauma patients, *J Am Coll Surg* 199:869–874, 2004.

Kertai MD, Boersma E, Westerhout CM, et al.: A combination of statins and beta-blockers is independently associated with a reduction in the incidence of perioperative mortality and nonfatal myocardial infarction in patients undergoing abdominal aortic aneurysm surgery, *Eur J Vasc Endovasc Surg* 28:343–352, 2004.

Khan SN, Stansby G: Cerebrospinal fluid drainage for thoracic and thoracoabdominal aortic aneurysm surgery, *Cochrane Database Syst Rev* 4:CD003635, 2003.

Miller DL, Deschamps C, Jenkins GD, et al.: Completion pneumonectomy: factors affecting operative mortality and cardiopulmonary morbidity, *Ann Thorac Surg* 74:876–883, 2002.

Ng J: Extrapleural pneumonectomy. In Slinger P, editor: *Principles and practice of anesthesia for thoracic surgery*, New York, 2011, Springer, pp 395–403.

Pedoto A, Amar D: Respiratory, renal, and cardiovascular postoperative complications. In Barbeito A, Shaw AD, Grichnik K, editors: *Thoracic anesthesia*, New York, 2012, Lange, pp 440–466.

Poldermans D, Boersma E, Bax JJ, et al.: The effect of bisoprolol on perioperative mortality and myocardial infarction in high-risk patients undergoing vascular surgery. Dutch Echocardiographic Cardiac Risk Evaluation Applying Stress Echocardiography Study Group, *N Engl J Med* 341:1789–1794, 1999.

Rahimtoola A, Bergin JD: Acute pulmonary embolism: an update on diagnosis and management, *Curr Probl Cardiol* 30:61–114, 2005.

Senior K: Aspirin withdrawal increases risk of heart problems, *Lancet* 362:1558, 2003.

Slinger P: Update on anesthetic management of pneumonectomy, *Curr Opin Anaesthesiol* 22:31–37, 2009.

Sugarbaker DJ, Jaklitsch MT, Bueno R, et al.: Prevention, early detection, and management of complications after 328 consecutive extrapleural pneumonectomies, *J Thorac Cardiovasc Surg* 128:138–146, 2004.

Van Mieghem W, Coolen L, Malysse I, et al.: Amiodarone and the development of ARDS after lung surgery, *Chest* 105:1642–1645, 1994.

Vaporciyan AA, Correa AM, Rice DC, et al.: Risk factors associated with atrial fibrillation after noncardiac thoracic surgery: analysis of 2588 patients, *J Thorac Cardiovasc Surg* 127:779–786, 2004.

第44章 肾上腺手术的并发症

Rajeshwari Subramaniam

病例概要 1

嗜铬细胞瘤

患者，女性，38 岁，主诉为近 1 年反复发作心悸、头痛、发汗，偶有右侧腹痛，近 2 月出现颈部肿胀。经检查，患者有严重高血压（220/130 mmHg）；颈前部有一个 3 cm 的甲状腺结节。腹部超声提示右侧肾上腺肿块。患者被收治入院接受进一步的评估、调整，拟行肾上腺肿块切除术。

病例概要 2

库欣综合征

患者，男性，45 岁，因进行性近端肌无力、下腰痛及全身水肿 6 周到内分泌科门诊就诊。经检查发现患者存在双侧肾上腺增生，皮质醇和促肾上腺皮质激素（adrenocorticotropic hormone，ACTH）水平升高，低钾血症和代谢性碱中毒。并且患者在住院期间病情迅速恶化，遂立即行急诊肾上腺切除术。

病例概要 3

Conn 综合征

患者，男性，56 岁，患有胆结石，发现无症状低钾血症（K^+ 浓度为 2.0 mmol/L）。有高血压病史，正在接受治疗。计算机断层扫描术（CT）结果显示左肾上腺肿瘤大小为 2.7 cm × 2.4 cm，患者被收治入院，拟择期行腹腔镜肾上腺切除术 + 胆囊切除术。

问题分析

定义

肾上腺疾病来源于皮质（产生过量皮质醇、盐皮质激素及雄激素）和髓质（产生过量儿茶酚胺及其代谢产物）。皮质相关疾病包括库欣综合征和 Conn 综合征（原发性醛固酮增多症），前者通常为双侧增生，后者通常由单个腺瘤引起。**库欣病**由垂体分泌 ACTH 促进肾上腺增生导致，伴有色素沉着。ACTH 来源于其他部位所致的**库欣综合征**（异位 ACTH）常伴有双侧肾上腺增生和严重皮质醇过剩症状。嗜铬细胞瘤是起源于神经嵴的肿瘤，可发生于交感神经干和肾上腺髓质的任何部位。通常将位于肾上腺髓质的肿瘤称为**嗜铬细胞瘤**，其他称为**副神经节瘤**。它们不仅分泌肾上腺素、去甲肾上腺素和多巴胺，其代谢产物甲氧基肾上腺素和甲氧基去甲肾上腺素可通过瘤内儿茶酚胺 -O- 甲基转移酶（catecholamine-O-methyltransferase，COMT）来代谢。去甲肾上腺素由苯乙醇胺 -N- 甲基转移酶

（phenylethanolamine-N-methyl-transferase，PNMT）发生甲基化作用，转变为肾上腺素。大部分嗜铬细胞瘤是单侧的。双侧肿瘤与先天性综合征有关，主要见于儿童。肾上腺外嗜铬细胞瘤（副神经节瘤）很少产生肾上腺素，可能是多发性或恶性的，与琥珀酰脱氢酶（SDH）基因亚基的基因突变有关。呈明显散发的嗜铬细胞瘤，高达 25% 的可能是遗传或家族性的。在嗜铬细胞瘤患者中发现有 5 个基因（RET 原癌基因，VHL 基因，NF1 基因，SDH 亚基 D 和 B）发生生殖系突变。

相当比例（10% ～ 30%）的嗜铬细胞瘤可表现为"偶发瘤"。这些患者可能尚未表现出任何症状，但在手术期间会出现严重的血压和心率波动。

肾上腺恶性肿瘤的发生与雄激素过量、皮质醇 / 盐皮质激素过量以及肿瘤的压力效应有关。

不管病因如何，几乎所有肾上腺肿瘤患者均出现了显著的继发性高血压。皮质醇 / 盐皮质激素分泌过多也会导致代谢紊乱，如高血糖、低钾血症和代谢性碱中毒等。

识别

嗜铬细胞瘤

高血压合并头痛、心悸、发汗等临床症状提示嗜铬细胞瘤。高血压可呈持续性，也可呈偶发性。嗜铬细胞瘤症状多样，可表现为高血压、心脏病、神经症状或代谢危象，有类似表现者须高度怀疑。儿茶酚胺过量产生是诊断嗜铬细胞瘤的第一步。血浆游离甲氧基肾上腺素等物质对嗜铬细胞瘤的诊断灵敏度最高，它的缺乏排除嗜铬细胞瘤。肿瘤的大小、位置与血浆游离甲氧基肾上腺素浓度呈良好的相关性。如果血浆游离甲氧基肾上腺素的含量超过血浆甲氧基肾上腺素和甲氧基去甲肾上腺素总和的 15%，则肿瘤很可能位于肾上腺。对肿瘤进行解剖定位可通过磁共振成像和 MIBG/DOTANOC-PET 扫描进行。

库欣综合征

糖皮质激素和盐皮质激素在皮质中合成，控制着包括葡萄糖稳态和 Na^+/K^+ 平衡在内的多种代谢过程。库欣综合征可由原发性肾上腺增生或异位来源 ACTH 刺激所致。肾上腺增生继发于垂体微腺瘤产生过量 ACTH，并导致库欣病。异位 ACTH 肿瘤导致肾上腺增生、色素沉着和皮质醇过量的特征。

库欣综合征的临床表现较突出，包括躯干肥胖、皮下脂肪薄、易淤伤、腹纹、近端肌无力、高血压及高血糖等。虽然临床表现明显，但监测到高浓度的血清皮质醇才能确诊，须实施地塞米松抑制试验和促肾上腺皮质释放激素试验。在不产生 ACTH 的肿瘤中，前者导致 ACTH 浓度下降至非常低的水平，而在原发性垂体疾病中后者会导致 ACTH 释放显著增加，但肾上腺肿瘤或异位 ACTH 患者则表现为阴性。

Conn 综合征

原发性醛固酮增多症（Conn 综合征）伴随低钾血症、代谢性碱中毒、高钠血症、严重高血压、肌无力、多尿和口渴，通常由孤立腺瘤引起。肾功能不全可继发于高血压。血清醛固酮浓度升高和血浆肾素浓度降低可确诊。Conn 综合征占所有继发性高血压病例的 0.5% ～ 3%。

肾上腺癌

肾上腺恶性肿瘤与性激素、皮质醇和醛固酮的过量分泌有关。临床表现为雄激素的男性化作用、库欣综合征的症状和体征以及醛固酮的过量产生（低钾血症和高血压）。通过放射学检查可进行诊断。

肾上腺皮质和髓质肿瘤在初步内科治疗后，控制症状，使代谢调节至最优状态，最终治疗方法仍是肾上腺切除术。

风险评估和启示

肾上腺切除术有很高的不良事件发生率。库欣综合征患者行双侧肾上腺切除术后，围术期死亡率可达 5% ～ 10%。此手术对患者的影响与患者个体的肾上腺病变、病因和手术过程相关（表 44.1）（见下文讨论）。

嗜铬细胞瘤：围术期启示

术前问题及准备

患者术前多为重度高血压，需进行评估和控制。心血管受累包括心肌缺血、心律失常或充血性心力衰竭（儿茶酚胺心肌病）。血液循环中的儿茶酚胺可导致严重的血管收缩，表现为面色苍白及血细胞比容增高。选择性 α - 受体阻滞剂为首选治疗药物，可同时控制血压和症状。酚苄明现已被多沙唑嗪和哌唑嗪取代。如增加 α - 受体阻滞剂剂量不能获得

表 44.1 肾上腺手术的围术期并发症

术前问题		
嗜铬细胞瘤	库欣综合征	Conn 综合征
高血压	高血压	高血压
心脏损害	高血糖症	低钾血症
血管收缩	代谢性碱中毒	
	低钾血症	
	困难气道，血管通路	
	骨质减少	
	免疫抑制	

术中并发症	
与疾病相关的并发症	与手术入路 / 技术相关的并发症
血流动力学不稳定：高血压 / 低血压 / 肺水肿 / 充血性心力衰竭	气腹相关的血流动力学改变
心律失常	血管损伤及出血
低钾血症	实质器官损害
代谢性碱中毒	膈肌损伤，气胸
葡萄糖稳态	肠道损伤

术后并发症	
与肾上腺切除相关的并发症	手术操作相关
低血压	肺部并发症
低血糖症	深静脉血栓形成
高钾血症	创面感染
类固醇 / 盐皮质激素依赖	

满意的血压控制效果，可适当加入钙通道阻滞剂和可乐定。随后可加入 β - 受体阻滞剂用于控制心率和心律失常。术前须做心电图、血压、心率及超声心动图检查。高血糖很常见，或需胰岛素治疗。此外，α - 受体介导的胰岛素抑制作用超越 β - 胰岛素释放作用，可导致嗜铬细胞瘤患者葡萄糖耐受不良。

术中高血压

在嗜铬细胞瘤患者中，大多数严重高血压发生于可引起交感神经刺激的麻醉诱导期（如喉镜检查、气管插管、口胃管或鼻胃管插入等）。使用迷走神经抑制剂可导致儿茶酚胺分泌，组胺释放或多巴胺受体阻滞，从而诱发高血压。这些药物包括氯胺酮、大剂量吗啡、阿托品、泮库溴铵、氟哌利多、甲氧氯普胺、氟烷和地氟烷等。在镇痛效果不佳的情况下，用力的外科消毒、摆放体位或切皮也可导致血压迅速上升。这些情况下的高血压是由交感神经末梢释放大量储存的儿茶酚胺所致，这种高血压一般可控制（如增加麻醉深度）。相比之下，气腹、直接操作或手术中挤压腺体可导致高血压危象，需要使用多种血管舒张药来控制。血浆去甲肾上腺素浓度高、肿瘤体积大、使用 α - 受体阻滞剂后重度直立性血压下降（>10 mmHg）、平均动脉压高于 100 mmHg 以及有症状的高血压，这些因素都被认为与术中严重的血流动力学不稳定有关。使用多沙唑嗪，术中血流动力学较稳定。家族性嗜铬细胞瘤往往存在更为严重的高血压。

术中严重高血压的后果

控制不佳或严重的术中高血压可导致心肌缺血、肺水肿或充血性心力衰竭。它很少发展为需要透析和呼吸机支持的多系统器官衰竭。据报道，气腹操作时严重的术中高血压和血管收缩可导致横纹肌溶解，术中儿茶酚胺危象可导致瞳孔散大和肺水肿。

术中高血压的处理

可使用酚妥拉明（10～20 mg）、硝普钠（0.01% 溶液滴定至起效）、硝酸甘油 [1 ～ 2 μg/（kg · min）] 和硫酸镁（30 ～ 50 mg/kg 推注，1 ～ 2 g/h 输注）治疗术中高血压。硫酸镁具有多种益处：抑制儿茶酚胺的释放，阻断儿茶酚胺对肾上腺受体的作用，是一种抗心律失常药。它也被证明对应激性心肌病有效，这种心肌病通常与嗜铬细胞瘤相关。据报道，尼卡地平（5 ～ 10 mg/h）和非诺多泮 [0.2 mg/（kg · min）] 已用于耐药患者。乌拉地尔输注（10 ～ 15 mg/h）已成功用于腹腔镜嗜铬细胞瘤切除术中预防血流动力学危象。最近发现，右美托咪定 [0.3～0.7 μg/(kg · h)] 有助于术中血流动力学的管理。

心律失常

在肿瘤切除过程中，常见室上性心律失常，偶可发生室性异位或心律不齐。0.5 mg/kg 艾司洛尔用于室上性心律失常，1 mg/kg 利多卡因用于室性心律失常，胺碘酮更适用于心肌收缩力受损的患者。拉贝洛尔（10 ～ 20 mg 推注）也可用于分泌肾上腺素为主的嗜铬细胞瘤患者。

低血压

持续性低血压是嗜铬细胞瘤肾上腺切除术后恢复室或重症监护室停留时间延长的最常见原因。术后低血压的原因有多种，包括 α- 肾上腺素受体的下调、长效 α- 受体阻滞剂的残留效应或术中给予血管扩张剂、对侧肾上腺抑制或血容量不足。极少数情况下，低血压可能在手术后持续 1 ～ 3 天。大多数患者在手术后 10 天内血压恢复正常。肿瘤大于 60 mm、尿肾上腺素水平大于每天 200 mg 和尿去甲肾上腺素水平大于每天 600 mg 是长期低血压的独立预测因素，需要术后给予儿茶酚胺支持。与酚苄明相比，使用多沙唑嗪术后低血压的发生率更高。血容量的增加可能并不预防低血压。药物通常选择去甲肾上腺素滴定（通常 4 ～ 20 μg/min），其他药物包括去氧肾上腺素（10 ～ 100 μg 推注或输注）、麻黄碱推注（5 ～ 10 mg），较少使用肾上腺素（1 ～ 10 μg/min）。难治性低血压可能还需使用血管加压素（0.1 ～ 0.4 U/min），但有心肌缺血的风险。

低血糖

嗜铬细胞瘤切除术后低血糖并不少见，可隐匿出现。这可能是因胰岛素反跳性分泌过多引起。术后短暂清醒或延迟苏醒后又出现嗜睡或昏迷，通常提示低血糖。这种情况的发生很罕见，因此定期监测血糖非常必要。

Conn 综合征：围术期启示

低钾血症和高钠血症是 Conn 综合征（原发性醛固酮增多症）的常见表现。严重代谢性碱中毒也很常见，应注意避免过度通气。钾替代治疗和螺内酯可能对低钾血症无效。低钾血症和碱中毒可增强和延长神经肌肉阻滞药物的作用。低钾可增加心肌兴奋性和术中心律失常的风险，并可因通气增强和七氟烷诱发的多尿而恶化。在需进行有创监测的 Conn 综合征患者中，术中对肾上腺的操作可使患者迅速释放儿茶酚胺，并常常伴有难治性高血压。多次动脉血气评估可指导呼吸机支持治疗。

原发性醛固酮增多症（Conn 综合征）患者实施肾上腺切除术后也可出现低血压，通过给予氟氢可的松可纠正。此外，术后约有 5% 的患者可发生高钾血症，通常伴有直立性低血压。其病因被认为是由于抑制了对侧肾上腺盐皮质激素的活性。补充盐皮质激素治疗效果显著。

库欣综合征：围术期启示

由于向心性肥胖、“水牛背”并且存在低氧血症，这些患者通常为困难气道。严重代谢性碱中毒常导致呼吸抑制和酸中毒、肺不张和低氧血症。由于肺顺应性差，可能发生术中通气困难从而加重现有的高碳酸血症和低氧血症。低钾血症是由盐皮质激素作用较弱引起的。近 80% 的库欣综合征患者患有糖尿病，因此在围术期控制血糖十分重要。血糖水平的升高与死亡率升高、感染率升高和住院时间延长息息相关。美国临床内分泌学家协会（American Association of Clinical Endocrinologists）和美国糖尿病协会（American Diabetes Association）的指南建议重症监护病房的血糖目标值为 140 ～ 180 mg/dl，围术期为 100 ～ 180 mg/dl。由于这类患者容易骨折和擦伤，进行体位摆放时要特别小心。血管穿刺置管和中心静脉穿刺尤其具有挑战性。最近一项对 300 多名患者进行的大型研究报告表明，接受肾上腺切除术的库欣综合征患者需常规类固醇替代治疗，并应在术前开始使用。

极少数情况下，皮质醇增多症可能难以治疗甚至危及生命，导致不受控制的全身水肿、代谢性碱中毒和低钾血症，须进行紧急肾上腺切除术。

肾上腺手术外科并发症

自 1992 年 Gagner 等发表文章以来，腹腔镜肾上腺切除术已成为肾上腺切除术的标准，开腹手术仅适用于 10 cm 以上的肿瘤或肾上腺恶性肿瘤。开腹手术可导致肺炎高发、再次气管插管、呼吸机脱机失败、脓毒症、心脏停搏、肾功能不全、伤口感染和 30 天高发病率等。腹腔镜路径具有高分辨率、放大率，止血效果好，减少血流动力学波动和出血量，术后疼痛轻，美观，行走和恢复快等优点。

气腹和血流动力学改变

早期研究报道，腹腔镜下嗜铬细胞瘤切除术因二氧化碳注入可引起严重高血压。然而后来的研究表明，腹腔镜路径有放大手术视野、显微操作、“切开部位远离肿瘤”等优点。“腹内压力低于 10 mmHg 与儿茶酚胺释放较少且血流动力学变化较小有关。”然而有报道，气腹开始后发生血管扩张剂难以控制的严重高血压和肺水肿，最终行开放手术。

血管损伤和出血

血管损伤是腹腔镜肾上腺切除术最常见的手术并发症，常累及下腔静脉 / 右肾上腺静脉，发病率在 0.7% ～ 5.4%。据报道，在腹腔镜肾上腺手术中，血液替代品的需求高达10%。气腹的压力可阻止较小的静脉出血，这可能在术后表现为血肿或血流动力学不稳定。

肠损伤

大多数肾上腺切除术期间肠损伤被发现时较晚（> 72 h），患者出现腹膜炎并且与高死亡率相关。

肝、脾和胰腺损伤

这些器官在每一侧都很容易受损（即右侧肾上腺切除术时肝易受损和左侧肾上腺切除术时脾和胰腺易受损）。

胸膜和膈肌损伤

气腹时腹内压升高，气体容易经烧伤或利器损伤造成的横隔小的病变进入胸膜腔。据报道，腹腔镜肾手术时此并发症的发生率为0.6%；目前尚无相应的肾上腺切除术发生率的数据报道。

气道压力的增加是麻醉科医师须注意的胸膜破裂的第一个信号，并且伴随呼气末二氧化碳的增加以及血氧饱和度和血压的逐渐下降。这些改变通常可伴有腹内高压，容易与继发于气腹的气管导管移位相混淆，可能导致诊断延迟。高度怀疑这种可能性的发生对及时诊断至关重要。胸膜腔内负压消失导致膈肌在每次释放压力时都翻滚进入腹腔（“软膈膜”征）。横膈膜裂口小可于内镜下缝合；大型气胸须肋间引流24 ～ 48 h。

腹腔镜肾上腺切除术的主要手术并发症

最近有报道称，腹腔镜肾上腺切除术出现了一系列罕见且严重的可危及生命的并发症，原因归结为外科医师缺乏经验或发生在大型转诊中心以外。包括完全横断肝门、结扎肝动脉、结扎输尿管、结扎肾动脉以及切除正常肾上腺。前两种情况，肝衰竭需要进行肝移植。第三和第四种情况的患者肾功能已丧失，最终需要进行肾切除术。

术后激素替代

接受类固醇治疗的患者中严重感染和住院时间延长较为常见。

肾上腺切除术后肺部并发症

多达85%的库欣综合征患者行开放性肾上腺切除术后会出现肺部并发症，如肺不张和肺炎等。而腹腔镜手术的应用极大地降低了肺部并发症的发生率。

库欣综合征的静脉血栓栓塞

库欣综合征患者行肾上腺切除术后，肺血栓栓塞的发生率明显升高，其原因可能为糖皮质激素诱发高凝状态，以及手术和肥胖。由于皮质醇相关的止血和溶纤维蛋白标志物的改变，库欣综合征患者表现出促凝表型，从而导致静脉血栓栓塞发生率增加，需进一步采取血栓预防措施。

总之，许多肾上腺切除术患者围术期并发症是由原发性疾病导致的。术前进行重点评估和优化、采用有创监测、术中积极控制血流动力学和代谢等可将发生率降至最低。手术并发症可能较轻微也可能呈灾难性，可通过经验丰富的外科医师在手术体量较大的转诊中心进行手术来尽量减少术后并发症。

（翟学花　译　倪丽亚　校）

延伸阅读

Agrawal R, Mishra SK, Bhatia E, et al.: Prospective study to compare perioperative hemodynamic alterations following preparation for pheochromocytoma surgery by phenoxybenzamine or prazosin, *World J Surg* 38:716–723, 2014.

Bittner IVJG, Gershuni VM, Mathews BD, et al.: Risk factors affecting operative approach, conversion, and morbidity for adrenalectomy: a single-institution series of 402 patients, *Surg Endosc* 27:2342–2350, 2013.

Brunt LM: Positive impact of laparoscopic adrenalectomy on complications of adrenal surgery, *Surg Endosc* 16:252–257, 2002.

Bruynzeel H, Feelders RA, Groenland THN, et al.: Risk factors for hemodynamic instability during surgery for pheochromocytoma, *J Clin Endocrinol Metab* 95:678–685, 2010.

Ferrau F, Korbonits M: Metabolic comorbidities in Cushing's syndrome, *Eur J Endocrinol* 173:M133–M157, 2015.

Gaujoux S, Bonnet S, Lentschener C, et al.: Preoperative risk factors of hemodynamic instability during laparoscopic adrenalectomy for pheochromocytoma, *Surg Endosc* 30:2984–2993, 2016.

Habbe N, Ruger F, Bojunga J, et al.: Urapidil in the preoperative treatment of pheochromocytomas: a safe and cost-effective method, *World J Surg* 37:1141–1146, 2013.

Iijima T, Takagi T, Iwao Y: An increased circulating blood volume does not prevent hypotension after pheochromocytoma resection, *Can J Anesth* 51:212–215, 2004.

James MF, Cronje L: Pheochromocytoma crisis: the use of magnesium sulfate, *Anesth Analg* 99:680–686, 2004.

Jano A, Domi R, Berdica L, et al.: Anesthetic considerations of Conn syndrome: a case presentation and mini-review: the anesthesiologist and Conn syndrome, *J Clin Med Res* 3:132–135, 2014.

Jyotsna VP: Role of bilateral adrenalectomy in adrenocorticotropic hormone dependent Cushing's syndrome, *Indian J Endocrinol Metab* 19(5):537–540, 2015.

Kiernan CM, Du L, Chen X, et al.: Predictors of hemodynamic instability during surgery for pheochromocytoma, *Ann Surg Oncol* 21:3865–3871, 2014.

Manetti L, Bogazzi F, Giovannetti C, et al.: Changes in coagulation indexes and occurrence of venous thromboembolism in patients with Cushing's syndrome: results from a prospective study before and after surgery, *Eur J Endocrinol* 163:783–791, 2010.

Namekawa T, Utsumi T, Kawamura K, et al.: Clinical predictors of prolonged postresection hypotension after laparoscopic adrenalectomy for pheochromocytoma, *Surgery* 159:763–770, 2016.

Sharma A, Subramaniam R, Misra MC, et al.: Anesthetic management of emergent laparoscopic bilateral adrenalectomy in a patient with a life-threatening cortisol crisis, *A&A Case Rep* 4:15–18, 2015.

Shen WT, Lee J, Kebebew E, et al.: Selective use of steroid replacement after adrenalectomy: lessons from 331 consecutive cases, *Arch Surg* 141:771–776, 2006.

Sood J, Jayaraman L, Kumra VP, et al.: Laparoscopic approach to pheochromocytoma: is a lower intra-abdominal pressure helpful? *Anesth Analg* 102:637–641, 2006.

Subramaniam R: Pheochromocytoma—current concepts in diagnosis and management, *Trends Anaesth Crit Care* 1:104–110, 2011.

Tahir A, McLaughlin K, Kline G: Severe hyperkalemia following adrenalectomy for aldosteronoma: prediction, pathogenesis and approach to clinical management—a case series, *BMC Endocr Disord* 16:43–50, 2016.

Tessier DJ, Iglesias R, Chapman WC, et al.: Previously unreported high-grade complications of adrenalectomy, *Surg Endosc* 23:97–102, 2009.

Thonangi RP, Bhardwaj M, Kulshreshtha B: A case report of reactive hypoglycemia in a patient with pheochromocytoma and its review of literature, *Indian J Endocrinol Metab* 18:234–237, 2014.

van der Zee PA, de Boer A: Pheochromocytoma: a review on preoperative treatment with phenoxybenzamine or doxazosin, *Neth J Med* 72:190–201, 2014.

第45章 类癌并发症

Kerri M. Wahl

病例概要

患者，男性，55岁，因小肠梗阻拟行紧急剖腹探查术。麻醉诱导方法为静脉推注芬太尼、利多卡因、丙泊酚和琥珀胆碱，吸入七氟烷与空气-氧气混合物以及静脉推注维库溴铵维持麻醉。手术过程中，患者出现严重低血压，且对加速输液、应用麻黄碱和肾上腺素无反应。患者的面部和颈部潮红。

问题分析

定义

类癌是一种神经内分泌肿瘤，原发于胃肠道（67.5%位于中肠：回肠、阑尾、直肠、胰腺）或肠外如肺、支气管（25.3%位于前肠）。原发性中肠类癌可转移至肝或区域淋巴结，且可能出现肠梗阻。它们可能不具有分泌功能，也可能与面部潮红、腹泻、心脏瓣膜纤维化和支气管收缩有关。肿瘤合成、储存和释放多达40种生物活性介质，其中最主要是血清素、5-羟色氨酸、组胺、缓激肽、速激肽和前列腺素。肝通常可使分泌至门静脉的介质失活。因此，类癌综合征是由于血管活性胺、多肽、蛋白质和前列腺素直接进入体循环。这可能发生在胃肠道肿瘤肝转移、原发性肝类癌和无门静脉引流的原发性肿瘤（支气管、卵巢、腹膜后）。在类癌细胞中，70%的色氨酸转化为5-羟色胺，然后在肝、肺和脑中通过单胺氧化酶代谢为5-HIAA（5-羟吲哚乙酸），并最终通过尿液排泄。5-羟色胺的吸收和储存也发生在血小板中。尿5-羟色胺通常保持正常水平或轻度增加。

类癌的发病率为每年10万人中1.2～2.1人，而尸检结果的发病率更高达8%。发病率最高的是非洲裔美国男性，4.5/10万人。75%～80%的类癌综合征患者为小肠肿瘤。小肠类癌患者发病年龄通常为50～60岁，最常见的是肿瘤的体积效应（如腹痛或梗阻）。大多数小肠类癌在发现时已有转移，约5%合并类癌综合征。5年总生存率为80%，伴远处转移者则下降至20%。

类癌综合征的急性加重可导致危及生命的类癌"危象"，引起严重的皮肤潮红、低血压或血压剧烈波动、昏迷、腹泻、精神错乱、支气管痉挛、心律失常以及高热。这些危象可由肿瘤活动、麻醉诱导和气管插管、镇痛不足、手术应激、药物引起的介质释放、化疗以及肝动脉栓塞引发。

识别

约10%类癌肿瘤患者存在类癌综合征，一般比较少见。临床医师通常通过患者临床表现怀疑是否存在类癌综合征，并通过鉴别原发灶、定位转移灶和检测血清素代谢副产物5-HIAA的尿排出量增加以确诊。通过5-HIAA阳性结果诊断类癌的敏感性为73%，特异性为100%。血清嗜铬蛋白A是一种由神经内分泌肿瘤分泌的糖蛋白，其诊断类癌的敏感性为80%，特异性为95%。神经内分泌肿瘤可通过免疫组化技术诊断。利钠肽（NT-proBNP）可作为诊断类癌心脏疾病的简便指标，随后可通过二维超声心动图加以证实。转移性疾病最常见的诊断方法是腹部CT增强扫描。沉积物表现为等密度、富集血管病变。用铟-111标记的生长抑素进行生长抑素受体显像也具有诊断意义。

类癌综合征的临床特征包括：

- 间歇性皮肤潮红、毛细血管扩张、发绀；
- 低血压/高血压；

- 腹泻和痉挛；
- 支气管痉挛；
- 类癌心脏瓣膜病。

患者的症状类型和严重程度差异很大。缓激肽和组胺可引起低血压和皮肤潮红，这是类癌综合征的标志。患者的面部、颈部和胸部可能会突然出现轻微的灼烧感和皮肤潮红，持续时间为 30 s 至 30 min。随着病情的进展，面部潮红持续时间延长，并可能向周围扩散和发绀，最终整个脸部呈现毛细血管扩张。这些症状可能伴有严重的低血压和心动过速。诱发因素包括某些食物（如牛油果、水果、坚果、甜瓜等）、咖啡和酒精、排便、情绪变化、机械刺激和麻醉因素。皮肤潮红还可能伴有出汗、喘息和呼吸急促。

5- 羟色胺可导致分泌性腹泻、腹部痉挛、支气管收缩、高血压和肠缺血。5- 羟色胺还可刺激成纤维细胞生长和纤维生成，而导致腹膜和心脏瓣膜纤维化。类癌心脏病的特征是由平滑肌细胞、肌成纤维细胞和上覆的内皮细胞层所组成纤维组织斑块样沉积物。沉积通常发生在心内膜的瓣膜尖部和瓣叶、心腔，偶尔也发生在肺动脉或主动脉的内膜。这些改变会导致严重的三尖瓣反流（tricuspid regurgitation，TR）、肺动脉瓣异常和右心内膜疾病。由于肺对体液物质的失活可保护左心，因此右心的瓣膜和心内膜最常受到影响。左侧心脏病并不常见，通常与支气管类癌或右向左心内分流有关。类癌心脏病发生于超过 50% 的类癌综合征患者，是此类患者发病和死亡的主要原因。超声心动图是诊断和量化 TR 的标准。生物标志物血清嗜铬蛋白 A 和 NT-proBNP（N-terminal probrain natriuretic peptide）的升高与 TR 的严重程度和总体死亡率相关。

严重难治性低血压的鉴别诊断包括以下几点：

- 5- 羟色胺诱发的类癌危象；
- 术前服用血管紧张素Ⅱ受体阻滞剂和血管紧张素转化酶抑制剂；
- 过敏 / 变态反应；
- 脓毒症伴或不伴休克；
- 未识别的容量减少或血容量不足；
- 肝硬化合并门脉高压症和体循环阻力低；
- 肾上腺功能不全；
- 依托咪酯、大剂量丙泊酚、错误用药；
- 腔静脉机械压迫；
- 右心室空气栓塞 / 栓子栓塞；
- 类癌心脏衰竭、冠状动脉缺血、心律失常；
- 内环境：低钠血症、高钾血症、代谢性 / 呼吸性酸中毒。

围术期低血压最常见的治疗方法包括核实血压，检查 SpO_2（血氧饱和度），减浅麻醉深度，静脉输液和单次注射升压药物（去氧肾上腺素、麻黄碱、肾上腺素或血管升压素）。对于初步治疗方法无效的低血压，临床医师须回顾患者的病史和手术操作；评估患者的面部潮红、皮疹、荨麻疹或支气管痉挛；确认静脉输液通畅程度。通常，最有可能的诊断将指导干预措施，其中可能包括加压输液、胶体、输血、类固醇或者经食管超声心动图（transesophageal echocardiography，TEE）进行心脏评估。以难治性低血压为特征的类癌危象可作为一种排除诊断。对于已知或疑似类癌的患者，术中严重低血压的最合适治疗方法是使用血管升压素、奥曲肽和输注液体。

风险评估

类癌发病率相对较高，但很少有症状。在没有治疗的情况下，恶性类癌综合征患者的中位生存期为 12 ～ 38 个月。局限性类癌的 5 年生存率估计为 75% ～ 93%。若心脏受累和合并有症状的右心衰竭（纽约心脏协会Ⅲ级或Ⅳ级），预后较差，其中位生存期不到 1 年。类癌心脏病患者的血清和血浆中 5- 羟色胺、血小板 5- 羟色胺和尿 5-HIAA 的值比无心脏受累的患者高 2 ～ 4 倍。CgA 和 NT-proBNP 水平也与总死亡率有关。CgA 正常的患者 5 年生存率为 81%，CgA 升高但 NT-proBNP 正常者为 44%，CgA 和 NT-proBNP 均升高者为 16%。

启示

麻醉可诱发类癌综合征患者的类癌危象。如前文所述，其特点是面部潮红、血压的急剧变化、支气管收缩、心律失常、神志不清或昏迷，这都可能危及患者生命。术前评估应包括病史、体格检查，对分泌性腹泻引起的血容量不足、营养不良、贫血和电解质失衡的评估。50% 以上的类癌综合征患者均合并类癌心脏病。因此，心脏评估应包括超声心动图、心电图和胸部 X 线片，尤其是对于 NT-proBNP 升高的患者更需要进行评估。

醋酸奥曲肽（Sandostatin）简化了类癌患者的围术期管理，被认为是治疗类癌症状和危象的标准方法。术前应该用奥曲肽类似物控制类癌的症状，并且加强围术期管理。围术期和术后经常需要大剂量的生长抑素。奥曲肽是一种生长抑素合成的八肽类似物，皮下给药后消除半衰期约为 1.5 h。奥曲肽 -LAR（每月注射一次）可通过与生长抑素 G 蛋白偶联受体的 sstr-2 亚型结合而阻止生物活性胺的释放。醋酸奥曲肽的药理作用类似于天然生长抑素，但它是一种更有效的生长激素、胰高血糖素和胰岛素的抑制剂。与生长抑素相似，它也能抑制黄体生成激素（luteinizing hormone，LH）对促性腺激素释放激素（gonadotropin-releasing hormone，GnRH）的反应，降低内脏血流量，抑制 5- 羟色胺、胃泌素、血管活性肠肽、促胰液素、胃动素和胰腺多肽的释放。奥曲肽具有广泛的作用，包括 QT 间期延长、心动过缓、传导异常、腹部痉挛、恶心和呕吐。尽管副作用持续大约 18 个月，但 80% 以上患者的症状都会得到缓解。胰岛素对高血糖的释放反应也受到抑制，这可能使肥胖患者或非胰岛素依赖型糖尿病患者的血糖管理更为复杂。不幸的是，奥曲肽并不能预防或延缓心脏瓣膜疾病。

管理

类癌患者的麻醉管理需要注意以下几点：

- 静脉输注奥曲肽治疗围术期类癌危象（诱导前 50 μg 静脉注射，术中静脉输注 100 μg/h；可在术前 12 h 开始持续输注并持续至术后 48 h；必要时可增加至 500 μg/h，如对肝转移瘤进行操作时）。
- 有创监测：有创动脉和中心静脉压力检测 /TEE；大口径静脉通路；液体加温。
- 对于术前超声心动图确定中度 / 重度 TR 或右心衰竭的患者应有麻醉预案。
- 避免使用肾上腺素、麻黄碱、去甲肾上腺素或钙，可能会引起肿瘤介质的释放。
- 谨慎使用小剂量的去氧肾上腺素。
- 静脉输注奥曲肽、液体和血管升压素治疗低血压。停止刺激肿瘤的手术操作。减浅麻醉深度。如果静脉输注奥曲肽对低血压无效，则考虑使用抑肽酶（激肽释放酶抑制剂）。
- 支气管痉挛：β - 受体激动剂可引起强烈的、持久的血管舒张。用静脉输注奥曲肽、抗组胺药和雾化吸入异丙托溴铵治疗。
- 部分肝切除 / 肝移植可能发生大量失血，这可能是因为病变的血管分布和 TR/PR 或右心病变导致的静脉压（肝静脉压）升高。
- 考虑用类固醇、H_1- 或 H_2- 受体拮抗剂和 5-HT_2 受体拮抗剂进行预处理。
- 术中类癌危象：面部潮红、持续低血压、支气管痉挛、酸中毒和室性心动过速。
- 避免因应激、诱导、插管、组胺释放药物、低血压、低温、拟交感神经药物和刺激肿瘤引起的介质释放。
- 全麻 / 胸段硬膜外 / 瑞芬太尼输注是理想的加速康复方案。
- 避免使用导致 QT 延长的药物。
- 术后治疗：监测介质释放的症状，输注奥曲肽 48 h（未被发现的转移灶仍可分泌多肽）；液体和电解质，急性疼痛管理；重症监护病房。

血流动力学的变化、麻醉剂或手术刺激可能促进不可预测的、无法控制的激素释放。这可能导致低血压或高血压危象和循环虚脱，此时传统强心和升压治疗通常没有效果。持续的血压监测是非常必要的，因为血压可能突然发生剧烈波动。如果已知患有类癌的患者出现严重低血压且对静脉输液无反应时，一线疗法为静脉注射奥曲肽随后持续静脉输注，而血管升压素静脉推注 / 输注为二线疗法。如果继续低血压，停止刺激肿瘤的手术操作，减浅麻醉深度，并考虑使用抑肽酶。拟交感神经药物常被使用，但可能会加重低血压，因为激活 α - 肾上腺素能可导致肿瘤进一步释放生物活性肽。去甲肾上腺素被证明可激活肿瘤中的激肽释放酶，导致缓激肽的合成和释放，反而导致血管扩张和加剧低血压。去氧肾上腺素或其他肾上腺素受体激动剂也可进一步触发生物活性肽的释放。

通过刺激去甲肾上腺素的释放和抑制其再吸收，5- 羟色胺增强了血管对儿茶酚胺的反应。它还可直接刺激突触后 α_1- 受体。由此导致的血压升高应接受标准治疗，如增加麻醉深度或使用拉贝洛尔、尼卡地平、硝普钠等药物。也可使用卡坦色林（2.5 ～ 5 mg 静脉推注随后 5 mg/h 静脉持续输注），它可阻断 5- 羟色胺、α_1- 受体和 H_1 受体。

类癌患者的治疗包括使用生长抑素类似物以

减少激素分泌和减轻症状；切除原发肿瘤；切除转移瘤或消融治疗（例如射频消融、冷冻治疗、动脉化疗栓塞）。在特定的病例中，肝移植可能是一种治疗方法。其他治疗选择包括间碘苄胍制剂（m-iodobenzylguanidine，MIBG）、干扰素-α 和化疗。心脏瓣膜置换手术适且于类癌心脏瓣膜病患者，但其发病率和死亡率较高。

（林省伟　译　孟　岩　校）

延伸阅读

Connolly H: Carcinoid heart disease. In Otto C, Yeon S, editors: *UpToDate*, 2017. Waltham, MA. Available at www.uptodate.com/contents.

Mancuso K, Kaye AD, Boudreaux JP, et al.: Carcinoid syndrome and perioperative anesthetic considerations, *J Clin Anesth* 23:329–341, 2001.

Powell B, Al Mukhtar A, Mills GH: Carcinoid: the disease and its implications for anaesthesia, *Contin Educ Anaesth Crit Care Pain* 11:9–13, 2011.

Strosberg J: Treatment of the carcinoid syndrome. In Tanabe K, Whitcomb D, Savarese D, editors: *UpToDate*, 2017. Waltham, MA. Available at www.uptodate.com/contents

第46章 腹腔镜手术的并发症

Katarzyna Luba

病例概要

患者，男性，75岁，既往有高血脂和高血压病史，拟行腹腔镜食管裂孔疝修补术。他除了口服治疗高血压药物（氯沙坦和氢氯噻嗪）外，已禁食12 h。在全身麻醉诱导期间，他的收缩压降至85 mmHg。麻醉科医师给予患者静脉输注乳酸林格氏溶液500 ml和静脉推注100 μg去氧肾上腺素后，其血压稳定。麻醉科医师进行动脉置管并告诉外科医师可以继续手术。在腹腔内注入二氧化碳（CO_2）后，将患者置于反向Trendelenburg（头高脚低）体位。血压突然下降，低于60 mmHg，然后动脉波形变成直线，不能触及颈动脉搏动。双侧有相同强弱的呼吸声。心电图（electrocardiogram，ECG）最初显示为正常窦性心律，但很快发展为窦性心动过缓伴ST段压低。静推1 mg肾上腺素和静脉输注1000 ml晶体溶液后，血压和心电图恢复正常，立即人工气腹放气，并将患者置于Trendelenburg（头低脚高位）。但是，麻醉科医师和外科医师决定取消手术并对患者进行彻底的心脏检查以排除冠状动脉问题。

问题分析

定义

尽管腹腔镜技术从伤口愈合时间、术后疼痛、住院时间、患者对伤口美观效果的满意度层面来说具有微创手术的优势，但对患者生理功能产生显著影响。人工气腹、Trendelenburg（头低脚高）体位或反向Trendelenburg（头高脚低）体位，用于产生气腹的CO_2的全身吸收以及全身麻醉的心血管影响，均会导致患者在腹腔镜手术时发生生理性变化。为了对腹腔镜手术进行安全的麻醉管理，麻醉科医师需要充分认识腹腔镜手术固有的副作用和并发症。

人工气腹建立时，腹内压增加导致胸腔受压，静脉回流减少，体循环和肺血管阻力增加，左心室壁张力增加。心排血量下降，主要发生在腹腔充气开始时。经食管超声心动图（transesophageal echocardiography，TEE）检查证实左心室舒张末期容量减少。然而，腹腔充气时胸膜腔内压的升高可导致心脏充盈压升高。Trendelenburg体位可以在一定程度上减轻人工气腹对静脉回流和心排血量的影响，但是反向Trendelenburg体位可能会大大增加这种影响，特别是同时合并低血容量和血管舒张时。

气腹常伴有急性神经内分泌反应。儿茶酚胺和血管升压素释放以及肾素-血管紧张素-醛固酮轴被激活，可导致体循环阻力增加。腹部充气期间，肾血流量、肾小球滤过率和尿量均会减少。

气腹对通气功能的影响包括降低肺顺应性、降低功能残气量以及通气/血流比例失调。Trendelenburg体位易导致形成肺不张。肺泡通气量降低和腹膜腔吸收CO_2会导致呼吸性酸中毒。$PaCO_2$的增加和Trendelenburg体位可增加脑血流量、颅内压以及眼内压，但这些影响的程度和临床意义目前尚不清楚。

腹腔镜手术期间发生的心律失常有多种原因。在腹腔充气初期，患者血流动力学影响最为严重时，最常发生快速性心律失常（窦性心律失常、心房和室上性异位心律和心动过速、室性异位心律、室性心动过速或心室颤动）。这些也可能是静脉气体栓塞的早期征兆。在建立气腹期间发生快速性心律失常可能由于高碳酸血症和相关的儿茶酚胺激增所致。缓慢性心律失常（窦性心动过缓、游走性房性起搏、交界性心律、房室心脏传导阻滞、心搏停止）可能是迷走神经反射介导的并继发于腹内压急剧增加，或由于严重的呼吸性酸中毒所致。无脉性电活动可能发生于极度低血压的情况，如当腹内压增加和反向 Trendelenburg 体位同时发生，严重阻碍静脉回流时。

气腹针（Veress 针）位置放置不正确可能会导致 CO_2 进入腹膜外。腹腔镜手术中皮下气肿的发生率在 0.4% ～ 2%。充入的 CO_2 可以延伸到纵隔和心包中。心包积气可能会产生心包压塞的临床表现。加压气体也可通过天然的腹膜-胸膜通路或膈肌意外损伤后进入胸膜腔，导致气胸。最后，在充气期间把 Veress 针意外置入血管内导致血管内气体栓塞。对行腹腔镜胆囊切除术的所有患者进行 TEE 检测，发现高达 2/3 的患者存在轻微的血管内气体栓塞。CO_2 迅速被吸收并且很容易通过肺部呼出，因此二氧化碳气体栓塞的后果可能不那么严重。CO_2 栓塞的致死剂量约为空气的 5 倍。但是，未意识到的血管内注气将导致大量的气体栓塞，这通常是致命的损害。

腹腔套管针的放置可能会意外导致肠穿孔或实质器官或血管损伤，导致严重的出血，但在初期可能会被忽视。在腹腔镜手术过程中，止血较为困难，且通常需要紧急转换为开放手术。在腹部充气之前放置胃管减压管，被认为可以降低 Veress 针或套管针引起胃穿孔的风险。

横纹肌溶解症是在极度 Trendelenburg 体位下长时间手术的罕见并发症。这种并发症可能是由于下肢抬高引起动脉灌注减少，下肢静脉受支撑物压迫和腹内压增加导致的股静脉引流障碍共同所致。

1999 年引入机器人手术，从另一层面增加了腹腔镜手术麻醉管理的复杂性。机器人体积庞大，占据了大部分手术室空间。它的手臂坚硬，在手术过程中任何患者体动都可能导致严重的损伤。一旦机器人对接就位，通常接触患者特别是气道会严重受限，且不再可能调整患者在手术台上的体位。因此，体位相关的伤害和意外丧失气道的风险增加。妇科和泌尿外科机器人手术需要极端的 Trendelenburg 体位和非常高的气腹压，因此对血流动力学和呼吸系统的麻醉管理的挑战更加严峻。长时间的极端 Trendelenburg 体位可能导致严重的面部和上呼吸道水肿。机器人手术中角膜磨损的发生率更高。

经腹腔镜手术的患者术后恶心呕吐发生率达 40% ～ 70%。由于膈肌刺激引起的术后疼痛通常局限于肩部、颈部或上腹部。

识别

通过加强对腹腔镜手术潜在并发症与手术操作的时间相关性的警惕和意识，有助于麻醉科医师迅速识别并处理这些经常发生的严重的甚至偶尔会危及生命的事件。

腹部充气和在手术开始时将患者置于 Trendelenburg 体位，可能会使肺部顺应性急剧下降和血流动力学不稳定。在腹腔镜手术期间，反向 Trendelenburg 体位和腹部充气压力的增加可能导致额外的血流动力学不稳定。密切监测血流动力学参数和通气力学参数，对患者出现任何动态变化做出快速反应，是麻醉管理过程中的精髓。

突发性低血压可能是低血容量和充气致腹内高压共同导致，尤其是在反向 Trendelenburg 体位下。同时也必须考虑其他可能的原因，如出血、心动过缓和张力性气胸，仅举几例作为参考。

在腹部充气时和充气后吸气峰压（peak inspiratory pressure，PIP）通常增加。由于膈肌活动受限和肺顺应性降低，在人工气腹建立期间气道压逐渐增加。但是，当气道压突然增加，应怀疑气胸，这可能是由膈肌损伤或经胸膜腔与充气的腹膜腔之间的天然通路或者肺气压性损伤导致。鉴别诊断应包括气管导管（endotracheal tube，ETT）阻塞或主干移位。肺部听诊，尝试手动通气，沿 ETT 放入吸引导管，纤维支气管镜检查和 $ETCO_2$ 波形分析等检测都可用于快速找到气道峰压急剧增加的原因。

二氧化碳波形图是腹腔镜手术中最有用的监测方法之一。它可能提供即将发生的灾难性事件的早期预警信号。$ETCO_2$ 突然部分减少可见于低心排血量或 ETT 的主干移位，但也可能意味着静脉空气栓塞、肺栓塞或心脏停搏。$ETCO_2$ 波形的突然完全消失通常表示回路断开、采样管阻塞、气道阻塞或拔管。

行腹腔镜手术的患者通常很少需要有创血压监测。然而，对于既往存在严重心肌或瓣膜功能障碍或呼吸系统疾病的患者，有创血压监测则非常有帮助。这有助于诊断和治疗显著的生理紊乱。有创血压监测也适用于极度肥胖的患者，这类患者在摆放腹腔镜体位后可能无法进行无创血压监测，例如双臂卷塞固定。经食管超声心动图对不同原因引起的严重血流动力学不稳定的紧急诊断具有价值，如低血容量、心肌缺血、心室功能障碍、静脉气体栓塞或肺栓塞。

风险评估

因为对患者的风险过高或者腹腔镜手术在技术上不可行，而导致绝对禁忌实施腹腔镜手术的情形很少。腹腔镜手术的相对禁忌证则较常见，包括腹腔镜手术在技术上具有挑战性和风险，或由于患者并存疾病引起的生理限制而不适合腹腔镜手术。

气腹可导致既往存在严重血流动力学损害的患者发生心脏停搏，例如休克、主动脉瓣重度狭窄、晚期心力衰竭或心包积液。严重的限制性肺病也不考虑行腹腔镜手术，例如严重脊柱侧凸或已行全肺切除术后，或有严重间质性肺病。肺不张和气腹致肺内分流增加可能导致危及生命的低氧血症。此外，受限制的肺容积不允许患者过度通气以代偿减少气腹期间的 CO_2 吸收。患者可能会出现极度高碳酸血症，导致术后通气障碍和患者无法拔管。用力呼气量小于 70% 且弥散能力小于 80% 可预示在腹腔镜手术过程中更严重的高碳酸血症。此外，对许多患有慢性限制性或间质性肺病的患者，缺氧和高碳酸血症会加剧肺动脉高压和右心室功能不全。患有肺气肿或严重阻塞性肺病的患者在行腹腔镜手术会增加气压伤和气胸的风险。

腹内压特别高的患者可能不适于行腹腔镜手术，其原因可能是广泛占位的肿瘤、腹腔间隔室综合征或大量腹水。腹腔镜手术的其他技术性的挑战包括妊娠、肠扩张、凝血功能障碍、腹壁感染以及既往广泛腹部手术。

在颅内压增高（脑肿瘤，脑积水，脑室分流）和极度肥胖的情况下，气腹和 Trendelenburg 体位为相对禁忌。当腹部充气，特别是与反 Trendelenburg 体位同时进行时，存在严重血容量不足、充血性心力衰竭或主动脉瓣狭窄的患者耐受性较差。当患者患有冠状动脉疾病，行腹腔镜手术会增加术中冠状动脉事件发生的风险。患有脑动脉疾病（包括颈动脉或椎动脉狭窄）的患者在难治性低血压发作期间有围术期缺血性卒中的风险。

腹腔镜手术的主要并发症主要来自于心脏事件和血管损伤。腹腔镜手术的死亡率约为 0.13%。心脏并发症占腹腔镜手术相关死亡的 25%。

启示

腹腔镜已成为几种外科手术（如胆囊切除术或胃旁路术）的金标准。腹腔镜手术通常在门诊进行手术。自 1999 年推出以来，机器人辅助的腹腔镜手术技术已成为泌尿科和妇科手术的首选方法。由于腹腔镜方法的普及和便利以及不断积累的腹腔镜手术技术经验，一些以前对腹腔镜手术的“绝对”禁忌证不再是其应用的阻碍。因此，腹腔镜手术所固有的并发症风险增加的患者已成为目前麻醉实践的常见挑战。麻醉科医师因此必须为行腹腔镜手术的患者在合理地选择、筛查和建议方面做好准备。麻醉科医师和外科医师必须完全熟悉在腹腔镜手术期间可能发生的正常生理的严重变化，并能够诊断和处理任何由此产生的并发症。

管理与预防

腹内压增高是腹腔镜手术中低血压的主要原因。腹内压增高会阻止静脉回流，并且可能通过在充气期间拉伸腹膜而引起迷走神经介导的反射性心动过缓。通过逐渐而非快速的充气可缓解气腹对静脉回流的影响。在腹腔镜手术前给予静脉输液可以纠正先前存在的血容量不足并预防严重的低血压。嘱患者在手术当天继续服用抗高血压药物，如利尿剂或血管紧张素转换酶抑制剂，可降低腹腔镜手术期间难治性低血压的发生率。充气后发生低血压时，应给予静脉输液，可增加静脉回流。心动过缓时，可应用抗胆碱能药物——格隆溴铵或阿托品治疗。如果患者即将发生心脏停搏，应使用肾上腺素，治疗极度心动过缓和低血压。减少反向 Trendelenburg 体位的程度可改善静脉回流。当患者出现在严重血流动力学不稳定的情况下，应将腹腔内压力降至 10 ～ 15 mmHg，或暂时释放气腹。如果给予静脉补液和减少腹部充气压力以及减小反向 Trendelenburg 体位的程度仍未能改善患者对气腹的耐受，则可能需要放弃腹腔镜技术。

腹腔内压力超过 15 mmHg 会降低前负荷并增加体循环阻力和后负荷。即使心排血量下降，血流动力学净效应可能是高血压，特别是如果患者处于 Trendelenburg 体位。积极治疗高血压会凸显静脉回流和心排血量的减少，并导致血流动力学不稳定。尼卡地平是一种快速可逆的动脉扩张剂，可能是治疗这种情况下的高血压的最佳选择。

腹腔镜手术期间患者出现的心动过速和高血压，是由于腹膜腔吸收 CO_2 引起的进行性高碳酸血症的交感神经刺激的表现。通过调节呼吸频率以增加分钟通气量，来控制 $PaCO_2$ 和 $ETCO_2$ 的增加。增加约 20% 的分钟通气量通常足以维持正常 CO_2。当腹膜外大量 CO_2 蓄积（例如皮下气肿或纵隔气肿）时，高碳酸血症可能难以纠正。在这种情况下，高碳酸血症可持续至手术结束后数小时。

张力性气胸是一种危及生命的急症。如果根据临床表现强烈怀疑张力性气胸，立即减压可防心肺不稳定加剧转变为心脏停搏。将大口径，至少 2 英寸长的静脉导管置于第二肋间水平的锁骨中线可紧急减压。快速识别双侧气胸并进行双侧减压至关重要。导管（或所有导管）应保持在与水密封系统连接的位置相平。同时，应立即停止并释放腹部气腹。应将胸腔穿刺导管留在原位直至停止正压通气。很少需要放置胸管，因为 CO_2 可迅速从胸膜腔吸收。术后连续的胸部 X 线片检测是必须检测的项目。

当怀疑静脉气体栓塞时提示应该紧急处理，不能延误。

应立即停止腹部充气，释放气腹，并将患者同时调整为 Trendelenburg 体位和右侧在上的体位。这将右心室流出道置于右心房的下方位置，可有助于释放滞留于右心室流出道的气泡。应开始使用 100% 氧气进行通气，如果使用氧化亚氮，应立即停止使用。静脉气体栓塞经常引起室上性心动过速，因此使用去氧肾上腺素作为一线药物可有助于治疗所导致的低血压。如果血流动力学不稳定变得更为严重，则使用肾上腺素和血管升压素。应尝试将多孔中心静脉导管置入右心房并抽吸气泡。如果发生心脏停搏，如果不进行右侧心脏栓塞气体抽吸，则胸外按压和心肺复苏可能无效。卵圆孔未闭（patent foramen ovale，PFO）存在于约 25% 的成年人群中，因此，必须牢记通过 PFO 可能会出现反常脑栓子或冠状动脉栓子。静脉气体栓塞后存活的患者，应评估患者的神经功能缺陷和心肌缺血情况。

在长时间的腹腔镜手术过程中，患者可能会形成深静脉血栓（Deep venous thrombosis，DVT），并且可能因肺栓塞（pulmonary embolism，PE）而使病情进一步复杂化。肥胖症和癌症患者 DVT 的风险增加。常规预防包括在手术前立即给予皮下肝素，并使用加压装置对下肢加压。超过 50% 的减肥外科医师对高风险患者术前放置下腔静脉（inferior vena cava，IVC）过滤器用于预防 PE。但目前尚未确定胃旁路手术前预防性置入 IVC 过滤器是否有效。

致谢

感谢 Shahar Bar-Yosef 博士对本章上一版的贡献。

（张晓秀 译 许 涛 校）

延伸阅读

Cockcroft JOB, Berry CB, McGrath JS, et al.: Anesthesia for major urologic surgery, *Anesthesiol Clin* 33(1):165–172, 2015.

Danic MJ, Chow M, Alexander G, et al.: Anesthesia considerations for robotic-assisted laparoscopic prostatectomy: a review of 1,500 cases, *J Robot Surg* 1(2):119–123, 2007.

Harris SN, Ballantyne GH, Luther MA, et al.: Alterations of cardiovascular performance during laparoscopic colectomy: a combined hemodynamic and echocardiographic analysis, *Anesth Analg* 83:482–487, 1996.

Hsu RL, Kaye AD, Urman RD: Anesthetic challenges in robotic-assisted urologic surgery, *Rev Urol* 15(4):178–184, 2013.

Jo YY, Lee JY, Lee MG, et al.: Effects of high positive end-expiratory pressure on haemodynamics and cerebral oxygenation during pneumoperitoneum in the Trendelenburg position, *Anaesthesia* 68:938–943, 2013.

Kaye AD, Vadivelu N, Ahuja N, et al.: Anesthetic considerations in robotic-assisted gynecologic surgery, *Ochsner J* 13:517–524, 2013.

Leonard IE, Cunningham AJ: Anesthetic considerations for laparoscopic cholecystectomy, *Best Pract Res Clin Anaesthesiol* 16:1–20, 2002.

Nguyen NT, Goldman CD, Ho HS, et al.: Systemic stress response after laparoscopic and open gastric bypass, *J Am Coll Surg* 194:557–566, 2002.

Rowland SP, Dharmarajah B, Moore HM, et al.: Inferior vena cava filters for prevention of venous thromboembolism in obese patients undergoing bariatric surgery: a systematic review, *Ann Surg* 261(1):35–45, 2015.

Sood J: Advancing frontiers in anaesthesiology with laparoscopy, *World J Gastroenterol* 20(39):14308–14314, 2014.

Struthers AD, Cuschieri A: Cardiovascular consequences of laparoscopic surgery, *Lancet* 352:568–570, 1998.

Wahba RWM, Tessler MJ, Kleiman SJ: Acute ventilatory complications during laparoscopic upper abdominal surgery, *Can J Anaesth* 43:77–83, 1996.

Whiteley JR, Taylor J, Henry M, et al.: Detection of elevated intracranial pressure in robot-assisted laparoscopic radical prostatectomy using ultrasonography of optic nerve sheath diameter, *J Neurosurg Anesthesiol* 27(2):155–159, 2015.

第 47 章 碎石术的并发症

Jerome F. O'Hara Jr.

病例概要

患者，女性，78 岁，在全身麻醉下行体外冲击波碎石术，既往有严重冠状动脉疾病病史。患者入医用水池 10 min 后心率由 78 次 / 分钟上升到 138 次 / 分钟，并且气管导管内可见粉红色泡沫液体。患者从水池中被移出，并且立即拍摄胸部 X 线片提示充血性心力衰竭。

问题分析

定义

体外冲击波碎石术（extracorporeal shock wave lithotripsy，ESWL）是通过冲击波在患者体内的传导来粉碎尿路结石。与第二代碎石机不同，第一代碎石机要求患者浸泡在医用水池中（图 47.1）。除了麻醉风险外，这种独特的环境还使患者处于水中浸泡以及冲击波释放能量的潜在不良反应中。

在 ESWL 过程中，一个机械性振动波穿过水后形成一次脉冲压力。到达患者时，冲击波再穿过患者的组织到达“靶区”，即包含结石的区域（图 47.2）。通过 X 线透视，使结石位置保持在目标区域内。当冲击波遇到不同密度的物体（如尿路结石）时，释放的能量将使结石碎裂成砂粒状，达到预期的治疗效果。然而，其他组织或植入的机械装置也可能会在治疗过程中受到破坏。为防止出现心律失常，碎石机可以在患者心脏周期的不应期同步触发冲击波。对于某些患者来说，浸泡产生的静水压力会显著损害心血管和肺的功能。

识别

冲击波能量的不良影响包括：

- 由心房或心室心律失常引起的循环不稳定；
- 对起搏器或植入式心脏复律除颤器的潜在损伤或因故障导致的损伤；

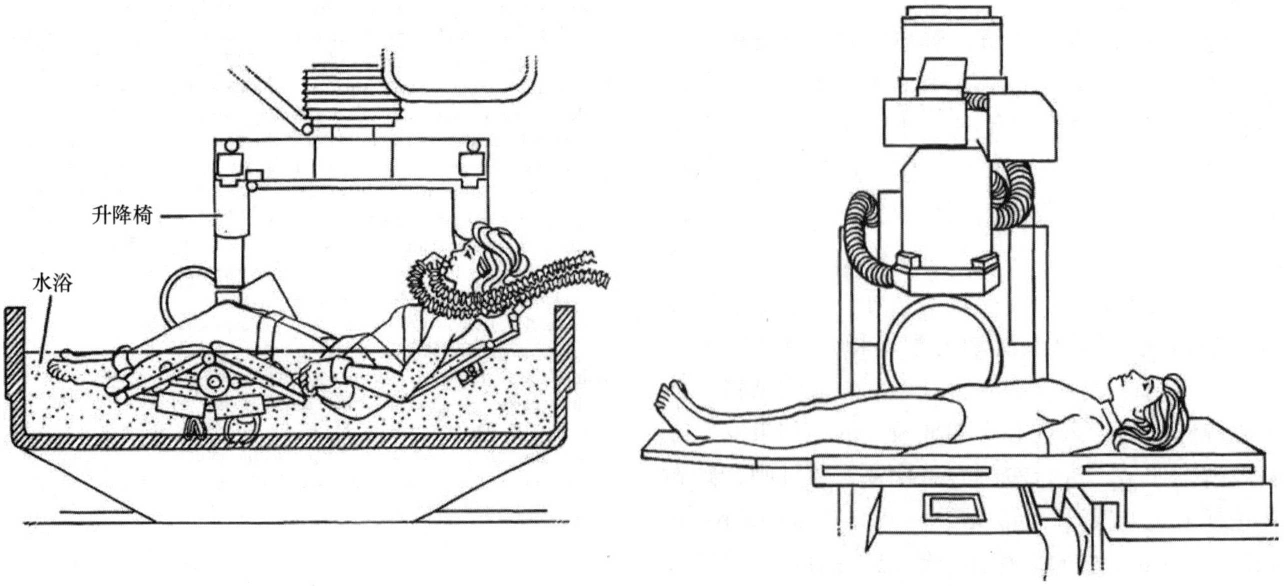

图 47.1　第一代碎石机，患者位于升降椅中，浸入水浴（左）。较新型二代碎石机（右）

- 肾周出血或腹腔内出血引起的低血压；
- 皮肤淤点和疼痛性淤斑，尤其是瘦弱患者；
- 镇静、镇痛不足引起的不适和体动。

浸没式碎石的不良影响包括：

- 升降椅压迫点造成的神经和肌肉骨骼损伤；
- 由水浴温度引起的体温过高或过低；
- 患者气道相对不易接近；
- 心血管和肺的变化（表 47.1）。

风险评估

如果冲击波指向错误或遇到尿路结石以外的组织，释放的能量可能会损伤患者。这些损伤包括：

- 肺挫伤和咯血，尤其是儿童，因为肺底和肾非常接近；
- 硬膜外麻醉时，如果空气进入硬膜外腔，会造成神经损伤；
- 钙化的主动脉瘤或肾动脉瘤可能受到损伤甚至破裂。

在一些患者中，与水浸相关的心血管和肺部变化可导致严重的并发症。例如，严重心室功能障碍的患者可发生急性充血性心力衰竭。严重的慢性阻塞性肺疾病患者在区域阻滞麻醉下可能无法维持足够的通气。ESWL 的绝对禁忌证和相对禁忌证列于框 47.1。

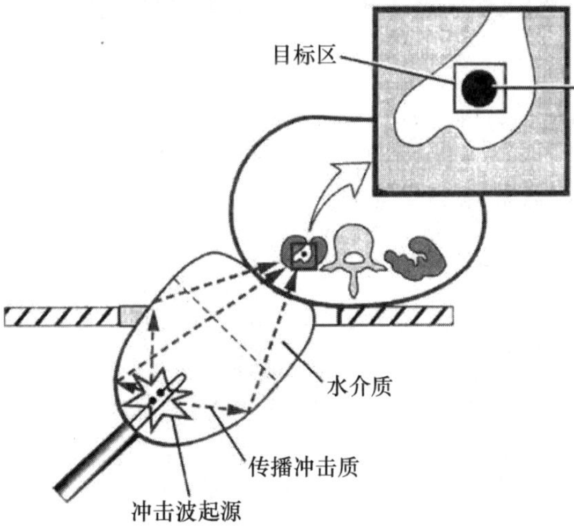

图 47.2 冲击波如何产生以及如何传递至肾结石的示意图

表 47.1 在碎石术期间人体被浸泡时的心肺变化

系统	变量	改变方向
心血管	中心血容量	增加
	中心静脉压	增加
	肺动脉压	增加
呼吸	肺血流量	增加
	肺活量	减少
	功能残气量	减少
	潮气量	减少
	呼吸频率	增加

Modified from Malhotra V：Anesthesia and the renal and genitourinary systems. In Miller RD，editor：*Anesthesia*. New York，Churchill Livingstone，1994，p 1961.

启示

为了避免 ESWL 过程中可能出现的并发症，麻醉科医师必须了解冲击波的产生和传导至患者的物理原理。在择期手术前评估需要麻醉的患者时，需要考虑某些风险。

管理

麻醉方式的选择取决于碎石机的类型和麻醉科医师的偏好。高功率冲击波（>18 kv）通常需要全身或区域麻醉，而低功率冲击波（<18 kv）通常只需要静脉镇静。

全身麻醉的优点是能够通过气管插管确保气道的安全，并提供更小、更稳定的潮气量。小而稳定的潮气量，可以最大限度地减少肾结石或输尿管结石的移位，确保它们保持在靶区内。区域麻醉允许患者自主调节升降椅的位置，而且在需要转移患者接受额外的泌尿外科手术时更为方便。脊髓或硬膜外麻醉需要 T4-T6 平面的感觉阻滞。

区域麻醉的潜在缺点包括：

- 建立麻醉需要较多时间；

框 47.1 体外震波碎石术的禁忌证

绝对禁忌证

肾结石远端梗阻
出血异常或使用抗凝药物
妊娠

相对禁忌证

钙化的巨大主动脉瘤或肾动脉瘤
未经治疗的泌尿系统感染
起搏器或植入式心律转复除颤器
病态肥胖

- 改变呼吸动力学；
- 可能感觉阻滞不全；
- 单次给药后无法追加剂量。

无论使用何种麻醉方式，ESWL 的恢复其实主要是麻醉的恢复。因此，ESWL 应按照门诊手术麻醉流程来处理。需要明确患者有无心肺基础疾病，并清楚这可能增加并发症发生的风险。虽然对于严重心肺功能损害的患者可能需要有创监测，但控制浸入的速度和深度同样重要。为了防止麻醉过程中出现撞击、压迫、臂丛神经或颈部损伤，需要合适的体位和填充缓冲物，尤其是在水浴时。

计划行 ESWL 治疗的某些患者需要考虑以下具体问题：

- 儿科患者通常需要接受全身麻醉，以便在手术过程中控制他们的体动。可以用泡沫塑料填充物来保护肺叶下段免受冲击波。
- 截瘫患者仍需要麻醉，因为其有自主神经反射亢进的风险。
- 碎石机可能无法承受病态肥胖患者的体重以及无法准确定位他们体内的结石位置。这必须在麻醉诱导前进行评估。
- 使用心律管理装置（cardiac rhythm management device，CRMD），即心脏起搏器或植入式心内除颤器（见第 16 章）的患者可以安全地进行 ESWL，但程序参数可能会发生变化。应采取下列步骤：
- 建议关闭患者的 CRMD 的自适应速率响应程序。
- 必须停用植入式心内除颤器，并用泡沫塑料遮挡，以保护其免受冲击波的损害，并且在手术后应对设备进行检查。这也适用于心脏起搏器。
- 必须明确安装 CRMD 的指征，以便团队做好处理此类心律失常的准备，尤其是在一些 CRMD 治疗功能（如治疗快速心律失常）已经被关闭的情况下。如果是这样，临时起搏器和体表除颤器必须处于备用状态。
- 对于有植入式 CRMD 设备的患者，在治疗前和治疗后都应该检测脉冲发生器的功能是否正常。

预防

麻醉科医师必须识别有 ESWL 相关并发症风险的患者，并在 ESWL 期间，特别是在水浴浸泡和冲击波治疗开始时，严密地监测患者的体位和血流动力学变化。为浸没于水中的患者建立和演练一套开放气道和心肺复苏的抢救流程是非常明智的。还应制订应急预案，使心脏不稳定患者从独立的或可移动的 ESWL 治疗室转运到重症监护病房的过程更为安全便捷。

（董　朋　译　陈元杰　校）

延伸阅读

American Society of Anesthesiologists Task Force on Perioperative Management of Patients with Cardiac Rhythm Management Devices: Practice advisory for the perioperative management of patients with cardiac rhythm management devices: pacemakers and implantable cardioverter-defibrillators, *Anesthesiology* 103:186–198, 2005.

Chung MK, Streem SB, Ching E, et al.: Effects of extracorporeal shock wave lithotripsy on tiered therapy implantable cardioverter defibrillators, *Pacing Clin Electrophysiol* 22:738–742, 1999.

Drach GW, Weber C, Donovan JM: Treatment of pacemaker patients with extracorporeal shock wave lithotripsy: experience from 2 continents, *J Urol* 143:895–896, 1990.

Liguori G, Trombetta C, Bucci S, et al.: Reversible acute renal failure after unilateral extracorporeal shock-wave lithotripsy, *Urol Res* 32:25–27, 2004.

Monk TG, Weldon BC: The renal system and anesthesia for urologic surgery. In Barash PG, Cullen BF, Stoelting RK, editors: *Clinical anesthesia*, 4th ed, Philadelphia, 2001, JB Lippincott–Williams & Wilkins, pp 1022–1025.

Morgan GE, Mikhail MS: Anesthesia for genitourinary surgery. In Morgan GE, Mikhail MS, editors: *Clinical anesthesiology*, Stamford, CT, 1996, Appleton & Lange, pp 601–610.

Saberski LR, Kondamuri S, Osinubi OY: Identification of the epidural space: is loss of resistance to air a safe technique? *Reg Anesth* 22:3–15, 1997.

Stowe DF, Bernstein JS, Madsen KE, et al.: Autonomic hyperreflexia in spinal cord injured patients during extracorporeal shock wave lithotripsy, *Anesth Analg* 68:788–791, 1989.

Vasavada SP, Streem SB, Kottke-Marchant K, et al.: Pathological effects of extracorporeally generated shock waves on calcified aortic aneurysm tissue, *J Urol* 152:45–48, 1994.

大量输血的并发症

第48章

Joanna David，*Perumal Tamilselvan*

病例概要

患者，男性，50 岁，因屋顶坠落伤被送至急诊室。入院时患者心动过速（120 次 / 分），血压正常（130/88 mmHg），伴有明显腹部膨隆，格拉斯哥昏迷评分（Glasgow Coma Scale）评分为 15，计算机断层扫描提示腹腔内出血。患者需行紧急剖腹手术，腹部打开时血压降至 60/30 mmHg。患者在 1 h 后止血成功，共需输注 6 个单位红细胞。

问题分析

定义

对于“**大量输血**”一词的定义，目前还没有达成共识。该定义旨在量化治疗大出血过程中所需的血液和血液制品。其中一些定义包括以下内容：

- 替换超过 150 ml/min 的失血量；
- 3 h 内替换超过 5 个单位的失血量；
- 24 h 内替换超过 10 个单位的红细胞；
- 24 h 内替换全身总血容量；
- 4 h 内替换总血容量的一半。

识别

大量输血及其相关并发症是由治疗急性失血所致，治疗过程中需要用晶体、非红细胞（red blood cell，RBC）胶体、血液和血液制品快速替换血管内容量。导致大量输血的最常见情况是严重创伤。其他情况包括以下：

- 胃肠道出血；
- 产科大出血；
- 大血管手术 / 损伤；
- 心脏手术；
- 肝手术 / 损伤；
- 颅面部手术；
- 根治性肿瘤手术；
- 骨科手术 / 脊柱重建手术。

有人指出，随着对出血及其相关凝血障碍的早期识别和积极治疗，使得血制品使用减少，大量输血的发生率正在下降。

增加和导致输血相关并发症发生的情况包括：

- 使用抗凝剂；
- 凝血因子缺陷（遗传、稀释或获得性凝血因子缺乏；凝血因子消耗；体外膜氧合和循环辅助装置）；
- 低体温；
- 使用血液回收器或自体血回输装置。

儿童以及年轻人对于血容量丢失量高达 30% 时仍具有较强的耐受性。他们低血容量的体征可能很轻微，包括心率小至中等幅度增快，脉压降低。

风险评估

任何需要紧急大量输血的患者都有发生大量输血相关并发症的危险。婴儿和新生儿由于自身凝血系统的不成熟，似乎面临着更大的风险。可能会发生以下并发症：

- 凝血功能障碍；
- 低体温；
- 酸中毒；
- 低钾血症或高钾血症；
- 低钙血症。

更完整的常见并发症清单见图 48.1。

启示

患者的预后取决于早期识别、失血的速度和严重程度以及及时的干预。新生儿和婴儿在凝血完整性方面的实验室结果超出了成人参考值范围 [尤其是凝血酶原时间（prothrombin time，PT）和部分凝血活酶时间（partial thromboplastin time，PTT）]。因此，对于成人来说正常的实验室值并不能代表新生儿的止血能力，必须谨慎参考。

管理

治疗的目标是维持血管内容量以及功能的完整，其中血液的携氧能力及凝血功能最为重要。在大量失血的情况，这些治疗目标只能通过输注全血或成分输血来实现。常用成分及用量见表 48.1。

大量红细胞输注或成分输血可能导致的并发症见框 48.1。

框 48.1 大量输血并发症

早期：
稀释性凝血功能障碍
酸碱紊乱
低温
高血钾 / 低血钾
枸橼酸盐超负荷（低钙血症）
输血相关循环超负荷（TACO）
溶血性输血反应
非溶血性发热反应
输血相关性肺损伤（TRALI）
过敏反应
细菌性脓毒症
微血栓或微聚颗粒形成导致急性呼吸窘迫综合征

后期：
输血相关疾病（细菌和病毒）
延迟性溶血反应
红细胞可塑性变化
移植物抗宿主病
输血相关的铁超载
输血相关的免疫调制

表 48.1 大出血时常用血液成分剂量

血液成分	大出血时使用剂量
红细胞	维持血红蛋白 >80 g/L（心血管疾病患者 >10 g/L）
新鲜冰冻血浆	15 ml/kg
冷沉淀	5 ～ 10 ml/kg（不超过 300 ml）
血小板	1 成人份
浓缩凝血因子	咨询血液科

稀释性凝血功能障碍

大量输血最常见的并发症是稀释性凝血功能障碍。大量扩容（晶体、白蛋白）、输注血液及血制品使得血液中凝血成分被稀释。持续稀释剩余血小板和凝血因子导致止血功能受损。早期使用新鲜冰冻血浆（fresh frozen plasma，FFP）可以预防稀释性凝血障碍。

消耗性凝血功能障碍

无明显稀释情况下也可能会发生止血失败。这种情况可能是由于纤溶亢进、抗凝血途径激活或血小板功能障碍所致。除了血小板减少症（血小板计数为 100 000/mm^3），凝血功能障碍很难得到及时的诊断。因此，血小板和 FFP 在大量输血中无需等待凝血功能障碍的明确诊断依据就必须使用。不管是婴儿还是成人都可以采用如下输血方案：

- 给予 0.3 U/kg 血小板以达到血小板计数超过 50 000/mm^3（如果有活动性出血，则需达到 100 000/mm^3）；
- 每输注 6 U 浓缩红细胞，给予 4U FFP；

成分替代输血的适应证以及特殊成分输注治疗的利弊见表 48.2 所示。婴儿和新生儿的血浆凝血因子浓度低于成年人，稀释性凝血功能障碍发展得更快，因此婴儿凝血因子替代治疗的阈值更低。

代谢紊乱

酸碱改变在血液收集和保存过程中就可能发生。新鲜采集的血液加入枸橼酸盐-磷酸盐-葡萄糖溶液后，其酸碱度降至 7.0；在接下来 21 天的存储时间里，pH 会下降至 6.84。pH 减少主要原因是二氧化碳分压增加，因为储存容器不允许其排出。

不建议使用碳酸氢钠纠正酸中毒（除非在严重酸中毒时作为临时措施）。治疗的主要方法是液体复苏和改善组织灌注。

低体温

大量输血常发生体低温，会导致凝血功能障碍。据创伤文献记载，如果患者的核心温度低于 32℃，无论创伤的严重程度如何，其死亡率都是 100%。大量未经加温过的晶体、不含红细胞的胶体、血液和血制品都会导致心脏停搏。可以通过在输液前加温

表 48.2 成分输血的适应证及其预期止血特点

成分	适应证	优点	缺点
浓缩红细胞	红细胞丢失相关的低血容量	随时可用（自体、同源、血液回收）；比血液替代品更有效率；维持或提升血容量及血液氧输送能力	稀释性凝血功能障碍；溶血反应；感染；稀有血型难以获得
新鲜全血	贫血；低血容量伴贫血；大量输血（新生儿）	与供体接触数量减少，尤其是新生儿；含功能性血小板和凝血因子；维持或提升血容量及血液氧输送能力	可利用性受限；溶血性输血反应
新鲜冰冻血浆	凝血功能障碍	能替代预计正常成人浓度的所有蛋白质凝血因子；在冷冻状态下普遍可用	使用时机受限；感染；某些因子的浓度在某些患者中可能不足（如纤维蛋白原）；可利用性受限（至少需要 30 min 解冻）
冷沉淀	凝血功能障碍；Ⅷ因子缺乏	高浓度的纤维蛋白原和Ⅷ因子	集合产品；有感染的风险；使用时机受限；可获得性低（并非所有血库都有）
血小板	血小板功能障碍；血小板减少症	增加血小板计数：1 U 增加血小板计数（20 ～ 40）$\times 10^9$/L	低血压；单捐赠者与多名捐赠者；感染；功能半衰期短

液体和监测患者温度来预防低体温。

高钾血症

高钾血症是由于快速输注库存的红细胞所致。随着细胞裂解，储存在血液中的钾浓度随之增加。尽管肾功能正常的患者很少表现出高钾血症及其相关的血流动力学后果，但肾功能不成熟的新生儿和婴儿，或肾功能不全的患者，应该接受洗涤红细胞。有时候在停止输注库存红细胞后，可能会出现看似矛盾的迟发性低钾血症。

低钙血症 / 低镁血症

低钙血症或功能性低钙血症发生于快速输注储存于枸橼酸盐的血液时。枸橼酸盐与钙和其他共价阳离子（如镁）结合成螯合物。输血过快可能导致低血压，尤其是输注浓缩血小板或 FFP 时。当患者出现低钙血症或枸橼酸盐毒性症状（手足抽搐、低血压、QT 间期延长、心肌收缩力下降、脉压差变窄）时，应该给予纠正。应检查血镁水平，必要时进行补充。

肺功能不全、多器官功能衰竭和全身炎症反应综合征

下列因素可能会导致肺部和其他器官受损：

- 肺血管系统微聚物形成和通透性增加；
- 炎症介质释放导致全身性炎症反应综合征；
- 人类白细胞抗原系统相关的免疫反应。

输血相关性肺损伤（transfusion-related lung injury，TRALI）通常发生在输血后 6 h 内，与输血相关性循环超负荷（transfusion-associated circulatory overload，TACO）难以鉴别。监测心排血量和 B 型利尿钠肽可能会有所帮助。

感染

大量输血会增加感染风险，无论是通过传染源的传播还是免疫反应的抑制。尽管人类免疫缺陷病毒（human immunodeficiency virus，HIV）、病毒性肝炎，西尼罗病毒和巨细胞病毒的传播风险很低，但每接受一个供体都会增加患者感染潜在致命疾病的可能性。极少数情况下，可能会发生血液制品的细菌污染。

溶血

溶血通常是由于 ABO 血型不相容，一旦发生，会导致灾难性的后果。最常见的原因是管理失误。在 Kell、Kidd 和 Lewis 系统中发现的抗体也可能引发溶血反应。因此，在给予任何血液制品之前应尽可能地进行完整的血型和交叉匹配。

血栓形成

标准静脉血栓预防应在止血后尽快开始，因为患者在大量出血后会出现促血栓形成状态。

减少输血需求的其他疗法和干预措施

自体血回输和血液回收装置

使用血液回收装置回收丢失的红细胞已经成为常态。处理冲洗回收的血液，并将浓缩的红细胞悬浮于生理盐水中。尽管这些装置减少了使用同源红细胞的需要，但它们会稀释所有止血成分。因此，当输血量接近或超过 1.5 倍血容量时，无论采用何种替代策略，对凝血功能进行实验室评估都是至关重要的。

新鲜全血

并非所有大量失血的患者都可以通过成分输血进行优化治疗。然而，在紧急情况下输注新鲜全血不切实际，且难以提供保障。此外，对捐赠血液中 HIV 的核酸检测不可能在 48 h 内完成，这也使得新鲜全血的安全性低于库存血液。尽管它在大量输血方面具有理论优势，然而这项技术在婴儿心脏手术人群之外尚未被研究过。

重组凝血因子Ⅶa

当患者已经使用了足够的替代疗法但仍然出血不止时，重组凝血因子Ⅶa 可用来治疗微血管出血。重组凝血因子Ⅶa 最初被开发用于治疗血友病，通过与组织因子相互作用促进损伤部位的止血。尽管目前还缺乏相关的临床对照试验，并且对其使用仍然存在争议，但它已被纳入创伤治疗方案。因此它只能用作紧急干预措施，且使用流程应摆放在位。重组凝血因子Ⅶa 半衰期短，需要每 2 h 重复（90 U/kg）使用，直到出血得到控制。其他药物，如抑肽酶，在心脏和骨外科文献中被报道为减少失血和输血需求的辅助药物，但已不再普遍使用。也有报道说，在没有血小板减少的情况下，成人外科手术患者的 PT 和 PTT 值可能会增加到对照值的 1.5 倍，临床上却没有表现出失血量增加或异常出血。

氨甲环酸

氨甲环酸是一种纤溶酶原激活剂，它的使用得到了 CRASH-2 试验的支持。给药方式为 1 g 静注，然后 8 h 内静脉输注 1 g。颅内出血的患者禁用。

凝血酶原复合物浓缩物

凝血酶原复合物浓缩物从人血浆中提取。它包含因子Ⅱ、Ⅶ、Ⅸ和Ⅹ，以及蛋白质 C 和蛋白质 S，并可紧急逆转华法林。剂量为 25 ～ 50 IU/kg。

抑肽酶

抑肽酶是丝氨酸蛋白酶抑制剂，用于减少与纤维蛋白溶解增加相关的失血，但是由于存在严重的安全问题，现在只用于心肌血运重建。

预防

成功治疗大量失血的患者需要以下措施：

- 对预计会出血的择期手术采取预防措施：
  - 术前纠正先前存在的凝血障碍（或在紧急情况下尽快纠正）；
  - 对缺铁性贫血患者术前使用促红细胞生成素和静脉或口服铁剂；
  - 早期控制出血（止血带、加压、手术）；
  - 术中使用血液回收和氨甲环酸。
- 血库支持（血液学专家和技师）。
- 实验检验科支持。
- 合理的员工配置（搬运工，跑腿者等）。
- 患者保温和温度监测：所有静脉和外科冲洗液均需加温，并使用外部保温装置。
- 监测急性输血反应。
- 使用人工或电子患者识别系统确保向正确的患者提供正确的血液或血液制品。

并发症的预防需要获得及时的血库资源，适当的管理设备和快速的实验室周转。仔细记录和报告所有输入液体（包括晶体、胶体和血液制品）的数量、类型和时间，以及向血库传达预期需求至关重要。另外，还需要一些人员跟踪细节、协助沟通、运输样本和耗材。

大多数医院实施了大出血处理方案，推进了适当血制品的获取速度，以及相关团队的功能。所有工作人员都能迅速了解自己的角色。大出血演习使工作人员能够在预期事件发生时对这一流程非常熟悉（图 48.1）。

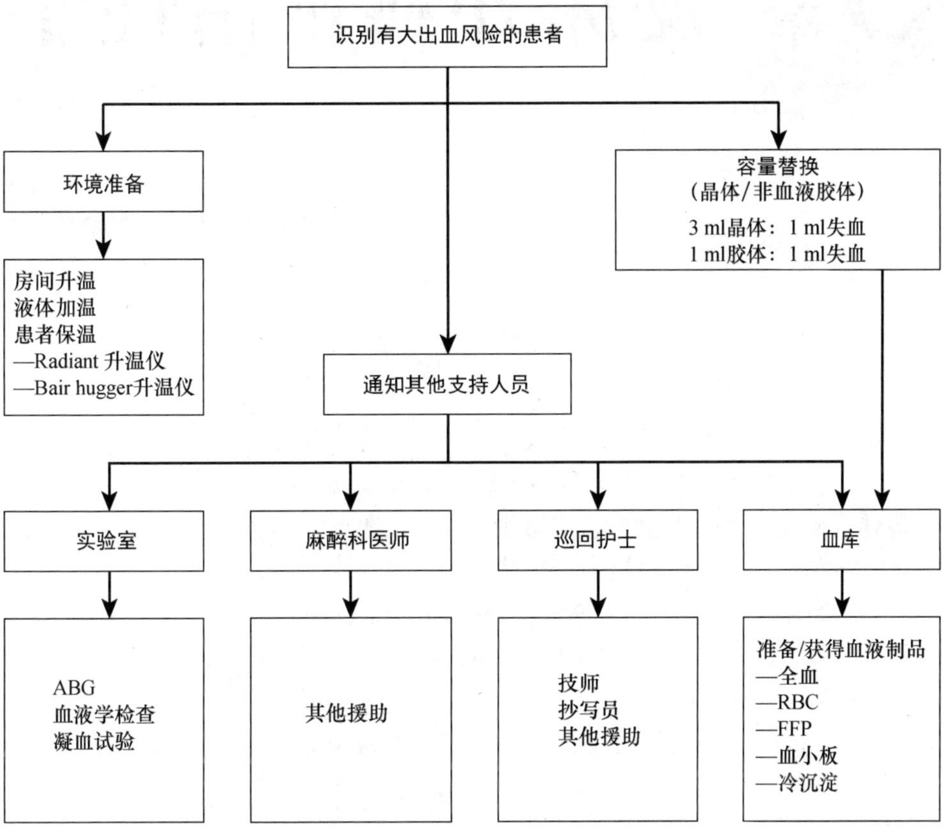

图 48.1 大量输血流程图。ABG，动脉血气；FFP，新鲜冰冻血浆；RBC，红细胞

（周 艳 译 陈 芳 校）

延伸阅读

Andrew M, Vegh P, Johnston M, et al.: Maturation of the hemostatic system during childhood, *Blood* 80:1998–2005, 1992.

Association of Anaesthetists of Great Britain and Ireland: Blood transfusion and the anaesthetist: management of massive haemorrhage, *Anaesthesia* 65:1153–1161, 2010.

Coté CJ, Liu LM, Szyfelbein SK, et al.: Changes in serial platelet counts following massive blood transfusion in pediatric patients, *Anesthesiology* 62:197–201, 1985.

Hardy JF, De Moerloose P, Samama M, et al.: Massive transfusion and coagulopathy: pathophysiology and implications for clinical management, *Can J Anaesth* 51:293–310, 2004.

Jurkovich GL, Greiser WB, Luterman A, et al.: Hypothermia in trauma victims: an ominous predictor of survival, *J Trauma* 27:1019–1024, 1987.

Levi M, Peters M, Buller HR: Efficacy and safety of recombinant factor VIIa for treatment of severe bleeding: a systematic review, *Crit Care Med* 33:883–890, 2005.

Manno CS, Hedberg KW, Kim HC, et al.: Comparison of the hemostatic effects of fresh whole blood, stored whole blood, and components after open heart surgery in children, *Blood* 77:930–936, 1991.

Murray DJ, Olson J, Strauss R, et al.: Coagulation changes during packed red cell replacement of major blood loss, *Anesthesiology* 69:839–845, 1988.

Sihler KC, Napolitano LM: Complications of massive transfusion, *Chest* 137:209–220, 2010.

第49章 泌尿外科根治性手术的并发症

Victoria L. McCormack, Adam Pichel

病例概要

患者，男性，44岁，既往高血压控制可，大量吸烟史，患者身体不适、体重减轻、无痛性血尿。计算机断层扫描（computed tomography，CT）显示右肾肿瘤伴血栓延伸至右肾静脉，并有少量血栓延伸至下腔静脉。拟行右肾血管栓塞术 + 右肾肿瘤根治术 + 腔静脉切开术 + 下腔静脉修复术。患者入院时呼吸困难，窦性心动过速。其动脉血气（arterial blood gas，ABG）分析如下：pH：7.47，PaO_2：9.2 kPa（69 mmHg），$PaCO_2$：3.9 kPa（29.25 mmHg），HCO_3：22，BE：-1.0。

肺动脉血管造影（CT pulmonary angiogram，CTPA）显示多个亚段肺栓塞。静脉给予肝素治疗，在手术前4 h停止使用。患者麻醉顺利，直至外科医师分离肾静脉至血液充满术野。有创血压78/48 mm Hg，心率120次/分钟，脉搏血氧饱和度89%，脉搏波形差。

问题分析

泌尿外科根治性手术患者的围术期管理中，出血风险和静脉血栓栓塞风险之间的关系通常存在矛盾。

定义

根治性这个术语通常用于描述手术切除恶性肿瘤，而不是良性病灶。邻近的解剖结构也会受到癌组织的影响而被切除。值得注意的是，这些手术越来越多地采用腹腔镜手术，因此预期并发症的发生率和性质将有所不同。

根治性膀胱切除术

对女性来说，根治性膀胱切除术包括切除膀胱、盆腔淋巴结、远端输尿管、尿道和阴道前壁。子宫、输卵管和卵巢有时会被切除。回肠膀胱术可作为手术的一部分。在男性中，这通常被称为**膀胱前列腺切除术**，因为切除的结构包括膀胱、前列腺、盆腔淋巴结、远端输尿管、输精管和精囊。它通常用于膀胱浸润性移行细胞癌。

根治性肾切除术

切除肾连同周围的整个肾前筋膜、肾周脂肪、同侧肾上腺和周围的淋巴管。绝大多数（约90%）的肾实质肿块为肾细胞癌（renal cell carcinoma，RCC），其余主要为移行细胞癌或儿童肾母细胞瘤。

根治性前列腺切除术

与经尿道前列腺切除术（transurethral resection of the prostate，TURP；见第52章）相比，根治性前列腺切除术是将整个前列腺、精囊、射精管和部分膀胱颈切除。大约90%的前列腺癌是腺癌。

腹腔镜根治性泌尿外科手术

可以通过开腹或腹腔镜手术来完成上述所有手术。腹腔镜手术并发症将在第46章详细讨论。与所有大手术一样，腹腔镜手术应注意患者的体位，避免神经损伤，预防压疮。考虑到手术技术对胸腔内压力的影响，需要考虑机械通气的方法。必须妥善处理良好的手术入路和理想的通气参数之间的关系。例如，侧卧位肾切除时，腹腔镜手术将气体注入腹膜内，以及极度的屈氏体位，都会影响呼吸功能。使用高吸气压力来处理可能会引起气压伤，因此接受术中允许性呼吸性酸中毒可能是一种合理的方法。

识别

病例概要提到了两个根治性泌尿外科手术的主要并发症：静脉血栓栓塞（venous thromboembolism，VTE）和大出血。

静脉血栓栓塞

患者的危险因素包括恶性肿瘤、高龄和吸烟史。除了一般危险因素外，还应特别关注肿瘤和血栓向肾静脉、髂静脉、下腔静脉和右心房的扩散程度。肾细胞癌腔静脉扩散的 Novick 分级描述了肿瘤或血栓扩散到肾静脉以外的程度。目前尚不清楚这一分级与预后或肺栓塞的可能性有何直接关系。4% ～ 10% 的肾细胞癌在发现时已有血栓扩散到下腔静脉（表 49.1）。

据报道，开放性泌尿外科手术的 VTE 发生率在 0.2% ～ 5%。腹腔镜泌尿外科手术的发生率在 0.3% ～ 4.8%。

静脉血栓栓塞的表现从无症状到呼吸困难、胸膜炎性胸痛、小腿疼痛和肿胀、咳嗽、咯血以及急性心力衰竭不等。后者可根据心血管损害程度分为**小面积**肺栓塞或**大面积**肺栓塞（pulmonary embolism，PE）。这类患者的检查应包括 12 导联心电图、胸部 X 线片、心肌酶谱测定和动脉血气分析，以及筛查血样。必要时可能还需要超声心动图和 CTPA（表 49.2）。

术中突发的肺栓塞可导致心动过速、血压降低和呼气末二氧化碳（$ETCO_2$）减少。术中经食管超声心动图成像（在一些中心常规使用）可实时证实肺栓塞。

表 49.1　RCC 患者腔静脉肿瘤扩散的 Novick 分级

1 级	血栓进入 IVC，但在肾静脉上方 <2 cm
2 级	血栓在肝内腔静脉以下
3 级	血栓累及肝内腔静脉，但低于横膈膜
4 级	血栓累及右心房

IVC，下腔静脉；RCC，肾细胞癌

表 49.2　静脉血栓栓塞的体征和症状

体征	症状
呼吸急促（70%）	呼吸困难（73%）
心动过速（30%）	胸痛（66%）
捻发音（51%）	咳嗽（37%）
低烧	恐惧 出汗

大出血

鉴于切除临近结构的解剖关系，在根治性泌尿外科手术中，大多数出血来自静脉。

Santorini 神经丛（如图 49.1）位于前列腺背面，在根治性切除腺体过程中易受损伤。

盆腔淋巴结切除可引起下腹部静脉出血，腹膜后淋巴结切除可引起 IVC 或周围静脉广泛出血。

据报道，在腹腔镜泌尿外科手术中，出血占所有并发症的 40%。开放根治性前列腺切除术的平均失血量约为 500 ～ 1000 ml，即使在手术量大、经验丰富的中心也是如此。在手术过程中需要保持临床警惕，而容积状态的评估是关键。常规监测可显示心动过速和低血压，同时要考虑到其他药物（如 β 受体阻滞剂、瑞芬太尼）的影响。ABG 分析可显示血红蛋白的急性下降或血清乳酸的升高，特别是如果静脉输注大量液体，会进一步加重术前贫血。

无创性心排血量监测设备越来越多地被用于特大肿瘤手术。这种监测仪使用患者**液体反应性**或特定的动态测量如**每搏量变异度**来检测早期可能继发于隐匿性出血的低血容量。

空气栓塞

应该注意的是，盆腔静脉开放时，存在空气栓塞的风险。当摆放 Trendelenburg 体位时，这种风险非常明显。它类似于肺循环的静脉血栓栓塞。大的空气栓塞可导致右心室流出道完全梗阻，引起严重的心血管损害、心律失常和心脏停搏。

尿脓毒血症

对于具有泌尿系疾病阻塞特征的患者，当术中行泌尿系统操作时，低级别细菌感染在临床上可能变得非常棘手。可能出现发热、心动过速、高碳酸血症和低血压。

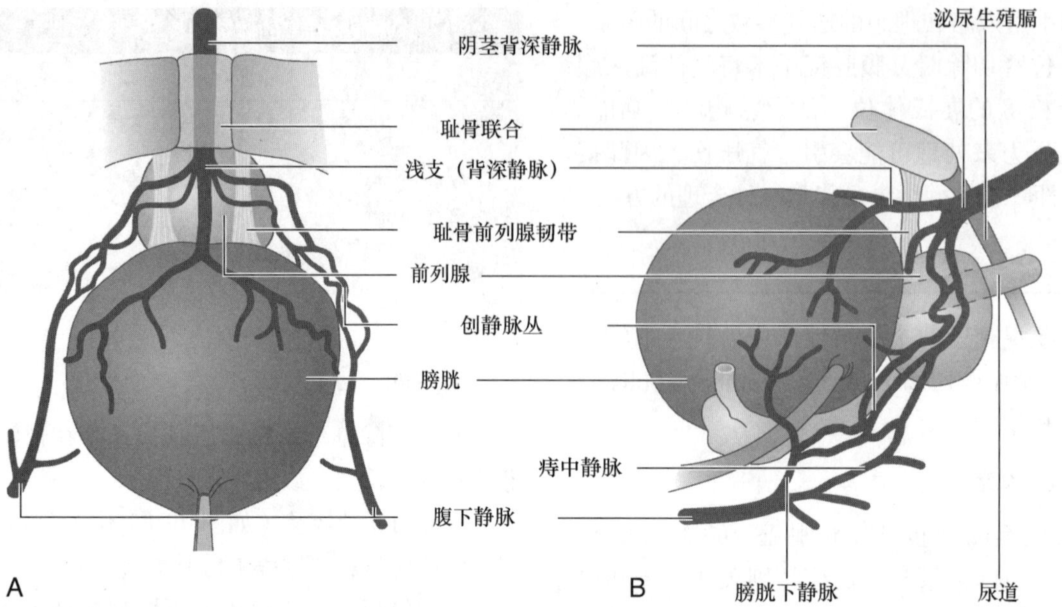

图 49.1 前列腺静脉流入 Santorini 丛，接受来自阴茎、前列腺、膀胱和精囊的血液。这个神经丛还与耻骨、阴部、深腹壁、闭孔和痔静脉相通［From Reiner WG，Walsh PC：An anatomical approach to the surgical management of the dorsal vein and Santorini plexus during radical retropubic surgery. *J Urol* 121（2）：198-200，1979.］

急性肾损伤

尽管急性肾损伤（acute kidney injury，AKI）不太可能在所有手术中发生，但在最漫长和复杂的手术中除外，应考虑其在围术期发生的可能性。尽管围术期危重症、贫血和围术期心血管并发症也可能对肾功能产生不利影响，但肾前性和肾后性梗阻的原因可能与泌尿外科患者相关。术中尽可能进行尿量监测，麻醉和术后护理时应考虑肾功能的术前参数。表 49.3 列出了急性肾损伤网络（Acute Kidney Injury Network，AKIN）鉴定 AKI 的标准。

风险评估

接受根治性泌尿外科手术的人群平均年龄为 60 岁。

表 49.3 急性肾损伤的 AKIN 分类 / 分级系统

阶段	血清肌酐的标准	尿量标准
1	血清肌酐增加 ≥ 0.3 mg/dl（≥ 26.4 μmol/l），或增加至基线水平的 150% ～ 200%（1.5 ～ 2 倍）	每小时 <0.5 ml/kg，持续 6 h 以上
2	血清肌酐从基线增加到 200% ～ 300%（2 ～ 3 倍）	每小时 <0.5 ml/kg，持续 12 h 以上
3	血清肌酐从基线增加到 >300%（>3 倍）（或血清肌酐≥ 4.0 mg/dl[≥ 354 μmol/L]，急性增加至少 0.5 mg/dl[44 μmol/L]）	24 小时低于 0.3 ml（kg·h）或 12 h 无尿

根治性前列腺切除术组可能相对没有并存疾病，因为高手术风险的患者中，放疗是一种替代治疗方案。由于治疗方案选择少，根治性膀胱切除术和肾切除术是患者的主要治疗方案。

一般注意事项

大手术需要对患者进行正确的评估，评估应考虑手术的复杂性、患者的并存疾疾、手术或保守治疗的紧迫性和预期寿命。考虑到手术的根治性，这可能包括对心肺功能的评估。手术评估由一个多学科小组审查，以确保良好的患者选择和允许术前内科治疗优化病情。一般来说，开腹手术切除较大的肿瘤比腹腔镜手术切除较小的肿瘤风险更大。年龄和术前肾功能是决定肾切除术后预后的重要因素。预期寿命较长的年轻患者可根据肿瘤部位选择保留肾单位的手术（例如，下极肿瘤部分切除肾）。这些操作可能更复杂，但最终在保护肾功能方面效果更好。

出血

易增加出血风险的手术因素包括既往手术史（如 TURP 或多次前列腺活检）或放疗使周围组织更脆弱或粘连。由于肿瘤的位置，手术入路可能更具挑战性，这应该通过术前影像学的彻底检查来确定。

静脉血栓栓塞

所有的癌症患者都被认为是 VTE 的高危人群。

因此，风险评估应考虑更多的因素，如 Novick 分级和平衡每种药物治疗的出血风险与 VTE 的风险。

启示

根治性泌尿外科手术通常老年患者居多，伴有大出血、静脉血栓栓塞或空气栓塞的风险，以及其他更普遍的大手术风险。一般风险包括体位不当造成的神经损伤、术后切口感染以及肺部感染或气胸等呼吸道并发症。对这些风险的评估、预防、认识和管理不善将造成重大威胁。

各报告的死亡率和发病率各不相同。一项对 11 010 名接受根治性前列腺切除术的男性患者进行的大型研究显示，总体死亡率为 0.5%。该研究还显示，20.4% 的患者在手术后 30 天内出现过一次或多次并发症。随着技术的进步和更多的治疗方法的提高，未来更多的高危患者可能会接受根治性泌尿外科手术。

管理

静脉血栓栓塞

出现 PE 的患者围术期应抗凝，综合考虑手术时机和既往肾功能（如静脉注射普通肝素或适当剂量的低分子肝素）来选择最合适的治疗方案。抗凝桥接治疗需要与手术小组商定和讨论，因为这可能影响到麻醉药物和麻醉方案（如硬膜外麻醉）的选择使用和管理。

在一些复杂的病例中，如肾细胞癌和扩散到 IVC 的病例，一些中心在透视下将充满盐水和造影剂的球囊插入 IVC，以捕捉操作肿瘤过程中脱落的栓子。在这种情况下，经食管超声心动图的术中成像是有用的。在某些情况下，考虑到血栓的位置，如果极有可能发生栓塞，则可以决定是否准备进行体外循环。

出血

治疗应以精细的外科技术、评估和以液体和血液制品复苏的形式对心血管参数做出反应为主。在病例开始之前，应讨论失血处理计划，并酌情估计失血量和进行交叉匹配。如果出现大出血，应启动大出血方案。对血红蛋白、血小板计数和凝血功能的动态测量（如血栓弹力图）进行逐个检测有助于指导围术期的决策。

现有的指南支持将氨甲环酸用于预测失血量大于 500 ml 的患者，以此作为限制自体输血的策略。此外，在考虑恶性肿瘤的情况下，也应考虑细胞修复，目前已解决细胞修复问题。然而，应该记住，如果要对肠道进行操作（例如，回肠膀胱成形术），此时应停止细胞修复以限制污染。对于肾细胞癌大面积扩张到 IVC 的患者，在**切皮**之前对肾进行血管栓塞有助于减少肾切除术时的失血。

空气栓塞

如果大量的空气进入循环，就有可能发生心力衰竭。必须立即采取支持措施，如提高吸入氧浓度。同样的，如果发生了心脏停搏，及时进行心肺复苏。为了使产生的空气栓子从肺流出道中排出，必须将患者置于头低左侧位。如果放置了中心静脉导管，则可从右心腔将空气抽出。为了防止进一步的空气栓塞，可用无菌液体冲洗手术区域。

尿脓毒症

术中管理多为支持性，应合理应用抗生素。在进行外科控制感染源时，需要使用血管升压药或强心药来支持循环。对于发生脓毒症的患者，可能需要术后加强监护治疗。

预防

急性肾损伤

识别与围术期 AKI 风险增加相关的患者特征，可对患者采取抢先治疗。美国一项大型前瞻性研究确定了接受普通外科手术的患者的 9 个危险因素。这些因素中有 6 个或以上的患者发生 AKI 的概率为 10%。

- 年龄大于 56 岁；
- 男性；
- 活动性充血性心力衰竭；
- 腹水；
- 高血压；
- 急诊手术；
- 腹腔手术；
- 术前肌酐大于 107 μmol/L；

- 糖尿病（口服降糖药或胰岛素控制）。

除了这些因素，避免或减少使用存在肾毒性药物是一个合理的方法。造影剂具有肾毒性，应使用尽可能低剂量的最小毒性的造影剂。如可能，术前应停止使用潜在的肾毒性药物（如血管紧张素转换酶抑制剂和非甾体抗炎药）。术前补液和术中注射 N- 乙酰半胱氨酸可作为中高危病例的预防措施。

术中必须在静脉输液治疗减轻肾前因素和使患者负荷过多损害其他系统之间取得平衡。例如，过度补液可能导致肺水肿，尤其是对心力衰竭患者。此外，极度的 Trendelenburg 体位和大量使用液体可能导致术后脑水肿。

术后，每日的肾灌注情况和谨慎的体液平衡将有助于此类患者的治疗。

尿脓毒症

手术部位感染（Surgical site infection，SSI）和尿脓毒血症是根治性泌尿外科手术的重要危险因素。SSI 使患者更可能需要危重治疗且住院费用几乎是普通住院费用的 2 倍。可通过评估患者因素、外科因素和潜在感染发病率来确定外科抗生素预防的益处。

除严格无菌手术技术外，还应考虑在**切皮**前 60 min 内，按照当地指南给予预防性抗生素。在大多数情况下，预防性使用抗生素应作为单一剂量，或最多在术后 24 h 内停止使用，而无需怀疑临床上有持续感染。给药时应考虑肾功能。大量失血需要追加抗生素治疗。

出血

在这些手术中预防大出血与其他大手术有很多共同之处。因此，正在进行的临床试验的结果，即在术前使用静脉注射铁制剂优化血红蛋白水平，可能会为实践提供参考依据。应根据具体情况考虑使用此类药剂。

避免静脉充血、胸内高压和高碳酸血症可能有助于减少静脉出血。考虑到可能引起的静脉充血，使用高容量稀释来减少血细胞比容可能并不恰当。应注意避免低体温及其凝血功能。

在某些合适的情况下，可以采用区域麻醉技术来减少手术失血。

静脉血栓栓塞

对于接受根治性泌尿外科手术的患者，应制定个体化预防静脉血栓栓塞的方案。如前所述，大多数患者具有 VTE 的高风险，可能已有 VTE。应根据患者的具体情况和手术时机来选择阻止血栓形成的治疗方法。

手术前必须计划好预防血栓迁移的外科干预措施，如使用充满盐水的球囊或心肺转流术（体外循环）。

致谢

感谢 Terri G.Monk 博士对本章上一版的贡献。

（戴柠宇 译 周 懿 校）

延伸阅读

American Urological Association: Best Practice Policy Statement on Urologic Surgery Antimicrobial Prophylaxis. Available at https://www.auanet.org, 2008 Accessed October 6, 2016.

Borthwick E, Ferguson A: Perioperative acute kidney injury: risk factors, recognition, management and outcomes, *BMJ* 341:c3365, 2010.
https://www.auanet.org
Chapman E, Pichel AC: Anaesthesia for nephrectomy, *Br J Anaesth*1–4, 2015.

Corris PA: A practical approach to the diagnosis of venothromboembolism, *Clin Med (Lond)* 1(4):274–281, 2001.

Crescenti A, Borghi G, Bignami E, et al.: Intraoperative use of tranexamic acid to reduce transfusion rate in patients undergoing radical retropubic prostatectomy: double blind, randomised, placebo controlled trial, *BMJ* 343:d5701, 2011.

Mehta RL, Kellum JA, Shah SV, et al.: Acute Kidney Injury Network: report of an initiative to improve outcomes in acute kidney injury, *Crit Care* 11(2):R31, 2007.

Novick AC, Kaye MC, Cosgrove DM, et al.: Experience with cardiopulmonary bypass and deep hypothermic circulatory arrest in the management of retroperitoneal tumors with large vena cava thrombi, *Ann Surg* 212(4):472–476, 1990. discussion 476-477.

Padhi S, Kemmis-Betty S, Rajesh S, et al.: Blood transfusion: summary of NICE guidance, *BMJ* 351:h5832, 2015.

Richards T, Clevenger B, Keidan J, et al.: PREVENTT: preoperative intravenous iron to treat anaemia in major surgery: study protocol for randomised controlled trial, *Trials* 16:254, 2015.

Ubee S, Kumar M, Athmanathan N, et al.: Intraoperative red blood cell salvage and autologous transfusion during open radical retropubic prostatectomy: a cost-benefit analysis, *Ann R Coll Surg Engl* 93(2):157–161, 2011.

Webb ST, Allen JSD: Perioperative renal protection, *Contin Educ Anaesth Crit Care Pain* 8(5):176–180, 2008.

脊柱手术的并发症

第50章

Jason D.Walls · Diana Ayubcba

病例概要

患者，男性，78岁，病态肥胖，体重指数（body mass index，BMI）43，有慢性心房颤动病史，服用达比加群（5天前停用）。因T8转移性肾细胞癌行椎体切除术和多节段融合术，术中联合躯体感觉诱发电位（somatosensory evoked potential，SSEP）和经颅运动诱发电位（transcranial motor evoked potential，tcMEP）多功能监测下以丙泊酚全凭静脉麻醉（total intravenous anesthesia，TIVA）。术中发生大量失血，需大量成分输血，SSEP和tcMEP整体降低，但通过过纠正急性贫血和低血压使其上升至基线水平。手术时间7 h，次日上午，患者在重症监护室（intensive care unit，ICU）拔管。苏醒后发现患者双侧视力突然丧失。

问题分析

神经损伤

定义

脊柱手术后的神经损伤似乎是罕见事件，但可能导致永久性和致残的结局。从创伤性损伤的固定到细致切除肿瘤，脊柱手术适应证各不相同，可导致不同形式的术后神经损伤，危及脊髓、单个神经根甚至臂丛终末神经。术后并发症可以从轻度感觉变化到更严重的中央脊髓综合征，布朗-塞卡（Brown-Sequard）综合征和四肢瘫痪。

识别

如果没有术中监测，脊柱手术的神经损伤直到患者麻醉清醒后才能发现，此时采取纠正措施往往为时已晚。然而，术中神经生理监测（intraoperative neurophysiologic monitoring，IONM）可以实时评估和监测即将发生的神经损伤。在神经结构有危险时，IONM会提醒外科医师，并促使其采取纠正措施。总的来说，IONM致力于提高脊柱手术的整体安全性，并防止严重神经损伤的发生。

IONM以多种不同的方式监测脊髓完整性，包括SSEP、tcMEP和肌电图（electromyography，EMG）。更具体地说，SSEP可持续监测周围神经受到刺激后上行背柱-内侧丘系感觉通路。然而，SSEP并不监测脊髓的前部，特别是皮质脊髓束。为了监测这些运动通路，在手术关键时刻间断性地检查tcMEP，方法是通过头皮电刺激，以刺激上肢和下肢的远端肌肉群。为了更全面地检查脊髓的完整性，tcMEP可以与持续的SSEP联合，以监测脊髓的前后两部分。最后，EMG，无论是自发的（自由运动的）还是触发的，都可以在神经根周围和椎弓根螺钉植入过程中进行更准确的监测。虽然tcMEP可以在神经根手术中监测运动功能，但肌群的大量重叠使其不能分辨特定的神经根，而EMG则可以实现这一功能。

虽然为提高安全性，IONM可实时评估神经完整性，但由于缺乏高质量的研究和随机对照试验，尚无临床应用的标准推荐。IONM的使用在复杂的脊柱手术中很常见，但在所有脊柱手术中的使用并不统一。虽然关于IONM改善临床结果的总体成本/效益分析仍然存在争议，但这种监测模式确实提供了术中神经完整性的反馈信息，能够降低术后神经损伤的发生率。

风险评估

在围术期脊髓损伤的各种病因中，手术创伤似乎是术后神经损伤的最大危险因素。损伤机制包括直接神经损伤、压迫、牵拉、硬体植入以及脊柱侧弯手术中明显脊柱形状改变。此外，围术期的其他因素也可能导致神经损伤，包括患者体位不当、肩带缠扎、低血压、失血和气道操作。

特别要注意的是患者已表现为颈椎不稳定或脊髓疾病。在这种情况下，气道操作时必须极其谨慎，以防止颈椎发生病理性移动。然而，大多数颈椎术后损伤并不是发生在颈椎不稳定的患者，而是发生在颈椎病患者，包括从解剖学异常至炎症病程导致的颈椎病（表 50.1）。这些情况降低了颈椎损伤的阈值，或是使气道管理更具挑战，增加了术中颈髓损伤的风险。术前应进行全面的评估以明确病情，在进行脊柱手术之前重新回顾影像学检查结果（即屈曲 / 伸展影像学，计算机断层扫描）。术前确定有风险的患者可以对其实施高级的监测和气道管理技术，以限制和预防加重神经损伤。

除了脊髓损伤外，某些情况还会增加围术期外周神经损伤的风险，包括糖尿病、肾疾病、甲状腺功能减退、酗酒、维生素缺乏和营养不良。在为这些患者选择合适的术中体位时，必须考虑周围神经损伤的风险和充分手术暴露的益处。

启示

脊柱手术中围术期神经损伤的预防涉及麻醉实施的许多方面，包括气道管理、IONM 和麻醉选择。颈椎不稳定的气道管理，无论病因如何，都需要精心准备和使用先进的设备。这些患者围术期脊髓损伤的风险很高，气道操作必须限制可导致严重脊髓压迫的颈椎病理运动。虽然对于成功的气管插管最安全的方法并没有明确的标准，但清醒下纤支镜插管仍然是最安全的方法。即使颈椎稳定的患者，当有显著的神经病理损伤时，气管插管也应根据体检结果和相关影像学检查，采用更先进的技术。研究表明，在颈椎有严重狭窄的患者中，即使是最轻微的颈部伸展也会增加损伤的易感性。

在使用 IONM 时，必须仔细制定具体的麻醉方法。目前实际使用的所有药物几乎都会干扰 IONM（表 50.2）。SSEP 和 MEP 均为多突触信号通路，需要依赖体内稳态才能发挥正常功能。SSEP 比 tcMEP 抗干扰性更强，如果用作单一的监测技术，可使用强效挥发性药物（大约 0.5 MAC）和肌肉松弛剂实施平衡全身麻醉。使用 tcMEP 时，无神经肌肉阻滞剂的 TIVA 似乎是最好的方法。挥发性麻醉药和 TIVA 均可安全用于 EMG，但必须避免使用神经肌肉阻滞药物。在行 IONM 时，关键的手术操作之前必须使患者达到稳定的麻醉状态。

表 50.1 术后颈椎损伤风险增加的病情

先天性异常	软骨发育不全，唐氏综合征，Klippel-Feil 综合征，神经纤维瘤病 1，小脑扁桃体下疝畸形，Morquio 综合征，先天性颈椎管狭窄
退行性变化	颈椎病，椎间盘突出，破坏性脊柱关节病
炎症性疾病	类风湿关节炎，强直性脊柱炎
感染性疾病	Grisel 综合征

出血

定义

严重失血可能是某些脊柱手术的主要并发症。尽管表现上已经止血，但手术止血不彻底仍可导致术中或术后出血。出血可导致严重和致命的并发症，如脊髓缺血。

对于脊柱外科来说，骨皮质剥脱和硬膜外静脉出血是术中出血的主要原因，在椎体切除术、多节

表 50.2 普通麻醉药物对脊柱手术中 IONM 的影响

药物名称	药物类型	对 SSEPs 的影响	对 MEPs 的影响
丙泊酚	GABA 激动剂	↓	↓
依托咪酯	GABA 激动剂	↑↑	—
咪达唑仑	苯二氮䓬类	↓	
氯胺酮	NMDA 拮抗剂	↑	—/↓
芬太尼	阿片类	—/↓	↓
瑞芬太尼	阿片类	—/↓	—/↓
舒芬太尼	阿片类	—/↓	↓
右美托咪定	α_2- 激动剂	—/↓	—/↓
异氟烷	吸入	↓↓	↓↓↓
七氟烷	吸入	↓↓	↓↓
地氟烷	吸入	↓↓	↓↓
N_2O	吸入	↓↓	↓↓

GABA，γ- 氨基丁酸；IONM，术中神经生理监测；MEP，运动诱发电位；NMDA，N- 甲基 -D- 天冬氨酸；SSEP，躯体感觉诱发电位。
Adapted from Rabai F，Sessions R，Seubert CN：Neurophysiological monitoring and spinal cord integrity. *Best Pract Res Clin Anaesthesiol* 30（1）：53-68，2016.

段脊柱内固定和融合手术中出血的风险最大。除了手术止血不彻底，凝血功能障碍和未控制的高血压是脊柱手术中出血的另外两种原因。

围术期凝血功能障碍有多种病因，包括体温过低，血浆凝血因子水平低，血小板减少，保证凝血和血小板功能正常的酶系统破坏，或纤维蛋白溶解亢进。

识别

出血导致循环容量减少，从而激活神经反射，支配心脏和其他器官的交感神经兴奋性增加。这种反应在围术期表现为心动过速、低血压、血管收缩和血液从非重要器官流出的重新分布。除了加强患者生命体征监测和体格检查外，麻醉科医师应与外科团队保持沟通以预测和治疗可能的失血，这一点也是极其重要的。

风险评估

术前全面的评估，包括病史、体格检查和实验室检查（如有必要），可提示围术期出血或凝血功能障碍的潜在危险因素。应询问患者已知的出血疾病、淤血、异常出血（鼻衄）、药物使用情况（氯吡格雷、阿司匹林、华法林、非维生素 K 拮抗剂、口服抗凝血剂和肝素）和营养缺乏。其他可能的危险因素包括既往脊柱手术史、每日饮酒量增加、高 BMI 值、既往使用非甾体抗炎药以及高龄。

根据患者的病史，术前可进行血小板计数、凝血酶原时间、部分凝血活酶时间和国际标准化比值等实验室检查。出血时间、活化凝血时间、纤维蛋白原水平和血栓弹性图通常是不必要的检查。对于有复杂遗传性出血疾病的患者，可能需要血液科进行会诊，以协助围术期凝血管理。

启示

出血可导致严重和致命的并发症，如脊髓缺血。在有脊髓损伤史的患者中，脊髓血流量的自我调节功能受损，增加了缺血的风险。此外，椎体移位或手术牵拉引起的外部压迫可进一步减少脊髓血流。出血导致的低血压与创伤性脊髓损伤后的神经功能恶化有关。

围术期视力丧失

定义

围术期视力丧失（perioperative visual loss，POVL）是一种罕见但具有破坏性的并发症。脊柱手术后 POVL 发生率仅为 0.03% ～ 0.2%，但俯卧位脊柱手术后 POVL 发生率最高，占所有报告病例的一半以上。患者俯卧位行脊柱手术时，三种不同的损伤机制可能导致 POVL：视网膜中央动脉阻塞（central retinal artery occlusion，CRAO）、缺血性视神经病变（ischemic optic neuropathy，ION）和皮质失明。目前为止，脊柱手术后 POVL 最常见的病因是 ION，其次是 CRAO。这两种情况将进一步讨论。

CRAO 导致术后失明，继发于对任何一只眼睛的直接外压，通常与头部位置放置不当有关。对眼睛的外部压迫会增加眼内压力，从而减少视网膜中央动脉的血流量，改变整个视网膜的氧供。CRAO 的其他罕见原因包括栓子和动脉血栓形成。

根据视神经损伤的解剖部位不同，ION 损伤分为两种类型。前 ION（anterior ION，AION）和后 ION（posterior ION，PION），分别发生在筛板的前部和后部。ION 的病因是多因素的，尚未完全了解。总的来说，在俯卧位脊柱手术后，PION 似乎比 AION 更常见。

识别

典型的 CRAO 表现为术后不久新发的单侧视力丧失。体格检查显示瞳孔对光反射消失。眼底镜检查显示视网膜变白和缺血，黄斑处有樱桃红斑点。同样，ION 在术后即刻出现，但通常表现为双侧无痛性视力丧失。AION 的临床表现不相同，可延迟数天发作。体格检查会发现传入性瞳孔障碍或对光反射消失。在 AION 中，眼底检查最初显示视神经盘水肿，视神经盘边缘模糊，可能伴有乳头周围裂片样出血，数周后进展为视神经盘苍白。在 PION，最初的眼底检查是正常的，但会进展到视神经盘苍白，数周后与 AION 无法区分。

风险评估

CRAO 引发 POVL 的风险与使用任何可能对眼睛施加压力的装置成正相关。因此，俯卧位时应避免使用马蹄形头枕和护目镜。

尽管 ION 的具体病因尚未明确，且很可能是多因素的，但 6 个独立因素增加了发生这种罕见并发症的风险（框 50.1）。然而，一些关于 ION 的报道中并未出现这些风险因素，这也表明 ION 损伤机制还未完全明了。俯卧位、术中血红蛋白的最低值以

框 50.1 脊柱手术后缺血性视神经病变的独立危险因素

男性
肥胖
使用 Wilson 框架
较长的麻醉 / 手术时间
估计失血较多
复苏时胶体液与非血液性液体的比例降低

及低血压似乎并不会单独增加 ION 的风险

启示

无论是来自 INO 还是 CARO，POVL 的预后都极差，视力几乎无法恢复，也没有有效的治疗方案。由于脊柱大手术后 POVL 的风险增加，在获取知情同意过程中应与患者讨论这一灾难性并发症。

气道损害

定义

脊柱手术后的气道损害包括需要紧急再插管或气管切开的情况。最近报道显示，多达 5% 的颈椎前路手术可能发生气道并发症，大约 1% 的病例需要再次插管。脊柱手术后气道损伤的病因是多方面的，包括咽喉或椎前软组织水肿、术后颈部血肿、脑脊液（cerebrospinal fluid，CSF）外漏、脓肿形成、植入物移位、甚至喉返神经损伤。此外，创伤性插管可能导致水肿、出血或气管损伤，可能导致气道阻塞。颈椎融合过程中超适应证使用骨形态生成蛋白可诱发强烈的炎症反应导致迟发性气道水肿。尽管病因不同，脊柱手术后气道损害必须得到识别和治疗，以避免气道梗阻、缺氧，以及最终不可逆转的脑缺血。

识别

术后气道损害患者可出现一系列症状，包括呼吸急促、呼吸困难、喘鸣、躁动或发绀。颈椎手术后气道症状可提示病因。喉头水肿引起的气道阻塞通常在术后 12 ～ 72 h 出现。术后 12 h 内的气道早期损害提示创面血肿。脓肿，脑脊液外漏和移植物故障时损害会延迟发生。

对于疑似气道受损的患者，必须进行重点体检并检查生命体征，包括脉搏血氧饱和度。头颈部解剖的评估应包括口腔和舌头的水肿以及颈部血肿。快速识别气道损害并采取纠正措施对安全避免术后缺氧至关重要。

风险评估

在颈椎手术后，最近的评论强调了患者自身、手术和麻醉因素都会增加术后气道损害的风险（表 50.3）。在比较所有因素时，术中手术因素对术后气道损害的影响最为显著。

启示

任何颈椎术后患者拔管前都应考虑术后气道损害的风险。应评估患者和手术危险因素，以及任何已知的困难气道史。如果对拔管后气道梗阻存在合理的担忧，术后应保留气管插管，并将患者送入 ICU 进行术后管理。有关安全拔管的最佳时间尚缺乏明确的指南或随机对照试验。目前的临床实践允许患者带管过夜。然而咽喉水肿可在术后 72 h 内发生，因此对于高危患者可能需要延长带管时间，直至度过这一高危期过后才能拔管。

管理

神经损伤

外科、麻醉和神经监测小组之间的术前沟通是预防严重术后神经损伤的第一步。脊柱手术前应就患者的体位、IONM 和麻醉类型达成一致。必须识别威胁脊髓完整性的疾病，并使用先进技术限制潜在的神经损伤。对于不稳定或稳定的慢性颈椎病患者，在未来的研究明确最佳和最安全的气管插管方法前，目前推荐使用纤维支气管镜插管来减少颈椎活动。即使是插管前的操作，包括抬下颏和托下颌，也会引起颈椎移位，必须谨慎使用。在紧急情况下，快速序贯诱导加手法保持中线稳定以及在可视喉镜

表 50.3 颈椎手术后气道损害的危险因素

患者	手术	麻醉
病态肥胖	>3 个椎体	多次尝试插管
阻塞性睡眠呼吸暂停	C2 ～ C4 水平	喉镜下声门暴露差
肺部疾病	失血量 >300 ml	
脊髓型颈椎病	手术时间 >5 h	
既往颈椎前路手术史	前 / 后路手术	

Adapted from Palumbo MA，Aidlen JP，Daniels AH，et al：Airway compromise due to laryngopharyngeal edema after anterior cervical spine surgery. *J Clin Anesth* 25（1）：66-72，2013.

下似乎是最佳的方法。

术中应维持血流动力学稳定，避免低血压，失血后容量复苏，以及持续监测患者的体位使患者术中保持稳定状态。当预计大容量复苏时，应考虑监测动脉压（Intraarterial blood pressure，IABP），以便快速纠正低血压，或根据临床需要诱发相对高血压。当 IONM 信号变化时，必须找出可逆的原因，包括低体温、低血压、使用强效吸入麻醉药、监测电极的技术问题，以及逆转高风险的手术操作。

出血

围术期出血或凝血需要立即干预。治疗的重点是使用合理的药物和血液制品来纠正任何可逆原因的凝血障碍。当凝血障碍需要血液制品进行纠正时，治疗方案包括新鲜冷冻血浆、血小板、冷沉淀、凝血酶原复合物浓缩液或重组因子Ⅶa。如果出血与血小板功能障碍有关，可给予去氨加压素。所有的液体和血制品在使用前都应加温。此外，应使用暖风毯或热灯对患者进行主动保温，进一步防止体温过低。

控制性低血压是另一种可用于减少择期脊柱手术中失血和输血需求的技术。这种方法的使用是基于临床判断，根据已有的并存疾病和脊柱手术的具体类型来评估患者的风险和收益。尼卡地平是一种动脉选择性血管扩张剂，在这种特殊用途上比硝普钠和硝酸甘油更受青睐。尽管动物模型表明，硝酸甘油在低血压时最有利于维持脊髓血流，但这一点尚未在人类得到证实。然而，低血压与创伤性脊髓损伤后的神经功能恶化有关，对于这类患者以及脊髓受压严重的患者控制性低血压应特别谨慎。

术中自体血回输是治疗出血的另一种有效方式。患者术中流出的血液会被回收、冲洗或过滤，并根据需要自体回输。然而，滤过型自体输血可能会出现纤溶和弥散性血管内凝血。细胞清洗系统去除可溶性物质也会导致凝血因子和血小板的丢失，从而导致凝血障碍。以前，化脓性感染和恶性肿瘤是相对禁忌证，但使用先进的过滤和清洗系统，自体血液回收已成为可能。

围术期视力丧失

目前对于 POVL 尚无有效的治疗方案。虽然缺乏循证支持，但获得有限成功的推荐包括纠正严重贫血、维持基础血压、抬高头部以减少眼眶周围水肿、甘露醇、高剂量类固醇和高压氧治疗。在未来的研究提供有效治疗办法前，POVL 的最佳治疗方法是预防。当怀疑 POVL 时，应立即请眼科会诊。

气道损害

脊柱手术后的气道损伤可以从轻微的症状发展到需要立即重新插管的紧急情况。从气道水肿、继发于近期融合手术后的颈部运动受限，到已知的颈椎疾病导致的困难气道，这些都使气管插管面临挑战。通常，应该考虑包括可视喉镜在内的高级气道设备，以提高首次插管的成功率。在这种可能存在困难气道的情况下，纤维支气管镜引导插管仍然是最安全的技术。

此外，如果无法保证气道安全，应在标准和高级麻醉技术下，使用外科气道设备进行紧急气管切开。如果气道阻塞是由颈部血肿所引起，手术伤口应重新打开，以便清除血肿，然后保护呼吸道。最终，医疗人员快速决策和坦诚沟通可以最快地利用可用设备将患者从术后气道阻塞中安全拯救出来。

预防

神经损伤

即使经过精心规划、合理的监测和标准的麻醉管理，脊柱手术后的神经损伤仍然有可能发生。不过，只要在围术期保持警惕，就可以及时发现和控制可预防的损伤。术前详细询问患者与脊髓疾病相关的病史可能会提醒整个团队该患者术后神经损伤风险高。术中使用纤维支气管镜技术进行保守和仔细的气道管理可以限制病理性颈椎移动。在关键的手术步骤，平稳的麻醉使得 IONM 和稳定的血流动力学得以实现。最重要的是，外科医师、麻醉科医师和神经监测小组之间的积极交流和坦诚对话可使患者在脊柱手术中得到最安全、有效的照护。

出血

如前所述，术前对患者进行全面的评估可以提示脊柱手术中出血的潜在危险因素，并采取合理的措施为大量失血做好准备。手术前必须开放足够多的大口径静脉通道，包括可能的中心静脉通路。IABP 监测在大量输血和频繁进行实验室检查以监测患者的凝血状况时较为有用。有必要进行血型和交叉配对以确保适当的血液制品可用。

围术期视力丧失

预防是脊柱手术中 POVL 的主要治疗手段。在高危患者或接受广泛脊柱手术的患者中，确切的预防措施尚未严格确定。维持较高的平均动脉压，降低胶体输注阈值，改变眼压，以及使用抗血小板药物和类固醇，尚未有文献证实会影响预后。目前对术中管理的推荐包括增加用于大容量复苏的胶体与晶体的比例，维持正常血压，连续监测血红蛋白，适当使用血管活性药，避免头低位以及分期进行复杂脊柱手术。为预防 CRAO，至少每 20 min 进行眼睛检查以预防眼睛受压和视网膜缺血。

气道损害

目前尚无经过证实的公式或循证指南可用来量化脊柱手术后气道损害的风险。根据已知临床危险因素保持高度警惕，以指导术后气道梗阻的预防性措施。高危患者应延迟拔管，带管进入 ICU。目前尚无共识指南指明患者应该保留插管的时间长短，临床专家应该指导拔管的决策。在高危患者中，气囊漏气试验可在拔管前提供一般信息。最近的报告显示，气囊漏气试验阳性可能是拔管后气道阻塞的先兆。然而，存在漏气对拔管后气道损害的预测价值较低。使用皮质类固醇似乎并不能预防脊柱手术后的气道水肿。最后，临床经验，患者已知的危险因素，以及困难气道的可能性，这些都是制定脊柱手术后拔管决策必须考虑的因素。

致谢

感谢 Michelle L · Lotto 博士对本章上一版的贡献。

（仁泽锋 译 曹 霞 校）

延伸阅读

Amiri AR, Fouyas IP, Cro S, et al.: Postoperative spinal epidural hematoma (SHE): incidence, risk factors, onset, and management, *Spine J* 13:134–140, 2013.

Edgecombe H, Carter K, Yarrow S: Anaesthesia in the prone position, *Br J Anaesth* 100:165–183, 2008.

Farag E: Airway management for cervical spine surgery, *Best Pract Res Clin Anaesthesiol* 30:13–25, 2016.

Hindman BJ, Palecek JP, Posner KL, et al.: Cervical spinal cord, root, and bony spine injuries: a closed claims analysis, *Anesthesiology* 114:782–795, 2011.

Kla KM, Lee LA: Perioperative visual loss, *Best Pract Res Clin Anaesthesiol* 30:69–77, 2016.

Lall RR, Lall RR, Hauptman JS, et al.: Intraoperative neurophysiological monitoring in spine surgery: indications, efficacy, and role of the preoperative checklist, *Neurosurg Focus* 33:E10, 2012.

Ochoa ME, Marin MC, Frutos-Vivar F, et al.: Cuff-leak test for the diagnosis of upper airway obstruction in adults: a systematic review and meta-analysis, *Intensive Care Med* 35:1171–1179, 2009.

Rabai F, Sessions R, Seubert CN: Neurophysiological monitoring and spinal cord integrity, *Best Pract Res Clinical Anaesthesiol* 30:53–68, 2016.

Roitberg B, Emechebe-Kennedy O, Amin-Hanjani S, et al.: Human recombinant factor VII for emergency reversal of coagulopathy in neurosurgical patients: a retrospective comparative study, *Neurosurgery* 57:832–836, 2005.

Rubin DS, Parakati I, Lee LA, et al.: Perioperative visual loss in spine fusion surgery: ischemic optic neuropathy in the United States from 1998 to 2012 in the Nationwide Inpatient Sample, *Anesthesiology* 125:457–464, 2016.

Yamada K, Abe Y, Satoh S, et al.: Large increase in blood pressure after extubation and high body mass index elevate the risk of spinal epidural hematoma after spinal surgery, *Spine* 40:1046–1052, 2015.

甲状腺手术的并发症　第51章

Senthil Nadarajan，Kavitha Kuntumalla

病例概要 1

患者，女性，55 岁，颈前部肿胀 5 年，行甲状腺次全切除术。既往有轻度活动后心悸史，睡觉时仰卧位有气短史，更喜欢侧卧位。她的声音有所改变，体格检查可触及突出的甲状腺。胸部 X 线片显示气管从中线向右轻度移位。间接喉镜检查显示双侧声带功能正常。

病例概要 2

该患者因多发结节性甲状腺肿进行了甲状腺次全切除术，术中平稳。术后 3 h 患者主诉呼吸困难。在检查时，患者稍有烦躁不安，可闻及轻度的吸气相喘鸣音。鼻导管吸氧 2 L/min 下脉搏血氧监测仪显示血氧饱和度为 94%，其他生命体征稳定。

问题分析：病例概要 1

甲状腺手术的范围可以从腺叶切除术到甲状腺全切除术（表 51.1）。孤立性甲状腺结节可行腺叶切除术或偏侧甲状腺切除术。甲状腺功能亢进（简称甲亢）最常见的原因是 Graves 病（Graves disease），其次是毒性甲状腺腺瘤和毒性多结节性甲状腺肿（multinodular goiter，MNG）。Graves 病的外科治疗涉及近甲状腺全切除术。然而，除甲状腺全切除术外，侵袭性甲状腺恶性肿瘤可能需要更广泛的颈部淋巴结清扫。

表 51.1　甲状腺手术的类型

甲状腺疾病	手术类型	潜在并发症
孤立性小结节	偏侧甲状腺切除术	喉部神经损伤风险低
孤立性毒性腺瘤	同侧腺叶切除术	甲状腺功能亢进
胸骨后甲状腺肿	甲状腺次全切除术	严重出血的风险，气道阻塞 可能需要胸骨切开入路
Graves 病	甲状腺全切除术	甲状腺功能亢进危象
侵袭性恶性肿瘤	甲状腺全切除术，颈部清扫术	喉部神经受伤 可能需要气管切开术
甲状舌管导管囊肿	甲状舌管导管囊肿切除术（Sistrunk 手术）	意外中损坏甲状软骨引起严重气道阻塞

术前评估

充分的术前评估和最佳的术前准备可以减少甲状腺切除术后的并发症。术前评估包括询问病史、体格检查、甲状腺功能检查、影像学和声带功能评估（表 51.2）。术前确保甲状腺功能处于正常状态非常重要。Graves 病是甲状腺功能亢进的常见原因，其次是毒性多结节性甲状腺肿（MNG）和毒性腺瘤。

降钙素水平升高可能提示甲状腺髓样癌。甲状腺髓样癌很少见，可能与多发性内分泌腺瘤 2 型（multiple endocrine neoplasia type 2，MEN 2）有关。所有患有 MEN2A 型或 MEN 2B 综合征的患者均应排除嗜铬细胞瘤的存在。

甲状腺功能亢进患者的识别和准备

甲状腺功能亢进患者可能突然出现体重减轻、心悸、频细震颤和甲状腺肿大。在开始治疗之前，必须对甲状腺功能亢进的病因做出正确诊断。甲状腺功能亢进患者围术期有发生甲状腺危象的风

表 51.2 术前评估

病史	评估气道受损（仰卧位呼吸困难） 评估甲状腺功能亢进 / 甲状腺功能减退的症状 药物治疗史包括抗血小板药 / 抗凝药 记住：嗜铬细胞瘤与甲状腺髓样癌的关系
检查	胸骨后甲状腺肿侵袭程度 寻找 SVC 阻塞的征象—面部潮红—Pemberton 征
血液检查	全血细胞计数（甲巯咪唑可能导致粒细胞缺乏症） 血型鉴定 甲状腺功能检查
影像学	胸部 X 线——气管偏离 CT 扫描——气管狭窄的解剖水平和程度
鼻内镜检查	对声带功能的评估
ECG（例如 AF）	评估节律，有无 LVH，缺血性改变
肺功能检查	在胸外气道阻塞（甲状腺肿）吸气气流减少
流量容积环	可区分潜在的哮喘还是甲状腺肿引起的局部压力效应

AF，心房颤动；CT，计算机断层扫描；ECG，心电图；LVH，左心室肥厚；SVC，上腔静脉

险，因此对甲状腺功能亢进患者进行充分的术前治疗非常重要。在甲状腺功能亢进症的术前治疗中，甲巯咪唑是最初使用的抗甲状腺药物，除了孕妇患者首选丙硫氧嘧啶以外。此外，可以使用 β - 受体阻滞剂来控制症状直至达到甲状腺功能恢复正常。在手术前 10 天开始服用无机碘以减少 Graves 病患者甲状腺的血管分布。患者应该每隔 4 周评估一次甲状腺功能。应监测中性粒细胞计数，因为甲巯咪唑可引起粒细胞缺乏症。甲巯咪唑可在手术当天停药。

风险评估

气道

必须进行全面的气道评估。应确定甲状腺肿大持续的时间和甲状腺肿块的大小。如果气道存在喘鸣，表明可能是由于甲状腺肿大导致气道变窄。长期患有甲状腺肿的患者有可能在术后发生气管软化，尽管这种情况很少见。

肿块体积增长迅速提示为恶性肿瘤。侵袭性甲状腺恶性肿瘤有可能侵犯喉返神经。因此，任何声音嘶哑的患者，应通过光导纤维喉镜或间接喉镜来确定声带的功能。

评估甲状腺肿大的胸骨后侵犯程度是非常重要。胸骨后的巨大甲状腺肿块可能会导致气道受压。通过颈部切口入路可能难以进行手术，少数可能需要开胸手术。这对气道管理有影响。仰卧位时呼吸急促或窒息感以及喜欢侧卧位可能表明胸骨后甲状腺肿压迫气管。

上腔静脉（superior vena cava，SVC）回流受阻是胸骨后甲状腺肿的一种罕见的并发症。抬高双臂时面部潮红和静脉充血表明上腔静脉阻塞（Pemberton 征）。影像学，特别是计算机断层扫描，有助于确定气道受压的部位和范围，有助于选择适当大小的气管导管。

颈部伸展活动良好是甲状腺手术体位摆放的必要条件。但是，如果术前颈部活动有限制，则要小心摆放体位。

管理

气道

全身麻醉并使用加强气管导管的气管插管是首选方案。必须考虑以下因素：神经完整性监测仪常用于术中近距离监测喉返神经，这需要使用肌电图（electromyogram，EMG）气管导管。此导管外径大，当巨大甲状腺肿块压迫气管，可能会给气管插管带来挑战。可视喉镜和塑形弧形导丝可有助于肌电图气管导管的放置。

可以考虑在局部麻醉下进行清醒的纤维支气管镜插管，例如颈部活动受限的患者，前提是无明显气道狭窄。有气道狭窄的患者最好避免使用纤支镜，该操作可能会有风险。

专家在气道阻塞的管理意见上有分歧。声门下气道阻塞的患者，可能无法插入气管导管。在这种情况下，由外科医师插入支气管硬镜可提供通气，可作为备用计划。此外，值得注意的是，在巨大甲状腺肿的情况下，气管造口术和环甲膜穿刺可能很难完成。与外科医师讨论管理计划非常重要。对于严重纵隔压迫的患者，进行股静脉插管和旁边准备好体外循环随时待用可能是最安全的选择。

预防

术中并发症

出血是甲状腺疾病比如 Graves 病和胸骨后甲状腺肿患者的严重并发症。通过抬高头部、使用胶带代替系绳来固定气管导管、控制低血压，可减少出血的可能性。术中使用基于瑞芬太尼输注的技术可减少神经肌肉阻滞的需求，并有助于外科医师对喉返神经损伤的监测。仔细的摆放颈部体位和支撑，以避免过度伸展，防止受伤和颈部疼痛。眼球突出症患者可能会出现磨损伤。因此，在润滑并贴上眼睑之后，使用适当的敷贴进行眼睛保护较为重要。地塞米松的使用降低苏醒期气道水肿的风险。甲状腺切除术中意外的气管穿孔是一种非常罕见的并发症。重要的是避免气管导管套囊的过度充气。在手术结束时 Valsalva 动作有助于外科医师查找任何漏气或出血。

围术期甲状腺危象

这种情况很少见，可在术中或术后数小时内发生。如果不及时诊断和处理，其死亡率很高。临床诊断是快速治疗的关键。未予充分治疗的甲状腺功能亢进患者存在严重风险。体温突然升高和明显的心动过速可能是甲状腺手术期间甲状腺危象的首要征象。可能会发生心律失常和心力衰竭（图 51.1）。

虽然肌肉僵硬和呼气末 CO_2 的快速上升是恶性高热的特征，但是很难鉴别诊断。治疗包括支持治疗和抑制甲状腺激素的合成、释放和外周作用。

苏醒和拔管

在自主呼吸恢复的患者中平稳清醒拔管是一种安全的方法。避免咳嗽非常重要，因为这可能会增加出血和血肿的风险。涉及颈部清扫的大面积手术之后，肿胀和水肿可能会导致气道受损。在这种情况下，拔管前观察气道并在放气后观察气管导管套管周围是否存在漏气。没有漏气可能表明气管软化。如果存在再插管困难的情况，应推迟拔管或考虑通过气道交换导管进行拔管。如果患者需要重新插管，气道交换导管可维持氧合并且还便于气管导管插入。

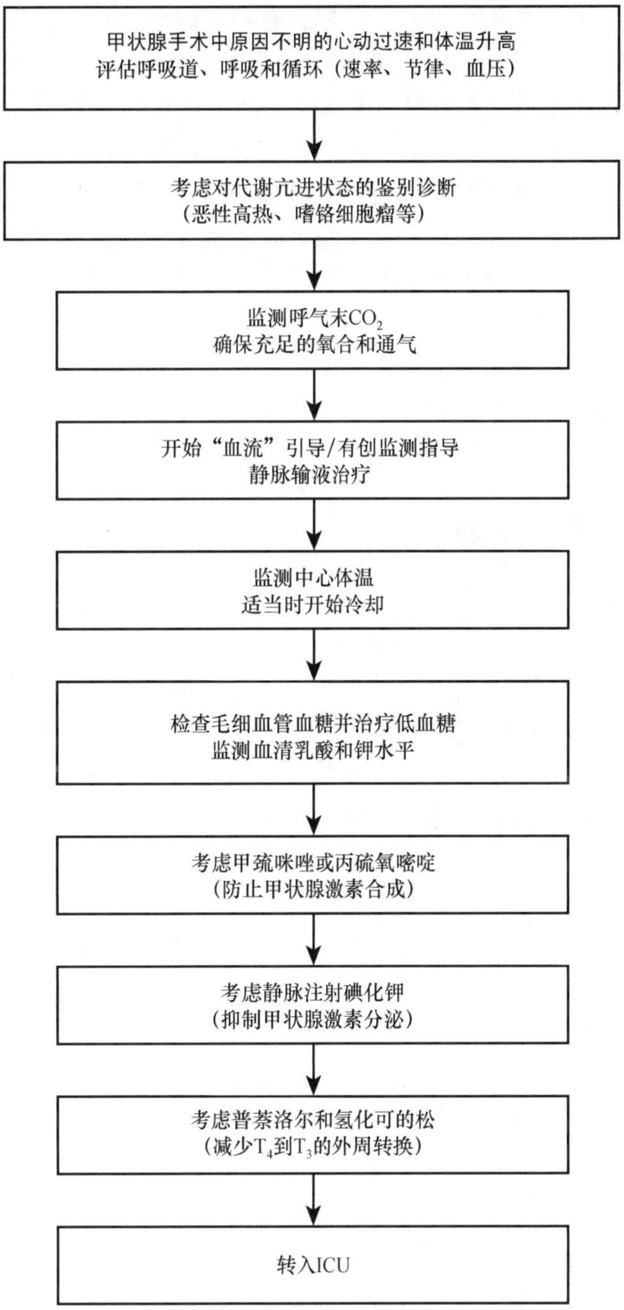

图 51.1 甲状腺功能亢进危象患者的治疗方法

问题分析：病例概要 2

气道阻塞和出现喘鸣音可能是由于甲状腺切除术后血肿、任何原因引起的喉头水肿、双侧喉返神经麻痹、气管软化或由低钙血症引起的喉痉挛。

管理与预防

血肿

在术后即刻阶段密切监测出血或血肿至关重要。

血肿可能发生在术后早期，有些可能会导致气道阻塞。针对性治疗方法是早期清除血肿。然而，带状肌群下方的血肿导致的室隔综合征可阻止静脉回流，导致喉咽水肿。这可能使再次气管插管变得困难。

评估呼吸道的通畅和呼吸的顺畅。患者坐起并开始高流量氧气。如果患者处于危险情况，应考虑在床边清除颈部血肿。紧急安排将患者转移到手术室进行血肿探查。此外，考虑静脉注射地塞米松和雾化肾上腺素，以减少喉头水肿。预计困难的插管，应寻求上级帮助，并使用一系列设备，包括视频喉镜和小直径气管导管，以确保气道通畅。

喉返神经麻痹

甲状腺切除术后，5% ～ 11% 的患者发生喉返神经（recurrent laryngeal nerve，RLN）麻痹，并且 RLN 是甲状腺切除术后第二常见的早期并发症。单侧 RLN 损伤导致外展性声带麻痹。受影响的声带位于旁正中位置。患者经常出现术后声音嘶哑。在大多数情况下，RLN 可恢复。

甲状腺切除术后的患者，双侧喉返神经麻痹发生率低于 0.1%。这导致在吸气时声带内收，出现气道阻塞和失声。这是甲状腺全切除术的罕见并发症，需要紧急气道管理。

低钙血症

短暂性低钙血症是甲状腺切除术中最常见的早期并发症，发生率约为 20% ～ 30%。低钙血症引起的喉痉挛导致的喘鸣非常罕见，其可能在术后 48 h 出现。低钙血症发生于创伤或甲状旁腺切除后。通过识别低钙血症症状，如麻刺感、口周区麻木，或面部抽搐进展为腕足痉挛来诊断低钙血症。心电图上可出现 QT 间期延长。持续气道正压可有助于缓解气道阻塞。依据患者的症状和血清钙离子浓度来滴定静脉注射葡萄糖酸钙量。之后可为改口服钙和维生素 D 并持续至少 10 天。

其他并发症

意外气管穿孔是甲状腺切除术中非常罕见的并发症。如果术中未能识别，症状可能会延迟至术后 1 周。气管壁损伤或缺血可能很少导致延迟性气管破裂。其可能表现为手术性肺气肿或纵隔气肿，需要及时处理。

甲状腺手术治疗甲状腺肿的并发症列于表 51.3。

表 51.3 甲状腺手术的并发症

手术中	甲状腺功能亢进危象（Graves 病） 出血（胸骨后甲状腺肿） 角膜磨损（尤其是眼球突出）
拔管时出现的并发症	气管软化症（罕见） 双侧喉返神经麻痹（双相喘鸣）
早期并发症	血肿（常见） 喉头水肿 短暂性低钙血症（20% ～ 30%） 引起喉痉挛的低钙血症（罕见）
晚期并发症	甲状旁腺功能减退 4% 甲状腺功能减退症 感染 气管穿孔（非常罕见）

致谢

感谢 Samuel A. Irefin 博士对本章上一版的贡献。

（张晓秀　译　严姝姝　校）

延伸阅读

Ahmed S, Clarke D, Vaughan RS, et al.: An unusual cause of stridor after thyroidectomy, *Anaesthesia* 57:578–583, 2002.

Atlas G, Lee M: The neural integrity monitor electromyogram tracheal tube: anesthetic considerations, *J Anaesthesiol Clin Pharmacol* 29(3):403–404, 2013.

Chen AY, Bernet VJ, Carty SE, et al.: American Thyroid Association statement on optimal surgical management of goiter, *Thyroid* 24(2):181–189, 2014.

Christou N, Mathonnet M: Complications after total thyroidectomy, *J Vasc Surg* 150(4):249–256, 2013.

Cook TM, Morgan PJ, Hersch PE: Equal and opposite expert opinion. Airway obstruction caused by a retrosternal thyroid mass: management and prospective international expert opinion, *Anaesthesia* 66(9):828–836, 2011.

Longbottom J, Macnab R: Thyroid disease and thyroid surgery, *Anaesth Intens Care Med* 15(10):458–464, 2014.

Mazeh H, Suwanabol PA, Schneider DF, et al.: Late manifestation of tracheal rupture after thyroidectomy: case report and literature review, *Endocr Pract* 18(4):e73–76, 2012.

Wootten CT, Goudy SL, Rutter MJ, et al.: Airway injury complicating excision of thyroglossal duct cysts, *Int J Pediatr Otorhinolaryngol* 73(6):797–801, 2009.

经尿道手术的并发症 第52章

Anuj Malhotra，Vinod Malhotra

病例概要

患者，男性，70 岁，平素体健，在腰麻联合镇静麻醉下行经尿道前列腺切除术（transurethral resection of the prostate，TURP）和经尿道膀胱肿瘤切除术（transurethral resection of a bladder tumor，TURBT）。血压 130/90 mmHg，心率 68 次 / 分，呼吸 16 次 / 分，血细胞比容 38%。手术进行 90 min 后，患者烦躁不安，血压 180/100 mmHg，心率 40 次 / 分，心电图显示 T 波压低。实验室检查如下：血细胞比容 27%，Na^+ 123 mEq/L，K^+ 3.0 mEq/L，Cl^- 95 mEq/L。

问题分析

定义

TURP 综合征是指在经尿道手术过程中，特别是 TURP，因血管内过度吸收低渗性膀胱灌洗液引起的一系列神经、心肺系统症状和体征的统称。清醒或者镇静状态下的患者，突发躁动不安时应高度怀疑 TURP 综合征。高血压提示血容量过多，反射性心动过缓是对血压升高相应的反应，T 波低平由灌注液中的甘氨酸导致，低钠血症是低渗灌洗液吸收的体征（表 52.1）。

血细胞比容降低最可能是由于失血和血液稀释共同所致。膀胱穿孔后亦可能出现心动过缓，在本病例中，患者的心动过缓是腹膜刺激导致的迷走神经反射，继发于任何渗出液，常伴有腹痛或肩痛和低血压。

表 52.1 用于 TURP 的低渗性灌洗液

溶液	渗透压（mOsm/kg）
水	0
2.5% 葡萄糖	139
3.5% 山梨醇	165
1% 尿素	167
1.2% 甘氨酸	175
2.7% 山梨醇和 0.54% 甘露醇	178
1.5% 甘氨酸	220
5% 甘露醇	275

识别

本案例阐述了经尿道手术的 3 个严重并发症：① TURP 综合征；②大出血；③膀胱穿孔。

TURP 综合征

TURP 综合征是由以下情况引起的一系列症状和体征：

- 循环超负荷；
- 水中毒或低渗透压；
- 低钠血症；
- 甘氨酸中毒；
- 氨中毒；
- 溶血；
- 凝血功能障碍。

这些症状和体征可能同时出现（表 52.2）。临床表现可进一步并发菌血症或败血症，引起寒战、低血压和心动过速。

大出血

大出血通常表现为手术出血，由于血液中含有大量的灌洗液，因此很难测量出血量。如果膀胱穿孔，可能发生隐匿性内出血。出血过多的临床体征包括低血压和反射性心动过速。然而在年龄相关性

表 52.2 TURP 综合征的病理生理及临床特点

病理生理学	临床特征
液体超负荷	高血压；心动过缓；心律失常；心绞痛；肺水肿和低氧血症；心室衰竭和低血压
水中毒或低渗透压	精神错乱和烦躁不安；抽搐或癫痫发作；昏睡或昏迷；瞳孔扩大或反射迟钝；视神经乳头水肿；脑电图低电压；溶血
低钠血症	中枢神经系统改变如上；心肌收缩力降低，QRS 波增宽；心电图导联低电压；心电图 T 波倒置
甘氨酸中毒	恶心呕吐；头痛；短暂性失明；光反射和调节反射丧失（眨眼反射保留）；心肌抑制；心电图变化
氨中毒	恶心呕吐；CNS 抑制
溶血	贫血；急性肾衰竭；发冷、皮肤湿冷；胸闷和支气管痉挛；高钾血症导致恶性心律失常或心动过缓
凝血障碍	严重出血；原发性纤维蛋白溶解；弥散性血管内凝血

窦房结功能障碍、使用 β-受体阻滞剂或高位脊髓麻醉的情况下，可能不会发生心动过速。

膀胱穿孔

膀胱穿孔在全身麻醉中很难被发现。可能发生非特异性低血压、心动过缓或心动过速。经验丰富的外科医师通常能立即发现膀胱穿孔。脊髓麻醉时，患者主诉腹部或肩部疼痛可有助于诊断。

风险评估

在美国，每年大约实施 40 万例 TURP。大约有 10% 的 65 岁以上男性需行 TURP，80 岁以上男性发病率升高到 20% ～ 30%。实施 TURP 的患者常合并以下的一种或多种情况：

- 心脏病；
- 高血压；
- 糖尿病；
- 慢性阻塞性肺疾病；
- 吸烟史。

围术期的发病率与相关疾病、年龄和脓毒症有关。非洲裔美国人和符合下列因素的患者，其发病率有所增加：

- 切除时间超过 90 min；
- 前列腺的重量超过 45 g；
- 急性尿潴留；
- 年龄大于 80 岁。

影响灌洗液吸收量的因素有：

- 切除时间；
- 前列腺大小；
- 灌洗液的静水压力；
- 静脉窦开放的大小和数量；
- 前列腺包膜是否完整。

在 TURP 中，慢性炎症、反复器械操作和留置 Foley 导管增加前列腺血管充血，导致出血和菌血症风险增加。前列腺体积大，切除时间长，使大量纤溶酶原激活物从前列腺组织中释放入血，导致原发性纤维蛋白溶解。前列腺组织和多发性微血栓也可能进入循环，导致弥散性血管内凝血（disseminated intravascular coagulation，DIC）。

TURBT 膀胱穿孔发生率 1%。如果膀胱肿瘤广基或带蒂，肿瘤大且呈脆性或浸润膀胱壁，则膀胱穿孔可能性高。膀胱慢性炎症、有放疗史或壁薄而扩张则更易穿孔。如果肿瘤位置增加切除难度，出血导致手术视野模糊，患者意外体动或咳嗽，或器械难以使用或损坏，这些都可增加穿孔的可能性。

启示

随着技术和监测的进步，TURP 的总死亡率稳步下降，由 1962 年的 2.5% 降至 2003 年的 0.1%。围术期发病率较高，为 7% ～ 20%。TURP 并发症会导致一定的病死率，包括 TURP 综合征、膀胱穿孔或脓毒症。15% 的患者发生一过性菌血症，其中 6% ～ 7% 进展为死亡率显著增高的败血症。由于这些并发症后果严重，故需积极治疗。

管理

TURP 综合征

立即积极治疗对患者生存至关重要。建议采取以下措施：

- 尽快结束手术。
- 静脉注射呋塞米 20 mg。
- 急查实验室检查：血细胞比容、血清电解质、肌酐、葡萄糖浓度；血浆渗透压（若可实施）；动脉血气分析和十二导联心电图。

- 开始或者持续输注生理盐水。如果血清钠浓度低于 100 mEq/l，低钠血症和低渗透压导致严重的中枢神经系统副作用，或心肌收缩下降导致的心血管衰竭时，可使用高渗盐水（3% 或 5%，输注速度小于 100 ml/h）。应注意过度或过速纠正低钠血症可能导致脑桥中央髓鞘溶解。
- 以 1 mg 递增剂量静脉注射咪达唑仑治疗抽搐或癫痫；如果癫痫持续发作，可添加巴比妥类药物。
- 胸部听诊和胸部 X 线片用以鉴别肺水肿。在肺水肿早期给予气管插管并机械通气。
- 必要时输注浓缩红细胞。
- 如果持续出血，应考虑 DIC 或原发性纤维蛋白溶解的可能性。给予晶体和血液制品治疗 DIC，维持血流动力学稳定和凝血功能正常。在原发性纤溶第 1 h 内，其对 6- 氨基己酸的效果良好，静脉注射 3 ～ 5 g，然后以 1 g/h 的速度持续静脉注射，直到出血得到控制。
- 进行有创监测，对症支持治疗，维持循环和肺功能稳定，防止肾衰竭。

膀胱穿孔

一旦发现膀胱穿孔，采取以下措施：

- 停止手术，采取止血措施。
- 静脉给予晶体液、血管收缩药和正心肌力药治疗低血压。
- 监测血细胞比容。如果持续活动性出血，立即输血。可能发生失血进入腹腔或后腹膜间隙的隐匿性出血。
- 通过膀胱尿道造影定位穿孔。

对于大多数穿孔，耻骨上膀胱造瘘术、留置 Foley 导尿管、置入输尿管支架（偶尔需要）即可。在某些情况下，可能需要立即剖腹探查来控制出血和修补穿孔。

脓毒症

立即积极治疗寒战和发热，静脉给予抗生素覆盖泌尿生殖系统菌群。必要时予以心血管支持治疗。

预防

TURP 综合征

采取以下预防措施：

- 将切除时间控制在 1 h 内；
- 切除过程中保持前列腺包膜完整；
- 保持灌注液距前列腺高度低于 60 cm；
- 监测术中和术后血电解质水平；
- 使用区域麻醉或联合轻度镇静或无需镇静，以便早期发现患者精神状态的变化。

膀胱穿孔；菌血症和败血症

避免膀胱过度膨胀、使用粗制滥造的器械、患者体动以及大范围切除前列腺组织或膀胱肿瘤。使用广谱抗生素预防菌血症和败血症。

单极 TURP、双极 TURP 和前列腺激光切除术

TURP 的传统金标准是使用单极电切设备，其发出的切割电流在局部穿过组织，最后通过接地电极片传出。因此，这项技术需要使用非电解质、低渗性灌注液来减少电流的分散，但是此类灌洗液被吸收可能会导致 TURP 综合征。双极 TURP 使用连续环路电极控制电流的输入和输出，使生理盐水可以作为灌洗液。Meta 分析显示这种技术避免了单极 TURP 可能发生的低钠血症和低渗透压，改善预后。但是如果大量的生理盐水通过开放的前列腺窦被吸收，仍然可以发生容量超负荷。

钬：钇–铝石榴子石（holmium：yttrium-aluminum-garnet，Ho：YAG）、光选择性大功率磷酸钛酰钾（potassium titanyl phosphate，KTP 或绿光）和绿光高性能系统（High Performance System，HPS）是 TURP 中最常用的三种激光系统。这些技术在治疗过程中形成凝血区，封闭前列腺静脉。生理盐水也可以作为膀胱灌洗液。与传统的 TURP 相比较，其主要优点是失血量小（仅为 50 ～ 70 ml）和灌注液吸收少，几乎可以消除 TURP 这两大并发症。它被推荐为抗凝患者手术的一种选择，并且由于 TURP 相关的风险较低，一些从业者已经不再强调使用区域麻醉作为首选。然而，由于治疗范围较小，手术时间较传统 TURP 要长，可能出现前列腺窝血凝块、术后前列腺碎片脱落等并发症，导致尿路梗阻。术中应佩戴防护眼镜，并采取排出烟雾的措施。

（钱 爽 译 席 鹏 校）

延伸阅读

Azar I: Transurethral resection of prostate. In Malhotra V, editor: *Anesthesia for renal and genitourinary surgery*, New York, 1996, McGraw-Hill, pp 93–109.

Barash PG, Cullen BF, Stoelting RK, et al.: *Clinical anesthesia*, 6th ed, Philadelphia, 2009, Lippincott Williams & Wilkins, pp 1365–1368.

Catalona WJ: Urothelial tumors of the urinary tract. In Walsh PC, Retik AB, Stamey TA, et al.: *Campbell's urology*, 6th ed, Philadelphia, 1992, WB Saunders, pp 1094–1158.

Gravenstein D: Transurethral resection of prostate (TURP) syndrome: a review of pathophysiology and management, *Anesth Analg* 84:438–446, 1997.

Hanson RA, Zornow MH, Conlin MJ: Laser resection of the prostate: implications for anesthesia, *Anesth Analg* 105:475–479, 2007.

Hawary A, Mukhtar K, Sinclair A, et al.: Transurethral resection of the prostate syndrome: almost gone but not forgotten, *J Endourol* 23:2013–2020, 2009.

Malhotra V: Anesthesia and renal and genitourinary systems. In Miller RD, editor: *Miller's anesthesia*, 8th ed, Philadelphia, 2015, Elsevier, pp 2217–2243.

Malhotra V: Transurethral resection of prostate, *Anesthesiol Clin North Am* 18:883–897, 2000.

O'Donnell AM, Foo ITH: Anaesthesia for transurethral resection of the prostrate, *Cont Med Ed Anaesth Crit Care Pain* 3(9):92–96, 2009.

O'Hara J: Anesthesia for select urologic procedures, *ASA Refresher Courses Anesthesiol* 39(1):115–119, 2011.

Reich O, Gratzke C, Bachmann A, et al.: Morbidity, mortality, and early outcome of transurethral resection of the prostrate: a multicenter evaluation of 10,654 patients, *J Urol* 180:246–249, 2008.

创伤手术的并发症

第53章

Maged Argalious

病例概要

患者，男性，23岁，因“右上腹枪击伤”急送至急救室，挣扎躁动、意识模糊。生命体征：心率119次/min，呼吸22次/分，收缩压70 mmHg。

问题分析

定义

创伤相关性损伤（trauma-related injury，TRI）是美国1～45岁人群死亡的首要原因，并在所有导致死亡的原因中位列第五。由于TRI主要影响的是年轻人，因此它是年龄低于75岁的人群寿命减少的主要原因。据世界卫生组织（World Health Organization，WHO）推测，TRI占15～45岁人群死亡原因的首位，并且预计到2020年，TRI将成为所有年龄组人群的第三大死因。

TRI患者对医疗保健服务系统提出了独特的挑战。他们往往有多个器官/系统受到损伤，需要资源密集型的医疗。此外，TRI还可能与许多慢性内科基础疾病发生不良相互作用。造成TRI的四大主要原因分别为机动车事故（包括小汽车、卡车和摩托车等）、跌倒、遭受袭击以及行走时被车辆撞伤。

许多创伤所致损伤可以避免。发生在成年人的车祸中，40%的汽车和卡车事故以及38%的摩托车事故涉及酒精或毒品使用。创伤分为故意伤害（如凶杀）和意外损伤，也可根据损伤的机制（如贯穿伤和钝器损伤等）来进行分类。得益于创伤相关医疗水平的提高，近年来与创伤有关的死亡人数有所下降。

识别

急性创伤患者的评估包括三个关键组成部分，即粗略评估、初步评估和二次评估。在此上述任何评估过程中可随时启动复苏。粗略评估往往只需要几秒钟，用于迅速确定患者病情是稳定、不稳定还是死亡。初步评估指迅速评估是否存在重要的、影响患者生存的功能性变化和指标。按照ABC进行评估，即**气道**（Airway）是否通畅以及**呼吸**（Breathing）和**循环**（Circulation）情况，随后进行简要的神经系统检查，优先处置颈椎损伤和可能出现的脑疝。由于在最初的60 min内识别并对危及生命的损伤进行快速干预可以提高患者的生存率和预后，因而粗略评估和初步评估也被称为诊疗的“黄金时段”。二次评估则需要对每个全身各解剖区域进行系统、全面的评估，可以发现之前被忽视的损伤，这其中的大部分属骨科问题，约可占到到3/4。根据二次评估的结果，可对患者进行针对性的进一步处置，例如立即送至手术室手术治疗、转送至影像科进一步诊断检查或送至ICU观察和治疗。

充分了解不同创伤机制所致损伤的不同特点，有助于早期预测和识别损伤。在明确诊断或完全排除诊断之前，切不能遗漏或忽略某种致伤因素可能导致的最严重的损伤，而往往许多创伤相关并发症直到术中才能被诊断出来（框53.1）。

钝性损伤除了导致局部的损伤外，还可以通过能量的传导转移到打击身体的其他部位。根据打击部位的不同和能量大小的不同，钝性损伤可能导致内脏破裂或组织破坏，包括多发性骨折等。而穿透性创伤则通常较局限在子弹或锐器进入体内的运行轨迹的周围。

风险评估

分类评分系统是基于体格检查结果以及患者的生理指标或损伤机制的参数而制定的。评分系统过去常用来决定转诊至创伤中心的患者模式。生存是

框 53.1 创伤患者的损伤及可能的围术期并发症

中枢神经系统
颈椎不稳或损伤以及可能的脊髓损伤
闭合性颅脑损伤伴颅内压增高
由于颅内压增高，可能发生脑疝
开放性颅骨骨折引起的脑疝

胸部和肺部
支气管插管
张力性气胸或血胸
纵隔气肿
肋骨骨折和可能出现的连枷胸
肺挫裂伤
支气管胸膜瘘
吸入性肺炎
支气管痉挛
气管支气管堵塞
长骨（如股骨）骨折并发的脂肪栓塞

心血管
心肌挫伤或心脏破裂
心脏压塞或心包积气
主动脉夹层或破裂
肺血管或腔静脉破裂
低血压：低血容量或神经源性低血压
低血容量性休克
空气栓塞

腹部
空腹脏器破裂或撕裂
肝裂伤
脾破裂

凝血系统
凝血障碍（尤其在大量输血时）
弥散性血管内凝血
原发性纤维蛋白溶解
溶血性输血反应

电解质或其他失衡
继发于枸橼酸中毒的低钙血症
高钾血症，低镁血症
酸碱失衡

其主要的结局变量。改良创伤评分（revised trauma score，RTS）是一种前瞻性的评分系统，其以两种形式存在：一种是设计用来作为分诊工具，另一类是用来评估住院患者的预后。RTS 可准确预测创伤性损伤后的死亡率，然而，目前却尚无明确的证据来支持其作为院外的主要分类工具或用来作为功能性结局和生活质量的预测指标。RTS 评分系统主要由格拉斯哥昏迷量表（Glasgow Coma Scale，GCS）评分、患者的收缩压和呼吸频率这三个项目构成，每项的分值从低到高记为 0 ～ 4 分（正常）。RTS 结果由各项分值加权并相加后得出，数值范围为 0 ～ 7.84（表 53.1）。数值越高表明预后越好。在当前世界范围内的众多创伤评分系统中，RTS 的使用最为广泛。

创伤所致的损伤和随后术中并发症的发生取决于损伤的模式。其影响因素包括年龄、性别、损伤部位的抗冲击性和固定程度、器官的解剖性保护和损伤的机制。

颈椎损伤高风险的患者包括：颈部疼痛或剧烈疼痛伴注意力分散的清醒患者，20% 的锁骨以上损伤的昏迷患者，中毒患者，以及有神经系统症状或体征的患者。颈椎损伤在远离颈部的穿透性创伤中并不常见。在清理颈椎之前，需要完善包含有全部 7 个颈椎和第 1 胸椎的前后位、侧位和开口位（示齿状突）平片。而即使在颈椎 X 线正常的患者，其韧带损伤的可能也只能通过计算机断层扫描（computed tomography scanning，CT）来加以排除。

不管是由于解剖性倾向还是实际的创伤，对潜在的困难气道的识别体现了麻醉科医师最为重要的角色之一。对不稳定性颈椎患者进行气管插管，可能会导致不可逆的脊髓损伤。

在创伤患者中，胃内容物误吸入肺的风险很高。创伤发生时，胃排空几乎停止，迟钝或昏迷患者的保护性气道反射受到损害。在清醒患者中，误吸的最大风险则发生在麻醉诱导和气管插管之间。肺误吸的死亡率为 5%。

表 53.1 改良创伤评分（RTS）

格拉斯哥昏迷量表（GSC）评分	收缩压（SBP，mmHg）	呼吸频率（RR，次 / 分）	分值
13 ～ 15	>89	10 ～ 29	4
9 ～ 12	76 ～ 89	>29	3
6 ～ 8	50 ～ 75	6 ～ 9	2
4 ～ 5	1 ～ 49	1 ～ 5	1
3	0	0	0

RTS 评分 =0.9368（GSC_c）+0.7326（SBP_c）+ 0.2908（RR_c）；其中 GCS 代表格拉斯哥昏迷量表评分，SBP 代表收缩压，RR 代呼吸频率，下标的 c 代表各项的分值。

Adapted from Champion HR，Copes WS，Sacco WJ，et al：Improved predictions from a severity characterization of trauma（ASCOT）over Trauma and Injury Severity Score（TRISS）：results of an independent evaluation. *J Trauma* 40：42-48，1996.

第一或第二肋骨骨折、连枷胸、纵隔增宽、大量血胸和肩胛骨骨折常与肺或血管损伤相关。在钝性创伤中，肋骨骨折是最常见的损伤，而血胸或气胸则多见于锐器造成的穿透性损伤。

对创伤患者进行复苏时，通常需要大量输注血液和血液成分，以及晶体和胶体容量替代治疗。对于难以控制的创伤性大量出血，应首先进行输血、成分血以及容量复苏。然后对出血的大血管进行明确的手术控制止血。然而，以大量输注成分血以达到止血目的会带来很大的风险。使用生理盐水可能导致高氯性代谢性酸中毒，而大量使用羟乙基淀粉则与凝血障碍和肾功能不全有关。

启示

颈椎损伤和误吸的风险决定了保护气道的方式。如时间允许，误吸预防治疗包括甲氧氯普胺、H_2 拮抗剂和枸橼酸钠，可有助于促进胃排空并降低胃 pH。多数到达手术室的患者穿戴颈托，因其尚未排除颈椎损伤。对于配合具有自主呼吸的患者，在清醒状态下经口咽部表面麻醉后使用光导纤维行经口气管插管。这是保护气道的选择之一。通常情况下应避免在患者清醒时进行经鼻插管，若患者存在颅底部或筛板骨折时，经鼻插管存在脑损伤的风险。然而，对于大面积口腔创伤患者，这可能是一个可行的选择。或者，这类患者还可以使用直接喉镜、视频喉镜（如 Glidescope）或睡眠状态下光导纤维引导技术，在静脉（IV）快速序贯诱导麻醉后进行插管。在进行诱导前，必须将患者颈托的前半部分移除，利用手法牵引使颈椎保持稳定。然后对患者进行预充氧，在快速序贯诱导期间向环状软骨施加压力，并选择上述方法中的一种进行气管插管（带套囊）。一旦气管导管套囊充气并确认有足够的通气和氧合，就可以释放环状软骨压力并将颈托的前半部分重新戴好。值得注意的是，环状软骨加压预防胃吸入有效性备受质疑，尤其在尚无证据的支持下使用这一技术。研究表明，高达 30% 的患者在插管时使用环状软骨加压（也称为 Sellick 手法）出现喉镜视野受损的情况。因此，环状软骨加压已不再作为 I 类推荐。

对于 TRI 患者的液体复苏，应将其分两个阶段：

- 早期：在活动性持续出血期间；
- 后期：出血控制后。

一些研究表明，在早期阶段，目标收缩压低于 100 mmHg，平均动脉压（mean arterial pressure，MAP）在 50 ～ 60 mmHg 之间的限制性复苏方案可提高持续出血患者的生存率。这种降压复苏方案有助于实现自发性止血，并减轻大量晶体可能会导致的稀释性凝血障碍。而过低的 MAP 可导致终末器官灌注不足，因此并不推荐进一步降低 MAP。

在早期“院外”阶段（例如战场受伤），通常采用损伤控制复苏，即基于预先建立的大量输血方案，经验性输注血制品和近似全血制品（例如，红细胞悬液-新鲜冷冻血浆-血小板以 1∶1∶1 的比例进行使用）。

如果上述早期阶段发生在“院内”环境，则可使用基于床旁黏弹性监测（并限制晶体的使用）实施流程图驱动-目标导向的止血复苏方案来使用血制品。

这些“目标导向方案”可在控制出血（晚期复苏）后继续进行，其最终目标是恢复正常的心排血量、血压、凝血功能、酸碱状态和核心温度，并达到可接受的红细胞比容的最低值。无论采用何种早期复苏方法（方案或目标导向），在复苏后期采用目标导向的治疗方案都是适用的，因为后期液体复苏旨在恢复所有器官系统的灌注，同时继续维持其重要的生理功能。

在膈肌以上开通足够的静脉输液通道非常重要。通过快速静脉输液装置，可以迅速地经静脉输注预热的液体、血液和血制品，从而快速恢复血管内容量。患者的容量状态、血流动力学稳定性和肺部并发症（如气胸）决定了哪些药物可用于全身麻醉的诱导和维持。在气道得到保护后，应建立中心静脉压和直接动脉压的监测。

动脉管路建立后，应立即抽取动脉血样并送检测定患者的氧合（PO_2）和通气（PCO_2）、pH 和血细胞比容。如不及时进行纠正，低血容量和酸中毒可导致不可逆的休克和死亡。创伤手术中大量输注全血和血液制品可能会造成一些并发症。这些并发症包括过多 / 不足的血制品替代、稀释性凝血功能障碍、枸橼酸钠中毒引起的低钙血症、低体温、酸碱平衡和电解质紊乱以及脓毒症导致的多器官系统衰竭。

对明确有颈椎或低位脊髓损伤的患者，应在损伤后 8 h 内经静脉注射大剂量甲泼尼龙（30 mg/kg），然后改为静滴维持 24 h[5.4 mg/（kg·h）]，这可能会促进神经功能恢复。

管理

气道

在进行气道管理时，麻醉科医师必须充分考虑到颈椎损伤、饱胃、患者不配合及预计插管困难等情况。对清醒患者使用直接喉镜辅助经口插管时需要先行表面麻醉，可能时刻需谨慎使用静脉镇静。对清醒或镇静的患者，也可在表面麻醉下使用纤维喉镜或纤维支气管镜技术来进行插管。或者也可在经静脉全身麻醉快速序贯诱导后，使用直接或视频喉镜或睡眠状态下光导纤维插管，以确保气道安全。在快速序贯诱导前充分预吸氧能够增加患者在脱氧饱和度之前可以耐受的呼吸暂停时间。

框 53.2 列出了创伤患者气管插管的一般适应证。外科气道的适应证包括：①插管失败；②疑似颈椎损伤的呼吸暂停的患者；③疑似颈椎损伤的面部创伤患者；④解剖结构受损的严重面部和喉部创伤。

颈部固定技术可能对影响喉部视野，从而增加困难插管的可能性。美国麻醉科医师学会困难气道管理工作组制定的流程图可适用于创伤患者（见第 27 章和第 139 章）。在建立外科气道或使用光纤导管引导插管时，诸如喉罩之类的装置可用作临时维持气道通畅的桥接手段。

外科气道的建立包括环甲膜切开术、经气管喷射通气和气管切开术。环甲膜切开术比气管切开术花费的时间少，因此是首选的手术方式。由于气管切开术需要患者颈部充分伸展，可能会加剧颈椎损伤。因此气管切开术更适用于喉部外伤和气管完全横断的患者。

框 53.2　创伤相关损伤中气管插管的适应证

- 心脏或呼吸骤停
- 气道阻塞或呼吸功能不全
- 气道保护（如头部损伤和格拉斯哥昏迷量表评分 <9）
- 需行深度镇静或镇痛甚至全身麻醉
- 复苏后缺氧或通气不足
- 需纯氧治疗的一氧化碳中毒
- 不配合或中毒患者，以利其完善诊断检查

Data from Mccunn M，Grissom TE，Dutton RP：Anesthesia for trauma. In Miller RD，editor：*Miller's anesthesia*，8th ed. Philadelphia，Elsevier，2015，pp 2423-2459.

呼吸

通气管理需要关注氧饱和度、呼气末二氧化碳浓度和气道峰压。一旦发生胃内容物误吸，治疗的方法包括增加吸入氧浓度，增加呼气末正压，使用支气管镜检并用生理盐水灌洗气道。压力限制通气模式可以降低气压伤的风险。如果出现气胸，应立即在锁骨中线第 2 肋间以针头穿刺进行减压，然后放置胸腔引流管。

循环

创伤患者出现的休克主要是由于排除其他病因的血容量不足所致，如梗阻性休克（由张力性气胸所致）或神经源性休克（由于脊髓横断或脊髓血管麻痹所致）等。要维持血流动力学的稳定，需要手术控制出血、迅速恢复循环血容量、纠正酸中毒和氧输送充足（血细胞比容）。在容量恢复的过程中，可使用升压药物来维持血压。

若失血量少于全身血容量的 30%，使用晶体液扩容即以足够，但通常还会加入胶体液。是否需要输注血液制品是基于患者的预计失血量、生命体征、活动性出血迹象和血细胞比容监测决定的。输血的触发标准已有所降低，当血细胞比容降低至 20% ～ 25% 时即可使用输血治疗。

因为 15 min 内便可提供相应血型的血液，因此目前临床上很少给患者输注 O 型、Rh^+（育龄妇女用 Rh^-）血。如可能，应行血型鉴定及交叉配血（需要 30 ～ 45 min）。延迟输血（或血制品）的概念是指让患者处于允许性低血容量状态，直至外科出血得到控制后才进行输血或血制品的复苏方法，这种临床实践方法尚未得到普遍的接受。

低体温

创伤患者在到达手术时通常出现低体温。提高手术室温度、使用空气压缩加温装置、预热静脉输注的液体和血制品、对吸入气体进行加湿处理、减少新鲜气流可有助于维持核心体温于 36℃甚至更高。低体温可降低心排血量和药物代谢、减弱免疫

反应。低体温亦可加剧血管收缩、心肌缺血、低血压、心动过缓、心律失常以及凝血障碍。在复温过程中，患者的氧耗会增加。

凝血功能障碍

创伤患者，尤其是那些疑似合并大血管损伤的患者，往往有明显的出血倾向。造成稀释性凝血功能障碍并导致出血的原因，主要在于止血成分缺乏（如纤维蛋白原、血小板、凝血因子等）、纤维蛋白溶解和弥散性血管内凝血。常规筛查弥散性血管内凝血指标（如凝血酶原时间、部分凝血活酶时间、血小板、纤维蛋白原、D- 二聚体等）或血栓弹力描记图来评估血凝块的形成和溶解，可用来指导纠正凝血功能障碍。新鲜冰冻血浆可以用于纠正凝血酶原时间异常。如果纤维蛋白原低于 100 mg/dl，则可使用冷沉淀。当存在活动性出血且血小板计数低于 100 000/mm^3 时可输注血小板。ε - 氨基己酸、氨甲环酸或抑肽酶可用于治疗原发性纤维蛋白溶解。

对于腹部创伤的患者，可经血栓弹力图指导，给予重组凝血因子Ⅶ a（rF Ⅶ a），能够更有效地纠正创伤相关的凝血功能障碍并减少血制品输注量。弥散性血管内凝血首先需要明确致病原因，然后给予凝血因子（新鲜冰冻血浆）、输注血小板和小剂量肝素（50 U/kg）。

预防

一级预防

公共安全运动必须强调酒后驾车的危害性。加强座位安全带和头盔使用立法。鼓励使用枪支锁，并严格执行枪支管理法。摩托车和驾驶安全课程以及儿童约束座椅亦可减少 TRI 和死亡。

二级预防

胜任工作、保持警醒的麻醉科医师，加上掌握创伤手术专业知识的外科医师，是创伤相关并发症二级预防的关键所在。麻醉–外科创伤救治小组必须有效运转，并与急诊、手术室和 ICU 的医护人员通力协作。医院影像科、检验科和输血科也应当能够提供所需的辅助支持。总之，上述所有部门的能力，及其有效部署，能够促进创伤患者的及时诊断和稳定，从而减少二次病死率的风险。

（王丽珍　译　费苗苗　校）

延伸阅读

Bracken MB, Shepard MJ, Holford TR, et al.: Administration of methylprednisolone for 24 or 48 hours or tirilazad mesylate for 48 hours in the treatment of acute spinal cord injury: results of the Third National Acute Spinal Cord Injury Randomized Controlled Trial. National Acute Spinal Cord Injury Study, *JAMA* 277:1597–1604, 1997.

Morrison CA, Carrick MM, Norman MA, et al.: Hypotensive resuscitation strategy reduces transfusion requirements and severe postoperative coagulopathy in trauma patients with hemorrhagic shock: preliminary results of a randomized controlled trial, *J Trauma* 70:652–663, 2011.

Yao D, Li Y, Wang J, et al.: Effects of recombinant activated factor VIIa on abdominal trauma patients, *Blood Coagul Fibrinolysis* 25:33–38, 2014.

第54章 连续神经阻滞：神经周围局部麻醉药输注

W. Michael Bullock，Stuart A. Grant

病例概要

患者，男性，62岁，行踝关节融合术在超声引导下放置内收肌管和腘窝-坐骨神经导管。手术麻醉使用0.5%罗哌卡因，术后镇痛选择0.2%罗哌卡因双导管持续给药。在术后恢复室时患者无痛感，但在术后第1天晚上，患者出现脚踝疼痛。双导管同时注射0.5%罗哌卡因，疼痛缓解。第2天，因患者出现下肢严重的运动阻滞，且在当天早晨理疗师声称在治疗过程中患者发生摔倒，外科医师发愁地联系了麻醉科医师。

问题分析

定义

这个病例概要提出了关于局部麻醉药（简称局麻药）的副作用及手术区域麻醉可能合并严重并发症的讨论。区域麻醉能提供高质量的镇痛，并最大限度地减少阿片类药物相关的副作用。尽管阿片类药物和手术并发症比区域麻醉并发症更为普遍，但区域麻醉的并发症也时有发生。

大量研究表明神经周围输注局麻药可以提供良好的镇痛。这种持续阻滞技术已被用于提供术中麻醉和术后镇痛。某些并发症是神经阻滞操作所特有的，例如锁骨上或锁骨下神经阻滞导致的气胸或腰丛阻滞导致的硬膜外扩散。本章不讨论神经阻滞特异性并发症，主要关注持续性外周神经阻滞的围术期并发症。

外周神经阻滞、神经周围置管和手术相关的各种并发症见表54.1。并发症的早期识别在后续治疗中至关重要。神经阻滞相关问题的识别应始于对病史和体格检查的详细关注。回顾病历中的全身用药或经外周神经导管用药的病历有助于缩小鉴别诊断的范围。此外，手术因素，包括但不限于患者术中体位、手术入路、术后包扎等，这些都可能是导致神经阻滞相关并发症的病因。

表54.1 外周神经阻滞、神经周围置管和手术相关发症

麻醉并发症	手术并发症
神经阻滞实施困难或导管置入困难	继发于术中体位神经损伤
神经阻滞注射时或置入导管时导致的疼痛	手术损伤：手术刀损伤、牵拉或止血带损伤
继发于局麻药的运动阻滞作用延长	压迫或缺血：术后外科敷料
针尖导致的神经损伤：神经失用，轴突断裂，神经断裂	压迫：术中血肿
局麻药或辅助药物导致的神经损伤；直接的神经毒性或继发性缺血	压迫：肢体缺血引起的间隔综合征或深静脉血栓形成
导管导致的神经损伤：导管置入或移除时导致的损伤或神经断裂	压迫：止血带过紧导致的术后疼痛
置管相关血肿导致的压迫	导管被误切
导管误入血管	术后外科感染
导管部分残留	
炎症性神经痛	
沿导管置管途径部位的感染	

识别

根据基本病理，外周神经导管的问题可以多种方式呈现。以下是包括神经损伤在内的神经系统并发症的临床特征：

- 停止局麻药输注后长时间运动阻滞；
- 停止给药后持续或恶化的触觉下降或感觉异常；
- 神经病理性疼痛；
- 肢体麻木或肢体感觉沉重或无力；
- 本体感受丧失。

以下是镇痛不足或缺血的临床特征：

- 患者的疼痛评分高或持续增加，不伴有麻木；
- 患者的疼痛评分高或持续增加，伴有麻木；
- 阿片类药物需求增加以及增加阿片类药物相关的副作用。

以下是感染性并发症的临床特征：

- 外周神经置管后 2 ～ 3 天的迟发症状；
- 导管置入部位的组织红肿；
- 导管置入部位疼痛和压痛；
- 白细胞增多和发烧。

这里将不再讨论局麻药中毒的临床特征，具体详见第 103 章。

风险评估

与全身麻醉和椎管内麻醉的风险相比，外周神经阻滞术后并发症发生率低。Auroy 和同事在一项前瞻性研究中报告了与区域麻醉相关的严重并发症的发生率，该研究使用了 103 730 例患者的数据。他们发现区域麻醉相关的心脏停搏和神经损伤发生率较低。与脊髓麻醉相比，区域麻醉后心脏停搏和神经损伤发生率降低至少 3 个标准差。虽然这些数据没有区分单次注射和连续外周神经阻滞，但总的来说，与椎管内麻醉相比，外周神经阻滞与神经损伤和心脏停搏等并发症相关性较小。

Brull 和他的同事在一篇报道中回顾了 32 项研究，结果发现中枢神经阻滞和外周神经阻滞的神经并发症发生率分别约为 0.4% 和 0.3%。然而，他们也注意到永久性的神经损伤在区域麻醉中并不常见。Bergman 和他的同事回顾性地调查了连续 405 例腋窝持续神经阻滞置管操作后的神经并发症，他们发现使用连续导管技术的神经并发症的发生率并不高于单次注射。Borgeat 和他的同事前瞻性地研究了肩外科手术中与肌间沟神经阻滞相关的并发症，发现导管技术和单次注射阻滞之间无差异。

留置导管可能存在感染和导管移入血管的潜在风险。与单纯口服镇痛药物相比，必须权衡好导管技术的风险与良好的镇痛效果的益处之间的关系。此外，尽管 Cuvillon 和同事在 208 根股神经导管中分离出 57% 的细菌定殖，但未发生临床相关感染并发症。在 Borgeat 研究的病例中有一例严重感染（脓肿），发生率为 0.1%，此外约有 0.7% 的患者出现浅表红斑（如前所述）。Boezaart 及其同事仅在最近的一些研究中报道了浅表皮肤感染（发病率 5%）。而移行入血管的病例仅在文献中查询到 1 例，因此该并发症的发生率尚不清楚。

随着长效酰胺类局麻药初次使用药物作用的消除，导管意外脱出或导管位置不正确是最常见的疼痛原因。这种情况可发生在 10% ～ 20% 的患者中，是目前为止最常见的持续外周神经阻滞并发症。此外，在工作良好的外周神经导管中输注低浓度局麻药的患者可能会突发剧烈疼痛。除了背景剂量输注之外，同时加上患者自控的快速推注量可以减轻突发性疼痛。如病例概述所示，临床科医师的挑战是权衡运动阻滞甚至局麻药中毒的风险与患者因止痛不足而产生的不适之间的关系。

术后跌倒的原因多样，包括下肢手术、年龄和肥胖。对于区域麻醉患者术后跌倒的发生仍存在一些争议。Wasserstein 及其同事和 Ilfeld 及其同事发现，持续股神经阻滞是全膝关节置换术后发生跌倒的独立危险因素。相反，Memtsoudis 及其同事回顾了一个包含 400 多家医院 19.1 万名患者的国家数据库后，发现区域麻醉与住院患者跌倒之间并无相关性。但他们未区分单针阻滞和导管置入阻滞。带有外周神经导管的患者必须多加强防护，麻醉科医师参与医院防跌倒项目的制订可有助于降低跌倒风险。

启示

神经系统并发症可导致肢体无力、慢性疼痛以及术后功能减退。谨慎的技术操作和患者选择是减少这些并发症发生的重要因素。较高浓度的局麻药产生的长时间运动阻滞可能会使早期下床延迟，但没有证据表明它会影响关节置换术后关节的长期功能。事实上与阿片类镇痛方案相比，接受硬膜外导管或者接受外周神经导管阻滞的患者，在接受人工膝关节置换术后 6 周恢复速度更快。阻滞失败会导致疼痛和患者满意度降低，很多时候会增加阿片类药物使用及阿片类药物相关副作用如呼吸抑制、瘙痒、恶心、呕吐和便秘。阻滞部位感染可能会导致不适、活动受限、可能会感染移植物和再次手术的风险。术后跌倒会增加患病率，延长住院时间及再次手术。

管理

病史与体格检查

对麻醉史和体格检查的关注是明确外周神经阻滞后神经损伤原因及促成因素的关键（框 54.1）。首先应检查输液细节，包括注药速率和患者推注功能。进行神经系统检查之前应停止输注，并给予足够的时间待阻滞消退。应使用患者疼痛模拟量表来评估患者疼痛。

框 54.1　相关病史和体格检查

病史

- 使用了何种阻滞方式？
- 阻滞技术是否困难？
- 注药是否困难（例如压力过高或“紧”）？
- 是否有局麻药添加剂（肾上腺素，地塞米松等）？
- 患者是否有解剖变异或异常？
- 患者是否在首次阻滞后功能恢复，而在再一次阻滞后功能丧失？
- 神经功能缺失是发生在单侧吗？
- 神经阻滞是在预期的神经阻滞范围内吗？
- 患者既往是否有神经系统疾病（例如先前存在的感觉异常，神经根或神经病变）？
- 患者是否有其他并存疾病，如神经肌肉疾病（Charcot-Marie-Tooth）、糖尿病、营养缺乏症（包括曾行减肥手术）、酒精滥用、化疗、慢性疼痛或其他神经病变？
- 患者是否服用可以导致目前现象的药物？
- 是否有手术因素导致了这种现象？
- 术后是否有任何影响因素，包括机械损伤或物理治疗，部分导致这一问题的出现？

体格检查

- 评估谵妄、痴呆或严重焦虑的总体精神状态
- 四肢的运动测试，以排除先前的双侧（例如糖尿病）或单侧（例如卒中）病变
- 四肢的感觉测试，以排除先前的双侧（例如糖尿病）或单侧（例如卒中）病变
- 触诊四肢的脉搏，以确定每个肢体的血供情况
- 检查导管置入深度是否恰当及是否存在明显的渗漏
- 检查导管部位是否有肿胀、触痛或红肿等症状
- 导管回抽确认是否有血液回流
- 检查外科敷料，包括夹板和铸件，确认压力和张力是否合适

进一步处理措施

详细的病史采集和神经系统的重点检查结果可指导进一步的处理。无论何种病因导致的术后疼痛都应尽早开始多模式镇痛，包括加巴喷丁和非甾体抗炎药，有相关禁忌证除外。图 54.1 中的流程图概述了基于主要并发症的处理措施和建议的治疗方式。麻醉科医师应全程密切关注患者的随访。

预防

了解手术过程中特有并发症的发生率至关重要。了解患者的具体病史，如糖尿病、慢性疼痛以及其他原有神经系统疾病，例如 Charcot-Marie-Tooth，对制定和实施麻醉亦很重要。一旦所有的手术因素和患者因素均已考虑到，则可以决定区域麻醉技术是否安全和恰当。

神经系统并发症

关于预防神经周围导管神经性并发症的证据很少，但在轻度镇静的患者中实施阻滞，降低注射压力，在患者感到疼痛时立即停止注射，都可能会降低神经损伤。使用钝性针尖和尖锐针尖的安全性经常存在争议，使用神经刺激和超声引导的讨论亦是如此。如果手术可能会导致神经损伤，术后应立即评估神经功能，一旦确认神经功能完好，既可放置空导管随后注射一剂药物实施镇痛。

在神经周围阻滞中使用较低浓度的药物可减少运动阻滞的发生。罗哌卡因比布比卡因能提供更好的感觉运动分离。置管时小心固定导管，通过导管推注一定剂量的局麻药可以减轻突发性疼痛，使用患者自控区域麻醉导管有助于降低术后疼痛的可能性。

患者并发症

手术前的病例选择和适当的术前讨论对于预防围术期并发症非常重要。麻醉科医师通过术前临床预约中心了解患者全面的病史和体格检查，以评估已有神经系统疾病或其他潜在的疾病。例如：神经周围置管可能不适合谵妄或痴呆的患者；神经阻滞

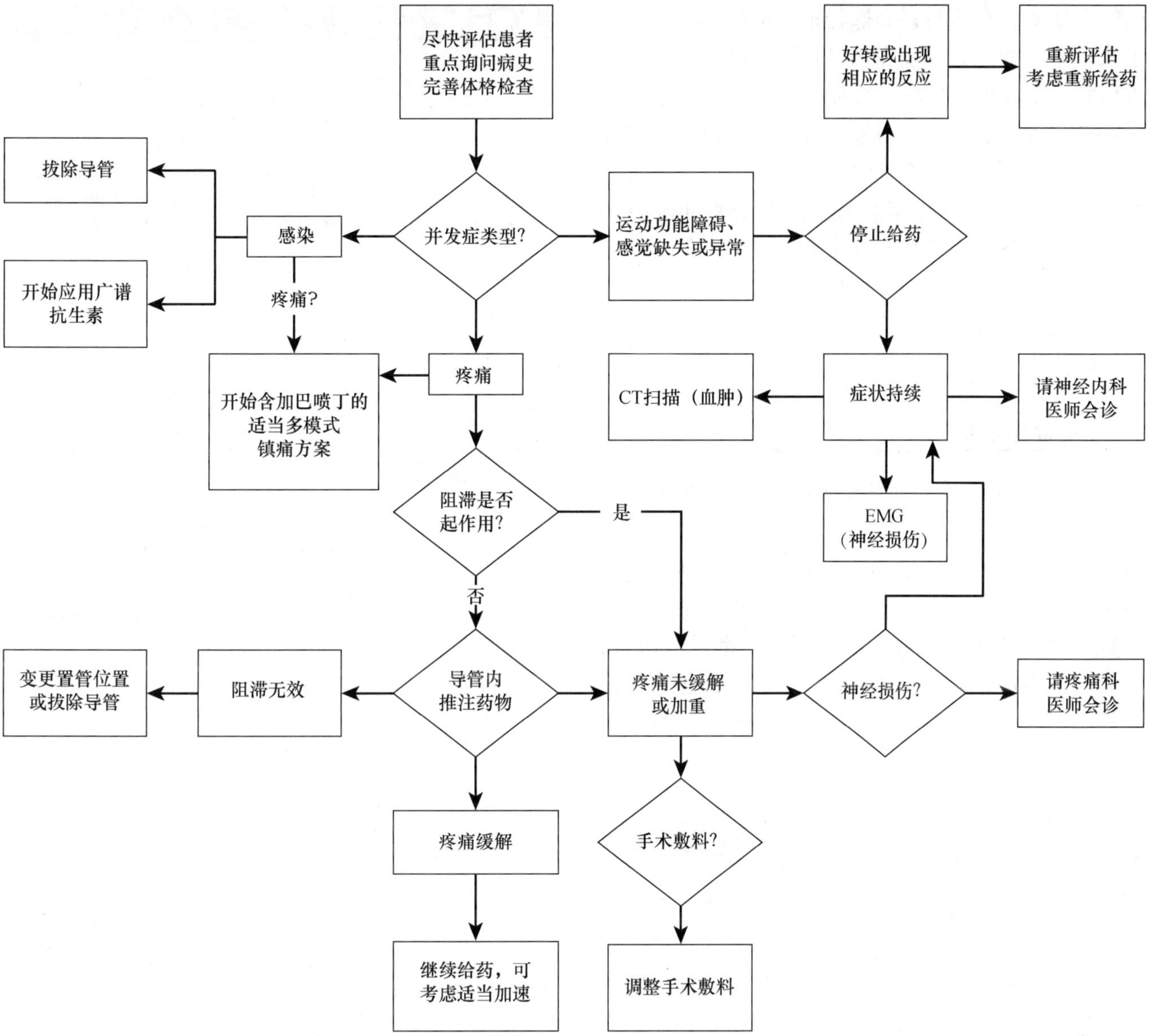

图 54.1　围术期区域麻醉及神经周围导管并发症的处理。CT，计算机断层扫描；EMG，肌电图

也不适合患有糖尿病或其他外周神经疾病的患者；患有严重焦虑症的患者可能需要在整个住院期间同时进行抗焦虑治疗，若治疗效果欠佳，则患者可能表现出更高的疼痛评分；患有慢性疼痛的患者应根据其家庭治疗方案进行治疗，以达到其原有疼痛控制水平，并应尽早转诊至本单位的疼痛服务机构；糖尿病患者通常不需要局麻药添加剂，特别是肾上腺素，这可能会严重影响患者的神经血管功能；应在手术前检查患者药物使用情况，尤其要注意抗凝剂和化疗药物。

麻醉和手术并发症

应提前安排好麻醉和手术方案，以避免神经损伤。一些麻醉科医师认为，超声引导与神经刺激和注射压力监测等技术相结合是神经损伤发生可能性最低的神经阻滞方式。外科医师和麻醉科医师应共同确认患者体位以避免对神经造成压迫或拉伸。在神经阻滞的情况下如果患者仍然有疼痛症状，有可能是外科敷料压迫。尽管尚无证据表明神经阻滞可以掩盖间隔室综合征引起的缺血性疼痛，但有间隔室综合征高风险的患者使用间隔室压力监测可预防严重损伤。

感染性并发症

恰当的皮肤准备可以减少感染性并发症的发生：在这方面，氯已定比碘制剂更有效。在使用氯已定时需要注意，在进行穿刺操作前，需确保氯己定已干燥。一方面是为了确保氯己定的消毒效果，另一方面氯己定有神经毒性，如果随导管渗入神经周围，可能会导致不良后果。另外，导管置入位点的选择很重要。例如，伴有血管翳的肥胖患者股神经置管很容易被感染。最佳医疗实践（best medical practice supports，BPS）建议所有外来物体置入人体时（包括神经导管）均应预防性使用抗生素。如果外科医师没有为患者处方抗生素，麻醉科医师则需要考虑预防性使用抗生素来防止神经周围导管的感染。

跌倒风险并发症

尽管区域麻醉会增加患者摔倒的风险，Memtsoudis及其同事研究证实，区域麻醉对于接受下肢手术并随后进行物理治疗的患者是安全的。助行器之类的活动辅助设备以及单人或多人辅助患者活动对于预防跌倒非常重要。住院患者应签署跌倒风险协议，门诊患者也应该有适当的拐杖、助行器或轮椅等辅助设备。医护人员应密切关注患者情况并提醒其不要单独行走。

总结

尽管有可能合并多种并发症，但只要麻醉科医师能够在合适的患者上进行正确的操作，神经周围置管是安全且有效的镇痛模式。特别是当与口服药物一起使用时，神经周围置管可以提供良好的镇痛效果。围术期问题的早期识别和有效管理对于预防进一步并发症至关重要。通过患者、麻醉科医师和外科医师三方之间的沟通，制订合理的围术期方案，这是手术成功的第一步，也是最重要的一步。

（李 岩 译 费苗苗 校）

延伸阅读

Auroy Y, Narchi P, Messiah A, et al.: Serious complications related to regional anesthesia: results of a prospective survey in France, *Anesthesiology* 87:479–486, 1997.

Bergman BD, Hebl JR, Kent J, et al.: Neurologic complications of 405 consecutive continuous axillary catheters, *Anesth Analg* 96:247–252, 2003.

Boezaart AP, De Beer JF, Nell ML: Early experience with continuous cervical paravertebral block using a stimulating catheter, *Reg Anesth Pain Med* 28:406–413, 2003.

Borgeat A, Dullenkopf A, Ekatodramis G, et al.: Evaluation of the lateral modified approach for continuous interscalene block after shoulder surgery, *Anesthesiology* 99:436–442, 2003.

Borgeat A, Kalberer F, Jacob H, et al.: Patient-controlled interscalene analgesia with ropivacaine 0.2% versus bupivacaine 0.15% after major open shoulder surgery: the effects on hand motor function, *Anesth Analg* 92:218–223, 2001.

Brull R, Hadzic A, Reina MA, et al.: Pathophysiology and etiology of nerve injury following peripheral nerve blockade, *Reg Anesth Pain Med* 40:479–490, 2015.

Brull R, McCartney CJL, Chan VWS, et al.: Neurological complications after regional anesthesia: contemporary estimates of risk, *Anesth Analg* 104:965–974, 2007.

Capdevila X, Barthelet Y, Biboulet P, et al.: Effects of perioperative analgesic technique on the surgical outcome and duration of rehabilitation after major knee surgery, *Anesthesiology* 91:8–15, 1999.

Cuvillon P, Ripart J, Lalourcey L, et al.: The continuous femoral nerve block catheter for postoperative analgesia: bacterial colonization, infectious rate and adverse effects, *Anesth Analg* 93:1045–1049, 2001.

Gillespie WJ, Walenkamp G: Antibiotic prophylaxis for surgery for proximal femoral and other closed long bone fractures, *Cochrane Database Syst Rev*(2)CD000244, 2000.

Grant SA, Nielsen KC, Greengrass RA, et al.: Continuous peripheral nerve block for ambulatory surgery, *Reg Anesth Pain Med* 26:209–214, 2001.

Ilfeld BM, Duke KB, Donohue MC: The association between lower extremity continuous peripheral nerve blocks and patient falls after knee and hip arthroplasty, *Anesth Analg* 111:1552–1554, 2010.

Memtsoudis SG, Danninger T, Rasul R, et al.: Inpatient falls after total knee arthroplasty: the role of anesthesia type and peripheral nerve blocks, *Anesthesiology* 120:551–563, 2014.

Tuominen MK, Pere P, Rosenberg PH: Unintentional arterial catheterization and bupivacaine toxicity associated with continuous interscalene brachial plexus block, *Anesthesiology* 75:356–358, 1991.

Wasserstein D, Farlinger C, Brull R, et al.: Advanced age, obesity, and continuous femoral nerve blockade are independent factors for inpatient falls after primary total knee arthroplasty, *J Arthroplasty* 28:1121–1124, 2013.

Yentur EA, Luleci N, Topcu I, et al.: Is skin disinfection with 10% povidone iodine sufficient to prevent epidural needle and catheter contamination? *Reg Anesth Pain Med* 28:389–393, 2003.

肢体止血带

第 55 章

H.David Hardman, Cody Rowan, Jay Schoenherr

病例概要

患者，女性，75 岁，在脊髓麻醉和静脉镇静下接受左膝关节置换翻修术。患者患有肥胖症，长期服用阿片类药物以缓解疼痛，并患有胰岛素依赖性糖尿病。在进行单次脊髓麻醉之前放置一个持续的收肌管导管用于术后疼痛控制。传统的矩形大腿止血带用于外科止血。肢体驱血后，袖带压力为 300 mmHg。手术顺利进行，止血带总时间为 2 h。脊髓麻醉作用消散后，术后第 2 天取出收肌管导管。随后，她主诉左腿麻木无力。

问题分析

定义

止血带常用于上下肢手术，以减少术中失血量。止血带的使用历史悠久，并发症发生率低（但不为零）。并发症可能有多种形式，从局部皮肤轻微撕裂到神经功能障碍（框 55.1）。神经、血管和肌肉组织的直接压迫以及缺血和再灌注，这些均是导致止血带并发症的病理生理基础。止血带使用后的术后神经功能障碍是一种明确但不常见的现象，且永久性影响非常罕见。全身影响可能发生，反映了肢体受压（如肺栓塞）或由于下方组织缺血所致全身炎症的直接影响。

框 55.1　止血带并发症

- 皮肤损伤
- 肌肉坏死
- 神经损伤
- 肢体缺血
- 自体输血
- 高血压
- 低血压
- 高碳酸血症
- 代谢性酸中毒
- 抗生素渗透受损
- 右心衰竭
- 低体温
- 深静脉血栓形成
- 肺栓塞
- 全身性血栓栓塞

动脉止血带广泛应用于上下肢手术和静脉局部麻醉。这种做法仍在继续，因为人们普遍认为，减少手术失血和创造不出血的手术视野所带来的好处超过了止血带相关并发症的风险。麻醉科医师必须意识到止血带相关组织损伤的潜在可能性，止血带充气和放气对全身的影响，以及在这些时候可能会发生的灾难性事件。

应该认识到，外科医师和麻醉科医师共同分担任何与止血带相关并发症的医学法律责任。文件记录应包括止血带的位置、敷料和巾单的使用、充气压力和持续时间。止血带压力与全身血压值的关系，长期充盈时间和总的血管阻断时间必须与外科医师小组沟通交流，并记录在麻醉单上。

局部损伤

对皮肤、肌肉、神经和血管的压力相关性损伤取决于止血带充气的压力及其持续时间。损伤是由直接压力造成的，但轴向拉伸和剪切力也可能导致损伤，特别是止血带的边缘。止血带远端缺乏动脉血流会导致缺血，引起进行性酸中毒、低氧血症和高碳酸血症。炎症介质的释放增加毛细血管通透性，引起组织水肿，加重缺血损伤，尤其是再灌注后。缺血 30 min 后可检测到超微结构的细胞变化，但缺血 2 h 以内是可逆转的。细胞内高能磷酸盐消耗逐渐发生。Na^+-K^+-ATP 酶依赖的离子交换泵的损伤可导致细胞外的钾泄漏和细胞内水肿。肌质网失去糖原，线粒体肿胀，髓鞘变性。如果不纠正缺血，就会发生细胞坏死。

受局部止血带压力影响的组织部位如下所述。

皮肤

对皮肤的创伤可能是由于皮肤和止血带之间不合适的敷垫造成的压力性坏死引起的，或者是由于止血带应用不当造成的摩擦灼伤所致。上肢皮肤皱褶丰富的肥胖患者皮肤损伤的风险增加。备皮溶液可能浸入止血带下的敷垫，导致全层的化学烧伤。

肌肉

肌细胞对压迫和缺血非常敏感。由于止血带长期充气或高压，损伤更为严重。通常情况下，止血带下的损伤最大。与之相关的缺血、水肿和微血管充血可导致止血带后综合征。症状包括僵硬、苍白和无力（不是瘫痪），并伴有主观肢体麻木。如果止血带在高压下长时间充气，可能发生横纹肌溶解。由于水肿和再灌注充血，止血带放气后可能会出现间隔室综合征。

周围神经

机械压力直接压迫止血带下的神经，袖带近端和远端边缘的剪切力也会造成神经损伤，从感觉异常到完全麻痹。远端缺血作用较小。止血带使用的时间对神经损伤的影响尚不清楚，据报道的引起瘫痪的止血带充盈时间短至 30 min。下肢神经损伤多累及坐骨神经。上肢与止血带相关的神经损伤似乎比下肢更常见，桡神经损伤比尺神经或正中神经损伤更常见。当止血带相关神经损伤发生在下肢时，坐骨神经最有可能受累。

局部神经损伤倾向于神经失用性损伤，结构损伤仅限于轴突周围的髓鞘，而不损伤轴突本身。神经失用性损伤倾向于自限性，具有良好的预后，在几天至数周内完全恢复。相反，轴突损伤涉及对轴突本身的损伤，一旦电兴奋性丧失，去极化不再发生，就会导致信号功能的丧失。这些损伤需要更长的时间才能恢复，因为轴突必须沿着结缔组织途径再生，有些损伤可能不能完全恢复。很少会出现永久性的神经缺损（表 55.1）。

血管系统

动脉和静脉，特别是假体移植（例如动静脉瘘、动脉旁路移植），很容易受到机械压迫造成的创伤性损伤。尽管直接动脉损伤很少见（0.03% ～ 0.14% 的发病率），破裂的动脉粥样硬化斑块可导致局部血栓形成或远端栓塞引起缺血。深静脉血栓（deep venous thrombosis，DVT）是下肢手术中常见的并发症，止血带与深静脉淤滞和血栓形成无关。相反，系统性高凝状态是由于止血带相关或手术疼痛引起的儿茶酚胺释放和血小板聚集。相比之下，止血带释放后的活动性出血可能因缺血引起的组织纤溶酶原激活物释放和纤维蛋白溶解而加重。

表 55.1　神经损伤特点

神经失用	髓鞘损伤 轴突完整 预后最好
轴突断伤	髓鞘和轴突受损 需要神经组织再生 恢复可能不完全
神经断伤	神经完全破坏 需要手术修复 预后不佳

全身效应

止血带充气和放气会产生全身性影响。其紊乱强度和持续时间与止血带充气时长、止血带覆盖肢体的大小和数量成正比。可观察到以下效应。

自体输血

肢体驱血和止血带快速充气，将血液分流到中央循环（自体输血），增加全身血管阻力。在双侧大腿止血带同时充气的情况下，自体输血的血液多达 800 ml。这会导致中心静脉压和收缩压的短暂升高，而后收缩压逐渐恢复到基线水平。在左心室功能受损的患者中，因循环超负荷和心脏停搏而引起的充血性心力衰竭已被报道。

高血压

止血带诱发高血压很常见。患者在止血带充气后 30 ～ 60 min 内出现心率、收缩压和舒张压升高，这种情况一直持续到止血带放松。平均动脉压增加的原因是：①血管床减少后全身血管阻力急剧增加；②止血带袖带充气前肢体驱血，会引起中央血容量急性扩张；③止血带压迫和肢体缺血引起的疼痛。该一系列生命体征变化的发生率与麻醉类型有关，从臂丛麻醉下的 2.5% 到全麻下的 67% 不等。皮肤机制可能是原因，例如局麻药混合物（eutectic mixture of local anesthetic agents，EMLA）可以减轻止血带的不适。在一项样本量有限的志愿者研究中，由于星状神经节阻滞在减少上臂止血带不适方面缺乏有效性，因此交感神经介导的通路可能性不大。止血带疼痛机制的主要假说是失去对无髓鞘、传导缓慢的 C 纤维的抑制。这些纤维通常被快速的 A- δ 有髓纤维所抑制，在止血带充气和机械压迫大约 30 min 后被阻断。

低血压

止血带放气后，血容量回流至下肢和缺血后反应性血管扩张，继而导致血压和中心静脉压下降。此外，随着再灌注，代谢物从缺血区释放进入到体循环有可能导致心肌抑制，并进一步降低血压。低血压通常有自限性（≤ 15 min）。

高碳酸血症

止血带释放后，由于缺血肢体的高碳酸性静脉血流出进入体循环系统，呼气末二氧化碳（$ETCO_2$）增加。$ETCO_2$ 峰值增加发生在止血带放气后的第 1 min，大约在 10 ～ 13 min 后恢复到基础水平。自主呼吸患者通过增加呼吸频率来控制。然而，那些机械通气的患者需要在 5 min 左右短暂增加 50% 的每分通气量，以维持血液正常碳酸状态。过度通气可以防止相关的脑血容量和颅内压增加，否则可能会对颅内高压患者有损害。

代谢性酸中毒

在离体肢体再灌注 30 min 左右，可观察到血清乳酸升高和 pH 降低。变化的程度与止血带充气的持续时间成正比。

血氧饱和度

动脉氧饱和度通常保持正常。然而，止血带释放后大量的失氧合的血液返回到中心循环时，混合静脉血氧饱和度暂时降低。

抗生素渗透受损

如果止血带在抗生素使用之前或使用期间加压，静脉注射的抗生素可能不会渗透到手术部位。抗生素使用与止血带充气加压之间的 5 min 间隔可能足以允许抗生素渗透。

核心体温

大多数患者体温在止血带使用期间仍保持正常。动脉压以上的止血带充气会暂时升高核心体温，而止血带放松则会使核心体温暂时降低。核心体温通常下降 0.7℃或更少，是由静脉血液从先前阻断的肢体进入全身循环所致。

深静脉血栓形成、肺栓塞或全身性血栓栓塞

这些潜在的灾难性并发症可能发生于下肢创伤和外科手术时，但术中很少发生。尽管经食管超声心动图的研究显示止血带释放后右心房栓塞的发生率高达 70%，但大多数栓子都很小，不太可能导致严重的发病率。然而，高凝状态和含有血栓的患者由于外伤或长期制动，此类风险增加。在这种情况下，人们认为血栓会在肢体驱血或止血带充气时驱出脱落。例如 DVT 或肺栓塞或全身栓塞这种灾难性事件更有可能发生在术后康复过程中。使用依诺肝素预防 DVT 可大大降低致命性肺梗死的发生率。然而，考虑到在止血带的充气和放气期间都有肺栓子和脑栓子的报道，麻醉科医师在这段时间里应特别警惕。应注意患者的神经状况以及动脉氧饱和度和 $ETCO_2$ 的任何突然、意外的变化。严重的肺栓子导致 $ETCO_2$ 的急剧降低，伴有心动过速和低血压，随后出现低氧血症和心肌缺血。右心室功能障碍也可能出现（另见第 65 章和第 142 章）。

识别

由于区域阻滞在下肢手术中的应用增加，使得术后疼痛评分明显降低，且患者可早期活动，如何区分与使用止血带有关的神经损伤和与区域麻醉有关的神经损伤？

止血带后综合征是与止血带使用相关最常见的问题。受影响的肢体轻度无力、主诉弥漫性麻木、肿胀、僵硬和轻微苍白通常在止血带放松后几个小时出现。此外，通过正常神经传导检查以及出现肌酸激酶（MM）的升高和肌球蛋白尿症，可以将肌肉的缺血性损伤与神经损伤区分开来。

如果止血带产生了压迫性神经损伤，就很难区分这种损伤和区域阻滞有关的损伤，特别是当止血带或止血带边缘与周围神经阻滞的部位重叠时。止血带相关神经损伤可以从感觉异常到受累肢体完全瘫痪。幸运的是，局部止血带相关的神经损伤通常为神经失用性，可完全康复，预后良好，尽管也可能发生轴突损伤。在这种情况下，恢复的预后取决于轴突损伤的程度，以及神经结缔组织结构是否完好无损（见表 55.1）。

术后应对受累肢体进行简单的神经学评估，并与术前检查进行比较。严重运动和感觉缺陷的证据需要神经科会诊和电生理诊断来确定损伤的位置和严重程度，以及恢复预后情况。在区域麻醉下，神经损伤的诊断可能会出现延迟，尤其是留置导管用于术后镇痛。

手术后即刻或延迟数小时后可能观察到急性间隔室综合征。止血带放气后发生反应性充血可能导致肢体肿胀的发生率高达 10%，有可能加重这一并发症，特别是使用包扎较紧的敷料或石膏。肢体通常会发生肿胀，肌肉僵硬，疼痛比预期的体检发现更为严重。当间隔室压力监测显示压力升高时，可证实该诊断。神经功能障碍也是一种常见的后遗症。

术后 Ⅰ 型或 Ⅱ 型复杂局部疼痛综合征可在术后数周或数月出现。先是灼痛和自主神经功能障碍，随后肢体出现营养不良改变。

止血带袖带摘除时皮肤损伤通常较为明显。可能存在淤斑、持续红斑、大疱形成或皮肤灼伤。

当袖带放松未导致肢体全部或部分再灌注时，应怀疑动脉损伤引起的血管功能不全。

风险评估

在高风险医疗事故环境中工作时，潜在术后神经损伤（postoperative nerve injury，PNI）可能会影响麻醉科医师对止血带诱发 PNI 高风险患者的麻醉方式的选择。框 55.2 列出了可能增加使用止血带并发症风险的因素。

动脉止血带的充气时间和压力的安全上限仍存争议。神经最容易受到机械压力的影响，而肌肉最容易受长时间缺血的影响。大多数临床医师建议尽可能缩短止血带充气时间，健康患者的止血带应以 2 h 为限；如果手术时间超过 2 h，止血带应每 2 h 放气一次，以允许肢体再灌注 10 min。即使止血带使用时间短，也可能发生肌肉损伤，尤其是袖带下方。老年创伤患者和周围血管疾病患者最易受到肌肉损伤。因此，应使用产生动脉压迫所需的最低压力。在正常血压，平均身高的成年患者，上肢的充气压力应为 200 mmHg，下肢的充气压力应为 250 mmHg。止血带压力应保持高于收缩压 50 ～ 150 mmHg 以上。用锥形压力袖带代替传统的矩形压力袖带会在较低的压力下产生动脉阻断，并可能减轻压力相关的组织损害。

框 55.2 可能增加止血带相关并发症风险的因素

止血带相关
未定期维修和检查压力精度的设备
双侧止血带同时使用
翻修、恶性肿瘤或其他需要长时间止血带的手术

血管性和代谢性
糖尿病
周围血管疾病
肥胖
雷诺病（Raynaud disease）
人工血管移植

凝血病
镰状细胞病和镰状细胞病携带者
原有凝血功能障碍
深静脉血栓的风险增加的患者

其他
周围神经病变
在手术前长期制动
创伤肢体伴有广泛的软组织损伤
局灶性感染
乳胶过敏（必须使用无乳胶止血带和管道）

启示

大多数与止血带相关的压迫性神经损伤都是神经失用（麻痹），损伤后数天到数周内可完全消失。治疗方法为物理治疗与病理性神经疼痛治疗相结合的姑息治疗。更严重的损伤，如轴突损伤或神经断伤，恢复病程不一，可为数月至数年的时间，即使是需要神经移植和神经转移的神经外科重建手术，也可能永远不会功能完全恢复。在最坏的情况下，可能会同时伴发复杂区域疼痛综合征（complex regional pain syndrome，CRPS）。

止血带后综合征所致的无力和肿胀会影响康复和伤口愈合。与压力有关的皮肤损伤增加了感染的风险。间隔室综合征对缺血性坏死和累及肌肉群的永久性挛缩有明显的风险。未识别的动脉供血不足可导致软组织和骨骼坏死。

在区域麻醉患者中，止血带疼痛和伴随的高血压可能需要丙泊酚或氯胺酮进行深度镇静，甚至全

身麻醉。单用阿片类药物通常无效。止血带放气引起低血压是可预期的，且常为自限性。如果机体不能自我调节，则使用液体冲击和小剂量的血管升压药物，直到低血压缓解。

大面积的肺栓塞会导致血流动力学不稳定、右心室劳损和心血管衰竭。非致命性栓塞可导致低氧血症，原因包括通气血流失调、心肌梗死，或者卒中（心内分流导致的反常性脑栓塞）。

管理

严重的神经损伤（明显的肢体运动无力或瘫痪）如果在 48 h 内无法解决，应转诊至神经科医师进行评估，以排除可治疗的手术相关原因，如压迫性血肿形成。后续的检查可包括止血带和手术部位的超声检查，以及磁共振成像（MRI）。更详细的电生理诊断，如神经传导检查（运动和感觉）和针电极肌电图，可在未缓解的严重损伤后立即进行，每隔 1 个月和 3 个月重复一次。止血带后综合征的治疗包括患肢抬高、伤口愈合监测、物理治疗和非阿片类镇痛药。与压力有关的皮肤损伤会根据需要进行治疗。水疱或化学烧伤需要烧伤护理，但在备皮之前，在止血带袖带远端涂上不可渗透的塑料屏障覆盖物以避免这些伤害。复杂区域疼痛综合征需要由一个综合性的慢性疼痛管理小组来管理，早期转诊至关重要。间隔室综合征是一种外科急症，需要筋膜切开术来给受累肌肉进行减压。

肢体动脉功能不全需要外科血管重建或溶栓治疗。经食管超声心动图可有助于术中肺栓子的诊断。肺栓子的治疗为支持性治疗，如有需要，可进行机械通气、氧疗、缩血管药物支持和心肺复苏。一些患者可能需要全身抗凝、溶栓治疗、外科血栓切除或介入放射学血栓清除术。脑栓塞可通过 CT 或 MRI 扫描诊断，治疗由神经外科医师和（或）介入神经科医师 / 放射科医师指导，用于血栓溶解、支架置入或疏通。

预防

正确筛选患者可以减少灾难性的并发症。在筛查高危 DVT 患者（长时间制动，高凝状态）时，如果发现血栓，应推迟择期手术。然而，使用造影剂增强的经胸超声心动图检查所有患者的心脏右向左分流并非物有所值，右向左分流是否会影响麻醉或外科治疗尚不明确。

1951 年首次描述了在手外科术中使用充气止血带止血的安全因素，后来 Braithwaite 和 Klenerman 于 1996 年修订了 Bruner 的 10 条规则。幸运的是，通过限制止血带最大压力和止血带充气时间，可以避免四肢手术中的大多数充气止血带并发症。虽然没有随机、对照、前瞻性的临床研究为我们提供循证指南，但有足够的动物研究和临床数据可以提出以下建议：

- 术前仔细筛选患者；
- 使用较宽的低压止血带袖带；
- 将止血带充气至防止出血所需的最低压力；
- 止血带缺血时间限制在 2 h 或更短；
- 设置最大止血带压力设置如下：手臂止血带，高于基线收缩压 50 ～ 75 mmHg；腿部止血带，高于基线收缩压 75 ～ 100 mmHg；
- 确保止血带下方有足够的衬垫；
- 使用屏障技术防止止血带袖口下有任何皮肤准备液；
- 如可能，交替使用两个止血带；
- 通过定期维护检查确保止血带的可靠性。

我们还可以做其他一些简单的事情来减少止血带相关的伤害，而不必等待研究和技术的进步。使用以下一般指南可能会导致止血带袖带压力比目前的常规临床实践使用压力低 30% ～ 50%：

- 使用锥形止血带袖带代替传统的矩形袖带。与传统的袖带相比，这种方法可以减少 23% 的肢体阻断压力。此外，它们更有效地将表面压力传递给深部组织，因为它们更接近符合肢体的形状。
- 通过多普勒或便携式超声检查确定肢体阻断压力来设置止血带压力。然后将止血带压力设置为高于肢体阻断压力 40 ～ 80 mmHg。
- 较宽的锥形袖带或袖带宽度与四肢周长之比大于 0.5 时，可产生略低于收缩压的阻断压。

将来，止血带相关的损伤可能会减至最小，并且可以延长止血带时间，如骨骼肌缺血预处理、更频繁的再灌注间隔、区域低温和缺血预处理相结合的技术。

（顾姣姣　译　严姝姝　校）

延伸阅读

Al-Ghamdi AA: Bilateral total knee replacement under tourniquet in a homozygous sickle cell patient, *Anesth Analg* 98:543–544, 2003.

Braithwaite I, Klenerman L: Burns under tourniquets—Bruner's ten rules revisited, *J Med Def Unions* 12:14–15, 1996.

Brull R, Hadzic A, Reina MA, et al.: Pathophysiology and etiology of nerve injury following peripheral nerve blockade, *Reg Anesth Pain Med* 40(5):1–12, 2015.

Bruner JM: Safety factors in the use of the pneumatic tourniquet for haemostasis in surgery of the hand, *J Bone Joint Surg Am* 33:221–224, 1951.

Duffy PJ: The arterial tourniquet. Available at http://www.uam.es/departamentos/medicina/anesnet/gtoa/hm1.html. Accessed May 18, 2016.

Estebe JP, Davies JM: Richebe, P: The pneumatic tourniquet: mechanical, ischaemia-reperfusion and systemic effects, *Eur J Anaesthesiol* 28(6):404–411, 2011.

Farah RS, Thomas S: Sympathetic blockade and tourniquet pain in surgery of the upper extremity, *Anesth Analg* 66:1033–1035, 1987.

Iwama H, Kaneko T, Ohmizo H, et al.: Circulatory, respiratory and metabolic changes after thigh tourniquet release in combined epidural-propofol anaesthesia with preservation of spontaneous respiration, *Anaesthesia* 57:588–592, 2002.

Kam P, Kavanaugh R, Yoong F: The arterial tourniquet: pathophysiological consequences and anaesthetic implications, *Anaesthesia* 56:53–54, 2001.

Lowrie A, Jones MJ, Eastley RJ: Effect of a eutectic mixture of local anaesthetic agents (EMLA) on tourniquet pain in volunteers, *Br J Anaesth* 63:751–753, 1989.

Murphy CG, Winter DC, Bouchier-Hayes DJ: Tourniquet injuries: pathogenesis and modalities for attenuation, *Acta Orthop Belg* 71(6):635–645, 2005.

Neal J, Barrington MJ, Brull R, et al.: The second ASRA practice advisory on neurologic complications associated with regional anesthesia and pain medicine: executive summary 2015, *Reg Anesth Pain Med* 40(5):401–430, 2015.

Tredwell S, Wilmink M, Inkpen K, et al.: Pediatric tourniquets: analysis of cuff and limb interface, current practice, and guidelines for use, *J Pediatr Orthop* 21:671–676, 2001.

Van Roekel HE, Thurston AJ: Tourniquet pressure: the effect of limb circumference and systolic blood pressure, *J Hand Surg* 10:142–144, 1985.

Wakai A, Winter DC, Street JT, et al.: Pneumatic tourniquets in extremity surgery, *J Am Acad Orthop Surg* 9(5):345–351, 2001.

Watson JC, Huntoon MA: Neurologic evaluation and management of perioperative nerve injury, *Reg Anesth Pain Med* 40(5):491–501, 2015.

Weiss SJ, Cheung AT, Stecker MM, et al.: Fatal paradoxical cerebral embolization during bilateral knee arthroplasty, *Anesthesiology* 84:721–723, 1996.

胎儿窘迫

第**56**章

James N. Bates

病例概要

患者,38 岁，初产妇，体重 120 kg，既往 2 型糖尿病病史且控制不佳。妊娠 35 周时出现胎膜破裂，体温 38.5℃。决定引产。产程中，产科医师声称电子胎心率监护仪提示出现胎儿窘迫（图 56.1），需要对患者施行紧急剖宫产术。

问题分析

定义

“**胎儿窘迫**（fetal distress）”是一个不精确的医疗术语，自 1998 年美国妇产科医师学会（American College of Obstetricians and Gynecologists，ACOG）于委员会上建议将“**胎儿窘迫**”替换为“**不安全的胎心率图**（nonreassuring fetal heart rate tracing）”后，其在医疗记录上的使用显著减少。尽管“**胎儿窘迫**”这一词语听上去不甚吉利，但通常胎儿娩出后多处于良好状态。根据 ACOG 的推荐，医疗记录中通常描述不安全胎心率都附加有发生诸如胎儿心动过缓、重复性晚期或变异减速以及变异性缺失等说明。然而，**胎儿窘迫**这一词语在交流患者病情时仍被频繁使用并表示情况十分危急。当麻醉科医师被呼叫协助处理胎儿窘迫时，首先应与产科医师沟通的部分内容就是明确母体与胎儿的状态、是否需要进行紧急分娩，因为这些因素在很大程度上决定了麻醉药物的选择。

识别

正确评估继续正常分娩对母体或胎儿的风险何时大于手术分娩，是产科医师在管理分娩患者时面临的巨大挑战之一。产科医师用于评估胎儿情况和预测分娩结局的工具有限。由于用法简单、实时连续、微创甚至无创且广泛可用，电子胎心率（fetal heart rate，FHR）监测是用于评估胎儿氧合的最基本的手段。该方法是对胎儿自身氧合和灌注情况进行

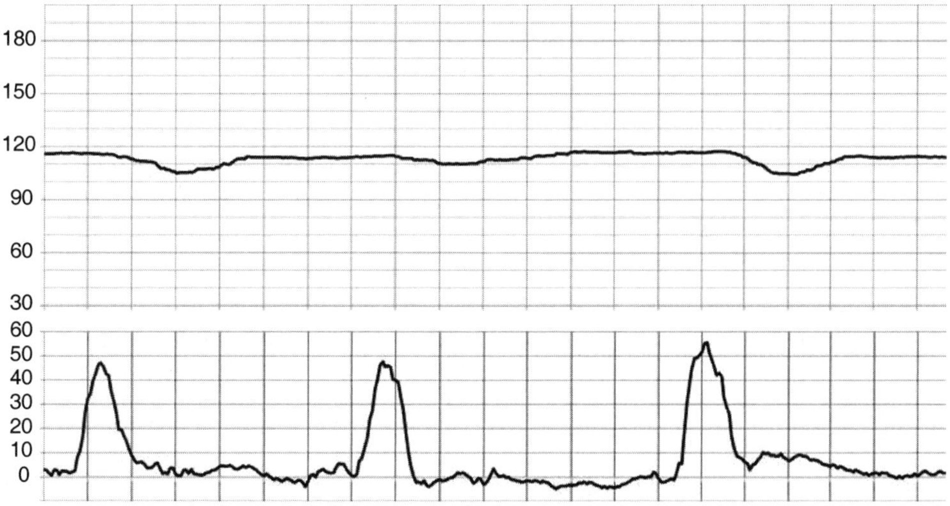

图 56.1 胎心率电子监护仪图显示胎心率基线缺乏变异性和周期性晚期减速，在第一次与第三次宫缩后尤为明显。该胎心率为Ⅲ类图形。图中网格间期为 1 分钟。上方描记图以每分钟次数显示胎心率曲线，下方描记图以 mmHg 表示宫缩压力波形

监测评估，因此它可反映多种信息，但同时也易受许多因素影响。影响胎儿中枢神经系统及自主反射的因素，如药物（例如阿片类药物、麻醉药物、交感或副交感神经调节剂如 β- 受体激动剂或阿托品等）、神经功能异常（如胎儿无脑畸形），或者可能改变测量指标的情况（如胎儿心律失常），都会使 FHR 监测的解读变得更加复杂。而另一方面，经过几十年的广泛使用与解读，目前积累了大量的不同类型胎心率与胎儿预后相关性的数据，使其成为了分娩中用于评估胎儿状况的最实用、最可靠的基本监测手段。

其他方法也可提供更多关于胎儿状态的信息，如：羊水中是否存在胎粪，FHR 对声音或头皮刺激的反应，从胎儿头皮中所得血液样本的血浆 pH，使用多普勒测速仪探测脐动脉中是否存在舒张血流的减少、缺失或逆流等。但这些手段都不能取代 FHR 监测的作用与价值。

FHR 监测发挥作用的理论基础是缺氧或窒息程度的增加会引起 FHR 模式发生特征性变化，但其中的调节机制尚未完全了解。最基本的原理是，压力与化学感受器对氧和二氧化碳的传入信号，经过脑干核、下丘脑中心以及大脑皮质的处理，产生交感、副交感以及体液信号来调节心率。

电子 FHR 监测仪记录了 FHR 和宫缩情况。基线 FHR 及变化情况可用于分析其与宫缩的关系。测量的 FHR 模式的主要特征（框 56.1）包括：心率基线，心率变异性，加速和减速（三种类型：早期减速、晚期减速和变异减速）。2008 年，为使 FHR 监测图的描述与解读全面标准化，美国引入了 FHR 图解读的三级系统（框 56.2）。依据观察到的波形特征以及预测价值，分为Ⅰ类（正常），Ⅱ类（不确定）和Ⅲ类（异常）。

风险评估

胎儿危象的发生率难以计算，因为如果出现胎儿窘迫时不加以干预可能会导致胎儿死亡或严重损伤，但采取适当的措施可降低甚至预防胎儿的损伤。加拿大的一项研究数据显示，每 1000 名活产婴儿中围产期死亡率为 0.67，而其中 0.09 被认为是可预防的（非严重早产或异常）。这可以代表对救治失败率的一种估计。与此相反，产妇的剖宫产率超过 30%，

框 56.1　胎心率特点

基线

正常基线胎心率为 110 ～ 160 次 / 分，超出此范围变化表示迷走或交感张力增加。

变异性

胎心率变异性是指胎心率波形出现波动，以前分为短间期（两次心搏间）和长间期（超过 1 分钟），但现已不再使用这种区分。正常胎心率变异性反映了胎儿大脑皮质、中脑、迷走神经和心脏传导系统的正常功能通路。

加速

胎心率突然增加，每分钟超过基线 ≥ 15 次，且持续 ≥ 15 s。

产前胎心率加速是对胎儿活动的一种反应，被视为胎儿健康的标志，是一种反应性非应激试验。

产时胎心率加速表明胎儿不存在明显的代谢性酸中毒。

减速

早期减速

- 明显可见，通常为对称性，胎心率逐渐减慢并恢复，与宫缩有关。
- 胎心率逐渐减慢定义为从开始至胎心率最低值所需时间 ≥ 30 s。
- 从减速开始到降至最低值来计算胎心率的减少量。
- 减速的最低值与宫缩的峰值同时出现。
- 大多数情况下，减速的起始、最低值和恢复分别与宫缩的开始、峰值和结束相对应。
  - 可能由轻度缺氧引起的迷走神经反射引起。
  - 并非预示着结局不良。

可变减速

- 明显可见胎心率突然出现减慢。
- 胎心率突然减慢是指从减速开始到降至最低点时间 < 30 秒，从减速开始到降至最低值来计算胎心率的减少量。
- 胎心率减慢 ≥ 15 次 / 分，持续 ≥ 15 s 且 < 2 min。
- 当可变减速与子宫收缩相关时，其起始、深度和持续时间通常随子宫收缩而发生变化。
  - 在第二产程中，脐带或头部受压可能引起压力或化学感受器信号改变，从而引起迷走神经反射。
  - 轻至中度（≥ 80 次 / 分）可变减速通常可耐受良好，但长期严重（< 60 次 / 分）减速可能导致胎儿损伤。

晚期减速

- 明显可见，通常为对称性，逐渐减慢并恢复，与宫缩有关。
- 胎心率逐渐减慢定义为至最低值所需时间 ≥ 30 s。
- 从减速开始到降至最低值来计算胎心率的减少量。
- 减速时程延迟，其最低值出现于宫缩峰值之后。
- 大多数情况下，减速的起始、最低值和恢复分别出现于宫缩的开始、峰值和结束之后。
  - 可能为胎儿对低氧的反应，但也可能反映存在心肌衰竭。
  - 若用于反映胎儿窒息的指标可能过于敏感，但结合胎心率变异性降低或缺失后，是提示胎儿存在损伤的可靠信号。

FHR，胎心率

Modified from Macones GA，Hankins GD，Spong CY，et al：The 2008 National Institute of Child Health and Human Development workshop report on electronic fetal monitoring：update on definitions，interpretation，and research guidelines. *Obstet Gynecol* 112（3）：661-666，2008.

框 56.2 三级胎心率的系统解读

Ⅰ类（正常波形）

Ⅰ类胎心率曲线包括以下所有特点：

- 基线心率：110 ～ 160 次 / 分
- 基线胎心率变异性：中度
- 晚期或变异减速：不存在
- 早期减速：存在 / 不存在
- 加速：存在 / 不存在

观察到此类心率时，强烈预示胎儿处于正常酸碱状态

Ⅱ类（不确定波形）

Ⅱ类胎心率曲线包括**所有非Ⅰ类或Ⅲ类胎心率**，Ⅱ类波形可能代表了临床治疗中所遇到的相当一部分，Ⅱ类胎心率曲线样本包括以下任何特点：

基线心率

- 心动过缓不伴有基线变异性缺失
- 心动过速

基线胎心率变异性

- 最小的基线变异性
- 缺乏基线变异性，不伴有周期性减速
- 显著基线变异性

加速

- 刺激胎儿后无诱导性加速

周期性或间断性减速

- 周期性出现变异减速伴有最小或中等基线变异性
- 持续较长的减速≥ 2 min 但 <10 min
- 周期性出现晚期减速伴中度基线变异性
- 变异减速伴其他特点，如缓慢回归基线，“超射”或“肩”部征

无法预测酸碱状态异常，但没有足够的证据将其归类为正常或异常

Ⅲ类（异常波形）

Ⅲ类胎心率曲线包括任一特点：

- 基线胎心率变异性缺失或出现以下任何情况：
- 周期性晚期减速
- 周期性变异减速
- 心动过缓
- 正弦波形

观察到此类心率时，预示胎儿处于异常酸碱状态，因此需要立即进行评估

Modified from Macones GA, Hankins GD, Spong CY, et al: The 2008 National Institute of Child Health and Human Development workshop report on electronic fetal monitoring: update on definitions, interpretation, and research guidelines. *Obstet Gynecol* 112 (3): 661-666, 2008.

而且过去 20 年的调查研究显示 2% ～ 10% 的剖宫产与胎儿窘迫或不安全胎心率相关。来自医疗成本和利用项目 2009 年和 2010 年全国住院患者抽样数据中，一项来自美国医院包含 1 475 457 个新生儿的 20% 抽样显示，10% 的新生儿被诊断为胎儿窘迫 [根据临床分类软件（Clinical Classifcations Software，CCS）代码 190 确定] 且其剖宫产率为 59%，而相比无该诊断的新生儿剖宫产率为 30%。在一份 2016 年的报告中引用了安全分娩联盟 2002—2008 年研究的数据显示，在初次剖宫产中 23% 以不安全胎心率曲线为指征。这些数据表示胎儿窘迫的诊断或不安全胎心率曲线并非少见，且其虽不能作为确凿证据但预示着较高的剖宫产可能。对于每一个被诊断为胎儿窘迫或不安全 FHR 曲线的病例，需要更多患者个体化信息以确定分娩的方式和紧急程度。

启示

未经纠正的胎儿严重缺氧最终会导致严重酸中毒，神经病学损伤包括癫痫、昏迷、肌张力减退、脑病或脑瘫以及最终死亡。

管理

对有临床征象的胎儿宫内缺氧，第一反应应当是立即进行宫内复苏，包括：吸氧，改变产妇体位（左侧或右侧卧位、膝胸位等），评估并治疗产妇低血压或低血容量，停用催产素并改善其他可能导致胎儿氧供不佳的情况。

统计数据表明，许多阴道分娩中记录有胎儿窘迫或不安全胎心率曲线，但大多数还是发生于剖宫产。目前尚不清楚有多少是根据首要目标是尽可能缩短“决定-切开”时间的真正的紧急剖宫产。但是显然，在许多出现胎儿窘迫的情况中，麻醉药物的选择不需要根据哪种技术可以提供最快的手术麻醉来决定。

当麻醉科医师被呼叫需要协助处理胎儿窘迫时，应对阴道分娩与剖宫产均做好准备，且必须决定选用哪种麻醉药物更为合适。出现包含有严重或长时间心动过缓的Ⅲ类胎心率曲线时，以及不稳定的母体情况如大出血或灾难性的子宫破裂等，需要立即手术介入。需行紧急剖宫产时，产科团队、麻醉团队以及患者之间的沟通很有必要。手术的紧急程度、母体的麻醉风险、麻醉对母体与胎儿产生的影响以及产科医师及患者的需求与期望，这些因素在选择

麻醉方式时都应予以考虑。

FHR 监测应当随转运持续监测到产房，如可能，当使用头皮电极时应使用到分娩。这一监测信息有助于指导麻醉药物的选择与管理。进入手术室后，若麻醉诱导前胎儿心动过缓出现缓解，产科医师可能会重新考虑是否行剖宫产，或者这也会影响继续手术是选择全麻还是椎管内麻醉的决定。

对每位患者必须仔细考虑全麻和区域麻醉的相对风险。全身麻醉诱导更加快速，但也和致命性或非致命性母体并发症的发生率升高相关。

若患者已存在有效的硬膜外置管，则可以此来实施手术麻醉。通常注射 15 ～ 20 ml 2% 利多卡因或追加 5 ml 3% 氯普鲁卡因足以产生 T4 平面的外科麻醉。硬膜外麻醉通常比脊髓麻醉起效慢，但可以加快。局麻药尤其是利多卡因中，通常添加肾上腺素（1∶200 000），它可以延长作用时间并增强阻滞效果，但是商业生产的含肾上腺素的利多卡因其 pH 低于单纯的利多卡因，会导致其起效较慢。为维持较高的 pH，肾上腺素可直接加入普通的利多卡因中，或可通过加入碳酸氢钠来调节 pH。每 10 ml 3% 氯普鲁卡因或 2% 利多卡因（含或不含肾上腺素）中加入 1ml 碳酸氢钠（8.4%），可通过增加非离子形式的药物比例来加速起效。一些研究报道，使用碱化的氯普鲁卡因或利多卡因达到外科麻醉效果所需的平均时间不超过 5 min。碱化氯普鲁卡因在所有硬膜外药物中起效最快，但原瓶装 3% 氯普鲁卡因与其起效速度相当，且可避免制备混合药物所需的时间，以及因仓促制药而带来的混合错误或污染的风险。如果没有准备好可用的碱化氯普鲁卡因及利多卡因，或者要避免混合药物，原瓶装制剂是个不错的选择。

0.5% 的布比卡因和 0.5% 的罗哌卡因均可为剖宫产提供较好的麻醉效果，但它们的起效速度远远慢于利多卡因和氯普鲁卡因，因此其在紧急剖宫产中使用较少。不推荐使用碳酸氢盐来碱化这些药物，因其会使药物容易产生沉淀。

若于产房中即决定对产妇行剖宫产术，在转送至手术室前可给予初始剂量的局麻药物。这样可以缩短达到外科麻醉效果的时间，降低需要改行全身麻醉的可能。然而，这也增加了发生副作用的风险（阻滞平面过高、低血压、需进行静脉注射等），因为与手术室环境相比，此时更加难以发现和处理。因此每位患者的相关风险与益处均需仔细权衡。

紧急或意外剖宫产时也应考虑脊髓麻醉。与硬膜外麻醉一样，分娩的紧急程度与在时间窗内提供外科麻醉的能力是做出麻醉选择的关键。在脊髓麻醉中，造成延迟最大的可能就是实施阻滞所需要的时间。麻醉科医师的操作技巧、患者的解剖结构、患者能够承受和维持必要体位的能力以及产科医师与患者对椎管内麻醉的接受程度等等，这些都是决定脊髓麻醉是否合适的因素。脊髓麻醉通常在给药后可迅速起效。通常在实施脊髓麻醉前，会静脉给予大量不含糖晶体液进行预补液，但《美国麻醉科医师协会（American Society of Anesthesiologists，ASA）实践指南》对产科麻醉的建议是，如果脊髓麻醉是患者最适合的方法，即使未完成预补液也不应推迟麻醉的实施。

若硬膜外麻醉与脊髓麻醉均不合适，则应选择全身麻醉。普遍认为，全身麻醉会增加产科患者发生严重并发症甚至死亡的风险。一项回顾性研究显示，与区域麻醉相比，行全身麻醉的产妇死亡率更高。由于在急诊手术和其他高风险手术中历来更倾向于采用全身麻醉，这些因素独立地增加了产妇的发病率和死亡率，因此研究结果可能存在偏差。但大多数研究者认为，大部分风险差异并不能由此得到解释。全身麻醉相关的发病率与死亡率在很大程度上与气道管理（比如插管失败、误吸或通气不足）有关。而区域麻醉通常可避免这些问题。与普通人群相比，产科患者发生此类问题的风险更高。据报道，产科患者插管失败率为 1/300，而普通手术患者为 1/2000。若胎儿窘迫患者于麻醉期间出现插管失败，胎儿的情况也应作为气道管理流程的一部分。若插管失败但可维持通气，且不存在胎儿窘迫，应苏醒患者，后续采用区域麻醉或清醒插管。然而，如果仍持续存在胎儿窘迫，在产妇可维持通气与氧合的前提下，首选使用面罩或喉罩进行吸入麻醉。

预防

早期诊断出可能会发生胎儿窘迫的高危患者可早期进行硬膜外置管。早期诊断Ⅱ类甚至Ⅲ类 FHR 曲线也可减少手术分娩的紧急决策。产科医师与麻醉科医师之间的良好沟通有助于确定最佳治疗并使母体与胎儿获得最好的结局。

致谢

感谢 Drenda.Bucklin 对本章上一版的贡献。

（徐 冰 译 侯 炯 校）

延伸阅读

American Society of Anesthesiologists Task Force on Obstetric Anesthesia: Practice guidelines for obstetric anesthesia: an updated report by the American Society of Anesthesiologists Task Force on Obstetric Anesthesia, *Anesthesiology* 106:843–863, 2007.

Devroe S, Van de Velde M, Rex S: General anesthesia for caesarean section, *Curr Opin Anesthesiol* 28:240–246, 2015.

Guglielminotti J, Wong C, Landau R, et al.: Temporal trends in anesthesia-related adverse events in cesarean deliveries, New York State, 2003–2012, *Anesthesiology* 123:1013–1024, 2015.

Kawakita T, Reddy UM, Landy HJ, et al.: Indications for primary cesarean delivery relative to body mass index, *Am J Obstet Gynecol* 215(4):e1–e9, 2016. 515.

Kozhimannil KB, Arcaya MC, Subramanian SV: Maternal clinical diagnoses and hospital variation in the risk of cesarean delivery: analyses of a national US hospital discharge database, *PLoS Med* 11(10):e1001745, 2014.

Macones GA, Hankins GD, Spong CY, et al.: The 2008 National Institute of Child Health and Human Development workshop report on electronic fetal monitoring: update on definitions, interpretation, and research guidelines, *Obstet Gynecol* 112:661–666, 2008.

Tsen LC: Anesthesia for cesarean delivery. In Chestnut DH, Wong C, Tsen LC, et al.: *Chestnut's obstetric anesthesia: principles and practice*, 5th ed, Philadelphia, 2014, Elsevier, pp 545–603.

第57章 异物误吸

Paul G. Firth

病例概要

一名 3 岁男童需行紧急硬质支气管镜检查，评估和取出疑似误吸的异物。由于咳嗽、喘息、轻度呼吸急促 1 周，先前使用支气管扩张剂和抗生素治疗，效果不佳。家长在回忆后称，在男童吃花生时，有一段时间的呛咳。胸部 X 线检查显示右边局灶性气体陷闭和肺气肿。

问题分析

定义

异物误吸是幼儿尤其是 1 至 4 岁儿童意外死亡的重要原因之一。大多数误吸物是食物或其他有机物质碎片，坚果（尤其是花生）和种子（尤其是葵花籽和西瓜籽）是最常见的误吸物。完全机械性气道阻塞或严重喉痉挛可导致突发死亡。如果异物不移除，幸存者可能会发展成肺炎或脓胸。如果由一个缺乏经验的临床医师在全麻下行支气管镜检查，从一个幼儿体内取出误吸的异物往往比较危险，全球报道的死亡率约为 0.4%。气道丧失、通气不足和缺氧是导致麻醉下死亡的主要因素。

识别

虽然支气管镜是最决定性的检查，但通常依靠结合病史、体格检查和影像学检查来进行诊断。

目击患者发生呛咳事件的病史可高度提示患者可能有异物误吸。尽管其阳性预测价值很高，但阴性预测价值却更低，因为许多误吸事件发生时并未被其照看人员所注意到。

频繁出现的体征和症状包括持续咳嗽、喘息（常在局部）和呼吸急促；发绀和喘鸣相对少见。

胸部 X 线片可能对气道内异物有提示作用。由于有机物是最常见的吸入物质，大多数吸入的物体射线可以穿透，相当一小部分的 X 线片显示为正常。常见异常由管腔堵塞所致，包括局部肺气肿和气体陷闭，或肺不张和渗出（图 57.1）。气胸和纵隔气肿相对少见。

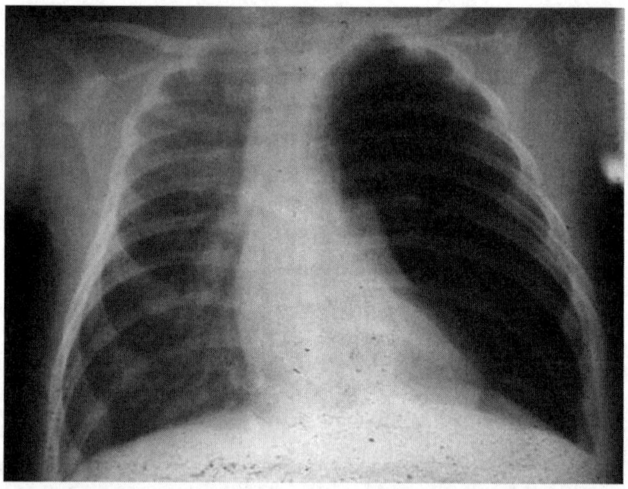

图 57.1 呼气末胸部 X 线片，显示射线可透过的支气管异物导致左侧肺气体陷闭（Courtesy Dr. Peter Masiakos，MD，Department of Surgery，Massachusetts General Hospital，Boston，MA.）

如果诊断不明确，CT 和仿真支气管镜（重新三维成像）也可用于检查呼吸道，然而辐射和成本问题限制了这种方法的应用。此外，硬质和软质支气管镜亦可用来确认或排除不明异物的存在。

风险评估

麻醉科医师应确定①误吸物嵌居位置，②误吸了何种物体，③误吸的时间。评估气体交换是另外一个重要的术前评估目标。

启示

大多数异物（>85%）嵌在支气管树，主要在右侧。卡在喉部或气管内的异物可能导致完全气道梗阻，通常应紧急取出。近端异物通常较为容易定位和移除，而远端异物可能需要更多时间来取出。远端异物会引起肺不张和肺炎，影响气体交换，使麻醉的实施更具挑战性。

当有机物体从气管壁上吸收液体后，会膨胀并造成进行性阻塞。如果异物卡在隆突上部，可能会导致延迟的完全性气道阻塞和致命的窒息。坚果油脂会引起明显的局部炎症。尖锐物体有时会刺穿气道，引起纵隔气肿或气胸，而正压通气可能会使症状加重。

异物误吸后的时间延误可能会影响取出难度和需要麻醉药物的时间。黏膜水肿、局部炎症和感染可能使异物取出更加困难和费时。

管理

支气管镜检查与显著的病死率相关，可能由导致问题的异物、支气管镜或麻醉药物（表 57.1）引起。麻醉科医师应确保气道通畅，通气充足；在气道阻塞、肺不张或肺炎可能损害气体交换的情况下，维持动脉氧合；并在支气管镜刺激期间防止咳嗽、呛咳和气道损伤。

异物可以用软质或硬质支气管镜取出，如果使用硬质支气管镜，氧合直接发生在镜下。静脉通道建立后，通过吸入麻醉药物完成诱导。对声带使用局部麻醉药进行表面麻醉，然后再置入硬质支气管镜。

表 57.1　移除气道异物时支气管镜检查和麻醉的并发症

并发症	注解
气道丧失	异物导致气管梗阻 异物掉入气管 喉痉挛 缺氧性心动过缓 心脏 / 呼吸骤停
通气不足	咳嗽 / 屏气 支气管痉挛 肺炎
气道撕裂伤	气胸 纵隔气肿 出血 支气管断裂
取出失败	气管切开术 胸廓切开术
喉部水肿	术后喘鸣 术后呼吸心脏骤停

维持麻醉的方式有多种，然而尚无被普遍接受的方法。全凭静脉麻醉是一种常见的方式，用丙泊酚 [200 ～ 400 μg/（kg·min）] 辅以阿片类药物，如输注瑞芬太尼 [0.05 ～ 0.2 μg/（kg·min）]。氧气中加七氟烷则是另一种常用的麻醉方法。

在实践中，在通气方面也有很大差异。控制通气和自主呼吸，或两者结合，都已被成功地运用。目前，尚不清楚哪种技术可更有效地防止术中低氧血症和咳嗽或呛咳。

如果使用软质支气管镜，可置入喉罩，并通过侧孔置入气管镜。支气管镜亦可通过气管插管进行。在吸入雾化利多卡因后，支气管镜通过鼻腔进入的方法亦有报道。然而，由于支气管镜和气道尺寸的限制，软质支气管镜并不能适用于所有患者。

术后必须密切观察患者气道阻塞和呼吸不畅情况。喉水肿可能会进展为完全性气道梗阻。根据术后临床情况决定患者出院的最佳时间。

预防

麻醉的基本目标是维持气道和通气，确保在最佳条件下取出异物。为达到这一目的，多种麻醉技术和方案可供选择。麻醉科医师、支气管镜检查者和助手的密切合作和明晰沟通，是确保安全取出气道异物的关键。

（郭品豪　译　薄禄龙　校）

延伸阅读

Chai J, Wu XY, Han N, et al.: A retrospective study of anesthesia during rigid bronchoscopy for airway foreign body removal in children: propofol and sevoflurane with spontaneous ventilation, *Pediatr Anesth* 24(10):1031–1036, 2014.

Fidkowski CW, Zheng H, Firth PG: The anesthetic considerations of tracheobronchial foreign bodies in children: a literature review of 12,979 cases, *Anesth Analg* 111(4):1016–1025, 2010.

Hu S, Dong HL, Sun YY, et al.: Anesthesia with sevoflurane and remifentanil under spontaneous respiration assisted with high-frequency jet ventilation for tracheobronchial foreign body removal in 586 children, *Pediatr Anesth* 22(11):1100–1104, 2012.

Huankang Z, Kuanlin X, Xiaolin H, Witt D: Comparison between tracheal foreign body and bronchial foreign body: a review of 1007 cases, *Int J Pediatr Otorhinolaryngol* 76(12):1719–1725, 2012.

Zhang X, Li W, Chen Y: Postoperative adverse respiratory events in preschool patients with inhaled foreign bodies: an analysis of 505 cases, *Pediatr Anesth* 21(10):1003–1008, 2011.

第58章 颅脑损伤

Armagan Dagal，*Arthur M. Lam*

病例概要

患者，男性，22岁，既往体健，因摩托车事故颅脑受伤，并伴有骨盆和股骨不稳定性骨折。他最初表现躁动挣扎，但很快就意识淡漠，格拉斯哥昏迷量表（Glasgow Coma Scale，GCS）评分为9分（E3V3M3；表58.1）。患者血压95/40 mmHg，心率100次/分。右侧瞳孔散大无反射。现场进行气管插管后该患者被转运至创伤中心。计算机断层扫描（CT）显示右侧大量硬膜外血肿伴中线移位。在输注2 L晶体后测得患者初始红细胞比容为32%，血压为130/80 mmHg，心率120次/分。该患者拟急诊行硬膜外血肿清除术，随后还要进行股骨、骨盆切开复位内固定术。

问题分析

定义

创伤性颅脑损伤（traumatic brain injury，TBI）是由于外部的钝性或穿透性的机械力对脑组织造成的一种获得性损伤。这种损伤可能会演变成短暂或长期的身体和社会心理认知功能的减弱。此外，TBI常常伴发其他颅外损伤。

发生率

TBI的发生率呈上升趋势。从疾病控制和预防中心（Centers for Disease Control and Prevention，CDC）估计，急诊科（emergency department，ED）的TBI就诊人数约250万人次/年。从这些病例中看，约87%（2 213 826）的患者接受了治疗并离开ED，另外11%（283 630）的患者住院治疗后出院，剩下2%（52 844）的患者死亡。

跌倒是非致命性TBI的主要原因（35%），其次是与机动车辆相关的伤害（17%）和头部受到物体的撞击或打击（17%）。总的来说，机动车交通事故是造成与TBI相关死亡的最常见原因，其次是自我伤害/自杀和跌倒。

TBI是40岁以下人群中致死和致残的最常见原因。过去的十年中，通过对疾病进程的理解加深以及技术水平的进步，TBI的死亡率降低了8.2%。

原发性损伤是指创伤直接引起的神经组织损伤，包括脑挫伤、弥漫性轴突损伤、硬膜外或硬膜下腔出血、脑实质内出血。**继发性损伤**是指在最初损伤后大脑出现的其他任何损害，导致进一步的神经元损伤。虽然脑缺血或缺氧是TBI后继发性脑损伤的最终原因，但全身性或局部性损伤，如颅内压（intracranial pressure，ICP）升高、全身性低血压和低氧血症等也常导致继发性损伤。

神经元死亡可能是由复杂的生化过程介导的，包括兴奋性氨基酸（如谷氨酸）的释放和细胞钙的内流。实际的细胞死亡本质可能是细胞坏死或凋亡。预防或减少继发性脑损伤是多数医疗管理策略的重点，无论是在手术室还是随后的重症监护病房

表58.1 格拉斯哥昏迷量表评分

睁眼		语言反应		运动反应	
自动睁眼	4	回答正确	5	能执行简单命令	6
呼唤睁眼	3.	言语错乱	4	对疼痛刺激能定位	5
疼痛刺激睁眼	2	用词不当	3.	对疼痛刺激能回缩	4
无反应	1	言语难以理解	2	疼痛刺激时肢体出现异常屈曲	3.
		无反应	1	疼痛刺激时异常伸展	2
				无反应	1

（ICU）都是如此。

TBI 通常与其他伤害有关（如病例概要所示）。因此，麻醉科医师可能需要参与患者最初的复苏，TBI 的外科干预（如硬膜下血肿的清除、去骨瓣减压术）和（或）剖腹探查术或伴随的骨折固定术，以及随后在 ICU 的处理。

识别

原发性颅脑损伤

意识、记忆、精神状态和（或）神经功能的改变与头部创伤相关时，临床医师会怀疑患者出现 TBI。TBI 的严重程度通常由 GCS 来评估，GCS 是对患者的最佳运动、语言和睁眼能力进行评分（表 58.1）。总分为 8 或更低提示严重的 TBI。使用 GCS 评估 TBI 患者减少了观察者间的变异性，并可以通过一系列检查来评估疾病的治疗效果或进展。然而，之前研究显示严重 TBI 具有异质性，不同致病机制的 TBI 表现出相同的 GCS 评分。此外，使用 GCS 作为预后指标尚有争议，GCS 评分仅适用于充分的心肺复苏后的患者，特别是伴有严重低血压或缺氧时。

除 GCS 外，还应检查瞳孔大小、对称性和对光反应。急性单侧血肿，同侧瞳孔扩张且无反应，提示小脑幕突出。相反，双侧瞳孔固定且散大提示严重的颅内高压，可能导致脑疝。

除了 TBI 外，生命体征也可以反映患者的整体临床状况。例如，低血压和心动过速可能是由于严重骨折隐匿性出血所致，高血压可能是由疼痛所致。生命体征的变化也可能反映 TBI 的性质。严重高血压可能是一种代偿现象，即在 ICP 升高时维持脑灌注压（cerebral perfusion pressure，CPP），CPP 是平均动脉压（mean arterial pressure，MAP）减去 ICP。严重的系统性高血压伴心动过缓是一种不祥之兆（库欣反射）。这预示着即将发生脑疝，需要立即进行治疗干预。

计算机断层扫描结果

颅脑计算机断层扫描（CT）对颅内出血和急性肿块的检测灵敏度很高。CT 结果提示 ICP 显著升高的诊断包括：

- 病灶大于 25 ml；
- 中线偏移 5 mm 或更大；
- 基底池或侧脑室受压；
- 钩状回的内侧移位。

继发性脑损伤

继发性脑损伤可由全身或大脑因素引起（表 58.2）。其中，低氧和低血压最有可能对 TBI 结局产生不利影响。但是原发性 TBI 的神经系统和全身表现可能掩盖了由脑缺氧或缺血引起的继发性损伤的表现。头颅 CT 异常时计算 CPP（需要有创动脉监测和 ICP 监测）有一定的作用，但是即使是正常的 CPP 也不能排除继发性缺血或脑缺氧的发生。

技术的进步使临床医生能够更好地洞察脑损伤及其功能变化。

脑灌注和氧合监测仪

颅内压监测仪

脑实质光纤探头或脑室内导管都可用于监测颅内压。通过连续动脉内压力监测，专业监护仪可连续显示 CPP（CPP=MAP-ICP），以此临床医师能对 CPP 进行优化管理。虽然最近的文献表明基于影像学结果、仔细的临床管理可以获得与基于 ICP 监测指导的临床管理的预后相似，但目前 ICP 监测仍然是 TBI 患者管理的基石，仍被认为是临床决策的金标准，根据 ICP 结果能够即时做出明断的临床决策。

颈静脉氧合监测

颈静脉球测氧导管（jugular venous bulb oximetric catheter, JBC）连续测量脑静脉血氧饱和度（$SjvO_2$）。脑灌注不足会增加氧摄取量，导致 $SjvO_2$ 降低，而无功能的脑组织摄取的氧却很少，导致 $SjvO_2$ 值过高（过度灌注）。因此，$SjvO_2$ 低于 55% 或大于 75% 与不良预后有关。$SjvO_2$ 导管特别适用于监测脑代

表 58.2　继发性脑损伤的风险因素

大脑因素	全身因素
颅内压增加	低血压
• 病灶体积扩大	低氧血症
• 高碳酸血症	贫血
• 低氧血症	低血容量
• 静脉受阻（颈托、体位不佳）	高血糖
• 全身低血压（代偿性脑扩张）	低钠血症
过度通气	低渗透压状态
创伤后血管痉挛（创伤性蛛网膜下腔出血）	凝血功能障碍
癫痫发作	发热

谢率（cerebral metabolic rate，CMR），特别是在采用控制性过度通气干预以减少全脑血流量（cerebral blood flow，CBF）从而降低ICP时。如果JBC乳酸浓度高于同时测得的动脉乳酸浓度，也可能显示无氧代谢增加。JBC的一个局限性是它只监测全脑CBF-CMR的平衡。小的区域缺血或梗死，$SjvO_2$值可为正常。所以临床医师对于JBC监测的最初热度很高，但后来该监测在许多临床情况下被脑组织氧分压测量所取代。

脑组织氧分压

脑组织氧分压（brain tissue oxygen tension，$PbrO_2$）传感器能对脑实质氧分压行连续测量。它能反映局部脑组织氧供和需求之间的平衡。正常$PbrO_2$在23～35 mmHg。低于20 mmHg的$PbrO_2$值代表脑组织氧合受损，也是应考虑予以干预的阈值。BOOST Ⅱ试验表明，在现有ICP/CPP指导的管理中增加$PbrO_2$监测，可显著缩短脑缺氧的持续时间和严重程度，同时死亡率降低10%，并且6个月的死亡率呈下降趋势，神经预后也有所改善。这是一种有创监测，要使其发挥最佳功能，就必须将其置于缺血风险最高的脑组织中，也就是缺血半暗带，但是这是一项很难完成的挑战。一种替代的做法是将它放置在额叶，与ICP监测仪结合使用。

近红外光谱

近红外光谱以反射光谱为基础，它测量从大脑中血红蛋白反射出来的光，从而得出区域的氧饱和度。它提供了关于血流灌注和代谢之间平衡的信息。一般认为，其正常范围在60%～75%之间，变异系数为10%左右。光反射的颅外污染是一种潜在的伪差来源。

经颅多普勒超声

经颅多普勒超声（transcranial Doppler ultrasonography，TCD）可评估脑血管阻力，显示颅内压升高时搏动增加，并可作为颅内循环抑制的确认性检查。最近的研究表明，用TCD连续监测血流速度，可以确定大脑自动调节功能最强的血压范围，从而实现最佳的血压管理。

微透析

微透析导管放置在脑实质中，用灌流液持续灌注大脑，取样少量液体（透析液），检测乳酸、丙酮酸、谷氨酸、葡萄糖和甘油的浓度。乳酸与丙酮酸的比值大于40表明脑供氧不足，葡萄糖供应不足，或潜在的神经元线粒体功能障碍。然而，采集和分析样品至少需要1 h的时间间隔，这一时间差妨碍了临床决策的实时性。目前，它本质上仍然是一种研究工具。

风险评估和启示

低氧血症和高碳酸血症

TBI患者发生气道梗阻和通气不足的风险增加。这些会导致低氧血症和高碳酸血症，从而引起脑血管扩张。后者可加重ICP的升高。

颅内压升高

急性占位性病灶会增加ICP，降低CPP。ICP增高可导致脑疝，造成灾难性后果。

全身性低血压和低血容量

成年人通常不会单独因为TBI失血而变得低血容量和低血压。相反，小儿在TBI时会失血过多，从而导致血压下降。其他损伤（如脾破裂、大的骨折）可使TBI患者血压降低，ICP增高的患者CPP进一步降低。代偿性高血压和心动过缓（库欣反射）伴ICP升高可使临床表现进一步复杂化。因此，在TBI患者中，正常血压和心动过速仍可与严重低容量同时存在，而后者可因体循环阻力增加（库欣反射）而表现得并不明显。而这种看似血压“正常”往往会误导医务人员产生已充分复苏的安全感。如果去骨瓣或血肿清除后ICP下降，则可能突然发生严重低血压或心脏停搏。

在所有与继发性脑损伤相关的因素中，全身低血压可能是危害最大的。在大脑自我调节受损的情况下，低血压必然导致CPP降低。即使大脑自我调节完整，但颅内顺应性降低，在低血压时患者CPP也有下降的风险。MAP的降低会间接扩张脑血管，维持脑血流，这会导致脑血流量和ICP增加。而ICP的增加进一步损害了CPP，导致代偿性脑血管进一步扩张。这种恶性循环被称为血管扩张剂级联反应（图58.1）

大脑自动调节受损

大脑的自动调节是一种稳态机制，它在较宽范围的MAP上维持大脑的几乎恒定的灌注。在正常成

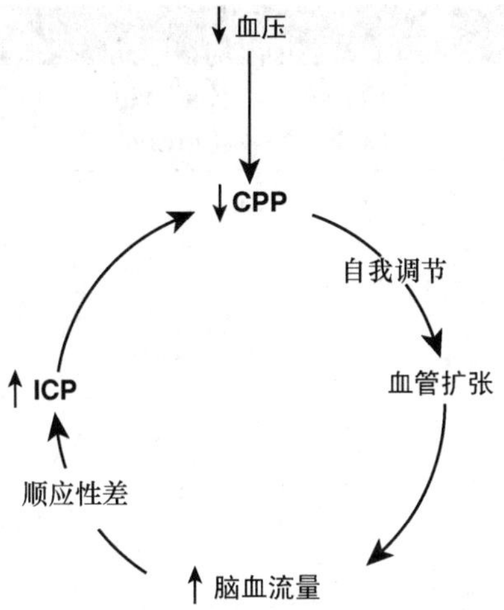

图 58.1 当自动调节完整时，血管扩张剂级联显示全身低血压与颅内血流动力学之间的潜在相互作用。当血压升高时，也会发生相反方向的级联。CPP，脑灌注压；ICP，颅内压

人中，这一范围为 60～160 mmHg。在 TBI 患者中，自动调节功能可能受损，虽然严重 TBI 患者的自动调节功能受损的频率较高，但临床上无法预测哪些患者会受到影响。即使是轻微的 TBI 也可能损害自动调节。如果是这样，CBF 与血压直接成正比。在严重 TBI 中，大脑自动调节功能的丧失与更差的结局相关。

凝血障碍

严重的 TBI 时受损的神经元会释放相当多的凝血活酶，从而导致凝血障碍，其程度可以从轻微到严重不等。凝血障碍可以增加手术的病残率和死亡率，也可使颅外手术取消或推迟，从而导致预后较差。

发热

发热会增加 CMR，增加缺血和神经损伤的风险，特别是当脑灌注处于边缘状态时。脑血容量随着体温的增加而增加，这是由于血流灌注与代谢偶联，这会加剧 ICP 升高。虽然人体研究并不能确定体温与 TBI 预后的关系，但动物和人类的研究都显示 TBI 脑梗死范围与发热有关。

高血糖

虽然尚无明确的因果关系，但 TBI 和卒中时的高血糖与不良预后有关。在动物实验脑缺血模型中，已证实高血糖的有害性。此外，一项前瞻性试验结果显示宽松血糖控制的危重病患者的预后比血糖严格控制的患者差。然而，严格血糖控制的患者易发生同样有害的严重低血糖。

液体和电解质异常

TBI 患者出现急性液体和电解质紊乱往往是由于液体管理不当。这也可能是由尿崩症引起的。低钠血症和过量的游离水会加重脑水肿，从而增加 ICP。容量治疗应使用等渗液，避免使用包括白蛋白在内的胶体。输血阈值仍有争议，但一般采用限制性输血的方法（表 58.3）。

合并颅外损伤

高达 10% 的 TBI 患者伴有脊柱损伤，如果患者需要紧急的神经外科治疗（如硬膜外或硬膜下血肿清除），脊柱评估往往会延迟。因此，在脊柱损伤评估完成前搬动患者应始终保护脊柱。TBI 患者还可能伴有未确诊的肢体和实质性器官损伤。

管理

有关一般管理目标的列表，请参阅框 58.1 的内容。

气道与通气

对于严重颅脑损伤的患者，尤其是 GCS 评分在 8 分或更低的患者，必须立即进行气管插管。建立明确的气道可以防止胃内容物的误吸，控制呼气末二氧化碳，并有助于患者的治疗和转运。

低氧血症（PaO_2<60 mm Hg）和高氧血症（PaO_2>300 mm Hg）均产生有害影响，应将 PaO_2 目标值时刻控制在正常范围。中度过度通气治疗（$PaCO_2$ 30～35 mmHg）仅作为一种暂时性的、挽救生命的干预措施，用于即将发生的脑疝，以等待确定性治疗，或利于实施神经外科手术。在其他情况下，$PaCO_2$ 的理想目标范围应为 35～45 mmHg。

麻醉药物

血流动力学的稳定性尤为重要，因此，需要合理地使用麻醉诱导药物。在颅脑损伤患者中，通常很少使用全诱导剂量。只要仔细滴定药物，并注意患者的反应，丙泊酚和依托咪酯都可以安全使用。两药均能降低 CBF 和 $CMRO_2$，降低 ICP。然而，依托咪酯在合并多处创伤的 TBI 患者中低血压不良风险较低。氯胺酮是有用的替代药物，其在控制通气环境下以及与其他镇静剂联合使用的安全性已经确定，因为研究未显示 ICP 有任何增加。应使用短

表 58.3 静脉输液

液体	渗透压（mOsm/kg）	胶体渗透压（mmHg）	Na^+（mEq/L）	Cl^-（mEq/L）	K^+（mEq/L）	Ca^{2+}/Mg^{2+}（mEq/L）	葡萄糖（g/L）
血浆	289	21	141	103	4～5	5/2	
晶体							
0.9% NS	308	0	154	154			
0.45% S	154	0	77	77			
3% HTS	1027	0	515	515			
7.5% HTS	2400	0	1200	1200			
23.4% HTS	8008						
LR	273	0	130	109	4	3/0	
D_5LR	527	0	130	109	4	3/0	50
D_5W[a]	252	0					50
D_5 NS[a]	586	0	154	154			50
$D_5$0.45% S[a]	406	0	77	77			50
Normosol/ 勃脉力	295	0	140	98	5	0/3	
甘露醇（20%）	1098	0					
胶体							
羟乙基淀粉（6%）	310	31	154	154			
白蛋白（5%）	290	19					
人血浆蛋白粉	270～300	?	145	100	0.25		

[a] 葡萄糖溶液的渗透压随着葡萄糖进入细胞而降低

D_5W，5% 葡萄糖；HTS，高渗盐水；LR，乳酸林格氏；NS，生理盐水；S，盐水

框 58.1 一般管理目标列表

- pH 7.35～7.45
- PaO_2 100～300
- $PaCO_2$ 35～40 mmHg
- 体温 36～37.5℃
- 收缩压 100～180 mmHg
- 颅内压 <20 mm Hg
- 脑灌注压 60～70 mmHg
- 脑静脉血氧饱和度 50～75 mmHg
- 局部脑组织氧分压≥ 20 mmHg
- 葡萄糖 120～180 mm Hg
- 血红蛋白 >7 g/dl
- 血小板≥ $75 \times 10^3/mm^3$
- 国际标准化比值≤ 1.4
- 钠 135～145 mmol/L

效肌肉松弛剂。琥珀胆碱是首选，琥珀胆碱禁忌时可使用罗库溴铵。

在 TBI 患者维持麻醉药物和技术方面有许多选择。如果挥发性麻醉剂的浓度保持在 1 个最低肺泡有效浓度（minimum alveolar concentration，MAC）以下，阿片类药物和挥发性麻醉剂是合适的组合。较高的浓度可能导致脑血管扩张，或"过度灌注"。全凭静脉麻醉是首选的麻醉方法，但丙泊酚是一种有效的间接脑血管收缩剂，可能需要血管加压药来维持血压。硫喷妥钠同样有效，但北美洲已不再有此药可用。最好避免使用氧化亚氮，因为它可以增加 CMR 和加重缺血，且它可能会加剧现有的颅内积气。值得注意的是，迄今为止麻醉诱导药物的神经保护作用还未在人体研究中证实。

维持足够的大脑灌注压

最新《脑创伤基金会指南》（Brain Trauma Foundation guidelines，2007）建议 CPP 维持在 50～60 mmHg 之间。为了维持 CPP，必须有良好的静脉通路，并且必要时必须补充血管内容量来进行液体复苏。不

应因为顾虑脑水肿加重而不进行足够的液体复苏。理想的液体复苏应以目标为导向，并密切关注 TBI 后第一个 96 h 内的液体平衡。

升压药和正性肌力药物常与液体复苏一起以维持 CPP。然而，需小心使用这些药物，因为他们可能会增加急性呼吸衰竭的风险。应监测血压和避免低血压（收缩压 <90 mmHg）。

缺血可能是继发性颅脑损伤的最终通路。尽管输血阈值尚有争议，理想的血细胞比容应在 21% ～ 25% 之间，以提供足够的氧供。如果急性硬膜下或硬膜外血肿的患者出现了库欣反应，手术减压可能会导致血压的急剧降低。该现象可根据临床结果来预测（如低 GCS 评分、CT 中线的明显移位、异常瞳孔大小），并且必须预先进行液体复苏。手术减压后，立即静脉输液和使用血管升压药或正心肌力药治疗低血压至关重要。

降低颅内压

颅内高压的定义是 ICP 持续高于 20 mmHg（>5 min）。为了优化 CPP，ICP 应低于 20 mmHg 来维持 CPP 处于 50 ～ 60 mmHg 之间。ICP 监测指征为复苏后昏迷的严重 TBI 患者（GCS 评分 <9）伴有颅脑 CT 异常或是符合下述三个标准中两个：年龄 >40 岁；收缩压 <90 mmHg；异常姿势。最近一项国际多学科共识会议建议那些基于临床和（或）影像学判断的 ICP 升高患者，应监测 ICP 和 CPP，以指导临床和手术干预措施。

甘露醇（0.25 ～ 1 g/kg）可有效减少脑组织体积和降低脑脊液量，两者共同导致 ICP 降低。在补充液体容量后给予甘露醇。相较于甘露醇来说，高渗性盐水（hypertonic saline，HTS）（3% 或 7.5%）反弹性水肿更少发生，效果更持久，全身副作用更少。但是最近的 meta 分析并未表明高渗性盐水可减少死亡率或者改善 ICP。

急性过度通气使大脑血容量减少，动脉二氧化碳分压每降低 1 mmHg，CBF 降低约 3%。大量的过度通气可能会发生脑缺血。动脉二氧化碳分压不应低于 30 mmHg，短时间内除外（如脑疝即将形成时）。相反，ICP 低于 20 mmHg 时，血二氧化碳分压应维持正常或轻度低二氧化碳血症（35 ～ 40 mmHg）。其他降低 ICP 的重要手段是轻度抬头和保持颈部中立位，以促进静脉回流和阻止静脉阻塞这个常被忽略的 ICP 升高原因。很多 TBI 患者戴有颈托，检查颈托以保证其并未阻止静脉回流；颈托太紧能够增加 ICP。同时要避免使用系绳固定气管导管。对于药物治疗反应差的 ICP 增高患者，可进行开颅减压术。

巴比妥类或丙泊酚抑制 CMR 可降低 ICP。出现爆发抑制或等电位脑电图时这些药物效果最佳。CMR 最大抑制时需要血管加压药来维持血压。TBI 患者常输注低剂量丙泊酚，因为这能够有效控制 ICP，并在需要时能够快速进行神经评估。然而，长期丙泊酚输注后可发生以心力衰竭和乳酸性酸中毒为特征的代谢综合征，尤其是儿童患者。

如果脑室尚未被压缩到无法置入导管的话，可进行侧脑室引流脑脊液来降低 ICP。腰穿置管引流也有成功的案例，但是该技术尚存在脑干疝的固有风险，所以并不提倡。

作为神经保护技术和 ICP 升高的治疗方法，轻至中度低体温（33℃）已被广泛研究。尽管其是否有神经保护的积极效果尚不可知，但其降颅压的作用是确定无疑的。为了有效降颅压，复温阶段必须积极治疗寒战和严密监测 ICP。

对药物治疗反应差的 ICP 升高患者需考虑开颅减压术（decompressive craniectomy，DC）。开颅减压术既是基本治疗措施（颅内血肿清除期间去骨瓣），也可是后续治疗措施（因 ICP 持续升高而去骨瓣减压）。该措施尚存争议，因为延长生存期需要以患者严重残疾和生活质量下降为代价。无论开颅减压术作为基本治疗措施还是后续治疗措施，目前都是当前临床试验的研究内容。

纠正凝血障碍和贫血治疗

创伤急性凝血病和 TBI 相关凝血病为已得到公认的临床现象，可导致显著的凝血功能衰竭。消耗性凝血功能障碍和内源性纤维蛋白溶解在创伤的急性凝血功能障碍进展中发挥着关键作用。TBI 患者会释放大量凝血活酶到血中，引起凝血过程紊乱。另外，大脑内皮细胞损伤激活血小板以及凝血级联反应，导致血管内血栓形成并消耗凝血因子。

凝血因子缺乏增加 TBI 患者手术相关的病残率。必须密切关注凝血功能，任何凝血因子的缺乏都必须积极补充。仅基于临床观察试验结果，一些外科医师主张早期补充血小板和凝血因子。

最近基于两项氨甲环酸（tranexamic acid，TXA）试验的meta分析表明TXA改善对颅内血肿的进展有统计学差异，但对预后的改善并无统计学差异。一项国际多中心3期临床试验（CRASH-3）正在进行中，以评估TXA对10 000名TBI患者的死亡和致残的影响。

贫血在TBI急性期很常见，50%的患者可出现贫血。目前可用的证据支持目标血红蛋白阈值水平为7～9 g/dl。TBI患者目标导向血红蛋白大于10 g/dl并不能改善神经功能的预后，但与血栓事件和严重出血损伤风险增加相关。

治疗高血糖

液体复苏时应避免使用含糖溶液，否则可能会引起高血糖，加重脑缺血损伤。目前的指南建议血糖保持在120～180 mg/dl。全麻患者需要经常评估血糖水平。

恢复正常体温

高温对缺血性脑损伤高风险患者无疑是有害的。低体温的有益影响似乎仍不明确。TBI的多项临床试验表明，低温尽管有可能改善ICP，在标准治疗的同时加用低温治疗受益甚少，据报道患者功能恢复较差。如前所述，当与其他降低ICP的技术（如DC、甘露醇、丙泊酚、巴比妥酸盐镇静）联合使用时，低温仍可提高药物治疗的效果。疗效可能会根据具体患者群体、损伤严重程度和损伤特征（局灶性或弥漫性）而异。体温过低可能会导致凝血功能紊乱，对已经有凝血功能紊乱风险的患者不应选择低温治疗。体温过低也会增加感染的风险，患者体温小于35℃可能造成$PbrO_2$血红蛋白氧解离曲线左移。考虑一些引起体温过低的不确定因素，除非用于控制ICP的升高，我们建议保持体温在略低于正常的温度范围（35～36℃）。

延迟非紧急的治疗操作以及TBI的全身影响

一般来说，对于严重创伤性脑损伤和ICP不稳定的患者，实施非神经外科手术的益处必须与大脑进一步损伤的风险相权衡。对于不稳定的TBI患者应延迟非紧急治疗。这些患者应该进入ICU，并进行复苏治疗，恢复凝血指标，控制ICP。重要的是，即使在没有直接颅外损伤的情况下，超过80%的严重TBI患者可能会出现严重的器官功能障碍，包括心血管、呼吸系统、免疫系统、血液系统和内分泌系统障碍等。全身性并发症影响早期治疗，且与预后差独立相关。

当病情危重患者的生理从初始创伤恢复后，此类患者可以使用外固定支架行损伤控制手术，以减轻对机体的进一步损伤。

病例概述中的管理

若有指征，应迅速评估患者的容量状态，并开始复苏。严重骨盆骨折可导致突然出血，应及时排查。可立即行介入放射学治疗实施血管内闭塞术。建立有创动脉血压监测，选择性放置中心静脉导管，但置管不应延误手术过程。应备好血液以随时输注。使用丙泊酚和阿片类药物实施全凭静脉麻醉是一种合理的麻醉方案。减压后可能发生低血压，手术和麻醉团队之间的良好沟通非常重要。应监测凝血功能，出现任何异常时应立即予以纠正。维持正常到轻度低的体温。应监测血糖，并根据需要进行治疗。如需要行损伤控制手术，术后最好直接将患者从手术室运送到神经外科危重监护病房进行下一步治疗。最后，ICP监测导管可放置或不放置，取决于脑部情况和是否行DC来决定。

（石亚平 译 李 博 校）

延伸阅读

Andrews PJD, Sinclair HL, Rodriguez A, et al.: Hypothermia for intracranial hypertension after traumatic brain injury, *N Engl J Med* 373(25):2403–2412, 2015.

Berger-Pelleiter E, Émond M, Lauzier F, et al.: Hypertonic saline in severe traumatic brain injury: a systematic review and meta-analysis of randomized controlled trials, *CJEM* 18(2):112–120, 2016.

Brain Trauma Foundation: American Association of Neurological Surgeons, Congress of Neurological Surgeons: guidelines for the management of severe traumatic brain injury, *J Neurotrauma* 24(Suppl 1):S1–S106, 2007.

Centers for Disease Control and Prevention: *Report to congress on traumatic brain injury in the United States: epidemiology and rehabilitation*, Atlanta, GA, 2015, National Center for Injury Prevention and Control, Division of Unintentional Injury Prevention.

Chesnut RM, Temkin N, Carney N, et al.: A trial of intracranial-pressure monitoring in traumatic brain injury, *N Engl J Med* 367(26):2471–2481, 2012.

Clifton GL, Miller ER, Choi SC, et al.: Lack of effect of induction of hypothermia after acute brain injury, *N Engl J Med* 344:556–563, 2001.

Coles JP, Fryer TD, Smielewski P, et al.: Incidence and mechanisms of cerebral ischemia in early clinical head injury, *J Cereb Blood Flow Metab* 24:202–211, 2004.

Coronado VG, Xu L, Basavaraju SV, et al.: *Surveillance for traumatic brain injury: related deaths—United States, 1997–2007*, Atlanta, GA, 2011, Centers for Disease Control and Prevention. Available at http://www.cdc.gov/mmwr/preview/mmwrhtml/ss6005a1.htm. Accessed November 1, 2016.

Dagal A, Lam AM: Head trauma: anaesthetic considerations and management. In Smith CE, editor: *Trauma anesthesia*, ed 2, Cambridge, 2015, Cambridge University Press, pp 364–381.

Dietrich WD, Bramlett HM: Therapeutic hypothermia and targeted temperature management in traumatic brain injury: clinical challenges for successful translation, *Brain Res* 1640(Pt A):94–103, 2016.

Faul M, Xu L, Wald MM, Coronado VG: *Traumatic brain injury in the United States: emergency department visits, hospitalizations, and deaths, 2002–2006*, Atlanta, GA, 2010, Centers for Disease Control and Prevention, National Center for Injury Prevention and Control. Available at http://www.cdc.gov/traumaticbraininjury/pdf/blue_book.pdf. Accessed Nov 1, 2016.

Gantner D, Moore EM, Cooper DJ: Intravenous fluids in traumatic brain injury, *Curr Opin Crit Care* 20(4):385–389, 2014.

Hlatky R, Furuya Y, Valadka AB, et al.: Dynamic autoregulatory response after severe head injury, *J Neurosurg* 97:1054–1061, 2002.

Junger EC, Newell DW, Grant GA, et al.: Cerebral autoregulation following minor head injury, *J Neurosurg* 86:425–432, 1997.

Kawaguchi M, Sakamoto T, Ohnishi H, et al.: Preoperative predictors of reduction in arterial blood pressure following dural opening during surgical evacuation of acute subdural hematoma, *J Neurosurg Anesth* 8:117–122, 1996.

Kolias AG, Adams H, Timofeev I, et al.: Decompressive craniectomy following traumatic brain injury: developing the evidence base, *Br J Neurosurg* 30(2):246–250, 2016.

Lam AM, Mayberg TS: Anesthetic management of patients with traumatic head injury. In Lam AM, editor: *Anesthetic management of acute head injury*, New York, 1995, McGraw-Hill, pp 181–221.

Lam AM, Winn HR, Cullen BF, et al.: Hyperglycemia and neurological outcome in patients with head injury, *J Neurosurg* 75:545–551, 1991.

Le Roux P, Menon DK, Citerio G, et al.: Consensus summary statement of the International Multidisciplinary Consensus Conference on Multimodality Monitoring in Neurocritical Care: a statement for healthcare professionals from the Neurocritical Care Society and the European Society of Intensive Care Medicine, *Intensive Care Med* 40(9):1189–1209, 2014.

Makarenko S, Griesdale DE, Gooderham P, et al.: Multimodal neuromonitoring for traumatic brain injury: a shift towards individualized therapy, *J Clin Neurosci* 26:8–13, 2016.

Marion DW, Puccio A, Wisniewski SR, et al.: Effect of hyperventilation on extracellular concentrations of glutamate, lactate, pyruvate, and local cerebral blood flow in patients with severe traumatic brain injury, *Crit Care Med* 30:2619–2625, 2002.

Quintard H, Patet C, Suys T, et al.: Normobaric hyperoxia is associated with increased cerebral excitotoxicity after severe traumatic brain injury, *Neurocrit Care* 22:243–250, 2014.

Rincon F, Kang J, Vibbert M, et al.: Significance of arterial hyperoxia and relationship with case fatality in traumatic brain injury: a multicentre cohort study, *J Neurol Neurosurg Psychiatry* 85:799–805, 2014.

Robertson CS, Hannay HJ, Yamal J-M, et al.: Effect of erythropoietin and transfusion threshold on neurological recovery after traumatic brain injury: a randomized clinical trial, *JAMA* 312(1):36–47, 2014.

Rosner MJ, Rosner SD, Johnson AH: Cerebral perfusion pressure: management protocol and clinical results, *J Neurosurg* 83:949–962, 1995.

Valadka AB, Hlatky R, Furuya Y, et al.: Brain tissue Po_2: correlation with cerebral blood flow, *Acta Neurochir Suppl* 81:299–301, 2002.

van den Berghe G, Wouters P, Weekers F, et al.: Intensive insulin therapy in the critically ill patient, *N Engl J Med* 345:1359–1367, 2001.

Vedantam A, Yamal J-M, Rubin ML, et al.: Progressive hemorrhagic injury after severe traumatic brain injury: effect of hemoglobin transfusion thresholds, *J Neurosurg* 125(5):1229–1234, 2016.

Wijayatilake DS, Sherren PB, Jigajinni SV: Systemic complications of traumatic brain injury, *Curr Opin Anaesthesiol* 28(5):525–531, 2015.

Zehtabchi S, Abdel Baki SG, Falzon L, et al.: Tranexamic acid for traumatic brain injury: a systematic review and meta-analysis, *Am J Emerg Med* 32(12):1503–1509, 2014.

第59章 血液稀释和血液保护

Bryan S. Ahlgren，Glenn P. Gravlee

病例概要

患者，男性，61岁，体重80 kg，拟行髋关节置换术，患者担心输血和传染病的传播，特别是人类免疫缺陷病毒（human immunodefciency virus，HIV），要求尽可能避免输注异体血。患者预捐了2个单位的自体血。术中出血量在2000 ml以上，在给予两个单位的自体血以后，血红蛋白水平7.5 g/dl，生命体征和尿量保持在正常范围内，预计术中还会有500 ml的失血。

问题分析

定义、识别和风险评估

自现代输血治疗开始以来，输注同源（又称异体）血液制品的并发症已得到公认。在引进冷藏和无菌塑料袋之前，细菌污染是相当普遍的。随后，病毒（如巨细胞病毒、乙型和丙型肝炎病毒、HIV和人类嗜T淋巴细胞病毒）的污染发病率越来越高。现在，西尼罗病毒和可能变异的克一雅病（Creutzfeldt-Jakob）已被列入了输血可能传播的病毒疾病的名单。幸运的是，在献血者筛查和血液成分检测方面的改进已将HIV和丙型肝炎传播的风险降低到1/100万以下，而乙型肝炎的传播风险则降到1/13.7万。巨细胞病毒在血液中仍然普遍存在，在使用临床免疫抑制剂的情况下，其传播更为普遍。然而，现在所有的血库在发放细胞血液成分之前，都会例行地对其进行减白处理，这大大减少了巨细胞病毒的传播风险。因此通过输血传播病毒是少之又少，细菌污染再次成为了风险最高的感染性并发症，约1/3万单位红细胞（red blood cell，RBC），1/（2000～3000）单位血小板，尽管实际临床感染率远低于这个数字（大约1/500万单位RBC和1/10万单位血小板）。血型不相容和过敏反应仍然很少见。

启示

相当多的证据支持输血可导致免疫抑制的严重后果，这增加了癌症复发的风险和受血者中细菌感染的风险。

大量失血和血液稀释也提出了一个问题，即在麻醉患者中，要使其血管内容量和生命体征在接受的范围内，合理的最低血红蛋白水平是多少？这是一个令人惊讶的复杂问题，但总的来说，健康的患者能够安全地耐受6 g/dl的血红蛋白水平。病情较重的患者可能需要10 g/dl的血红蛋白。

假设在病例概要中所描述的患者在其他方面是健康的，那么限制因素可能是失血速度和可预见性，因为如果突然发生额外的失血，需要有一定的安全边际。此外，必须考虑术后大量出血的可能性。因此，患者的血红蛋白浓度为7.5 g/dl，表明可能需要进行相应的输血，除非失血已得到有效控制。

管理

本节重点介绍可用的技术（表59.1）和可能减少或避免使用同源红细胞或血液成分治疗的自体输血技术的成分效益分析。

自体预输血

患者可在手术前42天内献血，这是现代抗凝剂和储存液的最大储存期。献血的频率和量取决于患者在维持足够的血红蛋白水平的同时，是否能够耐受连续的献血。一般情况下，患者在手术前2～4周

表 59.1 自体输血技术			
技术	成本	风险	可行性[a]
自体预输血	适度	低	有
急性等容性血液稀释	低	低	没有
术中回收	高	低	有
术后回收，未清洗	低	中	没有
术后回收，清洗	适度	低	有

[a] 针对病例概述中的患者

每周献血 2 个单位。捐赠的最低推荐血红蛋白水平为 11 g/dl。为了维持这一水平，患者需常规补充铁剂。促红细胞生成素可用于提高献血前血红蛋白水平，使患者捐献更多的单位。然而，每单位促红细胞生成素花费大约 800 美元是昂贵的。如果存在以下因素的组合，促红细胞生成素增加自体捐献前的作用可能是合理的：

- 术前准备时间较短（如肿瘤切除）；
- 不可能输注异体血（例如耶和华见证人）；
- 患者贫血；
- 预期手术失血量大（大于 2000 ml）。

自体预输血与其他自体输血技术（如术中采血）联合使用时，是避免同种输血最有效的方法。自体捐赠的成本效益差异很大，但往往达不到通常的疗效标准。由于这个原因，它的流行程度已经减弱。自体输血本身的住院风险约为 1/1.7 万，是社区健康人士献血的 12 倍。尽管血液是自体的，但是它的使用仍然会带来一些常见的同源输血风险，包括细菌污染或笔误导致输注血型不一致。与同种异体血液单位相比，自体血液单位通常需要相同的检测程序，但储存和鉴定程序就更为复杂，因此自体血成本较高。

急性等容性血液稀释

急性等容性血液稀释（acute normovolemic hemodilution，ANH）是指在麻醉诱导前或诱导后将血液取出，同时使用晶体或胶体进行等容置换。这项技术需要标准的麻醉检测仪（心电图、血压、脉搏血氧仪和体温），以及使用 14 或 16 号外周或中心静脉进行大口径静脉穿刺。将血液收集到标准枸橼酸盐-磷酸盐-葡萄糖贮血袋中。收集的血液可以安全地在室温下储存长达 8 小时，如果不输注则可以冻存。为确保血小板功能，室温下储存的全血应恒定搅拌（置于振荡器上）。

ANH 的基本原理是由于血液稀释，患者在手术中丢失的红细胞会更少。假设最低血容量仍可接受（大于 20%），且血管内容量也保持不变，则组织灌注将得到维持（或增强）。此外，由于血液黏度降低，氧供将足够。其他的临床优势包括低成本，储存简单，运输和记录保存的便利性。

如果容量替换不充分，急性等容血液稀释可能会导致血容量不足。此外，如果存在未确诊的病症，例如冠状动脉或颈动脉的严重狭窄，则血红蛋白浓度的强制性下降可能诱发未预计的终末器官缺血。统计分析强烈提示，除非采用相当极端的技术，如，血细胞比容从初始的 40% 血液稀释到 20% 或更低，否则减少失血的作用很小。通常，这相当于需要取出 6 ～ 10 袋 500 ml 的血袋。研究发现，在全髋关节置换术患者中，3 个单位的急性等容性血液稀释与等量的自体献血相比，同种异体输血量无差异。

术后血液回收

这项技术包括术后的血液回收和再输注。血液通过一个相对较大的过滤器收集，然后通过一个小孔过滤器重新注入。这种血液可以不经处理重新注入（“未清洗”），也可以与术中血液回收相同的方式清洗和浓缩。

再输注血液凝血因子和血小板含量很低，但纤维蛋白降解产物、游离血红蛋白和细胞因子等炎症产物的水平升高。在全髋关节置换术中，可能含有脂肪和骨针。因此许多临床医师只有处理过后才选择给患者输注回收血液。这种有争议的技术仅在术后失血量大（例如 >1000 ml）时才减少对同种异体血的需要，因为术后出血的血细胞比容通常在 15% ～ 20%。

术中自体血液回收

该方法是使用吸引器收集术野范围内的出血。血液中加入抗凝剂，然后被储存在一个滤过的容器中，一旦收集到足够的血液（通常大于 700 ml），就会进行清洗和浓缩处理，这样最终产品的红细胞比容通常在 55% ～ 70%。

由于术中回收自体血只保留了红细胞而不保留血浆和血小板，因此如果失血量接近或超过患者全身血容量，应预见到患者可能发生稀释性凝血障碍。如果遵循适当的程序和标准，并且血液没有被细菌污染，这种技术的风险很低。使用这种技术保存红细胞的能力在很大程度上取决于外科医师通过吸引器收集失血的能力。在这方面，全髋关节置换术是介于开腹手术和主动脉瘤修复手术之间的一个中间类别，其体腔中的血液容易被收集，更简单的手术，例如乳房缩小整形术，失血容易从术野流出到洞巾或被纱布吸收。

预防

通常，临床医师没有意识到患者在输血前能安全承受多少失血。这可以用下面的公式来估计：

$$ABL=V\times(H_i-H_d)/H_m$$

其中 ABL 是允许失血量，H_i 和 H_d 分别是初始和允许的血细胞比容；H_m 是 H_i 和 H_d 的平均值。假设血容量为 5600 ml×（80 kg×70 ml/kg），H_i 为 40%，H_d 为 25%，那么病例概要中的患者可以承受的失血量接近 2600 ml 且不需要输血治疗。ABL 与术中自体血回收效率成正比。

自体预输血

回顾过去，根据外科医师髋关节置换术的跟踪记录来预测病例概述中患者的失血量，那么患者应该接受铁治疗并在手术前 3 ～ 4 周预先捐赠 3 或 4 个单位自体血。如果患者原来的血细胞比容低于 40%，补充促红细胞生成素是合理的，尽管健康保险政策不包括用于此目的的促红细胞生成素的费用。

急性等容性血液稀释

该操作最常见的应用是在体重较小的患者（例如，<70 kg）中抽出 2 个单位和在体重较大的患者中抽出 3 个单位。如果术中失血量在 3000 ～ 6000 ml（这大约接近正常血容量的一半到全部），该方法可以节省 1 ～ 2 个单位的同种异体浓缩红细胞。如失血超过 6000 ml，该方法节约的红细胞单位数量逐渐减少（至 0.5 ～ 1 个单位）。

首先，收集大约 450 ml 的血液，然后将 500 ml 的胶体溶液或者大约 1500 ml 的晶体溶液注入患者体内，以维持血容量。低血压或心动过速意味着容量替代不足，只要患者能够耐受这个过程，那么这种交换会持续到预期值。建议定期检查红细胞比容或血红蛋白浓度，以重新评估预期值是否适当。8 h 内用血可以常温保存；否则，需要冷藏。

术中血液回收

在本病例中，术中血液回收可能是尊重患者不输血意愿的最佳方法。此外，该技术的有效使用倾向于替代了急性等容血液稀释的任何理论益处。或者说如果患者在其他方面完全健康，那么可以“耐受”低至 20% 的血细胞比容，然而考虑到患者的年龄，将血细胞比容降低到这个水平显然是不明智的。

术后血液回收

由于这种技术的成本较低，在病例概要中描述的患者术后大量出血的可能性高，因此术后血液回收是恰当的措施。由于伤口引流中含有各种不良成分，因此建议再输注前进行清洗。由于存在细菌污染可能性，因此除非在 8 h 内引流超过 500 ml，应该尽量避免使用这种策略。此后如果计划回输回收血液，应更换收集装置。

替代性血液保护技术

其他可能的血液保存方法列于表 59.2 中。如果患者其他方面完全健康，则可以实施适度的控制性降压。但对于一个 60 岁的患者来说，设置一个相对保守的较低的平均动脉压限制（70 mmHg 维持 1 ～ 2 h）需要谨慎。[a] 另一个合理的方法是如果有必要可以控制性降压将患者平均动脉压降低至术前基线水平的 20% 左右，可安全维持数小时。许多研究表明，氨甲环酸可以减少失血，降低并发症的风险，并且在关节成形术中减少异体输血的需要。

（钱 爽 译 万小健 校）

---

[a] 因为我们假设的患者是男性，年龄大于 60 岁，并且没有冠状动脉疾病或危险因素（高脂血症、高血压或吸烟史），另一种评估控制性降压（即维持冠状动脉灌注压所需的）最小可接受压力的方法是舒张压—左心室舒张压 =50 mmHg。在高龄、舒张期心力衰竭、有冠状动脉家族史、高血压、其他心脏疾病（均伴有一定程度的左心室舒张末期压力升高）的患者中应该维持更高的冠状动脉灌注压。

表 59.2 其他潜在的血液保护技术

技术	成本	风险	可行性[a]
控制性降压	多变	多变	可行性存疑，患者年龄是顾虑之一
预防应用氨甲环酸	中等	低	尚不明确；减少失血但价格昂贵
脊髓或硬膜外麻醉	低	低	利于血压控制；减少深静脉血栓形成

[a] 针对病例概述中的患者

延伸阅读

American Society of Anesthesiologists Task Force on Blood Component Therapy: Practice guidelines for blood component therapy, *Anesthesiology* 84:732–747, 1996.

Birkmeyer JD, Goodnough LT, AuBuchon JP, et al.: The cost effectiveness of preoperative autologous blood donation for total hip and knee replacement, *Transfusion* 33:544–551, 1993.

Goodnough LT: Red blood cell support in the perioperative setting. In Simon TL, Dzik WH, Snyder EL, et al.: *Rossi's principles of transfusion medicine*, 3rd ed, Philadelphia, 2002, Lippincott Williams & Wilkins, pp 590–601.

Goodnough LT, Despotis GJ, Merkel K, et al.: A randomized trial comparing acute normovolemic hemodilution and preoperative autologous blood donation in total hip arthroplasty, *Transfusion* 40:1054–1057, 2000.

Goodnough LT, Monk TG, Brecher ME: Autologous blood procurement in the surgical setting: lessons learned in the last 10 years, *Vox Sang* 71:133–141, 1996.

Jacobs MR, Palavecino E, Yomtovian R: Don't bug me: the problem of bacterial contamination of blood components—challenges and solutions, *Transfusion* 41:1331–1334, 2001.

Kuehnert MJ, et al.: Transfusion-transmitted bacterial infection in the United States, 1998 through 2000, *Transfusion* 41(12):1493–1499, 2001.

Wei Z, Liu M: The effectiveness and safety of tranexamic acid in total hip or knee arthroplasty: a meta-analysis of 2720 cases, *Transfus Med* 25(3):151–162, 2015.

Wu W-C, Rathore SS, Wang Y, et al.: Blood transfusion in elderly patients with acute myocardial infarction, *N Engl J Med* 345:1230–1236, 2001.

第60章 颅内动脉瘤再出血

Suneeta Gollapudy，Lois A. Connolly

病例概要

患者，男性，55岁，蛛网膜下腔出血12 h，拟行开颅手术结扎右前交通动脉动脉瘤，在麻醉诱导期间出现了急性高血压和心动过缓。

问题分析

定义

颅内动脉瘤是由湍流和血流动力学波动引起的动脉膨出。**动脉瘤再出血**定义为动脉瘤破裂，引起突然的临床恶化[清醒患者格拉斯哥昏迷量表（Glasgow Coma Scale，GCS）评分下降]，并伴随蛛网膜下腔、颅内和脑室内的出血。

再出血使颅内压（intracranial pressure，ICP）升高，导致脑灌注受损和神经功能恶化。多种并发症可随之出现（表60.1）。突如其来的蛛网膜下腔凝血块聚积阻塞了脑脊液（cerebrospinal fluid，CSF）通过蛛网膜下腔基底池的通道，导致急性脑积水。脑梗死可能是由于血肿引起脑损坏或颅内容物移位，伴随脑血管的损害。蛛网膜下腔出血量越大，ICP越高，脑血流量（cerebral blood flow，CBF）就越有可能减少，患者的神经系统状况会进一步恶化。蛛网膜下腔出血（subarachnoid hemorrhage，SAH）也损害了大脑自动调节功能，即大脑在平均动脉压（mean arterial pressures，MAP）50～150 mmHg之间保持CBF相对恒定的能力。

表60.1 蛛网膜下腔出血并发症

早期	晚期
血肿，ICP ↑，再出血，癫痫，脑积水	再出血，脑积水，血管痉挛，梗死，癫痫
神经麻痹，偏瘫，LOC下降	永久性偏瘫，认知障碍
心律失常	心肌梗死，肺炎，肝、肾功能不全
短暂BP ↑	持续BP ↑
视力减退	玻璃体出血
体液和电解质失衡	神经系统恶化，死亡

BP，血压；ICP，颅内压；LOC，意识水平

流行病学

在大多数西方人群中，颅内动脉瘤的总患病率为3.2%，颅内动脉瘤（intracranial aneurysm，ICA）破裂导致蛛网膜下腔出血（SAH）发生率为0.002%～0.016%。ICA破裂率为每年0.05%～6%，取决于动脉瘤的大小和位置。大部分（80%～85%）的ICA位于前循环，大于7 mm时有破裂倾向。既往有SAH患者的破裂风险是有症状未破裂动脉瘤患者的11倍。

SAH后再出血可能是灾难性的，幸存者的功能恢复不佳，预后不良，且死亡率大于60%。再出血的风险在最初的2～12 h内最大，出血后的24 h内高达13.6%，72 h内高达23%。事实上，超过1/3的再出血发生在症状出现后3 h内，近一半发生在6 h内，早期再出血比晚期再出血更严重。Van Donkelaard等认为，3～4级的Fisher量表分级（表60.2）是前驱症状出现后24 h内院内再出血的预警。此外，24 h内脑脊液引流与再出血独立相关。在他们的研究中，前驱症状出现后24 h内，医院内的累积再出血率为5.8%，在24～72 h内为1.2%。早期治疗破裂的动脉瘤可以降低再出血的风险。在治疗后脑动脉瘤再次破裂（cerebral aneurysm rerupture after treatment，CARAT）研究中，动脉瘤不完全闭塞预示复发性动脉瘤蛛网膜下腔出血（aneurysmal SAH，aSAH），发生出血的中位数为治疗后3天，但1年后很少发生。尽管有些动脉瘤需要再治疗，aSAH术后动脉瘤完全闭塞的患者5年内复

表 60.2 Fischer 量表（出血的 CT 表现）

组 1	未检测到血液
组 2	蛛网膜下腔出血扩散积聚厚度小于 1 mm
组 3	局部凝块和（或）垂直血液层厚度大于或等于 1 mm
组 4	弥漫性或无蛛网膜下腔血液，但存在颅内或脑室内血凝块

发 aSAH 的风险很低。在晚期接受最终治疗的患者中，动脉瘤在血管痉挛窗口期延迟闭塞与再出血的风险比动脉瘤早期闭塞更高。如果不治疗，50% 破裂的 ICA 在初始 SAH 后 6 个月内重新出血，大约 20% ～ 30% 破裂的 ICA 在初始 SAH 后 30 天内再出血。在随后的 5 个月内，另有 10% ～ 15% 的患者发生再出血。

术中动脉瘤破裂（intraoperative aneurysm rupture，IAR）的发生率为 6% ～ 8%，因不同的医疗机构而异，取决于动脉瘤的大小和位置。由动脉瘤形成的病因以及与麻醉、手术或其他干预有关的复杂因素相互作用共同决定。动脉瘤破裂和再出血的外科原因，按出现频率递减顺序排列分别是剥离、脑组织回缩、血肿清除、打开硬脑膜和蛛网膜。麻醉诱导可诱发 IAR（发病率 1% ～ 2%），预后极差，死亡率为 75%。大多数破裂发生在气管插管患者出现咳嗽时，这表明气道操作和由此产生的交感神经兴奋可能是原因之一。

识别

ICA 再出血的症状主要是由颅内出血所致。这是因为先前的 SAH 引起的粘连将动脉瘤与蛛网膜下腔隔开，以致新的出血都转至脑实质。

ICA 再出血后，清醒患者的意识水平（GCS 评分）恶化，患者出现局灶性神经功能缺损（失语症、偏瘫）、生命体征异常（高血压、心动过缓、心律失常、不规则呼吸）和体温升高。患者也可能会出现液体和电解质失衡（尤其是低钠血症），眼科检查可发现明显视网膜出血（框 60.1）。在重症监护室接受插管、镇静和密切监测的生命体征较差的患者可能已行脑室外引流。如果血压（blood pressure，BP）、瞳孔大小突然变化或新鲜血液从 CSF 引流管中流出，可行计算机断层扫描确认再出血。

如果在麻醉诱导期间或麻醉诱导后立即出现 ICA 再出血，患者血压会升高，心率可能会降低或不降低。重要的是要认识到 ICP 也会增加。此时，颅内多普勒超声可以诊断 ICA 的破裂，并监测治疗效果。术中 ICA 破裂较易发现。手术结束后再出血的信号是：麻醉后未能苏醒或术后觉醒后神经功能进一步恶化（例如意识水平下降，出现新的局灶性神经功能缺损或失语症）。

框 60.1 动脉瘤再出血的影响

- 直接脑损伤
- CSF 循环紊乱→脑积水
- 血肿、脑出血、脑室内出血引起的 ICP ↑
- CBF ↓导致的脑梗死
- 体液和电解质失衡
- 心律失常，BP ↑
- 呼吸功能受损

BP，血压；CBF，脑血流；CSF，脑脊液；ICP，颅内压

风险评估

首次 SAH（框 60.2）后，ICA 再破裂是神经功能恶化的主要原因之一。高血压是动脉瘤破裂和再出血的最重要的危险因素。再出血的可能性与患者术后收缩压直接相关。对于已经发生多次再出血的患者，进一步破裂和死亡的可能性要大得多。严重 SAH 分级差、动脉瘤治疗时间较长、入院时神经系统状态恶化、意识丧失、动脉瘤较大、前哨出血、收缩压大于 160 mmHg 以及症状出现 3 h 内接受血管造影的患者早期再出血的风险更高。遗传因素虽然与 ICA 的发生有关，但似乎与增加再出血的发生率无关。其他危险因素包括女性（再出血的发生率是男性的 2 倍）、身体状况差、高龄、脑后部 ICA、较高的颅内或脑室内血肿发生率以及异常凝血参数。怀孕期间，不稳定 ICA 再出血的风险为 33% ～ 50%。尽管 50% ～ 68% 的患者会死亡，但没有证据表明孕妇的再出血率与普通人群有差异。

启示

初次动脉瘤性 SAH 后的病理生理后遗症和再出血并发症相当严重。由于复发性出血通常比初次出血更严重，复发性出血的死亡率加倍至 80%，存活患者的病残率较高。血肿大小是影响结局的最关键因素（框 60.3）。硬膜下血肿大，计算机断层扫描显示中线移位较多，伴有颅内或脑室内出血的患者预

框 60.2 蛛网膜下腔出血后神经功能恶化的原因

再出血-颅内高压
血肿
脑积水
脑水肿
  癫痫发作
  脑膜炎
自动调节功能紊乱
二氧化碳反应障碍
酸碱平稳紊乱
体液和电解质紊乱
血管痉挛
迟发性缺血性损害
脑梗死——继发脑损伤
  低血压
  低氧血症
  高血糖症
  颅内高压（初次出血后）

框 60.3 急性蛛网膜下腔出血后死亡率的预测因素

与血肿大小直接相关的入院时临床状况或分级不佳
、意识水平下降
血压升高
再出血
迟发性缺血性损害（血管痉挛）
初次 CT 扫描下蛛网膜下腔血栓的厚度
基底动脉瘤
高龄
先前存在的内科疾病

后较差。

由于大部分再出血发生在第一次 SAH 后 6 ～ 24 h 内，因此早期干预以防止动脉瘤破裂（无论是通过外科夹闭或血管内弹簧圈栓塞）已成为治疗再出血的主要手段。因此，必须快速有效地完成再出血的诊断和治疗。此外，由于对 SAH 及其后遗症的经验增加，加上对患者治疗的改善，社区医院和专门从事 ICA 外科和血管内治疗中心必须保持良好的协作关系。

预防

美国心脏协会（American Heart Association，AHA）和神经重症监护学会（Neurocritical Care Society，NCS）于 2012 年发布了动脉瘤性蛛网膜下腔出血的管理指南，为 SAH 患者的治疗提供循证指南。再出血与高死亡率相关，预后及功能恢复差。再出血的最高风险发生在最初的 12 h 内。动脉瘤破裂的早期手术或操作治疗可降低再出血的风险。国际蛛网膜下腔动脉瘤试验（International Subarachnoid Aneurysm Trial，ISAT）提供了令人信服的证据，证明弹簧圈可以提供更好的临床效果，但脑实质内大血肿和大脑中动脉瘤应考虑夹闭手术。建立紧急神经生命支持包括迅速和早期识别 SAH、控制疼痛和焦虑、Hunt 和 Hess 或世界神经外科医师联合会评分、早期气道管理（包括因神经功能评分恶化而插管）、无法保护气道以及需要过度通气治疗颅内高压或低氧治疗。其他降低再出血风险的措施包括密切控制血压，维持脑灌注压，短疗程抗纤维蛋白溶解药早期治疗，以及预防癫痫发作。在一项使用氨甲环酸的前瞻性随机研究中，包括使用短期抗纤维蛋白溶解药（氨甲环酸）早期治疗，在 SAH 后立即给药时，早期再出血率和不良后果降低。

虽然癫痫发病率很低，但如果一旦发生了癫痫，结果可能是灾难性的。癫痫可导致动脉瘤再出血并且会导致 ICP 升高。AHA 和 NCS 建议在出血后立即预防性使用抗惊厥药物。然而，癫痫预防药物的常规应用仍然存在争议。预防性使用苯妥英钠与更差的认知预后独立相关。苯妥英钠和其他抗惊厥药与血管痉挛、迟发性脑缺血和发热有关。

初次 SAH 后的再出血治疗旨在维持脑灌注，减少颅内高压和容积，控制体循环血压，并降低动脉瘤壁的跨壁压力（MAP – ICP）。在这一背景下，优化大脑氧供取决于动脉血总的氧含量，需要维持正常的血红蛋白浓度和动脉血氧饱和度。

避免腰椎穿刺和 ICA 夹闭前快速脑室引流也可以防止再出血。然而，当颅内高压严重影响脑灌注时，这些措施有时被用来降低颅内压。

在夹闭 ICA 的操作过程中，亦有必要采取干预措施防止再出血。主血管近端临时性阻断用于降低 ICA 腔的肿胀，血压维持在患者正常血压范围偏高水平，以增强远端和侧支灌注。当然，如果在动脉瘤安全处置前临时取下血管夹，血压必须迅速恢复到患者较低的正常范围，以防止动脉瘤破裂。

对正常血压、正常血容量和甘露醇的治疗方案，一些神经外科医师增加了脑电波爆发抑制，并报道其具有益处。如果在暂时性 ICA 阻断前给予丙泊酚诱发爆发抑制，也可提供大脑保护。保持血糖正常和体温维持到 35℃也可以降低暂时性脑血管阻断引起的缺血性风险。

治疗

手术中或操作中动脉瘤破裂

很少有文献或数据能指导麻醉科医师如何立即处理手术或操作中动脉瘤破裂。Chowdhury 等围绕这些患者的管理提供了一篇很好的回顾述评。高血压是动脉瘤破裂的最重要的危险因素。当颅内压保持不变时，高血压会增加跨壁压力梯度（transmural pressure gradient，TMPG）。TMPG 的突然波动可导致破裂。如果血压突然升高或 ICP 突然下降，TMPG 会升高。因此控制血压和 ICP 至关重要。

监测和控制血压对于权衡脑卒中、高血压相关的再出血风险和维持脑灌注压很有必要。在麻醉诱导过程中，有必要应用有创动脉压监测以及药物控制高血压。注意可能导致血压急剧升高的围术期操作：插管、体位摆放、颅骨钉固定、切皮和切开骨膜。

虽然 AHA/NCS 指南认为血压低于 160 mmHg 比较合理，但尚不清楚降低再出血风险的最佳血压是多少。许多可滴定的抗高血压药物可供使用。尼卡地平是一种类似硝苯地平的二氢吡啶钙通道阻滞剂，是一种作用温和的常用降压药物。已有人研究使用尼卡地平控制蛛网膜下腔出血患者的血压。除了极少数短暂和容易解决的并发症，如低血压、心律失常和心动过速，尼卡地平似较安全。它对脑血管和冠状动脉更有选择性。本质上尼卡地平并不降低心肌收缩力。此外，静脉注射尼卡地平可降低动脉瘤性 SAH 患者迟发性脑动脉狭窄的发生率和严重程度。

拉贝洛尔是一种 α/β - 肾上腺素受体阻滞剂，常用于控制 SAH 患者的高血压。拉贝洛尔通过降低全身血管阻力来降低血压，对每搏量、心率和心排血量几乎没有影响。许多研究评价了拉贝洛尔与尼卡地平对血压的控制效果。Ortega Gutierrez 等发现，这两种药物在初次入院时对 SAH 和颅内出血的血压控制同样有效和安全，但为了更好地控制血压，可能需要两种药物的联合应用。然而，其他研究者发现尼卡地平更具优势。尼卡地平与拉贝洛尔相比，在治疗 SAH 患者时血压下降更快，治疗失败率也更低。

氯维地平是一种超短效的钙通道阻滞剂，是治疗的另一种选择。在所有动脉瘤性 SAH 患者中，氯维地平控制收缩压的时间不超过 22 min，并保持其在 70% 的时间内无严重并发症。氯维地平目前正在进行第 2 阶段的研究，以确定它是否会减少对血管痉挛的影响。

其他用于治疗血压升高的药物包括静脉推注 10 mg 的肼屈嗪或静脉注射 1.25 mg 的依那普利。曾经常用的硝普钠，现在已经被可滴定的新型降压药所取代。

在预防 TMPG 升高方面，控制 ICP 与控制高血压同样重要。ICP 可通过腰椎穿刺引流或脑室内螺栓测量，有助于平衡血压和 ICP，以维持脑灌注压（MAP－ICP），并指导血压管理。ICP 降低可能是由于快速注射甘露醇或硬脑膜开放前过度通气所致。从引流管中快速排出 CSF 也可能改变 ICP。少有数据表明 ICP 的变化是动脉瘤破裂的主要原因；然而，仍建议谨慎采用缓慢降低 ICP 的措施。

破裂动脉瘤的处理取决于动脉瘤术中破裂的时间。

硬脊膜切开前动脉瘤破裂

颅内动脉瘤破裂导致 ICP 突然升高和脑灌注风险增加，导致脑缺血和神经元损伤。管理目标是降低 ICP 并制定神经保护策略。

降低 ICP：过度通气，使用瑞芬太尼静脉麻醉、丙泊酚诱发爆发抑制。

神经保护策略：二级神经保护——控制血压，防止血肿扩大，优化组织氧合（脑氧合监测有助于指导过度通气），控制高血糖（避免血糖 >8.33 mmol/L），避免低血糖（血糖 <4.44 mmol/L）。

迄今为止，针对兴奋性毒性、氧化应激和炎症等过程的原发性神经保护治疗前景尚不明朗。

低温是降低脑代谢和稳定神经元膜电位的有效机制。国际动脉瘤手术低温试验（International Hypothermia for Aneurysm Surgery Trial，IHAST）评估了轻度全身低温是否可为开颅手术治疗脑动脉瘤破裂时保护大脑免受缺血损伤。IHAST 得出的结论是，与维持正常体温（目标温度 36.5℃）相比，轻度全身低温（33℃）不会改善神经系统预后，因此不应常规应用。但温度若高于正常值时，应立即降低体温。

外科及时抢救性夹闭动脉瘤是决定预后的关键因素。

栓塞术中脑动脉瘤破裂

术中动脉瘤破裂可导致血压突然大幅度升高，伴或不伴有心动过缓。

迅速拮抗肝素的抗凝作用：输注血小板，逆转抗血小板的活性。

减少脑代谢：使用静脉麻醉剂瑞芬太尼，丙泊酚诱发爆发抑制。

控制突然增加的 ICP：适度的过度通气、渗透性利尿。

血压控制：血压低于 160 mmHg——避免过度控制，因为可能导致脑缺血。

手术干预。

硬脊膜切开后脑动脉瘤破裂

打开颅骨和硬脑膜可以更好地处理术中脑动脉瘤破裂。大多数破裂发生在分离、血管夹置入、硬膜切开或牵引器置入过程中。

神经保护策略：使用静脉麻醉剂瑞芬太尼和丙泊酚诱发爆发抑制，优化组织氧合（脑氧合监测可能有助于指导过度通气），控制高血糖。

维持正常血压：过去曾提倡将平均动脉压迅速降低到 50 ～ 60 mmHg，但这种方法可能对脑灌注压产生不利影响，特别是在脑自动调节功能受损的情况下。应尽量减少低血压的程度和持续时间。

维持正常血容量：立即用血液制品、胶体（白蛋白）或晶体液替代丢失的血液，使血红蛋白保持在 8 ～ 10 g/dL。维持正常的血容量至关重要。

维持正常血糖和电解质平衡。

应用血管夹或短暂闭塞：操作起来可能比较困难，取决于动脉瘤破裂的时间。可以通过应用腺苷短暂阻止血流来实现。在瑞芬太尼和丙泊酚诱发爆发抑制作用时，腺苷的推荐起始剂量为 0.3 ～ 0.4 mg/kg。

术后治疗

术后早期阶段需要进行脑血管成像。再出血患者应留置气管插管，并在重症加强治疗病房接受与脑卒中相关的强化治疗。

在 ICA 得到控制后，患者可以接受脑血管痉挛的预防或治疗，如高血压、高血容量、血液稀释（“三 H 疗法”），而无需担心 ICA 再破裂。SAH 后的血管痉挛是发病率和死亡率的重要因素。尼莫地平的运用、维持正常血容量和避免低血压对于减少与血管痉挛相关的迟发性脑缺血至关重要。通常情况下，第一个症状是无法逆转的神经系统损害。经颅多普勒超声有助于进一步诊断评估和临床干预。如果患者因脑血管痉挛而出现神经功能恶化，则必须谨慎地进行三 H 疗法（见上文）。为了避免再出血，可将收缩压从 120 mmHg 适度增加到 150 mmHg，中心静脉压从 10 mmHg 增加到 12 mmHg，肺毛细血管楔压从 12 mmHg 增加到 16 mmHg。

致谢

感谢 Philippa Newfeld 博士对本章上一版的贡献。

（姚　寒　译　倪丽亚　校）

延伸阅读

Abd-Elsayed AA, Wehby AS, Farag E: Anesthetic management of patients with intracranial aneurysms, *Ochsner J* 14:418–425, 2014.

Adamczyk P, He S, Amar AP, et al.: Medical management of cerebral vasospasm following aneurysmal subarachnoid hemorrhage: a review of current and emerging therapeutic interventions, *Neurol Res Int* 2013, 2013. 10.1155/2013/462491.

Bendok BR, Gupta DK, Rahme RJ, et al.: Adenosine for temporary flow arrest during intracranial aneurysm surgery: a single-center retrospective review, *Neurosurgery* 69:815–820, 2011. discussion 820–821.

Chowdhury T, Petropolis A, Wilkinson M, et al.: Controversies in the anesthetic management of intraoperative rupture of intracranial aneurysm, *Anesthesiol Res Pract* 2014:1–10, 2014.

Connolly Jr ES, Rabinstein AA, Carhuapoma JR, et al.: Guidelines for the management of aneurysmal subarachnoid hemorrhage: a guideline for healthcare professionals from the American Heart Association/American Stroke Association, *Stroke* 43:1711–1737, 2012.

Darsaut TE, Jack AS, Kerr RS, et al.: International Subarachnoid Aneurysm Trial—ISAT part II: study protocol for a randomized controlled trial, *Trials* 14:156, 2013.

Elliott J, Smith M: The acute management of intracerebral hemorrhage: a clinical review, *Anesth Analg* 110:1419–1427, 2010.

Hillman J, Fridriksson S, Nilsson O, et al.: Immediate administration of tranexamic acid and reduced incidence of early rebleeding after aneurysmal subarachnoid hemorrhage: a prospective randomized study, *J Neurosurg* 97:771–778, 2002.

Hindman BJ, Bayman EO, Pfisterer WK, et al.: No association between intraoperative hypothermia or supplemental protective drug and neurologic outcomes in patients undergoing temporary clipping during cerebral aneurysm surgery: findings from the Intraoperative Hypothermia for Aneurysm Surgery Trial, *Anesthesiology* 112:86–101, 2010.

Kim S, Kim S, Park M, et al.: Effectiveness of nicardipine for blood pressure control in patients with subarachnoid hemorrhage, *J Cerebrovasc Endovasc Neurosurg* 14:84–89, 2012.

Lecours M, Gelb AW: Anesthesia for the surgical treatment of cerebral aneurysms, *Rev Colomb Anestesiol* 43:45–51, 2015.

Lee CZ, Gelb AW: Anesthesia management for endovascular treatment, *Curr Opin Anaesthesiol* 27:484–488, 2014.

Ortega-Gutierrez S, Thomas J, Reccius A, et al.: Effectiveness and safety of nicardipine and labetalol infusion for blood pressure management in patients with intracerebral and subarachnoid hemorrhage, *Neurocrit Care* 18:13–19, 2013.
Pong R, Lam AM: Anesthetic management of cerebral aneurysm surgery. In Cottrell JE, Young WL, editors: *Cottrell and Young's neuroanesthesia*, ed 5 Philadelphia, 2010, Elsevier, pp 218–246.
Rhoney DH, McAllen K, Liu-DeRyke X: Current and future treatment considerations in the management of aneurysmal subarachnoid hemorrhage, *J Pharm Pract* 23:408–424, 2010.
Van Donkelaar CE, Bakker NA, Veeger NJ, et al.: Predictive factors for rebleeding after aneurysmal subarachnoid hemorrhage: rebleeding aneurysmal subarachnoid hemorrhage study, *Stroke* 46:2100–2106, 2015.
Varelasa P, Abdelhak T, Corry J, et al.: Clevidipine for acute hypertension in patients with subarachnoid hemorrhage: a pilot study, *Int J Neurosci* 124:192–198, 2014.
Zhao ZX, Wu C, He M: A systematic review of clinical outcomes, perioperative data and selective adverse events related to mild hypothermia in intracranial aneurysm surgery, *Clin Neurol Neurosurg* 114:827–832, 2012.

第61章 颅内动脉瘤：血管痉挛和其他关注点

Ehab Farag，Alex M. Witek，Mark Bain

病例概要

患者，女性，58 岁，既往有高血压和 2 型糖尿病，长年吸烟，因剧烈头痛收治入急诊科。患者头部的计算机断层扫描（computed tomography，CT）显示蛛网膜下腔出血 Fisher 3 级，脑血管造影显示前交通动脉区域宽颈动脉瘤破裂。手术医师使用分流系统（管道栓塞装置）对患者的动脉瘤进行腔内弹簧圈堵塞。患者于术后 4 天出现偏瘫和精神状态受损，经颅多普勒检查显示，大脑前动脉的血流速度从入院时基础值 110 cm/s 增加至 170 cm/s。CT 血管造影（computed tomography angiography，CTA）显示颅内远端有小血管的痉挛，确诊该患者为脑血管痉挛和迟发性脑缺血。此外，磁共振成像（magnetic resonance imaging，MRI）显示患者存在多发性脑梗死灶。患者通过口服尼莫地平，维持正常血容量和诱导性高血压的方案以进行治疗。

问题分析

蛛网膜下腔出血

尽管脑卒中已从人类最常见死亡原因的第三位降至第四位，但颅内动脉瘤导致的蛛网膜下腔出血（subarachnoid hemorrhage，SAH）的死亡率并未下降，其中美国的年死亡率仍高达 9/10 万，全球每年约有 60 万名患者死于 SAH。颅内动脉瘤多发于女性，男女比例 1∶3，此外，女性患者更易患多发性动脉瘤。雌激素对促进正常内皮功能及其对血管结构的影响至关重要，绝经期雌激素下降导致 50 ～ 59 岁之间的女性出现 SAH 的高峰。男性患者比女性更早出现（未破裂和破裂的）动脉瘤。

与不良预后相关的因素包括高龄、入院时神经系统检查结果不佳，以及最初头部 CT 所见的出血量（Fisher 评分）。Fisher 量表有四个等级：1、2、3 和 4。其中 Fisher 3 级（CT 显示弥漫性蛛网膜下腔出血）本身与脑血管痉挛的发展显著相关。用于 SAH 患者评估的两个临床量表是 Hunt-Hess 评分和世界神经外科医师联合会评分（World Federation of Neurological Surgeons，WFNS）。Hunt-Hess 从 1 级表示仅有轻度头痛症状的正常人，至 5 级表示昏迷患者。WFNS 将格拉斯哥昏迷量表和局灶性神经系统体征结合起来，评分范围为 1 分至 5 分，分数越高，预后越差。

头部非增强 CT 在 12 h 内诊断 SAH 的敏感性为 98% ～ 100%，但在 24 h 时降至 93%，6 天时可低至 57%。如果 CT 扫描结果为阴性但根据临床表现怀疑患者有 SAH，则应进行诊断性腰椎穿刺。

应密切监测血压，并将最高收缩压控制在 150 ～ 160 mmHg 左右。发现 SAH 后 24 h 内再出血的风险可能为 15%，复发性出血死亡率约为 70%。因此，建议破裂的动脉瘤应早期治疗，以减少再出血，并使用诱导性高血压策略以改善脑血管痉挛。

颅内动脉瘤的治疗

鉴于早期再出血的风险，动脉瘤引起的 SAH 患者需要对动脉瘤进行治疗。颅内动脉瘤有多种治疗选择：显微手术夹闭包括进行开颅手术以将金属夹放置在动脉瘤的颈部（图 61.1）；腔内放置弹簧圈是 20 世纪 90 年代引入的夹闭术的替代方案，并且在过去的 20 年中弹簧圈手术的数量大大增加，具体做法是通过微导管将弹簧铂线圈送入动脉瘤的位置，然后释放弹簧圈，从而封闭动脉瘤囊（图 61.2）。与放置弹簧圈相辅的策略包括放置球囊和支架辅助技术，这些措施可以防止弹簧圈脱垂，并降低复发风险。近年来，分流支架已成为治疗动脉瘤的有用工具，可用于治疗以往难以夹闭或弹簧圈封堵的动脉瘤（图 61.3）。分流支架形成孔隙的概率要小于其他颅内支架，而孔隙形成会导致动脉瘤内的血流停滞，从而引起血栓形成，最终动脉闭塞；同时该支架可使所覆盖的分支血管通畅。

治疗方案的选择较为复杂，取决于多种因素，包括动脉瘤位置、动脉瘤形状、患者临床状态和并存疾病，以及患者和外科医师的偏好。虽然有三项随机研究比较了在治疗破裂动脉瘤中显微夹闭术和血管栓塞术的优劣，但是对于多数动脉瘤来说，仍没有足够的数据以得出有信服力的结论。国际蛛网膜下腔动脉瘤试验（International Subarachnoid

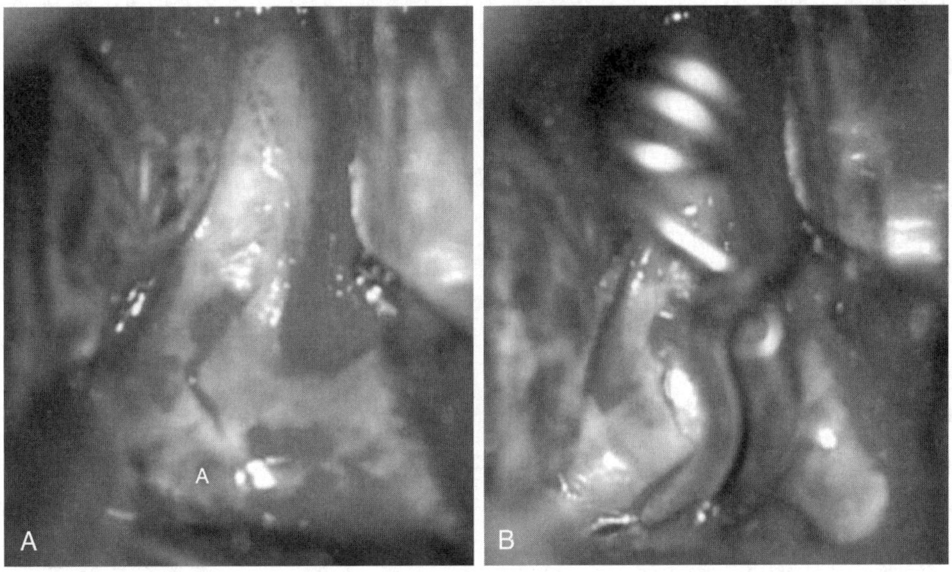

图 61.1 A，打开 Sylvian 裂隙后的显微外科视图显示位于大脑中动脉分叉处的动脉瘤（A）。**B**，将钛夹置于动脉瘤的颈部并封闭动脉瘤

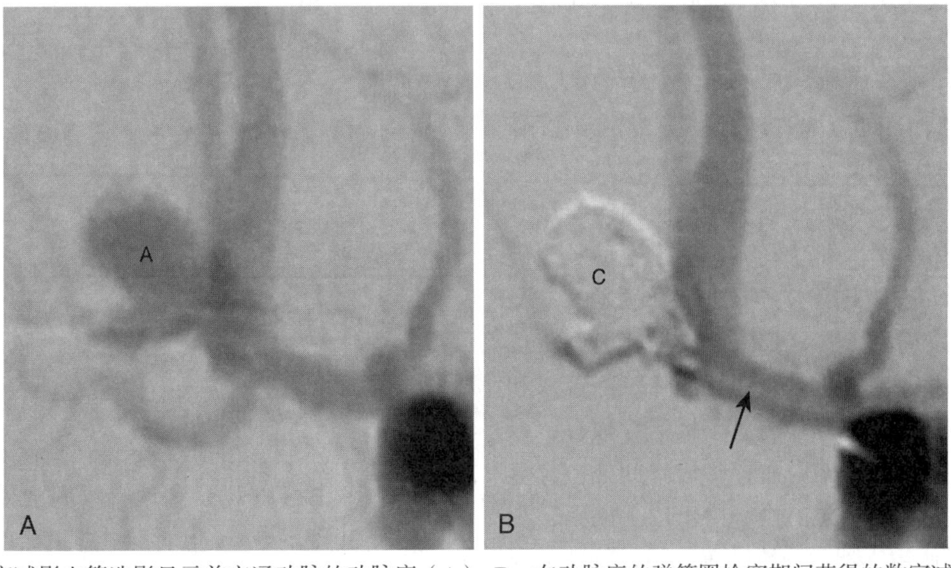

图 61.2 A，数字减影血管造影显示前交通动脉的动脉瘤（A）。**B**，在动脉瘤的弹簧圈栓塞期间获得的数字减影血管造影。微导管（箭头）已经置于动脉瘤中，铂弹簧圈（C）已经被填充到动脉瘤的圆顶中，此时动脉瘤不再显示造影剂

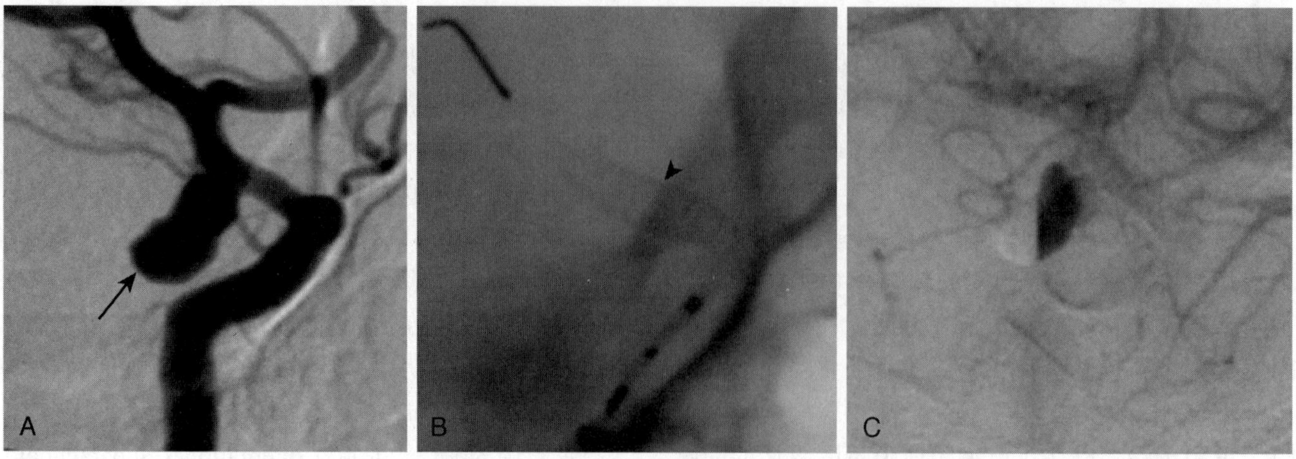

图 61.3 A，数字减影血管造影显示源自颈内动脉交通段的动脉瘤（箭头）。**B**，荧光镜视图显示管道栓塞装置（箭头）置于颈内动脉中，并覆盖了动脉瘤的颈部。**C**，放置管道栓塞装置后的数字减影血管造影显示经栓塞的动脉瘤内血流停滞

Aneurysm Trial，ISAT）是这些试验中最大的一项，发现接受弹簧圈治疗的患者的死亡率或对治疗的依赖率（11%）低于接受夹闭治疗的患者（14%）；然而，此项试验中只有 22% 符合条件的患者被随机分配。此外，对 22 个英国神经外科中心的 1644 名患者的死亡和临床结果进行的随访研究表明，接受弹簧圈栓塞患者的 10 年生存率优于接受夹闭治疗的患者。Barrow 动脉瘤破裂试验（Barrow Ruptured Aneurysm Trial，BRAT）报告在治疗后循环动脉瘤中，接受弹簧圈栓塞患者的预后优于接受夹闭术的患者，但是在治疗前循环动脉瘤中两种方法无差异。动脉瘤形态是一个重要的考虑因素，若动脉瘤颈部狭窄更倾向于使用血管内弹簧圈栓塞术。高龄、具有内科并存疾病和临床分级较差的患者也倾向于腔内治疗，因为开颅手术会增加这些患者出现相关不良事件的风险。

动脉瘤夹闭术往往是一种更加耐久的治疗方法，因为其复发率低、再治疗的可能性低。无论治疗破裂还是未破裂的动脉瘤，并发症的可能性是一个重要的考虑因素。对于经历开颅手术或腔内治疗动脉瘤的患者，常见的围术期并发症包括术中动脉瘤破裂和脑卒中。动脉瘤夹闭术需要进行开颅术，这会增加并发症的发病率，且延长患者的恢复时间。接受支架置入的患者（包括支架辅助的弹簧圈置入和分流装置置入）需要进行双抗血小板治疗数月，以防止上皮形成期间的支架内血栓形成。此外，分流装置植入不能立即防止再出血。由于以上原因，很少对 SAH 患者使用支架和分流装置，但在特殊情况下可能必须使用。

总之，治疗颅内动脉瘤有多种选择。尽管由于随机试验的选择偏倚和交叉，所以尚无法诠释夹闭手术和血管内栓塞手术孰优孰劣，然而对于破裂的后循环动脉瘤而言，弹簧圈栓塞手术似乎更有利。手术决策在很大程度上也依赖于术者的经验。

脑血管痉挛和延迟性脑缺血

延迟性脑缺血（delayed cerebral ischemia，DCI）是 SAH 后常见且严重的并发症。DCI 发生率约 20% ～ 40%，并且与脑梗死发生率和死亡率增加相关。DCI 通常由血管痉挛引起，血管痉挛是蛛网膜下腔动脉的可逆性狭窄。它通常发生在 SAH 后的第 3 天至第 15 天，在第 10 天达到高峰。约 70% 的血管痉挛可在血管造影扫描时观察到，但仅 20% ～ 30% 的患者会引发症状。因此，血管痉挛主要描述诊断性检查的结果，而 DCI 应该被用来描述临床症状出现恶化的情况，例如出现诊断 SAH（GCS 评分至少降低 2 分）后出现偏瘫、失语和意识改变。

血管造影引起的血管痉挛

血管造影时发现血管狭窄主要是由于蛛网膜下腔血凝块引起的血管收缩。尽管动脉纤维化、内皮增厚和血管顺应性降低持续发生，但是血管造影引发的血管痉挛总会消散。尽管在高达 60% ～ 70% 的 SAH 患者中可以观察到近端颅内血管的动脉狭窄，但只有 30% 的 SAH 患者会出现 DCI。值得注意的是，DCI 的发展取决于血管造影时血管痉挛的范围

和严重程度、先前存在的侧枝和吻合血流情况、脑代谢需求和血压。

迟发性脑缺血的病理生理学

遗传因素

纤溶酶原激活物抑制剂 -1（plasminogen activator inhibitor-1，PAI-1）是组织纤溶酶原激活物（tissue plasminogen activator，t-PA）的主要抑制剂，PAI-1 抑制纤溶酶原转化为活性纤溶酶。PAI-1 基因中的 4G 等位基因与较高的 PAI-1 水平相关，升高的 PAI-1 水平与 SAH 后的不良预后相关，因为它能促进微血栓形成。

内皮一氧化氮合成酶（endothelium nitric oxide synthetase，eNOS）27 VNTR（特别是“4a”等位基因）与动脉瘤引起的 SAH 的发生显著相关。eNOS T-786C SNP（特别是“C”等位基因）与脑血管痉挛的发生显著相关。

微血栓

SAH 后，实质微血管中血小板聚集诱导的微血栓已被确定为 DCI 的主要罪魁祸首之一。血小板活化的过程与蛋白酶（如基质金属蛋白酶 9）的释放有关，因蛋白酶可消化血管层中的胶原蛋白Ⅳ。值得注意的是，SAH 后数小时或数天，皮质和（或）实质内小动脉的收缩会促进血栓形成。

除了在 SAH 发生数小时内形成微血栓外，大动脉血管造影引起的血管痉挛还会介导内皮损伤，从而增强血小板聚集和微血栓形成。此外，SAH 后凝血系统的激活有助于终止出血，但也可在远端循环中产生更多的栓子。最后，对 SAH 患者来说，全身的高凝状态促进脑循环中微血栓的形成。

蛛网膜下腔出血和炎症

SAH 后，蛛网膜下腔内游离血红蛋白诱导了内皮细胞中细胞黏附分子的表达，从而促进白细胞向蛛网膜下腔的迁移，迁移的白细胞可诱导炎症发生，并且清除一氧化氮（nitric oxide，NO），影响 NO 介导的血管舒张。

在血红蛋白自氧化过程中形成的活性氧（reactive oxygen species，ROS）构成了发生脑血管痉挛的主要病因。ROS 将胆红素氧化为胆红素氧化产物，从而抑制 eNOS 和 NO 的产生。

触珠蛋白（haptoglobin，Hp）是一种铁循环蛋白，出血后可清除血管外游离血红蛋白。Hp 通过捕获释放的血红蛋白，并将其导向至表达 CD163 受体的巨噬细胞，内部消化游离血红蛋白，从而对抗血红蛋白的毒性作用。人类存在两个 Hp 的等位基因，因此有三种可能的基因型：Hp 1-1、Hp 1-2 和 Hp 2-2。Hp 2-2 可促进炎症反应，并被白细胞缓慢清除，这种作用极大地延长了 NO 的清除。因此，Hp 2-2 基因型的 SAH 患者发生症状性脑血管痉挛的风险更高。通过注射 L- 瓜氨酸以补充 NO，可防止 Hp 2-2 基因型的动物发生血管痉挛。

蛛网膜下腔内的血液和脂质过氧化会引发强烈的炎症反应。SAH 患者脑脊液中活化的白细胞会合成并释放内皮素 -1（endothelin-1，ET-1）和其他细胞因子，包括白细胞介素 -6，白细胞介素 -1β、肿瘤坏死因子 -α 和无氧自由基。SAH 后必定会激活细胞间黏附分子 -1（intercellular adhesion molecule-1，ICAM-1）和血管黏附分子 -1（vascular adhesion molecule-1，VCAM-1），它们能促使白细胞黏附到内皮，并进入蛛网膜下腔，诱导炎症反应。经颅多普勒诊断可见，脑脊液和血清 ICAM-1 和 VCAM-1 的浓度与血管痉挛的发展相关。布洛芬抑制 ICAM-1 和 VCAM-1 上调，其被发现可减少实验诱导的血管痉挛。然而，预防 ICAM-1 和 VCAM-1 上调所需的布洛芬剂量可产生全身毒性作用。在猴 SAH 的模型中，通过蛛网膜下腔植入布洛芬聚合物，局部药物浓度高，可控性好，从而阻止了血管痉挛的发展，且毫无局部或全身中毒的迹象。然而，尽管 SAH 后炎症反应是有害的，但是它在 SAH 后的修复过程中也起到有益的作用。

血脑屏障的破坏

SAH 后血脑屏障破坏可能导致大脑损伤，但也可能具有一定的益处。因此，急性血脑屏障的破坏会促使基质金属蛋白酶的激活，以促进后期的脑修复。

皮质扩散缺血

皮质扩散抑制（cortical spreading depression，CSD）已被认为是 SAH 后发生 DCI 的一个可能的机制。CSD 是脑灰质中的去极化波，以 2 ～ 5 mm/min 的慢速传播。这种大量细胞的去极化导致离子和神经递质的重新分布，形成一个循环，其终点为神经元的失活，继之出现皮质的短暂抑制。在正常大脑中，CSD 通常与局部脑血流量（cerebral blood flow，CBF）的增加以及氧供的增加相关。CBF 和氧供增加是提供离子泵驱动神经元复极化所需能量的必要手段。然而，SAH 后不再发生 CSD 相关的充血反应，从而导致 CBF 减少、氧供减少，诱发缺血区域的扩散。

尽管一些患者血管造影并没有发现血管痉挛，但是他们在脑动脉瘤破裂后行夹闭手术之后会发生与 CSD 集群相关的 DCI，CSD 集群的数量、持续时间与 DCI 的发展显著相关。

出现 CSD 的同时会伴随着细胞质钙离子的显著增加，使神经元线粒体去极化并通过钙单向转运体线粒体膜触发氧利用的增加。CSD 还激活糖酵解途径，增加皮质乳酸的产生。由于红细胞裂解，细胞外钾水平增加，直接使小动脉平滑肌细胞去极化，并通过电压门控钙通道促使细胞内钙离子增加，从而引起血管收缩。此外，镁可以保持神经元 N- 甲基 -D- 天冬氨酸（N-methyl-D-aspartate，NMDA）受体的激活，而神经元的去极化除 NMDA 受体上阻断的镁离子，该过程还增加了受体对少量间质谷氨酸增加的敏感性。谷氨酸与 NMDA 受体的相互作用促发钾和谷氨酸的释放，从而引发 CSD 的进一步扩散。蛛网膜下腔内血液可以迅速清除 NO 并促进 CSD 的发展。动脉低血压可延长 CSD 的持续时间，而高血压可降低 CSD 的持续时间。因此，SAH 后维持脑灌注压对于减轻 SAH 后 CSD 有害影响十分重要。

延迟性脑缺血的预测因子

增厚的蛛网膜下腔的血凝块、入院时临床状况不佳和发作时意识丧失会增加 DCI 的风险。高等强度的证据表明吸烟会增加 DCI 的风险，中等强度的证据表明糖尿病、全身炎症反应综合征、高血糖和脑积水也会增加 DCI 的风险。ET-1、IL-6 和脑脊液中某些凝血酶活化标记物可用于预测 SAH 后的 DCI。

延迟性脑缺血的诊断和管理

高达 50% 的 SAH 患者可在 3 ～ 14 天后出现延迟性神经功能恶化，仅有约 5% 的病例发生在第 10 天后。DCI 的临床诊断可能很困难，特别是镇静、机械通气的评分较差的患者。未临床诊断过的 DCI 患者可能表现为无症状，然而针对这些患者，CT 扫描可显示 10% ～ 20% 的脑梗死范围，MRI 可显示 23% 的脑梗死范围。脑梗死与预后不良密切相关，两种最常见的梗死原因是动脉瘤栓塞手术和 DCI。

入院时 WFNS 等级为 1 ～ 3 的老年患者，CT 上无 SAH 或少量的 SAH，他们发生 DCI 风险较低，因此其无需过频繁的监测。

血管造影

血管造影依旧是诊断血管痉挛的金标准，但它正在被 CT 血管造影（CT angiography，CTA）取代。诊断血管痉挛的最准确组合是通过 CTA 对狭窄的动脉进行定性导管血管造影，并结合 CT 灌注平均转运时间（血液灌注组织区域所需的平均时间）超过 6.4 秒，这种组合的准确性几乎与导管血管造影相似。

经颅多普勒超声

经颅多普勒超声（transcranial Doppler ultrasound，TCD）可用于筛查和诊断脑血管痉挛。TCD 显示大脑前动脉和大脑中动脉（middle cerebral artery，MCA）的血流流速在 120 ～ 130 scm/s 时提示轻度血管痉挛，在 140 ～ 170 scm/s 时提示中度血管痉挛，MCA 流速 180 scm/s 且 Lindegaard 比值（MCA 与颅外颈内动脉的平均流速比值）大于 3 为重度血管痉挛。

TCD 技术具有一些局限性，因为它仅用来评估少数大动脉，并且依赖于检查人员的技术水平（例如无法获得时间窗）。当血压增加时可能出现假阳性，动脉狭窄非常严重的病例可见假阴性（由于血流量低）。

脑电图和其他技术

连续脑电图非常有助于检测癫痫样放电，并指导医师对患者进行早期治疗。此外，相比于其他技术如 TCD 和血管造影术，脑电图中 α 波活动对其他波的相对变异性降低对诊断血管痉挛的敏感度为 100%，特异度为 50%。

近红外光谱是一种测量脑血饱和度的无创技术，可用于诊断 DCI。

氙（Xe）增强 CT 扫描技术也是一种有用的无创技术，用于测量局部脑血流量。平均 Xe-rCBF（Xenon-regional CBF）值若小于 32 mL/100 g/min，且在血管造影上确诊了血管痉挛，提示为血流动力学相关的血管痉挛，则可诊断为症状性血管痉挛。

有创性脑组织监测

脑微透析是一种有创监测方法，可用于判别和监测 DCI。脑缺血与升高的谷氨酸、甘油水平以及乳酸与丙酮酸的比例增加有关。若微透析探针插入缺血区域附近，以上化合物的变化可被检测到。

热扩散流量探针是另一种有创性技术，它可用于测量局部脑血流量（regional cerebral blood flow，rCBF）。通过该技术测得的 rCBF 的降低更具灵敏度，且可成为 DCI 的特异性标志物。

预防

系统性延迟脑缺血

西洛他唑

西洛他唑（Cilostazol）是磷酸二酯酶 -3 的选择性抑制剂，并发挥血管扩张和抗血栓形成作用。西洛他唑 100 mg 口服，每天两次，持续 14 天，能够改善出院时患者预后，其预后指标可通过分析改良排序量表（modified ranking scale，mRS）进行评定。西洛他唑的严重不良反应，如出血性并发症或难治性低血压未见报道。

克拉生坦

克拉生坦（Clazosentan）是一种选择性内皮素受体 -A 拮抗剂，经测试可降低血管痉挛相关死亡率。既往有三项大型随机对照试验，即克拉生坦对抗神经性缺血和梗死临床试验 -1，-2 和 -3（Clazosentan to Overcome Neurological Ischemia and Infarction，CONSCIOUS-1，-2 和 -3），目的是测试克拉生坦对脑血管痉挛的影响。CONSCIOUS-1 显示，克拉生坦可剂量依赖地减轻中度或重度血管造影相关的血管痉挛，15 mg/h 的剂量可降低 65% 的血管痉挛风险。CONSCIOUS-1 具前景的发现促使了研究者在后续试图研究 SAH 后行夹闭术（CONSCIOUS-2）和腔内手术（CONSCIOUS-3）使用克拉生坦对脑血管痉挛的影响。CONSCIOUS-2 未能证实克拉生坦能降低死亡率或新发脑梗死率和 DCI 的发生率，这些阴性结果导致在 CONSCIOUS-3 试验中仅入选 571 名患者后就被迫提前停止了试验。然而在 CONSCIOUS-3 试验中，与安慰剂组相比，服用克拉生坦（15 mg/h）可降低血管痉挛相关死亡率和全因死亡率（15% vs. 27%；p=0.007）。综上，需要进一步研究以充分了解克拉生坦在 SAH 患者中的潜在用途。

二十碳五烯酸

ω-3 脂肪酸如二十碳五烯酸（eicosapentaenoic acid，EPA）可降低血小板反应性，并具有血管舒张作用。EPA 在 SAH 患者行夹闭术后其治疗脑血管痉挛的功效已经得到证实。治疗组的症状性血管痉挛和脑梗死的发生率显著降低，但 EPA 对通过改良排序量表（mRS）评估的临床结果无统计学差异。

促红细胞生成素

促红细胞生成素（erythropoietin，EPO）已被证明可在使用数小时内增加脑血管痉挛患者的脑氧分压。EPO 刺激 eNOS，因此它增加了流向缺血区域的血流量，其可能的潜在机制为脑的自动调节和抗炎效力的恢复。

法舒地尔

法舒地尔是一种发挥血管扩张作用的 Rho 激酶抑制剂，它将症状性血管痉挛的相对发生率降低了 30%，血管造影性血管痉挛降低了 38%。该药物是日本的标准预防性治疗，因为尼莫地平尚未在日本获得批准。在一项随机对照试验中，法舒地尔和尼莫地平在临床血管痉挛发生率或 CT 低密度发生率方面无差异。然而，分析显示，法舒地尔组患者的临床预后（GCS 评分）在 1 个月后优于尼莫地平组。

肝素

肝素增强内皮细胞的多糖蛋白质成分的完整性，并增强内皮功能，从而发挥抗炎作用。此外，其抗凝作用使肝素成为预防 DCI 的有效疗法。与对照组相比，使用剂量为 8 U/（kg·h）的肝素显著降低了症状性血管痉挛，且在研究组中无出血性并发症的报道。

尼莫地平

尼莫地平是一种电压门控钙通道拮抗剂，可抑制钙进入平滑肌细胞和神经元。美国心脏协会/美国卒中协会（American Heart Association/American Stroke Association，AHA/ASA）的最新指南（Ⅰ类，证据水平A）推荐在SAH中预防性使用尼莫地平以降低DCI和其他不良预后的风险。尼莫地平改善SAH患者的功能性预后，但对减少血管造影性血管痉挛没有影响。其神经保护作用归因于它减弱细胞缺血后神经元钙增加的事实，钙超载会导致皮质扩散缺血和细胞死亡。尼莫地平通过降低血浆中的PAI-1水平来增加纤维蛋白溶解活性。它还抑制血小板功能，因其减少了血栓素B_2的释放。尼莫地平的服用应从转入重症监护室开始，每4 h口服60 mg，持续21天。

镁

镁是生理钙拮抗剂，因此发挥血管扩张作用。然而，使用静脉注射硫酸镁治疗动脉瘤性蛛网膜下腔出血（MASH-1和-2试验）的试验未能显示硫酸镁对脑血管痉挛的任何作用。

他汀类药物

他汀类药物通过脑内皮细胞一氧化氮合酶的表达以增加脑血流量。在使用辛伐他汀治疗动脉瘤性蛛网膜下腔出血（simvastatin in aneurysmal subarachnoid hemorrhage，STASH试验）中，患者口服40 mg或80 mg辛伐他汀，每天1次，连续21天，结果显示辛伐他汀未能降低DCI的发生率或改善6个月时的mRS评分。

白蛋白

白蛋白在体内具有多种生理功能。它通过对内皮糖萼的作用来维持血管屏障的完整性。它将红细胞产生的鞘氨醇-1磷酸（sphingosine-1 phosphate，S1P）转移到内皮细胞，S1P有助于维持内皮细胞之间的紧密连接，从而维持血管屏障的完整性。此外，S1P刺激内皮细胞产生NO。值得注意的是，白蛋白是血液中NO的主要载体。白蛋白有助于减少血小板聚集，因此有助于增加血液流向缺血区域。此外，它被认为是体内的主要抗氧化剂。因此，白蛋白在局灶性脑缺血的动物模型中具有神经保护作用。

白蛋白治疗蛛网膜下腔出血（albumin in a subarachnoid hemorrhage，ALISAH）试验显示，以1.25 g/（kg·d）的剂量使用25%人白蛋白可降低血管痉挛（结合TCD）、DCI和脑梗死的发生率。

尼卡地平控释植入剂

尼卡地平是一种钙离子拮抗剂。尼卡地平植入释放剂使用仅用于行手术夹闭的患者。延着暴露的血管使用4 mg的缓释球植入剂可降低SAH患者（Fisher分级3）行夹闭术后DCI的发生率。

诱发高血压

血流动力学三H疗法包括高血容量、高血压和血液稀释，以克服痉挛血管流动阻力的增加，数十年来这一直是治疗脑血管痉挛的主要方法。然而，诱导的高血容量或血液稀释会引起多种并发症，包括肺水肿、心力衰竭、脑水肿、低钠血症和与使用非白蛋白胶体溶液相关的凝血疾病。当患者出现DCI和脑血管痉挛时，最有效的方法是通过诱发高血压以增加脑氧合。在健康的大脑中，大动脉收缩或全身性低血压引起的血压下降，可通过机体小动脉的扩张而达到代偿，该过程可将组织灌注维持在正常范围。小血管的扩张可为组织提供代谢所需的营养。然而，该代偿机制在SAH中受损。因此，当患者存在DCI时，诱导性高血压是维持脑灌注的最有效方式。最近的推荐是严格维持等量体液，避免血容量过多。初始血红蛋白水平低于9 g/dl的患者建议输血。

对于升压药和正性肌力药难以治愈的难治性心力衰竭患者，主动脉内球囊反搏（intraaortic balloon pump，IABP）可改善血管痉挛SAH患者的心功能和CBF。可见于一些高龄或是一些神经源性的心肌顿抑的SAH后患者。IABP的使用可能引起同侧下肢缺血、感染、血小板减少，假性动脉瘤和主动脉夹层。患者有主动脉夹层或主动脉瘤的情况下，应绝对禁止使用IABP。在使用IABP的最初48 h内，通常不需要使用抗凝血剂，48 h后，建议进行低剂量肝素治疗。

蛛网膜下腔血液清除

已证实，蛛网膜下腔的血液量与脑血管痉挛发展呈正相关。蛛网膜下腔血液清除技术包括腰椎引流和溶栓剂的脑池冲洗，可能有助于降低脑血管痉挛和DCI的发生率。使用头部振动器或结合局部溶栓治疗的侧向旋转治疗，这些动力疗法可清除蛛网膜下腔的血液，从而降低 DCI 的发生率。

介入神经放射治疗

介入神经放射治疗被认为是处理内科难治性脑血管痉挛的救援措施。球囊血管成形术治疗效果的持续时间长，手术可在近端痉挛的血管（例如颈内动脉）中安全地进行，此外还包括大脑中动脉的 M1 和 M2 段；大脑前动脉的 A1 和 A2 段；大脑后动脉、椎动脉和基底动脉的 P1 和 P2 段。血管成形术主要并发症的发生率为 5%，其中血管破裂的风险占 1%。动脉内解除痉挛具有短暂的效应，但仅适用于更远端的弥漫性的血管痉挛。动脉内联合应用米力农和尼莫地平似乎具有良好的解痉作用。此外，动脉内应用钙阻滞剂如尼卡地平和维拉帕米作为扩张动脉血管的药物显示具有效果。罂粟碱不作为常用的血管扩张剂，因为其具有毒害作用，如增加大脑高血压的发生、失明和神经毒性。

新型治疗方案

他莫昔芬是一种乳腺癌化疗药物，在脊髓损伤、颅内出血、脑缺血、缺氧缺血性脑损伤等动物模型中具有神经保护作用。在大鼠 SAH 模型中，应用他莫昔芬可减轻炎症，并且大鼠未表现出有早期脑损伤的证据，例如皮质水肿和血脑屏障破坏。最引人注目的是，与对照组相比，他莫昔芬治疗的大鼠完全逆转了 SAH 引发的空间工作记忆功能障碍。

格列本脲是一种抗糖尿病药，可选择性抑制磺酰脲受体 1- 瞬时受体电位美拉他汀 4 型（sulfonylurea receptor 1-transient receptor potential melastatin 4，Sur1-TRPM4）通道，该通道与神经炎症有关。因此，格列本脲目前正应用于急性中枢神经系统损伤的Ⅱ期临床试验中。

超声可通过在血管壁中引发剪切应力，从而增强了内皮一氧化氮合成酶和神经元一氧化氮合成酶活性，扩张痉挛的脑血管，改善痉挛脑血管的血流。因此，MRI 引导的经颅超声被认为是治疗脑血管痉挛的一种方案选择。

癫痫发作和预防性抗惊厥药的使用

SAH 癫痫发作的危险因素是高龄患者（大于 65 岁）行 SAH 后的动脉瘤夹闭术、蛛网膜下腔厚血凝块、脑实质内血肿或梗死。使用抗惊厥药，特别是苯妥英，可能会加重 SAH 的预后。如果需预防性使用抗惊厥药，建议短程（3 ～ 7 天）用药。

心脏并发症

心脏和大脑通过脉管系统和神经紧密相连。一旦大脑因 SAH 受损，副交感神经功能障碍可能会引起心律失常，并导致炎性细胞因子释放，进入血管系统。受损心脏释放的炎症因子，可诱发脑部产生炎症反应。此外，过量脂肪组织会释放脂肪因子，会增加脑损伤后的神经炎症易感性。因此，在 SAH 期间，动脉粥样硬化和糖尿病可以动员免疫系统，并加剧炎症反应。

SAH 患者的心脏表现可包括心电图异常，如 QT 间期延长、T 波倒置、心律失常和左心室（left ventricle，LV）功能障碍。

Takotsubo 心肌病

应激性心肌病或 Takotsubo 心肌病（Takotsubo cardiomyopathy，TC）于 20 世纪 90 年代初在日本首次被报道。它的日本名称来自左心室特征性外观，在急性冠状动脉综合征的评估时，冠状动脉造影检查的心室造影发现：由于心室尖端节段的顿抑，左心室呈圆底窄颈状，心尖部变钝，形状类似日本章鱼陷阱（日语发音 takotsubo）。以上特征也解释了为什么 TC 也被称为“短暂的心尖气球综合征”。TC 的病理生理学假说认为 SAH 导致下丘脑损伤，促使心交感神经终端释放过量儿茶酚胺，从而引起心肌损伤。SAH 后 TC 的发生率介于 1% 和 6% 之间，主要影响绝经后的女性，表现为心肌酶的升高和 ST 段的偏离，包括心电图上不常见的 ST 段抬高和 T 波倒置。TC 的特征在于冠状动脉血管造影中表现为非阻塞性冠状动脉疾病。SAH 诱导的 LV 受损通常在 2 ～ 4 周内消退，且与不良后遗症无关。

针对 TC 主要采取支持性治疗，例如正性肌力支持、主动脉内球囊反搏和积极利尿。严重 TC 病例可能因左心室心尖血栓的形成而复杂化，此时针对患 TC 的 SAH 患者，是否需要进行抗凝治疗会成为左右为难的问题。

低钠血症

低钠血症在 SAH 患者中非常常见，多达 57% 的 SAH 患者发生低钠血症。低钠血症的临床表现包括轻度低钠血症的注意力不集中和步态紊乱、癫痫发作，急性重症低钠血症引起的脑水肿增加甚至死亡。低钠血症与几种急危病有关，特别是 1950 年首次描述的脑耗盐综合征（cerebral wasting syndrome，CSW）和抗利尿激素分泌不适当综合征（syndrome of inappropriate antidiuretic hormone，SIADH）。CSW 患者循环利钠尿肽水平升高，该激素可加速盐的肾性丢失和尿钠排泄，从而导致负钠平衡、低钠血症和血管内液体流失。SIADH 是由抗利尿激素分泌异常增加引起的，导致机体无法适当地排泄游离水，导致血容量过多。这两种疾病都与尿渗透压和尿钠浓度的不适当升高有关。因此，区分 SIADH 和 CSW 主要基于对患者体液状态和尿量的评估。

低钠血症的血钠浓度不能在 24 h 内矫正超过 12 ～ 24 mmol/L，以避免脑桥中央脱髓鞘。在低钠血症治疗期间维持正常血容量对于避免 DCI 至关重要，因此，应慎重对 SAH 患者限制液体。考尼伐坦（Conivaptan）是血管加压素受体拮抗剂，可用于治疗 SAH 患者因 SIADH 而引起的低钠血症，也可以使用盐酸地美环素（demeclocycline hydrochloride）。使用皮质类固醇（如氟氢可的松和氢化可的松）可有效地限制过量的尿钠排泄和低钠血症，特别是在 CSW 的情况下。此外，可尝试使用 3% 盐水来治疗低钠血症。

高钠血症

SAH 患者中高钠血症比低钠血症少见，这可能是血容量不足，或是使用高渗盐水 / 甘露醇治疗脑水肿的结果。若患者血容量不足且尿液低渗，尿崩症可能是高钠血症的另一个原因。

高血糖

对 SAH 患者实施宽松葡萄糖管理时，当葡萄糖浓度超过 220 mg/dl 时与感染风险增加有关。然而，发现若通过胰岛素输注以达到严格血糖控制（80 ～ 110 mg/dl），这会增加低血糖的发作，且与更多的血管痉挛有关，对患者 3 个月的临床预后更加不利。葡萄糖控制临床试验（Normoglycemia in Intensive Care Evaluation and Survival Using Glucose Algorithm Regulation，NICE-SUGAR 试验）发现使用胰岛素输注严格控制血糖会影响患者预后。因此，共识推荐是避免低血糖（血清 <80 mg/dl）并将血糖维持在 200 mg/dl 以下。如果使用微透析进行监测，可以调整血清葡萄糖以避免大脑低血糖。

肺部并发症

肺部并发症几乎占所有致命性内科并发症的一半，并且主要与治疗脑血管痉挛所使用的高血容量和血液稀释疗法有关。氧合受损是最常见的肺部异常，其定义是指肺泡和动脉的氧分压差大于 100 mm Hg，或动脉血氧分压与吸入氧浓度的比值（PaO_2 : FiO_2）小于 300，这样的患者约占所有 SAH 患者的 80%。氧合能力受损的主要原因是 SAH 患者常合并急性肺损伤（acute lung injury，ALI）和急性呼吸窘迫综合征。神经源性肺水肿也常见于 SAH 患者，通常是由于 SAH 患者早期体内的儿茶酚胺激增，从而影响肺血管内皮和心肌，这可能是 SAH 患者发生 ALI 的重要原因。

其他常见肺部并发症包括肺炎（15% ～ 20%）、充血性心力衰竭（8%）、气胸（3%）和肺栓塞。

对于并发症来说，预防胜于治疗。因此，预防措施包括预防医院获得性和呼吸机相关性肺炎、预防深静脉血栓形成、预防呼吸机相关肺损伤，对于预防 SAH 患者肺部并发症是必不可少的。应对正行机械通气的 SAH 患者常规使用具有呼气末正压的肺保护和小潮气量策略。至关重要的是，应保持控制 SAH 患者的血容量，避免液体超负荷，从而避免医源性肺水肿，并控制神经源性肺水肿。

结论

SAH 仅占所有卒中的 5%，但病死率高（40%），部分死亡原因是 DCI 和 SAH 后的神经系统并发症。SAH 影响心脏、肺和其他身体系统。早期识别和处理这些并发症将有助于改善患者的预后。

（谭可哲　译　卞金俊　校）

延伸阅读

Bonow RH, Silber JR, Enzmann DR, et al.: Towards use of MRI-guided ultrasound for treating cerebral vasospasm, *J Ther Ultrasound* 4(6):1–8, 2016.

Campi A, Ramzi N, Molyneux AJ, et al.: Retreatment of ruptured cerebral aneurysms in patients randomized by coiling or clipping in the International Subarachnoid Aneurysm Trial (ISAT), *Stroke* 38(5):1538–1544, 2007.

Chalouhi N, Zanaty M, Whiting A, et al.: Treatment of ruptured intracranial aneurysms with the pipeline embolization device, *Neurosurgery* 76:165–172, 2015.

Farag E, Ebrahim Z, Taul D, et al.: Perioperative management of intracranial aneurysm and subarachnoid hemorrhage, *Curr Pharm Des* 19:5792–5808, 2013.

Fiorella D, Woo HH, Albuquerque FC, et al.: Definitive reconstruction of circumferential, fusiform intracranial aneurysms with the pipeline embolization device, *Neurosurgery* 62(5):1115–1120, 2008. discussion 1120–1121.

Ghods AJ, Lopes D, Chen M: Gender differences in cerebral aneurysm location, *Front Neurol* 3:78, 2012.

Green DM, Burns JD, DeFusco CM: ICU management of aneurysmal subarachnoid hemorrhage, *J Intensive Care Med* 28(6):341–354, 2012.

Khurana VG, Sohni YR, Mangrum WI, et al.: Endothelial nitric oxide synthase gene polymorphisms predict susceptibility to aneurysmal subarachnoid hemorrhage and cerebral vasospasm, *J Cereb Blood Flow Metab* 24:291–297, 2004.

Koivisto T, Vanninen R, Hurskainen H, et al.: Outcomes of early endovascular versus surgical treatment of ruptured cerebral aneurysms: a prospective randomized study, *Stroke* 31(10):2369–2377, 2000.

Korbakis G, Prabhakaran S, John S, et al.: MRI detection of cerebral infarction in subarachnoid hemorrhage, *Neurocrit Care* 24:428–435, 2016.

Lucke-Wold BP, Logsdon AF, Manoranjan B, et al.: Aneurysmal subarachnoid hemorrhage and neuroinflammation: a comprehensive review, *Int J Mol Sci* 17:497, 2016.

Macdonald RL: Delayed neurological deterioration after subarachnoid hemorrhage, *Nat Rev Neurol* 10:44–58, 2014.

Molyneux AJ, Birks J, Clarke A, et al.: The durability of endovascular coiling versus neurosurgical clipping of ruptured cerebral aneurysms: 18 year follow-up of the UK cohort of the International Subarcahnoid Aneurysm Trial (ISAT), *Lancet* 385(9969):691–697, 2015.

Molyneux A, Kerr R, Stratton I, et al.: International Subarachnoid Aneurysm Trial (ISAT) of neurosurgical clipping versus endovascular coiling in 2143 patients with ruptured intracranial aneurysms: a randomised trial, *Lancet* 360(9342):1267–1274, 2002.

Molyneux AJ, Kerr RS, Yu LM, et al.: International subarachnoid aneurysm trial (ISAT) of neurosurgical clipping versus endovascular coiling in 2143 patients with ruptured intracranial aneurysms: a randomised comparison of effects on survival, dependency, seizures, rebleeding, subgroups, and aneurysm occlusion, *Lancet* 366(9488): 809–817, 2005.

Spetzler RF, McDougall CG, Zabramski JM, et al.: The Barrow Ruptured Aneurysm Trial: 6-year results, *J Neurosurg* 123(3):609–617, 2015.

Vajkoczy P, Horn P, Thome C, et al.: Regional cerebral flow monitoring in the diagnosis of delayed ischemia following aneurysmal subarachnoid hemorrhage, *J Neurosurg* 98:1227–1234, 2003.

Veldeman M, Höllig A, Clusmann H, et al.: Delayed cerebral ischemia prevention and treatment after aneurysmal subarachnoid hemorrhage: a systemic review, *Br J Anaesth* 117(1):17–40, 2016.

Vergouwen MDI, Frijns CJM, Roos YBW, et al.: Plasminogen activator inhibitor-1 4G allele in the 4G/5G promoter polymorphism increases the occurrence of cerebral ischemia after aneurysmal subarachnoid hemorrhage, *Stroke* 35:1280–1283, 2004.

Vergouwen MDI, Vermeulen M, Coert BA, et al.: Micro thrombosis after aneurysmal subarachnoid hemorrhage: an additional explanation for delayed cerebral ischemia, *J Cereb Blood Flow Metab* 28: 1761–1770, 2008.

Weiner MM, Asher DI, Augoustides JG, et al.: Takotsubo cardiomyopathy: a clinical update for the cardiovascular anesthesiologist, *J Cardiothorac Vasc Anesth*, 2016. [Epub ahead of print].

第62章 喉镜和显微喉镜

Joshua H. Atkins

病例概要

患者，肥胖男性 [体重指数（body mass index，BMI）=41]，62岁，有喉癌病史，拟行显微直接喉镜检查、食管镜检查和支气管镜检查，以评估最近正电子发射体层成像（positron emission tomography，PET）检查发现的阳性病变灶。既往患有慢性阻塞性肺疾病（吸家用氧气 2 L）、高血压、高脂血症、吸烟史（35 包年），因患喉癌曾接受过经口机器人手术和随后的放射治疗。他在外科诊所接受过鼻咽喉镜检查，结果显示没有明显的肿块、喉部水肿及瘢痕。在使用丙泊酚和瑞芬太尼全身麻醉诱导后，出现面罩通气困难，但仍足以维持氧饱和度大于 90%。气道立即移交给耳鼻喉科专科医师处理。使用 Jackson 外科喉镜无法看到喉部。继续行面罩通气，随后使用前联合镜进行暴露，以便将 4% 利多卡因喉气管喷洒器和金属吸引导管通过声门。通过金属吸引导管启用高频喷射通气（频率 120，驱动压力 22 psi，吸气时间为 40%，FiO_2 100%）。静脉推注 10 mg 麻黄碱治疗低血压（血压 90/50 mmHg）和心动过缓（心率 48 次 / 分），手术操作完成，未进行活检，无出血。外科医师将一根 6.0 的气管插管通过前联合镜插入，待患者完全清醒后拔除。困难气道标识戴好后，患者被转运至麻醉恢复室。

问题分析

术前评估

接受显微直接喉镜检查（microdirect laryngoscopy，MDL）及相关操作的患者通常有显著的并存疾病。通过对喉及相关癌症进行先进的诊断和治疗性干预，患者的预期寿命得到了提高。围术期医疗团队最大的担心是气道相关并发症，尤其是气道失去控制。越来越多曾接受过气道手术、放射治疗或手术与放射联合治疗的患者，到手术室进行活检或评估 PET 阳性复发率。喉部肿块可在全麻诱导后阻塞气道，阻挡声门视野，妨碍气管导管通过声门开口，或在喉镜检查时易损伤出血。放疗引起纤维化、水肿，导致组织活动度下降，这可能是影响声门暴露的关键。除了喉镜检查外，常规检查还包括食管镜检查和纤维支气管镜检查。气道解剖异常，尤其是放射治疗后喉部活动度降低，也可能给气管造口术或紧急环甲膜切开术带来困难。

管理

手术计划与管理

耳鼻喉科医师可在手术室麻醉诱导前患者清醒状态下，再次进行鼻咽喉镜检查以重新评估气道。虽然这不能像喉镜那样直接评判声门的暴露情况，但能提供有关水肿的程度和脆弱组织的范围、肿块大小和位置等信息，以及经鼻纤支镜插管用于紧急抢救的可行性。亦有推荐通过外部操作评估伸舌和甲状软骨处喉部的活动性。如果甲状软骨固定且颈部纤维化，则可能无法进行喉移位以使声门与管 / 喉镜视图对齐。应在诱导前确定急诊气管切开术的标志，包括环甲膜和低位气管。放射治疗后，这些标志可能难以触及或覆盖在炎性瘢痕组织中。超声逐渐成为识别环甲韧带的有效工具，尽管在放射治疗颈部的应用中尚未得到详尽阐述。在这种情况下应考虑“清醒暴露”喉镜检查，用 2% ～ 4% 利多卡因雾化吸入气道表面后，可以将视频喉镜轻轻地放入口腔中，如果能获得较好的视野就可以用这种方式插管，或者移除喉镜并诱导全身麻醉。在任何气道程序中，耳鼻喉科专家都应该在手术室中，包括“清醒暴露”和全身麻醉的诱导，外科气道工具车应在手术室内时刻处于备用状态。当发生插管困难但不存在通气困难时，可以考虑使用七氟烷进行吸入诱导。一旦通过维持自主呼吸达到足够的麻醉深度，外科医师或麻醉科医师就可以进行初步喉镜检查来评估气道。如果视野不足，则可以通过声门上气道（supraglottic airway，SGA）借助光纤插管或经口气道插管。由于之前的气道手术改变了解剖结构，SGA 可能更难定位或封闭，文献中很少有关于这个问题的指导。我们更倾向于在全身麻醉诱导后，外科医师直接进行手术喉镜检查，以尽量减少尝试的次数，并具备立即在床边抢救气道所需的专业能力。如果手术暴露 / 插管 / 喉镜检查困难，且外科医师认为水肿、声带功能障碍或肿瘤生长有可能恶化，则应考虑进行气管造口术以保护术后气道。否则，应在完全清醒后才能拔管，并且外科喉镜设备随时备用，耳鼻喉科专家必须在场。如前所述，针对气道评估和规划的详细的团队化协作对于减少这种情况下的气道并发症不可或缺。

除气道丧失外，由 MDL、支气管镜检查和食管镜检查引发的其他潜在并发症包括食管穿孔、气胸、牙齿损伤和血流动力学变化。食管穿孔非常罕见，而牙齿损伤较常见。患有马里兰牙桥的患者在喉镜悬吊时，即使使用了牙科防护装置，也可能特别容易受到这种损伤，因为在喉镜悬吊期间，牙桥上的压力会造成这种损伤。气胸常被认为是高频喷射通气的并发症，这是继发于高驱动压力（尤其是儿科或 Sanders 型注射器中）或者供氧通道关闭导致的过度充盈，导致呼吸叠加和压力相关的损害。在实施 MDL 时，后一种情况极不可能，因为在整个手术过程中可以直视声门。如果患者有严重的远端气管狭窄，仍可能发生呼吸叠加。Acutronic Monsoon 等自动喷射通风装置可降低此类并发症的风险。如果达到高压阈值，氧气输送管线末端的压力传感器将触发警报并关闭输送。驱动压力应限制在小于 2 个大气压（28.4 psi）以下，以限制气胸的风险。最常见的血流动力学变化是由刺激引起的高血压或与喉镜相关的迷走神经张力引起的心动过缓。丙泊酚是一种很好的药物，特别是与瑞芬太尼联合使用，可以抑制喉镜引起的交感神经反应。瑞芬太尼可能与心动过缓有关。麻黄碱、格隆溴铵和小剂量阿托品都是治疗影响血流动力学的严重心动过缓的合理选择。

激光消融术是治疗非恶性声带病变或乳头状瘤的常用方法。与此方法相关的主要风险包括气道着火以及对手术室内患者及医护人员的激光烧伤，包括眼睛损伤。患者和护理人员应佩戴防护眼镜，患者的眼睛和面部应覆盖湿毛巾。在激光使用期间，吸入氧浓度应降低到 30% 或以下。可考虑采用抗激光气管插管、金属吸引导管喷射通气或间歇性呼吸暂停技术。在镇静状态或局部麻醉下，在气道附近进行激光治疗时，应使用空气氧气混合器。如果发生激光相关的气道着火，应立即停止通气，移除易燃气道装置，并用生理盐水熄灭。然后进行面罩通气，并使用柔性支气管镜检查评估气道，以指导进一步的治疗。

预防

术后注意事项

应持续警惕以观察术后气道是否发生损伤。在床边通过体格检查和鼻咽镜检查可快速评估诸如喘鸣、呼吸短促或咯血等症状。手术室内的困难气道，要比在手术室外紧急情况下变得更具挑战性。充分的器械准备和沟通协调的管理细节将是关键因素。困难气道的标识设计（例如手环）和用于困难气道紧急再插管的书面方案亦应考虑。这也将有助于提高后续麻醉的安全性。

（沈　玲　译　朱科明　校）

延伸阅读

Atkins JH, Mirza N, Mandel JE: Case report: respiratory inductance plethysmography as a monitor of ventilation during laser ablation and balloon dilatation of subglottic tracheal stenosis, *ORL J Otorhinolaryngol Relat Spec* 71(5):289–291, 2009.

Atkins JH, Mandel JE, Weinstein GS, et al.: A pilot study of respiratory inductance plethysmography as a safe, noninvasive detector of jet ventilation under general anesthesia, *Anesth Analg* 111:1168–1175, 2010.

Biro P: Jet ventilation for surgical interventions in the upper airway, *Anesthesiol Clin* 28:397–409, 2010.

Bruins BB, Mirza N, Gomez E, Atkins JH: Anesthetic management for laser excision of ball-valving laryngeal masses, *Case Rep Anesthesiol* 2015:875053, 2015.

Hill RS, Koltai PJ, Parnes SM: Airway complications from laryngoscopy and panendoscopy, *Ann Otol Rhinol Laryngol* 96:691–697, 1987.

Klussmann JP, Knoedgen R, Wittekindt C, et al.: Complications of suspension laryngoscopy, *Ann Otol Rhinol Laryngol* 111:972–976, 2002.

Mason RA, Fielder CP: The obstructed airway in head and neck surgery, *Anaesthesia J* 54(7):625–628, 1999.

Siddiqui N, Arzola C, Friedman Z, et al.: Ultrasound improves cricothyrotomy success in cadavers with poorly defined neck anatomy: a randomized control trial, *Anesthesiology* 123:1033–1041, 2015.

第63章 心肺转流术后主要器官系统功能障碍

M. Tracy Zundel，*Paul S. Pagel*

病例概要

患者，老年男性，67岁，患重度主动脉瓣狭窄（主动脉瓣面积 $0.5\ cm^2$）、重度二尖瓣反流、冠状动脉疾病、左心室收缩功能障碍（射血分数30%）和慢性肾功能不全（血清肌酐浓度167 μmol/L）行主动脉瓣置换、二尖瓣成形术和双支冠状动脉旁路移植术（coronary artery bypass graft，CABG）。行心肺转流术（cardiopulmonary bypass，CPB；又称体外循环）时间为235 min。患者在最初尝试脱离CPB期间处于低血压（平均动脉压为40 mmHg）。经食管超声心动图显示心肌功能严重受抑制。重新启动CPB，开始静脉输注肾上腺素和去甲肾上腺素，尽管采取了这些干预措施，但第二次尝试脱离CPB仍未成功。经右侧股动脉置入主动脉内球囊泵，同时持续静脉泵注正性肌力药物支持，患者成功脱离CPB。患者需输注新鲜冰冻血浆、血小板和低温冷沉淀物后方可完成止血和关胸，随后被转移到ICU。术后患者需机械循环辅助和血管活性药物来维持适当的平均动脉压和心排血量。患者有躁动，需在麻醉苏醒后采用右美托咪定清醒镇静。术后血清肌酐浓度逐渐升高，患者最终需持续静脉至静脉透析治疗急性肾损伤。尽管吸入高浓度氧（PaO_2/FiO_2 比值<100）、采用肺保护性机械通气策略、允许性高碳酸血症、气道呼气末正压 $15\ cmH_2O$，但患者仍有持续的低氧血症。胸部X线影像符合急性呼吸窘迫综合征。患者术后第3天还发生了心房颤动。

问题分析

定义

机械效应和生理上的变化共同导致CPB相关器官系统的功能障碍。由于暴露于CPB装置，术中和术后严重的全身炎症反应介导了CPB不良生理后果，造成了对血流的阻碍、空气或颗粒物栓塞以及血管损伤。手术创伤、失血和低温共同导致了这种炎性反应。三种不同机制产生了由CPB导致的强烈促炎状态。首先，血液与外源性体外循环装置表面（如塑料管道和插管、氧合器组件）的相互作用通过生成促炎细胞因子（如白介素-6和白细胞介素-10、肿瘤坏死因子-α）、刺激补体级联反应，以及激活细胞毒性白细胞引起体液和细胞免疫反应。其次，放置和松开主动脉阻断钳导致的心肌缺血再灌注损伤，也造成了来自激活中性粒细胞的炎症介质和大量活性氧的生成。第三，CPB期间的灌注不足导致胃肠黏膜屏障损伤，从而促进细菌易位和免疫系统的激活。针对CPB的全身炎性反应从根本上改变了微血管灌注和血管内皮的功能完整性。这些作用导致终末器官血流受损，并伴随CPB后毛细血管通透性增强（图63.1）。

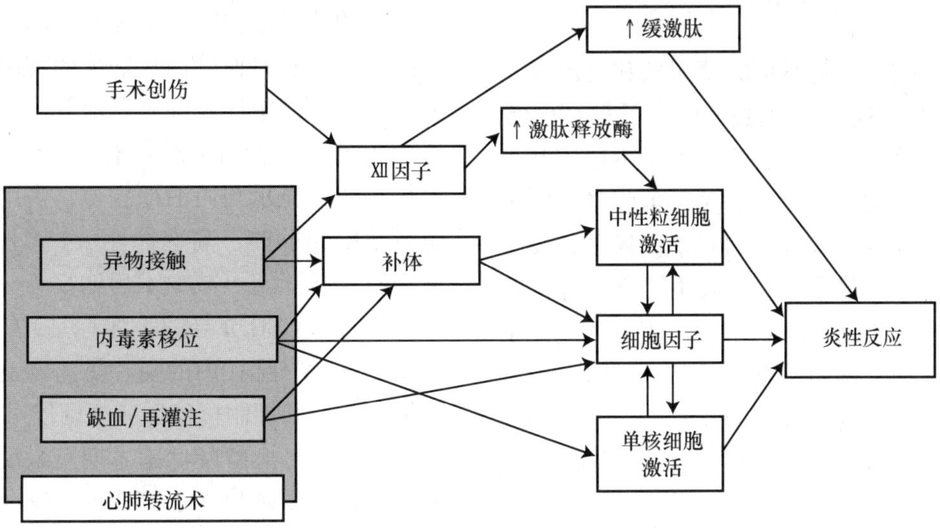

图 63.1 心肺转流术期间的炎症激活途径

识别

CPB 的机械并发症可导致灾难性损伤。动脉血流或静脉引流受阻、空气栓塞、急性主动脉夹层、主动脉斑块移位和栓塞、流入道和流出道错位是 CPB 主要的机械并发症（表 63.1）。CPB 炎性反应的临床表现可能更微妙，但最常见的原因是补体级联反应激活和促炎细胞因子生成所致的低血压和心肌、肺、肾、腹部脏器和中枢神经系统血管床的灌注不足。例如，CPB 后肾功能可能恶化，并随后进展为足够严重的急性肾衰竭，需要暂时或永久性（不太常见）血液透析。肺毛细血管内皮的通透性增加促进了肺水肿的发生，其特征是肺顺应性降低和气体交换受损。脑微血管中白细胞聚集所致的微血管阻塞对精神状态造成不利影响，产生谵妄，或引起无局灶神经系统病变的认知损害。可能发生伴有或不伴有房性或室性心律失常的心肌收缩力降低，从而进一步造成血流动力学不稳定、低血压、终末器官灌注不足和需血管活性药循环支持。

表 63.1 CPB 机械并发症的检测

并发症	检测
主动脉夹层	目视检测插管或主动脉 流入压力异常 外周动脉波形改变
主动脉斑块移位	胸部 X 线片检查 主动脉造影 经食管超声心动图或血管上超声心动图 直接触摸
静脉引流梗阻	检查头部和颈静脉 心肺转流术期间中心静脉压突发或意外改变
栓塞	经食管超声心动图 经颅多普勒 心肺转流术回路中气泡检测器 动脉过滤器
脑灌注不足	心肺转流术期间动脉压和流量监测 低温 混合静脉血氧饱和度监测 脑电图

由于 CPB 导致的损害主要通过全身炎性反应介导，临床体征和症状常常与其他炎症病因引起的体征和症状非常相似。而这种炎性反应的表现可能不是在所有器官系统中都能观察到。尽管存在 CPB 诱导的促炎状态，但不一定存在发热，白细胞计数可能保持在正常范围内。尿量可能减少但在沉淀物分析中不一定有急性肾小管坏死的证据。肺顺应性和气体交换的改变通常不具特异性，在严重程度上有变化，且通常类似于由其他病因引起的急性呼吸窘迫综合征。躁动、谵妄和认知受损可能也存在差异，但这些发现比局灶性神经功能缺损本身更常见。通常存在动脉压低下，由心排血量、体血管阻力降低所致，或两者兼而有之，但同样重要的是强调这种血流动力学紊乱在所有伴有 CPB 诱导的全身促炎状态的患者中并非始终存在。

风险评估

在行心脏手术的所有患者中，暴露于 CPB 总会引起某种程度的全身炎症，但 CPB 前存在或 CPB 期间发生的几种因素与临床相关的全身炎性反应有关。

术前因素

冠状动脉疾病、控制不良的糖尿病和之前存在左心室收缩功能障碍增加了促炎细胞因子对CPB反应的强度。这一反应与术后血流动力学不稳定和主要心血管不良事件的风险增加有关。术前肾功能不全也加剧对CPB的炎性反应，最可能的原因是减少促炎介质的清除。一般来说，伴有更严重并存疾病的患者在心脏手术期间暴露于CPB时更有可能产生更明显的炎症反应。例如，血浆促炎细胞因子浓度在接受心脏或肺移植的患者中明显较高，至少部分是因为存在难治性心力衰竭或终末期肺部疾病。

术中因素

CPB持续时间

包括全身炎性反应在内的CPB相关并发症的发病率和严重程度直接取决于CPB的持续时间。CPB持续时间与血浆白介素浓度、中性粒细胞黏附程度有关；这些因素增加了CPB后并发症的风险。血流量持续降低也导致与长时间CPB有关的终末器官损伤。例如，CPB期间腹部脏器灌注不足增加了胃肠黏膜的通透性，这种作用的不良后果（如肠梗阻、细菌移位、内毒素暴露）在CPB时间延长时更常见。同样，肺缺血再灌注损伤、肺血管内皮功能障碍和临床上显著的低氧血症随着CPB持续时间的增加更可能发生。

与CPB有关的因素

目前尚不清楚CPB期间采用的氧合器、泵或CPB回路或低温的程度是否影响所致炎性反应的程度和持续时间。例如，膜式氧合器引起的炎症比鼓泡式氧合器轻，但这种差异似乎未转化成临床上有意义的术后肺功能的改善。同样，未观察到基于CPB预充成分或CPB所用泵的类型对结果的明显影响。搏动性CPB血流与内毒素释放较少和较低的细胞因子浓度有关，但与连续血流技术相比，这些因素似乎并未显著影响临床结果。与低温CPB相比，中低温CPB增加了对CPB的炎性反应。相反，中低温停搏液减少了随后的炎症。

麻醉药物和技术

麻醉药发挥免疫调节作用，但这些作用对暴露于CPB患者的相对临床重要性仍未得到解决。挥发性麻醉药，包括七氟烷和异氟烷，在缺血再灌注损伤存在的情况下，降低了炎性细胞因子活性并减弱了中性粒细胞对血管内皮功能的细胞毒性作用。丙泊酚还可抑制中性粒细胞激活并可促进抗炎细胞因子的生成。尽管丙泊酚具有这些潜在的有益作用，但最近研究显示与丙泊酚相比，当用于心脏手术后患者清醒镇静时，高选择性 α_2 肾上腺素能受体激动剂右美托咪定可减少术后谵妄（一种神经系统并发症，常与CPB介导的炎症有关）的发病率和严重程度。包括吗啡在内的阿片类药物也可通过下调免疫细胞功能和抑制抗体反应来调控对CPB的炎性反应。胸硬膜外麻醉降低围术期应激反应，该技术基本上不影响细胞因子对CPB的反应。

输血

异体输血增加了对CPB炎性反应的强度。回收的纵隔血自体回输也增加炎性反应，因为这种血液中常含有高浓度促炎细胞因子。洗涤（血细胞回收器）设备可显著降低炎症介质的浓度，但通常洗涤后的血液中比自身循环中观察到存在更多的中性粒细胞。使用这些洗涤设备不影响CPB相关并发症的发生率。

启示

与CPB相关的全身炎症的影响可能是深远的。CPB导致中性粒细胞隔离进入肺部，导致肺上皮和内皮损伤。随之而来的肺血管内皮通透性增加引起间质和肺泡水肿，氧合下降和肺顺应性降低。肺功能检查显示结果变差，分别有12%和3%暴露于CPB的患者发生急性肺损伤。CPB持续时间和所致的肺损伤发病率和严重程度之间直接相关。术后神经功能障碍也与CPB的炎性反应有关。脑血管微栓塞、中性粒细胞活化导致的内皮损伤、一氧化氮代谢异常介导的脑微血管中血管运动控制功能障碍可能是导致神经损伤的机制。CPB后约有1/3和2/3的患者可能发生谵妄和认知功能损害，而局灶性神经功能缺损较少见（1%～3%）。术后认知功能受损可能是暂时的或永久的，与实际发病率相关，并对心脏手术后的生活质量有深远影响。

暴露于CPB的患者有7%～13%发生围术期肾功能障碍，显著增加了死亡风险，尤其是当需要血液透析时。CPB炎性反应导致急性肾损伤的具体机制尚不完全清楚，但缺血再灌注损伤和血管调节功能受损可能在这一病理生理过程中发挥重要作用。

CPB 后凝血功能障碍可能也与全身炎性反应有关。血小板功能障碍、补体和纤维蛋白溶解级联反应的激活以及促炎细胞因子浓度的升高与 CPB 的凝血障碍有关。值得注意的是，CPB 期间较低浓度的促炎细胞因子与心脏手术后失血减少有关。这些数据提供了 CPB 后发生的 CPB 介导的全身炎症与凝血功能受损相关的间接证据。

治疗

终末器官功能障碍的一级预防和二级支持疗法是治疗 CPB 后炎症状态的主要原则。为了实现这些目标，已经提出了许多可能有用的策略，但迄今为止还未确定单一的具体干预措施可明确地减轻 CPB 的炎性反应并降低相关的并发症和死亡率。

避免体外循环 / 主动脉阻断

非体外循环下 CABG 减轻但非完全消除与体外循环下 CABG 相关的全身炎症状态。然而，非体外循环下和体外循环下 CABG 在炎症方面的这一差异很可能无助于改善并发症和死亡率，因为最近几项大型随机临床试验表明，这两项技术导致的预后基本相同。

肝素涂层体外循环回路

肝素涂层体外循环回路减少了接触介导的补体、因子Ⅻ和中性粒细胞激活。白细胞过滤进一步增强了这些有益作用。临床试验表明，高危患者可能受益于这些干预措施，特别是长时间 CPB 和主动脉阻断时。

选择性胃肠去污染

早期临床试验结果提示术前口服非吸收性抗生素可降低胃肠道细菌易位所致的内毒素浓度，并可降低 CPB 后术后感染的风险。尽管这些初步结果很有希望，但这一方法与心脏手术患者的死亡率降低没有明确的联系。

血液滤过

采用血液滤过刻意将炎症介质从循环中去除可降低 CPB 介导的炎性反应的严重程度。血液滤过可减轻肾损伤和减轻 CPB 后肺部并发症的严重程度，但这项技术似乎并未显著影响整体结果。

皮质类固醇

在实验动物中进行的研究表明皮质类固醇可降低 CPB 对肺、心脏、肾和血液功能的炎症后果。在小型临床试验中，皮质类固醇也被证明可降低 CPB 后促炎细胞因子和内毒素的浓度。尽管有这些发现，围术期给予皮质类固醇未提供明显的临床益处，也未改善暴露于 CPB 的患者的预后。

支持疗法

减轻 CPB 炎症后果是支持疗法的核心。维持血流动力学稳定明显降低了后续缺血再灌注损伤的程度。建议采用肺保护机械通气法治疗 CPB 的不良肺部影响，避免肺泡过度膨胀、气压损伤和进一步的损害。与 CPB 相关的急性肾损伤可能需要血液透析直至肾功能改善。与其他透析技术相比，在心血管不稳定患者中持续静脉至静脉血液透析具有明显优势。高血糖需积极治疗（最常用静脉滴注胰岛素），使目标血糖浓度介于 6.11 ～ 10 mmol/L 之间，因为血糖浓度持续升高与心脏手术患者的并发症和死亡率有关。维持正常电解质，围术期使用 β_1 肾上腺素受体阻滞剂或临时左心房或双心房起搏可降低高危患者术后心房颤动的发生率。最后，重要的是强调脓毒症可能与 CPB 相关的全身炎症的临床表现密切相关。CPB 后出现血管扩张、低血压、肺毛细血管通透性增高伴低氧血症、急性肾功能不全、心肌功能不全不仅需要支持疗法，而且应及时检查全身感染情况。导管相关性脓毒症、纵隔炎、心内膜炎和肺部或尿道感染是术后心脏手术患者可能的感染源，应谨慎排除。

（徐业好　译　朱文忠　校）

延伸阅读

Anselmi A, Abbate A, Girola F, et al.: Myocardial ischemia, stunning, inflammation, and apoptosis during cardiac surgery: a review of evidence, *Eur J Cardiothorac Surg* 25:304–311, 2004.

Asimakopoulos G, Gourlay T: A review of anti-inflammatory strategies in cardiac surgery, *Perfusion* 18:7–12, 2003.

Chaney MA: Corticosteroids and cardiopulmonary bypass: a review of clinical investigations, *Chest* 121:921–931, 2002.

Laffey JG, Boylan JF, Cheng DCH: The systemic inflammatory response to cardiac surgery: implications for the anesthesiologist, *Anesthesiology* 97:215–252, 2002.

Paparella D, Yau TM, Young E: Cardiopulmonary bypass induced inflammation: pathophysiology and treatment. An update, *Eur J Cardiothorac Surg* 21:232–244, 2002.

Rady MY, Ryan T, Starr NJ: Early onset of acute pulmonary dysfunction after cardiovascular surgery: risk factors and clinical outcome, *Crit Care Med* 25:1831–1839, 1997.

第64章 纵隔肿块

Rebecca M. Gerlach，*Jerome M. Klafta*

病例概要

患者，男性，23岁，平素体健，拟行颈部纵隔镜检查以进行纵隔肿块组织学诊断。自述有3个月的疲乏和劳力性呼吸困难史，用于气短不能左侧卧位入睡。胸部CT显示右心房、升主动脉和肺动脉主干附近有一个10 cm × 8 cm × 5 cm的肿块，其他无异常。经丙泊酚和琥珀胆碱诱导后，患者插管顺利，但氧饱和度迅速降低。经积极手动通气后仍不能改善氧合，患者血压进行性下降。

问题分析

定义

患有前纵隔肿块的患者易发生潜在的、危及生命的并发症，因为这些肿块对邻近结构（上腔静脉、气管分叉或主支气管、肺动脉主干、主动脉弓和心脏）产生影响。前纵隔肿块患者麻醉的主要应注意以下三种潜在并发症：

- 气管支气管树受压或阻塞；
- 上腔静脉综合征；
- 心脏和肺血管受压。

此外，患者可因各种原因需接受麻醉或麻醉监护，包括：

- 胸内肿瘤切除术（原发或转移）；
- 淋巴结活检（用于组织诊断）；
- 中心静脉置管（用于化疗）；
- 胸内肿块活检（开胸或胸腔镜）；
- 任何其他手术，不论与纵隔肿块有关（如病理性骨折的开放复位和内固定）或无关（剖宫产）；
- 影像检查（儿童）。

虽然这些肿块被称为"前（纵隔肿块）"，但通常位于前纵隔、上纵隔和中纵隔的交汇处（图64.1）。

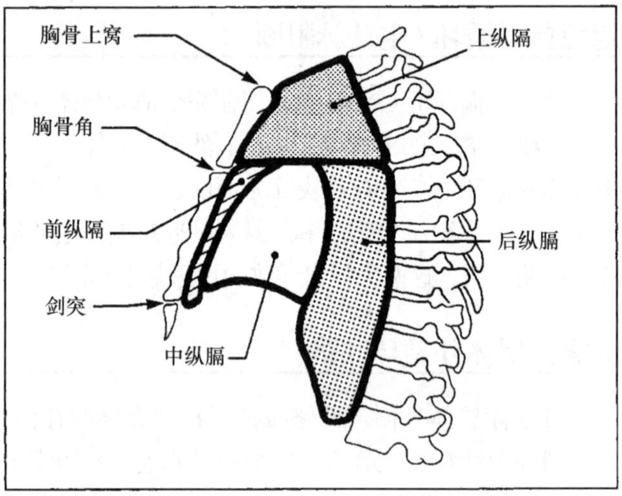

图64.1 纵隔分为上纵隔和下纵隔，下纵隔又分为前、中、后纵隔（From Benumof JL：*Anesthesia for thoracic surgery*，2nd ed. Philadelphia，WB Saunders，1995，p 39.）

识别

气管支气管树受压或阻塞

气管支气管树受压或阻塞是前纵隔肿块引起的三种潜在并发症中最常见的一种。对这样的受压或阻塞来说，既有静态的因素，也有动态的因素。动态因素只有在仰卧位（图64.2）、全麻诱导或使用肌松药后才能显现出来（表64.1）。典型情况包括在没有上气道阻塞情况下的面罩通气困难和插管成功后的通气困难。

术前特征可包括：

- 端坐呼吸、体位性呼吸困难病史；
- 胸部X线片显示巨大肿块，气道受压；
- 胸部CT扫描显示气道或其他结构受压（图64.3）；
- 流量-容积环显示呼气相和可能的吸气支中断（图64.4）。

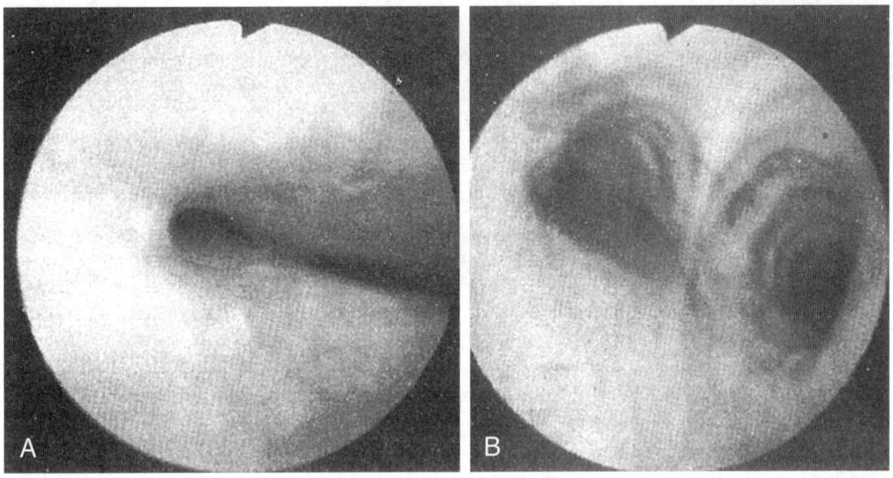

图 64.2 麻醉后的前纵隔巨大肿块患者仰卧位时下段气管的纤维支气管镜表现（A），几乎在前、后平面上完全阻塞气管。当患者取坐位（B）时，管腔看起来正常（From Prakash UBS，Abel MD，Hubmayr RD：Mediastinal mass and tracheal obstruction during general anesthesia. *Mayo Clin Proc* 63：1004-1011，1988.）

表 64.1 可能源于纵隔肿块的围术期并发症

并发症	表现	机制
气道受损	困难插管	SVC 阻塞引起上气道水肿
	上呼吸道梗阻	肿块压迫或手术损伤喉返神经引起声带功能障碍 / 麻痹
呼吸受损	气管支气管阻塞	气管和（或）主支气管变形、软化或动态塌陷导致困难通气 / 氧合
	肺水肿	左心房受压引起肺静脉压升高
血流动力学受损	前负荷减少	右心房、左心房或右心室受压影响心脏充盈
	右心室劳损或衰竭	右心室流出道或肺动脉受压引起右心室压力超负荷
	出血	外科操作后肿瘤出血，可能加剧 SVC 阻塞

SVC，上腔静脉

上腔静脉综合征

上腔静脉（superior vena cava，SVC）综合征是由于肿瘤受压或直接侵犯上腔静脉所致，具有如下特点：

- 面部或上肢水肿；
- 面部或上肢静脉扩张伴侧支循环；
- 呼吸系统症状（鼻塞、咳嗽、端坐呼吸）；
- 中枢神经系统影响（精神状态改变、头痛）；
- 胸部增强 CT 显示有明显的侧支循环。

心脏和肺动脉受压

心脏或肺动脉受压是一种罕见但危及生命的并

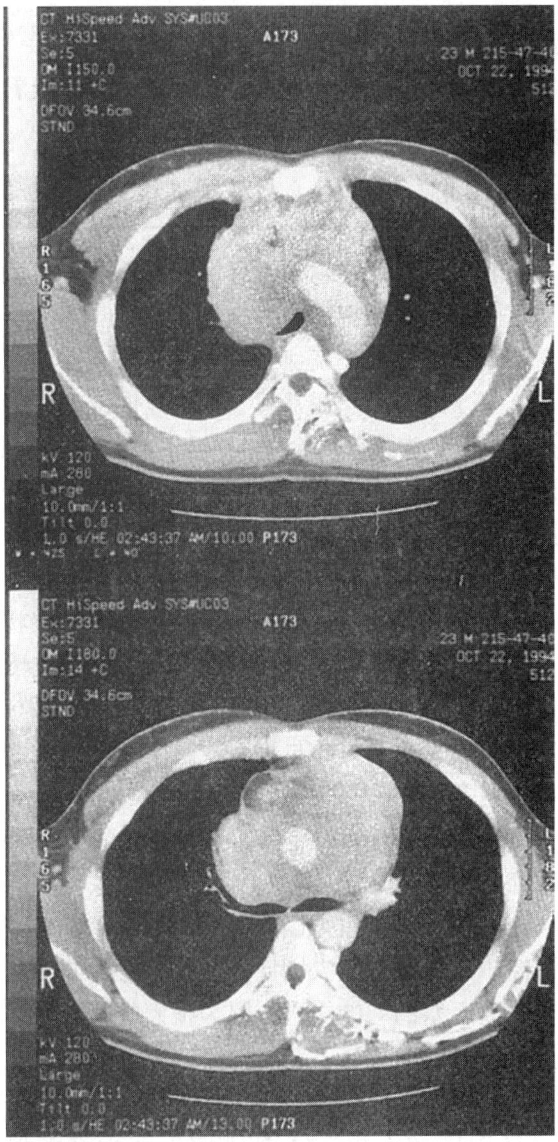

图 64.3 胸部 CT 扫描显示气管（上图）和主支气管（下图）水平的外源性压迫

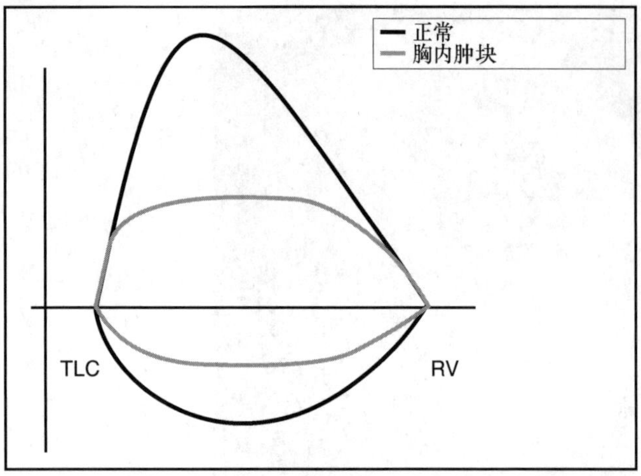

图 64.4 气道正常的患者和胸内肿块患者的流量-容积环。TLC，总肺活量；RV，残气量（From Pullerits J，Holzman R：Anaesthesia for patients with mediastinal masses. *Can J Anaesth* 36：681-688，1989.）

发症。Valsalva 动作试验有晕厥病史为强烈提示，至少应当在术前重点行超声心动图检查，专门查看是否存在来自心腔或肺动脉的外在压迫。

风险评估

一般来说，肿块越大，对生理的影响可能就越大。然而，识别哪些纵隔肿块患者在全身麻醉下有较高的围术期心肺并发症风险，这种前瞻性的能力通常有限，因为我们通常基于历史数据或病例衍生相关因素避免为预期风险最高的患者实施全身麻醉。在以儿童和成人为人群基础的研究中，局部麻醉和镇静通常是高危人群选择的麻醉方式，从而限制了有关全身麻醉安全性的结论。

围术期并发症高危患者分层的依据有：症状表现（严重体位性症状、喘鸣、发绀）；气管受压大于 50% 或相关支气管受压；心包积液；或 SVC 综合征。在成人中，有心包积液或阻塞性复合限制性肺疾病是围术期呼吸系统并发症最高发的相关因素。在儿童中，端坐呼吸、上身水肿、大血管受压和主支气管受压等表现与风险最高相关。

总的来说，儿童围术期并发症的发生率可能明显高于成人。与成人相比，婴儿和低龄儿童受外源性气道阻塞的影响更大，因为他们的气道可压缩性更强，也因为气道直径的微小减少会成比例地对气道的横截面积和阻力造成更大影响。在儿童中，建议气管横截面积（由 CT 测量）低于预测值的 50% ～ 66% 作为临界，低于临界值时应尽量避免全身麻醉。唯一与气管狭窄程度密切相关的症状是端坐呼吸。然而，它在预测术中气道塌陷方面的价值是值得怀疑的。气管受压大于 50% 的成人可能术中无气道塌陷，但术后呼吸道并发症的风险升高。

肺功能检测异常可作为判断气流受阻和并发症风险的替代指标。在儿童中，最大呼气流速低于预计值的 50% 对于检测气流受阻可能比单独气管横截面积更敏感。在成人中，阻塞性和限制性的混合模式表明肿块大到足以压缩肺实质和大气道；然而，CT 扫描可以更容易发现。流量容积环的呼气相变钝虽然在传统上认为是特异性表现，但并不能准确预测并发症。

启示

- 气管支气管树受压：
  - 不能通气或氧合，伴高碳酸血症或缺氧；
  - 可能的心搏骤停。
- SVC 综合征：
  - 如果手术部位涉及头部、颈部或上肢，易致出血过多；
  - 通过上肢静脉导管给药或输液不可靠；
  - 颈内或锁骨下中心静脉通路的相对禁忌证；
  - 可能的气道水肿。
- 心脏和肺血管受压：
  - 低血压或心血管衰竭。

治疗

气管支气管树受压

最好的办法是预防。但是，如果确实发生气管支气管树受压，则应尝试以下操作：

- 将患者的体位改为侧卧位或者半坐卧位。
- 恢复自主呼吸。
- 尝试推进气管内导管通过阻塞部位：
  - 考虑使用纤维支气管镜引导或气管导管交换器；
  - 考虑使用一个更小号的、柔韧性好的气管导管。
- 尝试使用硬式支气管镜绕过阻塞并通气。
- 通过股-股心肺转流进行氧合（如果未能在术前做好准备，不太可能有足够的时间成功实施）。

上腔静脉综合征

- 认识到相关的气道水肿对插管的影响，并在预见到插管困难时考虑清醒下纤维支气管镜插管；
- 抬高床头以降低静脉压力；
- 使用下肢静脉通路作为通往中心循环的更可靠的途径；
- 考虑使用利尿剂、类固醇或术前血管内 SVC 支架。

心脏和肺动脉受压

- 进行术中超声心动图检查以评估损伤程度；
- 将患者调整至受压最小的体位（侧卧位或甚至俯卧，任何患者术前认为是症状最轻的体位）；
- 根据需要使用液体、升压药和正性肌力药，维持静脉回流、肺动脉压和心排血量；
- 自主呼吸可能会有所帮助；
- 紧急实施心肺转流的计划（麻醉诱导前局部麻醉下股动静脉插管）。

预防

对于有明显血管、心脏或气道受累的患者，强烈建议术前放射治疗以缩小肿瘤或选用局部麻醉手术（如果可行）。术前放射治疗的一个潜在缺点是它可能掩盖组织学诊断并影响治疗。在一些治疗中心，CT 引导下经胸骨活检是一种可供选择的诊断技术。只有采取多学科方法（肿瘤学、放射肿瘤学、外科学和麻醉学），才能根据风险–受益比为治疗过程做出明智的决定。

麻醉计划和所需准备各不相同，取决于既定的手术（和手术方法）、患者症状的严重程度以及其他并存的情况和疾病。对于高危患者，应选择创伤最小的手术方案，麻醉计划尽可能选择局部麻醉和镇静。可保留患者自主呼吸的药物，如氯胺酮、右美托咪定或咪达唑仑，通常会有所帮助。当需要全身麻醉时，可遵循以下指南：

- 对于有任何症状或其他证据（如 CT 扫描）表明气道受压的患者，可以降低全身麻醉诱导前动脉置管的标准。可以在呼吸或血流动力学受影响的情况下提供实时的连续血压监测。
- 如果对气道塌陷有特别的担忧，诱导时应在手术室准备一个硬性支气管镜和外科主治医师一起使用。
- 在没有禁忌证的情况下（例如误吸风险、面罩通气困难），最好采用慢诱导全身麻醉（静脉注射或吸入）。保持自主通气直到确认建立有效的正压通气。如有需要，使用琥珀胆碱进行气管插管（除非有禁忌证）；其作用时效短，在肌松药不利于对患者建立通气时却是有益的。同时，应使用所需的最小剂量的琥珀胆碱（≤ 1.0 mg/kg）。
- 如果可行的话，可实施清醒、保留自主呼吸的纤维支气管镜插管。纤维支气管镜还可用于评估导管位置或动态气道塌陷。
- 应尽量做到插管和拔管过程非常平稳，因为过度咳嗽和紧张，既可加重气道阻塞，又可加重 SVC 综合征的症状。
- 如果需要中心静脉通路或监测（适应证与并存疾病相关），则应通过股静脉通路来实施。
- 即使是准备好的团队和预充好的泵，“备用”的心肺转流也不太容易及时建立以防止在气道阻塞或心血管衰竭的情况下发生灾难性的神经学损伤。在高危患者中，诱导前股血管置管是一种合理的方法。

（赵景昕　译　侯　炯　校）

延伸阅读

Bechard P, Letourneau L, Lacasse Y, et al.: Perioperative cardiorespiratory complications in adults with mediastinal mass, *Anesthesiology* 100:826–834, 2004.

Blank RS, de Souza DG: Anesthetic management of patients with an anterior mediastinal mass: continuing professional development, *Can J Anaesth* 58:853–859, 2011. 860–7.

Fabbro M, Patel PA, Ramakrishna H, et al.: CASE 5-2014 challenging perioperative management of a massive anterior mediastinal mass in a symptomatic adult, *J Cardiothorac Vasc Anesth* 28:819–825, 2014.

Hoerbelt R, Keunecke L, Grimm H, et al.: The value of a noninvasive diagnostic approach to mediastinal masses, *Ann Thorac Surg* 75:1086–1090, 2003.

Johnson D, Hurst T, Cujec B, et al.: Cardiopulmonary effects of an anterior mediastinal mass in dogs anesthetized with halothane, *Anesthesiology* 74:725–736, 1991.

Neuman GG, Weingarten AE, Abramowitz RM, et al.: The anesthetic management of the patient with an anterior mediastinal mass, *Anesthesiology* 60:144–147, 1984.

Shamberger RC, Holzman RS, Griscome NT, et al.: CT quantitation of tracheal cross-sectional area as a guide to the surgical and anesthetic management of children with anterior mediastinal masses, *J Pediatr Surg* 26:138–142, 1991.

Shamberger RC, Holzman RS, Griscome NT, et al.: Prospective evaluation by computed tomography and pulmonary function tests of children with mediastinal masses, *Surgery* 118:468–471, 1995.

Slinger P, Karsli C: Management of the patient with a large anterior mediastinal mass: recurring myths, *Curr Opin Anesthesiol* 20:1–3, 2007.

Stricker PA, Gurnaney HG, Litman RS: Anesthetic management of children with an anterior mediastinal mass, *J Clin Anesth* 22:159–163, 2010.

第 65 章 甲基丙烯酸甲酯

Bridget Perrin Pulos，*Nabil M. Elkassabany*

病例概要

患者，女性，75 岁，因股骨颈骨折拟行人工半关节置换术。患者既往有高血压、冠状动脉疾病、中度肺动脉高压和骨质疏松症病史，目前服用赖诺普利和氯吡格雷。患者采用全身麻醉诱导，手术进行顺利。在假体固定过程中，患者突发严重的低血压、低氧血症和心动过速。

问题分析

定义

甲基丙烯酸甲酯（methylmethacrylate，MMA）是一种用于骨科手术的加压骨水泥。它是由液态甲基丙烯酸甲酯单体与粉末状催化剂混合而成的聚合物。MMA 是用于全髋和全膝关节置换时的植入假体，以及用于股骨骨折时半髋置换术等手术。这种骨水泥经过发热反应，然后填充在假体和骨头之间的空隙中。

MMA 与骨水泥植入综合征（bone cement implantation syndrome，BCIS）有关。BCIS 是一种以低血压和组织缺氧为特征的潜在致命性疾病，并可能发展为肺动脉高压和右心室（right ventricula，RV）衰竭、意识丧失、心律失常，甚至心脏停搏。目前认为其发生可能与肺血管阻力增加导致右心室射血分数急剧下降和右心室扩张有关，扩张的右心室可能会挤压左心室，导致左心室充盈减少和心排血量降低（表 65.1）。该综合征可见于骨水泥固定、股骨钻孔、假体植入、关节复位或松止血带时。尽管 BCIS 具有众所周知的症状，但是目前还没有被广泛接受的标准化定义，该综合征的真实发病率尚不清楚，并可能存在一定程度的 BCIS 漏报。

2009 年，Donaldson 及其同事为了更好地描述与该综合征相关的发病率和危险因素提出了 BCIS 严重程度分类系统：1 级定义为中度缺氧或低血压；2 级定义为严重缺氧或低血压或意外意识丧失；3 级为循环衰竭，需要心肺复苏（表 65.2）。

表 65.1 骨水泥植入综合征的全身反应

器官系统	影响
心血管	随着肺血管阻力的增加，MAP 降低，每搏输出量减少，导致 RV 射血分数降低 肺动脉高压导致右心衰竭并最终左心衰竭 心律失常
肺	肺栓子导致肺动脉压增高和 V/Q 比例失调
血液	凝血级联的激活与血管舒张介质的释放 血小板聚集增加导致血栓的形成增加
中枢神经系统	精神错乱，意识丧失，如果患者有 PFO，则有可能出现反常的栓子和卒中

MAP，平均动脉压；PFO，卵圆孔未闭；RV，右心室；V/Q，通气 / 血流

表 65.2 Donaldson 等人对骨水泥植入综合征的严重程度分级

1 级	中度缺氧（动脉血氧饱和度 94%）或中度低血压（收缩压下降 >20%）
2 级	严重缺氧（动脉血氧饱和度 <88%）或严重低血压（收缩压下降 >40%）或意外意识丧失
3 级	需要心肺复苏的循环衰竭

2014 年，Olsen 和他的同事使用这个分类系统对 1016 名接受人工半关节置换术的患者进行了回顾性研究，发现 BCIS 的总发病率为 28%。1、2、3 级 BCIS 的发生率分别为 21%、5.1% 和 1.7%。重要的是，他们发现在出现 2、3 级 BCIS 患者 30 天的死亡率和远期死亡率显著增高。

BCIS 的病理生理机制尚不完全清楚，数个理论的提出提示不同的机制可能在其中发挥作用。其中

一种理论是单体介导的模型，循环 MMA 单体引起血管扩张，导致显著的血流动力学变化。MMA 被认为是一种外周血管扩张剂，但在骨科手术过程中的释放量比导致低血压实验模型中的量要小得多。更新的理论是涉及急性肺循环微栓塞的栓塞模型，这一模型认为，在固定和钻孔过程中髓内压力的增加会导致栓塞。这些栓子可能造成肺循环的机械性阻塞和血管内皮损伤，从而产生血流动力学变化，内皮的损伤导致血管活性介质的释放和血管张力的增加。术中应用经食管超声心动图（transesophageal echocardiography，TEE），可在右心房、右心室和肺动脉看到栓子雪花状影；一项研究显示骨水泥型比非骨水泥人工关节置换术的栓子负荷量更大。然而，栓塞模型也不能解释 BCIS 的所有方面，栓塞并不总是与血流动力学的改变有关，已有报道在不太可能发生大量栓塞的手术中（如经皮椎体成形术）使用 MMA 出现了低血压。在这些病例中看到的一些内皮损伤可能是各种炎症介质释放的结果，提示这些不同机制的相互作用可能是 BCIS 真正的病理生理过程。

与 MMA 的使用有关的职业暴露问题也存在。美国环境保护署（Environmental Protection Agency，EPA）规定，在 8 h 的工作时间内，职业性接触的上限为 1/10 000。急性暴露于极高水平的 MMA 可导致肝脏毒性和肺水肿。研究证实高剂量的 MMA 对小鼠有致畸作用，所以人们担心暴露在手术室 MMA 中可能对胎儿产生毒性影响。个人头部防护头盔和局部吸引器的使用可有助于最大限度地减少手术室中 MMA 的暴露。

诊断

BCIS 的特点是手术期间使用 MMA 后出现的低氧、低血压，或两者兼有。BCIS 的临床症状和体征与肺栓塞或脂肪栓塞相似（表 65.3）。在清醒患者，可以看到精神状态的突然改变或意识丧失。BCIS 的严重程度范围广泛，从动脉血氧饱和度瞬间而显著地下降到心脏停搏。如果有大的栓子栓塞肺部，呼气末二氧化碳可能会降低。栓子也可以引起皮肤淤斑和无尿，尽管这些可能是后期的症状。

表 65.3　骨水泥植入综合征的鉴别诊断

肺栓塞	脂肪栓塞
心肌梗死	快速性心律失常
卒中（神经认知改变）	其他导致肺动脉高压的心脏或肺疾病

风险评估

包括老年人、已有肺动脉高压或心脏病以及骨质疏松症等患 BCIS 风险较高的患者更能从有创监测中获益。增加 BCIS 风险的外科因素有病理性骨折、股骨粗隆间骨折和长骨干关节置换术。此外，麻醉科医师在如骨水泥固定、假体插入、关节复位或松止血带等关键手术过程时，应更加警惕。

管理

支持治疗是治疗 BCIS 的主要方法。出现严重症状的 BCIS 患者支持治疗包括：气管插管、有创动脉血压监测、中心静脉导管和（或）肺动脉导管进行有创监测、容量替代以及必要时使用血管活性药。在一些患者中，TEE 可用于指导与血管内容量状态和 RV 功能相关的管理。患者应以纯氧通气，可有助于最大限度地减少肺血管阻力的增加。

预防

对于风险最高的患者，应与外科医师讨论使用非骨水泥假体的可能性。如果这个方案不可行，也可能还有其他的外科技术，用来最大限度地减少栓子负荷量，如冲洗骨髓腔或骨质钻孔，以降低扩髓过程中的髓内压力。在高危患者中，使用动脉和（或）中心静脉进行预防性的有创监测很有必要，可有助于在发生 BCIS 时对患者进行管理。虽然这些措施不能预防 BCIS，但在整个过程中维持适当的容量状态能够优化患者以进行可能的进一步的复苏。

致谢

感谢 Kathryn P. King 博士对本章上一版的贡献。

（吴　昱　译　万小健　校）

延伸阅读

Clark DI, Ahmed AB, Baxendale BR, et al.: Cardiac output during hemiarthroplasty of the hip. A prospective, controlled trial of cemented and uncemented prostheses, *J Bone Joint Surg Br* 83:414–418, 2001.

Donaldson AJ, Thomson HE, Harper NJ, et al.: Bone cement implantation syndrome, *Br J Anaesth* 102:12–22, 2009.

Downes J, Rauk PN, Vanheest AE: Occupational hazards for pregnant or lactating women in the orthopaedic operating room, *J Am Acad Orthop Surg* 22:326–332, 2014.

Elmaraghy AW, Humeniuk B, Anderson GI, et al.: The role of methylmethacrylate monomer in the formation and haemodynamic outcome of pulmonary fat emboli, *J Bone Joint Surg Br* 80:156–161, 1998.

Ereth MH, Weber JG, Abel MD, et al.: Cemented versus noncemented total hip arthroplasty—embolism, hemodynamics, and intrapulmonary shunting, *Mayo Clin Proc* 67:1066–1074, 1992.

Fallon KM, Fuller JG, Morley-Forster P: Fat embolization and fatal cardiac arrest during hip arthroplasty with methylmethacrylate, *Can J Anaesth* 48:626–629, 2001.

Lafont ND, Kalonji MK, Barre J, et al.: Clinical features and echocardiography of embolism during cemented hip arthroplasty, *Can J Anaesth* 44: 112–117, 1997.

Olsen F, Kotyra M, Houltz E, Ricksten SE: Bone cement implantation syndrome in cemented hemiarthroplasty for femoral neck fracture: incidence, risk factors, and effect on outcome, *Br J Anaesth* 113: 800–806, 2014.

Orsini EC, Byrick RJ, Mullen JB, et al.: Cardiopulmonary function and pulmonary microemboli during arthroplasty using cemented or noncemented components. The role of intramedullary pressure, *J Bone Joint Surg Am* 69:822–832, 1987.

Pitto RP, Blunk J, Kossler M: Transesophageal echocardiography and clinical features of fat embolism during cemented total hip arthroplasty. A randomized study in patients with a femoral neck fracture, *Arch Orthop Trauma Surg* 120:53–58, 2000.

Rutter PD, Panesar SS, Darzi A, et al.: What is the risk of death or severe harm due to bone cement implantation syndrome among patients undergoing hip hemiarthroplasty for fractured neck of femur? A patient safety surveillance study, *BMJ Open* 4(6):e004853, 2014.

单肺通气

第66章

Danielle Shafiepour，Peter D. Slinger

病例概要

患者，男性，72 岁，因右上肺腺癌拟择期在机器人辅助下行右上肺叶楔形切除术。既往有稳定型冠状动脉疾病已行冠状动脉金属裸支架置入术和旁路移植术，高血压病史口服血管紧张素转换酶（angiotensin-converting enzyme，ACE）抑制剂治疗。术前肺功能检查显示：1 秒用力呼气量（forced expiratory volume in 1 second，FEV_1）占预计值的 85%，弥散容量占预计值的 56%，通气 / 血流比（ventilation/perfusion，V/Q）扫描右肺灌注为 65%。左双腔气管插管后，患者侧卧位，经支气管镜再次确认插管位置后实现肺隔离。在肺隔离 5 min 后，患者血氧饱和度开始下降，尽管采取改善单肺通气的氧合措施但患者氧饱和度仍在 30 min 时逐渐降至最低值 88%。

问题分析

定义与识别

在常规应用纤维支气管镜和对低氧性肺血管收缩的抑制作用较小的现代吸入麻醉药之前，单肺通气（one-lung ventilation，OLV）中经常发生低氧血症。虽然大多数需要 OLV 的患者在成功实现肺隔离后未发生严重的血氧饱和度降低，但仍有 1%～10% 的患者即使吸入纯氧仍发生严重的低氧血症。本病例也说明缺氧对麻醉科医师来说仍然是一个巨大的挑战。如本章所概述，了解 OLV 期间影响肺灌注的决定因素以及处理缺氧的系统方法将为麻醉科医师提供管理此类病例的策略。

在没有气管导管或支气管封堵器错位的情况下，OLV 过程中的缺氧主要是由于血液流经非通气侧肺发生分流所致。通过增加低 V/Q 比的额外区域，通气侧肺不张的发生进一步加重低氧血症。这些非通气区域的血流与通气肺段的血流混合在一起，导致 PaO_2 下降。有趣的是，在 OLV 期间，尚无普遍采用的最低饱和度阈值作为安全的下限；然而，一般情况下会接受 90% 的最低氧饱和度，而在无严重并存疾病的患者中可以耐受最长 80 s 的氧脱饱和。

OLV 期间最优的 V/Q 比值是通过最大化通气侧肺的灌注和非通气侧肺的肺血管阻力（pulmonary vascular resistance，PVR）来实现的。在 OLV 期间，许多因素在决定流经非通气侧肺的肺灌注比例方面起着作用，其中一些因素易受麻醉科医师的影响（图 66.1）。肺容积以双曲线方式影响 PVR；在极端时，PVR 增加而功能残气量（functional residual capacity，FRC）处于最低水平，这对于通气侧肺是理想的。在麻醉过程中，由于侧卧位的机械压迫和气体吸收，特别是在预充氧期间和 OLV 之前吸入纯氧后，肺不张易于发生在通气侧肺。因此，在没有正压来抵消这些因素的情况下，通气侧肺的呼气末容积趋向于残余容量。尽管维持呼气末正压（positive end-expiratory pressure，PEEP），一个 OLV 的猪模型显示，大部分通气侧肺在呼气末仍处于亚佳通气状态（图 66.2）。由于重力的影响，患者的体位是影响肺血流分布的另一个因素。最近的多项研究质疑了这种效应与其他特征相对对肺灌注分布的影响程度，表明由于血管床的基础结构，重力影响的前提是肺的非均匀性灌注。至少在某种程度上，侧卧位确实能因重力引起对通气侧肺的灌注增加，从而最大限度地减少分流。

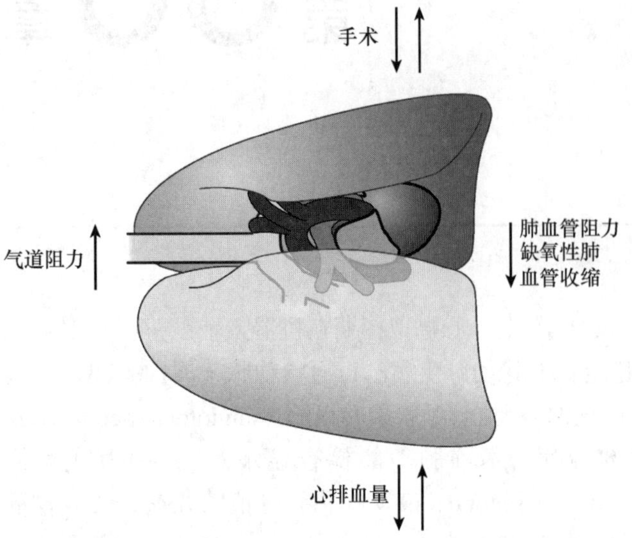

图 66.1 在侧位 OLV 期间影响肺血流分布的因素可根据相邻箭头的方向变化而定（From Slinger PD，Campos JH：Anesthesia for thoracic surgery. In Miller RD，editor：*Miller's anesthesia*，8th ed. Philadelphia，Elsevier，2015，pp 1942-2006.）

肺血管本身并非置身事外，相反，它在通过缺氧性肺血管收缩（hypoxic pulmonary vasoconstriction，HPV）来决定局部灌注方面起着积极的作用。在低肺泡氧分压时，肺动脉平滑肌收缩，通过肺血管床增加区域阻力，缺氧区血流重新分配。这一机制可改善 V/Q 比值，当肺组织的缺氧率在 30% ～ 70% 之间时最有效。这种反应开始迅速，平台期大约持续 20 min，随后 40 min 后开始进入延迟阶段。在实验环境中（向试验肺吸入 5% 的氧气），这种反应的幅度可使试验肺的肺血管阻力增加 3 ～ 5 倍，并使该肺的灌注减少 30% ～ 45%。关于是否存在预处理效应的问题，文献中存在争议，在重复暴露时，低氧反应的敏感性增加；这些结果的差异可能反映了实验条件的差异，如缺氧暴露的持续时间和再暴露前的时间间隔。ACE 抑制剂对 HPV 有抑制作用。

手术操作本身可能会影响肺血流的分布。虽然局部释放血管活性介质可能会对抗 HPV，但牵拉和机械性干扰肺血流可减少非重力依赖性（手术）肺的灌注。

风险评估

如前所述，大多数患者在吸入纯氧下使用双腔导管或支气管封堵器适当时，不会出现明显的低氧血症。框 66.1 中列出了可预测 OLV 期间的低氧饱和度的几个因素。

这些因素大多数与血液分流到非通气侧肺的比例直接相关。手术侧肺获得较高比例的通气或灌注以及对较大的右肺手术导致了相对较多的血液通过塌陷的肺而分流。仰卧位将消除重力对通气肺增加灌注的有利作用。

令人惊讶的是，OLV 时低血氧饱和度的风险与阻塞性气流受限成反比。已提出的机制包括非通气侧肺延迟塌陷，通气侧肺持续呼气末气流导致产生自动 PEEP，以及改变缺氧性肺血管收缩机制等。单肺通气前双肺通气（two-lung ventilation，TLV）的 PaO_2 水平是导致术中 OLV 发生低氧血症的最重要因素。当面临促进 V/Q 比值失衡如全身麻醉、正压通气、侧卧位等因素时，TLV 的 PaO_2 水平可作为呼吸系统优化 V/Q 比值能力的指标。

由于这些因素大多数在手术前即已知，这就使麻醉科医师能够为潜在的氧合困难做好准备，并应用预防措施来预防缺氧（见下文）。

预防

在大多数情况下，采用最佳的通气策略将有助于实现充分的氧合，并有助于减少急性肺损伤（acute lung injury，ALI）导致的术后缺氧，而 OLV 被认为是导致 ALI 的危险因素。虽然本章大部分讨论的是术中缺氧，但通气策略在减少 ALI 和术后缺氧方面的作用值得关注。OLV 时肺泡的损伤可能来源于气压伤、容积伤、塌陷肺泡序贯潮式复张引起的肺萎陷伤、炎症介质释放有关的生物损伤以及毛细血管切应力改变。Brassard 及其同事基于循证医学的 OLV 管理而提出了以下建议作为保护性策略：

1. OLV 之前的 TLV 期间：
   - 诱导时使用纯氧通气，提高诱导期间的安全界限；促进手术肺塌陷。
   - 在可能会发生去复张期间，如支气管镜检查之后，实施肺复张手法，应注意有关肺复张的最佳时机和压力仍未定论。
   - 根据理想体重（ideal body weight，IBW）使用 6 ～ 8 ml/kg 的小潮气量（volumes，V_t）。
   - 3 ～ 10 cmH_2O 的 PEEP。
2. OLV 期间：
   - 肺隔离后的手法复张。
   - 使用 4 ～ 6 ml/kg 的小潮气量（IBW）。

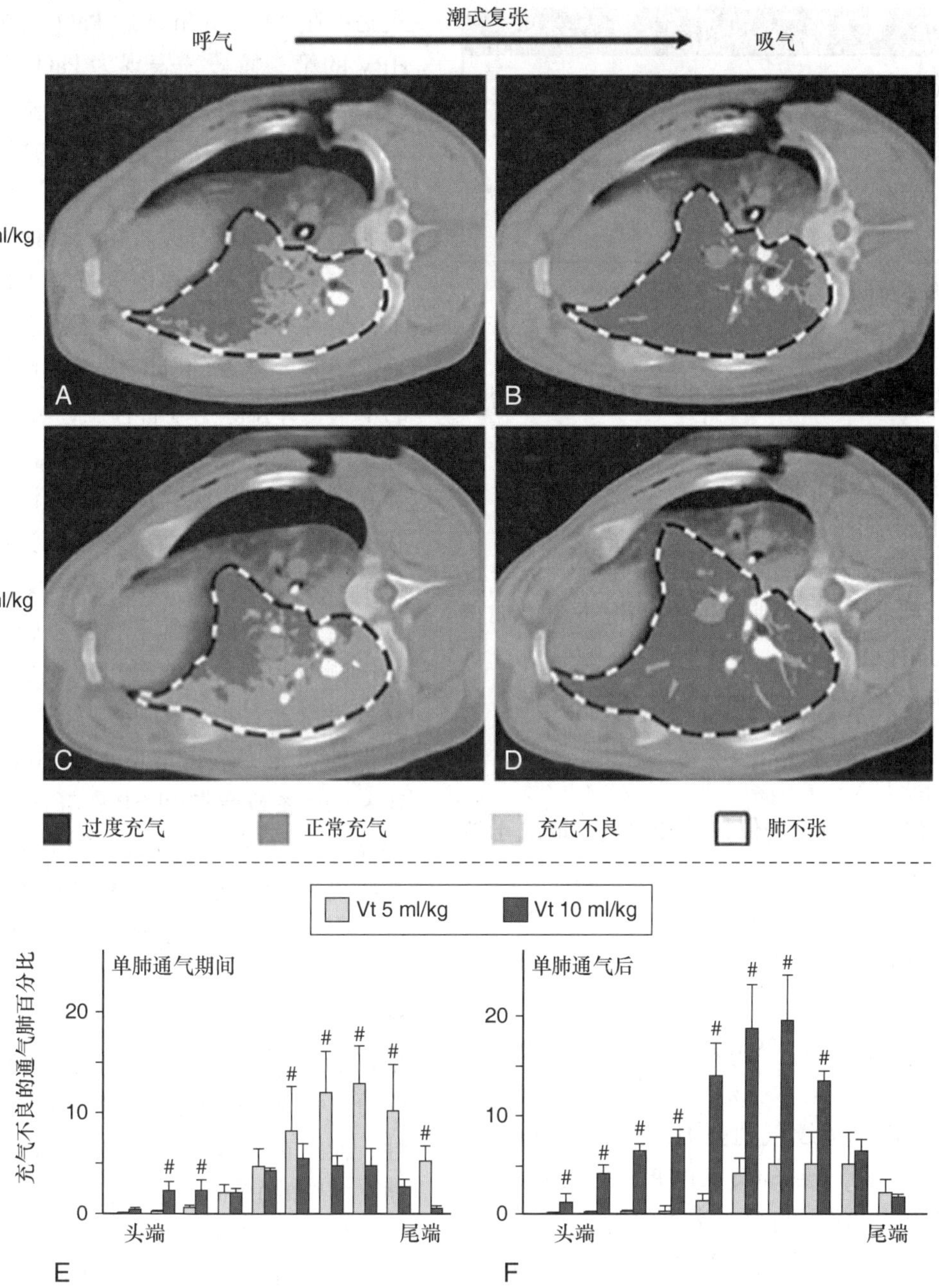

图 66.2 A-F，猪的 OLV 模型显示，PEEP 为 5 cmH_2O，潮气量分别为 5 ml/kg 和 10 ml/kg 时，呼气末仍有明显的肺泡塌陷。OLV 后较高潮气量（Vt）组出现更多的萎陷，这主要是由每次呼吸时潮式复张所致。（From Lohser J，Slinger P：Lung injury after one-lung ventilation：a review of the pathophysiologic mechanisms affecting the ventilated and the collapsed lung. *Anesth Analg* 121[2]：302-318，2015.）

- 维持峰值压力低于 30 cmH_2O，平台压力小于 20 cmH_2O。
- 使用 3 ～ 10 cmH_2O 的 PEEP。

请注意，虽然这在预防肺损伤方面有作用，但过低或过高的 PEEP 可能会加重缺氧。这可能是通过增加超过 FRC 的呼气末肺容量，从而增加 PVR 并使血液流向非通气侧肺而发生的。过低的 PEEP 可促进去复张和肺不张，增加通气侧肺的分流。

- 滴定 PEEP 以优化肺顺应性，并通过观察间断呼气流速来寻找存在自动 PEEP 的证据。
- 调整 FiO_2 以维持 SpO_2 在 92% ～ 96% 之间以避免氧中毒和肺不张，应注意大多数情况下 0.5 ～ 0.8 即已足够。
- 呼吸频率为 12 ～ 16 次 / 分，以避免呼吸频率过慢导致的高碳酸血症和 auto-PEEP，以及呼吸频率过快引起吸气和呼气时间缩短导致的呼

框 66.1 单肺通气时增加缺氧可能性的因素

术前 V/Q 扫描手术侧肺的通气或灌注率高
双肺通气时 PaO_2 较差，尤其是术中侧卧位通气时
右侧开胸
术前肺功能检查正常（FEV_1 或 FVC）或限制性肺疾病
单肺通气时仰卧位

FEV_1，1 s 用力呼气量；FVC，用力肺活量；V/Q，通气 / 血流比

吸机压力过高。

- 使用地氟烷或七氟烷维持麻醉，因为这些药物不会像过去的吸入药破坏 HPV 的程度高，而且可能有肺保护作用。

3. 手术侧肺的再膨胀：
   - 选择性单侧肺复张，以避免过度膨胀顺应性较好的非手术侧肺，在肺切除的情况下缓慢加压至 20 cmH_2O。
   - 使用最小的 FiO_2 进行肺复张，可以减轻再灌注损伤。
4. OLV 之后的 TLV：
   - 使用小潮气量维持的保护性肺通气（取决于切除范围）。
   - 由于双腔管（double-lumen tube，DLT）的阻力和新复张的肺易有肺不张倾向，维持 PEEP 和正压通气直到拔管。
   - 调整 FiO_2 至 92% ～ 96%，以避免高氧血症和肺不张。
   - 拔管后采用持续气道正压通气（continuous positive airway pressure，CPAP）预防高危患者的低氧血症和作为呼吸衰竭抢救措施。

除优化通气外，还应注意 OLV 过程中的循环。要了解 OLV 时心排血量和其对氧合的影响关系，应该先理解心排血量对灌注分布的影响以及其对混合静脉血氧饱和度（venous oxygen saturation，SvO_2）的影响。增加心排血量可导致肺血管床扩张并抵消 HPV，从而增加分流分数和恶化氧合。如果氧耗稳定，它还会增加 SvO_2，这在 OLV 中所见的有明显分流情况下可以改善氧合作用。总之增加和减少心排血量都将对氧合产生不利影响，因此应将其维持在正常水平。

管理

在 OLV 期间观察到的动脉氧合变化的典型模式是：在 20 ～ 30 min 后 PaO_2 为最低点，随之进入 HPV 的第二阶段，表现为 PaO_2 稳定或增加。如果发生突然或严重的氧饱和度下降，当务之急是恢复氧合，可能需要松开支气管堵塞器或双腔气管导管的套囊并以纯氧恢复双肺通气。肺隔离失败是可能的罪魁祸首，氧合改善后，可通过支气管镜进行确认。在某些情况下可能会选择不进行肺隔离继续手术；但许多胸科手术，如机器人和视频辅助胸腔镜手术，需要良好的肺隔离。一旦氧合恢复到可接受的水平，并排除了导管移位，可以应用其他技术。

由于心脏和大血管的操作，心排血量的急剧下降在术中并不少见，应该通过评估血压和与外科团队沟通来排除这种情况。可以尝试复张通气肺，因为高 FiO_2 和机械压迫常常导致肺不张；但必须注意的是，在对低位肺进行肺复张时，由于灌注向非通气侧肺转移，可能会出现短暂的饱和度下降。肺复张可以通过持续的压力（如 Brassard 及其同事所提倡的将压力缓慢地增加到 30 cmH_2O 并至少维持 10 s）或逐渐增加 PEEP 和峰压组成的周期性操作来完成。持续压力手法可能会对肺泡-毛细血管壁造成更大的损伤。可以考虑对通气侧肺增加额外的 PEEP，虽然通常建议的起始值为 5 cmH_2O，但通过 Ferrando 等描述的实施 PEEP 递减试验以寻求最大动态顺应性，可能会实现对 PEEP 精细的调控。如果持续存在缺氧，则应行动脉血气送检以保证通气充分，因为呼吸性碱中毒可能会损害 HPV 的有效性，而严重的呼吸性酸中毒可能会不成比例地增加通气侧肺的 PVR，同时加剧分流。

如果这些措施仍不能充分改善氧合，则应考虑将 CPAP 辅以氧气应用于非通气侧肺。这可以通过商品化的环路或简单的连接氧源的 PEEP 阀来实现。由于不张的肺泡需要较高的开放压力（>0 cmH_2O），对非通气侧肺实施肺复张手法后仅用 2 cmH_2O 的 CPAP 即可改善氧合。这在胸腔镜手术中需要短暂地中断手术操作，而即使少量的 CPAP 也可能会影响手术视野。间歇性吹氧至手术侧肺的其他方法亦有描述。方法之一是将一个标准的细菌过滤器连接到 DLT 的非通气腔上，并将氧气以 2 L/min 的流量连接到气体样品分析端口（图 66.3）。在 26 例开胸手术患者中，通过手动堵塞过滤器开口端 2 s，大约会有 66 ml 的氧气流入非通气侧肺，这并未对手术视野产生负面影响。

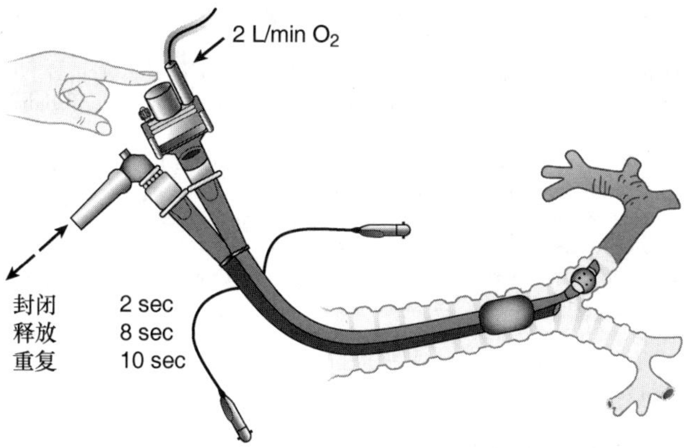

图 66.3 通过间歇短暂阻断与 DLT 非通气腔相连的抑菌过滤器，O_2 以 2 L/min 的速度流入过滤器上的气体采样口，可实现氧气间歇向非通气的肺内喷射（From Slinger P：*Principles and practice of anesthesia for thoracic surgery*. New York，Springer，2011.）

如果 CPAP 不能实施或不够有效，可采用多种方法对非通气侧肺进行部分通气。建议采用以下机制：

1. **肺节段选择性吹氧**（图 66.4）：将 5 L/min 的氧气连接到支气管镜上的吸引端口，操作者通过按下吸引扳柄选择性地向远离手术部位的手术侧肺部分吹氧。外科医师可以提醒麻醉科医师注意在显示器上观察到的任何过度膨胀现象。
2. **选择性肺叶塌陷**：将支气管封堵器引导到特定的肺叶支气管只阻塞特定的肺叶，这样就可以对该肺的其余部分进行通气。在插管时就必须将封堵器放在正确的肺叶支气管内。在某些情况下，这将干扰手术视野。

改善 V/Q 比值也可以通过机械性地限制手术侧肺的灌注来实现。可以让外科医师夹住手术侧肺动脉，但要记住，这代表着右心的后负荷急剧增加。

最后，分流程度可能受药物因素的影响。虽然现代挥发性麻醉药对 HPV 的影响不像以前的麻醉药那样严重，但限制在 1MAC 以下可能是有益的。应酌情停止使用全身性血管扩张剂，因为它们可以通过优先扩张更狭窄、非通气的肺的血管来增加分流。

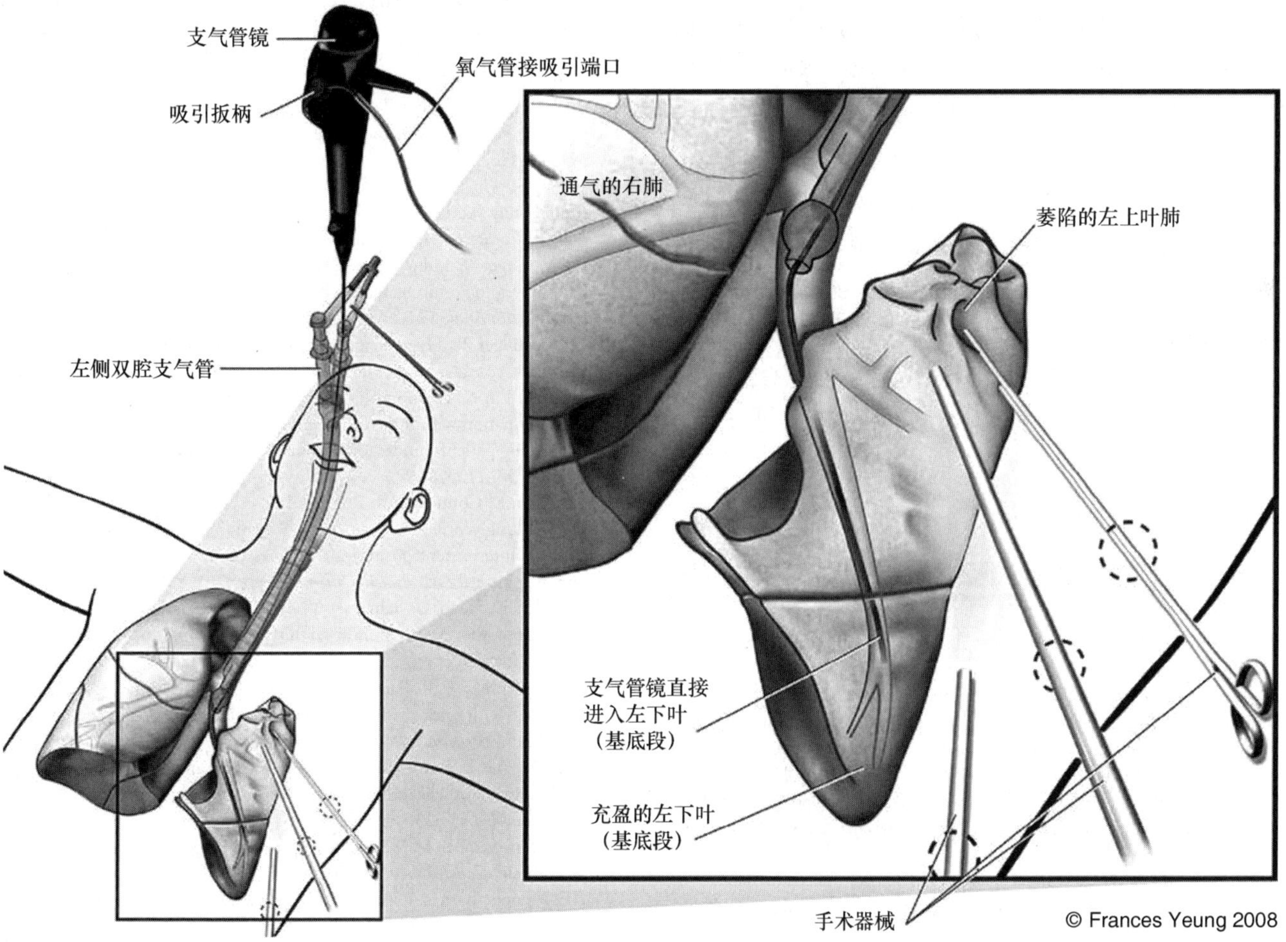

图 66.4 通过将 5 L/min 流量的氧气管连接到纤维支气管镜的吸引口，并在支气管镜进入合适的肺段后按下吸引扳柄，可以将氧气吹入指定的肺叶或肺段（From Slinger P：*Principles and practice of anesthesia for thoracic surgery*. New York，Springer，2011.）

吸入麻醉或复合使用全身性血管收缩剂亦被用于尝试选择性地扩张通气侧肺的血管床，以增强非通气侧肺 HPV 的效应。对吸入型一氧化氮（iNO）的研究正是基于这一目的，它是一种选择性肺血管扩张剂，虽然单独使用时不总是显示其对氧合的益处，但 20 ppm 的 iNO 和 4 μg/（kg·min）的静脉血管收缩药阿米替林联合使用可改善 OLV 期间的氧合。尽管根据这些结果尚不清楚每种药物的相对贡献程度，然而一项对 16 名患者的小型随机研究显示，单独使用阿米替林对 OLV 的 PaO_2 有显著的改善。这对于阿米替林来说是具有理论意义的，因为它以前是不允许作为呼吸兴奋剂在北美市场销售的。其他吸入性血管扩张剂包括前列环素（prostacyclin，PGI_2，flolan）和消除更为迅速的前列腺素 E_1（prostaglandin E_1，PGE_1）。在肺移植患者肺动脉阻断后首次肺植入（OLV 和灌注）中应用 PGE_1 的试验表明，PGE_1 通过优先扩张肺通气良好的肺血管床，从而改善了肺动脉压（pulmonary artery pressure，PAP），提高了 PaO_2/FiO_2 比值，同时减少通气侧肺内的分流。吸入 PGI_2 可以通过雾化直接送到呼吸机回路，与 iNO 一样，可降低心脏和肺移植患者的 PAP，它比 iNO 更便宜，是一种很有吸引力的替代方法。在一项病例研究中，吸入 PGI_2[50 ng/（kg·min）] 和静脉注射去氧肾上腺素可显著改善接受电视胸腔镜手术（video-assisted thoracoscopic surgery，VATS）的低氧血症患者的氧合。使用 PGI_2 益处包括允许具有临界肺功能的患者在更安全的情况下接受 OLV，并有助于减少肺移植受体者对心肺转流术的需求。

（吴 昱 译 杨宇光 校）

延伸阅读

Bindslev L, Jolin A, Hedenstierna G, et al.: Hypoxic pulmonary vasoconstriction in the human lung: effect of repeated hypoxic challenges during anesthesia, *Anesthesiology* 62(5):621–625, 1985.

Brassard CL, Lohser J, Donati F, et al.: Step-by-step clinical management of one-lung ventilation: continuing professional development, *Can J Anaesth* 61(12):1103–1121, 2014.

Campos JH: Effects on oxygenation during selective lobar versus total lung collapse with or without continuous positive airway pressure, *Anesth Analg* 85(3):583–586, 1997.

Della Rocca G, Coccia C, Pompei L, et al.: Inhaled aerosolized prostaglandin E_1, pulmonary hemodynamics, and oxygenation during lung transplantation, *Minerva Anesthesiol* 74(11):627–633, 2008.

Dorrington KL, Clar C, Young JD, et al.: Time course of the human vascular response to 8 hours of isocapnic hypoxia, *Am J Physiol Heart Circ Physiol* 273:H1126–H1131, 1997.

Douzinas EE, Kollias S, Tiniakos D, et al.: Hypoxemic reperfusion after 120 mins of intestinal ischemia attenuates the histopathologic and inflammatory response, *Crit Care Med* 32:2279–2283, 2004.

Ferrando C, Aguilar G, Piqueras L, et al.: Sevoflurane, but not propofol, reduces the lung inflammatory response and improves oxygenation in an acute respiratory distress syndrome model: a randomised laboratory study, *Eur J Anaesthesiol* 30(8):455–463, 2013.

Ferrando C, Mugarra A, Gutierrez A, et al.: Setting individualized positive end-expiratory pressure level with a positive end-expiratory pressure decrement trial after a recruitment maneuver improves oxygenation and lung mechanics during one-lung ventilation, *Anesth Analg* 118:657–665, 2014.

Glenny RW, Lamm WJ, Bernard SL, et al.: Selected contribution: redistribution of pulmonary perfusion during weightlessness and increased gravity, *J Appl Physiol* 89(3):1239–1248, 2000.

Hogue CW: Jr: Effectiveness of low levels of non-ventilated lung continuous positive airway pressure in improving oxygenation during one-lung ventilation, *Anesth Analg* 79:364–369, 1994.

Hurford WE, Kokar AC, Strauss HW: The use of ventilation/perfusion lung scans to predict oxygenation during one-lung anesthesia, *Anesthesiology* 64:841–845, 1987.

Katz JA, Lavern RG, Fairley HB, et al.: Pulmonary oxygen exchange during endobronchial anesthesia, effect of tidal volume and PEEP, *Anesthesiology* 56:164–169, 1982.

Khan TA, Schnickel G, Ross D, et al.: A prospective, randomized, crossover pilot study of inhaled nitric oxide versus inhaled prostacyclin in heart transplant and lung transplant recipients, *J Thorac Cardiovasc Surg* 138(6):1417–1424, 2009.

Kozian A, Schilling T, Schütze H, et al.: Ventilatory protective strategies during thoracic surgery: effects of alveolar recruitment maneuver and low-tidal volume ventilation on lung density distribution, *Anesthesiology* 114(5):1025–1035, 2011.

Ku CM, Slinger P, Waddell T: A novel method of treating hypoxemia during one-lung ventilation for thoracoscopic surgery, *J Cardiothorac Vasc Anesth* 37:432–436, 2009.

Lewis JW, Serwin JP, Gabriel FS, et al.: The utility of a double-lumen tube for one-lung ventilation in a variety of non-cardiac thoracic surgical procedures, *J Cardiothorac Vasc Anesth* 6:705, 1992.

Lohser J, Slinger P: Lung injury after one-lung ventilation: a review of the pathophysiologic mechanisms affecting the ventilated and the collapsed lung, *Anesth Analg* 121(2):302–318, 2015.

Lumb A, Slinger P: Hypoxic pulmonary vasoconstriction, physiology and anesthetic considerations, *Anesthesiology* 122:932–946, 2015.

Moutafis M, Liu N, Dalibon N, et al.: The effects of inhaled nitric oxide and its combination with intravenous almitrine on Pao_2 during one-lung ventilation in patients undergoing thoracoscopic procedures, *Anesth Analg* 85(5):1130–1135, 1997.

Raghunathan K, Connelly NR, Robbins LD, et al.: Inhaled epoprostenol during one-lung ventilation, *Ann Thorac Surg* 89(3):981–983, 2010.

Russell WJ: Intermittent positive airway pressure to manage hypoxia during one-lung anaesthesia, *Anaesth Intensive Care* 37(3):432–434, 2009.

Schwarzkopf K, Klein U, Schreiber T, et al.: Oxygenation during one-lung ventilation: the effects of inhaled nitric oxide and increasing levels of inspired fraction of oxygen, *Anesth Analg* 92(4):842–847, 2001.

Silva-Costa-Gomes T, Gallart L, Vallès J, et al.: Low vs high-dose almitrine combined with nitric oxide to prevent hypoxia during open-chest one-lung ventilation, *Br J Anaesth* 95(3):410–416, 2005.

Silva PL, Moraes L, Santos RS, et al.: Recruitment maneuvers modulate epithelial and endothelial cell response according to acute lung injury etiology, *Crit Care Med* 41:e256–e265, 2013.

Slinger P, Suissa S, Triolet W: Predicting arterial oxygenation during one-lung anaesthesia, *Can J Anaesth* 39:1030–1036, 1992.

Weir EK, Lopez-Barneo J, Buckler KJ, et al.: Acute oxygen-sensing mechanisms, *N Engl J Med* 353(19):2042–2055, 2005.

开放性眼球损伤

第 67 章

Alvaro Andres Macias

病例概要

患者，男性，35 岁，急诊室就诊，主诉在一建筑工地施工时左眼被钉子击中，伴有左眼疼痛和视力丧失。事故发生前 1 h，刚进食完午餐。

问题分析

定义

眼部损伤的最常见原因是异物（35%）、开放性损伤（25%）、挫伤（25%）和烧伤（15%）。大约 35% 眼部损伤发生于 17 岁以下患者。在美国，眼部损伤是单眼致盲的最常见原因。

识别

一般情况下，开放性眼球损伤的诊断可以通过病史和体格检查来判断。头部或面部的创伤，异物如金属或木屑，以及工业事故可在初期评估中即可判别。

对于任何遭受头部创伤的患者，必须评估其眼球和视力情况。

风险评估

眼科手术麻醉目的是提供麻醉和深度镇痛；避免咳嗽、干呕或呕吐；避免用力眨眼或哭泣。损伤性的眼内压增高（intraocular pressure，IOP）（框 67.1）可导致眼球开放患者的眼球内容物挤压。

框 67.1　可能增加眼内压的药物或因素

- 低氧血症、高碳酸血症、酸中毒
- 高血压
- 咳嗽、呕吐、喉镜检查、气管插管
- 环状软骨过度压迫
- 氯胺酮，琥珀胆碱
- 眼外肌张力增强
- 眼外内容物增多（肿瘤、出血）

除了眼球内容物的挤压外，与眼球开放损伤相关的最常见的危险和担忧是饱胃。这种危险不仅包括胃内容物误吸的可能性，还包括用于管理患者的药物或操作可能导致 IOP 增加。另一个值得关注的问题是眼内炎的发生。大多数指南建议眼睛受伤应在伤后 24 h 内进行修复。抗生素应尽早使用。

正常眨眼可使 IOP 较基线增加约 5 ～ 10 mmHg（正常 IOP 范围为 10 ～ 20 mmHg）。低氧血症可通过脉络膜动脉的血管扩张升高眼内压。持续性高血压可增加 IOP，而诱发低血压可降低 IOP。呕吐、咳嗽或“呛咳”可引起静脉系统充血，阻碍房水流出，增加脉络膜血容量，从而导致 IOP 急剧增加。这种压力的增加可能高达 30 ～ 40 mmHg。在麻醉效果欠佳的患者中，喉镜检查可使 IOP 增加 20 mmHg。

启示

麻醉诱导后，琥珀胆碱的使用可使 IOP 增加约 5 ～ 10 mmHg，持续约 5 ～ 10 min。在这段时间之后，IOP 恢复到基线。然而，开放性眼球的 IOP 相当于大气压。对于出现眼球破裂并接受琥珀胆碱进行插管的患者，目前尚无眼内容物挤压的报道。

治疗

术前应详细了解既往病史，并记录既往麻醉的任何反应。临床医师应采取措施减少和避免增加 IOP（框 67.2）。应避免使用大剂量麻醉药，因为它们可引起恶心和呕吐，并导致呼吸抑制和二氧化碳潴留，进而引起 IOP 升高。预防误吸可包括应用非颗粒性抗酸剂和甲氧氯普胺增强胃排空，以及应用

框 67.2 可能降低眼压的药物或因素

低体温
吸入性麻醉剂
过度通气（低碳酸血症、碱中毒）
眼外肌张力降低

H_2 受体拮抗剂提高胃液 pH、减少胃酸生成。

对于有前房损伤（异物）的患者，可以考虑眼球周围局部麻醉复合静脉镇静，但重要的是要记住，眼内阻滞会增加 IOP，进而增加眼内容物挤压的风险。在儿科病例中，首选全身麻醉。局部麻醉技术的使用取决于患者的情况、外科医师的意愿、相关的损伤以及开放性眼球损伤的严重程度。然而，全身麻醉通常是首选。患者应预充氧并避免面罩对眼睛的压力。虽然琥珀胆碱的使用是有争议的，但是使用瑞芬太尼 1 μg/kg、利多卡因 1 ～ 1.5 mg/kg 和诱导剂量的丙泊酚 1.5 ～ 3 mg/kg 或芬太尼 1 ～ 2 μg/kg 进行预处理可减轻 IOP 的升高。

在预充氧、压迫环状软骨和丙泊酚或硫喷妥钠诱导后，无需琥珀胆碱，使用非去极化肌松剂即可完成快速序贯诱导。罗库溴铵 1.2 mg/kg 可用于快速序贯诱导（从而将松弛时间缩短至约 60 s）。自从最近舒更葡糖在美国获得批准以来，罗库溴铵用于快速序贯诱导时所引起的长时间运动阻滞不再是一个问题。

氯胺酮对 IOP 的影响存在争议；然而，它可引起眼球震颤和眼睑痉挛，因此不应用于眼科手术。依托咪酯可降低 IOP，但可引起不可预测的肌阵挛，从而导致 IOP 升高。全身麻醉可以通过吸入性麻醉药或全凭静脉麻醉（total intravenous anesthesia，TIVA）技术来维持，这有利于避免术后恶心呕吐的发生。

术后拔管前应进行胃减压，口咽部吸痰，并给予 5- 羟色胺拮抗剂等止吐剂。静脉注射利多卡因（1.5 mg/kg）可减少苏醒期的呛咳。如果患者已禁食超过 8 h，可以考虑采用深麻醉下拔管技术。

预防

- 采取必要的预防措施，以防止咳嗽、紧张、呛咳和呕吐。
- 尽量减少高碳酸血症、缺氧和血压升高。
- 在确保患者安全的同时，尽量减少误吸的风险。
- 使用 H_2 受体拮抗剂、甲氧氯普胺和非颗粒抗酸剂预防术后恶心呕吐。

致谢

感谢 Stacey L. Allen 博士和 Ellen Duncan 博士对本章上一版的贡献。

（邓 瑜 译 周 懿 校）

延伸阅读

American Society of Anesthesiologists Committee: Practice guidelines for preoperative fasting and the use of pharmacologic agents to reduce the risk of pulmonary aspiration: application to healthy patients undergoing elective procedures: an updated report by the American Society of Anesthesiologists Committee on Standards and Practice Parameters, *Anesthesiology* 114(3):495–511, 2011.

Berry JM, Merin RG: Etomidate myoclonus and the open globe, *Anesth Analg* 69:256–259, 1989.

Boscia F, La Tegola MG, Columbo G, et al.: Combined topical anesthesia and sedation for open-globe injuries in selected patients, *Ophthalmology* 110(8):1555–1559, 2003.

Cook JH: The effect of suxamethonium on intraocular pressure, *Anesthesia* 36:359–365, 1981.

Cunningham AJ, Barry P: Intraocular pressure: physiology and implications for anesthetic management, *Can Anaesth Soc J* 33:195–208, 1986.

Gayer S: Rethinking anesthesia strategies for patients with traumatic eye injuries: alternatives to general anesthesia, *Curr Anaesth Crit Care* 17(3-4):191–196, 2006.

Konchiergeri HN, Lee YE, Venugopal K: Effect of pancuronium on intraocular pressure changes induced by succinylcholine, *Can Anaesth Soc J* 26:479–484, 1979.

Libonati MM, Leahy JJ, Ellison N: The use of succinylcholine in open eye surgery, *Anesthesiology* 62:637–640, 1985.

McGoldrick KE, Gayer SI: Anesthesia for ophthalmologic surgery. In Barash PG, Cullen BF, Stoelting RK, et al., editors: *Clinical anesthesia*, ed 7, Philadelphia, 2013, Lippincott Williams & Wilkins, pp 1373–1399.

Mehta MP, Choi WW, Gergis SD, et al.: Facilitation of rapid endotracheal intubations with divided doses of nondepolarizing neuromuscular blocking drugs, *Anesthesiology* 62:392–395, 1985.

Naguib M, Abdulatif M, Gyasi HK, et al.: Priming with atracurium: improving intubating conditions with additional doses of thiopental, *Anesth Analg* 65:1295–1299, 1986.

Peuler M, Glass DD, Arens JF: Ketamine and intraocular pressure, *Anesthesiology* 5:575–578, 1975.

Plaud B, Meretoja O, Hofmockel R, et al.: Reversal of rocuronium-induced neuromuscular blockade with sugammadex in pediatric and adult surgical patients, *Anesthesiology* 110(2):284–294, 2009.

Schwarz S, Ilias W, Lackner F, et al.: Rapid tracheal intubation with vecuronium: the priming principle, *Anesthesiology* 62:388–391, 1985.

Scott IU, McCabe CM, Flynn HW, et al.: Local anesthesia with intravenous sedation for surgical repair of selected open globe injuries, *Am J Ophthalmol* 134:707–711, 2002.

Taboada JA, Rupp SM, Miller RD: Refining the priming principle for vecuronium during rapid-sequence induction of anesthesia, *Anesthesiology* 64:243–247, 1986.

围术期心理创伤

第68章

Zeev N. Kain

病例概要

患者，男性，4岁，行腹股沟疝修补术。患儿在术前准备区，表现出既害怕又烦躁不安，拒绝离开母亲。与母亲分开时，大哭并试图摆脱麻醉科医师。术后1周，母亲报告患儿术后主要的行为变化，包括经常噩梦和发脾气。

问题分析

定义

对于儿童和父母来说，围术期往往是一个极其痛苦的时期。紧张、忧虑和担心的主观感受是儿童术前焦虑的主要表现。术前焦虑会刺激交感神经、副交感神经和内分泌系统，导致心率增快、血压升高和心脏兴奋性增加。这些表现都反映了孩子害怕与父母和家庭环境分离，失去控制；畏惧不熟悉的流程、手术器械和医疗操作。因此，在所有接受麻醉和手术的儿童中，高达65%的儿童在围术期出现极度焦虑和恐惧，就并不奇怪了。

儿童的术后行为比在术前准备区的行为更重要。临床医师和研究人员对患者术后心理反应早有认知，如一般性焦虑、夜间哭闹、遗尿、分离焦虑和发脾气。如果这些行为变化持续时间较长，并使儿童对后续医疗护理产生负面影响，或干扰其情绪和认知的发展，那么这些行为变化尤其值得关注。

识别

接受过麻醉和手术的儿童常表现出多种形式的焦虑。有些儿童明确地表达他们的恐惧，而另一些则通过行为表现出来。许多孩子看起来很害怕，显得焦躁不安，深呼吸，颤抖，停止说话或玩耍，或者开始哭泣。其他人可能会意外地弄湿自己，增加运动力度，并试图躲避医务人员。不同儿童不适应的行为表现可能差异很大。而最常见的还是分离焦虑，饮食紊乱，对医生和医院的恐惧增加，做噩梦和发脾气。

围术期焦虑与血清皮质醇、肾上腺素、生长激素和促肾上腺皮质激素水平升高有关。有报告显示心率加快和血压升高与焦虑行为评分之间存在显著相关性。术前焦虑通常与交感迷走神经介导的心率变异性中的迷走神经相对占优势相关。

风险评估

据报道，儿童术前焦虑的发生率为40%～60%。父母焦虑的儿童，害羞和拘谨的儿童，既往有手术史的儿童，既往接受过低质量医疗的儿童以及4～7岁儿童术前焦虑的发生风险增加。

有13%～40%的儿童在术后2周出现不适行为反应，如一般性焦虑、夜间哭闹、遗尿、分离焦虑和发脾气；这些儿童中有3%～20%在术后6个月仍持续表现出不良行为（图68.1）。只有0.8%的儿童出现更显著的行为改变，例如新发遗尿。值得强调的是，尽管大量儿童在术后即刻发生负面的行为反应，但这些变化的程度极其有限，只有少数儿童有持续、长期的不适行为反应。

在多因素模型中，儿童的年龄、气质基线、兄弟姐妹的数量、参加日托班和术前焦虑都是术后不适行为的独立预测因子（表68.1和68.2）。泌尿生殖手术的术后行为改变的发生率最高。鼓膜切开压力均衡术和鼓膜置管术后负面行为改变的发生率最低。

启示

术前焦虑可能对儿童和父母都造成困扰，并导

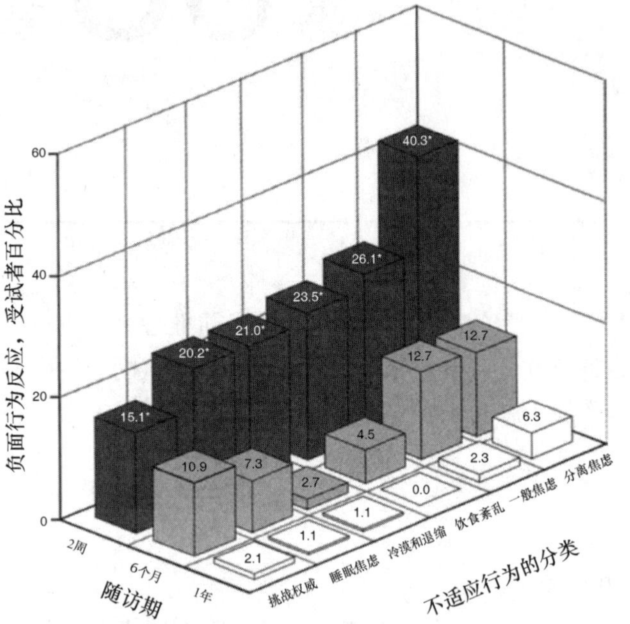

图 68.1 根据住院后行为问卷，负面行为反应的发生率随时间的变化情况。分离焦虑是患儿父母在 2 周（40.3%）和 6 个月（6.3%）报告的最常见的不适应行为。所有六个类别中的行为患病率从 2 周到 6 个月和 1 年显著下降（条形图中的数字代表总受试者的百分比）。*$P<0.05$（From Kain ZN，Mayes LC，O' Connor T：Preoperative anxiety in children. Predictors and outcomes. *Arch Pediatr Adolesc Med* 150[12]：1238-1245，1996.）

致术后即刻的负面行为反应。人们对影响儿童后续医疗护理反应和干扰正常发育的长期心理影响已有研究。尽管意见尚未统一，但有人认为术前焦虑可能会胃排空延迟和胃酸增加，因此，一些医生认为术前焦虑是吸入性肺炎的危险因素。术前焦虑还会增加麻醉苏醒期谵妄症状的风险，这与术后 24 h 内皮质醇和肾上腺素反应的改变相关。

管理

行为矫正和药物治疗是减少围术期焦虑的两项术前干预措施。

行为矫正

在麻醉诱导期间，父母陪伴可替代麻醉前用药。父母在场的潜在好处包括：

- 避免儿童尖叫和挣扎（分离焦虑）；
- 减少儿童在诱导期间的焦虑；
- 可能减少手术后长期行为影响。

反对父母在场的常见意见包括：

表 68.1 手术后 2 周负面行为改变的危险因素

预测变量	结果	相对风险（95%CI）
4 岁 vs. 6 岁	分离焦虑	9.4（1.2 ～ 39）
	一般性焦虑	3.3（1.1 ～ 7.8）
未办理日间病房登记 vs. 办理日间病房登记	分离焦虑	6.6（1.2 ～ 29）
术前准备区域非常焦虑的母亲 vs. 平静的母亲[a]	冷漠和退缩	6.6（1.6 ～ 19.1）
	睡眠焦虑	3.9（1.1 ～ 14）
	分离焦虑	3.4（1.2 ～ 6.7）
分离时非常焦虑的孩子 vs. 分离时保持冷静的孩子[b]	进食焦虑	4.2（1.3 ～ 8.7）
独生子与非独生子	分离焦虑	3.5（1.3 ～ 9.6）
易冲动的孩子与不易冲动的孩子[c]	一般性焦虑	2.7（1.1 ～ 6.8）

CI，可信区间。

[a]“非常焦虑”的定义为焦虑评分位于状态特质焦虑量表（STAI）状态子量表的上 25%；“平静”的定义为焦虑评分位于同一量表下 25%。

[b]根据临床焦虑评定量表进行测量。

[c]“易冲动”的定义为根据情绪、活动、社交、冲动仪器得出的冲动评分处于上 25%；“不易冲动”的定义为评分处于同一尺度的下 25%。

From Kain ZN，Mayes LC，O'Connor T：Preoperative anxiety in children. Predictors and outcomes. *Arch Pediatr Adolesc Med* 150（12）：1238-1245，1996.

表 68.2 手术后 6 个月负面行为改变的风险因素

预测变量	结果	相对风险（95%CI）
独生子与非独生子	一般性焦虑	3.0（1.4 ～ 6.9）
	分离焦虑	2.0（1.1 ～ 3.5）
	攻击性	2.0（1.1 ～ 4.1）
术前准备区域非常焦虑的儿童 vs. 平静的儿童[a]	进食焦虑	NA[b]
术前准备区域非常焦虑的母亲 vs. 平静的母亲[c]	睡眠焦虑	4.8（1.2 ～ 20.4）

[a]“非常焦虑”的定义为在维纳姆图像试验（Venham Picture Test）中焦虑评分位于上 25%；“平静”的定义为在同一测试中评分位于下 25%。

[b]NA 即 Not applicable（不适用）；由于 0 值为 0% vs. 17%，因此无法计算相对风险（$P=0.04$）。

[c]根据状态特质焦虑量表（STAI）状态子表进行测量。

CI，可信区间。

From Kain ZN，Mayes LC，O'Connor T：Preoperative anxiety in children. Predictors and outcomes. *Arch Pediatr Adolesc Med* 150（12）：1238-1245，1996.

- 扰乱手术室常规；
- 违背手术无菌原则；
- 造成手术室拥挤；

- 给麻醉科医师带来额外压力。

试验数据不支持常规使用此干预措施。虽然有早期的研究证明此举可减轻焦虑，但最近的研究表明，在麻醉诱导期间常规的父母陪伴并不总是有益的。受益的儿童如下：

- 4 岁以上的儿童；
- 性格害羞、拘谨的儿童；
- 父母能够保持镇定的儿童。

无论孩子年龄有多大或以前是否有过手术史（甚至包括那些在以前的手术前用过镇静药的儿童），大多数父母还是希望能够在麻醉诱导期间陪伴孩子。绝大多数麻醉诱导期间出现的父母都认为他们对孩子和麻醉科医师有所帮助。然而超过 90% 的父母都觉得在诱导期间感到一定程度的焦虑。虽然这具有临床意义，但是总的来说并不会对父母的健康产生较大影响。尽管现有数据表明麻醉诱导期间有父母陪伴仅对一些儿童有益，但是在美国这一比例依然在增加。关于父母是否应该在麻醉诱导期间陪伴儿童这一问题，我们应考虑所有可能的因素和情况。目前这方面的研究主要关注点在于父母在麻醉诱导过程中应该做什么，而不仅仅是他们是否应该在场。

药物应用

术前使用镇静药是一种有效且广泛使用的减少儿童焦虑的方法。其主要目的是使儿童在与父母分离时更加顺利且无焦虑。儿童麻醉前用药的详细讨论超出了本章的范围。下面仅列出常用药物。

咪达唑仑是目前最常用的术前用药。它起效和消除迅速，效果可预测，且不会引起心肺抑制。根据临床情况，可以通过任何途径给药。然而，当用于术前焦虑时，最常见的是口服（0.5 mg/kg）或经鼻给药（0.2 mg/kg）。当药物与调味糖浆或泰诺林混合并口服给药时，咪达唑仑可在 20 ～ 30 min 内提供良好的镇静和抗焦虑作用。尽管在鼻腔滴注中哭闹的发生率很高，但可在 10 min 内提供理想的效果。咪达唑仑也可以通过直肠给药（0.3 ～ 0.4 mg/kg），尽管年龄较大的儿童可能会拒绝这种给药途径。

氯胺酮作为不合作患儿的麻醉前用药或诱导药物尤其有效。当与可乐味软饮料混合并口服（6 mg/kg）时，氯胺酮可在 20 ～ 25 min 内提供可控的镇静作用。鼻腔给药途径在相似剂量下也可提供良好的镇静作用。

芬太尼为脂溶性药物，故无法作为口服的术前用药。然而，芬太尼棒棒糖可通过口腔黏膜吸收产生有效的术前镇静作用，便于吸入麻醉诱导的实施。然而，有研究报道经黏膜吸收的芬太尼（10 ～ 15 μg/kg）会引起面部瘙痒，并且相当多的儿童在使用后会发生围术期恶心和呕吐。

最后，我们需要强调的是，对所有儿童都常规应用麻醉前镇静药可能会导致药物成本增加，并且需要额外的护理人员以及在等候区设置适当的床位。因此，准确识别术前焦虑的高风险人群，并仅对这些儿童使用麻醉前镇静药更加重要。

预防

术前行为学准备项目可供预防使用，但常规提供这项服务的美国医院越来越少。这些项目包括儿童和家庭的术前教学，参观和使用玩偶进行角色扮演，让孩子熟悉一个令人焦虑的新环境。这样可以增强孩子的合作行为并减轻他们在术前准备区和手术室内的焦虑。大多数研究表明儿童的行为准备可以减少压力并增强应对机制，但仍有研究认为，这些准备工作可能会使年幼的孩子更敏感。

（刘洪君 译 王 薇 校）

延伸阅读

Brophy CJ, Erickson MT: Children's self-statements and adjustment to elective outpatient surgery, *J Dev Behav Pediatr* 11:13–16, 1990.

Kain ZN, Caldwell-Andrews AA, Maranets I, et al.: Preoperative anxiety, emergence delirium and postoperative maladaptive behaviors: are they related? A new conceptual framework, *Anesth Analg* 99:1648–1654, 2004.

Kain ZN, Caldwell-Andrews AA, Mayes LC, et al.: Parental presence during induction of anesthesia: physiological effects on parents, *Anesthesiology* 98:58–64, 2003.

Kain ZN, Caldwell-Andrews AA, Wang SM, et al.: Parental intervention choices for children undergoing repeated surgeries, *Anesth Analg* 96:970–975, 2003.

Kain ZN, Mayes LC: Anxiety in children during the perioperative period. In Borestein MH, Genevro JL, editors: *Child development and behavioral pediatrics*, Mahwah, NJ, 1996, Lawrence Erlbaum, pp 85–103.

Kain ZN, Mayes LC, Caramico L: Preoperative preparation in children: a cross sectional study, *J Clin Anesth* 8:508–514, 1996.

Kain ZN, Mayes LC, Caramico LA, et al.: Parental presence during induction of anesthesia: a randomized controlled trial, *Anesthesiology* 84:1060–1067, 1996.

Kain ZN, Mayes LC, O'Connor T: Preoperative anxiety in children. Predictors and outcomes, *Arch Pediatr Adolesc Med* 150:1238–1245, 1996.

Lumley MA, Melamed BG, Abeles LA: Predicting children's presurgical anxiety and subsequent behavior changes, *J Pediatr Psychol* 18:481–497, 1993.

Melamed BG, Dearborn M, Hermecz DA: Necessary considerations for surgery preparation: age and previous experience, *Psychosom Med* 45:517–525, 1983.

Vernon DT, Schulman JL, Foley JM: Changes in children's behavior after hospitalization, *Am J Dis Child* 111:581–593, 1966.

第 69 章 周围血管手术

Ronak Desai, Elizabeth W. Mburu

病例概要

患者，女性，74 岁，因间歇性跛行，日常活动受限，拟行右下肢血运重建手术。既往有长期的胰岛素依赖型糖尿病史、高血压、慢性肾病史以及吸烟史（吸烟指数为 50）。目前使用药物：卡维地洛、辛伐他汀、赖诺普利、胰岛素。自述爬两层楼出现慢性心绞痛，休息可缓解。多巴酚丁胺负荷超声心动图显示，负荷前后均有下壁基底段单节段心肌运动功能减退。拟行气管插管全身麻醉。手术可能会使用自身上肢血管作为移植材料。手术平稳进行 1 h 后结束，患者进入苏醒室。外科医师行血管多普勒超声检查发现旁路血管血栓形成，需再次进入手术室探查血管。

问题分析

定义

周围动脉疾病（peripheral arterial disease，PAD）以下肢动脉粥样硬化闭塞症为代表。PAD 与脑血管疾病、冠状动脉疾病一起，是动脉粥样硬化的三大综合征。在美国，至少 800 ～ 1200 万人受 PAD 困扰，有相当的发病率和致死率，使得患者生活质量降低。

糖尿病和吸烟是罹患 PAD 两大主要危险因素，其余公认的危险因素包括：高龄（>60 岁）、高血压和高脂血症。Fontaine 或 Rutherford 分级系统可用于评估患者临床症状严重程度，级别越高，疾病越严重。近期有关科学文献中较多使用 Rutherford 评分系统。两种分级方法均基于“截肢风险与血运重建益处比较分析”中所使用的缺血模型，因此，可能不能为糖尿病合并肢体受累的患者提供同样可靠的预测价值。

PAD 最常见的症状是间歇性跛行（intermittent claudication，IC），但也有多数患者没有症状或者出现 IC 以外的其他症状。

此外，此疾病谱的另一端为发生致命性的急性肢体缺血（acute limb ischemia，ALI）的患者，表现为静息痛、坏疽以及慢性、经久不愈的伤口。事实上，ALI 是多种复杂致病机制相互作用的结果，而不仅仅是因为动脉粥样硬化进展的原因。ALI 是指突发的（<2 周）肢体灌注减少威胁到肢体存活的一类疾病。肢体缺血严重程度取决于血管闭塞程度、远端肢体供血量、侧支循环形成情况。与慢性肢体缺血（chronic limb ischemia，CLI）相比，ALI 由于没有足够时间产生侧支循环以绕过闭失部位，导致肢体的存活能力受到严重威胁。

在美国，每年因 ALI 住院约 26/100 000 人，因 CLI 住院约 200/100 000 人。患有急性肢体缺血的患者均患有全身系统性疾病，其发生围术期死亡的风险是 CLI 患者的 3 倍（约 10% *vs.* 25%）。因此，及时准确的诊断对于保存肢体功能、降低死亡率尤其重要。为防止肢端完全缺血、组织进一步坏死，发生 ALI 的患者需在 6 h 内接受紧急血运重建。

ALI 的临床特点通常被归纳为方便记忆的 6P：感觉异常（paresthesia）、疼痛（pain）、脉搏消失（pulselessness）、苍白（pallor）、变温（poikilothermia，肢体温度与环境温度相等）、运动障碍（paralysis）。除运动障碍和感觉异常外，其余临床症状、体征均无特异性，且与血管闭塞程度相关性差。挤压受影响的肌肉出现疼痛，预示着其供血血管发生梗死且即将发生不可逆的组织损伤。若患者手指和（或）脚趾仍能活动、肢端感觉仍然存在，那么在 6 h 内紧急血运重建或许可以挽救缺血肢体。由于全身炎症反应和缺血再灌注损伤的影响，在严重缺血后 10 ～ 12 h 尝试血运重建往往会失败。

ALI 的病因大致可分为：①急性栓子（60%），栓子的 80% 来源于心脏，20% 来源于病变动脉；②肢体动脉（如腘动脉瘤）或旁路移植术后动脉内急性血栓形成（30%）。其他病因还有：血管损伤（钝性或穿透性）、灌注不良（主动脉夹层或无侧支的外周动脉发生夹层）、医源性损伤（手术、动脉内药物注射）、凝血障碍（如肝素诱导的血小板减少综合征）、脓毒症（特别是肺炎链球菌和脑膜炎链球菌所致）。值得注意的是，静脉坏疽易被误诊为 ALI。

目前 ALI 患者的治疗情况：25% 接受药物治疗，50% ～ 60% 接受血运重建手术，25% 需做截肢术。ALI 的治疗目标是挽救肢体，促进伤口愈合，减轻患者疼痛，降低心血管病风险，改善生活质量。由于此类患者随时面临着截肢的风险，因而多需紧急接受手术治疗。主-髂动脉栓塞型可采用腋-股动脉旁路术，远端动脉栓塞型可采用股-腘动脉旁路术重建血运。此外，手术能否成功、移植血管能否长期供血取决于移植血管的血流量、凝血功能、移植血管内术后是否发生动脉粥样硬化。围术期麻醉管理对于患者短期和长期预后均有重要影响。

识别

周围血管手术（peripheral vascular surgery，PVS），尤其是腹股沟以上的手术，属于高危手术。接受此类手术的患者，多合并有其他临床危险因素，会增加围术期心脏并发症的风险。因此务必密切关注患者心脏功能和代谢状态。这些危险因素 [根据修正的心脏风险指数（Revised Cardiac Risk Index，RCRI）] 包括：缺血性心脏病、充血性心力衰竭、脑血管疾病、术前需胰岛素治疗的糖尿病和血清肌酐大于 2 mg/dl 的病史。具有三个或三个以上危险因素的患者发生严重心脏并发症的风险为 5.4%。围术期心肌梗死（myocardial infarction，MI）的病理生理复杂，但主要原因是冠状动脉斑块破裂（Ⅰ型心肌梗死，T1MI）、心肌氧供需不平衡（Ⅱ型心肌梗死，T2MI）。所有活动性心脏疾病患者，包括不稳定型冠脉综合征、心力衰竭失代偿、严重的心律失常、严重心脏瓣膜疾病，都应在手术前接受评估和治疗。

风险评估

围术期心肌梗死是大血管手术后最常见的死亡原因。现有多项研究表明，围术期 MI 多发生于术后 48 h 内，常表现为无症状型 MI，但极易恶化为有症状型 MI，增加术后 30 天死亡率。血管紧张素转化酶抑制剂（angiotensin-converting enzyme inhibitor，ACEI）可能对于肾素-血管紧张素系统（renin-angiotensin system，RAS）诱发的动脉粥样硬化有保护作用。针对 RAS 的药物，如 ACEI、血管紧张素Ⅱ受体阻滞剂（angiotensin-Ⅱ receptor blocker，ARB）被广泛应用于降低血压。基于动物模型的最新研究表明，这些药物有减轻动脉粥样硬化的作用，且该作用与其降血压作用无关。一项纳入 9297 例 55 岁以上患者的心脏结果预防评估试验（the Heart Outcomes Prevention Evaluation，HOPE）显示，高血浆肾素活性是心血管事件和死亡率的主要预测因子，这就说明抑制 RAS 能使这类患者获益。

PAD 患者常被推荐服用一些降低心血管风险的药物，包括抗血小板药、β 受体阻滞剂、他汀类药物。高危患者（RCRI 指数评分≥ 3）服用阿司匹林、β 受体阻滞剂和他汀类药物治疗，围术期 MI 风险以及术后 30 天死亡率、术后 1 年死亡率均降低了 3 倍。此外，在这些患者中，因使用阿司匹林而引起的中度或严重出血的发生率并无明显增加。在术前和出院后接受抗血小板药和他汀类药物治疗，可改善血管手术患者术后 5 年的生存率。一项关注“周围血管手术出血并发症与抗血小板药物治疗 [阿司匹林和（或）氯吡格雷] 之间的关系”的大型前瞻性研究发现，在使用不同抗血小板药物治疗的患者中，因出血再次手术的风险没有显著差异。

2014 年美国心脏协会（American Heart Association，AHA）/ 美国心脏病学会（American College of Cardiology，ACC）/ 疾病控制和预防中心（Centers for Disease Control and Prevention，CDC）颁布的高血压指南推荐，无论年龄大小，高血压患者的目标血压都应≤ 139/89 mmHg。其他指南，如 JNC-8 则推荐，60 岁以上老年人目标血压应≤ 150/90 mmHg。根据 2015 年 Sprint 试验的结果，这种不太严格的建议可能会有所改变，这是一项超过 9000 名 50 岁以上患者加入的随机对照试验，由于随后的证据表明更积极地降压治疗，使目标血压达到 120/80 mmHg 可有效降低心脑血管事件的发生率和死亡率，该试验提前结束。一般来说，高血压Ⅰ期（收缩压 140 ～ 159 mmHg 或舒张压 90 ～ 99 mmHg）或高血压Ⅱ期（收缩压≥ 160 mm Hg 或舒张压≥ 100 mmHg）的患者应接受生活方式干预治疗，如 6 个月内未能有效控制血压，应开始接受噻嗪类利尿剂或联合使用 ACEI、ARB、钙通道阻滞剂中的一种进行治疗。

吸烟可加重血管炎症、加速动脉粥样硬化进程、最终导致血管旁路移植失败，因此，应鼓励患者戒烟。主动吸烟的远期结局包括增加截肢、MI 和死亡的风险。术前 4 ～ 8 周内开始戒烟的患者与术前未禁烟的患者相比，肺部并发症的发生风险并无差异。肺功能试验能更好地预测吸烟患者发生肺部并发症的风险。

麻醉监测

术中必要的监测项目包括：至少两导联的心电图，且需精确放置 V4 或 V5 电极位置、体表脉搏氧饱和度、呼吸末二氧化碳浓度监测、吸入麻醉药浓度监测、无创动脉压监测。某些患者，尤其是伴有症状或严重心血管疾病的患者（如：心力衰竭Ⅲ期或Ⅳ期、有症状的心律失常），需进行有创监测。有创监测包括：动脉置管、中心静脉压监测、经食管超声心动图以及肺动脉导管等。这些操作在麻醉诱导前、后实施均可。对于患有严重高血压、左心室功能障碍（射血分数≤ 0.35）或有症状的冠状动脉疾病患者，麻醉诱导前实施有创监测有利于麻醉科医师在麻醉诱导、气管插管、心血管负荷增加时，更严格地控制患者血流动力学变化。是否实施中心静脉压、肺动脉导管监测不应受麻醉方式选择（区域麻醉或全身麻醉）的影响。若患者外周血管不通畅或上肢静脉将用作手术移植导管时，应开放中心静脉通路。在全身麻醉中，经食管超声心动图可用于监测心脏功能和容量状态，尤其是对于血流动力学不稳定或存在心源性（房颤）或主动脉源性（不稳定斑块）血栓的患者。

治疗

麻醉方式的选择，主要应考虑外科血运重建手术的方法、患者对于麻醉和手术（通常需要几个小时）的耐受程度以及术前心肺危险因素。同时也要考虑到麻醉方式（区域麻醉与全身麻醉）对于血运重建成功率和围术期预后的影响。通常需考虑以下几个因素。

交感神经阻滞

此操作可增加血管床血容量，降低心脏前负荷，为维持正常心排血量，液体需要量相应增加，同时也可降低全身血管阻力。如果交感神经阻滞期间能降低心脏后负荷、减少心脏做功，则可改善全心和左心室功能。例如，胸段硬膜外麻醉引起的心交感神经阻滞，可通过降低心肌室壁张力、心率和后负荷来增加心肌氧供、减少心肌做功。因此，与对照组相比，此类患者更少出现心肌缺血相关的心电图表现。

交感神经阻滞也可改善应激导致的高凝状态、降低静脉血栓形成的概率。Tuman 及其同事报道，随机比较区域麻醉和全身麻醉移植血管失败率为 2.5% *vs*. 20%，这表明肢体血运重建术中选择椎管内麻醉有利于维持移植血管的通畅性和术后早期肢体的存活能力。

应激反应

区域麻醉可以减弱手术引发的机体应激反应。相较硬膜外阻滞，蛛网膜下腔阻滞者术中皮质醇，去甲肾上腺素以及总儿茶酚胺的水平更低，因而后者减轻神经内分泌应激反应效果更为显著。此外，机体代谢系统、免疫系统、神经内分泌系统均会发生明显的变化，如心肌氧供需不平衡、动脉血管收缩、高凝状态和纤维蛋白溶解状态、少尿、高血糖、水钠潴留、伤口感染、癌症复发、术后谵妄和认知功能障碍等，而区域阻滞可对上述变化产生有利的影响。且在下肢手术中，切皮前硬膜外给予局部麻醉药联合阿片类药物用于镇痛，对手术应激反应的抑制作用优于仅全身应用阿片类药物。

区域麻醉与全身麻醉

虽然周围血管疾病（peripheral vascular disease，PVD）手术相关的麻醉方法、药物选择、外科因素的对比研究较难进行，近期仍有几项前瞻性对照试验发现，采用椎管内麻醉与全身麻醉相比死亡率无差异（表 69.1）。其结果无差异可能是由于相较以往试验，

表 69.1 周围血管手术行区域麻醉与全身麻醉比较的研究总结

研究	病例数		围术期死亡率		心血管并发症		PVS 移植血管失败率		备注
	GA	RA	GA	RA	GA	RA	GA	RA	
Ghanami et al. 2013	4768	694	37.3%	34.0%	2.8%	2.2%	7.3%	7.2%	CLI 患者下肢旁路转流术预后不受麻醉方式影响，麻醉方式的选择取决于当地医院的技术和实践
Dodds et al. 2007	37	45	4%	0%	16%	11%	13%；16%（7 天，30 天）	0%；5%（7 天，30 天）	GA 手术组患者 7 天内再次手术率显著升高，差异具有统计学意义（P=0.02）
Singh et al. 2006	9757	503	—	—	1.8（1.32 ～ 2.48）（OR；95% CI）GA vs. RA		1.43（1.16 ～ 1.77）（OR；95% CI）GA vs. RA		GA 组心血管不良事件、移植血管失效率、二次手术率更高，住院时间、30 天内死亡率无统计学差异
Tuman et al. 1991	40	40	0	0	27	10	—	—	GA 术后硬膜外镇痛对比 GA 术后 PCA；对照组（N=40）随机选择 GA 患者（非 CV 手术），但无 PVD
Christopherson et al. 1993	51	49	3.9	4.1	7.8	8.2	21[a]	4[a]	EA 患者术后硬膜外镇痛，GA 患者术后 PCA 镇痛；11（GA）vs. 2（RA）患者术后进行再次移植或血栓切除术

CI，置信区间；CLI，慢性肢体缺血；GA，全身麻醉；OR，比值比；PVS，周围血管手术；RA，区域麻醉。
[a]，$P \leqslant 0.05$

这些近期试验围术期心血管系统管理做得更好。

术后持续区域镇痛，可提高移植血管的通畅性，减少再次移植手术、血栓切除术、截肢术的概率。表 69.1 中，有两项研究（Tuman 和 Christopherson）显示，单独采用全身麻醉与区域麻醉联合或不联合全身麻醉相比，术后移植物失败率有显著差异，而在其他研究中并没有发现这种差异。出现这种相反结果的原因可能是不同研究中采用的方法、移植血管类型、远端血管病变程度、辅助麻醉药物等方面存在差异。因此，接受 PVD 手术的患者中，区域麻醉方式对于早期移植失败风险最高的患者或因任何原因需再次手术者更有利。下肢血运重建术中，高凝状态和使用人工血管是血管移植失败的独立危险因素。

区域麻醉可改善一些促凝因素（如血小板功能、纤维蛋白原、纤溶酶原激活物抑制剂水平）。此外，血清检测证实的高凝状态与术后移植血管的长期通畅率较低有关，且会降低腹股沟以下血管旁路移植术后肢体的挽救率和生存率。然而，区域麻醉是否能防止移植血管内血栓形成仍存在争议。

虽然目前已对多种麻醉方式进行了评估，但是对于下肢血运重建手术，尤其是股-腘-胫动脉旁路术，仍不能确定何种麻醉方式最为适宜。尽管如此，一些内科和外科因素可能有助于确定某些特殊患者的最佳麻醉方式。手术时长即为一项重要考虑因素。由于使用患者自身静脉相较冻存的静脉或人工血管的短期和长期通畅率均更高，因此，手术医生往往需要花费相当长的时间来获取患者用于自身移植的静脉。多次血管血运重建术往往耗时更长，术式也更复杂。当然，耗时长的手术依然可以选用区域麻醉——可常规置入硬膜外导管持续给药维持麻醉。但是，患者可能不能耐受长时间的静脉镇静。术中采取改良的半坐卧位和背部支撑有助于减少患者不适或减轻甚至避免端坐呼吸的发生。

另一需要考虑的问题是，术中是否需要获取上肢静脉，尤其是进行第二次手术的患者。若术中涉及获取上肢静脉，就不能单独使用区域麻醉，但是可以考虑区域麻醉联合全身麻醉。

若决定为某位患者实施区域麻醉，必须考虑到其围术期抗凝治疗方案。美国区域麻醉与疼痛医学会指南中强调了抗凝治疗的影响，并就区域麻醉后出血的预防和治疗给出了建议。

目前，区域麻醉和全身麻醉相比，哪种麻醉方式在预防不良心血管结局、移植血管内血栓形成、降低死亡率方面更有优势尚不明确。有一项试验证明，气管内全身麻醉的患者相比接受椎管内麻醉的患者，术后更易发生肺炎。另一项研究表明，区域麻醉可降低老年人术后认知功能障碍发生率和死亡率，但仍需进一步试验证实。正如前所述，一些假说可以解释椎管内麻醉的患者预后更好，但这些机制尚未确认。因此，麻醉方式的选择应在与外科医师和患者沟通后，根据具体患者的情况而定。内科和外科因素，以及患者的诉求，均可帮助确定患者的最佳麻醉策略。

维持血流动力学目标

持续性心动过速是医生最不能容忍的血流动力学变化之一。务必查明并纠正其发生原因，譬如：手术刺激、大量或快速失血（常发生于血栓切除术中）。麻醉苏醒期是发生围术期心肌缺血的最常见时段，这可能与无意识或有意识的痛觉引起的高血压相关。拉贝洛尔、艾司洛尔可用于减弱增加心率的反应，也可与硝酸甘油、肼屈嗪、尼卡地平一起用于降血压或治疗心率恢复后仍然存在的心肌缺血。发生心动过速时，应首先考虑加深麻醉或使用 β 受体阻滞剂。全身麻醉中，心血管并发症高危患者可能受益于围术期使用 β 受体阻滞剂。血管手术后 48 h 持续控制心率有助于防止心肌缺血，可以显著减少和（或）消除高危患者术后出现 ST 段压低的情况。

液体管理

围术期的液体管理应依据患者及手术情况进行调整，以维持血流动力学稳定并尽量减少并发症。目前尚无足够证据证明在成人大手术中，开放性液体方案与目标导向液体方案孰优孰劣，但围术期结果更倾向于后者，尤其是考虑到肺炎和肾并发症的因素。开放性液体方案理论上可增加器官灌注，但增加了肺部感染和肺水肿的风险，延长了住院时间。对于接受大手术的患者，优化患者结局的最重要因素，不是只关注围术期绝对的输液量，而是应根据客观血流动力学监测指标为目标进行液体复苏，如监测心排血量、脉搏压变异度（pulse pressure variation，PPV），或经食管多普勒 FTc。通过动脉波形分析可获得机械通气患者的 PPV 或每搏量变异度。对行大手术的患者开放足够的静脉通路，以便快速给药或快速补液。

术中一旦发生出血，应输注晶体液或胶体液以维持血容量，必要时输注红细胞以维持足够的携氧能力。术前，应测定患者全血细胞计数、凝血酶原时间 / 国际标准化比值和部分凝血活酶时间。根据患者的理想体重、男性或女性的平均血容量按 65 ～ 75 ml/kg 计算，可粗略估算出患者能耐受的最大失血量。主动脉-双股动脉旁路术大出血的可能性更大，而腹股沟以下的血管旁路术则出血较少。定期评估患者血红蛋白浓度和凝血情况（血栓弹性图）有助于指导治疗。对于冠状动脉疾病高危人群，应维持血红蛋白浓度≥ 80 g/L 以维持心肌氧供。除非患者拒绝或有特殊禁忌证，否则应采取术中红细胞回收和自体血回输。

血管外科医师认为降低血液黏滞度有利于增加移植血管的血流量。因此，一定程度的贫血可能有利于移植血管的存活，但同时，也有减少重要脏器和组织氧供的风险。对于高危患者，术中维持血细胞比容在 28% 左右较为合理。

维持正常体温

围术期低体温对心血管会产生不利影响，因而，术中维持体温恒定是一个重要考虑因素。使用压缩空气加温毯、升高手术室室温、液体加温、呼吸环路加湿器和（或）采用低流量新鲜气流均可用于维持正常体温。

手术治疗

1998—2009 年间，美国医疗保险人群中 ALI 的发病率显著下降，而接受血管内治疗技术的患者比例显著增加。与此同时，ALI 患者 1 年截肢率下降。此外，尽管 ALI 患者院内死亡率下降，但 1 年死亡率并未改善。

然而，对于具有可接受手术风险的患者来说，外周肢体血管旁路术仍是一种补充疗法。移植血管常选用优质自体大隐静脉，但是移植血管 5 年失败率仍高达 30% ～ 50%。术后持续吸烟使移植血管失败率至少增加 3 倍，这说明戒烟对预防 PAD、维持移植血管通畅性具有重要意义。目前新兴的 CLI 治疗方式包括基因和细胞疗法，可促进血管再生和形成。

急性肢体缺血是涉及全身的系统性疾病，此类患者术后通常需要重症监护。考虑到围术期风险高、术前禁食时间短，全身麻醉诱导可采取快速序贯诱导，并压迫环状软骨，以防反流误吸。

麻醉诱导时，应优先选择血流动力学稳定性好的药物。缺血组织一旦恢复动脉供血，再灌注损伤可能引起循环和代谢紊乱。血管活性物质释放入血会导致全身性低血压和心肌抑制。为了纠正持续性低血压，可能需要使用正性肌力药和（或）持续输注血管加压药物。此外，术中应频繁监测患者动脉血气和钾离子水平，以早期发现异常。可静脉输注葡萄糖酸钙、碳酸氢钠和（或）胰岛素葡萄糖来纠正高钾血症和酸中毒。调整呼吸机参数防止呼气末二氧化碳增加。组织释放肌酸激酶造成的横纹肌溶解和肾损伤，应采用水化和碱化尿液来治疗。如果出现严重的肌肉坏死，可能需要进行截肢。

预防

一般认为，需行下肢 PVS 的患者均存在全身广泛性的动脉粥样硬化，且常并发冠状动脉疾病。因此对此类患者的围术期处理类似于对心脏病患者行非心脏手术的处理。应采取积极的预防策略：风险因素干预、药物治疗（如 β 受体阻滞剂、降脂药、抗血小板药）。抗血小板药物和区域麻醉可降低术后移植血管内血栓形成的发生率。心肌缺血、心肌梗死是 PVS 最主要的并发症，β 受体阻滞剂可降低心肌缺血和心肌梗死的风险。但是 β 受体阻滞剂不应在手术当天紧急开始使用，许多专家建议应至少术前 1 周使用，通过缓慢滴定法调整至最佳剂量，以免发生某些研究中观察到的围术期脑卒中现象。

目前，区域麻醉与全身麻醉相比，尚未明确何种麻醉方式更有利于降低死亡率、预防心血管不良事件的发生以及移植血管血栓形成。如上所述，一些假说机制可以解释区域麻醉的预后更好，但并未得到明确证实。因此，麻醉方式的选择应在与外科医师和患者沟通后，根据具体患者的情况而定。内科和外科因素以及患者的诉求可以帮助确定每位患者的最佳麻醉策略。

（李露茜 译 陈 芳 校）

延伸阅读

Attanasio S, Snell J: Therapeutic angiogenesis in the management of critical limb ischemia: current concepts and review, *Cardiol Rev* 17(3):115–120, 2009.

Baril DT, Ghosh K, Rosen AB: Trends in the incidence, treatment, and outcomes of acute lower extremity ischemia in the United States Medicare population, *J Vasc Surg* 60(3):669–677, 2014. e2.

Baser O, Verpillat P, Gabriel S, Wang L: Prevalence, incidence, and outcomes of critical limb ischemia in the US Medicare population, *Vasc Dis Manag* 10(2):E26–E36, 2013.

Becker F, Robert-Ebadi H, Ricco JB, et al.: Chapter 1: definitions, epidemiology, clinical presentation and prognosis, *Eur J Vasc Endovasc Surg* 42(S2):S4–S12, 2011.

Blaisdell FW, Steele M, Allen RE: Management of acute lower extremity arterial ischemia due to embolism and thrombosis, *Surgery* 84:822–834, 1978.

Breslow MJ, Parker SD, Frank SM, et al.: Determinants of catecholamine and cortisol responses to lower extremity revascularization. The PIRAT study group, *Anesthesiology* 79:1202–1209, 1993.

Caldicott L, Lumb A, McCoy D: Lower limb revascularization. In Caldicott L, Lumb A, McCoy D, editors: *Vascular anaesthesia: a practical handbook*, Oxford, 1999, Butterworth-Heinemann, pp. 198–224.

Callum K, Bradbury A: ABC of arterial and venous disease: acute limb ischaemia, *BMJ* 320:764–767, 2000.

Calvo-Soto P, Martínez-Contreras A, Trujillo-Hernández B, et al.: Spinal-general anaesthesia decreases neuroendocrine stress response in laparoscopic cholecystectomy, *J Int Med Res* 40:657–665, 2012.

Carson JL, Terrin ML, Noveck H, et al.: Liberal or restrictive transfusion in high-risk patients after hip surgery, *N Engl J Med* 365:2453–2462, 2011.

Christopherson R, Beattie C, Frank SM, et al.: Perioperative morbidity in patients randomized to epidural or general anesthesia for lower extremity vascular surgery, *Anesthesiology* 79:422–434, 1993.

Conte MS, Bandyk DF, Clowes AW, et al.: Results of PREVENT III: a multicenter, randomized trial of edifoligide for the prevention of vein graft failure in lower extremity bypass surgery, *J Vasc Surg* 43: 742–750, 2006.

Corcoran T, Rhodes JE, Clarke S, et al.: Perioperative fluid management strategies in major surgery: a stratified meta-analysis, *Anesth Analg* 114:640–651, 2012.

Cowart JB, Bates JT, Taylor AA: Perioperative management of cardiovascular risk in vascular surgery patients: what's new in 2014? *J Vasc Med Surg* 2:168, 2014.

Criqui MH, Fronek A, Klauber MR, et al.: The sensitivity, specificity, and predictive value of traditional clinical evaluation of peripheral arterial disease: results from noninvasive testing in a defined population, *Circulation* 71(3):516–522, 1985.

De Martino RR, Eldrup-Jorgensen J, Nolan BW, et al.: Perioperative management with antiplatelet and statin medication is associated with reduced mortality following vascular surgery, *J Vasc Surg* 59:1615–1621, 2014.

Desborough JP: The stress response to trauma and surgery, *Br J Anaesth* 85:109–117, 2000.

Devereaux PJ, Yang H, Guyatt GH, et al.: Rationale, design, and organization of the Perioperative Ischemic Evaluation (POISE) trial: a randomized controlled trial of metoprolol versus placebo in patients undergoing noncardiac surgery, *Am Heart J* 152:223–230, 2006.

Dodds T, Fillinger M, Walsh D, et al.: Clinical outcomes after lower extremity revascularization: a comparison of epidural and general anesthesia, *J Appl Res* 7:238–249, 2007.

Feringa HH, Bax JJ, Boersma E, et al.: High-dose beta-blockers and tight heart rate control reduce myocardial ischemia and troponin T release in vascular surgery patients, *Circulation* 114(Suppl):I-344–I-349, 2006.

Fleisher LA, Fleischmann KE, Auerbach AD, et al.: 2014 ACC/AHA guideline on perioperative cardiovascular evaluation and management of patients undergoing noncardiac surgery: a report of the American College of Cardiology/American Heart Association Task Force on Practice Guidelines, *Circulation* 130:e278–e333, 2014.

Frank SM, Beattie C, Christopherson R: Unintentional hypothermia is associated with postoperative myocardial ischemia. The Perioperative Ischemia Randomized Anesthesia Trial Study Group, *Anesthesiology* 78:468–476, 1993.

Ghanami RJ, Hurie J, Andrews JS, et al.: Anesthesia-based evaluation of outcomes of lower-extremity bypass procedures, *Ann Vasc Surg* 27:199–207, 2013.

Goodney PP, Beck AW, Nagle J, et al.: National trends in lower extremity bypass surgery, endovascular interventions, and major amputations, *J Vasc Surg* 50:54–60, 2009.

Hirsch AT, Duprez D: The potential role of angiotensin-converting enzyme inhibition in peripheral arterial disease, *Vasc Med* 8:273–278, 2003.

Kertai MD, Boersma E, Klein J, et al.: Long-term prognostic value of asymptomatic cardiac troponin T elevations in patients after major vascular surgery, *Eur J Endovasc Surg* 28:59–66, 2004.

Landesberg G, Shatz V, Akopnik I, et al.: Association of cardiac troponin, CK-MB, and postoperative myocardial ischemia with long-term survival after major vascular surgery, *J Am Coll Cardiol* 42: 1547–1554, 2003.

Lau WC, Froehlich JB, Jewell ES, et al.: Impact of adding aspirin to beta-blocker and statin in high-risk patients undergoing major vascular surgery, *Ann Vasc Surg* 27:537–545, 2013.

Lee TH, Marcantonio ER, Mangione CM, et al.: Derivation and prospective validation of a simple index for prediction of cardiac risk of major noncardiac surgery, *Circulation* 100(10):1043–1049, 1999.

Liem TH, Booij LH, Hasenbos MA, Gielen MJ: Coronary artery bypass grafting using two different anesthetic techniques: part 1: hemodynamic results, *J Cardiothorac Vasc Anesth* 6:148–155, 1992.

Marik PE, Monnet X, Teboul JL: Hemodynamic parameters to guide fluid therapy, *Ann Crit Care* 1:1, 2011.

Mason SE, Noel-Storr A, Ritchie CW: The impact of general and regional anesthesia on the incidence of post-operative cognitive dysfunction and post-operative delirium: a systematic review with meta-analysis, *J Alzheimers Dis* 22(Suppl 3):S67–S79, 2010.

McBride CM, Emmons KM, Lipkus IM: Understanding the potential of teachable moments: the case of smoking cessation, *Health Educ Res* 18:156–170, 2003.

McDermott MM, Greenland P, Liu K, et al.: Leg symptoms in peripheral arterial disease: associated clinical characteristics and functional impairment, *JAMA* 286(13):1599–1606, 2001.

Naidoo NG, Rautenbach PS, Kahn D: Acute lower extremity ischaemia. Acute lower limb ischemia is a surgical emergency, *Contin Med Educ* 31(6):201, 2013.

Nakagawa M, Tanaka H, Tsukuma H, Kishi Y: Relationship between the duration of the preoperative smoke-free period and the incidence of postoperative pulmonary complications after pulmonary surgery, *Chest* 120:705–710, 2001.

Nehler MR, Hiatt WR, Taylor LM: Is revascularization and limb salvage always the best treatment for critical limb ischemia? *J Vasc Surg* 37(3):704–708, 2003.

Norgren L, Hiatt WR, Dormandy JA, et al.: Inter-Society Consensus for the Management of Peripheral Arterial Disease (TASC II), *J Vasc Surg* 45:S5–S67, 2007.

Owens CD, Ho KJ, Conte MS: Lower extremity vein graft failure: a translational approach, *Vasc Med* 13:63–74, 2008.

Pierce ET, Pomposelli Jr FB, Stanley GD, et al.: Anesthesia type does not influence early graft patency or limb salvage rates of lower extremity arterial bypass, *J Vasc Surg* 25:226–232, 1997.

Raby KE, Brull SJ, Timimi F, et al.: The effect of heart rate control on myocardial ischemia among high-risk patients after vascular surgery, *Anesth Analg* 88:477–482, 1999.

Rogers RK, Hiatt WR: Pathophysiology and treatment of critical limb ischemia. February 11, 2013. Web October 11, 2015. Available at http://www.vascularmed.org/clinical_archive/Pathophysiology-Treatment-of-CLI_11Feb2013.pdf. Accessed December 12, 2016.

Rooke TW, Hirsch AT, Misra S, et al.: 2011 ACCF/AHA focused update of the guideline for the management of patients with peripheral artery disease (updating the 2005 guideline): a report of the American College of Cardiology Foundation/American Heart Association Task Force on Practice Guidelines: developed in collaboration with the Society for Cardiovascular Angiography and Interventions, Society of Interventional Radiology, Society for Vascular Medicine, and Society for Vascular Surgery, *J Vasc Surg* 58:2020–2045, 2011.

Rutherford RB, Baker JD, Ernst C, et al.: Recommended standards for reports dealing with lower extremity ischemia: revised version, *J Vasc Surg* 26:517–538, 1997. [Erratum J Vasc Surg 33:805, 2001.].

Scholl R, Bekker A, Babu R: Neuroendocrine and immune responses to surgery, *Internet J Anesthesiol* 30(3), 2012.

Singh M: Stress response and anesthesia: altering the peri and post-operative management, *Indian J Anaesth* 47(6):427–434, 2003.

Singh N, Sidawy AN, Dezee K, et al.: The effects of the type of anesthesia on outcomes of lower extremity infrainguinal bypass, *J Vasc Surg* 44:964–968, 2006.

Stone DH, Goodney PP, Schanzer A, et al.: Clopidogrel is not associated with major bleeding complications during peripheral arterial surgery, *J Vasc Surg* 54:779–784, 2011.

Tongers J, Roncalli JG, Losordo DW: Therapeutic angiogenesis for critical limb ischemia; microvascular therapies coming of age, *Circulation* 118:9–16, 2008.

Tuman KJ, McCarthy RJ, March RJ, et al.: Effects of epidural anesthesia and analgesia on coagulation and outcome after major vascular surgery, *Anesth Analg* 73:696–704, 1991.

Weitz JI, Byrne J, Clagett GP, et al.: Diagnosis and treatment of chronic arterial insufficiency of the lower extremities: a critical review, *Circulation* 94(11):3026–3049, 1996.

Willigendael EM, Teijink JA, Bartelink ML, et al.: Smoking and the patency of lower extremity bypass grafts: a meta-analysis, *J Vasc Surg* 42:67–74, 2005.

垂体瘤手术继发尿崩症 第70章

Chad D. Courtemanche，*Melissa A. Laxton*

病例概要

患者，男，58 岁，因蝶鞍上垂体泌乳素腺瘤，行经蝶窦垂体切除术。术后 10 h，尿量 >3 L/h，血钠 150 mEq/L。

问题分析

定义

尿崩症是一种由高渗血症引起的多尿、口渴和多饮为特征的综合征。神经源性或"中枢性"尿崩症由抗利尿激素（antidiuretic hormone，ADH）分泌不足所致，继发于下丘脑神经垂体轴的损伤。接近 90% 分泌 ADH 的神经元受损才会引发临床相关的多尿症状。肾性尿崩症则表现为肾对 ADH 的作用产生抵抗。妊娠期尿崩症常发生于妊娠晚期，并于产后 4 ～ 6 周消退。

ADH 的绝对不足导致尿液浓缩功能受损、多尿及脱水倾向。多数患者为不完全性神经源性尿崩症，仍保留有限的浓缩尿液和储存自由水的能力。然而，如果患者无法补充水分（如无意识，围术期禁食），则可发生高渗性脱水和高钠血症。高钠血症的症状和体征包括精神运动性兴奋、神经肌肉兴奋、嗜睡、昏迷和癫痫发作。

识别

在经蝶窦垂体切除术后 24 h，多达 70% 的成人患者会发生尿崩症。然而，该症状通常是一过性的，研究表明 20% 的患者出院时仍有尿崩症。围术期糖皮质激素替代治疗可促进多尿的发生。尿崩症的实验室检查结果如下：

- 24 h 尿量 >50 ml/kg；
- 尿渗透压 <300 mOsm/（kg · H_2O）；
- 尿比重 <1.010；
- 血浆渗透压 >300 mOsm/（kg · H_2O）；
- 高钠血症（血钠 >142 mEq/L）。

慢性多尿会使高渗性肾髓质浓度梯度被"冲洗掉"，导致尿液浓缩机制受损，从而加重多尿症状。只有排除多尿症的其他原因，才能充分诊断是原发性神经源性尿崩症或是肾性尿崩症（框 70.1）。

风险评估

如前所述，经蝶窦垂体切除术后，多达 20% 的患者出院时伴有暂时性尿崩症。然而，约 2% 的患者会发展为永久性尿崩症。与局限于鞍区的肿瘤相比，鞍上的大腺瘤术后发生尿崩症的风险更高。最近研究表明，与传统的经蝶窦直接入路相比，内镜下经蝶窦垂体瘤切除术可能会降低尿崩症的短期和长期发病率。肿瘤的分泌类型似乎对术后尿崩症的发生没有影响。

术后尿崩症分三种：暂时性、三相性和永久性。术后尿崩症通常于术后 12 ～ 24 h 发生，但数天至数周后才被诊断。约 70% 的患者是暂时性尿崩症，仅持续 3 ～ 5 天。少数患者可持续数周，然后逐渐消退。暂时性尿崩症常发生在局限于鞍区的垂体腺瘤切除术后。鞍上的垂体大腺瘤经颅切除术，或术中损伤垂体

框 70.1 多尿症的病因（除外原发性神经源性或肾性尿崩症）

化学利尿
甘露醇
尿素
放射造影剂
高血糖
呋塞米、噻嗪类利尿剂、利尿酸
急性肾衰竭
药物诱发的肾性尿崩症（如顺铂、锂）
去梗阻后利尿
复苏后利尿

柄近端后，易发生完全性或部分性尿崩症。某些病例可持续数年，随着神经元再生，症状才会改善或消退。

少部分患者（5% ～ 10%）术后表现为经典的三相反应。这种尿崩症最常见于严重头部创伤或广泛的鞍上肿瘤切除引起的垂体柄受损。初期的特点是ADH的释放突然停止，表现为多尿，常始于损伤后12 ～ 24 h，持续4 ～ 8天。此后进入抗利尿期，持续5 ～ 6天。此期表现为尿液浓缩，自由水重吸收后引起的血浆低渗透压和低钠血症。如果此期诊断延迟，可能会导致严重的低钠血症及伴随的并发症。低钠血症的症状包括恶心、头痛和癫痫发作。退化的神经垂体组织中储存的ADH过度释放可能是此期发生的原因。一旦储存的ADH释放完，尿崩症会频繁复发。症状通常持久，有时也会改善或消退。

启示

尿崩症患者无法浓缩尿液和保留水分。如不治疗，会导致血管内容量减少，心脏每搏量下降，机体通过增加心率来维持心排血量。灌注不足可表现为外周脉搏弱、直立性低血压、皮肤湿冷、呼吸浅快和意识水平降低。高钠血症可表现为癫痫发作和反射亢进。由于患者通常在术后数天内出院，仔细评估患者是否出现尿崩症的症状和体征是非常重要的。

治疗

鉴于围术期尿崩症以暂时性为主，一些轻度患者可口服液体治疗，特别是当患者可以配合，并且口渴机制完整时。然而，如果患者无法配合，合并低钾血症，以及担心肾髓质浓度梯度被"冲洗掉"，则可能需要更积极的治疗。

去氨升压素或血管升压素水剂可作为ADH的外源性替代剂。经蝶窦切除术后，通常每8 ～ 12 h皮下注射去氨升压素1 ～ 2 μg或去氨升压素250 ～ 500 ng缓慢静脉输注至少2 h。去氨升压素优先作用于V2受体，无血管升压素的收缩血管的作用，很少引起与V1受体相关的高血压或腹部痉挛。对于需要ADH长期替代的患者，可使用经鼻制剂和口服制剂。然而，由于患者对治疗的反应有很大的变异性，剂量必须个体化。

尽管去氨升压素是治疗慢性尿崩症的首选药物，但其作用时间长达12 ～ 18 h。对于常见的暂时性尿崩症，一些临床医师更喜欢用血管升压素水剂，因为其半衰期仅约20 min。血管升压素水剂是浓度为20 U/ml的溶液，作用峰值时间为1 ～ 2 h，作用持续时间为4 ～ 8 h。通常起始剂量为每4 ～ 6 h皮下或肌内注射2 ～ 5 U，或以0.25 ～ 1.0 μU/（kg·h）的速度开始输注。其他治疗药物有卡马西平、氯磺丙脲、氯贝丁酯和噻嗪利尿剂。

应仔细评估液体摄入量、尿量、尿渗透压和尿比重、血浆渗透压、血钠浓度以及体重，以指导血管升压素或去氨升压素的治疗。临床医师必须警惕抗利尿期发生的可能，此期激素替代治疗无效，并伴有水中毒。

预防

精细的手术切除是预防围术期尿崩症的最佳方法。麻醉科医师应高度怀疑尿崩症发生的可能，尤其当神经外科患者有鞍上垂体瘤或其他内分泌异常时。

致谢

感谢Patricia Petrozza博士对本章上一版的贡献。

（孟庆元　译　樊玉花　校）

延伸阅读

Adams JR, Blevins Jr LS, Allen GS, et al.: Disorders of water metabolism following transsphenoidal pituitary surgery: a single institution's experience, *Pituitary* 9:93–99, 2006.

Arafah BM, Nasrallah MP: Pituitary tumors: pathophysiology, clinical manifestations and management, *Endocr Relat Cancer* 8:287–305, 2001.

Barker II FG, Klibanski A, Swearingen B: Transsphenoidal surgery for pituitary tumors in the United States, 1996–2000: mortality, morbidity, and the effects of hospital and surgeon volume, *J Clin Endocrinol Metab* 88:4709–4719, 2003.

Carrau RL, Kassam AB, Snyderman CH: Pituitary surgery, *Otolaryngol Clin North Am* 34:1143–1155, 2001.

Fukuda I, Hizuka N, Takano K: Oral DDAVP is a good alternative therapy for patients with central diabetes insipidus: experience of five-year treatment, *Endocr J* 50:437–443, 2003.

Oiso Y, Robertson GL, Nørgaard JP, et al.: Clinical review: treatment of neurohypophyseal diabetes insipidus, *J Clin Endocrinol Metab* 98:3958–3967, 2013.

Rajaratnam S, Seshadri MS, Chandy MJ, et al.: Hydrocortisone dose and postoperative diabetes insipidus in patients undergoing transsphenoidal pituitary surgery: a prospective randomized controlled study, *Br J Neurosurg* 17:437–442, 2003.

Singer PA, Sevilla LJ: Postoperative endocrine management of pituitary tumors, *Neurosurg Clin North Am* 14:123–138, 2003.

Vance ML: Perioperative management of patients undergoing pituitary surgery, *Endocrinol Metab Clin North Am* 32:355–365, 2003.

Verbalis JG: Management of disorders of water metabolism in patients with pituitary tumors, *Pituitary* 5:119–132, 2002.

颅后窝手术

第71章

Diana Ayubcha，*Dimitry Y. Baranov*

病例概要

患者，女性，53 岁，接受颅后窝开颅手术以切除右侧听觉神经鞘瘤。术前症状包括耳鸣、发作性眩晕、头痛、面部不对称、协调和平衡丧失。外科医师拟使用乙状窦后入路，并计划仰卧抬高右肩位置和术中使用躯体感觉诱发电位（somatosensory evoked potential，SSEP）、脑干听觉诱发电位（brainstem auditory evoked potential，BAEP）、面部，舌下神经，辅助和肌电图（electromyography，EMG）。在手术期间，神经生理医师无法引发面神经的 EMG 活动。拔管后，患者右侧面部下垂。

问题分析

定义

颅后窝是一个体积小、顺应性低的隔室，包含许多极其重要的神经结构，这些神经结构在功能和病理方面具有独特的差异。传统上，在神经外科和神经麻醉文献中，关于颅后窝病理学相关内容的讨论被合并为一章，尽管有人可能认为这种方法可能是无意的，但可能具有误导性。对颅后窝中的各个解剖结构进行的每项手术都有其独特的挑战和潜在并发症的风险。为了设计和执行每个特定手术干预的围术期麻醉管理计划，需要对这些挑战深入了解，并与神经外科和神经生理学团队密切合作和沟通。考虑到在颅后窝中发现的病理情况十分广泛（框 71.1），提供必要的全面综述以解决这些手术麻醉管理的各个方面超出了本章的范围。然而，本章将介绍涉及预测、识别和管理颅后窝手术中麻醉围术期并发症的一些常见原则。

由于在有限的颅后窝空间内存在重要的神经元和血管结构，因此颅后窝手术对外科医师和麻醉科医师都提出了挑战。颅后窝包含重要的呼吸、血管舒缩和心脏控制中心，特别是在脑干内。除了形成脑干的中脑、髓质和脑桥外，颅后窝中还有小脑、后组颅神经和许多关键的血管结构。血管解剖结构包括椎基底动脉循环的动脉和穿过颅后窝的静脉窦，包括乙状窦、横窦和枕窦。对这些区域的操作，如手术牵拉时，可显著影响呼吸驱动、静息血管张力、血压和心率。该空间内体积的小幅增加，主要是由于术后血肿或水肿，可导致隔室压力快速升高，并随后发生危及生命的脑干压迫。术中目标旨在有利于手术入路，满足对神经组织和颅神经完整性的可靠神经生理学监测以及维持呼吸和心血管稳定性的要求。脑脊液（cerebrospinal fluid，CSF）通过脑导水管处特别狭窄。极小程度的阻塞也可导致颅内压显著增加。基于受影响的确切位置和结构不同，颅后窝病变患者的表现各不相同。例如，触及脑导水管的小病灶可能导致阻塞性脑积水，出现头痛症状和精神状态改变。同样，位于外侧脑桥的小病灶可能导致孤立的颅神经功能障碍。因此，在术前确定病变的确切位置以及结构受累以及所有相关的神经系统或系统损害是至关重要的。

识别

在讨论与颅后窝手术相关的并发症时，识别可能发生这些并发症的常见手术和其非危及生命的性质是十分重要的。在最近的 500 例病例回顾中，总并发症发生率低于 32%，其中绝大多数是脑脊液漏、脑膜炎、伤口感染和颅神经麻痹。脑积水和小脑血肿占所有手术并发症的一小部分，总死亡率低于 3%。大多数这些并发症不太可能与麻醉管理有关。

框 71.1 颅后窝病理学及手术方法

桥小脑角病变手术
- 神经鞘瘤
- 脑膜瘤
- 听神经瘤
- 颈静脉球瘤

微血管减压和血管手术
- 三叉神经痛
- 面肌痉挛
- 小脑后动脉动脉瘤
- 椎动脉 / 椎基底动脉瘤
- 基底动脉瘤
- 动静脉畸形

小脑病变手术
- 星形细胞瘤
- 蛛网膜囊肿
- 血管母细胞瘤
- 小脑凸性脑膜瘤
- 小脑动静脉畸形

岩斜区域手术
- 脊索瘤
- 脑膜瘤

轴向病变手术
- 成神经管细胞瘤
- 小脑星形细胞瘤
- 脑干胶质瘤
- 室管膜瘤
- 脉络丛乳头状瘤
- 皮样瘤

囊肿切除术
- 表皮样囊肿
- 蛛网膜囊肿

与手术操作或方法（如静脉空气栓塞）无直接关系的严重围术期并发症传统上被认为属于麻醉管理领域，并且非常罕见。虽然在颅后窝手术中血流动力学不稳定更常见，但暂时性血流动力学不稳定通常可以迅速得到治疗且不产生后果，不应被视为并发症。大多数麻醉并发症可分为广泛且相互重叠的类别：①与颅后窝手术定位有关的并发症；②未依据术中神经生理学监测提供足够的麻醉深度，以监测术中可能损伤的神经元通路的完整性；③与脑干血管运动中枢受压或刺激有关的严重血流动力学紊乱；④与血肿扩大和实质水肿有关的术后并发症，特别是对于有气道风险的患者。

颅后窝的手术暴露是公认的挑战。在临床上坐位和平卧位均有使用。在过去，由于 CSF 和血液因重力从手术区排出，坐位被视为可提供更好的手术暴露和解剖学定向，并可改善静脉引流，减少失血，膈肌运动自如，更容易进行气管插管和气道管理。然而，由于存在与此体位相关的潜在严重并发症以及医疗事故索赔的风险，此体位在许多中心已经不再采用。坐位开颅手术的并发症是众所周知的，包括静脉空气栓塞（VAE）、反常空气栓塞（PAE）、张力性气颅、舌和喉水肿、四肢瘫痪、外周神经损伤、严重的血流动力学不稳定和脑灌注减少。使用水平体位（例如侧卧、俯卧或躺椅位）可降低 VAE 和 PAE 的发生率，但也会带来其他挑战。经常使用的极度颈部屈曲以改善暴露可能导致颈髓缺血、巨舌症和气道水肿的风险增加。俯卧位导致腹内和胸内压力增加、静脉引流受损以及术后视力丧失的风险。如果不采取适当的措施来减轻手臂的拉伸和压缩，那么躺椅位和侧卧位可能导致臂丛神经损伤。所有这些体位都需要特殊设备和重要的专业知识和经验，但由于这些体位使用得越来越少，这种情况已经日益少见。听神经瘤切除术中最常见的方法是患者保持仰卧，使用沙袋使同侧肩部抬高。该位置与上述并发症的风险增加无关。关于每个体位的管理以及与之相关的并发症的全面讨论超出了本文的范围。而对 VAE 和 PAE 的监测模式和管理的描述将在本章节中予以讨论。任何需要使用这些体位进行手术的医师应提前做好充分的准备，包括与参与该手术的手术团队成员进行密切沟通。

为改善颅后窝手术中的神经功能保护而实施的神经生理学监测可能包括躯体感觉诱发电位（SSEP）、脑干听觉诱发电位（BAEP）和肌电图（EMG）。各种麻醉剂在不同程度上均影响神经生理学监测，需要适当的麻醉管理以提供最佳监测条件。如果不了解拟施手术的具体监测需求，可能会导致患者监测不充分，结果不理想。

在颅后窝手术中经常会出现严重的血流动力学不稳定。对脑干心脏和血管舒缩中心的手术刺激或损伤可导致快速且不可预测的血流动力学变化。极端心率和血压改变在手术操作中很常见，并且需要快速识别和治疗。需要记住的是，外科医师可能依赖于血压和心率的变化来早期发现重要脑干结构和颅神经的手术损伤。因此，必须在与外科同事协商的情况下进行血流动力学变化的预防性治疗。

最后，目前仍然没有针对脑干众多重要功能的术中监测仪器，例如气道维护、吞咽和呼吸控制等。颅后窝术后患者发生由于术后小水肿或血肿快速压迫脑干而导致的气道风险、呼吸系统受损和神经系统骤然恶化的风险增加。因此，必须预先制定麻醉管理方案，以便在拔管前对气道反射和神经系统状态进行可靠的评估。患者管理团队应讨论血流动力学参数的可接受范围、预计的神经元或延髓功能障碍以及在需要时解决气道保护和呼吸功能改变所需的措施。应事先讨论术后通气支持、插管或诊断性检查（例如血管造影、计算机断层扫描、磁共振成像），并且需根据这些讨论制订适当的计划并转发给 ICU 治疗组。

风险评估

了解目标病变的解剖位置、预设的手术流程以及术中涉及的实际结构都是颅后窝手术的关键要素。只有在了解个体患者的病史和体格检查、放射学评估以及与神经外科医师的讨论之后，才有可能进行风险评估。手术最大的风险与直接涉及脑干的肿瘤（例如，脑桥和髓质）、气道维持和保护所需的颅神经直接受累的病变、涉及面神经的病变以及患者的手术体位相关。在手术过程中遇到的实际事件是无法预测的，这对神经外科手术特别是颅后窝手术的全身麻醉提出了重大挑战。在开始任何颅后窝手术之前，至少应制订针对血流动力学不稳定、呼吸功能障碍、颅神经功能改变和静脉空气栓塞的诊断和管理计划。

启示

如前所述，接受颅后窝手术的患者面临的风险直接影响术前准备、监测方法和达到最佳围术期结局所需的麻醉技术。在手术前，必须仔细监测患者，并且非常小心地滴定镇静催眠药和镇痛药。术中风险主要是血流动力学不稳定和心血管衰竭。特别是对于涉及脑桥和髓质的手术，心率和血压的极端血流动力学变化可能导致患者不稳定。这种不稳定通常局限于直接手术操作时，但在临床上极为重要。静脉空气栓塞可引起血流动力学崩溃和心脏骤停，两者在所有颅后窝（和颅底）手术中可相继发生，即使在水平体位的患者中也可发生。必要时，应使用动脉置管和右心房导管。使用现代短效静脉制剂（全凭静脉麻醉），如丙泊酚、瑞芬太尼和右美托咪定等的麻醉方案对实施 SSEP 及颅神经 EMG 监测具有一定优势。目前，常用剂量的大多数麻醉药对 BAEP 影响较小。

管理

充分了解患者的病情和预计外科需求是管理的重要组成部分。未能理解颅后窝病变的具体位置和影响则会严重限制麻醉科医师提供最佳治疗和管理。整体麻醉管理类似于幕上病变手术。重点是准备好治疗突然和极端的血流动力学不稳定性，并确保在摆放体位时仔细注意细节，以避免与这些位置相关的多种并发症。

术后，为了确定是否需要持续监测和支持，应在患者清醒后专门评估与手术部位相关的所有颅神经和脑干功能。这要求麻醉方式可在手术结束时进行神经系统检查，优选在手术室中进行神经系统检查，然后再运送到重症监护室。而用于为神经生理学监测提供最佳条件的麻醉剂往往也能确保快速苏醒。

手术时程和颅后窝恶化的迹象和症状可能与幕上手术类似。对于幕上病变，恶化（通常由于肿块或脑积水扩大）通常会随着时间的推移而发展，因此连续监测较为合适。对于颅后窝手术，则可能发生快速的局部恶化，导致延髓功能丧失，呼吸停止或血流动力学崩溃。因此，必须在术后期间保持警惕。重要的是在拔管后重新评估气道，以便为术后可能出现的困难气道准备所有的必要设备。

预防

需要仔细评估患者并与外科医师讨论关于定位、影响和建议手术方法，以便对接受颅后窝手术的患者进行最佳管理。对常见的严重并发症有所预期，如术后 VAE 和气道或呼吸功能障碍，是麻醉管理的关键部分，因为这需要专门的监测技术。尽管与颅后窝手术相关的严重并发症在目前的外科手术中并不常见，但高度怀疑和持续警惕是围术期管理最重要的要素。

（蒋政宇 译 孟 岩 校）

延伸阅读

Dubey A, Sung WS, Shaya M, et al.: Complications of posterior cranial fossa surgery—an institutional experience of 500 patients, *Surg Neurol* 72(4):369–375, 2009.

Porter JM, Pidgeon C, Cunningham AJ: The sitting position in neurosurgery: a critical appraisal, *Br J Anaesth* 82(1):117–128, 1999.

Rath GP, Bithal PK, Chaturvedi A, Dash HH: Complications related to positioning in posterior fossa craniectomy, *J Clin Neurosci* 14(6):520–525, 2007.

产后出血

第 72 章

Joanna David，*Perumal Tamilselvan*

病例概要

患者，女性，29 岁，G4P2，娩出一名 4200 g 婴儿。由于体温升高和阴道流出的恶臭液体进行了催产。麻醉科医师在胎盘娩出后 2 h 被呼叫协助抢救，此时患者出现持续的低血压、心动过速且面色苍白。麻醉科医师到达时，被告知她的恶露比正常情况更重，阴道出现缓慢且持续的出血。

问题分析

定义

原发性产后出血（primary postpartum hemorrhage，PPH）定义为分娩后 24 h 内出血量达到 500 ml 或以上。PPH 可分为轻度（500 ~ 1000 ml）和重度（>1000 ml）。重度可进一步分为中重度（1000 ~ 2000 ml）和极重度（>2000 ml）。

大多数导致发病或死亡或使临床医师在管理中面临挑战的病例，失血量都超过 1000 ml。

尽管原发性 PPH 是产科出血最常见的形式，但不应忽视继发性 PPH。继发性 PPH 的定义为产后 24 h 至 12 周产道出血异常或过多。

识别

PPH 的发生率高达 10%。出血可以是明显的，如阴道出血或手术伤口出血。然而，出血也可以隐藏在子宫、软组织或腹膜内。患者可有如下表现：

- 焦虑、精神错乱或无反应；
- 低血压；
- 心动过速（注意使用 β 受体阻滞剂的患者可能表现为正常的心率或心动过缓）；
- 外周灌注不良；
- 少尿；
- 不明原因的代谢性酸中毒；
- 需要持续大量的液体输注来维持正常血压。

风险评估

大多数 PPH 患者没有明确的危险因素。具体的危险因素见表 72.1 和 72.2，这些危险因素可能导致直接失血或凝血功能障碍。其他危险因素包括以下

表 72.1　产后出血的主要危险因素

产前表现	PPH 的近似优势比（99% CI）
胎盘早剥	13（7.61 ~ 12.9）
胎盘前置	12（7.17 ~ 23）
多胎妊娠	5（3.0 ~ 6.6）
子痫前期 / 妊娠期高血压	4
既往有 PPH	3
种族	2（1.48 ~ 2.17）
肥胖（BMI>35）	2（1.24 ~ 2.17）
巨大儿（>4 kg）	2（1.38 ~ 2.60）
贫血（血红蛋白 <90 g/L）	2（1.63 ~ 3.15）
年龄 >40	1.4（1.16 ~ 1.74）
分娩过程中的显著危险因素	
剖宫产，急诊	4（3.28 ~ 3.95）
剖宫产，择期	2（2.18 ~ 2.80）
引产术	2（1.67 ~ 2.96）
胎盘滞留	5（3.36 ~ 7.87）
中外侧会阴切开术	5
手术助产的阴道分娩	2（1.38 ~ 2.60）
产程延长（12 h）	2
分娩时发热	2

BMI，体重指数；CI，置信区间；PPH，产后出血

表 72.2 产后出血病因与诱发因素的关系

病因	诱发因素
宫缩乏力	多胎妊娠，巨大儿，羊水过多，绒毛膜羊膜炎，产程延长，急产，催产，多胎产，使用宫缩抑制剂，使用强效吸入麻醉药
胎盘滞留	既往有胎盘滞留史，孕中期分娩，不正常的胎盘形成
创伤	急产，产钳助产，巨大儿
子宫内翻	宫缩乏力，脐带牵引不当，子宫畸形，不正常的胎盘形成

几点：

- 羊水过多；
- 急产；
- 催产；
- 多次分娩；
- 使用宫缩抑制剂；
- 吸入高浓度麻醉剂。

PPH 最常见的原因是宫缩乏力。足月时，通过胎盘脉管系统的血流量约为 600 ml/min。分娩后，控制出血的主要机制是子宫肌层的收缩。宫腔压塞可破坏前胎盘部位的血管。宫缩乏力会导致大量快速的血液流失。

胎盘滞留也是早期和迟发 PPH 的常见原因，尽管并非所有病例都会导致大量失血。滞留的胎盘碎片可能未被识别，因此出血可能是隐匿性的。既往有过胎盘滞留史或提前分娩病史的患者出现胎盘滞留可能性大。

所有产后宫缩正常但持续失血的患者均应考虑与分娩相关创伤导致的 PPH。创伤性出血可发生在以下部位：

- 阴道；
- 子宫颈；
- 子宫（剖宫产时处理不良，缝合线断裂）；
- 会阴（撕裂伤或会阴切开术）；
- 其他结构——阔韧带撕裂，卵巢动脉破裂。

子宫内翻是引起 PPH 的罕见原因，但可能是灾难性的。在所有存在明显低血压的 PPH 病例中，都应考虑到这个可能性。

启示

患者的预后取决于早期识别、失血速度和严重程度，以及及时的麻醉或产科干预。值得记住的是，PPH 是发生产后发病的主要原因，并且仍然是发达国家和发展中国家产妇死亡的五大原因之一。

管理

基础治疗

沟通

一旦患者发生产后出血，立即打电话寻求帮助，并通知高年资麻醉科医师和产科医师到场。还要通知血库、血液科医师和运输人员。确保抢救团队中有一个领导者和一个记录人员。

复苏

基本复苏遵循 ABCDE 模型。随着评估的进展，应对患者进行系统评估和支持。

- A：如果患者意识清醒，应给予高流量氧气。如果她的气道不能维持通畅，在气管插管前提供气道支持和氧合。
- B：如果需要，给予机械通气；同时监测脉搏氧饱和度。
- C：使用两根大口径静脉置管；采集血液进行分型、交叉配型和基础血液检查，包括静脉血气；静脉输注 2L 温热晶体液，若有指征应尽快输血；评估血压和心电图；控制出血，并在适当时抬高双下肢。
- D：检查患者的格拉斯哥昏迷量表（Glasgow Coma Scale，GCS）评分、瞳孔和血糖。
- E：全面评估患者情况；记录体温。

针对性治疗

这是一项多学科的工作，需要良好的沟通，并通过建立内部机制和演练得到帮助。

药物治疗

收缩子宫药物

子宫收缩乏力的主要治疗方法是使用子宫收缩药物。缩宫素是治疗和预防子宫收缩乏力的首选药物。预防性使用缩宫素使 PPH 的风险降低约 60%。在第三产程，预防性缩宫素以 5 ～ 10 IU 肌内注射，在剖宫产时 5 IU 缓慢静脉注射。缩宫素 10 IU 加于 0.9% 氯化钠注射液中静脉输注，有助于维持分娩后的子宫收缩。缩宫素输注时可引起血管扩张、低血压、恶心和面色潮红。

麦角生物碱是治疗子宫收缩乏力的二线药物，通常与缩宫素联合使用。麦角新碱主要通过 α- 肾上腺素能受体产生子宫强直性收缩。常规用量是 0.5 mg 肌内注射，一般在几分钟内起效，可以维持数小时。这类药物可能引起极端的高血压，尤其是高血压患者或同时接受升压药治疗的患者，严重的时候可以引起颅内出血、卒中或癫痫发作。

如果上述这些方法不能缓解子宫收缩乏力，15-甲基前列腺素 F_2（卡前列素）可用于难治性病例。但该类药物可引起支气管痉挛并改变肺通气 / 血流比值，导致低氧血症。常规的用量是 250 μg 肌内注射或宫内注射，每 15 ～ 30 min 重复一次，但总剂量不应超过 2 mg。另一种治疗 PPH 的前列腺素米索前列醇的安全性和有效性已被研究。标准剂量子宫收缩剂无反应的严重 PPH 经直肠给予 1000 μg 米索前列醇是有效的。最近几个病例报告描述了重组凝血因子Ⅶ a（20 ～ 40 μg/kg）在严重难治性 PPH 的患者中的成功应用。

宫缩抑制剂

这类药剂有助于子宫的松弛，并且在 PPH 发生的情况下，使得产科医师可进行人工剥离胎盘或恢复内翻的子宫。在血容量正常的患者中，静脉注射硝酸甘油（50 ～ 100 μg）可使子宫在 45 s 内松弛并持续约 60 s。硝酸甘油喷雾可作为静脉给药的替代方法，喷雾每经舌下喷一次均可释放约 400 μg 的硝酸甘油，使用时必须密切关注患者的血压。如果硝酸甘油无效或宫颈闭合（即不允许经阴道或其他手术操作），可能需要深度全身麻醉。在快速序贯诱导和气管插管后，强效吸入麻醉药可以使子宫松弛，但干预后应尽快停药。

纠正凝血功能

除了患者的复苏和麻醉剂的使用之外，麻醉科医师还负责纠正任何凝血功能的异常。这包括但不限于以下内容：

- 早期评估凝血功能和血液制品的需求量；
- 早期输注纤维蛋白原；
- 输注氨甲环酸；
- 与血液科医师保持联系，并按要求提供血样；
- 根据需要检查和输注红细胞悬液、血小板、新鲜冰冻血浆、冷沉淀和重组凝血因子Ⅶ a；
- 维持液体平衡。

这样做的目的是实现以下目标：

- 血红蛋白 >8 g/dl；
- 血小板计数 >75 × 10^9/L；
- 凝血酶原时间 <1.5 × 平均对照；
- 活化凝血酶原时间 <1.5 × 平均对照；
- 纤维蛋白原 >1.0 g/L。

手术治疗

为了达到止血的目的，可能需要手术干预。产科止血程序如下：

- 子宫外按摩（或剖宫产时宫内按摩），按摩时配合使用缩宫素；
- 人工剥离胎盘；
- 修复产道损伤；
- 宫腔填塞；
- Rusch 球囊导管压迫治疗；
- 剖腹探查术：术中判断是否需要行改良 B-Lynch 缝合术，是否需要行子宫切除术，是否需要行其他必要的术式；
- 处理子宫内翻；
- 如果在剖腹手术中无法确定出血点，可能需要介入放射治疗。

除了剖腹手术和大出血病例之外，大部分手术均可在区域麻醉下进行。阴道或会阴撕裂的修复也可以通过产科医师的局部浸润麻醉进行。

如果失血量很大和（或）持续失血，则需要全身麻醉，首选快速序贯诱导，压迫环状软骨行气管插管。

对于那些手术时间长且伴有大量失血的手术，可以使用区域麻醉，但一般不建议使用。

复苏后的治疗

产妇应转入产科高依赖病房（HDU）或重症监护病房（ICU）中持续监测生命体征直至稳定。并应根据当地指南进行定期评估。

预防

所有产妇在第三产程积极使用缩宫素应当成为

治疗标准。

如前所述，PPH 通常在没有预警的情况下发生。要预防相关的发病率和死亡率，就必须提高警惕，高度怀疑，并做好快速反应的准备。

使用早期预警评分，例如产科改良早期预警评分（Modified Early Obstetric Warning Score，MEOWS），使各级人员和有经验人员能够快速识别、评估、应对病情恶化的患者，从而促进早期复苏和生命支持。

应在分娩前识别存在产后出血风险的患者并进行会诊。当产妇准备分娩时，麻醉科会诊医师和产科工作人员必须在场。

如果产后出血风险很大（例如，存在胎盘植入的产妇），产妇应该被转到具有处理大出血的丰富专业知识和资源的机构，包括术中血液回收、介入放射学、适当的外科专业知识和加强治疗。产妇分娩时应确保相关科室的会诊医师和产科工作人员在场。

应该制订好主要的产科出血治疗方案，以迅速应对预料外的产后大出血。

在特定的患者群体（例如宗教团体：耶和华见证人）中，必须在预产和分娩时与患者沟通，以确定他们将接受哪些血液制品。这应该连同预立医疗指示一起在患者的病历中仔细记录。

（常永青 译 万小健 校）

延伸阅读

Boehlen F, Morales MA, Fontana P, et al.: Prolonged treatment of massive postpartum haemorrhage with recombinant factor VIIa: case report and review of the literature, *Br J Obstet Gynaecol* 3:284–287, 2004.

Crowley M: Postpartum hemorrhage. In Atlee JL, editor: *Complications in anesthesia*, Philadelphia, 1999, WB Saunders, pp 817–819.

El-Refaey H, Rodeck C: Post-partum haemorrhage: definitions, medical and surgical management: a time for change, *Br Med Bull* 67: 205–217, 2003.

Mayer D, Spielman F, Bell E: Antepartum and postpartum hemorrhage. In Chestnut DH, editor: *Obstetric anesthesia principles and practice*, ed 3, Philadelphia, 2004, Mosby, pp 668–682.

Papp Z: Massive obstetric hemorrhage, *J Perinat Med* 31:408–414, 2003.

Paterson-Brown S, Howell C: *Managing obstetric emergencies and trauma: the MOET course manual*, ed 3, Cambridge, UK, Cambridge University Press, 2014.

Royal College of Obstetricians and Gynaecologists: Postpartum haemorrhage, prevention and management (Green-top Guideline No. 52), 2009. Available at https://www.rcog.org.uk/en/guidelines-research-services/guidelines/gtg52/. Accessed May 24, 2016.

早 产

第73章

Amanpreet Kaur

病例概要

患者，女性，28岁，G2P1，估计胎龄为28周，出现新的有规律的子宫收缩。入院进行静脉补液和保胎治疗。

问题分析

定义 / 流行病学

2014年，疾病控制和预防中心（Centers for Disease Control and Prevention，CDC）的数据显示，早产率为9.57%。2012年的数据显示，美国有45万名早产儿；这意味着每9个新生儿中有1例是早产。早产的定义是妊娠不足37周的分娩。2010年，早产相关性死亡占新生儿死亡的35%，早产是导致儿童神经系统功能障碍的主要原因。其他还包括呼吸问题、喂养困难、脑瘫、发育迟缓、视力和听力障碍（框73.1）。目前产科的处理措施是尽可能延迟分娩。

识别

美国妇产科医师协会（ACOG）定义如下：

- **早产**（preterm labor），定义为在妊娠37周前出现有规律的子宫收缩。至少每10 min一次，伴宫颈扩张或宫颈管消失（表73.1）。
- 早产儿是指在妊娠37周前分娩的任何婴儿。
- 无论胎龄如何，任何出生时体重小于2500或1500 g的新生儿，均称为低出生体重（low-birth-weight,LBW）儿或极低出生体重（very-low-birth-weight，VLBW）儿。
- 妊娠29周时，超过90%的胎儿预估体重低于1500 g。
- 尽管在妊娠23周时存活率可能高达25%，但这些大多数都有明显的远期神经损伤。
- 从妊娠23周延迟分娩至31周可使新生儿存活率从25%提高到96%。

框73.1 早产的结局

- 呼吸问题
- 喂养困难
- 脑瘫
- 发育迟缓
- 视力问题
- 听力障碍

表73.1 早产常用术语的定义

术语	定义
早产	妊娠20～37周出现规则宫缩，10 min一次，宫颈检查改变
早产儿	妊娠37周前出生的婴儿
低出生体重儿	出生体重低于2500 g
极低出生体重儿	出生体重低于1500 g
胎膜早破	临产前胎膜破裂
早产胎膜早破	妊娠<37周发生胎膜破裂

风险评估

对早产患者的初步评估包括全面的查体，以排除可治疗的病情，比如急产，行盆腔检查排除胎膜早破。卧床休息、静脉补液、持续监测胎心率和宫缩描记几乎适用于所有情况。多数患者仅需卧床休息和补液。如果这些保守治疗无效，则须超声检查，必要时羊膜穿刺，以判断胎龄和胎儿成熟度。卵磷脂 / 鞘磷脂（lecithin/sphingomyelin，L/S）比值被视为胎儿成熟的标志。L/S比值大于2是胎儿肺成熟的标志。

一旦确诊，产科医师必须决定是否进行药物性保胎治疗。决定因素包括预估的胎龄、胎儿体重以及胎心率是否在安全范围。一般来说，胎龄在

20～34周之间，胎儿体重小于2500 g，且胎心率好，无胎儿窘迫，是保胎治疗的指证。有时，为了促进胎肺成熟，有必要等待24 h以完成两次剂量的地塞米松或倍他米松治疗。

目前常用的保胎药可能与麻醉药发生显著的相互作用。此外，早产可能会影响分娩途径（阴道或腹部）。

启示

理解药物干预以终止早产的机制、子宫收缩的生理基础和钙的作用非常重要。

目前对发动临产的过程尚未完全理解，更多理解的是子宫收缩的生理学。子宫肌层含有肌球蛋白和肌动蛋白，它们产生收缩力。子宫肌层内的自律细胞能够自发的产生收缩活动，并可通过细胞间连接扩散到整个子宫肌层。

钙发挥着关键作用。收缩前，钙通过肌质网释放或通过肌膜，细胞内钙浓度增加。钙与钙调蛋白结合，激活肌球蛋白轻链激酶。激活的肌球蛋白轻链激酶磷酸化肌球蛋白，然后与肌动蛋白结合。腺苷三磷酸（adenosine triphosphate，ATP）被肌球蛋白腺苷三磷酸酶（ATP酶）水解，导致肌动蛋白-肌球蛋白的滑动和子宫肌层收缩。细胞内钙浓度降低或肌球蛋白去磷酸化抑制肌动蛋白-肌球蛋白相互作用，导致舒张（框73.2）

级联反应为药物干预提供了许多靶点。刺激子宫平滑肌细胞膜上的β_2-肾上腺素能受体，可激活腺苷酸环化酶，将ATP转化为环腺苷酸（cyclic adenosine monophosphate，cAMP）。cAMP的增加降低了细胞内的钙离子浓度，抑制了肌球蛋白轻链激酶，降低了收缩活性而导致舒张（框73.3）。

框73.2 描述子宫收缩的流程图

子宫肌层的起搏细胞开始自发活动→钙通过肌质网释放或通过肌膜→细胞内钙增加→钙—钙调蛋白复合物→激活肌球蛋白轻链激酶→肌球蛋白磷酸化→肌球蛋白ATP酶水解ATP→肌动蛋白-肌球蛋白相互作用开始收缩。

框73.3 描述子宫舒张的流程图

肌质网摄取钙→细胞内钙减少→肌球蛋白去磷酸化→抑制肌动蛋白-肌球蛋白相互作用，引起舒张。

硫酸镁可能通过竞争结合部位降低细胞内游离钙浓度，减少子宫活动。还可能激活腺苷酸环化酶，增加cAMP的合成。

通过阻断细胞膜中的电压依赖性钙通道（或改变细胞内的摄取和释放机制），钙通道阻滞剂降低了肌层内游离钙的浓度。

前列腺素$F_{2\alpha}$和$E_{2\alpha}$是子宫活动的强效刺激物。分娩时，其在母体血液和羊水中的浓度增加。非甾体抗炎药可抑制前列腺素合成酶，从而抑制前列腺素的产生。

管理

目前所有可用的保胎药物并非都一定能成功保胎，因此很难比较这些药的有效性。每种方式都有副作用，因此可能限制其使用（表73.2）。保胎药包括硫酸镁、β_2-肾上腺素能受体激动剂、前列腺素合成酶抑制剂和钙通道阻滞剂（框73.4）。此外，一种新型药物缩宫素抑制剂阿托西班在欧洲也得到了应用。

表73.2 常见保胎药对母体和胎儿的副作用

保胎药	母体副作用	胎儿副作用
阿托西班	无至极小	可能增加围生期死亡
硫酸镁	剂量依赖性（见表73.3）	呼吸抑制，反射减退，音调减低胎心率变异度降低，生物物理评分降低
β_2-肾上腺素能受体激动剂	低血压，心排血量增加，高血糖，低钾血症，快速性心律失常，肺水肿	快速性心律失常
前列腺素合成酶抑制剂	可能影响母体凝血功能	胎儿动脉导管提前关闭，减少尿生成，羊水过少，肾衰竭
钙通道阻滞剂	低血压、反射性心动过速、头痛、恶心	极小

框73.4 常见的保胎药

硫酸镁
β_2-肾上腺素能受体激动剂
前列腺素合成酶抑制剂
钙通道阻滞剂

缩宫素抑制剂

阿西托班｛1-（3-巯基丙酸）-2-[3-（对乙酰苯基）-D-丙氨酸]-4-L-苏氨酸-8-L-鸟氨酸缩宫素｝是缩宫素受体拮抗剂。是一种与子宫肌层和蜕膜上缩宫素受体结合的缩宫素竞争性抑制剂。由于它不会改变子宫肌层对缩宫素的敏感性，所以产后子宫收缩乏力和出血的风险微乎其微。

二期和三期研究表明阿托西班是一种有效的保胎药。它对母体的副作用更少，胎盘屏障透过最少，不增加产妇分娩时的失血。在回顾性研究中，由于阿托西班组的围生期新生儿死亡率较高，因此阿托西班尚未获得美国食品药品监督管理局的批准。

尚无关于阿托西班与麻醉药相互作用的数据。然而，考虑到该药的血流动力学特征，我们不希望发生明显的相互作用。阿托西班在欧洲国家已得到广泛应用。

硫酸镁

镁剂因其成本低、严重副作用的发生率相对较低，是大多数中心首选的静脉保胎药。在神经肌肉接头，镁剂抑制乙酰胆碱的释放，降低突触后终板对乙酰胆碱的敏感性。硫酸镁可能通过竞争结合位点降低细胞内游离钙浓度，减少子宫收缩。还可能激活腺苷酸环化酶，增加 cAMP 的合成。

正常血清镁浓度范围为 1.6 ～ 2.4 mg/dl。治疗：初始静脉注射 4 ～ 6 g，之后以 1 ～ 2 g/h 的剂量维持。滴定并维持血清浓度在 4 ～ 8 mg/dl；尽管通常足以抑制子宫收缩，但这并不总能有效。

镁剂会引起周围血管扩张，尤其是在开始治疗时，产妇经常会感到温热、脸红和恶心。镁剂可能导致母体出现短暂性的心动过速和低血压。在较高的血清浓度下，还可观察到其他作用。镁的浓度低于 10 mg/dl 时，宽大的 QRS 波和 PR 间期延长并不常见，但在治疗浓度下也可出现。浓度为 12 mg/dl 或更高时，深反射消失。浓度为 18 mg/dl 可导致呼吸停止，浓度为 25 mg/dl 时可发生心脏停搏（表 73.3）。胎儿影响少见；有报道胎心率变异率降低，胎儿生理活动评分降低。母体长期接受镁治疗，新生儿有呼吸抑制、反射减弱和子宫张力下降的报道。

由于血管扩张，这些患者在椎管内麻醉时可能出现低血压。硬膜外或脊髓麻醉须在监测母体血压的条件下实施，推荐选择起效较慢的硬膜外麻醉。

表 73.3 血清镁浓度对母体的副作用

血清镁浓度（mg/dl）	母体的副作用
4 ～ 8（治疗浓度）	温热，脸红，恶心；短暂性心动过速和低血压
>10	宽大的 QRS 波和 PR 间期延长
>12	深反射消失
>18	呼吸抑制
>25	心脏停搏

当需要全身麻醉时，接受镁治疗的产妇对肌松药更敏感。使用琥珀胆碱后，需用肌松监测仪密切关注四个成串刺激，以指导肌松药的使用。由于肌松药的作用被扩大，再一次给药时应减小剂量。尽管治疗浓度的镁剂可以降低氟烷的最低肺泡浓度，但这并没有显著的临床意义。分娩后可能会出现宫缩乏力和产后出血。应及早发现并及时治疗。

β_2-肾上腺素能受体激动剂

利托君（羟苄羟麻黄碱）和特布他林（间羟叔丁肾上腺素）可用于保胎，然而仅羟苄羟麻黄碱被 FDA 批准用于抑制宫缩。羟苄羟麻黄碱通过持续静脉输注给药，并根据宫缩情况滴定。间羟叔丁肾上腺素可单次静脉或皮下给药，可迅速但短暂抑制子宫收缩，并可继续口服。

尽管减少宫缩仅需兴奋 β_2 受体，但这两类药物都有显著的 β_1-肾上腺素能效应，这是产生副作用的主要原因。β_2-肾上腺素能活性可引起血管扩张（导致低血压）和高血糖。直接兴奋 β_1 受体，增加心肌收缩力和心率，可增加心排血量，这可能对局部麻醉期间的低血压起到保护作用。β-受体激动剂治疗最显著的副作用与心脏相关。无论是心源性的还是非心源性的肺水肿，发生率高达 4%。通常通过限制静脉输液量来解决。心肌缺血也有报道，表现为胸痛和心电图改变；可以通过停药解决。快速性心律失常（母体和胎儿）时有发生。最后，这些患者还常伴有高血糖和低钾血症。

当需要麻醉时，最好停止治疗至少 60 ～ 90 min；不幸的是，这种延迟可能危及胎儿。为防肺水肿，应避免过度静脉输液，选择升压药（麻黄碱）维持母体血压。

前列腺素合成酶抑制剂

前列腺素 $E_{2\alpha}$ 和 $F_{2\alpha}$ 是子宫收缩的有效刺激物，

它们也会在临产期促使宫颈软化（“成熟”）。前列腺素合成酶抑制剂阻止花生四烯酸转化为具有活性的前列腺素。虽然这类药物都具有这种作用，但对于早产来说，只有吲哚美辛应用广泛。它可以口服和直肠给药，并持续数周。

与镁剂和 β-受体激动剂相比，吲哚美辛对母体几乎没有副作用。它可能会影响母体的凝血，但这似乎没有临床意义。对于止血功能正常的健康产妇，通常不需要进一步评估产妇凝血状态。

然而，这类药物对胎儿可能具有显著的作用。前列腺素合成酶抑制剂可能导致子宫内胎儿动脉导管提前关闭；这种影响似乎与胎龄有关，在妊娠 32 周前较少出现。吲哚美辛可能导致胎尿液减少，羊水减少，但很少导致新生儿肾衰竭。最后，在出生前子宫内给予吲哚美辛治疗后，新生儿的坏死性小肠结肠炎、颅内出血和支气管肺发育不良发生率增加。

钙通道阻滞剂

钙通道阻滞剂通过抑制钙离子内流，降低子宫肌层收缩力。硝苯地平被广泛应用于宫缩。舌下给药后迅速起效，并可口服维持治疗。

硝苯地平对母体的副作用一般较轻，其对心脏影响不大，常见血管扩张和血压下降。反射性心动过速、头痛和恶心可能与此相关。

预防

尽管积极治疗，通常却是保胎失败并进入产程。当分娩不可避免时，必须选择最佳的分娩方式。大多数产科医师认为胎儿存活的下限是妊娠 24 ～ 25 周。LBW、VLBW、臀位和小于 32 周胎龄，常规选择剖宫产。外科分娩目的是避免头部外伤和继发的颅内出血。估计胎龄小于 32 周且为臀位的胎儿在阴道分娩时容易出现脐带脱垂、肌肉损伤和头部夹闭。然而，必须权衡外科分娩对胎儿的优点与剖宫产导致母体损伤的缺点。

剖宫产时，硬膜外麻醉优于全身麻醉。大多数用于全身麻醉诱导和维持的麻醉药透过胎盘，对胎儿有抑制作用。硬膜外麻醉下行剖宫产的早产儿，其 1 min 和 5 min Apgar 评分高于全身麻醉。一些动物研究的数据表明，未成熟的大脑暴露于麻醉药，如丙泊酚、硫喷妥钠、氯胺酮和吸入麻醉药，可引起胚胎/新生动物出现显著的神经细胞凋亡，并导致功能性的学习障碍。在无胎儿窘迫的情况下，椎管内神经阻滞时对母体氧疗的作用仍有争议。

值得注意的是，除阿托西班外，分娩后保胎药的子宫松弛作用持续存在。根据治疗的持续时间和药物的半衰期，所有这些药物都可能导致术中子宫松弛。因此有必要积极的治疗，以恢复子宫张力和预防产后出血。应建立两个或多个大口径静脉通路。获取血型及交叉配血，同时配备恢复子宫张力的药物；包括缩宫素、甲氧西林、前列腺素 $F_{2\alpha}$ 拮抗剂和米索前列醇。

VLBW 儿如需进行阴道分娩，行硬膜外麻醉可使骨盆得到良好的松弛。子宫颈扩张无论是否伴有胎膜膨胀，应根据操作者的技术，尽可能选择侧位进行硬膜外麻醉。阴部阻滞或会阴局部浸润对生产疼痛没有帮助。椎管内镇痛可以降低母体儿茶酚胺的浓度，只要避免低血压，甚至可以改善子宫胎盘灌注。尽早开始硬膜外镇痛的一大优势是需紧急剖宫产时能迅速从分娩镇痛转变为外科麻醉。

然而，改善早产儿存活率最重要的是确保有经过培训的新生儿科医师在场进行复苏，并随时可转入新生儿重症监护室进行后续护理。综上所述，需要产科医师、麻醉科医师和新生儿科医师共同努力来改善产妇尤其是早产儿的预后。

致谢

感谢 Craig Palmer 博士对本章上一版的贡献。

（李路路　译　文平山　校）

延伸阅读

ACOG Practice Bulletin: Management of preterm labor, *Obstet Gynecol* 101:1039–1047, 2003.

Childress CH, Katz VL: Nifedipine and its indications in obstetrics and gynecology, *Obstet Gynecol* 83:616–624, 1994.

Goldenberg RL: The management of preterm labor, *Obstet Gynecol* 100:1020–1037, 2002.

Hack M, Fanaroff AA: Outcomes of children of extremely low birthweight and gestational age in the 1990s, *Early Hum Dev* 53:193–218, 1999.

Huddleston JF, Sanchez-Ramos L, Huddleston KW: Acute management of preterm labor, *Clin Perinatol* 30:803–824, 2003.

Lumley J: Method of delivery for the preterm infant, *Br J Obstet Gynaecol* 110(Suppl 20):88–92, 2003.

Palmer CM: Complications of labor. In Palmer CM, D'Angelo R, Paech MJ, editors: *Handbook of obstetric anesthesia*, Oxford UK, 2002, BIOS Scientific Publishers Ltd, pp 163–173.

Wilkins IA, Lynch L, Mehalek KE, et al.: Efficacy and side effects of magnesium sulfate and ritodrine as tocolytic agents, *Am J Obstet Gynecol* 159:685–689, 1988.

肺动脉高压

第 74 章

Andrew Roscoe

病例概要

患者，男性，55 岁，患终末期肺病，因普通间质性肺炎接受双肺移植术。术中对第二肺进行再灌注时，患者发生缺血再灌注损伤。患者出现急性移植物功能障碍、肺动脉高压和右心室衰竭。

问题分析

定义

肺动脉高压（pulmonary hypertension，PHT）指在静息状态下，右肺动脉平均压（mean pulmonary artery pressure，mPAP）≥ 25 mmHg。根据肺动脉楔压（pulmonary artery wedge pressure，PAWP），分为毛细血管前 PHT（PAWP ≤ 15 mmHg）和毛细血管后 PHT（PAWP>15 mm Hg）。

PHT 可依据 mPAP 分为轻度、中度、重度：

- 轻度：25 mmHg ≤ mPAP<40 mmHg；
- 中度：40 mmHg ≤ mPAP<55 mmHg；
- 重度：mPAP ≥ 55 mmHg。

mPAP 与心排血量（cardiac output，CO）、肺血管阻力（pulmonary vascular resistance，PVR）的关系如下：

$$mPAP=CO \times PVR$$

因此，CO 和（或）PVR 增加可导致 mPAP 增加。正常人肺循环血管顺应性高，CO 增加时，肺血管复张，PVR 可相应降低，使 mPAP 保持稳定。

对毛细血管后 PHT 患者，跨肺压（transpulmonary pressure，TPG）可用于识别高危患者：

$$TPG = mPAP-PAWP$$

毛细血管后 PHT 的患者早期 TPG 正常（<12 mmHg），但可发展为混合型毛细血管前和毛细血管后 PHT，此时伴 TPG 升高。由于 TPG 受心排血量的影响，PVR 可作为混合型 PHT 的更好的指标。正常 PVR 小于 3 伍德（Wood）单位 [<240 dynes/（$s \cdot cm^5$）]。

PHT 可根据病理学和病理生理学进行分类（框 74.1）。

识别

放置肺动脉导管（pulmonary artery catheter，PAC）的患者，易于诊断急性 PHT。

没有 PAC 时，经食管超声心动图（transesophageal echocardiography，TEE）可以辅助诊断。存在三尖瓣反流（tricuspid regurgitation，TR）时，基于连续波多普勒评估 TR 射流峰值速度（peak velocity of tricuspid regurgitation，V_{TR}），利用简化的伯努利方程估计收缩期肺动脉压（systolic pulmonary artery

框 74.1 肺动脉高压的临床分型

1 动脉性肺动脉高压
  1.1 特发性
  1.2 遗传性
  1.3 药物诱导性
1′ 肺静脉闭塞病
1″ 新生儿持续性肺动脉高压
2 继发于左心疾病的肺动脉高压
  2.1 收缩性心功能不全
  2.2 舒张性心功能不全
  2.3 瓣膜疾病
3 继发于肺部疾病和（或）低氧的肺动脉高压
  3.1 慢性阻塞性肺疾病
  3.2 间质性肺疾病
  3.3 限制性与阻塞性并存的肺疾病
  3.4 睡眠障碍
4 慢性血栓栓塞性肺动脉高压
5 多因素机制所致肺动脉高压
  5.1 血液系统疾病
  5.2 系统性疾病
  5.3 代谢性疾病

pressure，sPAP）：

$$sPAP=4V^2_{TR}+CVP$$

没有明显 TR 时，脉搏波多普勒（pulse-wave Doppler，PWD）可有助于评估肺动脉（pulmonary artery，PA）血流，测量 PA 加速时间（pulmonary artery acceleration time，PAAT），从而得出 mPAP：

$$mPAP=73-(0.42\times PAAT)$$

PA PWD 波形的形态亦可有助于区分是毛细血管前还是毛细血管后病因。此外，TEE 在快速诊断右心室衰竭和检测左心室功能障碍方面发挥关键作用。TEE 还可排除导致毛细血管后 PHT 的任何机械性原因，如肺静脉吻合术的狭窄。

风险评估

肺移植术后原发性移植物功能障碍（primary graft dysfunction，PGD）以肺水肿、低氧血症和 PHT 为特征表现。其在肺移植术后发生率高达 25%。风险因素包括：供体因素（年龄 > 45 岁、女性、头部创伤）、受体因素（肺动脉高压、体重指数 > 25）和手术因素（缺血时间延长、应用体外循环）。PGD 的发生与患者术后机械通气时间延长和早期死亡率增加有关。

发生 PHT 的非肺移植术后的患者中，75% 继发于左心衰竭。

启示

非心脏手术中，PHT 并非围术期心血管事件病死率风险评分的公认风险因素。但是，已确认患有 PHT 的患者发生围术期并发症的风险显著增加。中度 PHT 患者在接受非心脏手术时，病残率和死亡率分别高达 42% 和 7%。心脏外科手术中，PHT 是公认的预后因素之一，与患者围术期死亡率有明确的相关性。

管理

PHT 管理的原则是，优化右心室前负荷、增强右心室收缩力、维持右冠状动脉（right coronary artery，RCA）灌注压、采取降低 PVR 的措施。

右心室前负荷

当患者 PVR 增加、右心室功能障碍时，容量负荷增加不利于维持血流动力学稳定。右心室 Starling 曲线比左心室更平坦，因此前负荷增加会导致右心室扩张，而每搏输出量仅少量增加。右心室扩张会导致：

- 游离室壁张力增加，氧耗增加；
- RCA 灌注压降低，氧供减少；
- 三尖瓣环状扩张，导致三尖瓣关闭不全恶化，加剧容量超负荷；
- 心室壁向左移位，阻碍左心室舒张期充盈，左心室每搏输出量减少，导致体循环低血压。

正压通气可影响前负荷，尤其是气道压力高或应用呼气末正压（positive end-expiratory pressure，PEEP）纠正低氧血症时。

治疗包括应用利尿剂或血液透析降低前负荷，通常使中心静脉压（central venous pressure，CVP）低于 15 mmHg。

右心室收缩力

心室游离壁心肌过度拉伸或心肌血液灌注减少、氧供减少导致心肌缺血，都可能导致右心室收缩功能障碍。正性肌力药常用于提高右心室收缩力，但同时会增加氧耗并可能导致快速性心律失常，因此必须合理选用：

- 多巴胺 [5 ～ 10 μg/（kg · min）] 和肾上腺素可增强右心室收缩力，同时可维持体循环动脉压，对 PVR 几乎没有影响。
- 低剂量多巴酚丁胺 [5 ～ 10 μg/（kg · min）] 可增强右心室收缩性并改善右心室–肺动脉耦合。然而，当剂量升高时，其可通过 β_2 受体介导的体循环血管舒张导致 RCA 灌注压降低。
- 磷酸二酯酶 -3 抑制剂米力农具备一些颇具吸引力的特性，如：正性肌力和扩张肺血管，但可引起显著的体循环血管舒张，更适于治疗毛细血管后 PHT 和双心室衰竭。
- 钙敏化剂左西孟旦，一种强效的强心扩血管药，可改善右心室舒张功能，但也可显著扩张体循环血管。

右冠状动脉灌注

正常情况下，右心室的心肌在整个心脏周期内都有血液灌注。当 PA 压力接近体循环血压时，RCA

仅在心脏舒张期有血液灌注，且灌注量决定于体循环动脉压和右心室舒张压。在右心室容量超负荷、扩张，同时体循环动脉压降低时，心肌灌注量更少。主要治疗方法是确保维持足够的体循环血压：

- 去甲肾上腺素主要作用于 α_1 受体，引起血管收缩，但也有部分激活 β_1 受体的作用，增强 RV 收缩性，并已在一些研究中证明其可改善右心室-肺动脉耦合。
- 血管升压素作用于 V_1 受体，低剂量（<0.03 U/min）时引起肺血管扩张，高剂量时引起肺动脉和冠状动脉血管收缩，无正性肌力作用。可作为去甲肾上腺素的辅助用药以维持体循环动脉压。

降低肺血管阻力

降低 PVR 的基本措施包括避免缺氧、高碳酸血症和酸血症；保持正常体温；肺复张手法以减轻通气/血流（ventilation/perfusion，V/Q）比失调；小潮气量通气（PVR 在功能残气量时最小）；使用肺血管扩张剂（框 74.2）。

吸入性肺血管扩张剂，一氧化氮（nitric oxide，NO）和前列环素衍生物，可降低 PVR，而对体循环动脉压影响小。尽管其可改善肺血流动力学，但是否有利于预后仍待研究证实。

框 74.2　肺血管扩张剂

吸入

- NO
- PGI_2 类似物
- 米力农

静脉

- 硝酸甘油
- 腺苷
- PGI_2 类似物
- 多巴酚丁胺
- 米力农
- PDE-5 抑制剂

口服

- PDE-5 抑制剂
- PGI_2 类似物
- ET 拮抗剂
- 可溶性鸟苷酸环化酶（sGC）激动剂利奥西呱
- 肼屈嗪
- CCBs

CCBs，钙通道阻滞剂；ET，内皮素；PDE，磷酸二酯酶；PGI_2，前列环素

静脉用肺血管扩张药的缺点是对体循环具有显著的副作用，且可影响缺氧性肺血管收缩机制、加重 V/Q 失衡。钙通道拮抗剂有负性肌力作用，在 RV 功能障碍的情况下应避免使用。内皮素受体拮抗剂广泛用于治疗特发性 PHT 和慢性血栓栓塞性 PHT，但已证明可增加毛细血管后 PHT 的死亡率。

机械辅助循环

在传统药物治疗均无效时，可以考虑应用体外生命支持（extracorporeal life support，ECLS）提供临时辅助。若 PHT 仅由低氧血症所致，可应用静脉-静脉 ECLS 提供氧合，降低 PVR，从而改善右心室功能。若存在其他原因，可应用静脉-动脉 ECLS 可提供循环和呼吸支持。但是，ECLS 只能在病因可逆的情况下临时应用。

预防

减轻 PHT 对右心室功能影响以及严重程度的基本方法：

- 确保足够的氧合；
- 避免高碳酸血症；
- 避免酸血症；
- 维持正常体温；
- 小潮气量通气；
- 手法复张以减轻 V/Q 失调。

已有研究探讨在肺移植术、左心室辅助装置、肺切除术中预防性使用吸入 NO 的作用，但结果并不一致。

（李露茜　译　刘　毅　校）

延伸阅读

Ashes C, Roscoe A: Transesophageal echocardiography in thoracic anesthesia: pulmonary hypertension and right ventricular function, *Curr Opin Anesthesiol* 28:38–44, 2015.

Costanzo MR, Dipchand A, Starling R, et al.: The International Society of Heart and Lung Transplantation Guidelines for the care of heart transplant recipients, *J Heart Lung Transplant* 29:914–956, 2010.

Fox DL, Stream AR, Bull T: Perioperative management of the patient with pulmonary hypertension, *Semin Cardiothorac Vasc Anesth* 18:310–318, 2014.

Galie N, Humbert M, Vachiery JL, et al.: 2015 ESC/ERS Guidelines for the diagnosis and treatment of pulmonary hypertension, *Eur Heart J* 37:67–119, 2016.

Haddad F, Elmi-Sarabi M, Fadel E, et al.: Pearls and pitfalls in managing right heart failure in cardiac surgery, *Curr Opin Anaesthesiol* 29:68–71, 2016.

Hill NS, Roberts KR, Preston IR: Postoperative pulmonary hypertension: etiology and treatment of a dangerous complication, *Respir Care* 54:958–968, 2009.

Hoeper MM, Barbera JA, Channick RN, et al.: Diagnosis, assessment and treatment of non-pulmonary arterial hypertension pulmonary hypertension, *J Am Coll Cardiol* 54:S85–S96, 2009.

Hosseinian L: Pulmonary hypertension and noncardiac surgery: implications for the anesthesiologist, *J Cardiothorac Vasc Anesth* 28: 1064–1074, 2014.

Kanwar MK, Thenappan T, Vachiery JL: Update in treatment options in pulmonary hypertension, *J Heart Lung Transplant* 35:695–703, 2016.

Lang RM, Badano LP, Mor-Avi V, et al.: Recommendations for cardiac chamber quantification by echocardiography in adults: an update from the American Society of Echocardiography and the European Association of Cardiovascular Imaging, *J Am Soc Echocardiogr* 28:1–39, 2015.

Minai OA, Yared J, Kaw R, et al.: Perioperative risk and management in patients with pulmonary hypertension, *Chest* 144:329–340, 2013.

Porteous MK, Diamond JM, Christie JD: Primary graft dysfunction: lessons learned about the first 72 hours after lung transplantation, *Curr Opin Organ Transplant* 20:506–514, 2015.

Ramakrishna G, Sprung J, Ravi BS, et al.: Impact of pulmonary hypertension on the outcomes of noncardiac surgery, *J Am Coll Cardiol* 45: 1691–1699, 2005.

Rosenkranz S, Gibbs JS, Wachter R, et al.: Left ventricular heart failure and pulmonary hypertension, *Eur Heart J* 37:942–954, 2016.

Ventetuolo CE, Klinger JR: Management of acute right ventricular failure in the intensive care unit, *Ann Am Thorac Surg* 11:811–822, 2014.

球后阻滞

第 75 章

Wendy B. Kang

病例概要

患者，70 岁，拟在监护麻醉下行白内障超声乳化 + 人工晶状体植入术。既往有高血压，控制良好。有冠状动脉疾病、轻度肺气肿和肾功能不全。麻醉科医师行球后阻滞，同时静脉给予 1 mg 咪达唑仑镇静和语言安慰。5 min 后患者失去反应，心率为 35 次 / 分，且呼吸不规律，氧饱和度为 83%。

问题分析

定义

人口数量迅速增长的工业化国家，白内障手术仍然是最常见的外科手术。然而，可能是由于缺乏技术熟练度，或是术后当天患者的随访不及时，许多麻醉科医师并没有意识到与眼科区域麻醉相关的视力和危及生命的并发症。麻醉科医师必须意识到局部麻醉药（局麻药）注射到患者眼中所产生的罕见但可能致命的后果，以预测并发症并予以适当处理。

文献指出眼科麻醉临床实践向微创发展。自 1884 年 Knapp 在球后使用 4% 可卡因起，Atkinson 在 1936 年提倡了一种“现代”的方法，即眼眶内盲穿。1986 年，Davis 和 Mandel 提出球周技术。1992 年，Stevens 发表关于在眼筋膜下阻滞下白内障摘除术的文章。无需完全眼球运动抑制和镇痛的现代眼科手术中，结膜下和表面麻醉是有效的方法。

与其他区域阻滞相比，球后阻滞联合面神经阻滞能提供良好的运动抑制、麻醉和镇痛效果。其适应证包括：

- 内科并存疾病多的老年患者，避免全身麻醉；
- 需最佳手术条件的下列手术：白内障囊外摘除术、超声乳化术、人工晶状体植入术和开放式全眼球手术（例如玻璃体切除术、青光眼治疗、视网膜脱离修复）；
- 时间长、难度大的手术（如既往有眼科手术史）或患有硬性白内障或眼球震颤的患者。

球后阻滞的禁忌证包括：

- 对局麻药过敏；
- 已告知使用静脉镇静药物减少疼痛和无围术期知晓，患者仍拒绝；
- 无法配合的患者。

手术室团队应确定局部麻醉的禁忌证。“不配合”的患者包括精神障碍、青少年、痴呆、耳聋、严重肺气肿或充血性心力衰竭、过度焦虑、帕金森震颤、下肢不宁综合征或无法平躺。对于这些患者，选择区域麻醉复合最小剂量静脉镇静药和语言安慰，还是选择全身麻醉，应由眼科医师、麻醉科医师和患者应共同商讨决定。

还必须考虑凝血功能异常。有证据表明服用非甾体抗炎药、阿司匹林或华法林的患者可以安全地进行眼科手术。

识别

并发症

影响视力的损伤主要包括眼球、视神经、视网膜中央静脉和动脉以及这些结构周围肌肉的针刺伤。曾有发生差错（非手术）注射的报道。在眼球内注射麻醉药导致巩膜穿孔、玻璃体出血、玻璃体液体丢失和低眼压、视网膜红反射减弱和视网膜脱离。非术侧眼短暂性视力丧失，是局麻药注射到视神经鞘，通过蛛网膜下腔扩散至视交叉以及对侧视神经造成。视网膜中央静脉、动脉出血，造成血管阻塞，视神经受压和缺血。即刻、延迟和部分至完全视力丧失均有报道。上直肌和下直肌注射引起对抗肌肉之间收缩不协调，导致复视、垂直斜视和永久性肌病引起的持续斜视。结膜下血肿或前房积血，对视觉影响明显，但危害较小。

报道的出现危及生命并发症的麻醉技术有球后、球周甚至微创技术。直接蛛网膜下腔注射局麻药导致并可以即刻发生的脑干麻醉，以及严重高位脊髓麻醉需要心肺复苏治疗心动过缓或心脏停搏、呼吸暂停和低血压。当患者表现出轻微的意识模糊、对言语或疼痛刺激逐渐无反应、颤抖和痉挛发作、双侧眼神经麻痹和黑矇、偏瘫、四肢瘫、呼吸抑制和血流动力学不稳定等脑干麻醉（如前所述）缓慢发作的症状时，其诊断难度增加。急性肺水肿、三叉神经阻滞和“昏迷”，免疫功能低下患者出现严重眼眶蜂窝织炎，近视性葡萄肿和球后阻滞后结膜水肿均有报导。如果手术铺单已完成，除非麻醉科医师警惕并注意发现这些可能的并发症，否则诊断和治疗可能会延迟。应始终保证能获得足够的复苏能力，以防止死亡。

在球后或球周阻滞时，与眼心反射相关的心动过缓、心脏停搏或其他心律失常可能与脑干麻醉相混淆。眼球注射、眼球压迫、眼外肌牵拉、结膜牵拉或眼球牵拉刺激通过三叉神经的眼支传递到迷走神经。未经阿托品预处理的幼儿更易发生眼心反射。

以老年人为主的人群中，其他内科病因如心绞痛、控制不佳的高血压、心肌梗死的隐匿性发作或卒中，是必须鉴别的诊断。在没有眼部注射或眼压变化的情况下，血管迷走神经反射发作可以开始于静脉注射时。患有视网膜病变的糖尿病患者可能有低血糖或糖尿病酮症酸中毒的症状。恰当的麻醉前评估和患者状态优化可以减少部分围术期混杂因素。

区域麻醉并发症的发生率非常低。眼球穿孔发生率为 1/（1300 ～ 16 000），脑干麻醉发生率为 1/（300 ～ 500）（框 75.1）。英国最近一些观察性研究指出眼球穿孔发生率为 0.009% ～ 0.13%，脑干抑制发生率为 0.09% ～ 0.79%。在一项回顾性研究中，麻醉相关复视的发生率为 0.25%，其中球后阻滞占其中的 0.39%。

框 75.1 球后阻滞的并发症

- 球后或球周出血
- 眼球穿透或穿孔
- 视神经损伤导致视力改变，包括失明
- 中枢神经系统抑制导致脑干麻醉
- 严重的眼心反射
- 复视和眼肌不协调

不幸的是，尽管采用微创眼科技术，但危害患者安全和导致眼部损伤的事件仍有发生。2007 年一项针对英国常规眼科实践的前瞻性观察性研究估计，92% 的白内障手术在无镇静局麻下进行。在约 375 000 个局麻病例中，球周阻滞、眼筋膜下阻滞、球后阻滞、结膜下麻醉、表面麻醉和前房内局麻所占比例分别为 30.6%、42.6%、3.5%、1.7%、9.9% 和 11.0%。2009 年，英国白内障国家数据库审核统计 55 567 例手术，眼筋膜下麻醉使用最广泛。球周阻滞平均为 19.5%，球后阻滞降至 0.5%。与眼筋膜下使用钝性套管针相比，锋利穿刺针麻醉严重并发症风险显著增加。

微创技术允许焦虑的患者挤压眼睑或手术目标移动。当为眼球筋膜注射使用剪刀分离组织时，可发生眼球穿孔和后囊膜撕裂，需要进行眼前段玻璃体切割术。

解剖学因素

为了解用于眼科手术的球后阻滞和其他区域麻醉技术的并发症，有必要对眼部解剖结构进行简要回顾（图 75.1）。眼外肌肉环绕眼球并形成肌锥。外直肌由外展神经（第Ⅵ脑神经）支配，上斜肌由滑车神经（第Ⅳ脑神经）支配，其他肌肉由动眼神经（第Ⅲ脑神经）支配。鼻睫状神经、动眼神经、外展神经和视神经与视网膜中央动脉和静脉伴行，走行于眼球后方的肌锥内。重要的是，硬脑膜包绕视神经。

颅内三叉神经中的眼神经发出泪腺神经、额神经和鼻睫神经。前两个神经提供眶外和结膜的感觉。鼻睫神经分支支配眶内、角膜、巩膜、虹膜和睫状体。筛前神经是鼻窦神经的分支，被阻滞将导致鼻塞。

鼻睫神经的睫状神经节位于球后肌锥的顶点附近，因此它与视神经和视动脉有关。Edinger-Westphal 核的副交感神经纤维在神经节内伴随着动眼神经和突触，而 T1 的感觉和交感神经纤维继续穿过神经节。它的传出神经，即睫状短神经，向前行走，为眼球提供感觉，为虹膜提供自主运动功能。

技术

所有感觉神经和运动神经都可以通过晶锥注射（眼球后阻滞）或眼眶脂肪注射（球周阻滞）

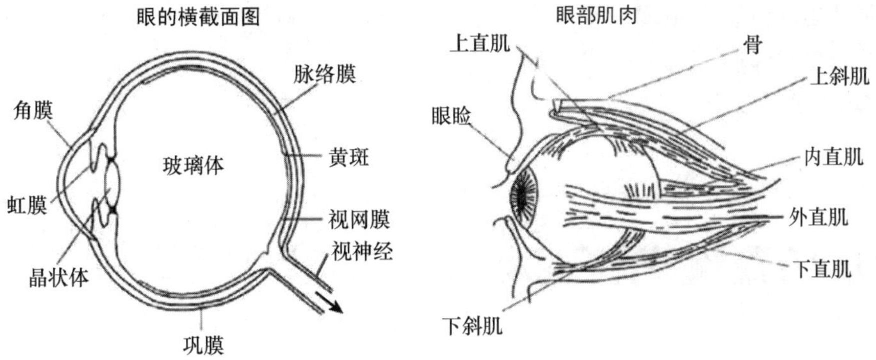

图 75.1　与球后阻滞性能相关的眼睛解剖示意图

阻断。球后阻滞由下眶缘进针，穿过眼球赤道部，然后向内向后进针。理想情况下，针尖在球后进入下直肌和外直肌间，在眼外肌形成的包裹空间内。在注射时，即使没有眼内压变化，眼球搏动性血流也会减少。患者整个过程中保持自然凝视、直视前方。

球后阻滞采用体表解剖标志和触觉定位。1995 年，一篇超声应用于球后阻滞的文章表明，针尖比操作者设想的更接近眼球。也许在侵入性眼科阻滞中，应常规应用超声引导外周神经阻滞。

风险评估

以下是与球后阻滞相关并发症的风险因素：

- 外科医师或麻醉科医师操作经验不足；
- 使用长度大于 35.0 mm 锋利的穿刺针，置入深度大于 25 mm；
- 近视眼球轴径长（细长的眼球）或轴径大于 24 mm；
- 由右利手医师行左侧下直肌注射；
- 使用过量的局麻药（≥ 4 ～ 5 ml），可能导致"筋膜间隙综合征"；
- 通过超声检测发现注射部位有葡萄肿；
- 多次注射；
- 过度焦虑或过度镇静状态下不配合的患者。

目前尚不清楚使用局麻药的类型或透明质酸酶的含量对并发症风险的影响。1999 年，英国一项观察性研究指出，所有眼科局部麻醉技术均出现罕见但严重的不良事件。在有严重不良事件的组中，利多卡因的使用显著减少。

启示

深部眼球注射技能可能因缺乏使用而日益减少。超声引导注射可能减少严重的视力和危及生命的并发症。

由于易于管理、快速实施、缺乏注射疼痛和并发症少，结膜下和表面麻醉的应用增加。但是眼球并不是固定的，即使在上直肌固定缝合和巩膜血管烧灼出现疼痛时，患者也必须合作。不合作或高度近视的患者，全身麻醉可能比球后或球周阻滞更安全。

管理

麻醉科医师对任何接受眼科手术患者的安全至关重要。保持与患者的沟通（如间歇性握手）与监测血压、心电图、呼末二氧化碳和脉搏血氧同样重要。

如果出现广泛的眼部出血或眼球穿孔，应由眼科医师指导进一步治疗。手术可以推迟或改变方式（如巩膜加压手术）。早期转诊至三级视网膜治疗可以减轻视力下降的灾难性后果。

麻醉科医师应该能够完成心肺复苏术。使用迷走神经抑制剂或抗惊厥药物进行气道管理和循环支持，直到患者恢复术前状态。

预防

了解眼部解剖结构及其与颅内结构的关系，不断致力于提高眼科区域麻醉技术，可以减少严重并发症的发生率。通过超声追踪穿刺针的位置可以保护眼及其神经血管和肌肉结构。使用 2.5 ～ 3 cm 短而钝的穿刺针和小剂量（3 ～ 4 ml）的局麻药是明智的。穿刺针置入深度（<25 mm）应尽量小，一旦出现剧烈疼痛就停止置入，可以降低眼球或硬脑膜穿刺的可能性。在穿刺过程中，眼睛应保持在自然

凝视或略向下和向外凝视位置。患者必须配合。使用语言安慰以尽量减少对静脉镇静的需求，加强监测将提升患者和眼球相关的安全。

（杜兆宁 译 周 懿 校）

延伸阅读

Bellucci R: Anesthesia for cataract surgery, *Curr Opin Ophthalmol* 10:36–41, 1999.

Birch AA, Evans M, Redembo E: The ultrasonic localization of retrobulbar needles during retrobulbar block, *Ophthalmology* 102:824–826, 1995.

Canavan KS, Dark A, Garrioch MA: Sub-Tenon's administration of local anaesthetic: a review of the technique, *Br J Anaesth* 90:787–793, 2003.

Davis DB, Mandel MR: Efficacy and complication rate of 16,224 consecutive peribulbar blocks: a prospective multicenter study, *J Cataract Refract Surg* 20:327–337, 1994.

Davis DB, Mandel MR: Posterior peribulbar anesthesia: an alternative to retrobulbar anesthesia, *Cataract Refract Surg* 12:182–184, 1986.

Edge R, Navon S: Scleral perforation during retrobulbar and peribulbar anesthesia: risk factors and outcomes in 50,000 consecutive injections, *J Cataract Refract Surg* 25:1237–1244, 1999.

Eke T, Thompson JR: Serious complications of local anaesthesia for cataract surgery: a 1 year national survey in the United Kingdom, *Br J Ophthalmol* 91:470–475, 2007.

Eke T, Thompson JR: The national survey of local anaesthesia for ocular surgery. II. Safety profiles of local anaesthesia techniques, *Eye* 13:196–204, 1999.

El-Hindy N, Johnston RL, Jaycock P, et al.: The cataract national dataset electronic multicenter audit of 55 567 operations: anaesthetic techniques and complications, *Eye* 23:50–55, 2009.

Gómez-Arnau JI, Yangüela J, González A, et al.: Anaesthesia-related diplopia after cataract surgery, *Br J Anaesth* 90:189–193, 2003.

Gross A, Cestari DM: Optic neuropathy following retrobulbar injection: a review, *Semin Ophthalmol* 29(5-6):434–439, 2014.

Gunja N, Varshney K: Brainstem anaesthesia after retrobulbar block: a rare cause of coma presenting to the emergency department, *Emerg Med Australas* 18:83–85, 2006.

Hamilton RC: A discourse on the complications of retrobulbar and peribulbar blockade, *Can J Ophthalmol* 35:363–372, 2000.

Jacobi PC, Dietlein TS, Jacobi FK: A comparative study of topical vs retrobulbar anesthesia in complicated cataract surgery, *Arch Ophthalmol* 228:1037–1043, 2000.

Kallio H, Paloheimo M, Maunuksela E-L: Haemorrhage and risk factors associated with retrobulbar/peribulbar block: a prospective study in 1383 patients, *Br J Anaesth* 85:708–711, 2000.

Kwinten FA, de Moor GP, Lamers R: Acute pulmonary edema and trigeminal nerve blockade after retrobulbar block, *Anesth Analg* 83:1322–1324, 1996.

Nicoll JMV, Acharya PA, Ahlen K, et al.: Central nervous system complications after 6000 retrobulbar blocks, *Anesth Analg* 66:1298–1302, 1987.

Nouvellon E, L'Hermite J, Chaumeron A, et al.: Ophthalmic regional anesthesia: medial canthus episcleral (sub-Tenon) single injection block, *Anesthesiology* 100:370–374, 2004.

Ripart J, Lefrant J-Y, Vivien B, et al.: Ophthalmic regional anesthesia: medial canthus episcleral (sub-Tenon) anesthesia is more efficient than peribulbar anesthesia: a double-blind randomized study, *Anesthesiology* 92:1278–1285, 2000.

Rüschen H, Bremner FD, Carr C: Complications after sub-Tenon's eye block, *Anesth Analg* 96:273–277, 2003.

Schrader WF, Schargus M, Schneider E, et al.: Risks and sequelae of scleral perforation during peribulbar or retrobulbar anesthesia, *J Cataract Refract Surg* 36:885–889, 2010.

Stevens JD: A new local anesthesia technique for cataract extraction by one quadrant sub-Tenon's infiltration, *Br J Ophthalmol* 76:670–674, 1992.

Taylor G, Devys JM, Heran F, et al.: Early exploration of diplopia with magnetic resonance imaging after peribulbar anaesthesia, *Br J Anaesth* 92:899–901, 2004.

Thind GS, Rubin AP: Local anaesthesia for eye—no room for complacency, *Br J Anaesth* 86:473–476, 2001.

Wadood AC, Dhillon B, Singh J: Inadvertent ocular perforation and intravitreal injection of an anesthetic agent during retrobulbar injection, *J Cataract Refract Surg* 28:562–565, 2002.

Wearne MJ, Flaxel CJ, Gray P, et al.: Vitreoretinal surgery after inadvertent globe penetration dural local ocular anesthesia, *Ophthalmology* 105:371–376, 1998.

小儿镇静

第76章

Mary Landrigan-Ossar，Joseph P. Cravero

病例概要

患儿，女性，10岁，肥胖伴有扁桃体肥大及睡眠呼吸暂停史，将接受磁共振成像（magnetic resonance imaging，MRI）检查，由该院儿科重症监护医师负责为其镇静。首先为患儿推注2.5 mg/kg丙泊酚，然后以200 μg/（kg·min）泵注。患儿入睡后被置于检查平台上，MRI扫描10 min后，其脉搏血氧饱和度从98%降至86%。看上去尽管存在呼吸运动，但呼气末二氧化碳监测却没有读数。

问题分析

定义

镇静可被描述为一种意识水平低下的持续状态。美国儿科学会（American Academy of Pediatrics，AAP）、美国麻醉科医师协会（American Society of Anesthesiologists，ASA）和美国医院评审联合委员会（the Joint Commission，TJC）已对镇静深度的标准化定义达成一致，包括**轻度镇静**、**中度镇静**、**深度镇静**和**全身麻醉**。镇静状态和患者反应性的定义见表76.1。镇静状态或深度与并发症相关，主要取决于正常气道/血管张力和保护性反射被抑制的程度。深度镇静抑制气道张力、保护性反射、呼吸动力和心功能的可能性更大，可能导致较大风险的并发症。

镇静是一个连续状态，而患者对镇静药物的反应不可预测。因此，医务人员应具备能力解救那些比预期镇静更深的患者。比如，使用药物以实现轻度镇静的医务人员，必须具有解救中度镇静患者的技能；拟实施深度镇静的医务人员，必须具有从全身麻醉状态解救患者的技能。儿童中多数与镇静相关的不良事件，与呼吸道功能受损或呼吸功能丧失有关，因此最重要的技能是及时识别通气不足并具备高级气道管理的能力。在临床实践中，大多数儿童需要深度镇静以满足长时间的诊断或治疗过程。因此，推荐使用指南来指导深度镇静过程。

大量研究证据充分地记录了镇静不良事件（并发症），特别是在儿科镇静研究联合会（Pediatric Sedation Research Consortium，PSRC）的一份报告中。这份超过30 000例患者的前瞻性观察报告，记录了镇静相关并发症包括（但不限于）呼吸暂停、气道阻塞、喉痉挛、缺氧、苏醒延迟和误吸，还有少数患者出现低血压和心动过缓（表76.2）。虽然严重

表76.1 患者对轻度、中度或深度镇静的预期反应

	轻度镇静[a]	中度镇静[b]	深度镇静[c]
患者反应	对语言刺激反应正常	对语言刺激及轻触觉有回应	对重复性或疼痛刺激有反应
呼吸道	无影响	不需要干预	可能需要干预
自主呼吸	无影响	充足	可能存在通气不足
心血管功能	无影响	通常能维持稳定状态	通常能维持稳定状态

[a] 药物诱发的类似于抗焦虑的状态；
[b] 药物诱发的意识水平低下，类似于清醒镇静；
[c] 药物诱发的意识水平低下，患者不易被唤醒源
Modified from the American Society of Anesthesiologists. Available at http://www.asahq.org.

不良事件的发生率很低，但数据证实儿童镇静涉及意识改变，而这与保护性反射的部分或完全丧失以及中枢神经系统和心肺生理学的巨大变化密切相关。

表 76.2 儿科镇静研究联合会并发症记录：30 000 例镇静患者诊疗过程中及术毕时并发症的前瞻性研究

	每 10 000 人中发生率	*N*	95%CI
并发症			
死亡	0.0	0	0.0 ~ 0.0
心脏停搏	0.3	1	0.0 ~ 1.9
误吸	0.3	1	0.0 ~ 1.9
低体温	1.3	4	0.4 ~ 3.4
镇静期间发生未预计的惊厥	2.7	8	1.1 ~ 5.2
喘鸣	4.3	11	1.8 ~ 6.6
喉痉挛	4.3	13	2.3 ~ 7.4
镇静期间新发哮鸣音	4.7	14	2.5 ~ 7.8
变态反应（皮疹）	5.7	17	3.3 ~ 9.1
静脉相关并发症	11.0	33	7.6 ~ 15.4
长时间镇静	13.6	41	9.8 ~ 18.5
苏醒延迟	22.3	67	17.3 ~ 28.3
呼吸暂停（未预计）	24.3	73	19.1 ~ 30.5
分泌物（需要吸引）	41.6	125	34.7 ~ 49.6
呕吐（非 GI 因素）	47.2	142	39.8 ~ 55.7
氧饱和度低于 90%	156.5	470	142.7 ~ 171.2
不良事件总数	339.6(1/29)	1020	308.1 ~ 371.5
计划外的治疗			
使用拮抗剂（未预计）	1.7	5	0.6 ~ 3.9
气道原因麻醉紧急会诊	2.0	6	0.7 ~ 4.3
收治入院（镇静相关）	7.0	21	4.3 ~ 10.7
气管插管（未预计）	9.7	29	6.5 ~ 13.9
经口建立气道（未预计）	27.6	83	22.0 ~ 34.2
球囊-面罩通气（未预计）	63.9	192	55.2 ~ 73.6
计划外治疗总数	111.9(1/89)	336	85.3 ~ 130.2
诊疗过程中存在的情况			
镇静不足，无法满足诊疗	88.9(1/338)	267	78.6 ~ 100.2

CI，置信区间；GI，胃肠道

From Cravero JP，Blike GT，Beach M，et al：Incidence and nature of adverse events during pediatric sedation/anesthesia for procedures outside the operating room：report from the Pediatric Sedation Research Consortium. *Pediatrics* 118（3）：1087-1096，2006.

TJC 和美国医疗保险与医疗补助服务中心（Centers for Medicare and Medicaid Services，CMS）均已意识到，应由麻醉科医师作为各级镇静 / 麻醉管理专家，两个组织都要求由麻醉科制定涉及所有患者（包括成人与儿童）镇静的策略，旨在为每个机构中进行镇静 / 麻醉的患者提供统一的标准化管理。

识别

合理的监测对于发现呼吸道梗阻或循环系统稳定性的变化至关重要。AAP 和 ASA 根据镇静深度制定了适当的监测标准（表 76.3）。对深度镇静患者，推荐监测心电图、血压和脉搏血氧饱和度。呼吸监测可能最为重要，可以通过多种设备或技术完成。最常用的是阻抗容积描记术、直接观察、心前区听诊（或放大呼吸音）以及呼气末二氧化碳监测。目前，二氧化碳监测得到广泛运用，因其可用于多种镇静场合（包括远离患者的场所），可反映气体交换而不仅仅是胸壁运动。使用二氧化碳监测可在低氧血症发生前及早发现并纠正通气失调。

另外，仅靠仪器监测并不能发现并发症。由一

表 76.3 识别镇静相关并发症的指南

	中度镇静	深度镇静
监测方式	脉搏氧饱和度—持续监测 心率—持续监测 呼吸频率—每 15 min 意识水平—每 15 min 血压—每 15 min	脉搏氧饱和度-持续监测[a] 心率—持续监测 呼吸频率—每 5 min 意识水平—每 5 min 血压—每 5 min[b]
记录	脉搏氧饱和度—每 15 min 心率—每 15 min 呼吸频率—每 15 min 意识水平—每 15 min[c] 血压—每 15 min	脉搏氧饱和度—每 15 min 心率—每 5 min 呼吸频率—每 5 min 意识水平—每 5 min 血压—每 5 min
人员	既能观察患者情况，又能参与诊疗过程	专注观察患者情况，不能参与诊疗过程
设备	脉搏氧饱和度仪 血压监测设备	脉搏氧饱和度仪 血压监测设备 心电图仪、除颤仪（备用）

[a] 注意是否给氧及如何给氧；

[b] 由于血压测量会干扰诊疗过程，如果其他生命体征稳定，可减少血压测量次数；

[c] 在某些过程中，如磁共振成像或计算机断层扫描，如果唤醒患者会妨碍扫描，那么对意识水平的评估可能不实用。

名专职监护人员跟踪仪器输出数据和记录趋势，是镇静并发症预防和管理的关键。这名监护人员必须接受培训，能识别出潜在不利情况，做出合理反应使患者恢复到安全基线。模拟教学是一个有用工具，既可教授基本及高级镇静技能，也可检验对不良事件处理方法的效果。

镇静通常不会随着诊疗完成而结束。患者仍应在设备齐全、人员齐备的苏醒区进行监护，并执行与全身麻醉恢复相一致的严格统一的出室标准。

风险评估

Coté 等的里程碑式研究发现，与镇静有关的最严重并发症涉及以下一个或多个因素：

- 同一个人为患儿执行镇静和诊疗操作；
- 复苏期间药物残留作用与监测不力；
- 缺乏对药物相互作用的理解和药物剂量使用错误；
- 让患儿父母在家中给予其镇静类药物，但随后无人观察小儿呼吸道梗阻的迹象。

调查人员对镇静事故进行了详细分析，发现约 2/3 事故发生在年龄小于 6 岁儿童中，一半以上接受了不止一种镇静剂。该研究还发现不良事件与所有给药途径（口服、直肠、鼻腔、肌肉、静脉、吸入）相关。12 例患者在前往医疗机构途中（2 例患者在家接受镇静治疗）或出院后（10 例患者）发生不良事件或出现不良结局。所有出院后发生不良事件的患者，均接受过长效镇静药物治疗。

来自儿科镇静研究联合会的系列镇静并发症的评估研究中，Cravero 等证实了接受镇静治疗的高风险儿科亚群的存在。这些患者包括低龄、ASA Ⅲ或Ⅳ级、肥胖以及使用丙泊酚等强效镇静剂的患者。一些高危诊疗如支气管镜检查和上消化道检查也被纳入其中。严重的不良事件与特定的镇静实施者类别无关。作者认为，其研究数据中严重不良事件的发生率相对较低，这是协同镇静服务的结果，既能够识别高危患者，还可提供良好监测、质量改进流程和团队合作。

由于术后相关并发症数据已趋于完整，Malviya 等观察了儿童在水合氯醛镇静下行超声心动图的恢复情况。与标准离室条件相比，使用基于患者在催眠环境中连续 20 min 保持清醒的能力，并结合密歇根大学镇静量表的离室条件，患者平均离室时间晚 75 min。这一研究表明，延长观察时间（可能在低一级观察单元）可能会提高长效药物用于儿科镇静的安全性。

综上所述，所有关于镇静的文献均明确认为，镇静风险可随患者亚群和诊疗过程的不同而发生变化。因此，需要对镇静的儿童进行系统评估，以显著降低麻醉相关的发病率和死亡率。

启示

仅靠说服婴幼儿和许多儿童配合诊疗操作是不可能的，这便需要药物控制。多年来，人们为实现这一目标使用了很多药物，包括巴比妥类、水合氯醛、丁酰苯类药物、阿片类药物、吩噻嗪类药物、苯二氮䓬类药物和镇静类药物，如丙泊酚和右美托咪定。其中部分药物或药物联合应用时，对小儿镇静安全性和有效性的信息非常缺乏。当镇静策略趋向于深度镇静时，更是如此。

由于没有足够数量的麻醉科医师可为儿童诊疗过程提供所需的镇静，许多患儿由儿科专科医师在操作中实施镇静。由非麻醉科医师提供的丙泊酚镇静引发关注和讨论，即其是否具备使用这种药物的资质。麻醉科医师过去曾试图限制非本专业人员使用丙泊酚及开展深度镇静。最近，急诊医师和其他非麻醉科医师已开始使用丙泊酚或其他药物提供深度镇静，该做法得到了 PSRC 大规模研究的支持。这些研究表明，至少在已确定的镇静程序范围内，深度镇静可由麻醉学专业之外的从业人员安全实施。ASA 已发布非麻醉科医师提供深度镇静和使用丙泊酚的指南。教育和培训这类人员是麻醉科医师的职责。事实上，TJC 和 CMS 也已认识到镇静中麻醉监测在医疗操作中的重要性。无论使用何种药物，镇静都需要由经过合理培训的医师和（或）护士提供，通过培训他们知晓如何使用此类药物，并能够识别和治疗其并发症。

管理

各类患者的长时间安全镇静需要一个健全体系，包括患者选择、术中管理、不良事件预防及合理复苏。如前所述，AAP 于 1985 年首次为院内、院外儿科患者制定镇静指南。该指南于 1992 年修订，此后又进行了两次 ASA 实践指南的扩增，并经历多次修订，最近一次修订为 2016 年。

实施镇静的系统性方法意味着以一种方式整合管理，即采取多种制约措施，使重要信息不会丢失，并在即将发生紧急情况前做出反应。对于小儿患者的镇静，这种方法涉及许多重要的组成部分：

- 所有患者都必须接受同等程度的监护，且必须建立统一标准，以确定哪些患者需要麻醉科医师监护，哪些患者可以转移给其他专家。主要考虑的因素有年龄、ASA 分级、气道解剖、肥胖以及心脏或呼吸系统疾病等内科并存疾病。
- 充分回顾患者病史、体格检查（包括详细的呼吸道检查）、当前使用药物、变态反应及既往内外科记录，并由各种监管机构授权。
- 严禁在家中给予镇静，小儿在用药前必须接受医疗监护。
- 镇静前，确保大小及型号适合的气道管理设备可用，同时备好急救药物，如阿片类及苯二氮䓬类药物的拮抗剂，提供正压通气设备，其氧气储备的使用时间至少能维持 1 h。
- 镇静期间对患者的监测应与患者镇静水平相适应（见表 76.3），记录监护数据以便其他从业人员能了解其镇静过程。
- 对不良事件和紧急情况的应急措施应尽可能标准化，特别是在启动应急呼救和困难气道管理上。此类事件的模拟教学，有助于解决医疗体系中的潜在问题。
- 镇静后患者的苏醒应与全身麻醉患者苏醒标准一致，离室标准也应标准化。
- 镇静项目应参与正在进行的安全审查和质量改进工作，不仅要跟踪不良事件，而且应从患者及其家属角度追踪镇静的质量及体验。

预防

与小儿镇静相关并发症的预防和干预措施已有详细介绍。Coté 等及 PSRC 研究数据清楚地概述了提供安全镇静监护的关键能力。镇静实施者（无论其专业或背景）必须能够识别通气不足或呼吸暂停。他们必须能够开放气道、清理阻塞物，并且能够提供通气支持及循环支持。预防并发症最重要（也是最成功）的策略是确保所有镇静实施者都经过专业培训并具备这些关键技能。

在许多机构中，指定“镇静团队”是确保镇静安全有效从而预防并发症的有效方法。当镇静小组获得适当资源时（理想情况下有一个中心操作室），相同的镇静过程可用于接受各种诊疗的患者。镇静团队可凭借培训和经验，共同制定技术规范，以促进安全镇静并提高患者、家属和医师满意度。在独立实践前，对这些团队的培训课程应包括课堂式教学，完成关键能力的模拟和实践训练。

麻醉科医师在预防镇静并发症方面起着至关重要的作用。当麻醉科没有人员为儿童实施镇静时，应为来自其他专业的人员提供镇静教育、培训、支持和持续监督。不管由谁来提供小儿镇静服务，所有机构的镇静安全性和质量必须保持一致。此外，应由一名行政主任负责所有的镇静 / 麻醉，逻辑上应由麻醉科主任承担。

病例总结

该病例概要阐明了本章的关键概念。首先，需要进行镇静前评估并认识到与麻醉相关的风险因素。患者有多种气道阻塞的危险因素，包括肥胖和阻塞性睡眠呼吸暂停。此外，在不能靠近患者时，可将呼气末二氧化碳监测作为合理的监测手段。最后，没有二氧化碳监测时，可通过胸壁运动来识别气道阻塞等并发症。干预和预防更严重的后果，只能由镇静实施者来完成，他们需具备识别并发症及开放气道进行干预的能力。对镇静实施者合理的培训及系统监督，可让磁共振扫描下潜在的危急并发症化险为夷。

（文　岑　译　李　黛　校）

延伸阅读

American Academy of Pediatrics; American Academy of Pediatric Dentistry, Coté CJ, et al.: Guidelines for monitoring and management of pediatric patients during and after sedation for diagnostic and therapeutic procedures: an update, *Paediatr Anaesth* 18(1):9–10, 2008.

American Society Anesthesiologists: Statement on granting privileges to non-anesthesiologist physicians for personally administering or supervising deep sedation. Approved by the House of Delegates on October 18, 2006, and amended on October 17, 2012. Available at www.asahq.org.

American Society of Anesthesiologists Task Force on Sedation and Analgesia by Non-Anesthesiologists: Practice guidelines for sedation and analgesia by non-anesthesiologists, *Anesthesiology* 96(4):1004–1017, 2002.

Beach ML, Cohen DM, Gallagher SM, et al.: Major adverse events and relationship to nil per os status in pediatric sedation/anesthesia outside the operating room: a report of the Pediatric Sedation Research Consortium, *Anesthesiology* 124(1):80–88, 2015.

Biber JL, Allareddy V, Gallagher SM, et al.: Prevalence and predictors of adverse events during procedural sedation anesthesia-outside the operating room for esophagogastroduodenoscopy and colonoscopy in children: age is an independent predictor of outcomes, *Pediatr Crit Care Med* 16(8):e251–e259, 2015.

Blike GT, Christoffersen K, Cravero JP, et al.: A method for measuring system safety and latent errors associated with pediatric procedural sedation, *Anesth Analg* 101(1):48–58, 2005.

Centers for Medicaid and Medicare Services (CMS): Publication 100–07: State Operations Manual. Available at https://www.cms.gov.

Coté CJ, Karl HW, Notterman DA, et al.: Adverse sedation events in pediatrics: analysis of medications used for sedation, *Pediatrics* 106(4):633–644, 2000.

Coté CJ, Notterman DA, Karl HW, et al.: Adverse sedation events in pediatrics: a critical incident analysis of contributing factors, *Pediatrics* 105 (4 Pt 1):805–814, 2000.

Couloures KG, Beach M, Cravero JP, et al.: Impact of provider specialty on pediatric procedural sedation complication rates, *Pediatrics* 127(5):e1154–e1160, 2011.

Cravero JP, Blike GT, Beach M, et al.: Incidence and nature of adverse events during pediatric sedation/anesthesia for procedures outside the operating room: report from the Pediatric Sedation Research Consortium, *Pediatrics* 118(3):1087–1096, 2006.

Cravero JP, Beach ML, Blike GT, et al.: The incidence and nature of adverse events during pediatric sedation/anesthesia with propofol for procedures outside the operating room: a report from the Pediatric Sedation Research Consortium, *Anesth Analg* 108(3):795–804, 2009.

Deitch K, Miner J, Chudnofsky CR, et al.: Does end tidal CO_2 monitoring during emergency department procedural sedation and analgesia with propofol decrease the incidence of hypoxic events? A randomized, controlled trial, *Ann Emerg Med* 55(3):258–264, 2010.

Hollman GA, Banks DM, Berkenbosch JW, et al.: Development, implementation, and initial participant feedback of a pediatric sedation provider course, *Teach Learn Med* 25(3):249–257, 2013.

The Joint Commission (TJC): The Joint Commission comprehensive accreditation and certification manual. Oak Brook, IL, Joint Commission Resources, 2014.

Lalwani K, Michel M: Pediatric sedation in North American children's hospitals: a survey of anesthesia providers, *Paediatr Anaesth* 15(3):209–213, 2005.

Lightdale JR, Goldmann DA, Feldman HA, et al.: Microstream capnography improves patient monitoring during moderate sedation: a randomized, controlled trial, *Pediatrics* 117(6):e1170–e1178, 2006.

Mace SE, Barata IA, Cravero JP, et al.: Clinical policy: evidence-based approach to pharmacologic agents used in pediatric sedation and analgesia in the emergency department, *J Pediatr Surg* 39(10):1472–1484, 2004.

Mallory MD, Baxter AL, Yanosky DJ, et al.: Emergency physician-administered propofol sedation: a report on 25,433 sedations from the Pediatric Sedation Research Consortium, *Ann Emerg Med* 57(5):462–468, 2011. e1.

Malviya S, Voepel-Lewis T, Ludomirsky A, et al.: Can we improve the assessment of discharge readiness? A comparative study of observational and objective measures of depth of sedation in children, *Anesthesiology* 100(2):218–224, 2004.

Malviya S, Voepel-Lewis T, Tait AR: A comparison of observational and objective measures to differentiate depth of sedation in children from birth to 18 years of age, *Anesth Analg* 102(2):389–394, 2006.

Scheier E, Gadot C, Leiba R, et al.: Sedation with the combination of ketamine and propofol in a pediatric ED: a retrospective case series analysis, *Am J Emerg Med* 33(6):815–817, 2015.

Scherrer PD, Mallory MD, Cravero JP, et al.: The impact of obesity on pediatric procedural sedation-related outcomes: results from the Pediatric Sedation Research Consortium, *Paediatr Anaesth* 25(7):689–697, 2015.

Tobin CD, Clark CA, McEvoy MD, et al.: An approach to moderate sedation simulation training, *Simul Healthc* 8(2):114–123, 2013.

Waugh JB, Epps CA, Khodneva YA: Capnography enhances surveillance of respiratory events during procedural sedation: a meta-analysis, *J Clin Anesth* 23(3):189–196, 2011.

第77章 脊髓损伤

Tod B. Sloan，Antoun Koht

病例概要

患者，男性，32岁，因驾驶摩托车事故被甩向路边而被送往急救室。患者反应轻度迟钝，呼出气体有酒精味，C5皮段以下感觉和运动功能消失，其他神经系统体格检查不能很好配合。颈椎侧位X线片难以鉴别骨损伤或半脱位。生命体征显示低血压（90/40 mmHg）、心动过缓（50次/分）、呼吸困难、口腔温度36.2℃。之后被送往急诊手术室进行开放性胫骨骨折的修复。

问题分析

定义

脊髓损伤（spinal cord injury，SCI）通常伴随神经功能障碍，伴有或不伴有脊柱破裂。在受伤后不久常需要麻醉下进行复苏或手术干预。同样，在慢性脊髓损伤患者手术时也需要麻醉处理。对于近期发生的医源性脊髓损伤患者（如脊柱侧弯矫正手术、主动脉重建手术）也需要麻醉下进行手术。急性脊髓损伤常伴随外伤，脊髓损伤出现的大多数问题是神经功能丧失的结果，并且可随时间的推移而进展。

早期识别脊髓损伤对降低或预防晚期严重并发症的发生很重要。在急性阶段，损伤水平远端的脊髓是无功能的（如反射消失、肌无力）。胸交感神经传出减少可导致脊髓休克综合征，其特点是由于迷走副交感神经张力亢进而引起低血压和心动过缓。脊髓损伤后几天到8周，未受伤脊髓节段中的脊髓反射开始恢复，但其不再接受高级中枢的控制（如头侧脊髓、脑干、大脑），这会导致失控的脊髓反射、肌肉痉挛，最终可致肌挛缩。这些改变可区分急性脊髓损伤与慢性损伤，并能了解急性和慢性期之间伴随的神经生理学差异。

识别

所有多发伤患者均应行急性脊髓损伤的评估，尤其是颈部不适主诉或有神经系统异常的患者，昏迷、低血压和反射消失患者，以及任何伴有明显的低血容量性休克而无代偿性心动过速的患者。大多数创伤性急性脊髓损伤发生在活动度较大的颈椎和胸腰椎区域，尤其是颈椎。颈椎侧位X线片（C1～C7）和前后位张口X线片通常可证实骨损伤。然而，在多达30%的病例中，不稳定的颈椎损伤经常被漏诊。因此，需要临床症状结合计算机断层扫描或磁共振成像来识别所有颈椎损伤。急性脊髓损伤也可不伴随韧带或骨性损伤，尤其在儿童中，这被称为“无放射学影像异常性脊髓损伤”（spinal cord injury without radiographic abnormality，SCIWORA）。

急性脊髓损伤进行评估包括以下内容：

- 受伤的节段；
- 受伤后的时间；
- 存在脊柱不稳定；
- 神经损害的程度和类型；
- 合并损伤（尤其是头部损伤）和健康问题。

脊髓损伤节段通常与损伤性质和损伤部位有关，由神经系统检查初步诊断，并由影像学确诊。急性脊髓损伤的节段决定了其潜在的并发症及其对治疗方式的影响。多达20%的患者（80%为颈椎损伤患者）存在超过一个节段的损伤。

脊髓损伤后的时间通常从创伤事件本身或神经检查中发现即可轻易判断。由于早期治疗可以减轻不可逆损伤的程度，因此早期识别急性脊髓损伤很重要。随着时间的推移，损伤会逐步加重（见下文）。

识别脊柱不稳定性（尤其是颈椎）对患者的体位和肢体活动，包括气道管理和气管插管，都是非常重要的，而脊髓损伤也可不伴有骨或韧带的不稳定（例如脊柱血肿和脓肿、术中损伤、儿童创伤）。最后，神经功能损害的程度和类型决定了潜在的神经功能后遗症。

风险评估

某些外科手术与急性脊髓损伤的风险密切相关。脊柱矫正手术的神经损伤风险约为 1%～4%。然而，严重后凸畸形的矫正手术脊髓损伤风险接近 75%，脊髓肿瘤切除风险也很高。胸主动脉相关手术也存在很高的神经损伤风险（见第 79 章）。在外科患者中，通过术中监测（感觉和运动诱发电位）可早期发现损伤并进行纠正，以免损伤进程（通常为局部缺血）引起的不可逆性损害。

所有外伤患者都应怀疑是否伴有急性脊髓损伤。重大创伤患者发生急性脊髓损伤的风险为 2.6%，头部外伤患者发生相关脊髓损伤的风险为 4% ～ 5%。创伤性急性脊髓损伤每年发生率约（12 ～ 53）/1 000 000，男性居多（4∶1），最常发生的位置在 C4 ～ C6，其次是 T11 ～ L2。损伤发生最常见的原因是机动车事故，往往与饮酒或药物滥用有关，老年人摔倒和落水事故也是其重要原因。在颈椎损伤患者中，约 25% 出现四肢瘫痪，40% 无残留神经损伤，而大约 35% 的患者则伴随一定程度的神经损伤。

无好转的急性脊髓损伤患者可发展为慢性脊髓损伤。对于昏迷的患者，需要进行详细的病史询问和神经学检查来区分慢性脊髓损伤与脑损伤。脊髓损伤机制的深入了解及其后续治疗的进一步完善使其总死亡率从第一次世界大战时期的 80% 下降到 20 世纪 80 年代早期的 2% 以下。

启示

脊髓损伤的并发症由脊髓损伤的区域决定，包括损伤节段及特殊的综合征。脊髓完全损伤时（相当于脊髓横断）其并发症的发生率最高，其特征为损伤节段以下的所有神经功能丧失。对于高位脊髓损伤（C4 ～ C6），肺功能检查显示总肺容量、肺活量、呼气储备容量和用力呼气容量下降，而残余肺容量增加。肺活量是衡量肺损伤的一个很好的指标，当肺活量小于 15 ml/kg 时，患者通常需要气管插管和辅助呼吸。

多种因素可导致通气障碍，67% 的急性脊髓损伤患者在损伤后的前几天会发生通气功能障碍（框 77.1）。急性脊髓损伤患者在仰卧位时呼吸更通畅，这是因为腹部内容物对膈肌的支撑可使膈肌在呼气和吸气时移动范围更大（除非胃肠胀气阻碍横膈运动）。气道分泌物和肺不张也是呼吸功能障碍的常见因素。慢性脊髓损伤患者可通过肋间肌肉和腹部肌肉收缩增强而改善通气。

急性颈椎脊髓损伤时，由于心脏和血管的交感神经张力丧失，心血管功能发生明显改变。随后静脉扩张可导致相对低血容量和前负荷的减少，外伤性或外科性失血则会加重这种情况。外周血管扩张降低了全身血管阻力，前负荷及全身血管阻力的降低会导致一种称为脊髓性休克的低血压状态。心脏交感神经支配的丧失（支配区域 T1 ～ T4/T5）导致在低血容量或失血时不能代偿性增加心肌收缩力和心率，由此产生迷走神经张力亢进从而增强了潜在的心动过缓和逸搏心律。这些情况的发生可因血压突然升高（即颈动脉弓反射亢进）或气道操作所致，可能需要使用阿托品或放置临时 / 永久起搏器。除了可能会发生心动过缓和低血压，急性脊髓损伤患者还面临急性心力衰竭和肺水肿的风险。实验表明，脊髓损伤时由于儿茶酚胺激增，以及后负荷迅速增加，可能会导致心肌损伤。

慢性脊髓损伤患者心血管系统则相对稳定。然而，当损伤节段在 T7 以上时，T7 以下的感觉刺激可能会引起过度性交感神经反射（即自主反射亢进），可引发强烈的血管收缩、心动过缓和高血压急

框 77.1　急性脊髓损伤中影响通气功能的因素

胃扩张和肠梗阻对膈肌运动的限制
吸入性肺炎
呼气储备及咳嗽能力降低，继发于腹肌（T2 ～ L1）和肋间肌（T1 ～ T11）功能的丧失
长骨骨折后脂肪栓塞
胸部外伤（肋骨骨折、肺挫伤、气胸、血胸）
膈神经脊髓输入段障碍（C3 ～ C5），无法控制膈肌运动
因头部创伤、酒精或药物引起的意识不清
头部创伤导致神经性水肿
继发于心血管功能障碍的肺水肿

症（见第 85 章）。

除了心血管功能障碍，急性脊髓损伤还伴有其他类型的损伤（框 77.2）。由交感神经介导的血管张力变化导致的体温调节受损，可出现非恒温状态并无法控制出汗。骨骼肌去神经化可致神经肌肉连接的超敏反应和不成熟受体的出现，可使去极化肌肉松弛药（如琥珀胆碱）介导钾的过度释放。这种情况开始于 6 ～ 12 h，24 ～ 48 h 达到高峰但通常不至于产生并发症，后逐步减弱直到慢性脊髓损伤的肌萎缩，其影响消除。一般认为在急性脊髓损伤 1 年后使用琥珀胆碱是安全的，然而最近的研究表明，这种病理改变可能是终身的。在创伤性急性脊髓损伤中，患者可能伴有相关的损伤（如头部损伤伴颅内高压；胸部、腹部或骨科损伤）。慢性脊髓损伤相关的其他症状还包括以下情况：

- 肾衰竭（由反复尿路感染或淀粉样变性引起）；
- 药物或酒精滥用或依赖（由抑郁或疼痛综合征引起）；
- 压疮。

同样在慢性脊髓损伤中，损伤节段下方的脊髓反射可能会导致不受控制的肌肉挛缩。急性和慢性脊髓损伤的患者都容易发生深静脉血栓（颈椎损伤患者高达 80% ～ 85%）。因此，肺血栓栓塞是急性脊髓损伤患者死亡的常见原因，这种情况可能需要放置腔静脉滤器。

治疗

急性脊髓损伤患者的首要任务是保护呼吸道，

框 77.2 急性脊髓损伤相关性损伤

心血管功能障碍（脊髓休克）
体温调节受损（变温）
神经肌肉接头超敏反应
头部创伤（颅内压升高）
胸部外伤（气胸、心脏挫伤）
心肌损伤
吸入性肺炎
气胸、纵隔气肿
颈部外伤伴呼吸道血肿
长骨骨折伴失血和脂肪栓塞
肾衰竭
肌肉挛缩
深静脉血栓形成及肺血栓栓塞

确保足够的氧合和通气，并提供循环支持。并存其他损伤和预防继发性缺血性脊髓损伤，需要进一步的处置。不稳定的脊柱需要通过牵引固定好体位直到神经评估结束。牵引可导致进一步的损伤，包括椎间盘突出、C1 ～ C2 韧带松弛或强直性脊柱炎。

气道的保护是重中之重。理想状态下，可控的清醒经鼻插管（如果无禁忌证）可减少颈部活动，并能在插管期间观察神经功能变化。如果需立即使用直接喉镜行气管插管，保持中线稳定（非牵引）可以减少颈椎运动的幅度。如果面部外伤不能进行经口插管，可能需要建立外科气道（气管切开或环甲膜切开术）或经气管通气。对于头部外伤患者，应尽量避免经鼻插管，除非能排除颅底骨折。

建立气道后，必须保证充足的氧供和通气。继发于急性脊髓损伤、低血容量和创伤引起的交感神经张力丧失的任何低血压都应通过静脉输液来保证足够的心排血量和血压。有时可能需要放置肺动脉导管，尤其是四肢瘫痪患者，因为过多的液体可致肺水肿。血管收缩剂（如多巴胺、麻黄碱、去氧肾上腺素）在扩容无效时用于增加心血管动力（注意去氧肾上腺素可能更有利，它是 α 肾上腺素能受体激动剂，通过收缩外周血管床，既能增加体循环血管阻力，又能增加心脏前负荷）。另外，必要时也可能需要使用正性肌力药物，因为急性脊髓损伤可能引起伴随血压增高的心肌损伤，这是由下行交感通路机械性压迫导致短暂、爆发性自主神经放电所致。暂时性心动过缓可通过使用阿托品或 β 肾上腺素能受体激动剂治疗，对持续性心动过缓或逸搏心律患者可给予起搏治疗。大剂量甲泼尼龙的治疗效果目前仍存争议（见下文的讨论）。

体位的突然改变可引起体位性低血压（头朝上）或肺水肿（头朝下），这是由于心血管代偿功能失调所致。临床医师应监测患者体温，使用保温毯或根据需要调节环境温度。原因不明的低血压也可能来源于未发现的腹腔内或腹膜后出血。

大约 2/3 的创伤性急性脊髓损伤患者均合并其他部位的严重损伤。特别值得关注的是胸腹部损伤，它可能由于感觉丧失或头部损伤而不易察觉。在急性脊髓损伤患者中，胸腹损伤的发生率高达 25% ～ 50%。脊髓损伤后并发症发生与损失后医疗护理有关，如胃糜烂、深静脉血栓形成和肺栓塞。

急性脊髓损伤的急诊手术通常是针对脊髓以外

的损伤。然而，对于牵引复位失败（如存在关节绞索）或存在骨折碎片嵌入椎间盘甚至侵入脊髓时，则可能需要进行紧急脊髓手术。该手术的麻醉处理包括维持脊髓充分的灌注。维持平均血压大于 85 mmHg，中心静脉压维持在 5 ～ 10 mmHg，动脉氧分压大于 100 mmHg，维持正常的血糖和血碳酸水平，则预后较好。此外，确保充分的自主通气功能恢复后再拔管。术后可能需要机械通气支持。由于需要再次进行颈部操作，急性颈椎损伤患者不适宜再次紧急插管。

如果急性脊髓损伤与近期的脊柱或主动脉手术有关，治疗时间与预后密切相关。一些外科医师认为在这种时候使用类固醇，如甲泼尼龙或地塞米松，并尽可能在数小时内摘除脊柱内固定或探查椎管内血肿。如果需要手术，则有必要实施电生理监测（感觉或运动诱发电位）以防止进一步的脊髓损伤。

慢性脊髓损伤患者常常因为压疮或肾结石需进行麻醉手术。根据手术部位和神经损伤程度，局部麻醉、区域麻醉或全身麻醉都可以选择。然而，许多 T7 以上损伤的慢性脊髓损伤患者（85%）在不使用麻醉或仅使用局部麻醉的情况下，易出现自主反射亢进及相关高血压，而区域麻醉和全身麻醉可以阻断这种现象。除了去除诱因，可能还需使用强效血管扩张药来治疗此症状。虽然硬膜外阻滞在泌尿外科或普外科手术不如蛛网膜下腔阻滞效果佳，但在分娩中应用广泛。由于肌肉挛缩或体位均能影响通气功能，对慢性脊髓损伤患者的体位变化需要预先考虑。慢性脊髓损伤患者常出现血容量浓缩（60 ml/kg），易发生直立性低血压。对于慢性脊髓损伤患者，其他可能需要使用麻醉的治疗操作包括放置脉冲发生器刺激膈神经或脊髓（分别用于改善通气功能或控制疼痛），以及鞘内给予巴氯芬治疗痉挛。

预防

一旦发生急性脊髓损伤，应尽力避免由于低氧血症、脊髓灌注受损及骨撞击等因素造成的二次损伤。急性脊髓损伤后是否应该使用大剂量类固醇目前尚存在争议，因为它似乎并不能改善神经功能，而且患者使用可出现明显的不良反应。对于穿透性腹部损伤患者不建议使用类固醇，因为可能会造成椎管内肠道菌群的感染。对急性脊髓损伤进行及时的干预，如行脊髓手术或减轻压迫等，都可减轻损伤程度。术中减少急性脊髓损伤的措施包括在术中全程和术后即刻维持正常的血压、动脉血二氧化碳分压和血糖浓度。最后，通过感觉和运动诱发电位监测脊髓功能可以减少任何对脊髓额外的（医源性）损伤，特别是在脊髓减压和脊柱融合操作时。

目前的重点工作是通过康复和功能辅助，尽可能地恢复神经功能。同时，提高脊髓再生能力的相关研究也正在进行中。

（文　岑　译　费苗苗　校）

延伸阅读

Chiles BW, Cooper PR: Acute spinal injury, *N Engl J Med* 334:514–520, 1996.

Gil K: Anesthesia for spinal cord injury surgery. In Mongan P, Soriano S, Sloan T, editors: *A practical approach to neuroanesthesia*, Philadelphia, 2013, Wolters Kluwer, pp 148–191.

Gupta R, Bathen ME, Smith JS, et al.: Advances in the management of spinal cord injury, *J Am Acad Orthop Surg* 18(4):210–222, 2010.

Lee TT, Green BA: Advances in the management of acute spinal cord injury, *Orthop Clin North Am* 33:311–315, 2002.

Martyn JA, Richtsfeld M: Succinylcholine-induced hyperkalemia in acquired pathologic states: etiologic factors and molecular mechanisms, *Anesthesiology* 104(1):158–169, 2006.

O'Dowd JK: Basic principles of management for cervical spine trauma, *Eur Spine J* 19(Suppl 1):S18–S22, 2010.

Rozzelle CJ, Aarabi B, Dhall SS, et al.: Management of pediatric cervical spine and spinal cord injuries, *Neurosurgery* 72(Suppl 2):205–226, 2013.

Schouten R, Albert T, Kwon BK: The spine-injured patient: initial assessment and emergency treatment, *J Am Acad Orthop Surg* 20(6):336–346, 2012.

Stahel PF, VanderHeiden T, Finn MA: Management strategies for acute spinal cord injury: current options and future perspectives, *Curr Opin Crit Care* 18(6):651–660, 2012.

Vanderhave KL, Chiravuri S, Caird MS, et al.: Cervical spine trauma in children and adults: perioperative considerations, *J Am Acad Orthop Surg* 19(6):319–327, 2011.

Wilson JR, Forgione N, Fehlings MG: Emerging therapies for acute traumatic spinal cord injury, *CMAJ* 185:485–492, 2013.

Woodring JH, Lee C: Limitations of cervical radiography in the evaluation of acute cervical trauma, *J Trauma* 34:32–39, 1993.

第 78 章 热烧伤患者

Katarzyna Luba

病例概要

作为当班麻醉科医师，烧伤科住院医师预约急诊四肢筋膜切开术。患者为 40 岁流浪汉，于昨晚从失火的车库中救出并收治入烧伤病房。患者在失火现场时被发现时没有反应，血液中酒精含量过高，80% 体表面积（total body surface area，TBSA）的深度烧伤。患者予呼吸支持治疗：容量控制模式，吸入氧浓度为 0.8，呼气末正压通气（positive end-expiratory pressure，PEEP）为 15 cmH_2O，潮气量为 400 ml。当准备转运患者至手术室（operating room，OR）时，发现患者气道峰压高。由于担心患者在转运期间及在手术室可能会因胸部顺应性降低导致无法进行有效的通气和供氧，向主治医师汇报了病情，主治医师决定进行胸腹焦痂切除术。

问题分析

定义

烧伤可由包括热、电流、腐蚀剂或腐蚀性化学物质引起。损伤的严重程度取决于组织破坏的程度和深度。热烧伤是由于皮肤、黏膜及皮下组织与热源接触的时间较长而引起的损伤。热烧伤的严重程度与热源的温度、接触时间长短和接触面积的大小成正比，与皮肤的厚度和接触面的血液供应成反比。化学烧伤是由蛋白质变性、脱水或腐蚀等化学反应而引起的。电烧伤是电流在身体表面的两个点间形成电弧而引起的外部损伤，或由于热量沿血管和神经传导而引起的深度损伤。二次热烧伤可能是由电流的电弧点燃衣服引起的。

识别

美国每年发生的烧伤人数估计在 100 万～ 200 万之间。每年有近 50 万人因烧伤接受治疗，其中 4 万～ 8 万人住院治疗，3500 人～ 5000 人死亡。大多数烧伤患者都在综合医院急诊科就诊而非专门的烧伤中心。大烧伤患者早期临床治疗最大的挑战是气道和通气管理、开放静脉通路、液体复苏和疼痛控制。

决定烧伤的严重程度因素包括：**占全身体表面积**（total body surface area，TBSA）的百分比、烧伤的深度以及是否存在吸入性损伤。燃烧的面积使用“九分法”（图 78.1）或 Lund-Browder 图（图 78.2）来估算。Lund-Browder 图为一图表，阐述了身体各

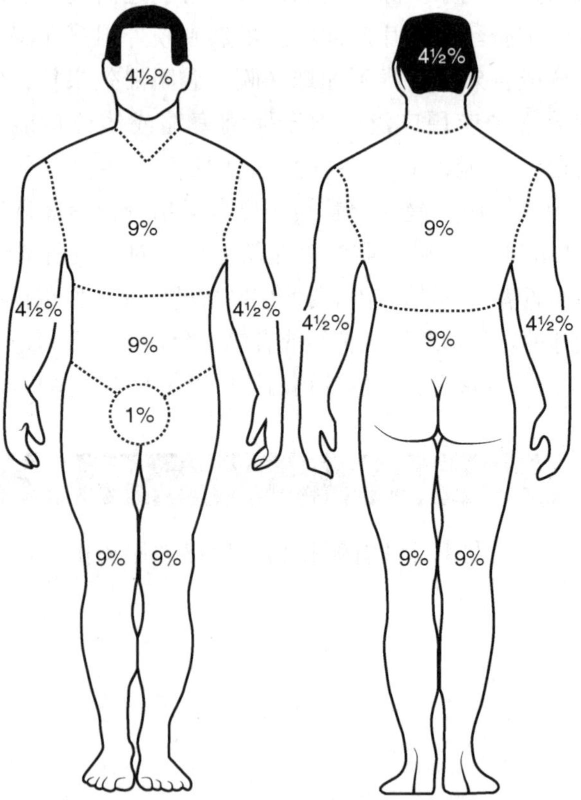

图 78.1 体表面积估算法：“九分法”

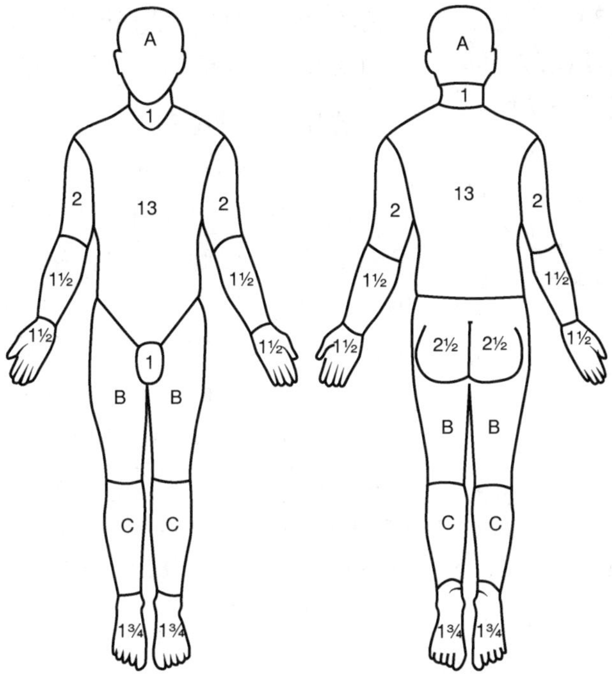

忽略小的红点

■ 部分厚度损伤 (PTL)

■ 全层厚度损伤 (FTL)

部位	% PTL	% FTL
头		
颈		
前躯干		
后躯干		
右手臂		
左手臂		
臀部		
会阴部		
右腿		
左腿		
总烧伤面积		

受生长影响的身体表面积的相对百分比							
区域	0	1	5	10	15	成人	年龄
A=½ 头	9½	8½	6½	5½	4½	3½	
B=½ 大腿	2¾	3¼	4	4½	4½	4¾	
C=½ 小腿	2½	2½	2¾	3	3¼	3½	

图 78.2　估计全身体表面积百分比：伦德–布劳德表

个部位面积的年龄变化，因此它更适合于评估儿童烧伤面积。烧伤深度分为Ⅰ度、Ⅱ度、Ⅲ度，取决于是表皮、部分还是全层皮肤损坏。

Ⅰ度烧伤（如：晒伤）仅限于表皮层，表现为皮肤完整的红斑，可能有疼痛，但无需特殊处理即可愈合。Ⅱ度烧伤，或部分烧伤，部分累及真皮层，形成水泡和潮湿，病灶有渗液，受压变白，并且感到非常疼痛。Ⅱ度烧伤需要进行特殊处理，包括植皮。Ⅲ度烧伤，或全层烧伤包括累及整个真皮层甚至达皮下组织。

Ⅲ度烧伤呈白色蜡状，常伴有红色小点（即热凝血红蛋白）。因为感觉神经末梢被破坏，所以Ⅲ度烧伤不会感到疼痛。如果不积极治疗，Ⅲ度烧伤会留下瘢痕，导致严重的毁容和瘢痕挛缩；因此，Ⅲ度烧伤应尽早清除和植皮以保证功能完整。不适当的治疗，尤其是液体复苏不充分，可能会将Ⅱ度烧伤转化为Ⅲ度烧伤。Ⅳ度烧伤用于描述累及深层结构的烧伤，如肌肉、筋膜和骨骼。

20% ～ 35% 住院烧伤患者存在吸入性损伤，并且 60% ～ 70% 的烧伤死亡与并发吸入性损伤相关，因此尽早识别吸入性损伤至关重要。如果燃烧的环境是一个密闭空间，特别是患者出现意识丧失或中毒等，则应怀疑存在吸入性损伤。体格检查时如发现：面部烧伤、嘴唇和口腔黏膜水泡、鼻毛或面部毛发烧焦、炭质痰、吞咽困难、声音嘶哑、呼吸急促、肋间收缩、啰音和喘息，均表明有可能发生吸入性损伤。随后可能表现为早期缺氧。胸部 X 线片检查在感染或肺不张发生前可能是正常的。纤支镜检查可发现气道黏膜的碳质碎片、红斑或溃疡。

风险评估和启示

烧伤病理生理学

大烧伤会引起广泛且严重的病理生理改变。在烧伤早期，烧伤引起的组织破坏会激活细胞因子介导的全身炎症反应，其特征是毛细血管通透性增加和组织水肿。当烧伤面积大于 25% TBSA 时，会出现全身水肿。由于广泛的毛细血管渗漏和烧伤表面液体渗出而导致血管内液体的丢失，皮肤脱落，可迅速导致休克以及组织、器官灌注不足。烧伤休克的发生不仅是因为血管内容量的减少，还因为全身和肺血管阻力的增加（由于儿茶酚胺和加压素的释放）和直接的心肌抑制。烧伤休克期的生化改变包括血液浓缩、乳酸酸中毒和混合静脉氧饱和度下降。休克导致肾小球滤过率降低，肾素-血管紧张素-醛固酮系统激活，表现为急性少尿。低体温是由于真皮的体温调节功能丧失导致的。

烧伤 48 ～ 72 h 内，毛细血管渗漏消失，水肿明显减轻。开放性烧伤伤口继续丢失水分。休克期之后是高代谢期，此阶段表现为氧耗增加、二氧化碳产生、蛋白质分解代谢增加和胰岛素抵抗。这一阶段的血流动力学特征为心排血量增加、心动过速和外周循环阻力降低。由于分布容积和间隙增加，大烧伤患者对大多数药物的需求增加，包括镇静剂、阿片类药物、神经肌肉阻滞剂和抗生素。急性进展期的严重脓毒症加重了高代谢状态。此外急性呼吸窘迫综合征（acute respiratory distress syndrome，ARDS）也可能会出现。

烧伤迟发的后果包括持续的炎症状态、免疫抑制和严重的蛋白质分解代谢，直至烧伤伤口愈合。创面感染是烧伤面积大于 60% TBSA 烧伤患者死亡的主要原因。必须对烧伤感染进行早期和反复的清创，以最大限度地提高患者的生存率。

全层烧伤在烧伤部位形成坚硬的焦痂。在烧伤的早期阶段痂下水肿形成时，四肢环形焦痂可导致间隔室综合征。积极的液体复苏对于烧伤休克的管理至关重要，但也可能会促进筋膜间隔室综合征的发展。未被识别的筋膜间隔室综合征可能导致广泛的肌肉坏死、横纹肌溶解，继发急性肾损伤和四肢受损。为了避免继发性缺血性损伤，我们应密切监测受伤肢体，一旦发现环形焦痂形成必须及时行切开术。躯干环形焦痂可导致胸部顺应性显著下降并干扰通气功能。这种焦痂也需要早期行切开术以实现有效的通气支持。

电烧伤常常导致广泛的深层软组织损伤，从而导致对液体复苏的需求量显著增加。骨骼电阻最大，因此电流通过骨骼时会释放较高的热量并对骨骼周围的深部肌肉造成巨大的损伤。深部肌肉损伤可导致水肿、间隔室综合征、肌肉坏死和横纹肌溶解。广泛的肌肉坏死引起的肌红蛋白尿可导致急性肾衰竭。电击常引起心律失常和心肌损伤，类似于心肌挫伤。

腹腔间隔室综合征

毛细血管通透性增加（脓毒症、创伤、烧伤）的情况下，大量液体复苏会导致腹膜后、肠系膜、肠道水肿和腹腔内高压（intraabdominal hypertension，IAH），表现为肺顺应性逐渐下降，对液体复苏无反应的少尿，低血压和酸中毒。如果没有及时治疗，可能会迅速发展为致腹腔间隔室综合征（abdominal compartment syndrome，ACS），伴随急性肾衰竭、通气困难、肠缺血和多器官系统衰竭（multiorgan system failure，MOSF）而死亡。对此类临床情况（如严重烧伤）应保持高度怀疑，监测腹内压和限制液体复苏的总量可以预防 ACS 发生。

腹内压超过 20 mmHg 时提示有 IAH 发生。治疗方法包括深度镇静、允许性高碳酸血症、胸腹切开术、神经肌肉阻滞和腹水引流。如果保守治疗不能阻止 IAH 的进展，可能需要紧急开腹减压来预防 ACS。

吸入性损伤

吸入性损伤的原因有：①吸入蒸汽和（或）热气烫伤面部和上呼吸道；②烟雾的有毒成分对气管、支气管和肺间质造成化学损伤；③一氧化碳中毒破坏氧气运输过程；④吸入氰化物抑制氧利用。吸入性损伤与烧伤相关的发病率和死亡率显著相关。面部和上呼吸道烫伤可导致面部、舌头、会厌和声带严重水肿，并可迅速导致气道阻塞。气道水肿可延迟出现数小时，它可能是由积极的液体复苏引起的。高度警惕和反复评估呼吸功能可能有助于预防致死性气道梗阻的出现。

吸入烟雾会导致气管支气管的化学损伤。来自室内火灾的燃烧产物，如盐酸、硫酸、甲醛、丙烯醛、氨和光气都可以对气管、支气管和肺泡产生损害。黏膜纤毛运动障碍会影响细菌、黏液和组织碎片的清除。表面活性物质受损及小气道堵塞可迅速导致肺不张发生。ARDS 可能会持续进展，尤其是在烧伤合并 MOSF 的情况下。其机制包括来自烧伤部位的炎症介质释放、液体复苏的效应以及感染等。

吸入的烟雾中含有一氧化碳（carbon monoxide，CO）和氰化物可导致全身毒性。CO 与血红蛋白氧合位点的亲和力高达 200 倍。CO 的结合降低血红蛋白的携氧能力，导致组织缺氧。这也导致血红蛋白的氧解离曲线左移。CO 中毒的非特异性临床症状，包括躁动、意识模糊、精神状态受抑制和昏迷，对症状的高度怀疑有助于准确诊断。正常脉搏血氧仪不能区分碳氧血红蛋白和氧合血红蛋白。在吸氧状态下，CO 中毒患者的 PaO_2 可能是正常的。CO 中毒的诊断是通过测定动脉血中碳氧血红蛋白的水平或通过测定血红蛋白的携氧能力来确定的。碳氧血红蛋白水平大于 15% 说明存在 CO 中毒。浓度大于 40% 会导致严重的神经功能损伤和昏迷。浓度大于 60% 会导致严重的脑缺氧损伤。呼吸室内空气时，碳氧血红蛋白的半衰期是 4 h。给予 100% 氧气可将碳氧血红蛋白的半衰期缩短至 1 h。有人提出高压氧疗法可减少 CO 中毒的神经后遗症。然而，目前高压氧治疗 CO 中毒并没有可靠的疗效。

氰化物是由燃烧含氮物质产生的。对于代谢性酸中毒、高乳酸血症、充分给氧条件下混合静脉氧饱和度增加的患者，应怀疑氰化物中毒。氰化物通过与线粒体细胞色素氧化酶结合，阻碍了细胞利用氧气将丙酮酸代谢为腺苷三磷酸过程从而阻断氧化磷酸化的最后一步。腺苷三磷酸只能通过无氧代谢产生，导致乳酸酸中毒。混合静脉氧饱和度升高说明线粒体中毒和细胞无法利用氧气。氰化物浓度大于 20 ppm 被认为是有毒的。浓度为 100 ppm 可导致癫痫发作、昏迷、呼吸衰竭和死亡。

在过去几十年中，烧伤相关死亡率有所改善。这得益于认知度的提高和复苏技术的进步，烧伤创面的早期切除和植皮，伤口覆盖、麻醉和危重治疗方法的进展，感染的早期诊断和积极治疗，积极的营养支持，特别是早期和连续的肠内营养。现有数据支持将严重烧伤的治疗效果与是否早期转诊到烧伤专科病房联系起来。在小型中心和综合医院中，大多情况下不具备治疗严重烧伤患者所需的专业知识、人员和设备。在烧伤中心住院患者的死亡率大约为 4%。一项大型分析结果表明预测烧伤死亡的 3 个危险因素包括有：年龄大于 60 岁、烧伤面积超过 40% TBSA 和吸入性损伤。死亡率与以上危险因素数量呈函数相关。

治疗和预防

严重烧伤的患者应首先被看作多发伤患者进行治疗。治疗应从受伤现场开始，根据《高级创伤生命支持指南》进行创伤评估。这包括基本的 ABC[气道（airway）、呼吸（breathing）、循环（circulation）] 应用，心肺复苏的启动以及对并发损伤的评估。转入烧伤中心的患者中，多达 7% 同时存在非烧伤损伤。全面的创伤评估应该从急诊科开始，并在转移到专门的烧伤中心途中以及在进入烧伤中心之后持续进行。

气道管理

气道和呼吸功能的评估是初始评估的重点。上呼吸道热损伤会导致水肿，后续积极的液体复苏可快速加重水肿并引起气道梗阻。气道热损伤患者一般应尽早插管，以免水肿造成插管困难。在儿科患者中，由于气道直径较小，气道水肿发展到气道阻塞可能非常迅速。在患者被转移到不同的机构（如烧伤中心）之前，即使没有明确的指征，也应考虑提前插管。严重的气道水肿应在局部麻醉下采用纤支镜插管，同时保留自主呼吸。在所有儿科患者和大多数成人中，纤支镜插管时很有必要给予充分镇静。不损害咽肌张力和自主通气的镇静剂，如氯胺酮和右美托咪定，是较佳选择。

烧伤后即刻的患者应被视作饱胃。在烧伤患者的后期治疗中，由于肠道水肿、脓毒症和阿片类药物的使用等，延迟了胃排空，也使得反流误吸风险持续存在。烧伤患者由于面部水肿、疼痛、渗出物、局部抗生素和敷料等使面罩难以贴合，难以或无法进行面罩通气。替代插管技术，如清醒纤支镜插管或声门上气道的使用，可避免面罩通气。

由于胶带无法粘住烧伤的皮肤，使面部烧伤患者气管导管（endotracheal tube，ETT）意外脱出的风险增加。其他的固定方法包括在患者头部周围系上柔软的环形带，用金属丝或外科缝线将 ETT 固定在牙齿上，或将 ETT 缝合在牙龈上。

液体管理

烧伤休克和 MOSF 只能通过迅速而积极的液体复苏来预防。Parkland 公式是美国用于估算烧伤患者液体需要量最常用的公式之一。这个公式建议在烧伤后的 24 h 内使用晶体，随后使用胶体。目前建议是在烧伤后 24 h 内补充胶体。考虑到用生理盐水

（0.9% NaCl）复苏时存在高氯酸血症风险，乳酸林格氏液（Lactated Ringer's solution，LR）是首选的晶体液。LR 中应添加 5% 葡萄糖以预防儿童低血糖。

根据 Parkland 公式计算，在烧伤后第一个 24 h 内的体液复苏量估计值为每千克体重 4 ml 乘以烧伤面积占总体表面积的百分比 [4 ml/（kg·%TBSA 烧伤）]。例如，一名 70 kg、烧伤 80% TBSA 的患者在最初 24 h 内需要 22 400 ml 晶体。在烧伤后的前 8 h，应给予所需总量的一半，然后重新评估和计算复苏量。

大量液体复苏加重了烧伤相关组织水肿，并有腹腔间隔室综合征和环形烧伤的四肢间隔室综合征的危险。虽然积极的液体复苏对严重烧伤患者救治至关重要，但复苏液体量需要不断重新评估和滴定到最低限度，以保持尿量在 0.5 ～ 1 ml/（kg·h）[儿童 2 ml/（kg·h）] 之间。对于大面积、全层烧伤、相关创伤或电烧伤患者，以及初始复苏延迟的患者，实际液体需求量可能远远超过估计的复苏量。吸入性损伤的存在使得液体需求量增加了 50%。

麻醉管理

术前评估

烧伤患者常用的手术干预措施包括早期减压手术，如肢体筋膜切开术和开腹减压术，早期和延迟清创和烧伤创面植皮，重建手术，以及一般的支持性手术，如气管切开、胃造口术或建立透析通路。

术前评估应确定烧伤的时间、范围和目前情况、当前的复苏计划和给予的液体总量、上呼吸道损伤和水肿、是否存在吸入性损伤、呼吸状态和通气参数、烧伤并发症（如脓毒症和 MOSF）以及重症监护计划和目标。与手术团队讨论手术计划，对于评估手术时间和失血量、计划必要的静脉通道、有创监测和血液制品的准备至关重要。

通气与氧合

烧伤常可导致呼吸衰竭。吸入性损伤的患者需要早期插管，以保证气道通畅和肺部引流，并可应对镇静和镇痛后继发的呼吸抑制。由于吸入损伤会导致气道黏膜脱落，显著增加了 ETT 堵塞的风险，因此需要积极的肺部吸引。胸部环形烧伤和由积极的液体复苏而引起的腹内压增加可导致胸部顺应性下降。吸入性损伤可并发肺不张和肺炎，导致通气血流比例失调及缺氧。随着二氧化碳生成增加，烧伤的高代谢阶段需要通气支持以保证较高的分钟通气量。严重烧伤，无论是否伴有吸入性损伤，通常会合并脓毒症和包括 ARDS 在内的 MOSF。肺损伤患者建议采用潮气量不超过 6 ml/kg 体重的肺保护性通气策略以及小于 30 cmH_2O 的气道压力，并且需要高水平的 PEEP 和 FiO_2 维持必要的氧合。

在从烧伤病房或 ICU 到手术室的转运过程中，吸入性损伤和 ARDS 患者可能面临严重缺氧的危险。在转运前，应在病床边进行人工通气试验，检验患者对人工通气的耐受性。一些患者可能需要使用能够产生高水平 PEEP 的转运呼吸机来维持足够的氧合。麻醉机必须与 ICU 中使用的机器具备相同的通气功能。

失血与静脉通路

烧伤创面的切除伴有严重的失血。由烧伤伤口到完整的组织，清创面积通常较大，而且通常难以量化丢失的血液量。有研究表明，每切除 1% TBSA，失血量为循环血容量的 2.6% ～ 3.4%。在大面积烧伤创面清除过程中，必须始终注意血容量状态、血红蛋白水平以及组织灌注的代谢指标（pH、血清乳酸水平、混合静脉饱和度）以指导输血和进行液体复苏。早期给予新鲜冰冻血浆以防止烧伤患者在创面切除时大量失血是合理的。如果患者出现难治性低血压、低体温、凝血功能障碍或代谢性酸中毒，应终止伤口清创并分期进行。

如果预期可能会出现大量失血，必须建立大口径静脉通道。建立静脉通路具有挑战性，因为浅表静脉被烧伤破坏，因此通常需要通过烧伤组织进入深静脉或中心静脉（肘静脉、股静脉、颈内静脉或锁骨下静脉）。超声引导对深静脉定位和中心静脉导管的安全放置非常有帮助。静脉导管需要缝合固定，特别是当静脉通路位于手术区域时。

监测

对于大面积烧伤患者来说，放置标准的监护仪，如心电图电极、血压袖带和脉搏血氧仪是一项挑战。心电图电极和脉冲血氧仪探头无法黏附在烧伤表面，可能需要用外科钉固定在组织上。放置脉搏血氧仪的位置，除了手指和脚趾外，还包括鼻、舌头、耳朵和嘴唇。可能无法获得未受损的位置放置四肢血压袖带，并且可能需要将无菌袖带小心地放置在植皮的伤口区域上。或者可以通过烧伤部位放置动脉管路并缝合固定。脉压变化对监测和管理血容量很有帮助。在严重烧伤的早期、脓毒症患者中，或在大面积烧伤创面切除过程中预计会出现大量失血时，应考虑放置动脉导管进行持续血压监测和采血。

低体温

烧伤患者由于中枢体温调节机制的功能失调和烧伤后皮肤体温调节功能的丧失，容易发生低体温。烧伤创面清理过程中的低体温会加速血液流失和分解代谢反应。手术室保持正常体温的方法包括将手术室温度调高到 30℃以上；使用加热灯、液体加热器、保温毯以及将吸入气体加温加湿；并用绝缘材料包裹患者的头部和四肢。严重低体温（<35℃）应及时终止手术。

药理学

烧伤会改变大多数药物的药动学和药效学。在急性烧伤后期，由于心排血量和器官灌注量的减少，肝和肾对药物的代谢和清除减少，患者可能对麻醉中使用的许多药物的敏感性增加。在随后的高代谢阶段，随着心排血量的增加，流向肾和肝的血液也增加，许多药物的清除率增加，因此需要调整剂量。

全身水肿增加了大多数药物的分布容积。分布容积的增加和清除增加导致烧伤患者对麻醉中使用的大多数药物（镇静剂、阿片类药物、抗生素、肌肉松弛剂）的敏感性降低。此外，烧伤患者可对苯二氮䓬类和阿片类药物迅速产生耐受，因此需要增加药物剂量。

烧伤明显改变了神经肌肉阻滞药的药理学特点。损伤后 24 h 内，神经肌肉接头外乙酰胆碱受体增加。烧伤后第一天给予琥珀胆碱可引起高钾血症导致心搏骤停。烧伤患者在完全康复后 1 年内应被视作为琥珀胆碱禁忌证。而对非去极化肌松药的敏感性降低是多因素的。这与神经肌肉接头外和未成熟型乙酰胆碱受体数量增加，肝、肾清除率增加以及 α_1- 酸性糖蛋白（一种急性期反应物）的结合增加有关。

致谢

感谢 Avery Tung 和 Michael F. O’Connor 两位医生对本章上一版的贡献。

（解 健 译 刘 征 校）

延伸阅读

Benson A, Dickson WA, Boyce DE: Burns, *BMJ* 332:649–652, 2006.

Bittner EA, Shank E, Woodson L, et al.: Acute and perioperative care of the burn-injured patient, *Anesthesiology* 122:448–464, 2015.

Buckley NA, Juurlink DN, Isbister G, et al.: Hyperbaric oxygen for carbon monoxide poisoning, *Cochrane Database Syst Rev* 4:CD002041, 2011.

Demling RH: Smoke inhalation injury, *New Horiz* 1:422–434, 1993.

Han T-H, Greenblatt DJ, Martyn JA: Propofol clearance and volume of distribution are increased in patients with major burns, *J Clin Pharm* 49: 768–772, 2009.

Han T-H, Martyn JA: Onset and effectiveness of rocuronium for rapid onset of paralysis in patients with major burns: priming of a large dose, *Br J Anaesth* 102(1):55–60, 2009.

Ryan CM, Schoenfeld DA, Thorpe WP, et al.: Objective estimates of the probability of death from burn injuries, *N Engl J Med* 338:362–366, 1998.

Sheridan RL, et al.: *ABLS provider's manual*, Chicago, 2001, American Burn Association.

Sheridan RL, Schulz JT, Ryan CM, et al.: A 35-year-old woman with extensive, deep burns from a nightclub fire, *N Engl J Med* 350:810–821, 2004.

Tung A: Management of burns. In Hall J, Schmidt G, Wood L, editors: *Principles of critical care companion handbook*, New York, 1998, McGraw-Hill/Appleton & Lange, pp 801–822.

Young CJ, Moss J: Smoke inhalation: diagnosis and treatment, *J Clin Anesth* 5:377–386, 1989.

Yowler CJ: Recent advances in burn care, *Curr Opin Anaesth* 14:251–255, 2001.

第79章 胸主动脉瘤

Justin Tawil

病例概要

患者，男性，80 岁。既往有腹主动脉瘤（abdominal aortic aneurysm，AAA）修补术史，1 h 前突然出现背痛。患者表现为警醒、发汗、心动过速和高血压，给予吸氧、硝酸甘油和吗啡。计算机断层扫描（computed tomography，CT）发现胸腹主动脉瘤（thoracoabdominal aortic aneurysm，TAAA）。左肾无血流。建立粗大的外周静脉通路，控制血压后疼痛缓解。该患者合并多种内科疾病，包括高血压、慢性阻塞性肺疾病（chronic obstructive pulmonary disease，COPD）、慢性肾病和糖尿病。

问题分析

定义

严重的主动脉疾病分为四种：动脉瘤、夹层、破裂和缩窄。缩窄，即动脉变窄，是典型的儿科疾病，通常在成人前就得到识别和治疗。复发性狭窄和近端动脉瘤可能需要在成年后进行干预。动脉炎、动脉粥样硬化和创伤很少引起获得性缩窄。

遗传性结缔组织疾病引起先天性主动脉病变，如 Marfan 综合征、Ehlers Danlos 综合征和 Loyes Dietz 综合征等。这些疾病使主动脉壁结构薄弱，易产生动脉瘤、夹层和破裂。其他与 TAAA 相关的疾病包括高血压、吸烟、多囊肾、使用类固醇和动脉炎（梅毒、巨细胞动脉炎、白斑病）。动脉瘤通常是指直径大于 4.5 cm 或是其正常尺寸的两倍以上的主动脉扩张。动脉瘤可能是真性的，如管壁包含所有三层（内膜、中膜和外膜），也可能是假性的。动脉瘤分类根据 Crawford 分型（图 79.1）。TAAA 是一种进行性疾病，根据大小和病因，每年的生长速度为 0.05 ～ 0.3 cm。如果动脉瘤变大，根据 LaPlace 定律，血管壁张力变大，破裂的风险增加。动脉瘤多半继发于血管内膜的急性撕裂。

主动脉夹层是主动脉壁内膜撕裂，血液从真腔泵入中膜或外膜形成假腔，如果撕裂到外膜，就会发生主动脉破裂。内膜瓣将假腔和真腔分开。由于没有流出道，任何血液进入假腔都会继续撕裂内膜。如果假腔扩大，就会压迫真腔，并可能中断流向分支动脉的血流。

主动脉夹层的定义依据 DeBakey 分型和 Stanford 分型（图 79.2）。破裂或夹层是动脉瘤进展的最终结果。夹层的解剖结构可能简单也可能复杂，复杂的夹层会导致器官或肢端灌注不良，或在控制血流动力学后，疼痛仍然存在。

无论之前有无动脉瘤，当发生剧烈活动或减速损伤时，会自发出现主动脉破裂。医源性破裂可能发生在修复性操作过程中，或少数发生在气道操作中，比如气管插管。主动脉破裂代表主动脉整层撕裂，以至于血液直接泵入邻近空间。动脉破裂通常是致命的，但也可能在出血之前被邻近结构包裹、血肿生成或间隔室压力升高。

识别

快速而特异的诊断可以挽救生命。如果不予治疗，其死亡率每小时递增 1%，48 h 后升为 50%。由于其罕见且多变的症状类似于更常见的疾病（冠状动脉疾病、胆囊炎、肾盂肾炎），多达 38% 的急性主动脉疾病患者可能会漏诊。表 79.1 列出了夹层的症状。患者很少出现典型的撕裂、游走性背痛、低血压和灌注不良综合征。许多动脉瘤是偶然发现的。巨大的胸主动脉瘤可伴有声音嘶哑、吞咽困难、呼

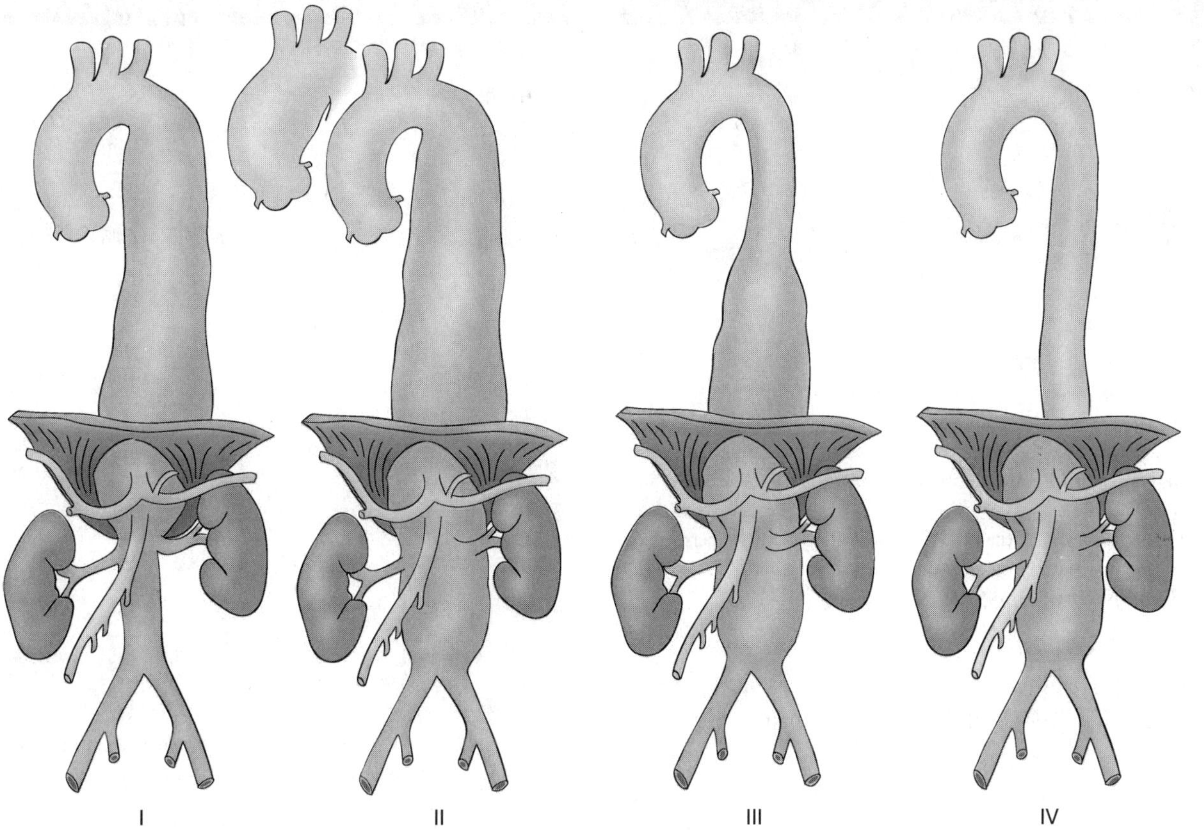

图 79.1 主动脉瘤的 Crawford 分型（From Norris EJ，Frank SF：Anesthesia for vascular surgery. In Miller RD，editor：Anesthesia，5th ed. Philadelphia，Churchill Livingstone，2000，p 1870.）

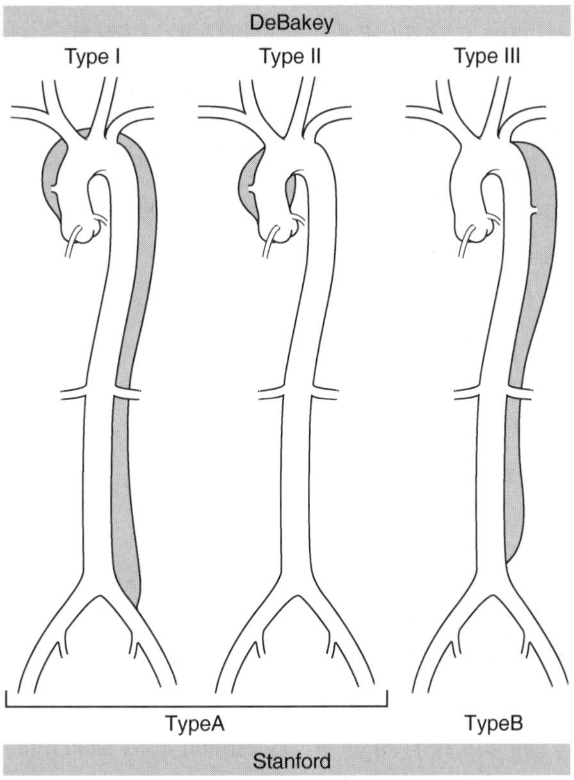

图 79.2 主动脉夹层的 DeBakey 分型（Ⅰ型，Ⅱ型，Ⅲ A 型和Ⅲ B 型）和 Stanford 分型（A 型和 B 型）（From Ibe R，Baig K，Chukwuemeka A：Surgery of the thoracic aorta. *Surgery [Oxford]* 30[1]：28-31，2012.）

表 79.1 急性夹层的症状和体征

诊断	尸检[b]	28%
神经系统	截瘫[a]	3%
	晕厥[b]	13%
	无痛[b]	6%
心血管系统	胸 / 背痛[a]	85%
	低血压[a]	A 型：27% B 型：3%
	仅有腹痛[b]	5%
肾	急性肾损伤[a]	60%

[a] Gallo A，Davies RR，Coe MP，et al：Indications，timing，and prognosis of operative repair of aortic dissections. *Semin Thorac Cardivasc Surg* 17：224-235，2005.

[b] Tsai TT，Trimarchi S，Nienaber CA：Acute aortic dissection：perspectives from the International Registry of Acute Aortic Dissection（IRAD）. *Eur J Vasc Endovasc Surg* 37：149-159，2009.

吸困难或心律失常。

影像学是快速做出特异性诊断的重要工具。紧急治疗需要有关解剖范围、定位、分支动脉灌注、渗血、破裂和压塞的信息。证实有内膜瓣的存在可以诊断夹层。无创成像已取代主动脉造影进行诊断。目前，增强 CT 已成为首选工具，因为它无创、快速，且在大多数中心都可应用。磁共振成像（magnetic resonance imaging，MRI）确实比 CT 特异性更强，但它应用不普遍，且耗时长、成本高。胸部 X 线片显示纵隔增宽对诊断夹层来说既不敏感也不特异，但可能有助于增加对有症状患者的怀疑度。经食管超声心动图（transesophageal echocardiography，TEE）具有与 CT 和 MRI 相同的特异性。术中经常使用 TEE 来定位近端内膜瓣，以评估手术的成功率，为远端循环支持装置（distal circulatory support devices，DCS）确定主动脉真腔的正确钢丝引导通路，并指导血流动力学的管理。但是经胸超声心动图不太适合用于诊断 TAAA。

风险评估

患者的基础病史中通常有多种并存疾病（表 79.2）。在几乎所有的系列报道中都有一个共识，年龄较大、病情较重的患者，围术期任何时候出现过血流动力学不稳定、灌注不足、急诊或长时间手术的患者总体预后要差得多。Crawford Ⅱ型和Ⅲ型患者通常年龄较大，病情更为严重，并存疾病较多，

表 79.2 胸腹主动脉瘤 / 夹层基线群体参数

短暂性脑缺血发作[a]	15%
卒中[b]	5%
颅内出血[b]	2%
男性[c]	66%
高血压[a, c, d]	70% ~ 80%
既往有过 CT 下手术史[c]	16% ~ 21%
既往有过夹层或动脉瘤修复术史[c, e]	2% ~ 25%
冠状动脉疾病[a, c, d]	40% ~ 70%
冠状动脉旁路移植术后或支架放置后[a]	33%
近期使用可卡因[c]	0.5% ~ 37%
高脂血症[a]	43%
吸烟[a]	63%
慢性阻塞性肺疾病[a, d]	33% ~ 41%
慢性肾衰竭（肌酐≥ 1.5）[a, d]	14% ~ 18%
糖尿病[a, c]	4% ~ 7%

[a] Kulik A，Castner CF，Kouchoukos NT：Outcomes after thoracoabdominal aortic aneurysm repair with hypothermic circulatory arrest. J Thorac Cardiovasc Surg 141：953-960，2011.

[b] Estrera AL，Miller CC，Goodrick J，et al：Update on outcomes of acute type B aortic dissection. Ann Thorac Surg 83：S842-S845，2007.

[c] Tsai TT，Trimarchi S，Nienaber CA：Acute aortic dissection：perspectives from the International Registry of Acute Aortic Dissection（IRAD）. Eur J Vasc Endovasc Surg 37：149-159，2009.

[d] Hnath JC，Mehta M，Taggert JB，et al：Strategies to improve spinal cord ischemia in endovascular thoracic aortic repair：outcomes of a prospective cerebrospinal fluid drainage protocol. J Vasc Surg 48：836-840，2008.

[e] Baril DT，Carroccio A，Ellozy SH，et al：Endovascular thoracic aortic repair and previous or concomitant abdominal aortic repair：is the increased risk of spinal cord ischemia real ？ Ann Vasc Surg 20：188-194，2006.

且预后最差。破裂的年度风险随着动脉瘤体积的增加而升高，4 cm 时为 5%，5 cm 时为 6%，6 cm 时成倍增加至 14%。

总体的死亡率难以评估，各类报道之间差异很大，且可能被低估。60% 的研究患者出现转诊，且大部分地方的尸检属于选择项目，许多死亡患者出现统计缺失。复杂的 B 型夹层死亡率约为 50%。非择期手术时死亡率增加 9 倍。

主动脉修复对全身器官系统都有影响，有关结局的小结见表 79.3。关于出血、卒中、脊髓缺血（spinal cord ischemia，SCI）、肾衰竭和胃肠道的损伤，通常在早期就会注意到。呼吸衰竭、心脏事件、感染和营养状况具有长期的重要影响。根据患者特

表 79.3 胸腹主动脉修复的结局

开放修复	住院死亡率[a, b]	选择性的：3% ～ 12% 非选择性的：20% ～ 45%
	1/5/10/20 年生存率[a, b]	85%/78%/72%/23%
	10 年内未再次手术[b]	60%
	卒中[a, c]	2% ～ 5%
	颅内出血[c]	2%
	脊髓缺血[a, b, c, d]	选择性的：0% ～ 8% 急诊的：15% ～ 40%
	气管造口[b]	11%
	充血性心力衰竭[b]	9%
	心肌梗死[c, e]	1% ～ 2%
	心房颤动[c]	15%
	急性呼吸窘迫综合征[c]	14%
	急性呼吸衰竭[c, f]	12% ～ 20%
	新发血液透析[b, c, f, g]	7% ～ 14% 幸存者中 4%
	深静脉血栓 / 肺栓塞[b]	5%
	胃肠道出血 / 肠系膜缺血[b, f, h]	0% ～ 9%
	脓毒症[b]	5%
介入修复	6 个月死亡率[b]	15%
	卒中[b, i]	3%
	脊髓缺血[b, I, j, k]	0% ～ 8% 腹主动脉瘤修复术后：14%
	血液透析[b]	3%

[a] Achneck HE，Rizzo JA，Tranquilli M，et al：Safety of thoracic aortic surgery in the present era. *Ann Thorac Surg* 84：1180-1185，2007.
[b] Kulik A，Castner CF，Kouchoukos NT：Outcomes after thoracoabdominal aortic aneurysm repair with hypothermic circulatory arrest. *J Thorac Cardiovasc Surg* 141：953-960，2011.
[c] Estrera AL，Miller CC，Goodrick J，et al：Update on outcomes of acute type B aortic dissection. *Ann Thorac Surg* 83：S842-S845，2007.
[d] Coselli JS，LeMaire SA：Tips for successful outcomes for descending thoracic and thoracoabdominal aortic aneurysm procedures. *Semin Vasc Surg* 21：13-20，2008.
[e] Svensson LG，Kouchoukos NT，Miller DC，et al：Expert consensus document on the treatment of descending thoracic aortic disease using endovascular stent-grafts. *Ann Thorac Surg* 85：S1-S41，2008.
[f] Aftab M，Coselli JS：Renal and visceral protection in thoracoabdominal aortic surgery. *J Thorac Cardiovasc Surg* 148：2963-2966，2014.
[g] Gallo A，Davies RR，Coe MP，et al：Indications，timing，and prognosis of operative repair of aortic dissections. *Semin Thorac Cardiovasc Surg* 17：224-235，2005.
[h] Tsai TT，Trimarchi S，Nienaber CA：Acute aortic dissection：perspectives from the International Registry of Acute Aortic Dissection（IRAD）. *Eur J Vasc Endovasc Surg* 37：149-159，2009.
[i] Buth J，Harris PL，Hobo R，et al：Neurologic complications associated with endovascular repair of thoracic aortic pathology：incidence and risk factors. A study from the European Collaborators on Stent/Graft Techniques for Aortic Aneurysm Repair（EUROSTAR）Registry. *J Vasc Surg* 46：1103-1111，2007.
[j] Baril DT，Carroccio A，Ellozy SH，et al：Endovascular thoracic aortic repair and previous or concomitant abdominal aortic repair：is the increased risk of spinal cord ischemia real ？ *Ann Vasc Surg* 20：188-194，2006.
[k] Greipp RB，Greipp EB：Spinal cord perfusion and protection during descending thoracic and thoracoabdominal aortic surgery：the collateral network concept. *Ann Thorac Surg* 83：S865-S869，2007.

定的危险因素，外科医师可能是确定器官保护优先顺序的最佳人选。辅助麻醉和外科技术已被用来改善主要结果。通常不单独研究相关技术，且缺乏个体化措施的高质量数据。

神经系统事件，特别是脊髓缺血和卒中，是主动脉术后的可怕结果。卒中可能更常见于腔内介入治疗，因为逆行导丝和导管增加了栓塞的风险。卒中和操作时间、女性、肥胖相关。卒中和低温停跳的时间相关，超过 40 min，卒中的发生率显著增加。据报道在之前的冠状动脉旁路移植术中，明确在无左侧优势椎动脉或左乳内动脉的情况下，支架覆盖左锁骨下动脉是安全的。随着时间的推移，停循环和腔内技术进一步降低了卒中的风险。

脊髓缺血及其引起的瘫痪或轻瘫可能会即刻发生，麻醉苏醒后就能观察到，也可能在发作前的检查正常，但延迟发作。延迟性脊髓缺血通常发生在低血压之后，可能由手术或胃肠道出血、疼痛治疗、全身炎症反应综合征（systemic inflammatory response syndrome，SIRS）、脓毒症或心脏原因引起。出现症状后进行脑脊液（cerebrospinal fluid，CSF）引流仅部分有效。在紧急情况下，脊髓缺血的风险可能高达 40%。SCI 降低患者生活质量、增加护理费用，且一年死亡率为 70%。一系列措施已被采取以降低 SCI 的风险。缺血是由于代谢的供需失衡所造成。这种失衡源于多种因素（原有血管疾病、必须性外科缺血、血管痉挛、颅内压增高、再灌注后水肿），因此及时找出原因并加以治疗并不容易。

各种合理的外科、药理学、血流动力学、脑脊液引流和监测技术提供了可能的干预措施的无限组合。诱发电位需要特别考虑，并可能使麻醉预案复杂化。虽然运动诱发电位（motor evoked potential，MEP）能较好地监测脊髓前角，但躯体感觉诱发电位（somatosensory evoked potential，SSEP）通常反映了脊髓血流的显著变化，并能很好地预测缺血。这些监测的使用变化多样，但可以提供最佳的实时神经保护。

在一些研究中，在影像引导下的肋间动脉再植入、血液回流或诱发电位降低了 SCI 的发生，但尚未得到广泛证实。这种变异性可能是由于缺血时间的增加以及额外的复杂技术所致。多达 5% 的再植入患者术后出血需要再次手术。另有报道表明立即结扎肋间动脉能改善 SCI。这项技术可以防止缺血

时来自脊髓的窃血 / 回流。这可能解释了为什么腔内手术治疗的患者脊髓缺血发生率并不高，因为肋间动脉被覆盖。经脊髓前动脉进入脊髓的侧支血流来自椎动脉、锁骨下动脉、肋间动脉、腰动脉和腹下动脉（图 79.3）。动物研究表明如果有侧支循环，完全性脊髓截断是可存活的。不幸的是，这些血管网在动脉粥样硬化、高血压患者中受到破坏。阻断时引起的高血压会增加侧支循环。

需特别注意根大动脉（Adamkiewicz），通常发自 T10。尸检报告显示它更常起源自腰椎水平（70%）。这解释了为什么既往有腹主动脉瘤修复史的患者脊髓缺血的发生率特别高。脊髓缺血风险增高也与急诊手术、围术期低血压、肥胖、糖尿病、高龄、长时间支架修复、髂外损伤、腹下或锁骨下动脉闭塞和肾衰竭有关。

脑脊液引流能够降低颅内压并改善灌注压和脊髓缺血的预后。脊髓和脑灌注压由如下公式计算：灌注压 = 平均动脉压（MAP）- 中心静脉压（CVP）或颅内压（ICP）中的较高值。这表明如果颅内压低于中心静脉压，那么它再降低也没有益处。这也提示对于高血压的治疗，静脉扩张可能比动脉扩张更有益。

冠状动脉疾病、高风险手术和极度的生理性应激可导致心肌缺血、心肌梗死和心力衰竭。阻断期间增加的体循环阻力（systemic vascular resistance，SVR）通过升高左心室舒张末期压力及增加氧耗降低冠状动脉灌注。联合使用麻醉性镇痛药、巴比妥类、艾司洛尔和硝酸甘油控制血压能增加冠状动脉血流并降低左心室每搏做功，其对自身调节的影响小于直接的动脉扩张剂。心律失常很常见，但报道的严重的心脏事件低于预期。

呼吸衰竭是罹病和死亡的主要原因。吸烟、

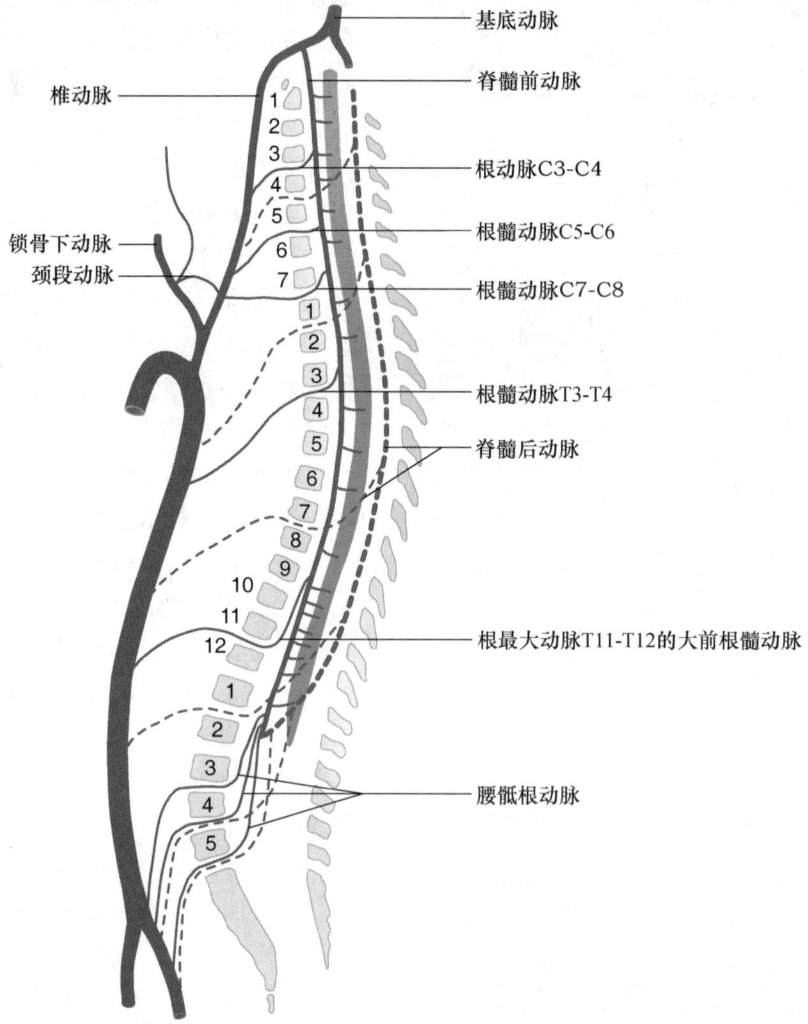

图 79.3　脊髓的血液供应（From Marijic J，El-Magharbel I，Weiss L，et al：Anesthesia for patients with thoracic aortic disease. In Leung J，editor：*Cardiac and vascular anesthesia*：*the requisites in anesthesiology*. Philadelphia，Mosby，2004，p 180.）

COPD、机械通气及输血输液引起的肺损伤很常见。开胸术切口大且疼痛，需要小心处理使肺不张得到最妥善处置。急性呼吸窘迫综合征、长时间通气和呼吸机获得性肺炎增加了这些患者术后病程的复杂性。弥散性血管内凝血、制动、SIRS 和易发生血栓的输注均会导致肺栓塞。

慢性肾病在这类人群中很常见。胸腹主动脉瘤疾病通常引起肾血管缺血，存在急性肾衰竭和新发血液透析的最高风险。多达一半的突发性急性肾衰竭的患者会发生多器官功能衰竭及死亡。增强 CT 用于诊断及术后监测，增加了额外的风险。多数已发表的研究使用不太敏感的肾损伤筛查工具，其结果可能被低估。

腹腔动脉、肠系膜上动脉疾病或肠系膜下动脉疾病所导致的内脏受累在血管病变中并不罕见。对这些血管的阻断或栓塞以及覆盖，会出现手术性缺血。缺血引起酸中毒，导致血流动力学紊乱。内脏缺血和胃肠道出血引起的死亡不常见，但也曾有过报道。术中机械灌注、动脉成形和序贯阻断可能会降低这些风险。

启示

主动脉弓部病变主要为外科疾病，但并不完全如此。内科治疗、阻断和缝合、远端循环支持和腔内技术会导致不同的并发症，取决于患者自身的解剖和生理状况。患者可能会出现需要细致处理或紧急的情况。一些患者相对没有希望，例如那些切开前完全停搏的，但是对患者和疾病的理解能够指导并优化治疗。

管理

所有主动脉疾病患者的初始治疗都集中在血流动力学的管理上。那些患有简单夹层的患者需要进入重症加强治疗病房严格控制血压。大部分患者（73% ～ 90%）仅通过内科治疗即可成功治愈。因为介入治疗死亡率高，不复杂的夹层和偶然发现的动脉瘤大多数会选择内科治疗。内科治疗患者入院后的死亡率约为 1%。内科治疗主要考虑减少主动脉管壁的压力。积极控制血压和心率已被证实可降低动脉瘤的扩张速度和破裂风险。β 受体阻滞剂，尤其是拉贝洛尔已被研究得很透彻，通常作为一线治疗药物使用。

有巨大动脉瘤、复杂夹层或持续症状不缓解的患者需要手术干预。如果有这些特征，其发病率和死亡率增加，即手术干预的风险超过保守治疗。这类患者自然病程的风险极高，于 2 名接受治疗的患者 5 年后存者为 1 例。

关于 TAAA 的治疗，不同外科医师和机构之间差别很大。医生之间经常就特定患者选择何种治疗方法产生争论。治疗方法包括心胸手术、血管手术、放射或心脏介入手术，医生之间也时常产生分歧。尚无随机对照试验可以明确定义最佳治疗实践。无论开放手术还是腔内手术，对于患者的长期生活质量的结局并无差异。

决定干预对象和何时进行干预是十分复杂的。尽管已发表了基于动脉瘤大小的指南，但很浅显且不充分。许多动脉夹层和破裂在指南建议干预之前即已发生。个体自然病程的风险必须与预期的干预结果进行权衡。所选择的修复方法、团队技能和使用的辅助设备在评估中均应着重考虑。对于腔内和开放手术，文献所提示的短期和中期结果都很不错。年龄和结缔组织疾病也在决策中起着重要作用。大多数结缔组织病患者比较年轻，手术修补需要的时间更久，而且通常被排除在腔内治疗之外。20 多年来已充分证明了，开放手术修复持久耐用性。但是高龄或高风险患者，尤其是合并严重肺疾病的患者，可能从腔内修补中获益更大。医疗机构对于治疗结局的认识需要关于风险和收益更有意义的讨论。因此，即使风险较低的患者也应尽早转诊到具有良好转归的大型中心，因为这些外科医师能够提供个体化的全面治疗。

Orr 及其同事就腔内支架选择和其技术差异进行了非常好的回顾。新型支架和释放装置持续拓展了适应范围，并使并发症得到改善。支持者声称腔内技术的好处是手术时间更短、操作时间更快、失血更少、避免全身麻醉以及开胸手术。

腔内治疗需要保留相关的分支动脉。早期直管型移植物需要避开重要结构，或者依靠流向重要脏器的侧支血流。较新型分支和开窗型移植物具有更多的灵活性。制造商已经能够根据患者的具体解剖结构制造支架。但是解剖因素依然限制了腔内技术在某些患者中的应用。因为移植物要求主动脉的某些部分必须是正常的结构以作为“着陆区”。通道和主动脉血管的大小和路径必须足够大、足够直，以充分容纳这些工具。

腔内技术特定的并发症包括移植物塌陷、内漏、移位、打折和通道血管的损伤。内漏，或动脉瘤体内和动脉压力 / 血流之间的流通，是多种原因导致的结果。腔内修复需要更频繁的监测成像，额外的步骤也很多。移植物 10 年后的长期的持久耐受性如何尚无明确的文献报道。

麻醉管理

开放性 TAAA 的手术治疗是麻醉中最大的挑战。TAAA 手术是高风险手术。要在高危人群中实施成功的麻醉，需要完美地应用一系列操作技巧，控制生理的巨大变化，并考虑到每个器官系统的损伤。不同的医生和机构之间的技术差异很大。手术和麻醉团队之间应明确沟通手术步骤，主要的风险因素和计划的辅助手段。

初始评估主要集中于气道、血流动力学以及手术预案。在紧急情况下，通过言语安慰、使用抗焦虑药和严密控制血流动力学来保证安全，对于降低术前动脉破裂的风险至关重要。然后对患者进行预给氧和标准化监测。

圆椎以下 L3-L5 水平的脑脊液引流时，最好在清醒下置管以减少神经损伤。引流管应采用封闭敷料覆盖。血性引流液不是引流或手术的禁忌证，但可能会增加硬膜外血肿的风险，尤其是肝素化的患者。患者体位改变或转运时应夹闭脑脊液引流管，以防止意外引流。

诱导前应在外周静脉放置大口径静脉导管并行动脉置管。手术可能要分离或阻断左锁骨下动脉，所以最好选择右上肢进行动脉监测。通过股动脉监测中心动脉压可有利于远端循环支持。对一些患者而言，在诱导前也可以开放中心静脉通路（有或无 Swan-Ganz 导管）。

在预给氧后，诱导时需关注高血压的预防。芬太尼滴定可阻滞交感神经，通常会出现心率降低，这是有助于患者的反应。任何低血压都不应矫枉过正。插管应按照病史和体格检查的提示进行。简言之，需要应用肺隔离技术用以改善术野暴露并减少撑开器的损伤。当患者处于危急状况时（通常在大量输血后），麻醉科医师需将双腔管在术后换成单腔气管导管。有研究报道动脉瘤破裂发生在气道操作之后，在术前应根据影像学和症状进行评估。

患者的通常体位是右侧半卧位，手术入路通过左侧开胸，切口向下延伸至中线。在摆放体位过程中，应注意受力点和避免臂丛神经受损。更换体位后，应检查导管和脑脊液引流的通畅情况。

高级的神经监测决定了麻醉的维持。脑脊液引流是一项有创操作，其并发症的发生率为 5%，包括头痛、神经损伤、硬膜下血肿、脑脊液漏、脑膜炎、导管折断和颅内出血。有些机构在没有诱发电位变化的情况下不实施脑脊液引流操作，而有些机构则会根据目标颅内压值每小时引流 5 ～ 20 ml，直至排除脊髓缺血。如果脑脊液中发现血液，就应该夹闭引流管直至影像学查明血液的来源。体温降低至目标 32 ～ 34℃。药物辅助也可以采用。

应备好正性肌力药物、β 受体阻滞剂、升压药、血管扩张剂、抗心律失常药、胰岛素、电解质、体内 / 体外除颤仪。TEE 和肺动脉导管有助于优化血流动力学并监测缺血。在阻断时，阻断近端的体循环阻力会增加。髂动脉上阻断影响最为剧烈。有远端循环支持或原有腋动脉旁路的患者对阻断的反应降低。在阻断前，体温和脊髓引流应处于目标值，采用合理的措施如吸入麻醉维持、输注艾司洛尔和硝酸甘油，芬太尼和苯巴比妥类将收缩压降低至 90 ～ 100 mmHg。进行阻断应与这些步骤相配合。应尽可能减轻左心室的负担并密切观察。轻度过度通气和输注碳酸氢盐可以控制酸中毒。尽管动脉阻断，但阻断部位的静脉回流仍然存在，因此 CVP 和 ICP 均增加。在此期间，MAP 应控制在 80 ～ 110 mmHg 之间。TEE 和多次血气分析可有助于这一关键时刻的监测。

在阻断松开之前，麻醉减浅，MAP 应维持在上限。并准备好推注用血管收缩药物、钙和碳酸氢盐。缓慢松开阻断使患者面临最大限度的动脉扩张、酸中毒和缺氧代谢物。松开前的容量负荷有助于充盈驱空的动脉系统。

TAAA 手术可能导致任何部位的快速失血。使用肝素、手术、低体温、纤维蛋白溶解和 DCS 均会导致出血过多。应备好血液制品、细胞保护装置和快速输血装置。术中输血几乎是普遍现象，因此预备的血液、血浆、血小板和冷沉淀的范围应为 5 ～ 10 个单位。在大出血的情况下，目标导向输血和监测国际标准化比值、纤维蛋白原、全血细胞计数和血栓弹力图可能会有一定的用途。

肾保护包括提供灌注压力和心排血量，同时避免肾毒性药物。冷晶体灌注和远端循环支持可减少开放手术中的缺血性损伤。静脉注射染料和尿液排泄之间的时间可预测术后肾功能恢复。应当监测尿量和膀胱温度。

（沈怡佳 译 刘 佳 校）

延伸阅读

Acher CW, Wynn MM: How we do it, *Cardiovasc Surg* 7:593–596, 1999.

Achneck HE, Rizzo JA, Tranquilli M, et al.: Safety of thoracic aortic surgery in the present era, *Ann Thorac Surg* 84:1180–1185, 2007.

Aftab M, Coselli JS: Renal and visceral protection in thoracoabdominal aortic surgery, *J Thorac Cardiovasc Surg* 148:2963–2966, 2014.

Baril DT, Carroccio A, Ellozy SH, et al.: Endovascular thoracic aortic repair and previous or concomitant abdominal aortic repair: is the increased risk of spinal cord ischemia real? *Ann Vasc Surg* 20:188–194, 2006.

Biglioli P, Roberto M, Cannata A, et al.: Upper and lower spinal cord blood supply: the continuity of the anterior spinal artery and the relevance of the lumbar arteries, *J Thorac Cardiovasc Surg* 127:1188–1192, 2004.

Buth J, Harris PL, Hobo R, et al.: Neurologic complications associated with endovascular repair of thoracic aortic pathology: incidence and risk factors. A study from the European Collaborators on Stent/Graft Techniques for Aortic Aneurysm Repair (EUROSTAR) Registry, *J Vasc Surg* 46:1103–1111, 2007.

Chiesa R, Tshomba Y, Melissano G, et al.: Hybrid approach to thoracoabdominal aortic aneurysms in patients with prior aortic surgery, *J Vasc Surg* 45:1128–1135, 2007.

Coselli JS, LeMaire SA: Tips for successful outcomes for descending thoracic and thoracoabdominal aortic aneurysm procedures, *Semin Vasc Surg* 21:13–20, 2008.

Dick F, Hinder D, Immer FF, et al.: Outcome and quality of life after surgical and endovascular treatment of descending aortic lesions, *Ann Thorac Surg* 85:1605–1613, 2008.

Estrera AL, Miller CC, Goodrick J, et al.: Update on outcomes of acute type B aortic dissection, *Ann Thorac Surg* 83:S842–S845, 2007.

Gallo A, Davies RR, Coe MP, et al.: Indications, timing, and prognosis of operative repair of aortic dissections, *Semin Thorac Cardiovasc Surg* 17:224–235, 2005.

Gega A, Rizzo JA, Johnson MH, et al.: Straight deep hypothermic arrest: experience in 394 patients supports its effectiveness as a sole means of brain preservation, *Ann Thorac Surg* 84:759–767, 2007.

Greipp RB, Greipp EB: Spinal cord perfusion and protection during descending thoracic and thoracoabdominal aortic surgery: the collateral network concept, *Ann Thorac Surg* 83:S865–S869, 2007.

Hansen CJ, Bui H, Donayre CE, et al.: Complications of endovascular repair of high-risk and emergent descending thoracic aortic aneurysms and dissections, *J Vasc Surg* 40:228–234, 2004.

Hnath JC, Mehta M, Taggert JB, et al.: Strategies to improve spinal cord ischemia in endovascular thoracic aortic repair: outcomes of a prospective cerebrospinal fluid drainage protocol, *J Vasc Surg* 48:836–840, 2008.

Kulik A, Castner CF, Kouchoukos NT: Outcomes after thoracoabdominal aortic aneurysm repair with hypothermic circulatory arrest, *J Thorac Cardiovasc Surg* 141:953–960, 2011.

Lemaire SA, Jones MM, Conklin LD, et al.: Randomized comparison of cold blood and cold crystalloid renal perfusion for renal protection during thoracoabdominal aortic aneurysm repair, *J Vasc Surg* 49:11–19, 2009.

Miller 3rd CC, Porat EE, Estrera AL, et al.: Number needed to treat: analyzing of the effectiveness of thoracoabdominal aortic repair, *Eur J Vasc Endovasc Surg* 28:154–157, 2004.

Orr N, Minion D, Bobadilla JL: Thoracoabdominal aortic aneurysm repair: current endovascular perspectives, *Vasc Health Risk Manag* 10:493–505, 2014.

Schepens MA, Kelder JC, Morshuis WJ, et al.: Long term follow-up after thoracoabdominal aortic aneurysm repair, *Ann Thorac Surg* 83:S851–S855, 2007.

Singh S, Hutton P: Anaesthesia for thoracic and thoraco-abdominal aortic disease—part 1: basic sciences, presentation and pre-operative preparation, *Curr Anaesth Crit Care* 17:101–107, 2006.

Singh S, Hutton P: Anesthesia for thoracic and thoraco-abdominal aortic disease—part 2: anaesthetic management and neuroprotection, *Curr Anaesth Crit Care* 17:109–117, 2006.

Svensson LG, Kouchoukos NT, Miller DC, et al.: Expert consensus document on the treatment of descending thoracic aortic disease using endovascular stent-grafts, *Ann Thorac Surg* 85:S1–S41, 2008.

Tsai TT, Trimarchi S, Nienaber CA: Acute aortic dissection: perspectives from the International Registry of Acute Aortic Dissection (IRAD), *Eur J Vasc Endovasc Surg* 37:149–159, 2009.

Zierer A, Moon MR, Melby SJ, et al.: Impact of perfusion strategy on neurologic recovery in acute type A aortic dissection, *Ann Thorac Surg* 83:2122–2129, 2007.

第80章 违禁药物摄入

Casey D. Bryant，Jeffrey S. Kelly

病例概要

患者，男性，25岁，在翻车事故中意外受伤，双侧胫骨开放性严重骨折急需要修复手术。据了解患者曾经在现场失去知觉。患者目前处于警觉但无定向力状态，格拉斯哥昏迷量表评分为14分，还表现出说话含糊不清和结膜充血。患者承认在事故发生前饮酒并服用了安非他明。患者血流动力学稳定，在完成初级和次级检诊（包括对头部、颈椎、胸部、腹部和骨盆CT检查）后进行彻底的创伤评估，排除了其他重大损伤。生命体征如下，血压110/50 mmHg，脉搏124次/分，呼吸频率24次/分，体温37.1℃，吸室内空气时脉搏血氧饱和度为100%。重要的实验室结果包括血细胞比容24%，pH 7.27，BE-10 mEq/L，血液酒精含量279 mg/dL。

问题分析

定义和识别

接触违禁药物的情况很常见，例如2013年，毒物控制中心共接到310万个电话。这些接触违禁药物电话中急性暴露占88%，非故意接触占80%，经口服用占79%，服用单一药物占89%，儿童暴露占57%，在私人住宅接触毒物占91%。尽管2013年这类病例中有近70%是在医疗体系之外处理的，但仍有601 642名患者就诊，228 230名患者住院治疗，99 117名重症监护患者和2 113人死亡。鉴于毒物控制中心的信息可能低估了违禁药物使用及不良事件的实际发生情况，因此以上数据更让人震惊。2013年死亡人数最多的药物（按频率降序排列）分别为镇痛剂、兴奋剂/街头毒品（海洛因、甲基苯丙胺和可卡因）、心血管药物、抗抑郁药和镇静剂/催眠药/抗精神病药。

风险评估

大多数违禁药品摄入往往遵循两种模式中的一种。小于12岁儿童通常无意中服用少量单一药物，很少出现病残或死亡。相比之下，青少年和成年人通常会有意地摄入较多的多种药物，从而导致更高的病残率和死亡率。

有关成人药物过量的数据显示大约50%病例同时摄入乙醇，而在相同比例的创伤病例中酒精明显干扰了最初的临床评估。2013年在美国与酒精相关的机动车事故造成近1/3（31%）的交通事故死亡，相关损失超过590亿美元。此外，据报道约18%的机动车司机死亡与使用酒精以外的药物有关。

因此，临床医师应高度怀疑青少年和成人创伤患者存在某种急性药物中毒，并应在最初的病史采集、体格检查和诊断检查期间评估是否有患者滥用药物的证据。这些重要的病史包括服用违禁药物名称、服用量、服用时间、服用以来的体征和症状、既往的医学和精神病史（包括自杀意图）、现在药物治疗史，以及过敏史和创伤史（意外偶然或自残行为）。由于患者在急性中毒情况下，病史采集往往是不可靠或不完整的，其他来源的补充病史（例如公共安全人员、家庭、医疗记录、地区药房、地方毒物控制中心和国家麻醉药品数据库）可能有助于诊断中毒。鉴于中毒或创伤环境中患者的病史通常较不明确，临床医师必须对患者进行快速、系统和全面的体格检查。应采取适当的保护预防措施，防止自身中毒（例如皮肤接触有机磷杀虫剂）。评估应首先关注ABC[气道（airway）、呼吸（breathing）和循环（circulation）]，积极干预任何发现的异常情况。

其他评估因素如下：

- **呕吐反射**：对过量摄入违禁药品患者的气道保护和可能的误吸有影响，但对临床医师评估是否需要插管和格拉斯哥昏迷量表的作用甚微。
- **核心温度异常**：可能涉及多种病因，包括违禁药品（水杨酸盐、兴奋剂）、环境和感染原因。
- 神经功能检查异常：发现中枢神经系统功能障碍（如意识混乱、昏迷或谵妄），临床医师应积极安排患者进行影像检查，如 CT 或磁共振成像，以评估其他潜在原因，如颈脊髓损伤、缺血性卒中或颅内出血。
- **药物滥用的意外伤害**：应检查患者穿刺伤口、针迹和鼻中隔穿孔。
- **体征和症状**：摄入某些违禁药品可能的典型表现包括异常生命体征、精神状态的改变、瞳孔变化和多种可能归因于特定药物种类的已知药理性质的多种杂项效应。具体违禁药品的范例见表 80.1。

实验室的评估应基于疑似摄入（即药物水平、血液酒精水平），并应考虑过量服用对乙酰氨基酚和水杨酸等情形。尿液药物筛查有时会提供有关可能摄入毒物的诊断线索，尽管结果通常无法及时获得，而且不同机构检测到的物质也不尽相同。

如病例概要所示，同时存在创伤和中毒可能会干扰对每个个体的准确评估。出现贫血、心动过速和代谢性酸中毒时的正常血压和脉压可能反映了部分被安非他明相关血管收缩掩盖的低血容量性休克。

管理

绝大多数急性中毒患者在给予适当的支持治疗后，都能得到满意的治疗效果，重点是积极的早期干预，以保护重要器官功能。最初的努力应该集中在维持稳定的、通畅的气道，维持适当的通气和氧合，稳定心血管功能，就像在其他紧急医疗情况下一样。所有精神状态抑郁的患者，如果存在缺氧，应给予吸氧治疗；如果临床担心阿片类药物过量，应考虑静脉注射纳洛酮；如果指尖血糖水平较低，应静脉注射葡萄糖。即使怀疑缺乏硫胺素的患者也应尽早纠正低血糖，因为最近的文献不支持在葡萄糖前给予硫胺素以避免诱发 Wernicke 脑病的经典做法。怀疑是违禁药品引起的强直性癫痫发作，最好

表 80.1 常见的中毒症候群

综合征	常见的临床症状	违禁药品
抗胆碱能	心动过速、发热、皮肤干燥、尿潴留、肠梗阻、瞳孔散大、谵妄、癫痫发作	抗组胺药、吩噻嗪类、三环抗抑郁药、抗精神病药、阿托品、东莨菪碱、曼陀罗、金刚烷胺
胆碱能	心动过缓、发汗、尿失禁或大便失禁、呕吐、瞳孔缩小、中枢神经系统抑制、虚弱、筋膜炎、喘息	抗过敏药物、鹅膏菌、巴氯芬、有机磷酸盐和氨基甲酸酯杀虫剂、毒扁豆碱、溴吡斯的明、依酚氯铵、某些菌类
拟交感神经（兴奋剂）	心动过速（心动过缓伴有纯 α 受体激动剂）、高血压、瞳孔散大、盗汗、瘙痒、发热、妄想、偏执、不安、躁动	可卡因、安非他明、非处方的解充血药（伪麻黄碱、苯丙醇胺、去氧肾上腺素）
麻醉性镇痛药	精神状态抑郁、通气不足、瞳孔缩小、肠梗阻、低血压、心动过缓	阿片类药物
镇静催眠药	困乏、口齿不清、精神状态抑郁、呼吸抑制、共济失调、体温过低	苯二氮䓬类、巴比妥类、乙醇、抗精神病药、抗惊厥药
5- 羟色胺	发热、盗汗、潮红、腹泻、反射亢进、震颤、肌阵挛、牙关紧闭	选择性血清素再摄取抑制剂、曲唑酮、氯丙咪嗪、美哌替啶、美沙酮、右美沙芬、利奈唑胺、曲马多等
致幻剂	幻觉、精神病、偏执、恐慌、发烧、瞳孔散大	可卡因、安非他明、大麻素、苯环吡啶（五氯苯酚）、麦角酸二乙胺（迷幻药）、抗组胺药
锥体外系	震颤，僵直，斜视，斜颈，舞蹈症，震颤，反射亢进	典型和非典型抗精神病药

Data from Hoffman RS，Howland MA，Lewin NA，et al.，editors：*Goldfrank's toxicologic emergencies*，10th ed. New York，McGraw-Hill，2015；and Levine M，Brooks DE，Truitt CA，et al.：Toxicology in the ICU：part 1：general overview and approach to treatment. *Chest* 140：795-806，2011.

使用苯二氮草类药物治疗，其剂量往往高于传统癫痫发作所需要的剂量。静脉注射巴比妥类药物是可以接受的第二类药物，因为它们具有 γ-氨基丁酸（GABA）-激动剂活性。鉴于中毒和创伤患者酒精滥用的发生率都很高，应及早监测酒精戒断情况，并根据需要适当启动苯二氮草类药物治疗。

最终中毒处理通常涉及早期（在适当情况下）使用特定的解毒剂和净化技术。胃肠道的净化主要围绕活性炭展开，活性炭被认为可以吸附潜在违禁药品。应该尽可能尽早实施（最好是在摄入后 1 h 内），并且仅对精神状态良好或气道安全的患者。目前只建议对摄入危及生命的药物如卡马西平、达普酮、苯巴比妥、奎宁或茶碱的患者重复使用活性炭。阿司匹林过量重复使用木炭仍有争议，但可能被临床医师考虑。其他更有历史意义的净化技术，如胃排空（使用吐根糖浆或洗胃）和使用渗透性泻药减少胃肠道吸收时间，由于一直缺乏基于循证文献支持，一直没有被应用。吐根糖浆已经被完全抛弃，洗胃的风险限制了它的使用，只有在极其罕见的和在胃肠内有大量未吸收的情况下，由经过适当培训和有经验的技术人员在摄入后尽早开始使用洗胃。支持使用大量等渗透性泻药进行全肠道灌洗的证据也不充分，但可考虑用于摄入肠内包衣/缓释药物、非法药物包或未吸附到活性炭上的物质（如锂、铁、钾）的情况。在临床影响程度较大时，可进行血液透析违禁药品（如水杨酸、锂、二甲双胍）（表 80.2、框 80.1 和 80.2）。

病例概要中所述患者使用安非他明后出现的体征和症状可被同时出现的其他症状所掩盖，如中枢神经系统抑制（即乙醇）作用、长骨骨折导致的血容量不足以及低温环境暴露。安非他明典型药理表现与弥漫性高肾上腺素能状态一致，包括高血压、心动过速、高热、出汗、瞳孔缩小和多动。精神症状可能包括躁动、偏执和幻觉。具体的治疗方法是使用苯二氮草类药物进行“药理学冷却”（例如，根据需要静脉注射安定 10 mg，并仔细滴定，直到患者平静下来）。治疗的目标是①减少躁动，用 GABA 激动剂治疗强直性阵挛性癫痫；②积极进行物理降温，处理明显的高热；③在横纹肌溶解病例中，以 1～2 ml/（kg·h）的尿量为目标，启动等渗性晶体静脉补液；④使用尼卡地平或硝普钠等药物控制对苯二氮草类镇静反应不佳的严重高血压。硝普钠应谨慎使用，因为长期滥用安非他明会导致类似慢性高血压的血管内容量相对减少。与嗜铬细胞瘤和可卡因滥用一样，在安非他明滥用时使用 β 受体阻滞剂可能会导致 α 肾上腺素能受体的无对抗性激活而加重高血压。在纠正某些安非他明同系物引起的低钠血症时应谨慎。仅在一些被认为是由于严重低钠血症导致的危及生命的情况（如癫痫发作），才使用 3% 的生理盐水。

表 80.2 精选中毒解毒剂

药物	解毒剂
阿片类药物	纳洛酮
苯二氮草类药物	氟马西尼（服用慢性苯二氮草类药物患者易诱发癫痫发作）
抗胆碱能类	毒扁豆碱（咨询毒理学家）
胆碱酯酶抑制剂	阿托品、磷定（杀虫剂）
钙通道阻滞剂	氯化钙、胰高血糖素、考虑高剂量胰岛素治疗
β-受体阻滞剂	胰高血糖素，考虑大剂量胰岛素治疗
地高辛	地高辛特异性抗体
对乙酰氨基酚	N-乙酰半胱氨酸
甲醇	甲吡唑、乙醇
乙二醇	甲吡唑、乙醇
异烟肼	维生素 B_6
氰化物	硝酸戊酯、亚硝酸钠、硫代硫酸钠、羟钴胺素
高铁血红蛋白	亚甲蓝
铁	去铁胺

Data from Brooks DE，Levine M，O'Connor AD，et al：Toxicology in the ICU：part 2：specifc toxins，Chest 140：1072-1085，2011；and Hoffman RS，Howland MA，Lewin NA，et al，editors：*Goldfrank's toxicologic emergencies*，10th ed. New York，McGraw-Hill，2015.

由于患者缺乏明显的安非他明相关症状，故对这位患者的最终治疗仅仅是积极的支持性治疗。他在术后被收治可进行远程监测的区域，该区域配备训练有素的人员，专门培训复杂创伤患者的治疗。对酒精抽搐的体征和症状进行了监测，但对于这个年龄段的患者，明确的戒断则相对少见。

预防

进行前瞻性的对照试验来评估违禁药品摄入引起的并发症是不合伦理的。流行病学研究、回顾性数据和病例报告提供了对特定违禁药品摄入后果的

框 80.1 中毒处理：活性炭

适应证

单剂量：在无禁忌证且预期疗效改善的情况下，服用与活性炭结合的药物或毒素。

多剂量：服用与活性炭结合的药物或毒素，且①预期吸收阶段会延长，②潜在毒性巨大，③患者已摄入危及生命的卡马西平、达普酮、苯巴比妥、奎宁或茶碱。重复服用阿司匹林过量仍有争议。

剂量[a]

初始剂量（单次或多次）

成人和儿童：1 g/kg 体重或活性炭与药物的比例为 10∶1，以较大者为准。

大剂量使用：如果容易实施大剂量活性炭或患者耐受性好，可有指征使用 2 g/kg 体重。

重复剂量[a]

成人和儿童：0.5 g/kg 体重，每 4 ～ 6 h 一次，持续 12 ～ 24 h，根据所摄入药物的剂量和剂型而定（偶尔可有指征使用较大剂量和较短的给药间隔）。

操作

向粉状物料中加入 8 份水；所有配方，包括预先包装的浆液，在饮用或通过口胃管或鼻胃管灌注之前，应摇匀至少 1 min，形成短暂稳定的悬浮液。

如果患者呕吐了一定量的活性炭，如果病情可以的话，应该重复。小而频繁的剂量或持续鼻胃给药可能耐受性更好，可能需要给予止吐剂。

如果使用鼻胃管或口腔胃管进行多次给药，则在吸引剩余的活性炭并取出该管之前，应留出时间让最后一次给药通过胃，因为这可能会妨碍活性炭的吸入。

禁忌证

有误吸危险且气道未受保护的患者。

腐蚀性摄入（活性炭在这些情况下作为吸附剂是无效的，可能会在烧伤区域积聚，干扰内镜检查）。

肠梗阻（多次给药禁忌）。

不良反应

吸入性肺炎。

呕吐。

胃肠黏膜模糊不清（内镜检查）。

便秘。

[a] 可以口服或通过口胃管或鼻胃管给药

Adapted from Hoegberg LCG，Gude AB：Techniques used to prevent gastrointestinal absorption. In Hoffman RS，Howland MA，Lewin NA，et al，editors：*Goldfrank's toxicologic emergencies*，10th ed. New York，McGraw-Hill，2015.

充分见解。因此，预防毒性后遗症需要进行全面、系统的临床评估，并熟悉所摄入药物的具体药理学、药效学和药代动力学。

（常馨宁 译 王恒跃 校）

框 80.2 中毒处理：全肠灌洗

一般适应证

使用聚乙二醇电解质灌洗液进行全肠道灌洗，可能有助于处理中毒和过量。①摄食含有肠衣 / 缓释药物、非法药物包或活性炭吸附能力不强的物质（如锂、铁、钾）；②需要或有必要快速清除整个胃肠道，避免呕吐或引起液体或电解质紊乱。

特定的适应证

缓释剂中毒

缓慢溶解物质（如铁片、油漆片、牛黄、混凝土）

“人体包装”或“人体填塞”吞服的毒品包（例如海洛因、快克、可卡因）

未被活性炭吸附的药物或毒素（如锂、铁、钾）

剂量[a]

成人：1 ～ 2 L/h，持续 4 ～ 6 h，或直至直肠流出物清澈

儿童：25 ～ 40 mL/（kg·h），持续 4 ～ 6 h，或直至直肠流出物清澈

注：如果涉及活性炭吸附性药物或毒素，应在全肠冲洗之前和期间使用活性炭；止吐药如甲氧氯普胺或 5- 羟色胺拮抗剂可以使用

禁忌证

胃肠道病理（如肠梗阻、穿孔、梗阻）

腐蚀性摄入

有吸入性肺炎风险的患者

不良反应

直肠瘙痒

呕吐（特别是快速给药）

腹胀

活性炭功效下降

活性炭中毒素的解吸

[a] 可以口服或通过鼻胃管给药

Data from Hoegberg LCG，Gude AB：Techniques used to prevent gastrointestinal absorption. In Hoffman RS，Howland MA，Lewin NA，et al.，editors：*Goldfrank's toxicologic emergencies*，10th ed. New York，McGraw-Hill，2015；and Levine M，Brooks DE，Truitt CA，et al.：Toxicology in the ICU：part 1：general overview and approach to treatment. *Chest* 140：795-806，2011.

延伸阅读

American Academy of Clinical Toxicology and European Association of Poisons Centres and Clinical Toxicologists: position paper: cathartics, *J Toxicol Clin Toxicol* 42:243–253, 2004.

American Academy of Clinical Toxicology: European Association of Poisons Centres and Clinical Toxicologists: position statement and practice guidelines on the use of multi-dose activated charcoal in the treatment of acute poisoning, *J Toxicol Clin Toxicol* 37:731–751, 1999.

Benson BE, Hoppu K, Troutman WG, et al.: Position paper update: gastric lavage for gastrointestinal decontamination, *Clin Toxicol (Phila)* 51: 140–146, 2013.

Blincoe LJ, Miller TR, Zaloshnja E, et al.: *The economic and societal impact of motor vehicle crashes, 2010 (Revised). (Report No. DOT HS 812 013.)*, Washington, DC, May 2015, National Highway Traffic Safety Administration.

Brooks DE, Levine M, O'Connor AD, et al.: Toxicology in the ICU: part 2: specific toxins, *Chest* 140:1072–1085, 2011.

Chyka PA, Seger D, Krenzelok EP, et al.: Position paper: single-dose activated charcoal, *Clin Toxicol (Phila)* 43:61–87, 2005.

Hoegberg LCG, Gude A-B: Techniques used to prevent gastrointestinal absorption. In Hoffman RS, Howland MA, Lewin NA, et al.: *Goldfrank's toxicologic emergencies*, 10th ed, New York, 2015, McGraw-Hill Medical, pp 83–96.

Hoffman RS, Howland MA, Lewin NA, et al.: *Goldfrank's toxicologic emergencies*, 10th ed, New York, 2015, McGraw-Hill Medical.

Hoffman RS, Howland MA, Lewin NA, et al.: Principles of managing the acutely poisoned or overdosed patient. In Hoffman RS, Howland MA, Lewin NA, et al.: *Goldfrank's toxicologic emergencies*, 10th ed, New York, 2015, McGraw-Hill Medical, pp 30–37.

Höjer J, Troutman WG, Hoppu K, et al.: Position paper update: ipecac syrup for gastrointestinal decontamination, *Clin Toxicol (Phila)* 51:134–139, 2013.

Jang DH: Amphetamines. In Hoffman RS, Howland MA, Lewin NA, et al.: *Goldfrank's toxicologic emergencies*, 10th ed, New York, 2015, McGraw-Hill Medical, pp 1030–1041.

Jones RK, Shinar D, Walsh JM: *State of knowledge of drug-impaired driving. (DOT HS 809 642.)*, Washington, DC, 2003, National Highway Traffic Safety.

Levine M, Brooks DE, Truitt CA, et al.: Toxicology in the ICU: part 1: general overview and approach to treatment, *Chest* 140:795–806, 2011.

Mowry JB, Spyker DA, Cantilena Jr LR, et al.: 2013 annual report of the American Association of Poison Control Centers' National Poison Data System (NPDS): 31st annual report, *Clin Toxicol (Phila)* 52:1032–1283, 2014.

National Center for Statistics and Analysis: *Alcohol-impaired driving: 2013 data. (Traffic Safety Facts. DOT HS 812 102.)*, Washington, DC, December 2014, National Highway Traffic Safety Administration.

Schabelman E, Kuo D: Glucose before thiamine for Wernicke encephalopathy: a literature review, *J Emerg Med* 42:488–494, 2012.

Thanacoody R, Caravati EM, Troutman B, et al.: Position paper update: whole bowel irrigation for gastrointestinal decontamination of overdose patients, *Clin Toxicol (Phila)* 53:5–12, 2015.

心肺转流术的常见故障排除

第81章

John R. Cooper，Jr.

主动脉根部插管并发症：急性主动脉根部夹层

病例概要

患者，男性，75岁，既往钙化性主动脉瓣狭窄病史，拟行主动脉瓣膜置换术。麻醉诱导、胸骨劈开及灌注导管置入均顺利。主动脉荷包缝合及插管位置佳，但主动脉管壁薄且已钙化。当开始心肺转流术（cardiopulmonary bypass，CPB）时，动脉插管压力增加，全身血压（桡动脉压力）降低，主动脉出现急性扩张并变蓝。

问题分析

定义

急性主动脉夹层是主动脉插管转流的严重并发症，虽罕见，但随时可能发生，即便术者经验丰富也不能避免。若未能及早诊断，将导致严重的后果，需要高度警惕。另外，主动脉夹层也可发生在CPB期间或主动脉插管拔出后。

主动脉夹层的产生是由于高压下的血液进入主动脉壁中膜造成的。在此病例中，主动脉插管意外放置于主动脉中膜而非真腔内，则当CPB开始时，压力增加导致夹层。

此外，对升主动脉的操作（例如，主动脉阻断钳放置，顺行灌注心脏停搏液或近端旁路移植）也可增加急性主动脉夹层的风险。其他增加急性主动脉夹层风险的诱发因素包括主动脉壁变薄的情形，如下：

- 囊性动脉中层坏死或其他遗传相关的组织脆弱；
- 与衰老相关的弹性或中层变性；
- 管壁组织变薄脆，类似于狭窄后管壁扩张（主动脉瓣狭窄）；
- 动脉粥样硬化。

主动脉夹层也可在术中或术后ICU期间自行发生。

识别

术中夹层发生时，通常出现突发的、无法解释的平均动脉压降低和静脉回流减少，泵管测量的动脉压力急剧升高，主动脉根部变蓝和扩张。如果夹层剥离扩大到其他大动脉，则可能出现心肌缺血、主动脉瓣关闭不全或两者兼具，也可能存在器官灌注不足（包括少尿和双侧瞳孔不对称）的体征。如果使用经食管超声心动图，夹层可在检查胸主动脉时显而易见（图81.1）。

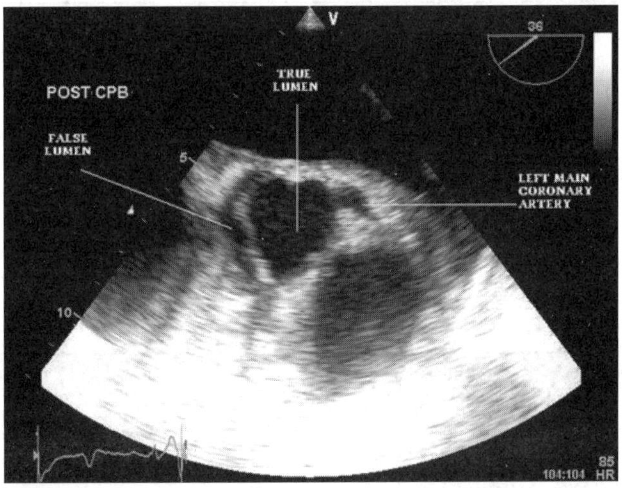

图81.1 位于主动脉瓣远端升主动脉的经食管超声心动图，显示术中主动脉夹层真假腔，夹层沿心脏停搏液注入方向顺行剥离

管理

一旦确认术中急性夹层，必须立即停止CPB。随后，外科医师必须重新调整或重新替换主动脉插管，使其位于主动脉弓更远端的真腔内或更多时改为股动脉插管。术中急性主动脉夹层几乎都需要手术修复，如果冠状动脉口受损，应行冠状动脉再植术。

预防

插管期间可能有效降低主动脉夹层风险的措施包括：

- 插管时严格控制血压（避免高血压）；
- 导管与主动脉呈直角插入，以防止组织剥离；
- 特别注意将导管尖端定位在主动脉的真腔中；
- 主动脉阻断钳使用和移除时适当降低血压；
- 使用无创主动脉阻断用具，并尽可能少用；
- 体外循环灌注师持续监测动脉导管压力。

无名动脉或颈动脉高灌注

病例概要

患者，女性，58岁，CPB下行冠状动脉旁路移植术，动静脉插管顺利，麻醉科医师注意到患者右侧面色苍白。进一步检查显示右颈动脉震颤。

问题分析

定义

灌注泵流量可被直接泵入颈动脉或无名动脉而不是主动脉，由于高灌注压或阻挡动脉血量的内膜瓣的作用，可出现脑水肿或动脉破裂。

识别

无名动脉插管的表现包括同侧面部苍白、瞳孔扩张和结膜水肿。左桡动脉或股动脉可监测到低血压，但右桡动脉可能显示高血压。

管理

必须重新确认插管位置，并采取相应措施减少脑水肿，如给予利尿剂或将患者头部抬高。

预防

使用短的带凸缘的主动脉插管通常可有效预防插管太深。主动脉插管后和CPB开始时，麻醉科医师可检查双侧颈动脉搏动有无震颤，但这可能不能可靠地检测由颈总动脉或无名动脉高灌注引起的问题。对于特定类型的插管，经食管超声心动图可有效确认其位置。

灌注泵静脉回流受阻

病例概要

患者，男性，60岁，主动脉和右心房插管顺利后，启动CPB。此时，泵-氧合静脉储存器容量迅速减少，使灌注泵不能够维持正常的流速。在回路中增加容量并不能解决问题，患者面部和颈部可见明显的静脉充血。

问题分析

定义

静脉回流至泵-氧合器受阻可能有以下几个原因：

- 静脉插管或管道内存在大气泡产生的“气塞”；
- 腔静脉夹闭套线未移除；
- 外科医师胸腔内抬起心脏；
- 静脉插管型号偏小；
- 右心房存在血栓或肿瘤；
- 插管扭曲或错位（最常见）。

当使用两根插管时，上腔静脉插管可能置入奇静脉中，若导管向头侧置入过深，则可能置入无名静脉。下腔静脉插管可以置入肝静脉。在此案例中，单根管插入下腔静脉过深，使得上腔静脉回流受阻。

识别

静脉回流至泵-氧合器不畅导致静脉储血器血量减少是首要征象。如未立即减少泵流量，将会导致静脉储血器排空，从而引发动脉空气栓塞。中心静脉压增加；面部、颈部有明显的静脉充血，进而发展到结膜水肿。此外，右心引流不畅可能导致右心室扩张和左心室压迫，这些变化通过直接观察或肺动脉压、左心房压力升高的证据可识别出来。

管理

在未找到静脉回流受阻的原因之前应减少泵流量。外科医师可通过逐渐升高并敲击气泡下方的管路来推动“气塞”通过静脉管路。错位的静脉管路必须重新放置。只有建立起充分的静脉回流且静脉储血器中的容量恢复后，才能继续进行全流量 CPB。

预防

外科医师应检查静脉管路是否有大气泡，并确认静脉管路位置合适，然而细微的置管错位并不能排除。麻醉科医师应定期检查患者的面部、颈外静脉和结膜是否有静脉高压的征象。由于中心静脉导管尖端可能低于阻塞位点，所以监测中心静脉压可能无法检测到上腔静脉阻塞。

大量气体栓塞

病例概要

患者，女性，65 岁，行二尖瓣置换术，主动脉和腔静脉插管顺利，启动 CPB。在阻断主动脉前，外科医师将一根引流管通过左上肺静脉插入左心房。最初，血液正常地流向静脉储存器，但随后方向逆转，大量空气进入心脏和全身循环。

问题分析

定义

全身性气体栓塞是 CPB 相关的最常见且严重的不良事件，并在很大程度上是可预防的。主要原因包括以下内容：

- 从空的或几乎空的氧合储血器中泵出涡流空气；
- 滚轴泵管路逆转使气体进入引流管或动脉插管中；
- 导管脱开、泄漏、氧合器破坏或动脉泵近端的管路阻塞，伴空气夹带进入或空腔形成；
- 心内血回收贮血器逐渐形成正压，产生逆行气流进入心脏或主动脉；
- 心脏停搏液灌注系统向主动脉根部注入空气；
- 氧合器中存在血栓或泵头失控；
- 心脏排出空气前开始泵血，打开搏动心脏的左心或存在右向左分流（即卵圆孔未闭）时打开搏动心脏的右心；
- CPB 期间氧合器或管路断开或破裂；
- CPB 结束时未能夹闭主动脉管路，若泵头意外重启则会导致空气进入。

识别

通常动脉插管中的空气显而易见，也可能出现心肌或其他器官缺血的迹象。少数情况下，动脉压监测管路中抽出空气可证实存在空气栓塞。

管理

如果气栓量很大，发现后必须停止 CPB，将患者置于大角度 Trendelenburg 体位（头低脚高位），移除主动脉插管，并重新预充 CPB 管路。首先逆行灌注上腔静脉（图 81.2），然后在低温下重启 CPB，并增加灌注压和使用纯氧。随后，可采取药物干预以减少脑损伤，包括甘露醇、类固醇和巴比妥类药物。术后干预包括高压氧治疗、头高脚低位、轻微过度通气、控制性低体温，并预防高血糖和低钠血症。

预防

体外循环灌注师必须维持氧合储存器中安全的血量。目前操作标准要求必须使用低水平报警和气泡探测器。当静脉回流可能受阻时，外科团队必须保护好静脉管路并在出现静脉回流受影响的任何时间应及时与灌注师沟通。其他可能的措施包括：

- 离心泵；
- 动脉管路过滤器；
- 带有单向保护阀的开放式空气-气泡过滤器；
- 可折叠的储液器；
- 左心引流管路上安装单向阀。

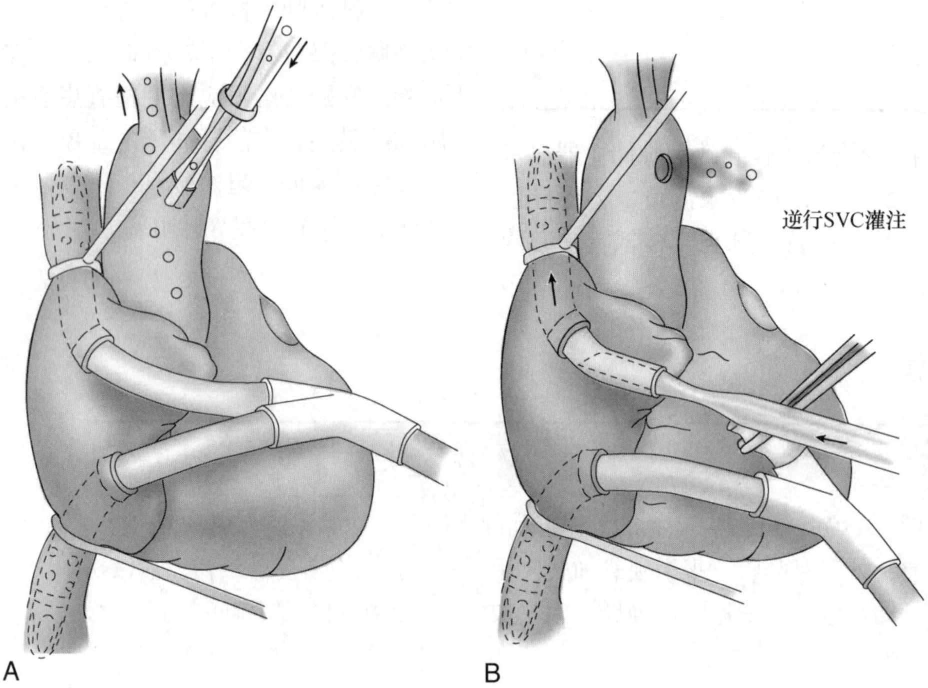

图 81.2 A，大量空气栓子通过主动脉插管（圆圈代表主动脉根部）。**B**，取出主动脉插管，排出空气（圆圈），并插入分流的上腔静脉（SVC）导管中。在 20℃下以 1200 ml/min 的流速进行逆行灌注 1～2 min，使空气离开主动脉插管部位（From Mills NL，Ochsner JL：Massive air embolism during CPB：causes，prevention and management. *J Thorac Cardiovasc Surg* 80：713，1980.）

机械泵或氧合器故障

病例概要

患者，男性，68 岁，CPB 下行二尖瓣置换联合冠状动脉旁路移植术。CPB 启动 5 min 后，麻醉科医师观察到主动脉管路中血液呈现深色，即时血气分析显示动脉血氧分压（arterial oxygen tension，PaO_2）。

问题分析

定义

动脉灌注氧饱和度低的原因可能是供气系统或氧合器本身的故障，或由患者的特征或病理生理导致。

机械泵故障是低 PaO_2 的第四个原因，这可能是由于电力或机械故障、管道破裂或断开、气泡或储液器液位检测器自动关闭造成的。失控的泵头还可能将泵流量调到最大。如果滚轴泵的阻塞设置不当，严重的反流将会导致前向的血流减少、低血压和代谢性酸中毒。

识别

氧合器失效会导致动脉管路中的血液颜色变深，并产生严重的血管舒张。氧合器破裂时可见血液泄漏至加热–冷却器水中。随着机械泵失灵和低 PaO_2，可观察到患者低血压，代谢性酸中毒甚至可能溶血。

管理

如果怀疑氧合器失灵，应从动脉流入管路抽取血液行血气分析，灌注师应增加氧流量并确定机械泵流量充足。此外，应采取以下措施：

- 仔细检查气体回路，包括气源、所有连接管道、气体管路过滤器和麻醉挥发罐；
- 检查氧合器是否有适当的血量并检查装置外壳是否有泄漏或裂缝；
- 检查静脉和动脉管路是否与患者连接准确；
- 确保患者有足够的肌松、合适的体温和麻醉深度。

如果心脏尚在搏动，则考虑将血泵至肺循环中以进行额外的氧合并继续使肺部通气，直到主动脉管路中的血液动脉化为止。必要时也可能需要更换氧合器，这将是一个复杂的操作。

如果机械泵存在故障，可使用手摇曲柄直到替代完成或更换好管路。在泵头失控的情况下，必须拔掉电源，并将管道切换到不同的滚动头。如果流量低或连续几分钟无流量，并且患者不能立即脱离 CPB，则应降低患者体温，并使用冰帽和冰沙对头部和心脏实施进一步保护。

预防

首先，始终保持警觉是至关重要的。使用机械泵动脉血氧饱和监测仪、氧分压分析仪或两者同时使用有助于问题的发现。另外，备用设备应始终处于可用状态。

氧合器或回路中形成血栓

病例概要

患者，男性，60 岁，行主动脉冠状动脉搭桥术和腹主动脉瘤修补术。脱离 CPB 后，在修复腹主动脉瘤的同时，使用 CPB 回路进行血液回收和再输注。1 h 后，当通过主动脉管路供血时，在氧合器中发现大的血凝块。患者活化凝血时间大于 400 s。

问题分析

定义

该不良事件会阻碍体外循环的流量，引起大量气体栓塞，并阻碍气体交换。原因包括肝素化不足，血液在旁路管路中停滞（例如在循环停止期间无血液流动），以及在 CPB 期间添加非肝素化血液制品。

识别

回路中可见血凝块最为可靠，但若观察到氧合器排出空气或动脉插管压力高也提示可能存在大的血凝块。

管理

如果可能的话，停止 CPB 并使用不同批号的肝素对患者进行再次肝素化。如果患者不能立即脱离 CPB，则应开始低温治疗并行胸内心脏按压。氧合器可能需要更换，必要时应遵循大量空气栓塞的治疗方案。

预防

手术团队应保证患者充分肝素化，并监测长时间手术的患者，同时应检查回路和动脉管路过滤器中是否有血凝块。加入回路的任何血液制品均应肝素化处理，即使实验室检查显示肝素化充分，也应避免 CPB 回路中的血液停滞。

（王 晓 译 吉 栋 校）

延伸阅读

Gravlee GP, Davis RF, Hammond J, et al.: *Cardiopulmonary bypass and mechanical support: principles and practice*, Philadelphia, 2015, Lippincott Williams & Wilkins, pp 66–275, pp 275–313.

Hensley Jr FA, Martin DE, Gravlee GP: *A practical approach to cardiac anesthesia*, ed 3, Philadelphia, 2013, Lippincott Williams & Wilkins, pp 513–556.

Mills NL, Ochsner JL: Massive air embolism during cardiopulmonary bypass: causes, prevention, and management, *J Thorac Cardiovasc Surg* 80:708–717, 1980.

Mora CT: *Cardiopulmonary bypass: principles and techniques of extracorporeal circulation*, New York, 1995, Springer-Verlag, pp 302–307.

第三部分

术中药物和潜在并发症

第82章 抗生素

Huong Le，Timothy E. Morey

病例概要

患者，男性，23 岁，从马上摔下来后拟行开放性胫骨骨折复位固定。在术前暂停核查时（time-out），外科医师要求在切皮前给予患者 1 g 万古霉素。给予丙泊酚和琥珀胆碱后成功气管插管，用七氟烷、N_2O 50%/O_2 50% 和芬太尼 2 μg/（kg·h）维持麻醉。万古霉素给药 4 min 后，患者出现心血管虚脱。

问题分析

定义

麻醉科医师经常给手术患者进行抗生素预防，以确保患者从手术治疗改进项目（即 SCIP-Inf 1）中获益。由于这个原因，麻醉科医师应该对围术期使用抗生素的适应证、剂量、并发症以及抗生素与麻醉药物和其他药物的相互作用有充分的了解。抗生素具有各种各样的副作用，并与许多麻醉辅助药物相互作用（表 82.1）。抗生素占自报告药物变态类别的大部分。由于这些原因，麻醉科医师必须了解和预测使用抗生素可能出现的并发症。

万古霉素是一种糖肽类抗生素，常用于骨科、神经外科和血管外科的细菌预防，是对青霉素类抗生素和头孢菌素过敏的患者或携带耐药微生物患者的替代抗生素。当使用万古霉素后出现危及生命的反应时，必须考虑超敏反应的可能性。万古霉素给药可引起多种超敏反应，其中两种为“红人”综合征（red man syndrome，RMS）和过敏反应。

红人综合征

RMS 或“红颈”综合征表现为低血压、皮肤潮红、红斑、荨麻疹、瘙痒和斑丘疹，好发于面部、颈部、手臂和胸部。症状群可能表现较轻，也可能严重到危及生命的程度。体征最早可在输液开始后 4 ～ 10 min 出现，也可在持续输注 1 h 内出现。万古霉素的一个不寻常的特征是它能够通过尚不清楚的剂量依赖性机制使嗜碱性粒细胞和皮肤肥大细胞的组胺释放量增加 1 倍。虽然临床上与手术室过敏反应难以区分，但 RMS 不涉及免疫球蛋白 E（immunoglobulin E，IgE）致敏。以前它被描述为一种类过敏反应，目前在文献中被描述为非 IgE 免疫过敏反应。诊断主要依据：①排除术中其他可能引起低血压的事件；②心血管不稳定与万古霉素输注的时间关系以及组胺释放的其他表现，如口周、眼周、面部水肿；③支气管组胺受体刺激引起支气管痉挛；④缺氧继发于组胺诱导抑制缺氧性肺血管收缩和后续形成肺分流。应注意可能增强 RMS 症状的其他组胺诱导药物（表 82.1）。作为免疫肥大细胞激活的标志物，胰蛋白酶释放在万古霉素诱导的类过敏反应中不会出现。组胺释放量的测定通常不切实际，因为组胺浓度在发病后 5 min 达到峰值，释放后 1 h 内恢复到基线水平。

释放的组胺引起外周血管扩张，同时增加心排血量、每搏量和肺动脉血压。但外周血管扩张是最突出的生理特征，可引起严重低血压和心血管虚脱。随着后来检测的推进、组胺释放的增加和低血压的加重，治疗方案变得更加积极。治疗措施包括：

- 停止或减慢万古霉素输注；
- 给予静脉推注液体；
- 停止或降低能引起低血压的其他药物的浓度（如麻醉药和硝普钠）；
- 给予 H_1 抗组胺药（如苯海拉明）；
- 如果有支气管痉挛，考虑吸入 β 受体激动剂；

表 82.1 常用的预防性抗生素的并发症

抗生素	并发症 常见	偶尔	罕见
氨基糖苷	肾毒性 耳毒性 神经肌肉阻滞增强	皮疹 恶性、呕吐 电解质紊乱	周围神经炎 过敏反应
头孢菌素	肌注时疼痛	恶心 药物热 腹泻 静脉炎 风疹	过敏反应 低血压 支气管痉挛 血管性水肿
克林霉素		腹泻 假膜性结肠炎 皮疹 金属味 抑制神经肌肉传导 神经肌肉阻滞增强	过敏反应 心脏停搏 红斑 粒细胞减少 血小板减少
红霉素	静脉注射导致静脉炎 肌注时疼痛	恶心、呕吐 腹泻 假膜性结肠炎	长 QT 综合征 发热 皮疹 嗜酸性粒细胞增多症
甲硝唑	恶心、呕吐 金属味 饮酒导致的双硫仑样反应	舌灼痛 尿道 / 阴道烧灼痛 黑尿 皮疹	抽搐 共济失调 周围神经病变 脑病 小脑功能障碍
青霉素 G，氨苄西林		皮疹 药物热 腹泻 白细胞减少症	过敏反应 支气管痉挛 血管性水肿 电解质紊乱 间质性肾炎
磺胺甲噁唑甲氧苄啶（SMZ-TMP）		皮疹	多形性红斑 腹泻 再生障碍性贫血 中性粒细胞减少症 血小板减少症
万古霉素	静脉炎 肌内注射时疼痛剧烈	“红人”综合征 “疼痛痉挛”综合征 低血压 过敏反应 肾毒性 耳毒性	中性粒细胞减少症

Adapted from Cheng，EY，Nimphius N，Hennen ER：Antibiotic therapy and the anesthesiologist. *J Clin Anesth* 7：425-439，1995.

- 严重低血压时，使用血管升压药（如麻黄素、去氧肾上腺素和肾上腺素）；
- 在发生心脏停搏时，启动高级心脏生命支持。

免疫球蛋白 E 介导的过敏反应

万古霉素致心血管虚脱的潜在原因可能与 IgE 介导的过敏反应有关。过敏反应的体征包括快速发病的病态皮疹或荨麻疹、麻疹、潮红、血管性水肿、呕吐、腹泻、鼻结膜炎和心动过速。这些症状可持续 48 h。由于这些体征在覆盖手术单和镇静或全身麻醉的患者身上更难发现，以前接触过万古霉素的患者出现低血压和支气管痉挛时，应立即考虑将 IgE 介导的过敏反应视为原因（框 82.1）。先前接触过万古霉素的患者会产生万古霉素特异性 IgE，并且在重复给药时，致敏的肥大细胞释放组胺、白三烯 C_4 和前列腺素 D_2。细胞因子如肿瘤坏死因子 α 和白细胞介素 4、5、6、8 和 13 等可随着炎症反应级联的升级而放大 Ⅰ 型超敏反应。细胞毒性 T 细胞可能参与了病态皮疹的发病机制。血清 β- 胰蛋白酶水平是 IgE 交联肥大细胞脱粒的标志物，应在反应开始后 1 ～ 2 h 内进行检测。血清总胰蛋白酶水平（α- 原胰蛋白酶和 β- 胰蛋白酶）高于 25 μg/L，比基线水平增加 2 ng/ml 或 135%，或总胰蛋白酶峰值与 β- 胰蛋白酶峰值之比大于 10，提示存在 IgE 介导的过敏反应。至少应在初次抽血后 2 天抽取另一份血样进行比较，因为胰蛋白酶水平预计将在 12 ～ 14 h 内恢复到基线值。

框 82.1　术中过敏反应 / 万古霉素不良反应 / 组胺诱导剂的体征

术中过敏反应体征
低血压
支气管痉挛
心动过速（可被 β 受体阻滞剂所掩盖）
心血管虚脱
红斑
血管性水肿

万古霉素的不良反应
线性免疫球蛋白 A（IgA）大疱性皮肤病
DRESS[a] 综合征
肾毒性
耳毒性
中性粒细胞减少症
粒细胞缺乏症
血小板减少症
静脉炎
免疫性血小板减少症

组胺诱导剂
抗生素（例如环丙沙星，万古霉素）
巴比妥酸盐
吗啡或哌替啶
泮库溴铵或阿曲库铵
琥珀胆碱苄基异喹啉化合物
血浆扩容剂（如右旋糖苷、尿素交联明胶）
放射性造影剂

[a] 有嗜酸性粒细胞增多和全身症状的药疹

治疗方案应针对所表现的症状，包括以下内容：

- 停止万古霉素输注；
- 根据反应的严重程度，给予的肾上腺素初始剂量由最初的 10 μg 迅速增加到 200 μg；
- 给予静脉液体；
- 停止或降低其他能引起低血压的药物浓度；
- 给予 H_1 抗组胺药（如苯海拉明）和 H_2 抗组胺药（如雷尼替丁）治疗荨麻疹和血管性水肿；
- 如果发生支气管痉挛，考虑吸入 β 受体激动剂；
- 考虑使用皮质类固醇来减轻支气管痉挛和防止后期休克；
- 在心脏停搏的情况下，启动高级心脏生命支持；
- 与变态反应学专家一起对皮肤试验进行随访（针刺试验和皮内试验；血清特异性 IgE 和放射性过敏吸附试验的敏感性较低）；
- 清楚地记录患者的病史，并和患者讨论。

治疗

在万古霉素给药后严重低血压的鉴别诊断中，麻醉科医师必须区分 RMS 和过敏反应，因为各自治疗方法的差异会影响患者的预后。RMS 是更常见的综合征，据报道，在 14% 的儿童和 80% ～ 90% 的志愿者使用 1 g 万古霉素 1 h 后出现了 RMS。

一般来说，当同时使用万古霉素和挥发性麻醉药（即麻醉诱导后输注万古霉素）时，与 RMS 相关的低血压风险更大，因为这两种药物都可能降低血压。此外，与 RMS 相关的万古霉素输注过程中的低血压在麻醉患者中比非麻醉患者更常见。有趣的是，菌血症、病情危重状态、恶性肿瘤和糖尿病可能会降低心血管不良反应的发生率和严重程度，部分原因是之前的疾病、围术期应激和鱼精蛋白给药已导致组胺耗尽。相比之下，围术期过敏反应是一种罕见的事件，但其死亡率高达 9%。在麻醉过程中发生的超敏反应中，大约 70% 是由 IgE 介导的。肾上腺素作为治疗 Ⅰ 型超敏反应的一线药物，能够稳定肥大细胞，抑制组胺释放，降低组胺相关的血管舒张和毛细血管通透性。对于 RMS 相关的严重低血压患者，肾上腺素适宜用于心血管支持。

预防

对于有万古霉素 RMS 或 I 型超敏反应史的患者，使用替代抗生素是预防这些反应的首选。奎奴普丁 / 达福普汀是一种大环内酯类-林肯酰胺链霉素，对耐甲氧西林金黄色葡萄球菌（methicillin-resistant *Staphylococcus aureus*，MRSA）和耐甲氧西林表皮葡萄球菌具有体外杀菌作用；其还可用于成人治疗由金黄色葡萄球菌（甲氧西林敏感）或化脓性链球菌引起的复杂皮肤和皮肤结构感染。利奈唑胺是一种噁唑烷酮，对链球菌、万古霉素耐药肠球菌和 MRSA 有活性。有证据表明，它比万古霉素更有效地治疗皮肤和软组织感染的患者，包括那些 MRSA 引起的感染。

对于经历严重 RMS 或出现过敏反应但又需要万古霉素治疗的患者，已制订万古霉素脱敏方案，使该患者群体能够安全地接受万古霉素静脉注射。这种治疗围绕着肥大细胞对万古霉素逐渐脱敏，通过逐渐增加这种抗生素的血清浓度，可以在 24 h 内完成急性患者的脱敏。当然，这一预防方案是为受过敏威胁的患者保留的，如果希望进行手术预防性万古霉素治疗，则需要在手术前制订计划。每次万古霉素输注都必须重复该方案，包括使用抗组胺药和皮质类固醇。有证据表明，在预防和治疗这些患者的组胺释放方面，H_1 和 H_2 抗组胺药的结合使用优于单独使用 H_1 抗组胺药。在围术期，万古霉素可在麻醉诱导前后安全使用。麻醉科医师将小心谨慎地努力遵循有关万古霉素输注持续时间的推荐，特别是在风险较大的患者（如儿童）或即使是轻度低血压也不能耐受的患者（如主动脉狭窄的患者），并了解药物的其他副作用（见框 82.1）。血流动力学受抑制时需要及时发现和治疗，以避免潜在的危及生命的心血管虚脱。

（杨迪迪　译　王恒跃　校）

延伸阅读

Galvão VR, Giavina-Bianchi P, Castells M: Perioperative anaphylaxis, *Curr Allergy Asthma Rep* 14:452, 2014.

Greenberger PA, Ditto AM: Chapter 24: Anaphylaxis, *Allergy Asthma Proc* 33:S80–S83, 2012.

Healy DP, Sahai JV, Fuller SH, et al.: Vancomycin-induced histamine release and "red man syndrome": comparison of 1- and 2-hour infusions, *Antimicrob Agents Chemother* 34:550–554, 1990.

Lieberman P: The use of antihistamines in the prevention and treatment of anaphylaxis and anaphylactoid reactions, *J Allergy Clin Immunol* 86:684–686, 1990.

Macy E, Poon K-YT: Self-reported antibiotic allergy incidence and prevalence: age and sex effects, *Am J Med* 122:778, 2009. e1-7.

Mertes PM, Malinovsky JM, Jouffroy L, et al.: Reducing the risk of anaphylaxis during anesthesia: 2011 updated guidelines for clinical practice, *J Investig Allergol Clin Immunol* 21:442–453, 2011.

Myers AL, Gaedigk A, Dai H, et al.: Defining risk factors for red man syndrome in children and adults, *Pediatr Infect Dis J* 31:464–468, 2012.

Renz CL, Laroche D, Thurn JD, et al.: Tryptase levels are not increased during vancomycin-induced anaphylactoid reactions, *Anesthesiology* 89:620–625, 1998.

Yue J, Dong BR, Yang M, et al.: Linezolid versus vancomycin for skin and soft tissue infections, *Cochrane Database Syst Rev* 7:CD008056, 2013.

第83章 止吐药

Mahmoud I. Wagih

病例概要

患者，女性，30 岁，拟作为日间手术行宫腔镜检查。患者既往无相关病史。使用甲氧氯普胺 10 mg、昂丹司琼 4 mg、丙泊酚 / 芬太尼静脉诱导，七氟烷维持麻醉。术后患者出现了顽固性呕吐，从而延长了从麻醉后监护病房到出院的时间，在随后的 48 h 内，她只能通过持续不断联合使用止吐药来控制病情，这导致她非计划住院治疗。

问题分析

定义

三分之一的患者会发生术后恶心呕吐（postoperative nausea and vomiting，PONV），有一些手术的发病率更高（妇科手术发生率为 45%，高危人群发生率达 80%）。PONV 是大多数手术患者认为的围术期经历的最糟糕的事情（疼痛只排在第二位）。在日间手术时代，由严重 PONV 引起的计划外过夜或再入院对运筹和经济的影响可能是严重的。PONV 预防和治疗措施的方法既不一致，效果也各不相同。

识别

非麻醉性因素，如机械性肠梗阻、药物因素和颅内压升高，可在围术期引起恶心和（或）呕吐。由于这些因素的病理生理学和治疗方法不同，因此需要单独考虑。

防治 PONV 有预防和治疗两方面，需要采取药理学和非药理学措施。几乎所有的止吐药都是中枢性受体激动剂 / 拮抗剂（甲氧氯普胺在外周发挥作用）。

了解它们的作用机制对认识它们的各种不良反应至关重要。

风险评估

最近的文献述评改变了对 PONV“传统”危险因素的认识。

患者相关因素

患者年龄（3 ~ 50 岁）与 PONV 存在较强的关联性。大量证据表明，女性和曾经发生过 PONV 是很大的危险因素。而吸烟患者 PONV 发生风险降低。

过去很多因素曾被认为会引起 PONV，但最近的文献综述却对其中一些提出质疑，如美国麻醉科医师协会提出的体格状况、围术期禁食时间、鼻胃管的使用、早期肠内摄入 / 禁食时间、焦虑、偏头痛、体重指数、月经周期等。

手术因素

腹部盆腔手术与 PONV 的发生风险增高相关（胆囊切除术、妇科手术和腹腔镜手术）。

对于儿科患者，斜视手术以及手术时间超过 30 min 的手术发生 PONV 的风险最高。但几乎没有证据来证明 PONV 还存在其他独立的危险因素。

麻醉相关因素

全身麻醉（持续时间和麻醉深度）与 PONV 之间存在很强的关联性。早期研究显示麻醉过程中挥发性药物、阿片类药物和氧化亚氮可能会导致 PONV。麻醉科医师的经验水平和神经肌肉阻断剂的使用与 PONV 并无相关性。

治疗

鉴于止吐药的不良反应（从头痛到尖端扭转型室速的个案报道）和 PONV 产生的后果（患者满意度差、计划外入院和医疗并发症），强烈建议应通过客观的 PONV 风险评估系统为高风险的患者制订有针对性的治疗方案。

降低 PONV 基线风险的一般措施

早期识别高危患者很有必要。不同的健康系统采用评分方法来评判 PONV 的发生率。

避免全身麻醉和明确可引起 PONV 的药物是一种有效的预防措施。对于有严重 PONV 病史的患者，最好采用全凭静脉麻醉。如果必须采用全身麻醉，诱导时尽可能使用丙泊酚。氧化亚氮的使用正在逐渐减少，尤其是日间手术比例较大幅度增加的情况下，PONV 显著增加了患者的治疗复杂性。使用其他模式镇痛以节省阿片类药物的镇痛技术正逐渐成为标准做法，包括区域阻滞技术、非甾体抗炎药、环氧合酶 -2 抑制剂和治疗神经病理性疼痛的传统药物。充分水化和低血压的及时治疗，不仅是良好的标准治疗，而且两者都能显著降低 PONV 的发生风险。关于是否常规预防性使用止吐药物的争论目前仍在继续。考虑到对患者和医疗卫生系统的影响，必须对副作用的发生率和可用性 / 负担能力进行权衡。现有证据表明常用的预防用药的效果相近，联合用药比单药治疗更有效。

干预措施

尽管低危患者可能不需要再采取额外的治疗措施，但高危患者可受益于预防性治疗，两组患者均应将止吐策略整合至围术期治疗计划中。

以下是对不同类别止吐药物的总结。

5– 羟色胺（5–HT_3）受体拮抗剂

该类药物包括昂丹司琼、多拉司琼、格拉司琼、托派司琼、拉莫司琼和帕洛诺司琼。它们通常对治疗呕吐比对恶心更加有效，因此为了最大限度地提高疗效，在手术结束时给药会更好。但它们可能会带来一系列不良反应，如头痛、肝酶升高、便秘和 QT 间期延长（剂量相关）。但临床上很少有被证实与 5-HT_3 受体拮抗剂使用有关的显著心律失常病例。总的来说，由于不良反应的发生率低使其在临床得到了广泛的应用。多拉司琼已退出美国市场。

神经激肽 –1 受体拮抗剂

这些药物是一种最新的止吐药物，在引入治疗化疗引起的恶心和呕吐后，这些药物逐渐开始应用于术后恶心呕吐的治疗。已成熟使用的药物有阿瑞匹坦、卡索匹坦和罗拉匹坦。

它们的作用时间较长（48 ～ 72 h），因此在麻醉诱导时即可使用。它们的不良反应相对较轻，包括头晕、虚弱和非特异性的轻微症状，目前尚无心血管不良反应的记录。

糖皮质激素

地塞米松和甲泼尼龙已被用于治疗 PONV。考虑到它们的药代动力学特征（主要是作用时间），它们多在麻醉诱导后使用，如果初始剂量无效，不建议再追加。最近的研究表明，大剂量地塞米松（8 mg）更有效。已证实其对患者恢复（包括疼痛控制）有积极影响。

短期使用的不良反应较为有限。磷酸盐制剂会引起严重的会阴瘙痒和疼痛（发生率 50%，女性多于男性）。地塞米松单次给药后 6 ～ 12 h 血糖升高，因此血糖控制不稳定的糖尿病患者应相对禁忌使用。

丁酰苯类

氟哌利多和氟哌啶醇是用于治疗 PONV 的两种主要的丁酰苯类药物，在手术结束时使用是有效的。因其不良反应，仅在挽救治疗时才推荐使用。

氟哌利多延长 QT 间期的模式及程度类似昂丹司琼，是最为严重的不良反应，美国食品药品监督管理局（Food and Drug Administration，FDA）2001 年对氟哌利多提出黑框警告。大剂量氟哌利多具有镇静作用。氟哌啶醇 QT 间期延长的发生率较低，但 FDA 并不批准其用于治疗 PONV。

抗组胺药

茶苯海明、美克洛嗪、赛克力嗪（英国）可用作止吐药，然而关于其应用的最佳时间却没有一致定论。它们的不良反应与其抗胆碱能特性相关（心动过速、视物模糊、幻觉、偶发尿潴留），特别多见于老年人。镇静为其另一种常见不良反应。

抗胆碱能药物

东莨菪碱经皮吸收制剂是该类药物的主要制剂。该药的贴剂有效作用时间可达 24 h，因此它可以在手术前晚或当天使用。其不良反应一般较轻，包括视力障碍和头晕。

抗多巴胺药物

吩噻嗪类药物如丙氯拉嗪和奋乃静已不再用作抗精神病药物。考虑到潜在的严重不良反应（和剂量相关），应联合使用其他药物治疗 PONV 或者作为挽救治疗药物使用。该类药推荐治疗 PONV 的剂量产生的镇静效果与安慰剂相当。此外，这类药物不良反应还包括发生率低的抗精神病药物恶性综合征和抗胆碱能反应。

甲氧氯普胺（胃复安）

最近的证据显示甲氧氯普胺在治疗剂量内（10 mg）的疗效较差。当剂量增加到 30 mg，疗效会提高，但仍低于同等剂量的其他药物组。然而锥体外系不良反应的发生率随着剂量的增加而显著增加（NNH 为 140）。

针灸

最近的文献综述表明，使用不同的针灸方式进行 P-6 刺激与较低的 PONV 发生率和较低的急救治疗需求有关。无论是成人还是儿童，无论是有创还是无创性的针灸疗法，均能维持这种效果，并且不依赖于刺激的时机。正中神经的神经肌肉刺激（尤其是强直刺激模式下）也显示出类似的效果。

（徐业好　译　查燕萍　校）

延伸阅读

American Society of Anesthesiologists Task Force on Acute Pain Management: Practice guidelines for acute pain management in the perioperative setting: an updated report by the American Society of Anesthesiologists Task Force on Acute Pain Management, *Anesthesiology* 116:248–273, 2012.

Apfelbaum JL, Silverstein JH, Chung FF, et al.: Practice guidelines for postanesthetic care: an updated report by the American Society of Anesthesiologists Task Force on Postanesthetic Care, *Anesthesiology* 118:291–307, 2013.

Carlotto A, Hogsett VL, Maiorini EM, et al.: The economic burden of toxicities associated with cancer treatment: review of the literature and analysis of nausea and vomiting, diarrhoea, oral mucositis and fatigue, *Pharmacoeconomics* 31(9):753–766, 2013.

Ekinci O, Malat I, Işıtmangil G, et al.: A randomized comparison of droperidol, metoclopramide, tropisetron, and ondansetron for the prevention of postoperative nausea and vomiting, *Gynecol Obstet Invest* 71:59–65, 2011.

Fero KE, Jalota L, Hornuss C, et al.: Pharmacologic management of postoperative nausea and vomiting, *Expert Opin Pharmacother* 12:2283–2296, 2011.

Flake ZA, Linn BS, Hornecker JR: Practical selection of antiemetics in the ambulatory setting, *Am Fam Physician* 91(5):293–296, 2015.

Gan TJ, Diemunsch P, Habib AS, et al.: Consensus guidelines for the management of postoperative nausea and vomiting, *Anesth Analg* 118:85–113, 2014.

Haiderali A, Menditto L, Good M, et al.: Impact on daily functioning and indirect/direct costs associated with chemotherapy-induced nausea and vomiting (CINV) in a U.S. population, *Support Care Cancer* 19(6):843–851, 2011.

Myklejord DJ, Yao L, Liang H, et al.: Consensus guideline adoption for managing postoperative nausea and vomiting, *WMJ* 111:207–213, 2012.

抗组胺药：H_1 和 H_2 受体阻滞剂

第 84 章

Michael Feduska

病例概要

患者，男性，90 岁，既往有多发梗死性痴呆病史，因血尿接受膀胱镜检查，术后在麻醉后恢复室出现意识混乱和躁动。术前给予咪达唑仑，诱导时给予芬太尼和丙泊酚，出现红斑后静注苯海拉明 50 mg。

问题分析

定义

基于与 4 种已知受体亚型（H_1，H_2，H_3，H_4）的相互作用，抗组胺药可分为四种不同的类型。H_1 和 H_2 受体阻滞剂或“拮抗剂”实际上是反向激动剂，与受体结合后促使其向非激活状态转变。组胺受体位于多个部位，包括平滑肌、外分泌腺和中枢神经系统（central nervous system，CNS）。第一代 H_1 抗组胺药在毒蕈碱受体、α 肾上腺素受体和 5-羟色胺受体上也具有活性。H_1 抗组胺药的主要用途包括治疗过敏性鼻炎、过敏性结膜炎和荨麻疹；预防高敏反应；治疗晕动病；以及作为睡眠辅助药物。

H_1 抗组胺药被改良后用来增加对 H_1 受体的特异性，并减少不良反应。第二代 H_1 抗组胺药不会引起与其前一代相同程度的抗胆碱能症状，而且透过血脑屏障的能力有限，从而减弱对 CNS 的作用。现在第二代 H_1 抗组胺药是治疗过敏症状的首选药物。

H_1 受体活性不影响组胺刺激所产生的胃酸。这促使了 H_2 受体亚型的发现以及 H_2 抗组胺药的研发。H_2 抗组胺药可以阻断肠嗜铬细胞释放组胺，从而阻止壁细胞分泌胃酸。H_2 抗组胺药可预防和治疗轻度消化性溃疡、胃食管反流病和应激性溃疡（表 84.1）。

表 84.1　常见抗组胺药

第一代 H_1 抗组胺药	第二代 H_1 抗组胺药	H_2 抗组胺药
茶苯海明	西替利嗪	西咪替丁
苯海拉明	地影雷他定	法莫替丁
多西拉敏	非索非那定	雷尼替丁
羟嗪	左西替利嗪	尼扎替丁
美克洛嗪	氯雷他定	芦帕他定
异丙嗪		

识别

由于对毒蕈碱受体的作用，第一代 H_1 抗组胺药的抗胆碱能作用占主导地位。抗胆碱能作用的症状包括散瞳、CNS 紊乱、红斑、高热和尿潴留。这种抗胆碱能类中毒症状可以通过“瞎如蝙蝠，疯如帽匠，红如甜菜，热如野兔，干如骨头”来助记。治疗剂量即可引起轻度 CNS 的改变，出现镇静、认知障碍、过度兴奋伴意识混乱和好斗（特别是儿童患者）。治疗剂量苯海拉明引起的肌张力障碍已有报道。与第二代药物相比，第一代 H_1 抗组胺药具有更强的 CNS 效应和抗胆碱能效应。

症状的严重程度因剂量而异，但文献报道的毒性阈值尚不明确。过量使用仅见于将第一代 H_1 抗组胺药用作自杀或致幻的患者中。这些患者可能出现躁动或幻觉，随后出现癫痫、昏迷、呼吸抑制、横纹肌溶解和心律失常。

H_2 抗组胺药副作用包括腹泻、便秘、肌痛和嗜睡等症状。在老年人群中，静脉注射 H_2 抗组胺药后出现了 CNS 的变化，如谵妄和幻觉。快速静脉给药可导致低血压（表 84.2）。

表 84.2 抗组胺药不良反应

系统 / 器官	第一代 H_1 抗组胺药	第二代 H_1 抗组胺药	H_2 抗组胺药
心血管	心动过速、QT 延长、低血压	N/A	低血压、房室传导阻滞、心动过缓
中枢神经系统	镇静、意识混乱、癫痫、肌张力障碍、散瞳、昏迷	对认知影响极小	嗜睡、头痛、谵妄
肺	N/A	N/A	肺炎发病率增加
胃肠 / 代谢	腹泻、恶心呕吐、便秘、体重增加、发热	腹泻、恶心 / 呕吐、便秘	腹泻、便秘、肝功能检测指标升高、肝炎
泌尿生殖系统	尿潴留	影响极小	阳痿
血液系统	N/A	N/A	全血细胞减少、血小板减少、粒细胞缺乏

风险评估和启示

评估术后躁动的原因时，在考虑 H_1 抗组胺药的同时还必须注意患者的基本精神状态、每日用药方案、术中用药和手术风险因素。使用异丙嗪或苯海拉明治疗术后恶心、呕吐、荨麻疹或轻微变态反应，与其他遗忘药物的影响一起发挥作用，可延长认知功能恢复。儿科患者、老年患者和肝或肾功能障碍患者发生 CNS 变化的风险增加。围术期应仔细监测尿量和输液量。术后尿潴留的原因是多方面的，包括患者疾病病理、手术操作和治疗药物。

多种第一代 H_1 抗组胺药可引起 QT 延长，并可诱发尖端扭转型心动过速。苯海拉明与钠通道阻滞有关，导致心脏 0 相动作电位降低，诱发宽大 QRS 波型心动过速。

第二代 H_1 抗组胺药被认为“无镇静作用”，对 CNS 的作用并不明显，抗胆碱能副作用也很小。应注意监测认知功能障碍，特别与具有相似副作用的药物联合使用时，如单胺氧化酶抑制剂和三环类抗抑郁药。与第一代药物相比，第二代 H_1 抗组胺药过量不会引起严重 CNS 反应和心脏毒性。

H_2 抗组胺药西咪替丁可通过抑制 CYP 酶易发生药物之间的相互作用，雷尼替丁相对弱一些。西咪替丁对细胞色素 P450（CYP3A4）有微弱的抑制作用，导致血浆中依赖 CYP450 代谢的药物（华法林、苯妥英、茶碱、丙戊酸）浓度升高。H_2 抗组胺药引起的罕见病例包括血小板减少症、全血细胞减少症和粒细胞缺乏症。

管理

对 H_1 拮抗剂的抗胆碱能效应的处理以缓解症状为目标。当出现尿潴留时需行膀胱超声检查，以排除尿量减少的其他原因。首先应尝试直接插入导尿管，在反复发生尿潴留时应放置 Foley 导尿管。必要时可寻求泌尿科会诊。

术后谵妄可以通过多次重新定向、一对一的监测和在适当的时候与家人接触来进行治疗。苯二氮革类药物可用于治疗躁动，但应避免在治疗效果不明确的任何高危人群中使用。氟哌啶醇在给药前，应先使用 12 导联心电图（electrocardiogram，ECG）评估 QT 间期。

应通过 12 导联心电图评估心律失常，并采用高级心脏生命支持方案进行治疗。碳酸氢钠可有效治疗苯海拉明所致宽大 QRS 波型心动过速。

虽然罕见，血小板减少症和全血细胞减少症与法莫替丁相关，特别是在重症监护病房环境中。H_2 抗组胺类药物与血小板减少症的相关性提示很有必要监测血小板计数。

预防

预防此类药物副作用的最好方法是避免在高危人群中使用。如必须使用，则应限制肝肾功能障碍、有精神病史和极端年龄患者的剂量。

致谢

感谢 Habibi 博士和 Riley 博士对本章上一版的贡献。

（尹光敏 译 文平山 校）

延伸阅读

Ecker RD, Wijdicks EF, Wix K, et al.: Does famotidine induce thrombocytopenia in neurosurgical patients? *J Neurosurg Anesthesiol* 16(4):291–293, 2004.

Jones AW: Perspectives in drug development and clinical pharmacology: the discovery of histamine H_1 and H_2 antagonists, *Clin Pharmacol Drug Dev* 5(1):5–12, 2016.

Mahdy AM, Webster NR: Histamine and antihistamines, *Anaesth Intensive Care Med* 12(7):324–329, 2011.

Scharman EJ, Erdman AR, Wax PM, et al.: Diphenhydramine and dimenhydrinate poisoning: an evidence-based consensus guideline for out-of-hospital management, *Clin Toxicol (Phila)* 44(3):205–223, 2006.

Sharma AN, Hexdall AH, Chang EK, et al.: Diphenhydramine-induced wide complex dysrhythmia responds to treatment with sodium bicarbonate, *Am J Emerg Med* 21(3):212–215, 2003.

Simons FE: H_1-antihistamines: more relevant than ever in the treatment of allergic disorders, *J Allergy Clin Immunol* 112(Suppl 4):S42–S52, 2003.

Simons FE, Simons KJ: Histamine and H_1-antihistamines: celebrating a century of progress, *J Allergy Clin Immunol* 128(6):1139–1150, 2011. e4.

Skidgel RA, Kaplan AP, Erdös E: Histamine, bradykinin, and their antagonists. In Brunton L, Chabner B, Knollman B, editors: *Goodman and Gillman's the pharmacological basis of therapeutics*, ed 12, New York, 2011, McGraw-Hill, pp 911–936.

第 85 章 自主神经反射亢进

Kof M. Kla，Lorri A. Lee

病例概要

患者，男性退伍军人，34 岁，10 年前在战争中有过 C5 完全性脊髓损伤，在清醒镇静下行膀胱镜检查及输尿管支架植入术。患者手术过程中血压骤然升至 260/120 mmHg，窦性心动过缓，心率为 42 次 / 分，主诉头痛和视物模糊，表现烦躁，意识混乱。

病例分析

定义

自主神经反射亢进，又称自主神经反射障碍，是一种与颈胸段脊髓损伤（spinal cord injury，SCI）相关的临床综合征。自主神经反射亢进发作通常急性起病且反应剧烈，表现为脊髓损伤水平以下刺激引起的血压急剧升高，血压升高可伴发心动过缓或心动过速（偶发）。自主神经反射亢进发作的临床标准包括收缩压增加基础值 20% 以上，且伴发至少一种以下症状：出汗、寒战、鸡皮样外观、面色潮红或头痛。自主神经反射亢进发作，轻则无症状，重则伴发高血压危象，可危及生命。自主神经反射亢进发作时，脊髓损伤水平以下的疼痛刺激会导致交感兴奋，且不再像正常患者一样受副交感神经抑制作用。脊髓损伤水平以下的交感兴奋会导致广泛的外周循环和内脏血管收缩，会引起轻度到严重的高血压。

无论患者有无感觉，自主神经反射亢进均可由脊髓损伤水平以下的疼痛刺激触发。这种刺激包括空腔脏器如肠或膀胱的扩张和收缩，其中膀胱扩张是自主神经反射亢进的最常见诱因。胃食管反流病、胃炎、胆结石、粪便嵌塞、痔疮、留置导尿管阻塞、泌尿系统手术操作、妊娠、分娩和外科手术都可能诱发自主神经反射亢进。其他诱因甚至包括痉挛、温度变化、性交、骨折以及髋关节脱位。

识别

患者在脊髓损伤水平以下，有肌张力增加、肌痉挛、立毛肌收缩等交感神经活动增加的表现。患者在脊髓损伤水平以上可能有皮肤潮红、出汗、鼻塞、头痛、心动过缓或心律失常等症状。这些症状原因在于脊髓损伤部位头端的主动脉弓或颈动脉窦压力感受器感受到血压升高后激活副交感神经系统。副交感神经系统激活引起脊髓损伤水平以上的血管舒张，对抗交感神经激活引起的脊髓损伤水平以下的血管收缩。自主神经反射亢进表现可以从无症状到严重症状不等，更凶险的症状包括呼吸困难和胸痛（急性左心室后负荷增加引起），视物模糊、头痛和意识模糊（血压急剧升高，超过脑血管自主调节上限且无法代偿导致）（框 85.1）。

风险评估

接诊脊髓损伤的患者时，认识到自主神经反射亢进的风险对麻醉管理的安全至关重要。尽管许多患者在脊髓损伤平面以下几乎很少有痛觉，手术或器械的刺激依然可以导致自主神经反射亢进发作。自主神经反射亢进发作通常发生在脊髓损伤的慢性期，一般是在脊髓损伤 1 个月以后，但也有在脊髓损伤后几周内发生的病例报告。自主神经反射亢进通常发生在脊髓 T6 平面或以上，因为绝大多数交感神经传出纤维发自脊髓 T5 ～ T6 平面以下。约有 20% ～ 70% 的 T6 或 T6 以上的脊髓损伤患者会有自主神经反射亢进的表现。与不完全性脊髓损伤相比，完全性脊髓损伤患者更容易发生自主神经反射亢进，脊髓损伤平面高的患者通常症状更严重。损伤平面在 T10 平面以下的脊髓损伤患者通常不太可能发生

框 85.1 自主神经反射亢进的症状、体征和后遗症

脊髓损伤水平以下的症状

立毛肌收缩
苍白
痉挛

脊髓损伤水平以上的症状、体征和后遗症

恶心
出汗
寒战
头痛
鼻塞
面色潮红
呼吸困难
意识模糊
视物模糊
胸痛
高血压（收缩压升高超过基础血压的 20%）
窦性心动过缓
窦性心动过速
心律失常
心脏停搏
心脏传导阻滞
缺血性心电图改变
癫痫发作
高血压脑病
出血性或缺血性脑卒中
心肌梗死
急性左心衰竭
肺水肿

自主神经反射亢进，因为在这个平面以下的交感神经发出很少。

手术部位也是诱发自主神经发射亢进的重要因素。手术部位在脊髓损伤平面以上，自主神经反射亢进的风险较低，但是脊髓损伤平面以下的导尿管阻塞刺激或其他刺激可能导致其发作。分娩时的子宫收缩可引起强烈的交感神经兴奋，此类患者也较易发作自主神经反射亢进。

启示

血压升高可能危及生命，若不及时治疗，可能导致癫痫发作、心肌梗死或急性左心衰竭，后负荷急剧增加导致的肺水肿、高血压脑病、出血性或缺血性脑卒中，甚至死亡。分娩期间的自主神经反射亢进会危及胎儿和母体，强烈的血管收缩会导致子宫胎盘功能不全和胎儿缺氧。

管理

自主神经反射亢进的最佳管理方案为充分认识自主神经反射亢进发作的风险并采取适当的预防措施。所有医护人员提高警惕性，准备好非药物治疗和药物治疗方案。

非药物治疗

自主神经反射亢进的一线治疗方法是识别和消除诱因。如果外科操作诱发并且血压已达危险值，外科医师需暂停操作（如膀胱镜检查时先暂时排空膀胱），同时加深麻醉、控制血压。改变患者体位，使其处于直立位，静脉容量增加，可以达到体位性血压下降。这种处理方法在手术室中不容易做到，但在苏醒室可能是一种有效的非药物治疗方法。解除约束装置或绑带也能增加静脉血容量，起到降低血压的作用。然而，以上策略可能收效甚微。实施这些策略的同时，积极开展药物治疗恶性高血压。当无法找到诱因时，或诱因清除后血压仍保持较高水平，则应开始使用抗高血压药物进行药物治疗。

药物治疗

当消除诱因、加深麻醉及非药物治疗无法降压或无法识别诱因时，就需要药物降压。用于治疗自主反射性血压升高的降压药最好应选择起效迅速且作用时间短的药物。手术室常见药物包括硝酸甘油、艾司洛尔和尼卡地平。硝酸甘油有多种给药方式（静脉、舌下含服、舌下喷雾或经皮给药）。硝酸甘油起效迅速且作用时间短，适用于清醒或麻醉的患者。当硝酸甘油与西地那非联用时，可导致严重低血压，甚至降低狭窄冠状动脉的血流量。因此，在使用硝酸甘油时，应避免使用西地那非。尼卡地平和艾司洛尔起效迅速且作用时间短；但应注意，β 受体阻滞剂会加重自主神经相关性高血压引起的反射性心动过缓。手术室内常用的抗高血压药物还包括拉贝洛尔和肼屈嗪，这两种药物的作用时间都较长，当诱因消除后仍可能导致长时间低血压。此外，应警惕拉贝洛尔也可能导致恶性心动过缓。无论选择哪种药物，都应易于获得，且不延误对高血压的治疗。

预防

多达 90% 的脊髓损伤患者在局部麻醉或无麻醉的情况下手术，会出现自主神经反射亢进。一项研究监测了脊髓损伤 T7 平面以上的患者手术期间的血压。接受镇静、局部麻醉或无麻醉的患者，术中血压均明显高于基础血压，接受全身麻醉的患者术中则无明显的血压波动，而接受脊椎麻醉的患者术中血压明显低于基础血压。此外，79% 接受镇静、局部麻醉或无麻醉的患者术中出现高血压，只有 23% 全身麻醉的患者和 7% 脊椎麻醉的患者术中出现高血压。椎管内麻醉在预防自主神经反射亢进方面优于全身麻醉，但阻滞平面不易评估，既往的脊柱内固定植入物也会加大椎管内麻醉的穿刺难度。

全身麻醉还是椎管内麻醉或者神经阻滞都应尽力维持足够的麻醉深度，并维持良好的术后镇痛效果。如果是手术刺激诱发的自主神经反射亢进，可以通过吸入麻醉药、阿片类药物和（或）丙泊酚加深麻醉。如果患者留置硬膜外导管或周围神经阻滞导管，可以导管内给药追加局部麻醉药。如果追加局部麻醉药无效，可能需要改全身麻醉来缓解自主神经反射亢进。

医学和康复科学的进步使更多脊髓损伤病史的女性患者能够怀孕和分娩，这些患者在分娩期间有自主神经反射亢进的危险，无论是顺产、引产或剖宫产，都可以采用脊椎麻醉、硬膜外麻醉或全身麻醉。当脊椎麻醉或硬膜外麻醉用于分娩时，麻醉平面至少要到达 T10 水平才可以阻断来自盆腔器官的手术刺激，这才是预防自主神经反射亢进最可靠的方法。脊髓损伤平面较高的孕产妇，推荐采用连续血压监测和心电监测。高危患者或合并并发症的患者可以采用有创动脉血压监测。分娩后子宫持续收缩，因此产后早期，持续硬膜外给药十分必要。

苏醒及术后管理

全身麻醉苏醒按常规进行，拔管应符合指征。在区域或椎管内麻醉下实施手术的患者可在手术结束后进入苏醒室。无论麻醉类型如何，术后应常规监测血压，因为当全身麻醉和（或）局部麻醉的效果消退时，会诱发自主神经反射亢进。为避免触发自主神经亢进发作，术后数日内应继续行连续硬膜外或周围神经导管给药镇痛。围术期团队成员应知悉自主神经反射亢进的风险，保持警惕，并能提前识别和诊治自主神经反射亢进，最好能避免其发生。

感谢

感谢 C. Lee Parmley 和 Steven J. Allen 博士对本章上一版的贡献。

（赵景昕 译 吴 倩 校）

延伸阅读

American College of Obstetrics and Gynecology: ACOG committee opinion. Obstetric management of patients with spinal cord injuries. Number 275, September 2002. Committee on Obstetric Practice. American College of Obstetrics and Gynecology, *Int J Gynaecol Obstet* 79(2):189–191, 2002.

Consortium for Spinal Cord Medicine: Acute management of autonomic dysreflexia: individuals with spinal cord injury presenting to health-care facilities, *J Spinal Cord Med* 25(Suppl 1):S67–S88, 2002.

Cross LL, Meythaler JM, Tuel SM, et al.: Pregnancy, labor and delivery post spinal cord injury, *Paraplegia* 30(12):890–902, 1992.

Curt A, Nitsche B, Rodic B, et al.: Assessment of autonomic dysreflexia in patients with spinal cord injury, *J Neurol Neurosur Ps* 62(5):473–477, 1997.

Eltorai IM, Wong DH, Lacerna M, et al.: Surgical aspects of autonomic dysreflexia, *J Spinal Cord Med* 20(3):361–364, 1997.

Graham GP, Dent CM, Evans PD, et al.: Recurrent dislocation of the hip in adult paraplegics, *Paraplegia* 30(8):587–591, 1992.

Gunduz H, Binak DF: Autonomic dysreflexia: an important cardiovascular complication in spinal cord injury patients, *Cardiol J* 19(2):215–219, 2012.

Hawkins Jr RL, Bailey HR, Donnovan WH: Autonomic dysreflexia resulting from prolapsed hemorrhoids. Report of a case, *Dis Colon Rectum* 37(5): 492–493, 1994.

Ishikura F, Beppu S, Hamada T, et al.: Effects of sildenafil citrate (Viagra) combined with nitrate on the heart, *Circulation* 102(20):2516–2521, 2000.

Karlsson AK: Autonomic dysreflexia, *Spinal Cord* 37(6):383–391, 1999.

Khastgir J, Drake MJ, Abrams P: Recognition and effective management of autonomic dysreflexia in spinal cord injuries, *Expert Opin Pharmacother* 8(7):945–956, 2007.

Krassioukov A, Warburton DE, Teasell R, et al.: A systematic review of the management of autonomic dysreflexia after spinal cord injury, *Arch Phys Med Rehabil* 90(4):682–695, 2009.

Krassioukov AV, Furlan JC, Fehlings MG: Autonomic dysreflexia in acute spinal cord injury: an under-recognized clinical entity, *J Neurotrauma* 20(8):707–716, 2003.

Lambert DH, Deane RS, Mazuzan Jr JE: Anesthesia and the control of blood pressure in patients with spinal cord injury, *Anesth Analg* 61(4):344–348, 1982.

McGillivray CF, Hitzig SL, Craven BC, et al.: Evaluating knowledge of autonomic dysreflexia among individuals with spinal cord injury and their families, *J Spinal Cord Med* 32(1):54–62, 2009.

McGregor JA, Meeuwsen J: Autonomic hyperreflexia: a mortal danger for spinal cord-damaged women in labor, *Am J Obstet Gynecol* 151(3):330–333, 1985.

Teasell RW, Arnold JM, Krassioukov A, et al.: Cardiovascular consequences of loss of supraspinal control of the sympathetic nervous system after spinal cord injury, *Arch Phys Med Rehabil* 81(4):506–516, 2000.

巴比妥酸盐：卟啉病 第 86 章

Nicolas N. Algarra，*Christoph N. Seubert*

病例概要

患者，女性，24 岁，因恶心、呕吐和腹痛，拟接受剖腹探查术。患者焦虑，既往史值得注意的是 2 年前行剖腹探查术阴性。血压 150/90 mmHg，脉搏 105 次 / 分；体格检查提示腹部压痛。电解质水平和白细胞计数正常。询问家族史时，患者称其母亲可能患有卟啉病。

问题分析

定义

了解诱发性卟啉病的基本缺陷，及其与麻醉和手术应激的相关作用，可以预防卟啉病的急性发作。

卟啉病为一类异质性的遗传疾病组，因酶的缺乏加上环境的诱发刺激可以产生急性发作，加上血红素合成中间产物的蓄积，可引起轻微到危及生命的症状。尽管卟啉病可根据其遗传缺陷为基础进行分类（图 86.1），临床简单分为可诱发性 / 急性和不可诱发性 / 慢性的分类法依然有其实用性。以分类中的后者为例说明，卟啉病最常见的形式是迟发性皮肤卟啉病（porphyria cutanea tarda，PCT）。除了患者皮肤脆性增加，PCT 与丙肝、人类免疫缺陷病毒或酒精滥用有关，无麻醉方面的顾虑，也不受限于药物的选择。相反，所有急性 / 诱发性卟啉病患者都有发生卟啉危象的危险，尤其是在围术期。在围术期用药、需要手术的病情、应激和（或）禁食可能会诱发卟啉病急性发作。如果这种疾病发作得不到治疗或未被识别，它可以是致命的。相反，控制诱发因素和（或）迅速的治疗，可避免或减缓疾病发作，并使手术得到安全实施。因此急性卟啉病是重要的麻醉问题。

卟啉的合成在所有细胞中都存在，在骨髓和肝中尤为重要。卟啉是参与氧的利用、运输和储存的蛋白质的重要组成部分。这些蛋白质包括呼吸链中普遍存在的细胞色素氧化酶、肝细胞色素 P450 酶以及血红蛋白等氧的储存和转运蛋白。卟啉的合成涉及一系列酶（图 86.1）。卟啉合成关键酶的基因在基因组中复制，允许肝和骨髓中血红素合成的过程中单独调控。在肝中，大多数血红素用于生成细胞色素 P450 酶。因此，血红素合成和 P450 产生以协同的方式进行调控。

四种急性卟啉病是急性间歇性卟啉病（acute

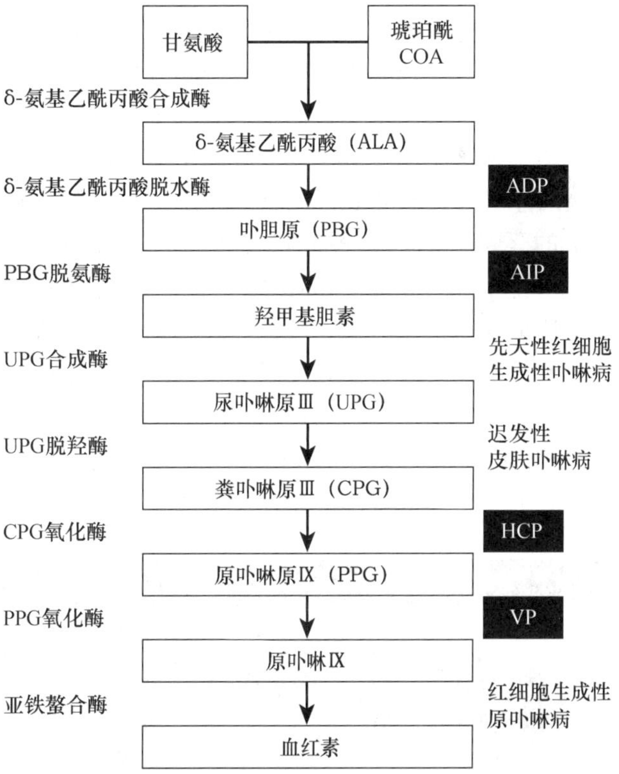

图 86.1　人血红素生物合成途径。催化这些步骤的酶在左边，由缺陷酶引起的卟啉病在右边。急性卟啉病见图中黑色方块。ADP，δ-氨基乙酰丙酸脱水酶卟啉病；AIP，急性间歇性卟啉病；HCP，遗传性卟啉病；VP，混合性卟啉病

intermittent porphyria，AIP）、混合性卟啉病（variegate porphyria, VP）、遗传性卟啉病（hereditary coproporphyria, HCP），和 δ-氨基乙酰丙酸脱水酶卟啉病（acid dehydratase-deficient porphyria，ADP）。造成急性卟啉病的基因缺陷是功能缺失突变，通常会使酶活性降低一半。这种减少是由于遗传模式是隐性的罕见的 ADP 或显性伴可变外显率所致，包括三种更为常见的急性卟啉病（表 86.1）。尽管不同分型卟啉病肝缺陷酶在血红素合成途径中的位置有所不同（图 86.1），但这四种疾病都可能出现急性发作，其症状和治疗相似。目前还不清楚为什么慢性或红细胞卟啉病中的酶缺陷不会导致急性发作。HCP 和 VP 可引起皮肤中多余卟啉的蓄积，紫外线刺激可引起皮肤起水泡和瘢痕。

识别

由于症状非特异性和多变，诱发性卟啉病的急性发作在围术期难以识别。典型症状和发作的频率见表 86.2。青春期前很少发作，成年后也很少复发。持续数天，以剧烈、稳定、难以定位的腹痛为特征。疼痛的强度与物理检查结果阴性形成鲜明对比，有时会导致急诊剖腹探查。恶心、呕吐和肠鸣音减弱是常见的症状，但临床表现不明显，通常无发热、白细胞增多和（或）腹部压痛。诱发性卟啉病的急性发作可累及外周神经系统，表现为近端加重的运动无力。这种症状在腹痛消退后偶尔出现，可能类似 Guillain-Barré 综合征，但脑脊液中没有特征性白蛋白升高。颅神经和感觉神经可能受到影响，神经系统可能累及呼吸延髓麻痹及死亡的进展。在四分之一的患者中，中枢神经系统也可能以精神症状的形式参与其中，例如焦虑、幻觉和（或）妄想。全身性癫痫发作可能是中枢神经系统受累的神经学表现，或由抗利尿激素分泌不当和（或）呕吐引起的严重低钠血症的表现。如果怀疑是急性卟啉病，可以通过筛选和定量卟啉前体 δ-氨基乙酰丙酸和尿液中的胆色素原来确诊。日光可将无色的卟啉原转化为卟啉，导致尿液颜色变暗，由红变紫。症状的缓解通常很快，但乏力可能持续数天或数月。

对于无症状的患者，围术期诊断急性卟啉病则主要依赖于详细的家族史。由于是常染色体显性遗传病，许多疑似病患都知道血缘亲属中有被诊断为急性卟啉病。相反，实验室检查可能为阴性结果，因为患者的代谢状况已经得到了代偿。因此，对间歇发作卟啉病的阳性诊断应由专家进行。（信息可在美国卟啉基金会找到，网站：http://www.porphyriafoundation.com 或南非开普敦大学：http://porphyria-professionals.uct.ac.za/）。

风险评估

急性卟啉病的流行情况（表 86.1）难以估计，因为多达 80% 的潜在患者在其一生中可能从未经历过急性发作。据估计，AIP 在北美洲的流行率约为 1∶10 000，但在北欧或北欧后裔中可能达到 1∶1000。临床上，它占急性间歇性发作的 3/4。VP 普遍较少，除了在南非的荷兰后裔中，那里有超过 20 000 个病例是由一对移民夫妇引起的。HCP 很少见，估计流行率为 1∶100 0000。ADP 目前则仅报告 7 例。

对风险评估来说，比患病率更重要的是急性发作总是原因多样。即使既往曾经暴露于诱发卟啉病发作的药物而未发作也不排除诊断为急性卟啉病。因此，如果一系列症状（表 86.2）可能符合急性卟啉病发作的症状，那么则应该高度怀疑。

表 86.1 急性 / 诱发性卟啉病

分类	发病率	遗传	脑脊髓交感神经系统症状	光敏性
δ-氨基乙酰丙酸脱水酶卟啉病（ADP）	极其罕见	常染色体隐性	++	-
急性间歇性卟啉病（AIP）	1∶10 000 斯堪的纳维亚更高	常染色体显性	+++	-
遗传性卟啉病（HCP）	罕见 1∶1 000 000	常染色体显性	++	++
混合性卟啉病（VP）	1∶300 000 南非更高	常染色体显性	++	++

表 86.2 卟啉危象的症状

症状		
周围神经系统	感觉运动	腹部疼痛 运动近端加重虚弱，可能涉及颅神经和呼吸肌肉
	自主神经	心动过速 高血压
中枢神经系统	精神病学	焦虑 幻觉 偏执
	内分泌	SIADH
	神经系统	癫痫
其他方面	恶心 / 呕吐 低钠血症	
实验室检查	尿中 ALA 和 PBG 升高 尿液在光照下会变成暗红色 / 粉红色	

ALA，δ-氨基乙酰丙酸；PGB，卟胆原；SIADH，抗利尿激素分泌失调综合征

启示

未能诊断和治疗卟啉病急性发作可导致死亡率高达 10%。这种失误不仅延长了发作时间，而且使患者面临进一步发病的危险：

- 由于葡萄糖摄入量的减少，肝血红素合成进一步上调；
- 累及运动神经并涉及呼吸肌和颅神经；
- 残留的轻瘫，即使在发作恢复后仍然存在；
- 癫痫发作，可能使用卟啉药物治疗；
- 暴露于进行其他支持性治疗的卟啉药物；
- 不必要的手术。

管理

对卟啉病患者的围术期治疗不只是避免使用巴比妥酸盐。术前评估应确定是否存在正处于急性发作的症状。事实上，正如在病例概要中所示，手术可能没有必要进行，内科处理应关注卟啉危象的治疗。在无急性发作的情况下，麻醉处方应包括非卟啉药物。具体细节以及减少急性发作风险的其他措施将在后面讨论。如果术前评估提示卟啉病急性发作，应当住院并采取对症和特异性治疗。

围术期急性卟啉病发作

急性卟啉病发作的具体治疗包括 3 种干预措施：给予血红素和葡萄糖（因为它们都能抑制 δ-氨基乙酰丙酸合成酶，从而纠正代谢异常）；明确诱发因素并去除，从而降低酶的诱导。临床应用的血红素（Panhematin，Ovation Pharmaceuticals，Deerfield，IL）含有碱性血红素，来源于经过处理的人类红细胞。它是一种冻干粉末，最好在白蛋白中溶解应用，形成稳定的溶液，减少血栓性静脉炎和抗凝。根据发作的严重程度，给药剂量为 3 ～ 4 mg/kg，持续 4 天。输入的血红素使肝的亚铁血红素储备恢复并通过提供负反馈调节过程纠正血红素的合成途径（图 86.1）。鉴于卟啉病急性发作的死亡风险和严重或长期神经系统症状的可能性，应尽早开始使用血红素治疗。葡萄糖以每天 300 ～ 400 g 剂量的治疗效果比血红素差，但已被证明可以减少卟啉前体的排泄。此外，禁食和低碳水化合物饮食可诱发急性发作。虽然葡萄糖在肠内给药是有效的，但急性发作时的恶心和肠道运动减弱使肠外给药更为可行。仔细评估患者应用的药物（表 86.3）以明确和去除诱发因素应作为最基本的要求。由于导致急性发作的因素众多，因此不可能完全消除诱发因素。

支持性治疗应关注与疾病发作相关的症状。疼痛应使用阿片类药物进行治疗。电解质失衡应得到纠正。颅神经受累可能需要预防误吸，而呼吸肌受累可能需要机械通气或至少在重症监护病房密切监测。癫痫发作是一个特殊的挑战，因为巴比妥酸盐、苯妥英和其他一些抗癫痫药物是急性发作的强效触发剂。应排除低钠血症是否为原因，咪达唑仑或氯硝西泮可以安全地终止癫痫发作活动。

急性卟啉病患者的麻醉处理

评估卟啉病的用药安全性颇为困难。一方面，药物是急性发作最常见的诱发因素；另一方面，并非所有卟啉病易感患者接触药物都会导致这种发作。关于卟啉病患者药物安全性的信息有以下 3 个来源，按临床适用性降低的顺序排列：①真实的病例提示时间先后相关或因果关系；②诱导卟啉病的动物模型；③细胞培养。后两种来源往往夸大了药物对患者的风险，并且常常是信息冲突的来源。（更详细的药物信息和安全及潜在不安全药物清单可在以下

表 86.3 急性卟啉病患者用药的安全性[a]

不安全 / 避免	使用谨慎 / 避免	可能安全
巴比妥类	酮咯酸	阿片类
依托咪酯	大环内酯类	神经肌肉阻滞剂
苯妥英	四环素类	格隆溴铵（胃长宁）
丙戊酸	喹诺酮类	阿托品
琥珀酰胺	肼屈嗪	新斯的明
吡唑啉酮	钙通道阻滞剂	纳洛酮
克林霉素		咪达唑仑
红霉素		氟马西尼
多西环素		氧化亚氮
磺胺类		挥发性麻醉药
胺碘酮		局部麻醉药
		普鲁卡因胺
		β 受体阻滞剂
		东莨菪碱
		苯海拉明
		去氧肾上腺素
		昂丹司琼

[a] 注意：此列表不完整。未上市药物不能被认为是安全的。这些分类旨在提供指导，而不是取代处方医师的临床判断。有些药物是根据临床经验分类的，不管包装说明书中是否有警告。应使用最少数量的必要药物治疗卟啉类疾病。有关详细信息，请参阅本文。

网站找到：http://www.drugs-porphyria.org/ 或 http://www.porphyriafoundation.com/drug database。）例如，挥发性麻醉剂在动物模型中是卟啉源性药物，但是临床经验表明氟烷和异氟烷可安全使用。因此，许多药物可以谨慎使用，前提是它们是有指征并且潜在收益大于风险。

对卟啉病患者的麻醉方案，应避免已知可诱发急性发作的药物。表 86.3 总结了这些情况。同样，应考虑对卟啉病患者安全的合适药物（表 86.3）。丙泊酚可选择作为全身麻醉的诱导药物，而巴比妥酸盐和依托咪酯应避免使用。目前尚无关于右美托咪定在卟啉病中的安全使用的足够数据。舒更葡糖已成功用于急性卟啉病发作。肌肉松弛药和阿片类药物可安全使用。临床上，虽然七氟烷和地氟烷的数据有限，但挥发性药物可在临床安全使用。局部和区域麻醉可安全地用于卟啉病患者，尽管在急性发作期间，自主神经不稳定、精神症状、虚弱和低血容量可能出现相对禁忌证。临床经验表明，酰胺类和酯类局部麻醉药均为安全的药物，即使利多卡因可增加了组织培养中 δ-氨基乙酰丙酸合成酶的活性。

预防

急性卟啉病患者围术期急性发作的预防需要所有医护人员的精心规划和良好沟通。术前一晚入院可预防性给予葡萄糖，从而最大限度地减少术前禁食的影响。安慰和术前用药可以缓解焦虑和压力。应尽量减少药量，并应评估每种药物诱发急性发作的风险。由于可能会在诱发事件发生后的 3 ~ 5 天延迟发生卟啉危象，出院指南应在术后患者的可汇报主诉中强调可能存在卟啉危象的症状。症状的检查应包括尿卟啉前体 δ-氨基乙酰丙酸和卟啉原的筛查和定量。这样一套综合的措施可使急性卟啉病患者安全实施手术。

（程 芳 译 马 宇 校）

延伸阅读

Balwani M, Desnick RJ: The porphyrias: advances in diagnosis and treatment, *Blood* 120(23):4496–4504, 2012.

Findley H, Philips A, Cole D, et al.: Porphyrias: implications for anaesthesia, critical care, and pain medicine, *Contin Educ Anaesth Crit Care Pain Adv*, February 27, 2012. http://dx.doi.org/10.1093/bjaceaccp/mks009. [Epub ahead of print].

Karim Z, Lyoumi S, Nicolas G, et al.: Porphyrias: a 2015 update, *Clin Res Hepatol Gastroenterol* 39(4):412–425, 2015.

Pischik E, Kauppinen R: An update of clinical management of acute intermittent porphyria, *Appl Clin Genet* 8:201, 2015.

Stein P, Badminton M, Barth J, et al.: Best practice guidelines on clinical management of acute attacks of porphyria and their complications, *Ann Clin Biochem* 50(Pt 3):217–223, 2013.

钾离子平衡紊乱

第 87 章

Richard J. Novak

病例概要

低钾血症

患者，老年男性，70 岁，患有高血压病，因肠梗阻在全身麻醉下行急诊手术。患者每日常规口服氢氯噻嗪。术前血清钾离子浓度为 3.4 mEq/L。术中因少尿给予 10 mg 呋塞米静脉注射。1 h 后，患者排尿 900 ml，心电图显示新的 U 波，每分钟出现 5 个室性期前收缩。复测血清钾离子浓度为 2.8 mEq/L。

高钾血症

患者，女性，55 岁，患终末期肾病，拟行左侧股腘动脉搭桥重建术。术晨患者通过左前臂动静脉瘘透析。术前血清钾离子浓度为 5.6 mEq/L。在手术开始第 4 h 股动脉阻断释放，心电图出现高尖 T 波，QRS 波幅增宽。复测血清钾离子浓度为 7.0 mEq/L。

钾离子在心肌细胞等兴奋性细胞的静息膜电位中起重要作用，钾离子平衡的紊乱可引起致命的心律失常。低钾血症在住院患者中发生率高达 20%，可使患者死亡风险增加 10 倍，主要由它导致的心律失常和心血管事件所致。据报道，1% ～ 10% 的住院患者可出现高钾血症，其中 10% 患者可出现钾离子浓度大于 6.0 mEq/L 的严重高钾血症。在终末期肾病死亡病例中，高钾血症占 2% ～ 5% 的比例。

围术期血清钾离子浓度异常较常见，识别和治疗低钾血症和高钾血症是重要的技能。维持整个机体内钾离子的平衡是通过钾离子的摄入与钾离子经肾或胃肠排出之间的平衡来实现。钾离子是细胞内主要的阳离子。人体超过 98% 的钾离子分布于细胞内，主要在肌细胞中。人体内钾的总储量为 50 mEq/kg，因此，70 kg 的人体大约含有 3 500 mEq 的钾离子。正常血清钾离子浓度为 3.5 ～ 5.3 mEq/L。正常细胞内钾离子浓度大约是血清内浓度的 30 ～ 40 倍。细胞膜中的 Na^+，K^+-ATP 酶能主动地将钠离子泵出细胞外，同时将钾离子泵入细胞内，从而维持细胞膜两侧钾离子的比例。

任何细胞内外钾离子浓度比例变化都比细胞外血清中测定的钾离子浓度更值得关注。细胞内外钾离子浓度比例的急性变化比慢性变化更危险，最主要的风险是对心脏电生理的影响，可导致心律失常和心肌收缩力下降。正如前面两个病例概要所示，伴发急性血清钾离子减少或增加的临床病史至关重要。

低钾血症

问题分析

定义

第一个病例概要举例说明了慢性低钾血症并发急性低钾血症。慢性低钾血症与体内钾总储存量和测定的血清钾离子浓度水平的减少有关，而细胞内外钾离子浓度比例保持正常。呋塞米利尿可引起肾排钾致体内钾丢失，血清钾离子从 3.4 mEq/L 降至 2.8 mEq/L。这种急性低钾血症导致细胞内外钾离子浓度比例的变化，导致静息电位增大，细胞膜超极化，易发生心律失常。

识别

在清醒患者中，血清钾离子浓度小于 3 mEq/L

时最常见的症状是虚弱和易疲劳。其他症状与心血管、中枢神经系统、神经肌肉、肾或机体代谢功能有关（框 87.1）。在全身麻醉下，患者心电图改变、心排血量下降、对升压药的反应降低，可能是低钾血症的最初表现。心电图异常改变或如第一个病例的急性利尿的临床场景，提示临床医师应检测血清钾离子浓度并对低钾血症进行确诊。低钾血症的心电图变化可能包括（图 87.1）：

- U 波的出现；
- T 波倒置或者低平，ST 段弓背下移；
- QRS 波群振幅增大；
- 房性或室性期前收缩；
- 伴有严重的低钾血症、室上性心动过速、心房颤动、心房扑动，以及潜在的室性心动过速或心室颤动。

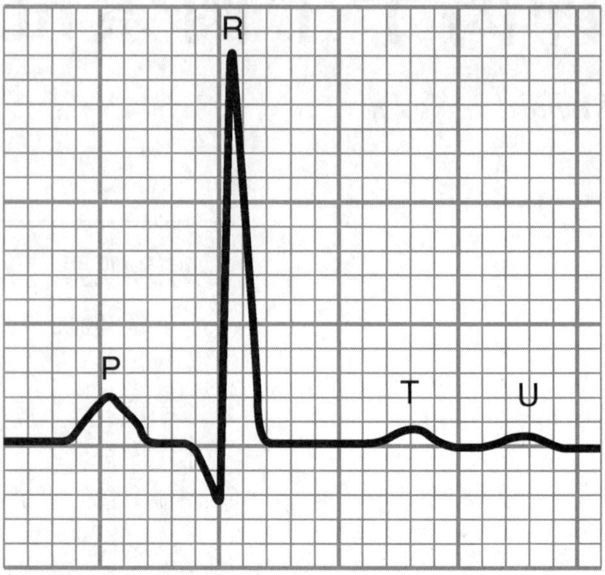

图 87.1　心电图改变伴血清钾离子浓度急性下降。注意 T 波的平坦和 U 波的出现

风险评估

低钾血症的原因列在框 87.2。这些包括酒精中毒或营养不良导致的口服摄入量不足，腹泻过度导致的胃肠道钾流失，噻嗪或袢利尿剂导致的肾钾流失，糖皮质激素或盐皮质激素过量，以及过度透析导致的钾流失。急性碱中毒、β_2- 儿茶酚胺受体激动剂或胰岛素治疗可导致钾离子从细胞外向细胞内转移。

框 87.1　低钾血症的症状或影响

心血管
降低心肌收缩力
电传导异常
直立性低血压和对血管升压药反应降低
洋地黄中毒的风险增加

肌肉和中枢神经系统
虚弱和易疲劳
意识混乱和抑郁
呼吸抑制（血清钾离子 <2.5 mEq/L）
周围神经病变和反射减弱
神经肌肉阻断药作用增强
横纹肌溶解（血清钾离子 <2.0 mEq/L）

肾和胃肠
多尿症；尿液浓缩能力降低
胃肠蠕动迟缓

新陈代谢
葡萄糖耐受不良
增强低镁血症和低钙血症

框 87.2　低钾血症的原因

饮食摄入量不足
营养不良
酗酒

胃肠道丢失
腹泻
呕吐

肾丢失
利尿治疗
糖皮质激素过量
盐皮质激素过量
镁缺乏
过度透析

钾离子向细胞内转移
急性呼吸性或代谢性碱中毒
β_2- 儿茶酚胺受体激动剂
增加胰岛素水平

启示

病例概要中第一例患者在血清钾离子浓度为 2.8 mEq/L 时发生心律失常。血清钾离子浓度低至何种程度会发生心律失常目前还不能够确定。任何低钾离子水平的临床意义取决于以下因素：

- 患者的内科并存疾病；
- 钾离子的缺乏是急性还是慢性；
- 低钾血症的原因；
- 计划的手术或操作；

- 预约的手术是否紧急；
- 任何紧急手术或麻醉都可能带来钾离子额外的急性平衡紊乱。

低钾血症的主要风险是对临床有重要影响的心律失常。细胞外与细胞内钾离子浓度比值的急性降低，增加了可兴奋细胞的跨膜钾离子浓度梯度和跨膜电位，可刺激心肌细胞的自动去极化，或者引起折返性心律失常。

管理

随着血清钾离子水平的缓慢下降，如在病例概要中第一例患者术前钾离子浓度为 3.4 mEq/L，快速钾替代治疗的风险大于慢性钾离子消耗的风险。术前低钾血症给临床医师带来了两个问题：①手术继续进行还是推迟；②如何治疗低钾血症。

是否进行麻醉和手术

在两项研究中，术前轻度至中度慢性低钾血症（钾离子 =2.6 ～ 3.4 mEq/L）与非心脏手术中较高的术中心律失常发生率无关。对于低钾血症患者是否进行手术和麻醉取决于血钾变化的剧烈程度和临床病情。对低钾血症患者进行手术或麻醉的考虑包括以下几点：

- 低钾血症持续时间；
- 计划手术的紧迫性和严重程度；
- 存在其他相关生理性或代谢性失衡；
- 低钾血症可能加重的其他内科并存疾病；
- 存在肾功能不全、未控制的高血压、心力衰竭或冠状动脉疾病。

当检测到血清钾离子浓度较低时，出现异常的实验室钾离子值应进行重复检测。如果确诊低钾血症，合理的非心脏手术术前处理如下：

- 若血清钾离子浓度低于 2.5 mEq/L，应取消除急诊手术外的所有手术，尤其是心电图出现变化的患者。在推迟手术期间，应确定低钾血症的原因，并补充钾治疗。
- 若血清钾离子浓度在 2.5 ～ 3.0 mEq/L，患者出现任何低钾血症心电图异常变化，应延迟手术，查明低钾的原因，行补钾治疗。如果建议的手术是紧急或急诊手术，手术可以继续进行并在术中静脉补钾治疗，术中监测钾离子水平，监测低钾血症或高钾血症相关心律失常。
- 若血清钾离子浓度在 3.1 ～ 3.5 mEq/L，若无超过 0.5 mEq/L 以上的急剧下降，且无低钾血症的心电图异常改变，则进行手术及麻醉的风险较小。例外情况可能包括有严重心脏病史的患者，如急性心肌梗死、心力衰竭、急性儿茶酚胺过量或洋地黄中毒。

低钾血症的治疗（框 87.3）

钾离子应从细胞外进入细胞内，并储存在细胞内，因此过快的钾离子替代比较危险。当患者为慢性低钾血症，且不是紧急或急诊手术时，建议口服补充氯化钾（氯化钾）数周。经典的口服氯化钾剂量为每天 40 ～ 100 mEq。在肾功能正常的情况下，机体总储存量每减少 100 mEq，血清钾离子下降约 0.27 mEq/L。低钾血症术前准备，从钾离子 3.4 mEq/L 补充到钾离子 4.4 mEq/L，在数天的时间内可能需要 400 mEq 或者更多的氯化钾。

术中低钾血症伴心电图改变和室性期前收缩需要紧急治疗。静脉注射氯化钾的速度通常不超过 10 ～ 20 mEq/h。如果急性大量钾丢失（例如本文病例概要里的急性利尿），并伴有心律失常，静脉注射氯化钾可高达 20 mEq/h。快速氯化钾灌注治疗必须持续监测心电图，并应经常重复测定血清钾离子浓度。

对低钾血症的治疗包括纠正碱中毒和停用加重病情的药物（例如排钾利尿剂、β 受体激动剂或胰岛素）。在低钾血症的治疗过程中，某些条件和药物

框 87.3 低钾血症的治疗

纠正潜在原因

停用利尿剂

纠正碱中毒

停止 β 受体激动剂和胰岛素的应用

非紧急钾替代治疗

口服氯化钾，每天 40 ～ 100 mEq

紧急钾替代治疗

氯化钾静脉注射，10 mEq/h（每小时最大 20 mEq 的替代速率），可经中心静脉导管注射并行连续心电图监测。经外周血管注射氯化钾浓度不超过 40 mEq/L。经中心静脉给药氯化钾浓度可增加到 20 mEq/100 ml

会导致补充的钾离子进入细胞内的转运延迟，导致血清高钾血症。这些条件包括糖尿病患者、酸血症、肾小管酸中毒，以及患者接受血管紧张素转换酶抑制剂、β 受体阻滞剂或非甾体抗炎药治疗。

低镁血症可伴有低钾血症，并通过影响钾离子储备而加重低钾血症。低镁血症常见于慢性酒精中毒、急性心肌梗死、腹泻、恶病质、营养不良或饥饿的危重患者。应测量这些患者的镁水平，有指征时应补充镁。

第一个病例的治疗概要包括术中以 10 mEq/h 的速度输注氯化钾，每小时复查血清钾离子。如果心电图变化持续不减或出现更多的心律失常，可通过中心静脉以 20 mEq/h 的速度给予补充氯化钾。与低钾血症本身相比，静脉补钾过快可导致更为严重的心律失常。

预防

临床医师需要了解引起低钾血症的各种原因，尤其要警惕危重患者或服用排钾利尿剂的患者。临床医师应熟悉低钾血症的心电图变化，并根据指征监测和治疗这些钾离子浓度降低的患者。

高钾血症

问题分析

定义

高钾血症定义为血清钾离子浓度高于 5.3 mEq/L。第二例病例概要中，高钾血症的病因是术中长时间血管重建后肾功能不全伴下肢缺血。血清钾离子浓度的升高至关重要，因为它可导致严重的心律失常、传导障碍和心肌收缩力降低。

识别

高钾血症几乎没有早期症状，诊断需要高度警惕。由于高钾血症使细胞膜部分去极化，清醒的患者可能表现为肌无力。高钾血症的最初诊断通常是在常规血钾测量中检测到钾水平升高，可伴有或不伴有心电图异常。与血清钾离子浓度升高相关的心电图改变包括以下内容（图 87.2）：

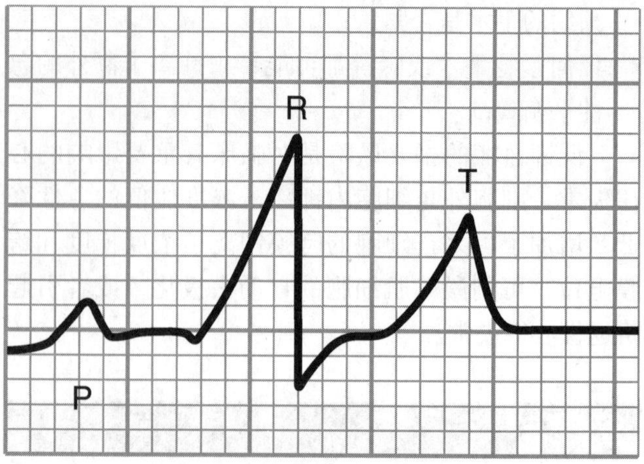

图 87.2 心电图改变伴血清钾离子浓度急性升高。T 波高尖，QRS 波增宽，P-R 间期延长。随着血清钾离子浓度进一步升高，QRS 波和 T 波融合，使心电图呈现正弦波状

- 窄而尖的 T 波；
- P-R 间期延长，P 波振幅减小；
- 随着高钾血症的加重，QRS 波群逐渐增宽。

随着严重高钾血症的加重，P 波消失，与 T 波融合的 QRS 波群变宽，心电图呈现正弦波状。这种节律可发展为室性心动过速、室性纤颤或心脏停搏。

风险评估

高钾血症的原因列于框 87.4。肾衰竭患者发生

框 87.4 高钾血症的原因

摄入量增加

医源性过量氯化钾治疗

输注库存浓缩红细胞

肾排泄减少

急 / 慢性肾功能不全

保钾利尿剂

原发性醛固酮减少症：肾上腺功能不全

继发性醛固酮减少症：血管紧张素转换酶抑制剂、血管紧张素受体阻断剂、非甾体抗炎药、肝素

细胞内至细胞外释放钾

酸中毒

重大创伤或组织坏死

大面积烧伤

横纹肌溶解

溶血反应

缺血后再灌注和细胞死亡（例如肠梗阻、主动脉阻断后释放）

患有骨骼肌肌肉疾病、重度烧伤、多发性创伤、肌肉失神经支配或上运动神经元损伤的各类患者使用琥珀胆碱

高钾血症并发症的风险最高。接受保钾利尿剂和钾替代治疗的患者也是高危人群。因为在血液保存过程中可能会导致钾蓄积，大量输血可导致高钾血症。在医院环境中过量或意外的医源性静脉注射氯化钾导致患者因急性高钾血症而死亡。

酸中毒加剧高钾血症。pH 急剧下降 0.1 会导致血清钾离子浓度增加 1.0 mEq/L，这是由于细胞内钾离子外流至细胞外所致。围术期代谢性酸中毒的原因包括出血、脓毒症、心脏疾病或过敏性休克继发的低灌注。围术期呼吸性酸中毒是由于通气不足所致。

大量细胞坏死或细胞膜破裂导致钾渗漏和高钾血症，例如严重创伤、大型Ⅲ度烧伤、横纹肌溶解和溶血。主动脉阻断释放后缺血区域再灌注或肠缺血再灌注释放钾。任何并发的缺血性代谢性酸中毒都会加重由此引起的高钾血症。

琥珀胆碱使肌肉去极化导致血清钾离子浓度瞬间升高约为 0.45 mEq/L，这在临床上可能对已有高钾血症具有重要意义。琥珀胆碱是神经肌肉疾病、肌肉疾病、急性损伤后引起广泛的骨骼肌去神经支配、偏瘫、上运动神经元损伤或严重烧伤患者的禁忌。这些条件改变了细胞膜钾通道开放的动力学，使钾通道保持开放更长的时间，这可能引发危及生命的高钾血症。

启示

高血钾症主要的围术期风险是危及生命的心脏并发症，包括以下几点：

- Ⅰ、Ⅱ、Ⅲ度房室传导阻滞；
- 心动过缓或心脏停搏；
- 室性或房室交界性逸搏心律；
- 室性心动过速或心室颤动；
- 心肌收缩力下降。

急性钾离子水平升高引起心律失常的发病率高于慢性钾离子水平升高。

管理

高钾血症的治疗取决于变化的剧烈程度和临床病情。决定是否进行手术或麻醉取决于以下因素：

- 高钾血症持续时间；
- 择期手术的紧迫性和严重性；
- 存在其他生理或代谢失衡；
- 由于高钾血症而加重的并发的内科并存疾病；
- 存在肾功能不全、未控制的高血压、充血性心力衰竭或冠状动脉疾病。

高钾血症的治疗没有确定的钾离子浓度目标值，临床心电图改变与钾离子浓度值相关性不一致。一项对终末期肾病、术前钾离子水平高于 6 mEq/L 的患者研究表明，由于透析治疗，手术和麻醉期间未出现不良结果。高钾血症伴心脏传导障碍、心律失常或心肌收缩力下降是临床急症，有必要对其进行持续的心电图监测和紧急治疗（框 87.5）。

葡萄糖酸钙或氯化钙可拮抗钾离子升高对心肌细胞膜的作用，从而降低高钾血症对心肌的影响。静脉注射葡萄糖和胰岛素可使钾离子向细胞内转移而迅速降低血清钾离子浓度。β_2 肾上腺素受体激动剂如沙丁胺醇也使钾离子在细胞内重新分配。

呋塞米通过肾排泄降低体内钾含量。聚苯乙烯硫酸酯钠盐（降钾树脂）或 Patiromer 新型口服钾结合剂通过患者胃肠道排泄减少体内钾含量。后两种药物的作用较慢。血液透析每小时可去除 25 ～ 30 mEq/L 的钾离子，适用于严重肾衰竭患者或严重心功能障碍患者。反复测量血清钾离子浓

框 87.5　高血钾症的治疗

稳定心肌细胞膜电生理效应

葡萄糖酸钙，10 ml 10% 溶液 3 ～ 6 g 静脉注射 2 ～ 3 min；或 3 ～ 4 ml 的 10% 氯化钙溶液，持续静脉注射 2 ～ 3 min（1 ～ 3 min 开始起效，持续 30 ～ 60 min；如心电图异常无变化，可重复剂量给药）

使钾离子向细胞内转移

短效胰岛素（10 ～ 20 U）加入 50 ～ 100 ml 50% 葡萄糖静脉注射（10 ～ 20 min 开始起效，30 ～ 60 min 达到高峰，持续 4 ～ 6 h）

沙丁胺醇 10 ～ 20 mg，加入 4 ml 生理盐水，雾化吸入 10 min 以上（30 min 开始起效，90 min 达到高峰，持续 2 ～ 6 h）

从体内去除钾离子

阳离子交换树脂从胃肠道缓慢清除：聚苯乙烯硫酸酯钠盐（降钾树脂）15 ～ 30 g 口服（完全有效可能需要 24 h；可能需要每 4 ～ 6 h 重复一次剂量）；或 Patiromer 4.2 ～ 8.4 g 口服，每天 1 ～ 2 次

呋塞米

通过低钾溶液行血液透析

度，避免治疗过度引起低钾血症。

在第二个病例概要中，心电图异常的初始治疗包括静脉注射葡萄糖酸钙，然后注射胰岛素/葡萄糖和吸入沙丁胺醇。应检查动脉血气，纠正任何酸中毒。术后反复透析将是最终的治疗方法。

预防

临床医师应了解高钾血症的各种原因，对于慢性肾衰竭患者尤其要警惕。临床医师应熟悉高钾血症的心电图变化，监测高危患者血清钾离子浓度。高尖T波出现在房室传导阻滞、心动过缓、心律失常或心肌收缩力下降等更为严重的并发症之前。对于钾离子浓度升高的患者，应避免补充钾、使用保钾利尿剂、酸中毒和使用琥珀胆碱。

（赵 莉 译 唐念中 校）

延伸阅读

Caruso LJ, Caruso JM: Sodium, potassium, and magnesium. In Lobato EB, Gravenstein N, Kirby RR, editors: *Complications in anesthesiology*, Philadelphia, 2008, Lippincott Williams & Wilkins, pp 461–473.

Edwards MR, Grocott MPW: Perioperative fluid and electrolyte therapy. In Miller RD, et al.: *Miller's anesthesia*, ed 8, Philadelphia, 2015, Elsevier, pp 1767–1810.

Epstein M, Pitt B: Recent advances in pharmacological treatments of hyperkalemia: focus on patiromer, *Expert Opin Pharmacother* 17(10):1435–1448, 2016.

Fleischer LA, Mythen M: Anesthetic implications of concurrent disease. In Miller RD, et al.: *Miller's anesthesia*, ed 8, Philadelphia, 2015, Elsevier, pp 1156–1225.

Hirsch IA, Tomlinson DL, Slogoff S, et al.: The overstated risk of preoperative hypokalemia, *Anesth Analg* 67(2):131–136, 1988.

Mégret F, Perrier V, Fleureau C, et al.: Changes in kaliemia following rapid sequence induction with succinylcholine in critically ill patients, *Ann Fr Anesth Reanim* 31(10):788–792, 2012.

Mount DB: Fluid and electrolyte disorders. In Kasper D, et al., editors: *Harrison's principles of internal medicine*, ed 19, New York, 2015, McGraw-Hill Education, pp 295–312.

Seifter JL: Potassium disorders. In Goldman L, Schafer AI, editors: *Goldman-Cecil medicine*, ed 25, Philadelphia, 2016, Elsevier, pp 755–762.

Vitez TS, Soper LE, Wong KC, et al.: Chronic hypokalemia and intraoperative dysrhythmias, *Anesthesiology* 63(2):130–133, 1985.

Wetherton AR, Corey TS, Buchino JJ, et al.: Fatal injection of potassium in hospitalized patients, *Am J Forensic Med Pathol* 24(2):128–131, 2003.

鞘内阿片类药物

第 88 章

Reza Salajegheh，*Bhiken I. Naik*

病例概要

一名健康的 26 岁产妇因婴儿臀位行剖宫产手术，麻醉方式采用脊椎麻醉，注射药物 1.6 ml，含 0.75% 高比重布比卡因（12 mg）和不含防腐剂的吗啡（0.3 mg）。手术过程顺利，新生儿的 Apgar 评分在出生后 5 min 和 10 min 均为 9 分。产妇在恢复室观察 2 h 后转送回病房。术后 6 h，产妇静脉注射苯海拉明 50 mg 治疗全身瘙痒，术后 7 h，静脉注射异丙嗪 25 mg 治疗呕吐。术后 10 h，患者主诉仍有持续性瘙痒和呕吐，表明苯海拉明无效。

问题分析

定义

鞘内注射阿片类药物能够为术中和术后提供有效镇痛。阿片类药物和局部麻醉药通常联合使用以减少两者的用量，从而限制其副作用。由于单剂量吗啡可提供长达 24 h 的镇痛，通常选用吗啡进行鞘内注射。鞘内注射阿片类药物的副作用包括早期和晚期的呼吸抑制、恶心呕吐、瘙痒、镇静和尿潴留（表 88.1）。

早期的呼吸抑制发生在鞘内注射阿片类药物后的 2 h 内，并被认为是由于血管对药物的吸收和再分布所致。延迟性呼吸抑制通常发生在鞘内注射的 6 ～ 12 h，被认为是由于阿片类药物在脑脊液中向头侧扩散。同样，恶心呕吐也是由于脑脊液中的阿片类药物向头侧扩散刺激了第四脑室的极后区。镇静与脑脊液中阿片类药物扩散到丘脑、边缘系统和大脑皮质。二氧化碳麻醉的高碳酸血症可加重镇静。尿潴留是由于骶部副交感传出神经的排尿抑制，膀胱逼尿肌松弛并无法舒张尿道括约肌。

接受鞘内阿片类药物注射的患者经常发生全身或局部瘙痒。**瘙痒**是一种不愉快的感觉，患者想要或反射性地进行搔抓。它通常先出现在鼻子、眼睛和面部区域，可能与三叉神经脊束核中阿片类受体相对浓度较高有关。值得注意的是，与全身应用相比，这种情况更常见于硬膜外或鞘内注射。虽然其机制尚未完全了解，但不认为组胺释放是一个致病因素。

识别

患者鞘内注射阿片类药物最严重的并发症是呼

表 88.1　鞘内注射药物并发症的原因及治疗

并发症	原因	治疗
早期呼吸抑制	血管快速吸收和再分布	机械通气，纳洛酮
晚期呼吸抑制	脑脊液向头侧扩散至脑干呼吸中枢	机械通气，纳洛酮
瘙痒	未知（不可能是由于组胺释放）	纳洛酮，抗组胺药（存在争议），混合型阿片受体激动-拮抗剂
恶心呕吐	脑脊液向头侧扩散至第四脑室内的呕吐中枢或化学感受器触发区	纳洛酮，止吐药，氟哌利多，东莨菪碱透皮贴剂
尿潴留	抑制骶副交感神经的传出	纳洛酮（大剂量），留置导尿管
镇静	脑脊液向头侧扩散至丘脑、边缘系统或大脑皮质；高碳酸血症	纳洛酮

吸抑制，但具有临床意义的呼吸抑制少于 0.5%。瘙痒虽然不会威胁生命，但仍然是患者最常见的主诉，可引起患者的极度不适，其发生率在产后患者为 83%，而非妊娠患者为 69%。对患者而言，在某些情况下，产生的瘙痒可能比疼痛更加令人不适。

鞘内注射阿片类药物引起瘙痒的确切机制，目前虽然尚未完全阐明，但已有几种学说。其中一种学说指出，瘙痒和伤害感受器有关，并通过这种途径传导信号。伤害感受器和瘙痒都是由 C 纤维传导的，前列腺素能增强这种传导信号。鉴于 C 纤维的小直径无髓鞘属性，瘙痒和伤害性感受都可以通过体表摩擦得到缓解。这和疼痛的闸门学说相一致，认为当粗大有髓鞘的 Aβ 感觉纤维活动增强时能调节丘脑投射神经元，可减少由小直径无髓鞘的 C 纤维传导的伤害性（和潜在的瘙痒）刺激。另一种学说认为，脊髓背角上的伤害特异性神经元抑制了脊髓丘脑束上的瘙痒特异性神经元。我们可以发现随着痛觉的增加，瘙痒产生的抓痕明显减少。加用阿片类药物会减弱这种抑制，引起瘙痒感增加。其他学说还包括 5- 羟色胺通路学说，但其具体机制未知。目前发现，脊髓背角和延髓中的三叉神经脊髓束中含有高浓度的 μ 受体和 5- 羟色胺受体。三叉神经脊髓核被认为是对面部感觉传入进行整合的“瘙痒中心”。研究表明使用昂丹司琼和丙泊酚能缓解瘙痒，而它们对 5- 羟色胺通道的活性具有非常强烈的非竞争性抑制作用，结果支持这个学说。总而言之，目前尚没有一个统一的学说能够完全解释阿片类药物引起的瘙痒。

尽管有效预防和处理瘙痒仍颇具挑战，对治疗选择和已知作用机制的准确理解对于确保围术期患者最佳的满意度非常重要。

风险评估

慎重选择患者进行鞘内注射阿片类药物是非常重要的。应当与患者讨论关于出现瘙痒的可能性及患者对此副作用的耐受程度。产妇在鞘内注射阿片类药物后发生瘙痒的风险较高，发生率为 60% ～ 100%。相比之下，骨科患者的发生率为 30% ～ 60%。

脂溶性阿片类药物如芬太尼和鞘内注射吗啡相比瘙痒的持续时间较短，可能是因为前者的全身吸收增加。毫不奇怪，随着鞘内阿片类药物的剂量增加，瘙痒的发生率也会增加。鞘内同时使用局麻药能减少鞘内阿片类药物的用量，在获得合适的镇痛同时减少了瘙痒的严重程度。然而，鞘内使用肾上腺素可能通过局部血管收缩减少阿片类药物的全身吸收，使脑脊液中浓度增加而加重瘙痒。

管理

对椎管内阿片类药物引起瘙痒的治疗仍然是一项重大挑战，其主要目标是必须权衡这些药物的镇痛和瘙痒副作用。传统认为，抗组胺药能够用来治疗阿片类药物引起的瘙痒，然而，H_1 受体阻滞剂治疗中枢性瘙痒的作用有限。有时候，第一代抗组胺药的镇静副作用还会被误认为有改善症状作用。

多种药物已被证实可用来有效治疗阿片类药物引起的瘙痒，然而，其有效性和证据等级各不相同。这些包括阿片受体拮抗剂、混合型激动剂–拮抗剂、5- 羟色胺受体拮抗剂、非甾体抗炎药（nonsteroidal antiinflammatory drugs，NSAIDs）、丙泊酚和多巴胺受体拮抗剂。

有强有力的证据支持阿片受体拮抗剂，如纳洛酮。研究发现，由于纳洛酮相对半衰期较短，持续注射对预防其血浆浓度变化最有效。注射低剂量的纳洛酮 [<2 μg/（kg·h）] 能治疗瘙痒又不影响有效镇痛，效果非常理想。

混合型阿片受体激动–拮抗剂（如纳布啡、布托啡诺）已被证实对阿片类药物引起的瘙痒有效，但可能会增加镇静的风险。此外，对儿童瘙痒的治疗效果尚不明确。

也有研究表明静脉注射 5- 羟色胺受体拮抗剂如昂丹司琼（0.1 mg/kg）能减少鞘内阿片类药物引起瘙痒的程度和发生率。5- 羟色胺受体拮抗剂对鞘内注射亲脂性阿片类药物的效果较差。

有一些尚存争议的证据表明 NSAIDs 能够减少瘙痒，一项研究表明经直肠给予双氯芬酸治疗有效，而另一项研究则表明给予塞来昔布 200 mg 治疗无效。丙泊酚在治疗鞘内阿片类药物引起瘙痒的研究结果也不一致。

预防

预防阿片类药物引起的瘙痒应从鞘内注射阿片

类药物之时开始。使用辅助用药能够尽可能减少达到最佳镇痛效果时所需要的鞘内阿片类药物剂量。经常评估并采取多模式积极治疗以尽可能减少瘙痒的发生和严重程度。

（沈怡佳 译 熊源长 校）

延伸阅读

Andersen HH, Elberling J, Arendt-Nielsen L: Human surrogate models of histaminergic and non-histaminergic itch, *Acta Derm Venereol* 95:771–777, 2015.

Ballantyne JC, Loach AB, Carr DB: Itching after epidural and spinal opiates, *Pain* 33:149–160, 1988.

Borgeat A, Stirnemann HR: Ondansetron is effective to treat spinal or epidural morphine-induced pruritus, *Anesthesiology* 90:432–436, 1999.

Chaney MA: Side effects of intrathecal and epidural opioids, *Can J Anaesth* 42:891–903, 1995.

Colbert S, O'Hanlon DM, Galvin S, et al.: The effect of rectal diclofenac on pruritus in patients receiving intrathecal morphine, *Anaesthesia* 54:948–952, 1999.

Ganesh A, Maxwell LG: Pathophysiology and management of opioid-induced pruritus, *Drugs* 67:2323–2333, 2007.

Hindle A: Intrathecal opioids in the management of acute postoperative pain, *Contin Educ Anaesth Crit Care Pain* 8:81–85, 2008.

Kumar K, Singh SI: Neuraxial opioid-induced pruritus: an update, *J Anaesthesiol Clin Pharmacol* 29:303–307, 2013.

Lee LH, Irwin MG, Lim J, et al.: The effect of celecoxib on intrathecal morphine-induced pruritus in patients undergoing caesarean section, *Anaesthesia* 59:876–880, 2004.

Osenbach RK, Davis EA: Spinal cord stimulation for the treatment of chronic intractable pain. In Smith H, editor: *Current therapy in pain*, Philadelphia, 2009, Elsevier, pp 547–556.

Paus R, Schmelz M, Bíró T, et al.: Frontiers in pruritus research: scratching the brain for more effective itch therapy, *J Clin Invest* 116:1174–1186, 2006.

Rockford MA, DeRuyter ML: Perioperative epidural analgesia. In Smith H, editor: *Current therapy in pain*, Philadelphia, Elsevier, 2009, pp 78–84.

Szarvas S, Harmon D, Murphy D: Neuraxial opioid-induced pruritus: a review, *J Clin Anesth* 15:234–239, 2003.

Torn K, Tuominen M, Tarkkila P, et al.: Effects of sub-hypnotic doses of propofol on the side effects of intrathecal morphine, *Br J Anaesth* 73:411–412, 1994.

Warwick JP, Kearns CF, Scott WE: The effect of subhypnotic doses of propofol on the incidence of pruritus after intrathecal morphine for caesarean section, *Anaesthesia* 52:270–275, 1997.

第89章 氯胺酮

Madhuri S. Kurdi

病例概要

患者，女性，22岁，拟急诊行阑尾切除术。术前血流动力学稳定，给予脊椎麻醉。手术取腹部切口，入腹后，患者大叫疼痛，麻醉科医师予氯胺酮（2 mg/kg）静脉注射后让外科医师继续手术。推注剂量后不久，患者出现数秒钟的呼吸抑制和呼吸暂停，行间歇正压通气后缓解。一段时间后，手术医师抱怨腹肌紧张，无法继续手术，要求加深肌松。此时患者四肢紧绷、牙关紧闭、血压和心率略有上升。口腔出现分泌物。立即清除其口腔分泌物并静脉注射（静注）格隆溴铵（0.02 mg/kg），患者随之出现喉痉挛，氧饱和度下降。麻醉科医师给予静脉注射琥珀胆碱 1.5 mg/kg，并行气管插管，术中应用维库溴铵维持肌肉松弛。手术结束时给予肌松拮抗后拔除气管导管。患者进入苏醒室，交接班后不久，患者反复呈现面色潮红，出现咂嘴动作，腼腆地四周张望，并反复呼喊："什么？那是什么？你在哪儿？" 她的哭声给苏醒室所有工作人员及其他患者带来不安。而且她多次试图从手术车上起身，最后自行拔除鼻胃管并一阵呕吐。麻醉科医师和苏醒室医师立即静脉注射咪达唑仑（0.05 mg/kg）和昂丹司琼（0.15 mg/kg），才使其停止躁动。

问题分析

定义

氯胺酮是苯环利定的衍生物，具有多种药理学特点，包括分离麻醉、镇静、僵住、深度躯体镇痛、遗忘、支气管扩张和交感神经系统激活。氯胺酮临床应用广泛，包括术前镇静，单独作为麻醉药使用或者作为辅助用药、围术期镇痛药物、操作镇静中的镇静药物以及疼痛治疗中镇痛兼抗抑郁药物。虽然氯胺酮具有很好的安全性，但因其独特的不良反应也会引起一些并发症（表 89.1）。

识别

这一病例展示了氯胺酮应用的典型并发症：①心动过速和血压升高；②骨骼肌张力增高；③唾液分泌增加；④喉痉挛；⑤苏醒期反应现象；⑥恶心和呕吐。

心动过速和血压升高

注射氯胺酮可导致中枢介导性交感张力增加，促使肾上腺髓质释放儿茶酚胺，间接性引起心率增快、血压升高，但这种心动过速和高血压发作较短。如果患者未在术前使用镇静药物，术中使用临床剂量的氯胺酮可使心率增快约 15% ～ 25%，收缩压升高约 20 ～ 40 mmHg（相比麻醉前升高 10% ～ 50%），舒张压升高幅度略低。通常注射后 3 ～ 4 min 内血压稳定上升，随后 10 ～ 20 min 内下降至正常范围。

骨骼肌肌张力增加

氯胺酮静脉注射后初期症状最为明显，之后逐渐消失。

呼吸抑制 / 呼吸暂停

正常剂量的快速给药、非常规大剂量给药以及合用辅助性镇静药时可能发生呼吸抑制或暂停。由

表 89.1 氯胺酮的并发症

术中 / 输液期间	术后 / 停止输液后	长期和重复使用 / 致幻应用
血压和心率增加 口腔和气管支气管分泌物增多、喉痉挛、气道梗阻 骨骼肌肌张力增加（角弓反张、体位异常、肌阵挛）、无目的运动 ICP 和 IOP 轻微升高、癫痫发作、眼球震颤、短暂性复视 短暂性呼吸暂停、呼吸抑制、呃逆 危重症患者和严重应激患者应用大剂量氯胺酮时产生负性心血管效应（直接心脏抑制）	苏醒期反应 恶心、呕吐	出血性膀胱炎、肾积水、乳头坏死 腹部痛性痉挛（“K”型痉挛） 肝酶轻度短暂升高 神经认知障碍、记忆力和注意力受影响、情绪反应迟钝、语言能力受损 药物耐受 停药后戒断综合征伴精神障碍、药物依赖

ICP，颅内压；IOP，眼压

于中枢神经系统的药物浓度远超正常水平，快速静注氯胺酮 1 ～ 2 min 后可致一过性呼吸抑制。如果联合使用咪达唑仑，呼吸暂停的可能性更大。

喉痉挛

唾液分泌增加可导致喉痉挛。肌内注射（肌注）氯胺酮导致喉痉挛的发生率增加，尤其是儿童（上呼吸道感染、气道异常、气道手术操作的儿童），以及接受高剂量肌注的成人。虽然每次喉痉挛的发作时间较短，但其可能反复出现并很难处理。

恶心和呕吐

通常发生于苏醒期。此时，患者处于警醒状态，并可自行清理呼吸道。

苏醒期反应

因为氯胺酮会导致类似精神病的不良反应，使得麻醉苏醒较为复杂。这种苏醒反应是继发于氯胺酮对听觉和视觉中继核的抑制，从而对听觉和视觉产生了错误的感受或理解。苏醒反应的严重程度和类型不同，一般在数小时内消退。患者常见临床表现包括躁动、愉悦或不愉悦的幻觉、意识混乱、欣快、定向力障碍、感觉和知觉错觉、噩梦（术后 3 ～ 30 天）、谵妄、兴奋、攻击性行为、灵魂出窍感、感觉异常、短暂妄想、感觉有光穿透身体、彩色视觉、身体部分的形状或大小变形，关于身体一致性的新体验如感觉身体是由干木 / 塑料 / 泡沫橡胶制成的，与某人 / 环境融为一体，感觉精力充沛，有四处运动和与人交流的强烈冲动，单音节词的喃喃而语，肢体麻木感，失去时间和身份感，“傻笑”面容，带有疏远或隔阂感，消极主义，怀有敌意，以及重复性的运动行为。6.3% 的患者为轻度的复苏躁动，仅 1.4% 的患者具有临床意义。其鉴别诊断包括酒精性颤抖性谵妄，颅脑外伤引起的谵妄，老年人术后认知功能障碍、术后谵妄、阿托品引起的谵妄，以及儿童因七氟烷、异氟烷、地氟烷引起的术后谵妄。

风险评估

麻醉剂量氯胺酮能引起血流动力学改变，但亚麻醉剂量下这种改变无法测量。唾液分泌的增加在儿童中和大剂量使用时尤为明显。氯胺酮相关的喉痉挛和呼吸抑制或暂停为短暂性，在儿童中的发生率分别为 0.3% 和 0.8%。与儿童相比，成人使用氯胺酮的呕吐发生率更高（5% ～ 15%），青春期早期是呕吐发生的高峰年龄。大剂量静脉注射、麻醉剂量和肌注常与呕吐的高发生率相关。苏醒期反应的发生率为 3% ～ 100%，儿童为 5% ～ 15%，其中 15 ～ 65 岁的成人患者发生率约 30% ～ 50%，女性高于男性。口服氯胺酮较少出现苏醒期反应。患有精神病和已确诊为精神分裂症的患者精神反应发生率较高。氯胺酮的精神症状存在量效关系。当静脉注射剂量大于 0.3 mg/kg 时，拟精神疾病症状增加。术中出现高碳酸血症，更易加重颅内压（intracranial pressure，ICP）和眼内压（intraocular pressure，IOP）升高等并发症。任何剂量的氯胺酮均可发生眼球震颤和复视。据文献报道，在健康和癫痫患者中作为术前用药或者麻醉诱导药静注或肌注氯胺酮均可诱发癫痫。然而，氯胺酮不仅能诱发癫痫也有抗惊厥作用。

启示

氯胺酮的心血管刺激作用可导致：气管插管对

血流动力学的不良反应增加；影响术中控制性低血压，特别是在给药后的 15 min 内；术野受到严重影响；舌血管瘤出现威胁生命的充血，继而阻塞气道；合并高血压、心血管疾病和血管内动脉瘤的患者产生灾难性影响。氯胺酮给药后肌张力增加，增加外科医师的手术难度，特别是腹腔和胸腔手术。氯胺酮导致的唾液分泌增加可引起喉痉挛和气道阻塞，使得气管导管固定困难，并影响纤支镜插管时的视野。有时临床医师会把患者无目的的肢体运动、肌肉僵硬、心率和血压升高、唾液分泌增加和喉痉挛误诊为麻醉过浅，而加大氯胺酮的使用剂量，这会进一步加重并发症的发生。由于氯胺酮有时会影响气道通畅和导致呕吐，应避免用于俯卧位和饱胃的患者。氯胺酮可增高眼压，产生眼球震颤现象，故应禁用于青光眼和开放性眼外伤患者。无论对患者本身还是麻醉科医师、外科医师、苏醒室医师、相邻患者和其他亲属，苏醒期反应都会让他们感到恐惧和不安，并可能对手术部位和引流管造成损害。

管理

在临床中，氯胺酮耐受性良好。大多数并发症为短暂发作并可有效处理（表 89.2）。

表 89.2 氯胺酮引起的并发症的预防和控制

并发症	预防	管理
心动过速和血压升高	• 丙泊酚、咪达唑仑、右美托咪定、可乐定、β 受体阻滞剂、吸入麻醉剂与低剂量氯胺酮联合给药 • 适量的地西泮、咪达唑仑、阿片类药物-东莨菪碱合剂 • 使用连续氯胺酮微量输注	• 通常短暂 • 如果棘手，注射 β 受体阻滞剂（如 IV 美托洛尔）或增加麻醉药剂量，如七氟烷、地氟烷、氟烷、丙泊酚、右美托咪定
唾液分泌增加	• 预防性应用阿托品 20 μg/kg 术前 30 min IM 或诱导时 IV 阿托品 10 ～ 20 μg/kg 或格隆溴铵 0.004 mg/kg	• 吸引 • 止涎剂，如静注阿托品 0.02 mg/kg，格隆溴铵 0.01 ～ 0.02 mg/kg
喉痉挛和气道阻塞	• 减少 / 预防分泌物 • 避免 3 个月以下儿童单纯使用氯胺酮 /URTI 患者 / 机械性刺激咽部的操作 • 避免大剂量 IM	• 给予纯氧，注射琥珀胆碱并辅助通气
呼吸抑制 / 暂停	• 在 60 s 内缓慢注射氯胺酮	• 呼吸囊面罩加压增加氧合
恶心和呕吐	• 同时应用丙泊酚 • 甲氧氯普胺 / 昂丹司琼	• IV 昂丹司琼 0.1 mg/kg，IV 甲氧氯普胺 0.1 mg/kg
苏醒期反应现象	• 术前静脉注射咪达唑仑（0.03 mg/kg）、异丙嗪、氟哌啶醇、阿片类药物、阿片类药物与东莨菪碱合剂、阿片类药物与氟哌利多合剂 • 避免快速应用大剂量的氯胺酮 • 使患者在光线柔和、安静的环境下苏醒 • 麻醉方案含有丙泊酚、硫喷妥钠、吸入麻醉药、右美托咪定 • 选择合适的患者、对潜在并发症提前进行讨论并提出积极的建议 • 使用 *S*（+）氯胺酮 • IV 咪达唑仑 0.07 mg/kg，直至麻醉结束	• 滴定给予苯二氮䓬类药物如咪达唑仑、地西泮、劳拉西泮 • 如果长期应用氯胺酮，口服、皮下注射氟哌啶醇或皮下咪达唑仑 • 小剂量的硫喷妥钠 • 拉莫三嗪 • 通常在几小时内消退；偶尔 24 h 后复发
颅内压升高（ICP）	• 避免在 ICP 升高和自主通气的人群中使用	• 实施控制通气 / 过度通气
惊厥	• 始终术前预先或术中同时给予苯二氮䓬类药物如咪达唑仑、地西泮	• 停止使用氯胺酮 • 给予 IV 苯二氮䓬类药物 / 巴比妥酸盐
肌张力亢进	• 同时使用苯二氮䓬类药物 • 避免在腹部、胸腔内手术中作为唯一的麻醉剂	• 给予 IV 肌肉松弛剂和 IPPV • IV 咪达唑仑 0.05 mg/kg

IPPV，间歇正压通气；URTI，上呼吸道感染；IM，肌注；IV，静注

预防

如果对患者和手术操作仔细选择，对患者进行合理的监测，由麻醉科医师给药，滴定给药以减少用药量，并合理应用预防性药物（如格隆溴铵）和苯二氮䓬类药物如咪达唑仑（表 89.2），则可减少氯胺酮诱导的并发症。

（阮林星　译　李晓菲　校）

延伸阅读

Baduni N, Sanwal MK, Jain A, et al.: Recurrent episodes of intractable laryngospasm followed by laryngeal and pulmonary oedema during dissociative anaesthesia with intravenous ketamine, *Indian J Anaesth* 54:364–365, 2010.

Cromhout A: Ketamine: its use in the emergency department, *Emerg Med* 15:155–159, 2003.

Dolansky G, Shah A, Mosdossy G, et al.: What is the evidence for the safety and efficacy of using ketamine in children? *Paed Child Health* 13:307–308, 2008.

Dundee JW, Wyant GM: Ketamine. In *Intravenous anaesthesia*, New York, 1988, Churchill Livingstone, pp 135–159.

Gorlin AW, Rosenfeld DM, Ramakrishna H: Intravenous sub-anaesthetic ketamine for perioperative analgesia, *J Anesthesiol Clin Pharmacol* 32:160–167, 2016.

Green SM, Roback MG, Kennedy RM, et al.: Clinical practice guideline for emergency department ketamine dissociative sedation: 2011 update, *Ann Emerg Med* 57:449–461, 2011.

Jaap V, Elske S, Marije R: Intravenous anesthetics. In Miller RD, Cohen NH, Eriksson LI, et al., editors: *Miller's anesthesia*, Philadelphia, 2015, Elsevier, pp 821–914.

Kolawole IK: Ketamine hydrochloride: a useful but frequently misused drug, *Niger J Surg Res* 3:118–125, 2001.

Kurdi MS, Theerth KA, Deva RS: Ketamine: current applications in anesthesia, pain, and critical care, *Anesth Essays Res* 8:283–290, 2014.

Niesters M, Martini C, Dahan A: Ketamine for chronic pain: risks and benefits, *Br J Clin Pharmacol* 77:357–367, 2014.

Rewari V, Ramachandran R: Ketamine: present status in anesthesia practice. In Sehgal R, Trikha A, editors: *Yearbook of anesthesiology—5*, New Delhi, 2016, Jaypee Brothers Medical Publishers(P) Ltd, pp 170–180.

第 90 章 镁

Richard C. Month

病例概要

患者，女性，23 岁，孕 34 周 3 天，重度先兆子痫，紧急送往手术室在全身麻醉下行剖宫产术。该患者术前正在输注镁剂治疗先兆子痫。常规使用丙泊酚和罗库溴铵快速序贯诱导后，顺利分娩，45 min 后患者仍持续处于深度肌松状态（4 个成串刺激 0/4，无强直后易化）。在手术室等待 30 min，无任何改善，患者带气管导管回到 ICU，6 h 后拔管。

问题分析

定义

镁平衡

镁是人体内含量第四丰富的阳离子，总量约 2000 mEq。正常血清镁（Mg^{2+}）浓度介于 1.4 ～ 2.1 mEq/L 之间，相当于 1.7 ～ 2.5 mg/dl（单位换算见表 90.1）；然而，血清 Mg^{2+} 浓度与全身总贮量之间的相关性较差，仅占不到总量的 1%。十二指肠和空肠是 Mg^{2+} 的主要吸收部位（每天 8 ～ 9 mEq）。通过胃肠道分泌从体内流失的 Mg^{2+} 相对恒定（每天 2 mEq）。相反，由于近端肾小管和髓袢（亨利袢）能重吸收 Mg^{2+}，在低镁血症时，肾显著影响 Mg^{2+} 的丢失。

细胞内的作用

镁是许多重要的细胞酶（如腺苷酸环化酶、Na^+，K^+-ATP 酶）的关键辅助因子。此外，镁化合物与三磷酸腺苷可作为调节肌肉收缩和松弛的酶促反应的底物。镁还通过拮抗钙和调节几种钾电流来调节细胞功能（框 90.1）

表 90.1　镁化合物和血清浓度的单位转换

化合物	单位转换
硫酸镁（$MgSO_4$）	1 g=8.13 mEq Mg^{2+}
氧化镁（MgO）	1 g=46 mEq Mg^{2+}
醋酸镁（$MgC_4H_6O_4$）	1 g=9.35 mEq Mg^{2+}
氯化镁（$MgCl_2$）	1 g=9.75 mEq Mg^{2+}
血清浓度（所有化合物）	1 mg/dl=0.83 mEq/L=0.415 mmol/L

血清 Mg^{2+} 浓度的变化影响多个器官系统。例如，高镁血症时通过直接与 Ca^{2+} 竞争来抑制平滑肌收缩，增加前列环素的释放，降低交感神经刺激后儿茶酚胺的释放，从而引起血管平滑肌松弛。在运动神经肌肉连接处，Mg^{2+} 的增加抑制突触前 Ca^{2+} 释放，从而抑制乙酰胆碱释放，进而降低了肌纤维膜的兴奋性。在心脏中，Mg^{2+} 的减少抑制自律性和房室传导来减慢心率。高镁血症还降低了早期后除极的幅度，以对抗触发性心律失常（见下文）。在大脑中，增加的 Mg^{2+} 通过阻断与 *N*- 甲基 -D- 天冬氨酸（*N*-methyl-d-aspartate，NMDA）受体相关的神经元钙通道起到抗惊厥作用。

治疗作用

镁的输注可以治疗触发性室性心律失常。心脏手术中也可作为心房颤动的辅助治疗，早产时作为

框 90.1　镁对细胞功能的影响机制

Ca^{2+} 拮抗

调控肌质网对 Ca^{2+} 的处理

通过细胞膜通道抑制 Ca^{2+} 流入肌细胞

调节第二信使系统（即腺苷酸环化酶–腺苷单磷酸）

与 Ca^{2+} 竞争肌动蛋白上的高亲和力位点

K^+ 电流

提高 Na^+，K^+-ATP 酶的功能

阻断外向 K^+ 电流，导致内向矫正 K^+ 电流增加

介导内向整流特性

保胎药，并可预防先兆子痫发作。

通过静脉注射镁，使血清 Mg^{2+} 浓度加倍，可减少低镁血症时的自律性或触发性室性心律失常（如尖端扭转性室速、洋地黄室性心律失常）的发作频率。这种输注可能会增加内向整流钾电流，以降低早期后除极的振幅，后者是尖端扭转性室速的触发因素。镁对洋地黄引起的室性心律失常的作用机制包括：改善 Na^+，K^+-ATP 酶功能，以及降低由于细胞内 Ca^{2+} 升高导致的延迟后去极化幅度。然而，大多数室性心律失常都是传导折返所致，静脉注射镁效果不明显。相反，术前 β 受体阻滞剂和钙通道拮抗剂辅以镁治疗可减少心脏术后患者心房颤动的发生。心肺转流引起的血液稀释和利尿剂治疗可导致低镁血症。

提高血清 Mg^{2+} 浓度已广泛应用于产科。血清镁水平增加 4 ～ 6 mEq/L 时可直接松弛平滑肌减少子宫活动。此外，镁输注是治疗先兆子痫的首选方法，因为镁输注可降低全身血管阻力（通过抑制血管平滑肌收缩和减少交感刺激后儿茶酚胺释放），并降低癫痫发作的风险（通过抑制 NMDA 受体和通过增加血流避免局部缺血）。最后，镁在有早产风险的患者中，被用于神经保护和避免胎儿脑瘫。

识别

低镁血症

血清 Mg^{2+} 浓度的变化通常易被忽略，它与其他血清电解质一起发生变化，如钙和钾。低镁血症最好的诊断方法是了解与之相关的病情（如长期酗酒、利尿剂或洋地黄疗法）。仅仅是低镁血症不会导致心电图改变；但与之相关的钙和钾的紊乱可能会导致这种改变。

高镁血症

使用镁剂与出现不良反应的时间相关性通常可诊断高镁血症。消化道疾病患者会导致镁吸收增加，肾功能不全导致镁排泄减少，大剂量的泻药、抗酸剂或含镁盐的镇痛剂可能导致显著的高镁血症。在这些情况下，镁给药时间的相关性往往不甚明显。

高镁血症也可以通过其不良反应的逐步发展模式来诊断，然后通过血清 Mg^{2+} 的测量来确认。高镁血症可产生以下副作用：

- 全身血管扩张；
- 嗜睡；
- 肌肉无力；
- 呼吸抑制；
- 窦性心动过缓；
- 房室传导阻滞；
- 心脏停搏。

表 90.2 列出了高镁血症的常见副作用以及这些副作用首次出现时血清 Mg^{2+} 的相关浓度。值得注意的是，根据相关代谢紊乱的不同，特定个体出现明显不良反应时的血清浓度会有所不同。

风险评估

低镁血症

低镁血症的发生率在怀疑有血清电解质异常的人中为 470/1000。在接受利尿剂和洋地黄治疗的充血性心力衰竭患者中占 7% ～ 37%。在酗酒者中占 30% ～ 40%。

高镁血症

高镁血症的发生率在怀疑有血清电解质异常的人中为 57/1000。肾可显著降低镁的再吸收，因此在镁持续输注治疗心律失常、宫缩或先兆子痫时呼吸和心脏骤停非常罕见。为防止高镁血症的副作用，

表 90.2　血清镁浓度与全身效应的关系

浓度（mEq/L）	全身效应
<0.8	心律失常可能对治疗无效 与低钙血症相关时：定向障碍、肌肉抽搐、舞蹈运动、癫痫发作
1.4 ～ 2.1	正常范围
3 ～ 4	潮红 P-R 间期增加 7% ～ 13% QRS 增宽 0% ～ 11% Q-T 间期无改变
5 ～ 6	血压轻微下降 心率轻度增加 FEV_1 和 FVC 下降 10%
10	适应和会聚反射减弱而导致的视力模糊
20	呼吸停止 房室传导阻滞 进行性 QRS 增宽和心动过缓
>25	心脏停搏

FEV_1，第 1 秒用力呼吸容积；FVC，用力肺活量

肾功能不全的患者最好避免服用镁。

启示

镁缺乏所致的自律性或触发性活性增加，显然有必要补充镁剂。输注镁降低急性心肌梗死的风险仍有争议，目前仍在研究中。镁用于早产安胎似乎是 β 受体交感神经疗法的一种安全替代方法，尽管可能无效。与苯妥英钠相比，镁在预防先兆子痫孕妇癫痫方面更有效。非去极化肌肉松弛药通过减少释放至运动终板的乙酰胆碱，与镁发挥协同作用。

管理

识别低镁血症和高镁血症是治疗的关键。低镁血症可通过口服或胃肠外治疗。表 90.1 给出了用于治疗低镁血症的各种含镁制剂的元素含量。对于肾功能正常的患者，可以在 30 min 至 1 h 内静脉注射 16 ～ 32 mEq 的硫酸镁进行快速纠正，或 8 ～ 24 h 进行缓慢纠正。

由于血清 Mg^{2+} 含量不到身体总镁储存量的 1%，低镁血症患者需要多次给予镁剂以补充全身储备。相反，高镁血症的治疗包括：

- 去除所有潜在的体外镁的来源；
- 当患者呼吸停止时，予以插管和通气支持；
- 予以呋塞米和无镁盐溶液，增加肾镁排泄量；
- 氯化钙（5 ～ 10 mEq，每 5 ～ 10 min）对抗高镁血症；
- 使用含镁量低的透析液进行透析。

预防

对高镁血症最好的预防方法是不给肾衰竭患者提供含镁盐或化合物。含镁化合物包括：

- 泻药（如枸橼酸镁）；
- 抗酸剂（如氧化镁）；
- 止痛药（如缓释阿司匹林）；
- 镁补充剂。

在给有胃肠道紊乱（如麻痹性肠梗阻、溃疡性结肠炎、十二指肠溃疡穿孔）的患者使用泻药期间，可能会发生大量的镁吸收。

（李路路 译 李 博 校）

延伸阅读

Dube L, Granry JC: The therapeutic use of magnesium in anesthesiology, intensive care and emergency medicine: a review, *Can J Anaesth* 50: 732–746, 2003.

Ducceschi V, Di Micco G, Sarubbi B, et al.: Ionic mechanisms of ischemia-related ventricular arrhythmias, *Clin Cardiol* 19:325–331, 1996.

Euser AG, Cipolla MJ: Magnesium sulfate for the treatment of eclampsia: a brief review, *Stroke* 40:1169–1175, 2009.

Hazelrigg SR, Boley TM, Cetindag IB, et al.: The efficacy of supplemental magnesium in reducing atrial fibrillation after coronary artery bypass grafting, *Ann Thorac Surg* 77:824–830, 2004.

Kelepouris E, Agus ZS: Hypomagnesemia: renal magnesium handling, *Semin Nephrol* 18:58–73, 1998.

Surawicz B: The interrelationship of electrolyte abnormalities and arrhythmias. In Mandel WJ, editor: *Cardiac arrhythmias: their mechanisms, diagnosis, and management*, Philadelphia, 1995, JB Lippincott, pp 89–109.

磁共振成像

第91章

Herodotos Ellinas

病例概要

患儿，4岁男孩，恶心、呕吐、持续10日伴中耳炎发作，需行头颅磁共振成像（magnetic resonance imaging，MRI）来评估可能的颅内病变。麻醉科医师被请求会诊以评估和协助实施麻醉。

病例分析

定义

MRI是一种无创性的诊断成像方式，可以产生精确的人体影像。它没有电离辐射，本身不产生任何已知的生物学损害。MRI成像原理是：原子核在强磁场中吸收射频能量脉冲，然后这些脉冲以无线电波的形式发射出来，再重新生成计算机处理后的影像。磁场强度一般在0.2～3 tesla（T）之间，虽然最高可达7 T（磁场强度7 T目前用于研究目的）。但在获得多层图像时，要求患者在一个小空间内静止不动。MRI比计算机断层扫描需要更长的时间成像，因此，患者的任何动作都会降低图像质量。事实上，患者位置的变化都会影响扫描磁场的均匀性，检查可能需要45 min到2 h，单序列需要3～10 min。扫描时噪音大，空间受限，无法活动，部分患者产生幽闭恐惧症。也有患者出现局部或全身体温升高，磁场强度可能会导致意外伤害。

MRI工作区域分为4块，根据核磁周围强度与安全性划分：

1. 区Ⅰ—公众自由出入区域；
2. 区Ⅱ—接待区，由磁共振室员工监督管理；
3. 区Ⅲ—限制区，仅限部分公共和员工出入；
4. 区Ⅳ—磁共振检查区。

识别

成年患者和大部分6岁以上的儿童在接受MRI检查时都能配合且平卧。耳机和音乐的应用使MRI成像成为耐受性较好的操作。然而，一些特定患者可能需要麻醉才能完成检查（框91.1）。

风险评估

框91.2列出了MRI检查常见的一些禁忌证。它们或与磁铁作用引起磁化物体移动或温度升高有关，或与射频脉冲和磁梯度产生感应电流有关。强磁场对未出生胎儿的影响尚不清楚，但已有报道阐述了对其听力损害和致畸性的担忧。根据患者的病情，除非有绝对适应证，医生应避免在妊娠早期对患者进行MRI检查。MRI扫描可能对永久性彩妆和文身

框91.1 磁共振成像镇静/全身麻醉适应证

- 极幼小、焦虑/躁动不安的患者
- 口服抗焦虑药失败的患者
- 幽闭恐惧症的患者
- 有严重并存疾病的患者（如阻塞性睡眠呼吸暂停、胃食管反流病）
- 长期研究（需多次扫描）
- ICU患者

框91.2 磁共振成像的绝对禁忌证或相对禁忌证

- 动脉瘤夹
- 心脏起搏器[a]
- 植入心律转复除颤器（ICD）[a]
- 植入人工耳蜗[a]
- 植入电子设备（如胰岛素泵）
- 硬膜外导管（某些为MRI专用如Flex Tip plus）[a]
- 植入金属假体且接近重要器官
- 神经刺激器[a]
- 阴茎假体
- 节育装置

[a] 关于MRI安全性的产品类别，咨询设备生产商

患者造成皮肤刺痛、烧伤和肿胀。

因为患者处在一个狭小空间，空间视野受限，麻醉风险也增加。胃食管反流病、癫痫发作或颅内压升高会影响麻醉药物的选择。其他可能出现的问题列于框 91.3。

启示

监视器必须适合在 MRI 检查室中使用。它们应为非铁磁性，且电缆能屏蔽电磁干扰（光纤比较理想）。为了避免影响图像质量的射频干扰，需要对信号进行滤波。尽管有专门的技术，一些问题仍然存在（表 91.1）。

所有的麻醉设备，包括脉搏血氧仪、静脉输液杆、麻醉转运车，也应该为非铁磁性。已有 MRI 适用的麻醉机、喉镜（锂电池）和听诊器可供使用。任何带有变压器的设备都必须远离磁场。气瓶必须为铝质。如果实施吸入麻醉，则应采用合适的气体回收系统。MRI 适用的蒸发罐可能含有少量的铁磁材料，须安装在麻醉机或呼吸机上，否则不应带入 MRI 检查室。磁场强度大于 5 高斯（标记在 MRI 检查室地板上）的区域周围不应包含任何含铁磁性物体。

框 91.3　与磁共振成像相关的潜在问题

- 麻醉设备故障
- 监测设备故障
- 麻醉设备干扰图像质量
- 固定不牢的铁磁性物体高速抛射损害
- 电子设备故障
- 肾性系统纤维化（急性或严重肾功能不全患者）

表 91.1　磁共振成像中的监测问题

监测	问题
心电图	T 波和 ST 段经常改变，MRI 扫描周期缺乏定性信息；心电图电线可能引起烧伤；为了避免烧伤，需要特殊的心电图电极
血氧饱和度	故障；探头升温可能引起烧伤；使用光纤连接患者最为理想
二氧化碳分析	需要较长的管路，导致二氧化碳波形出现长时间的上抬，实时测量有所延迟，呼吸速率和趋势仍然有用
体温	需要光纤传感器
血压	无创：应选用塑料接头连接袖带和软管 有创：使用光纤系统和不含铁的传感器进行测压

管理

与任何麻醉诱导一样，麻醉实施流程应遵守美国麻醉科医师协会监测标准。为避免监测导线出现问题，建议尽可能将导线放置靠近 MRI 磁场长轴正中。监护仪及导线也应该放置在患者身边距离磁场最远处，避免导线缠绕或交叉。具体麻醉方法取决于患者的年龄和并存疾病（框 91.4）。

蒸发罐可在 MRI 环境中正常使用。采用新型非铁磁性的静脉输液泵可在 5 高斯磁场强度下正常使用，并可在控制室进行远程监测。含铁磁的输液泵可以配合加长输液管使用。

通常患者需要使用造影剂（钆），由于造影剂诱发肾性系统纤维化的风险高，急性或严重肾功能不全的患者应谨慎使用。

如果患者来自 ICU，必须特别小心，确保所有导线和传感器都经过严格屏蔽，含铁磁性物体都被移除（例如 Foley 导尿管夹）。电线应拉直以防止灼伤。如果发生心脏停搏，应立即启动心肺复苏，并将患者从磁场中移出，转运至配备有复苏设备的指定区域。复苏小组成员必须保证在Ⅳ区外（磁共振检查区以外），以避免磁场意外开启，造成抛掷物带

框 91.4　磁共振成像的麻醉选择

小儿镇静

水合氯醛口服剂量（儿童 <3 岁），75 ～ 100 mg/kg，适合 1 h 左右的检查

右美托咪定单次静推：1 μg/kg，维持 1 ～ 2 μg/(kg·h)

戊巴比妥静注：2.5 ～ 5 mg/kg（最大单次剂量 100 mg）

丙泊酚单次静注：2 ～ 3 mg/kg，静脉维持 150 ～ 200 μg/（kg·min）

苯二氮䓬类药物用于成人镇静和抗焦虑

咪达唑仑、劳拉西泮或地西泮口服或静脉注射

适用于合并内科疾病较少，气道易于控制的患者

苏醒迅速；恶心或呕吐极少发生

气管插管全身麻醉

吸入麻醉或丙泊酚输注

适合年龄极小患者或胃食管反流病、饱胃或颅内压升高患者

喉罩通气保留自主呼吸的全身麻醉

吸入麻醉或丙泊酚输注

来人员损伤。

如果发生火灾或意外或者有意关闭磁场，应遵循规程，避免对患者和工作人员造成伤害，关闭核磁扫描仪可能会生成氦和产生高温，导致磁共振室内火灾和可能发生窒息。

预防

为了防止 MRI 检查室的并发症，必须了解 MRI 禁忌证（框 91.2）。影像科和麻醉科医师从一开始就可用的麻醉和监测设备进行充分沟通，对于预评估高危患者至关重要。参与 MRI 检查的麻醉科医师应意识到在这个独特的环境中可能出现的所有潜在的技术问题，应基于现有指南进行安全教育，并根据技术的进步持续改进。

致谢

感谢 Hind M. Gautam 博士和 Christopher M.B 博士对本章上一版的贡献。

（徐 航 译 吴 倩 校）

延伸阅读

American Society of Anesthesiologists: Practice advisory on anesthetic care for magnetic resonance imaging: an updated report by the American Society of Anesthesiologists Task Force on Anesthetic Care for Magnetic Resonance Imaging, *Anesthesiology* 122:495–520, 2015.

Bulas D, Egloff A: Benefits and risks of MRI in pregnancy, *Semin Perinatol* 37:301–304, 2013.

Dempsey MF, Condon B: Thermal injuries associated with MRI, *Clin Radiol* 56:457–465, 2001.

Dill T: Contraindications to magnetic resonance imaging, *Heart* 94:943–948, 2008.

Henrichs B, Walsh RP: Intraoperative MRI for neurosurgical and general surgical interventions, *Curr Opin Anesthesiol* 27:228–252, 2014.

The Joint Commission: Preventing accidents and injuries in the MRI suite. Issue 38, 2008.

Kaplan RF, Cravero JP, Yaster M, et al.: Sedation for diagnostic and therapeutic procedures outside the operating room. In Coté CJ, Lerman J, Anderson BJ, editors: *A practice of anesthesia for infants and children*, ed 5, Philadelphia, 2013, Elsevier, pp 993–1013.

The Medicines and Healthcare Products Regulatory Agency (MHRA): DB2007(03), Dec 2007.

Menon DK, Peden CJ, Hall AS, et al.: Magnetic resonance for the anaesthetist. Part I. Physical principles, applications, safety aspects, *Anaesthesia* 47:240–255, 1992.

Nazarian S, Hansford R, Roquin A, et al.: A prospective evaluation of a protocol for magnetic resonance imaging of patients with implanted cardiac devices, *Ann Intern Med* 155:415–424, 2011.

Peden CJ, Menon DK, Hall AS, et al.: Magnetic resonance for the anaesthetist. Part II. Anaesthesia and monitoring in MR units, *Anaesthesia* 47:508–516, 1992.

Zimmer C, Janssen MN, Treschan TA, et al.: Near-miss accident during magnetic resonance imaging by a “flying sevoflurane vaporizer” due to ferromagnetism undetected by handheld magnet, *Anesthesiology* 100:1329–1330, 2004.

第 92 章 肌肉松弛药

Constance L. Monitto

病例概要

患者，男性，2 岁，接受腹股沟疝修补术。在使用氧气、氧化亚氮和七氟烷吸入诱导期间，发生了喉痉挛，随即在肌内注射琥珀胆碱治疗。之后在心电监护仪上观察到宽 QRS 波的心动过速。

问题分析

定义

所有神经肌肉松弛药都可能引起并发症；然而，琥珀胆碱（succinylcholine，SCh）导致严重并发症的可能性最大。尽管这些并发症限制了其常规应用，但因其无与伦比的起效速度、短暂的作用时间以及在尚未获得静脉通道时可经肌肉给药等特点，在小儿麻醉中仍发挥着作用。这些特性保证了其在紧急插管和保守处理无效的喉痉挛治疗中的有效性。

与儿童使用 SCh 相关的显著并发症包括：

- 心律失常；
- 胃内压、眼内压和颅内压升高；
- 横纹肌溶解和肌红蛋白血症；
- 非预期的作用时间延长；
- 咬肌痉挛；
- 恶性高热（见第 195 章）。

非去极化肌松药（nondepolarizing muscle relaxants，NDMRs）按化学结构通常分为氨基甾体类（如泮库溴铵、维库溴铵、罗库溴铵、瑞库溴铵）或苄异喹啉类化合物（如右旋筒箭毒碱、美维库铵、阿曲库铵、顺阿曲库铵）。NDMRs 的并发症包括严重肌无力和肌肉松弛残余导致的呼吸功能障碍（见第 95 章）。曾有报道在重症监护病房长期输注氨基甾体类肌肉松弛药后发生长期肌病。还观察到危及生命的过敏反应和支气管痉挛。然而，NDMRs 最常见的副作用是组胺释放、胆碱能效应和毒蕈碱样效应。这些反应均不是小儿患者所特有的。

识别

去极化肌肉松弛药

尽管十甲季铵是 20 世纪 40 年代末引入临床的第一种去极化肌肉松弛药，但它已不再用于临床患者，因此本次讨论仅限于 SCh。由于琥珀胆碱在结构上与连接在一起的两个乙酰胆碱分子相似，所以它初期会激活神经肌肉接头处的乙酰胆碱受体。随后，尽管乙酰胆碱增加，但琥珀胆碱依然占据着这些受体，直到其从受体解离后被局部假性胆碱酯酶水解。

使用 SCh 后患者常出现心律失常，最常见的是窦性心动过缓或交界性心律。心动过缓是因 SCh 同乙酰胆碱一样会引起心脏的副交感神经兴奋。婴儿和儿童的心排血量很大程度上依赖于心率，这种窦性心动过缓会导致婴儿和儿童显著的低血压。同样对于依赖心房按时收缩以增加心室充盈的患者（如肥厚型、扩张型、限制型心肌病或致心律失常性右心室发育不良；见第 39 章），这种交界性节律也会造成显著影响。此外，在所有年龄的患者中均报道了 SCh 给药后出现的心脏停搏。危及生命的室性心律失常提示存在严重的横纹肌溶解、高钾血症或恶性高热，但是发生率较低。

琥珀胆碱可引起胃内、眼内和颅内压的升高，这是由于肌肉筋膜收缩、脑血流和代谢升高所致。

给药后，相当比例的儿童中可检测到横纹肌溶解和肌红蛋白血症。虽然有些患者可检测到肌红蛋白尿，但在绝大多数情况下，SCh 导致的横纹肌溶解预后良好。然而，在高危人群中，包括先天性肌肉疾病或对恶性高热敏感的患者，由于相关的电解质紊乱、肾衰竭或弥散性血管内凝血，SCh 导致的横纹肌溶解可能危及生命。

丁酰胆碱酯酶基因杂合子或纯合子遗传异常（假性胆碱酯酶缺乏）的患者接受 SCh 后，可能会发生神经肌肉阻滞作用的延长（见第 98 章）。由于短效非去极化肌松药美维库铵（不再在美国销售）也通过丁酰胆碱酯酶代谢，因此使用它也可能发生这种反应。

咬肌痉挛（或牙关紧闭）的特点是咬肌张力过度增加，导致给予 SCh 后不能张口。详细的调查表明，咬肌张力通常会在给予 SCh 后上升。因此，牙关紧闭可能代表了一种给予正常剂量 SCh 的极端的情况。因此，单凭咬肌强直不能诊断恶性高热。第 195 章讨论了恶性高热的识别和处理。

非去极化肌肉松弛药

术中对神经肌肉阻滞剂过敏是一种罕见但严重的并发症。尽管有时很难诊断，但临床症状包括：用药后出现潮红、低血压、心动过速和支气管痉挛。

某些苄异喹啉类肌肉松弛药会引起组胺释放，表现为皮肤潮红、低血压和心动过速。另外泮库溴铵可引起心率增快和血压升高，这与其阻断毒蕈碱 M_2 受体迷走作用相关，也与阻断神经元再摄取去甲肾上腺素相关。

1999 年，在临床实践中引入氨基甾体类 NDMRs 瑞库溴铵后，报告了危及生命的支气管痉挛发作，其特征为严重的通气困难和无法测出的呼气末二氧化碳，以及一些因不可逆的支气管痉挛而导致的死亡。随后的实验室研究表明，临床相关浓度的瑞库溴铵可能会因毒蕈碱样气道效应导致支气管痉挛，2001 年该药撤市，距 FDA 批准该药上市还不到 2 年。

风险评估

琥珀胆碱

迷走神经介导的心律失常，包括窦性或房室交界区性心动过缓、窦性停搏和一过性心搏停止，可发生于多达 40% ～ 60% 的儿童单次静脉给予 SCh 后，但很少发生在肌内注射后。与成人一样，重复给药可能导致更频繁和更严重的缓慢性心律失常。

急性或进行性去神经损伤（如脊髓横断、周围神经病变、脑卒中）、广泛的组织损伤（如烧伤、挤压伤）、长时间制动或神经肌肉疾病的患者，由于钾释放过多，可导致恶性室性心律失常，甚至给予 SCh 后出现心脏停搏。这些疾病与神经肌肉接头外乙酰胆碱受体数量的增加有关。患者的许多情况在麻醉诱导前就已明确，但患有进行性神经肌肉疾病的男孩而言并不总是如此。例如，杜氏肌营养不良影响了大约 1/3600 男孩。虽然男女均可携带该突变的致病基因，但由于其为 X 连锁隐性基因，在临床上女性很少受到影响。实验室检测可以识别出生时携带突变基因的儿童，但如果是由自发性生殖细胞突变引起，可能要等到孩子长大并出现症状时才能做出诊断。

从历史上看，通过检测血清肌红蛋白升高多达 40% 氟烷麻醉的儿童出现横纹肌溶解，有 8% 的儿童伴有肌红蛋白尿。一些病例报告中也描述了恩氟烷、异氟烷或七氟烷麻醉的病例中发生横纹肌溶解。横纹肌溶解虽然在儿童患者中比在成人中更常见，但对绝大多数儿童而言预后良好。然而，合并肌病的儿童可表现为危及生命的高钾血症、心律失常、急性肾损伤和弥散性血管内凝血。由于儿童潜在的肌病可能未被诊断出来，因此有报告称 SCh 给药后健康的儿童也可发生心脏停搏。

丁酰胆碱酯酶 / 假性胆碱酯酶在肝合成。尽管包括肝衰竭在内的多种疾病可能导致正常假性胆碱酯酶的循环浓度显著降低，但正常酶浓度降低远较基因缺陷酶的影响小。大约每 3000 名患者中就有 1 人会出现假性胆碱酯酶的隐性遗传变异，这种变异可导致在给予 SCh 或美维库铵后，神经肌肉阻滞时间明显延长。

咬肌痉挛的发生频率仍存在争议。一些研究显示其发病率为 1%，而另一些研究却从未报道过其发生。1994 年 Hannallah 和 Kaplan 报道称，使用氟烷和琥珀胆碱麻醉的儿童中，有 4.4% 松弛不完全，0.2% 的出现咬肌强直，但未观察到牙关紧闭（无法张开下颌）。SCh 导致的咬肌痉挛与恶性高热之间的相关性还存在争议。然而，该问题确实值得关注，因为从北美恶性高热组选择的病例中，50% 的咬肌痉挛儿童恶性高热筛查试验阳性（肌肉活检）。在这些患者中，大约有 10% 在围术期出现了恶性高热的临床症状。因此，对严重的咬肌痉挛患者临床医师必须提高警惕。

非去极化肌肉松弛药

神经肌肉阻滞剂过敏反应的真实发生率难以准

确量化。据报道，每 10 000 ～ 20 000 例麻醉中就有 1 例发生过敏反应，其中 50% ～ 70% 被认为与神经肌肉阻滞剂有关。不同患者群体的发生率不同，但给予 SCh 和罗库溴铵后的过敏反应可能更常见，给予维库溴铵或苄基异喹啉类 NDMRs 后的发生频率较低。是否有药物暴露史与过敏反应发生无关。有变态反应史或过敏史的患者可能更容易发生 NDMRs 引起的组胺释放（表 92.1）。

启示

琥珀胆碱

缓慢性心律失常通常是良性的和自限性的，或者对迷走神经疗法有反应。但是，如果它们持续存在或影响到血流动力学，则可能需要干预。与之相反的是，给予 SCh 后出现的恶性室性心律失常和心脏停搏，此时钾过量释放，预计死亡率高达 60%，需要及时诊断和治疗。

由于儿童的肌肉质量有限，SCh 引起的肌震颤导致的胃内压变化较小，因此临床意义不大。眼内压升高是一过性的，但对术中需要打开眼球的患者而言，可能有临床意义，因为它们可能导致玻璃体内容物的挤压。

横纹肌溶解很少有长期的影响，除非是肌病患者，其后果可能是可怕的。

非典型假性胆碱酯酶的患儿接受琥珀胆碱治疗，最终能恢复神经肌肉的功能，没有后遗症。短期内，他们可能需要呼吸机辅助通气，直到有足够的力量来维持足够的通气，但长期的影响更多与遗传和对疾病的认识相关。

咬肌痉挛通常没有什么直接的影响，因为痉挛局限于咬肌。但是，如果患者有恶性高热的风险，对儿童和家庭未来的影响是巨大的。

非去极化肌肉松弛药

术中 NDMRs 的过敏反应是一个严重的问题，死亡率约为 3% ～ 6%。会引起组胺释放的 NDMRs 最好避免用于哮喘、严重的右向左分流或瓣膜狭窄的患者。由于可能发生心动过速，对于心动过速可能导致严重后果的患者（如严重的二尖瓣、三尖瓣或主动脉瓣狭窄；冠状动脉狭窄或异常的左冠状动脉；提前出现的青少年冠状动脉疾病），最好避免应用泮库溴铵。

管理

琥珀胆碱

特别对婴儿而言，持续性或不利于血流动力学

表 92.1 儿童肌肉松弛药的插管剂量、主要清除率和副作用

肌肉松弛药	插管剂量（IV mg/kg）	主要清除方法	胆碱能效应	组胺释放
琥珀胆碱	2 ～ 3（婴儿） 2（儿童） 4（IM）	血浆胆碱酯酶	刺激	罕见
美维库铵	0.2 ～ 0.4	血浆胆碱酯酶	没有效果	+（剂量 >3 × ED_{95}）
阿曲库铵	0.3 ～ 0.5	酯水解；Hofmann 消除	没有效果	++（剂量 >3 × ED_{95}）
顺式阿曲库铵	0.15 ～ 0.2	酯水解；Hofmann 消除	没有效果	最少
维库溴铵	0.1 0.4（快速序列）	肝	没有效果 没有效果	没有 没有
罗库溴铵	0.6 1.0（快速序列） 1.0 IM（婴儿） 1.6 IM（儿童）	肝	没有效果	没有
d- 筒箭毒碱	0.3 ～ 0.6	肾	没有效果	+++
泮库溴铵	0.1	肾	阻滞 ++[a]	没有

[a] 会导致交感神经刺激

IM，肌内注射；IV，静脉注射

的缓慢性心律失常可用阿托品或者（在更危急的情况下）胸外按压、肾上腺素和（或）起搏治疗。心律失常伴高钾血症可用心肺复苏、碱化、钙剂和葡萄糖-胰岛素治疗。复苏成功的时间可能会延长，极端情况下可能需要体外循环，至少要到钾通过排泄或透析消除后。

NDMRs 预处理可以减轻眼内压或颅内压的升高，通过减少脑血流和代谢的干预也可以改善颅内压的升高。

对于未被发现的横纹肌溶解，大多数患者不需要特殊治疗。对于肌病患者，可能需要充分的心脏复苏，并促进肌红蛋白的排泄（如呋塞米、甘露醇）。

临床上疑似假性胆碱酯酶缺乏的儿童需要通气支持，直至神经肌肉功能恢复，有时甚至持续到给予神经肌肉阻滞剂后的 4 ～ 8 h。随后应测定假性胆碱酯酶的绝对活性以及地布卡因和氟化物的数值，以指导今后的麻醉管理。

单纯的咬肌痉挛通常不需要特殊处理，因为痉挛会在几分钟内消失。报告表明，在进行麻醉和手术时，仔细记录二氧化碳图和患者体温，充分的水合和监测血清电解质、酸碱平衡状态、肌红蛋白和肌酸磷酸激酶水平能保证临床的安全性。因为单凭咬肌强直不能诊断恶性高热，所以不需考虑改为非触发的麻醉药。但是，如果出现持续强直、代谢率增加或恶性高热的症状，则应中止手术，并可能需要进一步的检测。

非去极化肌肉松弛药

过敏反应的常规管理包括尽可能去除过敏源，抑制介质的产生和释放（例如给予类固醇），以及调节介质作用的干预措施。这些可能包括阻断组胺能、使用 β_2 受体激动剂治疗支气管收缩以及静脉输液和给予肾上腺素，以降低支气管高反应性并支持循环。实验室检查包括过敏反应时和 6 周后血清类胰蛋白酶、组胺和（药物特异性）免疫球蛋白 E 水平检测。

组胺释放引起的低血压可用静脉补液和血管升压药来治疗。与低血压无关的症状性心动过速的治疗可能包括加深麻醉、使用阿片类药物和 β 受体阻滞剂。

预防

琥珀胆碱

在最终被诊断为肌病的所谓健康儿童中，SCh 导致的横纹肌溶解、心脏停搏和死亡时有报道，因此 1993 年，药品制造商试图禁止儿童常规使用 SCh。为了回应麻醉科医师的抗议，他们意识到这种药物仍然有其独特的属性，FDA 召开了一次公开委员会会议，会上出现了对 SCh 的折衷标签（图 92.1）。然而，由于只有在高危患者（不能总是在术前确诊）中避免使用 SCh 才能预防危及生命的高钾血症，因此专家建议应避免在婴儿和儿童中常规使用琥珀胆碱。婴儿和儿童用药仅推荐用于紧急控制气道。

考虑到其他选择，已研究了罗库溴铵的肌肉给药，但其作用持续时间明显长于琥珀胆碱，而且插管条件并不令人满意。因此，当无法获取静脉通路时，不认为其是可接受的替代品。然而，当静脉输注时，最近的 Cochrane 综述发现，在接受改良快速序贯诱导的儿童和给予 1.2 mg/kg 罗库溴铵的成人之间，静脉输注罗库溴铵和 SCh 的插管条件没有差异。尽管 SCh 因其作用时间短而被认为具有优越性，但由于舒更葡糖钠自 2008 年起在澳大利亚和欧洲上市，FDA 于 2015 年底批准其在美国使用，所以目前这种局限性没有那么重要。舒更葡糖钠是一种 γ- 环糊精，通过将药物封装在其中央核内来逆

黑框警告

罕见健康儿童患者出现急性横纹肌溶解伴高钾血症，随后出现室性心律失常、心脏停搏和死亡，伴有未确诊的骨骼肌肌病；最常见的是杜氏肌营养不良。在健康的儿科患者（最常发生在 8 岁以下）和青少年中，给药数分钟内如果出现 T 波高尖 和心脏停搏。应开始治疗高钾血症；静脉推注 Ca^{2+}、碳酸氢盐和葡萄糖（含胰岛素）、过度通气。当出现恶性高热症状时，应采用适当的治疗措施。在需要稳定气道的情况下（例如，喉痉挛、困难气道、饱胃或在尚未获得静脉通道时可经肌肉给药），保留其用于儿科患者的紧急插管。

图 92.1　关于氯化琥珀胆碱（Anectine）与高钾性心脏停搏之间关系的黑框警告【From Anectine（succinylcholine chloride）— drug summary. PDR.net，2016. Available at http://www.pdr.net/drug-summary/Anectine-succinylcholine-chloride-680. Accessed June 16，2016.】

转氨基甾体类（罗库溴铵和维库溴铵）的神经肌肉阻滞作用。这种非共价键能在 3 min 内逆转罗库溴铵的作用，在与琥珀胆碱类似的时间框架内，使紧急逆转神经肌肉阻滞的可能性成为可能。

非去极化肌肉松弛药

由于阿曲库铵有组胺释放的特性，在临床实践中已被其代谢产物顺阿曲库铵所取代，顺阿曲库铵的药效是前者的 1.5 倍，即使在非常高的剂量下也不会释放组胺。同样，使用罗库溴铵或维库溴铵可排除泮库溴铵给药后出现的高动力效应。

（顾士杰 译 刘 佳 校）

延伸阅读

Bowman WC: Neuromuscular block, *Br J Pharmacol* 147(Suppl 1):S277–S286, 2006.

Brandom BW, Fine GF: Neuromuscular blocking drugs in pediatric anesthesia, *Anesth Clin North Am* 20:45–58, 2002.

Brown TC: Aspects of depolarizing neuromuscular blockers: decamethonium and suxamethonium, *Paediatr Anaesth* 23:868–870, 2013.

Burgoyne LL, Anghelescu DL: Intervention steps for treating laryngospasm in pediatric patients, *Paediatr Anaesth* 18:297–302, 2008.

Davis PJ, Bosenberg A, Davidson A, et al.: Pharmacology of pediatric anesthesia. In Davis PJ, Cladis FP, Motoyama EK, editors: *Smith's anesthesia for infants and children*, Philadelphia, Elsevier, 2011, pp 179–261.

Donati F, Bevan DR: Neuromuscular blocking agents. In Barash PG, Cullen BF, Stoelting RK, et al., editors: *Clinical anesthesia*, Philadelphia, 2009, Lippincott Williams & Wilkins, pp 498–530.

Hannallah RS, Kaplan RF: Jaw relaxation after a halothane/succinylcholine sequence in children, *Anesthesiology* 81:99–103, 1994.

Jahr JS, Miller JE, Hiruma J, et al.: Sugammadex: a scientific review including safety and efficacy, update on regulatory issues, and clinical use in Europe, *Am J Ther* 22:288–297, 2015.

Jooste E, Klafter F, Hirshman CA, et al.: A mechanism of rapacuronium-induced bronchospasm: M2 muscarinic receptor antagonism, *Anesthesiology* 98:906–911, 2003.

Kaplan RF, Uejima T, Lobel G, et al.: Intramuscular rocuronium in infants and children: a multicenter study to evaluate tracheal intubating conditions, onset, and duration of action, *Anesthesiology* 91:633–638, 1999.

Larach MG, Rosenberg H, Gronert GA, et al.: Hyperkalemic cardiac arrest during anesthesia in infants and children with occult myopathies, *Clin Pediatr (Phila)* 36:9–16, 1997.

Meretoja OA: Neuromuscular block and current treatment strategies for its reversal in children, *Pediatr Anesth* 20:591–604, 2010.

Meakin GH: Role of muscle relaxants in pediatric anesthesia, *Curr Opin Anaesthesiol* 20:227–231, 2007.

Rajchert DM, Pasquariello CA, Watcha MF, et al.: Rapacuronium and the risk of bronchospasm in pediatric patients, *Anesth Analg* 94:488–493, 2002.

Reddy JI, Cooke PJ, van Schalkwyk JM, et al.: Anaphylaxis is more common with rocuronium and succinylcholine than with atracurium, *Anesthesiology* 122:39–45, 2015.

Tran DT, Newton EK, Mount VA, et al.: Rocuronium versus succinylcholine for rapid sequence induction intubation, *Cochrane Database Syst Rev* 10:CD002788, 2015.

笑气：神经毒性

第93章

Ka Chun Suen，*Daqing Ma*

病例概要

一名7周大的婴儿因胆道闭锁行Kasai手术。患儿接受异氟烷和氧化亚氮治疗，手术过程顺利。术后5天，患儿出现低血压、反射减退和呼吸暂停。计算机断层扫描显示严重的脑萎缩，婴儿尿中检测到同型半胱氨酸。

问题分析

定义

氧化亚氮（N_2O），又称笑气，1772年由John Priestly首次发现。1798年，Thomas Beddoes创立气动研究所，旨在研究气体药物的使用。Humphry Davy是该研究所的助理，他注意到吸入N_2O后，智齿引起的爆发疼痛减轻了。他后来出版了一本关于N_2O的书，书中提及：氧化亚氮在使用过程中似乎能够降低身体疼痛，因此可能在没有大出血的外科手术中具有广泛使用的优势。但是，他的发现在当时并没有被广泛接受。之后，美国牙科医师Horace Wells在看到Gardner Quincy Colton接受N_2O时没有感觉到受伤的腿的疼痛后，也注意到了N_2O的麻醉作用。Wells后来要求在吸入N_2O的同时摘除他的牙齿，他说这是一次无痛的手术经历。然而，Wells在麻省总医院的一次演示中却没有表现出同样的效果。直到大约20年后，Colton重新引入使用N_2O的改进装置，N_2O的使用才普及。

识别

N_2O是一种无色、有甜味的气体，作为麻醉剂使用已经超过150年（表93.1）。目前为止，它因其最低肺泡浓度（minimal alveolar concentration，MAC）为104%而被认为是效能最低的吸入麻醉剂。由于这个特性，N_2O常被用作额外的吸入剂，以增强麻醉效果。有证据表明，50%氧气预处理的N_2O可提高七氟烷的诱导速度。N_2O的血气分配系数相对较低，只有0.47，这使得血液和气体的分压能够快速平衡。因此，N_2O的起效速度相对较快。此外，N_2O还具有“第二气体效应”，它可以提高其他气体麻醉剂的起效速度。例如，同时使用N_2O可提高地氟烷的起效速度。这种“第二气体效应”是由于N_2O的脂溶性低于氮，从而使N_2O迅速扩散到血液中，导致肺泡空间内挥发性麻醉剂浓度增加，从而加快起效速度。N_2O不与血红蛋白结合，能在血液中自由运输。因此，这种吸入麻醉药在人体中的清除很快。

表93.1 N_2O的理化性质

沸点	-88℃
分子量	44
最低肺泡浓度	104%
血气分配系数	0.47
脂肪：血液分配系数	2.3
颜色	无色
气味	甜味

Data from Brown SM，Sneyd JR：Nitrous oxide in modern anesthetic practice. *BJA Educ* 16（3）：87-91，2015；Becker DE，Rosenberg M：Nitrous oxide and the inhalation anesthetics. *Anesth Prog* 55（4）：124-131，2008.

作用机制

虽然N_2O已经使用了一个多世纪，但它的作用机制尚未完全清楚。作为一种麻醉剂，N_2O与γ-氨基丁酸A型（γ-aminobutyric acid type A，$GABA_A$）、*N*-甲基-*D*-天冬氨酸受体（*N*-methyl-*d*-aspartate receptor，

NMDA）和 α- 氨基 -3- 羟基 -5- 甲基 -4- 异噁唑丙戊酸受体（α-amino-3-hydroxy-5-methyl-4-isoxazole-propinate receptor，AMPA）等不同受体和通道相互作用。但是，N_2O 对 $GABA_A$ 通道的增强作用很弱甚至没有。N_2O 拮抗 NMDA 和 AMPA 受体，抑制其突触后电流的作用，因此被认为是 N_2O 的主要作用部位。作为一种镇痛剂，N_2O 与阿片受体的不同亚型结合。N_2O 竞争性地抑制 μ 阿片受体，而非竞争性地抑制 κ 阿片受体。

对心血管系统的影响

N_2O 对心率和动脉压的影响很小，但它通过激活交感神经，抵消轻微的心肌收缩抑制作用。尽管 N_2O 对不同生理参数的影响最小，但其对心血管系统的安全性影响最近受到质疑。有证据表明，术中给予 N_2O 可增加心肌缺血的发生率，这与患者同型半胱氨酸水平的增加有关。ENIGM-Ⅰ试验研究了与使用 N_2O 相关的不同并发症，结果表明，接受 N_2O 治疗的患者心肌梗死（myocardial infarction，MI）有增加的趋势。ENIGM-Ⅰ试验的后续研究证实了这一点，使用 N_2O 后 MI 的风险增加。尽管如此，ENIGM-Ⅱ研究，一项关于 N_2O 对围术期心血管不良事件风险影响的大型多中心随机对照试验，相较于 ENIGM-Ⅰ试验，提示使用 N_2O 者的死亡率或卒中发生率没有增加。

对呼吸系统的影响

N_2O 对呼吸系统的影响也很小，不会影响每分通气量或引起支气管扩张。

风险评估

用于小儿麻醉

N_2O 在临床中具有麻醉、镇痛、抗焦虑等多种功能。因此，它是小儿患者的普遍选择。N_2O 已被证明作为镇痛药可安全有效地用于不同的儿科手术中。等分子的笑气和氧气混合物（equimolecular mixture of oxygen and nitrous，EMONO）因其镇痛和抗焦虑特性，可以安全应用在儿童患者各类操作，包括腰椎穿刺、骨髓抽吸、纤维支气管镜检查和伤痕修复。小儿患者的严重不良事件（如气道阻塞和氧饱和度降低）中只有 0.2% 的儿科患者与 N_2O 给药相关，大多数不良事件是恶心、呕吐和亢奋。

小儿患者使用 N_2O 的神经毒性

尽管 N_2O 具有安全的特性，神经毒性仍是主要的关注问题。体内研究表明，与其他年龄段的大脑相比，老年大脑和围产期大脑更容易受到神经毒性的影响。在生命的早期，不同物种经历了至关重要的大脑发育。突触发生是神经元发生凋亡以及突触成熟和发育的过程。突触发生在大鼠出生后的前 2 周，但人类是从怀孕的第 3 个月到出生后的 2 年左右。有证据表明，N_2O 能在幼鼠的大脑皮质、海马和丘脑等多个部位引起广泛的神经细胞凋亡，造成认知损伤，导致长期记忆和学习障碍。Shu 及其同事发现，在缺氧条件下，用 N_2O 和异氟烷预处理 7 天龄的大鼠会导致抗凋亡因子 Bcl-2 的降低和海马中最显著的促凋亡因子 p53 的增加，同时观察到细胞色素 C 水平的增加，这是激活细胞凋亡的关键因素。N_2O 也能引起 c-fos 水平的升高，c-fos 是组织损伤的神经元标志物，也能引起细胞内细胞器的肿胀，如后扣带回和胼胝体后皮质的线粒体和内质网。出生后第 5 ～ 6 天，暴露于 N_2O 和异氟烷混合物中的恒河猴也能看到类似的效果，其中颞回、海马和额叶皮质中可以观察到神经细胞凋亡。值得注意的是，在恒河猴中 N_2O 影响大脑的位置不同于大鼠。这可能是由大鼠和恒河猴大脑发育的时间进程不同造成的。少量在人类子宫内的临床研究证明，怀孕期间使用 N_2O 可能导致脑积水和脑膨出，并与肌张力的增加有关。

N_2O 引起的神经毒性机制

尽管尚未完全了解神经毒性的原因，但有证据表明，这是由于 N_2O 拮抗位于具有 GABA 通道的神经元上的 NMDA 受体所致。它可引起大脑某些部位的乙酰胆碱（acetylcholine，ACh）的异常释放。在生理条件下，NMDA 促进 GABA 能神经元的抑制作用，从而抑制 ACh 的释放。然而，使用 N_2O 时，NMDA 受体的作用会被抑制，从而释放 ACh，反过来影响大脑的某些区域，包括基底神经节。

另一个原因是吸入 N_2O 可导致同型半胱氨酸水平升高。N_2O 不可逆地与维生素 B_{12} 中的钴原子结合，维生素 B_{12} 是甲硫氨酸合成酶的辅助因子，其主要作用是将同型半胱氨酸转化为甲硫氨酸。甲硫氨酸合成酶功能的损害导致同型半胱氨酸水平增加。同型半胱氨酸可以作为 NMDA 受体的激动剂，作

用时间比 N_2O 的拮抗时间更长，可导致呼吸、心血管和神经系统并发症以及死亡。此外，同型半胱氨酸与 NMDA 受体的结合也诱导细胞内 Ca^{2+} 的释放，这反过来导致活性氧物质的释放（包括超氧化物），损害大脑几乎所有的区域。

管理与预防

虽然有大量的临床前证据表明 N_2O 具有神经毒性，特别是在低龄人群中，但临床数据仍然缺乏。因此，需要更多的临床研究来加深我们的理解。麻醉科医师旨在寻找无副作用的理想吸入麻醉剂来取代 N_2O。氙气和右美托咪定是一种 α_2 肾上腺素能受体激动剂，可能不具神经毒性，但仍需临床研究进行确认。在此之前，N_2O 的使用仍然存在争议，一些作者建议避免使用它，而其他人主张继续使用它。

（姚　寒　译　余喜亚　校）

延伸阅读

Akaike A, Katsuki H, Kume T, et al.: Reactive oxygen species in NMDA receptor-mediated glutamate neurotoxicity, *Park Relat Disord* 5(4): 203–207, 1999.

Annequin D, Carbajal R, Chauvin P, et al.: Fixed 50% nitrous oxide oxygen mixture for painful procedures: a French survey, *Pediatrics* 105(4): E47, 2000.

Badner NH, Beattie WS, Freeman D, et al.: Nitrous oxide-induced increased homocysteine concentrations are associated with increased postoperative myocardial ischemia in patients undergoing carotid endarterectomy, *Anesth Analg* 91(5):1073–1079, 2000.

Badner NH, Drader K, Freeman D, et al.: The use of intraoperative nitrous oxide leads to postoperative increases in plasma homocysteine, *Anesth Analg* 87(3):711–713, 1998.

Becker DE, Rosenberg M: Nitrous oxide and the inhalation anesthetics, *Anesth Prog* 55(4):124–131, 2008.

Brown SM, Sneyd JR: Nitrous oxide in modern anaesthetic practice, *BJA Educ* 16(3):87–91, 2015.

Davy H: *Researches, chemical and philosophical, chiefly concerning nitrous oxide*, London, 1800, Biggs and Cottle for J Johnson.

Dobbing J, Sands J: Comparative aspects of the brain growth spurt, *Early Hum Dev* 3(1):79–83, 1979.

Ermens AA, Refsum H, Rupreht J, et al.: Monitoring cobalamin inactivation during nitrous oxide anesthesia by determination of homocysteine and folate in plasma and urine, *Clin Pharmacol Ther* 49(4): 385–393, 1991.

Fassoulaki A, Staikou C: Pretreatment with nitrous oxide enhances induction of anesthesia with sevoflurane: a randomized controlled trial, *J Anaesthesiol Clin Pharmacol* 31(4):511–516, 2015.

Fauroux B, Onody P, Gall O, et al.: The efficacy of premixed nitrous oxide and oxygen for fiberoptic bronchoscopy in pediatric patients: a randomized, double-blind, controlled study, *Chest* 125(1):315–321, 2004.

Felmet K, Robins B, Tilford D, Hayflick SJ: Acute neurologic decompensation in an infant with cobalamin deficiency exposed to nitrous oxide, *J Pediatr* 137(3):427–428, 2000.

Gall O, Annequin D, Benoit G: Adverse events of premixed nitrous oxide and oxygen for procedural sedation in children: urothelial malignant disease and Chinese herbal nephropathy, *Lancet* 358(9292):1514–1515, 2001.

Georgiev SK, Baba H, Kohno T: Nitrous oxide and the inhibitory synaptic transmission in rat dorsal horn neurons, *Eur J Pain* 14(1):17–22, 2010.

Giovannini MG, Mutolo D, Bianchi L, et al.: NMDA receptor antagonists decrease GABA outflow from the septum and increase acetylcholine outflow from the hippocampus: a microdialysis study, *J Neurosci* 14: 1358–1365, 1994.

Goerig M: Schulte Am Esch J: History of nitrous oxide—with special reference to its early use in Germany, *Best Pract Res Clin Anaesthesiol* 15(3): 313–338, 2001.

Hapfelmeier G, Haseneder R, Kochs E, et al.: Coadministered nitrous oxide enhances the effect of isoflurane on GABAergic transmission by an increase in open-channel block, *J Pharmacol Exp Ther* 298(1):201–208, 2001.

Hollmen AI, Jouppila R, Koivisto M, et al.: Neurologic activity of infants following anesthesia for cesarean section, *Anesthesiology* 48(5):350–356, 1978.

Hornbein TF, Eger 2nd EI, Winter PM, et al.: The minimum alveolar concentration of nitrous oxide in man, *Anesth Analg* 61(7):553–556, 1982.

Kalikiri P, Gajraj RS, Sachan S: Nitrous oxide induced elevation of plasma homocysteine and methylmalonic acid levels and their clinical implications, *J Anesthesiol* 8(2), 2003.

Kim SH, Price MT, Olney JW, et al.: Excessive cerebrocortical release of acetylcholine induced by NMDA antagonists is reduced by GABAergic and $alpha_2$-adrenergic agonists, *Mol Psychiatry* 4(4):344–352, 1999.

Lafon-Cazal M, Pietri S, Culcasi M, Bockaert J: NMDA-dependent superoxide production and neurotoxicity, *Nature* 364(6437):535–537, 1993.

Lane GA, Nahrwold ML, Tait AR, et al.: Anesthetics as teratogens: nitrous oxide is fetotoxic, xenon is not, *Science* 210(4472):899–901, 1980.

Leslie K, Myles PS, Chan MT, et al.: Nitrous oxide and long-term morbidity and mortality in the ENIGMA trial, *Anesth Analg* 112(2):387–393, 2011.

Leslie K, Myles PS, Kasza J, et al.: Nitrous oxide and serious long-term morbidity and mortality in the evaluation of nitrous oxide in the gas mixture for anaesthesia (ENIGMA)-II trial, *Anesthesiology* 123(6):1267–1280, 2015.

Lu LX, Yon JH, Carter LB, et al.: General anesthesia activates BDNF-dependent neuroapoptosis in the developing rat brain, *Apoptosis* 11(9): 1603–1615, 2006.

Luhmann JD, Kennedy RM, Porter FL, et al.: A randomized clinical trial of continuous-flow nitrous oxide and midazolam for sedation of young children during laceration repair, *Ann Emerg Med* 37(1):20–27, 2001.

Ma D, Wilhelm S, Maze M, et al.: Neuroprotective and neurotoxic properties of the "inert" gas, xenon, *Br J Anaesth* 89(5):739–746, 2002.

Myles PS, Chan MT, Leslie K, et al.: Effect of nitrous oxide on plasma homocysteine and folate in patients undergoing major surgery, *Br J Anaesth* 100(6):780–786, 2008.

Myles PS, Leslie K, Chan MT, et al.: Avoidance of nitrous oxide for patients undergoing major surgery, *Anesthesiology* 107(2):221–231, 2007.

Ori C, Ford-Rice F, London ED: Effects of nitrous oxide and halothane on mu and kappa opioid receptors in guinea-pig brain, *Anesthesiology* 70(3):541–544, 1989.

Pasarón R, Burnweit C, Zerpa J, et al.: Nitrous oxide procedural sedation in non-fasting pediatric patients undergoing minor surgery: a 12-year experience with 1,058 patients, *Pediatr Surg Int* 31(2):173–180, 2015.

Reynolds IJ, Hastings TG: Glutamate induces the production of reactive oxygen species in cultured forebrain neurons following NMDA receptor activation, *J Neurosci* 15(5 Pt 1):3318–3327, 1995.

Sanders RD, Xu J, Shu Y, et al.: Dexmedetomidine attenuates isoflurane-induced neurocognitive impairment in neonatal rats, *Anesthesiology* 110(5):1077–1085, 2009.

Savage S, Ma D: The neurotoxicity of nitrous oxide: the facts and "putative" mechanisms, *Brain Sci* 4(1):73–90, 2014.

Selzer RR, Rosenblatt DS, Laxova R, et al.: Adverse effect of nitrous oxide in a child with 5,10-methylenetetrahydrofolate reductase deficiency, *N Engl J Med* 349(1):45–50, 2003.

Shu Y, Patel SM, Pac-Soo C, et al.: Xenon pretreatment attenuates anesthetic-induced apoptosis in the developing brain in comparison with nitrous oxide and hypoxia, *Anesthesiology* 113(2):360–368, 2010.

Shu Y, Zhou Z, Wan Y, et al.: Nociceptive stimuli enhance anesthetic-induced neuroapoptosis in the rat developing brain, *Neurobiol Dis* 45(2): 743–750, 2012.

Taheri S, Eger EI: A demonstration of the concentration and second gas effects in humans anesthetized with nitrous oxide and desflurane, *Anesth Analg* 89(3):774–780, 1999.

Tsze DS, Mallory MD, Cravero JP: Practice patterns and adverse events of nitrous oxide sedation and analgesia: a report from the Pediatric Sedation Research Consortium, *J Pediatr* 169:260–265.e2, 2016.

Wakita M, Kotani N, Yamaga T, et al.: Nitrous oxide directly inhibits action potential-dependent neurotransmission from single presynaptic boutons adhering to rat hippocampal CA3 neurons, *Brain Res Bull* 118: 34–45, 2015.

Yamakura T, Harris RA: Effects of gaseous anesthetics nitrous oxide and xenon on ligand-gated ion channels. Comparison with isoflurane and ethanol, *Anesthesiology* 93(4):1095–1101, 2000.

Yon J, Daniel-Johnson J, Carter L, et al.: Anesthesia induces neuronal cell death in the developing rat brain via the intrinsic and extrinsic apoptotic pathway, *Neuroscience* 135(3):815–827, 2005.

Zou X, Liu F, Zhang X, et al.: Inhalation anesthetic-induced neuronal damage in the developing rhesus monkey, *Neurotoxicol Teratol* 33(5): 592–597, 2011.

非巴比妥类麻醉药

第 94 章

Kristen Burton，Gaurav Malhotra

病例概要

患者，男性，53 岁，75 kg，既往有控制不良的高血压及非胰岛素依赖型糖尿病病史，2 天前因从梯子上跌落拟行股骨骨折外固定术。自事故发生后，患者已经禁食并使用乳酸林格液（75 ml/h）维持输液。患者无已知的药物过敏史，平日家中服用氢氯噻嗪、赖诺普利和二甲双胍。患者进入手术室心率 96 次 / 分，血压 105/50 mmHg，给予鼻导管吸氧（2 L/min）SpO_2 98%。麻醉诱导时，给予芬太尼 150 μg、利多卡因 80 mg、丙泊酚 150 mg 和维库溴铵 8 mg，患者经过简单的面罩通气后行气管插管。诱导后血压 65/43 mmHg，心率 108 次 / 分。给予 100 μg 初始剂量的去氧肾上腺素和 10 mg 麻黄素无明显反应。最终，在输注 1 L 晶体液后患者的血流动力学趋于平稳。

问题分析

定义

除氯胺酮（详见第 89 章）以外，非巴比妥类麻醉药还包括咪达唑仑、右美托咪定、依托咪酯和丙泊酚。咪达唑仑和右美托咪定更常用作镇静–抗焦虑药，通常作为其他诱导药物的辅助用药。依托咪酯和丙泊酚均用于静脉（intravenous，IV）诱导，但对于血流动力学不稳定或有血流动力学不稳定风险的患者，依托咪酯更优于丙泊酚。

识别

作用机制

苯二氮䓬类药物、丙泊酚和依托咪酯均通过与中枢神经系统的主要抑制性神经递质 γ- 氨基丁酸（γ-aminobutyric acid，GABA）的相互作用而发挥作用。咪达唑仑则通过促进与 GABA 受体的结合来提高氯离子通道的开放，引起细胞膜超极化，从而对神经功能产生抑制作用。

右美托咪定是一种 α_2 受体激动剂，能够激活蓝斑和脊髓导致交感神经系统传出减少（去甲肾上腺素和肾上腺素），并通过减少环磷酸腺苷使细胞超极化。

依托咪酯是咪唑衍生物，同样能够引起神经元细胞膜超极化，从而使网状激活系统失活。依托咪酯也可能增加 GABA 受体的可用性。

丙泊酚是一种烷基酚，其作用机制可能与作用于中枢神经系统的 GABA 受体，提高氯离子通道开放频率有关。因此丙泊酚同样也有神经抑制作用。

药物代谢动力学

咪达唑仑是短效的苯二氮䓬类药物，在缓冲酸性介质中（pH=3.5）可溶于水，在体内生理性 pH 条件下具有高度亲脂性。咪达唑仑起效迅速、蛋白质结合率高。由于该药体内再分布和肝代谢，因而其作用持续时间短暂；然而由于咪达唑仑通过肾排泄，故对于肾衰竭患者其作用时效可能会延长。

右美托咪定是一种具有亲脂性和高蛋白结合率的咪唑类复合物，起效迅速、药物再分布后作用持续时间短暂。右美托咪定经肝代谢，因此在肝功能受损患者中应谨慎使用。其无活性代谢产物主要通过肾排泄，右美托咪定在晶体液中稀释，可以给予负荷剂量输注超过 10 min，然后以维持剂量输注。

依托咪酯为水溶性，并可溶于 35% 丙二醇中。其短暂的作用时间与初始分布（3 min）后的再分布有关。依托咪酯通过肝代谢，其不具活性的代谢产物由肾（85%）和胆汁（13%）排出体外。随着患者年龄的增加其清除率下降。尽管在肝硬化患者中其清除率仍正常，但药物的分布容积和消除半衰期却加倍。

丙泊酚为高度亲脂性药物，可配制于大豆油-蛋黄-卵磷脂乳剂中，其药效学特性取决于药物的血浆浓度。成人的丙泊酚诱导剂量为 1 ～ 2.5 mg/kg，此时血液浓度为 2 ～ 6 μg/ml。即使长时间输注丙泊酚后，苏醒也很迅速，通常血浆浓度在 1.0 ～ 1.5 μg/ml 时患者即可苏醒。丙泊酚的稳态血药浓度通常与输注速率成比例，由于其代谢清除迅速，故静脉输注即时半衰期（context-sensitive half-time）受输注持续时间的影响很小，该药的生物转化在肝中进行，但其清除超过了肝血流量，表明在体内存在着肝外代谢，尤其以肺部最为显著。代谢产物由尿液排出，肝或肾功能障碍不会降低本体的药物清除。

丙泊酚、右美托咪定、依托咪酯和咪达唑仑的其他药代动力学数据见表 94.1。

风险评估

当应用非巴比妥类麻醉药物作为全身麻醉诱导或镇静时，有数种药物可供选择，包括咪达唑仑、右美托咪定、依托咪酯、丙泊酚和氯胺酮（见第 89 章）。最常用的药物是丙泊酚，因为其起效迅速、恢复快、且无严重的副反应。然而，当选择这些非巴比妥类药物静脉诱导时，必须考虑患者是否存在或可能存在以下任何一种情况：

- 低血容量或循环休克；
- 心血管疾病；
- 呼吸功能不全；
- 中枢神经系统损害或损伤；
- 肝或肾损害以及任何相关的药代动力学影响因素；
- 药物的相互作用；
- 需注意的困难气道或其他需要清醒插管及保留自主通气的情况，包括颈椎失稳或巨大的纵隔肿块。

咪达唑仑

咪达唑仑对人体血流动力学参数几乎没有影响（表 94.2），0.2 mg/kg 的咪达唑仑对于有心血管疾病的患者为安全剂量。任何心率的增加可能是由每搏输出量和血压的适度下降所引起的反射性反应，以及抗焦虑所引起的交感张力降低。低血容量可加重上述效应。相反，咪达唑仑可以引起呼吸暂停并降低对二氧化碳（CO_2）的通气反应，尤其是在推注给药后更甚。咪达唑仑通常与阿片类药物（如芬太尼）联合用于镇静，因其能够增强咪达唑仑对呼吸的影响，故对于接受这类药物联合治疗的患者必须密切监测患者是否有呼吸功能不全的症状。

其他的考虑因素包括：

- 脑氧耗轻度减少，伴少量或不伴有脑血流量的减少。
- 颅内压（intracranial pressure，ICP）的轻度降低。
- 维持脑自动调节功能。
- 眼内压（intraocular pressure，IOP）大幅下降。
- 缩短癫痫发作的持续时间，提高其发作阈值。
- 意识丧失较慢，认知功能恢复的恢复期较长。
- 麻醉诱导时可能有咳嗽、呃逆、骨骼肌不自主运动的反应。

表 94.1 丙泊酚、依托咪酯、咪达唑仑、右美托咪定的药代动力学参数

	药物			
参数	丙泊酚	依托咪酯	咪达唑仑	右美托咪定
分布半衰期（min）	2 ～ 8	起始：3 后期：29	3 ～ 10	大约 6
消除半衰期（h）	0.5 ～ 1.5	2 ～ 5	1 ～ 4	2 ～ 3
生物转化	肝；肝外（肺部）	肝	肝	肝
代谢产物	无活性	活性极弱	无活性	无活性
排泄	肾	肾（85%）；胆汁（13%）	肾	肾；粪便（4%）
静脉诱导剂量	1 ～ 2.5 mg/kg	0.2 ～ 0.5 mg/kg	0.1 ～ 0.2 mg/kg	0.5 ～ 1 μg/kg 超过 10 min
静脉维持剂量	50 ～ 150 μg（kg · min）	2.5 ～ 10 μg（kg · min）	0.05 ～ 0.1 μg（kg · min）	0.2 ～ 0.7 μg（kg · h）

表 94.2 丙泊酚、依托咪酯、咪达唑仑和右美托咪定的血流动力学、呼吸和其他效应

参数	药物			
	丙泊酚	依托咪酯	咪达唑仑	右美托咪定
心率	↓	0/ ↑	0/ ↑	↓
平均动脉压	↓ ↓	0/ ↓	0/ ↓	单次推注时短暂↑ 维持输注时↓
体循环阻力	↓ ↓	0/ ↓	0/ ↓	↑ / ↓同上
平均肺动脉压	0	0/ ↑	0	0/ ↓
心脏指数	↓ ↓	0/ ↑	0/ ↓	↓
每搏输出量	↓ ↓	0/ ↓	0/ ↓	↓
心肌收缩力	0/ ↓	0/ ↓	0/ ↓	0
呼吸暂停	↑ ↑ ↑	↑	↑ ↑	0
对 CO_2 的通气反应	↓ ↓ ↓	↓	↓ ↓	0
支气管扩张	+COPD	0	0	+ 静脉用药
恶心、呕吐	减少	增加	极少	极少
镇痛	极少	极少	极少	辅助用药时适度镇痛
注射痛	严重	可能	极少	极少

COPD，慢性阻塞性肺病

右美托咪定

右美托咪定是高选择性 α_2 肾上腺素受体激动剂，然而快速的推注给药会引起血管收缩，伴有压力感受器介导的心动过缓，这是由于大剂量时 α_1 受体的交叉反应所致。右美托咪定的交感神经作用主要与维持治疗有关，除了镇静和抗焦虑作用外，还可导致低血压和心动过缓。因此，对于基础血压低、血容量不足、心动过缓或有心脏传导阻滞的患者、自主神经功能失调的患者、高龄以及服用房室结阻滞剂的患者，应慎用右美托咪定。长时间输注右美托咪定突然停药可能会出现反跳性高血压。当作为唯一用药时，右美托咪定对呼吸系统的抑制作用最小。除了镇静和抗焦虑作用，右美托咪定能够保留患者的自主呼吸，这使其成为在担心困难气道时采取清醒 / 镇静下纤支镜插管的理想药物。

其他考虑的因素包括：

- 用于区域麻醉和全身麻醉辅助药物时的镇痛作用；
- 用作全身麻醉补充药物时可以减少麻醉药物的需求；
- 降低 ICP，减少脑血流量和脑耗氧量；
- 降低 IOP；
- 减轻寒战；
- 其抗交感作用可能对心脏手术有利；
- 用于儿童可有助于预防苏醒期谵妄。

依托咪酯

依托咪酯不影响交感神经活性和压力感受器的反射功能。对于伴或不伴有心脏疾病的患者，依托咪酯能够可靠地维持血流动力学稳定，维持心肌氧供需比。在失血性休克的模型中，与硫喷妥钠相比，依托咪酯与生存率的增加有关。然而，一些研究表明，依托咪酯的心血管抑制作用与丙泊酚相似。有研究提示依托咪酯可增加危重患者因肾上腺皮质功能抑制而导致的死亡风险。最后，与咪达唑仑相比，依托咪酯不太可能会引起呼吸暂停，或减少对 CO_2 的通气反应。

其他考虑因素包括：

- 无镇痛作用；
- 增加了恶心呕吐的发生率；
- 外周静脉注射痛；
- 长期的输注甚至可能是单一剂量即可能引起临床显著的肾上腺皮质功能抑制；

- 可引起肌阵挛和骨骼肌不自主运动，预先使用阿片类药物或苯二氮䓬类药物可减弱上述现象；
- 延长癫痫发作时间，因此可用作电休克疗法；
- 降低脑血流和脑代谢率（cerebral metabolic rate，$CMRO_2$）；
- 可降低 IOP 和 ICP，但可被肌阵挛、瞳孔放大或咳嗽所抵消。

丙泊酚

丙泊酚具有强烈的心血管抑制作用。由于心肌抑制和血管舒张，它可使平均动脉压降幅高达 40%。静脉回心血量和体循环阻力的降低使得前负荷和后负荷均降低，这是由于丙泊酚降低交感神经张力，直接松弛血管平滑肌所致。丙泊酚的负性肌力作用则是由于 Ca^{2+} 内流受抑制导致心肌细胞内 Ca^{2+} 可利用率降低，但心肌氧供需平衡仍可得到维持。丙泊酚还会破坏急性出血时的血管收缩反射。

丙泊酚产生剂量依赖性的呼吸抑制，且随着阿片类药物和苯二氮䓬类药物的使用而增强。此外，它极有可能损害对 CO_2 的通气反应并导致呼吸暂停（见表 94.2）。连续输液可减少潮气量和呼吸频率。丙泊酚具有扩张支气管的作用，并可降低反应性气道疾病患者术中支气管痉挛的发生率。

其他考虑因素包括：

- 静脉刺激和注射痛（利多卡因有助于减轻疼痛）；
- 止吐、止痒和抗焦虑；
- 脂肪乳剂促进细菌生长；
- 诱导时咳嗽、打嗝及骨骼肌的不自主运动；
- 降低脑耗氧量、血流量、ICP 和 IOP；
- 对癫痫发作阈值无影响；
- 无镇痛作用；
- 长时间（>48 h）给予患者大剂量［>4 mg/(kg • h)］丙泊酚输注时存在丙泊酚输注综合征的风险：表现为代谢性酸中毒、横纹肌溶解、心律失常、心肌和肾衰竭、脂肪肝和死亡；年轻和危重患者的风险增加；
- 有报道会出现神经兴奋性延迟的副作用，包括可能引起癫痫发作、幻觉和角弓反张。

启示

合并心血管疾病或低血容量患者，常规诱导剂量的丙泊酚会增加心血管虚脱和心肌缺血或梗死的风险。如前所述，对于低血容量的患者，丙泊酚的心血管抑制作用更加显著。如可能，在诱导前应尽可能对患者进行容量复苏。对于严重低血容量或血流动力学受损的患者，任何诱导药物应谨慎滴定使用，以减轻对血流动力学的影响。已达到维持终末器官灌注的目的。

管理

选择合适的非巴比妥类静脉诱导药物必须考虑以下问题：

- 重视失血或其他原因的血管内容量耗竭导致的低血量或低血压，采用晶体液或胶体液恢复前负荷；
- 根据患者的并存疾病和容量状态，预估诱导过程中需要的血管活性药物；
- 考虑有创监测的需要，如动脉置管、中心静脉压和经食管超声心动图；
- 优化通气和氧合；
- 潜在困难气道管理、巨大纵隔肿块或颈椎不稳的患者，考虑在诱导过程中保留自主呼吸的必要性；
- 评估是否需要进行快速或改良的快速序贯插管；
- 考虑是否需要避免 ICP 或 IOP 大幅增加。

低血容量和气道管理

诱导的目标包括确保气道安全，改善氧供，恢复血容量，维持患者血流动力学稳定。快速序贯诱导对于降低误吸的风险可能很有必要。如有困难气道、颈椎不稳定者或纵隔肿块较大，则有清醒插管的指征。如前所述，右美托咪定在提供镇静和抗焦虑的同时能够保持自主通气，因而在这种情况下经常使用。静脉麻醉药的选择取决于其心脑血管和药代动力学效应（表 94.1 和表 94.2）。在本文所讨论的药物中，对于严重低血容量或失血的患者，依托咪酯可能是用来降低急性心血管虚脱风险的最安全的药物。但无论选择哪种药物，当出现明显出血或血容量减少时，必须减少用药剂量并仔细滴定。

颅内压增高或眼内压增高

咪达唑仑、依托咪酯和丙泊酚可有效地降低 ICP，而氯胺酮则会增加 ICP。然而，使用咪达唑仑后的缓慢苏醒则会影响术后早期神经功能的评估。

右美托咪定对 ICP 的影响最小。

咪达唑仑、右美托咪定和丙泊酚可降低 IOP。依托咪酯具有同样的作用，但可被其引起的肌阵挛、瞳孔扩大、咳嗽所抵消。氯胺酮则增加 IOP。

肾上腺功能抑制

依托咪酯的使用与人体的肾上腺功能抑制有关。即使是单一剂量也可以抑制皮质醇的生成，因此危重患者必须谨慎使用。

预防

为了避免使用非巴比妥类静脉诱导药物时出现并发症，需要注意以下问题：

- 如有指征，应进行容量补充和给予足够的血液或血液制品。
- 选择合适的静脉麻醉诱导药物。考虑其起效和苏醒时间，对镇静、镇痛、冠状动脉和脑组织灌注、体循环血压、心肌和大脑氧耗、呼吸暂停的发生，以及对 ICP 和 IOP 的影响。
- 缓慢滴定和调整诱导剂量。谨慎的滴定通常可以防止患者血压突然发生有害的变化，患者可能需要缩血管药物以平稳度过诱导期。静脉诱导药物的剂量应根据患者的年龄、理想体重和肝肾功能来进行调整。
- 各种静脉麻醉诱导药物的副作用及相对禁忌证。

病例概要中描述了患者在有高血压病史情况下出现了低血压。患者为长骨骨折，住院期间可能经口摄食过少。这类患者血容量耗竭的风险很高，如本例所示，在使用标准诱导剂量的丙泊酚后，存在严重低血压的风险。如果在诱导前就意识到这一点，适当的晶体或胶体复苏，以及谨慎滴定丙泊酚的剂量，可能有助于减轻这种心血管虚脱。同时，还应预料到患者可能需要使用血管活性药物。

（时　鹏　译　卞金俊　校）

延伸阅读

Kam PCA, Cardone D: Propofol infusion syndrome, *Anaesthesia* 62(7):690–701, 2007.

Lundy JB, Slane ML, Frizzi JD: Acute adrenal insufficiency after a single dose of etomidate, *J Intensive Care Med* 22(2):111–117, 2007.

Mackey DC, et al.: Adrenergic agonists and antagonists. In Butterworth JF, Mackey DC, Wasnick JD, editors: *Morgan and Mikhail's clinical anesthesiology*, ed 5, New York, 2013, McGraw-Hill Education, pp 239–254.

Reves JG, Glass PSA, Lubarsky DA, et al.: Intravenous nonopioid anesthetics. In Miller RD, editor: *Miller's anesthesia*, ed 6, Philadelphia, 2005, Churchill Livingstone, pp 317–378.

White PF, Eng MR: Intravenous anesthetics. In Barash PG, Cullen BF, Stoelting RK, et al.: *Clinical anesthesia*, ed 7, Philadelphia, 2013, Lippincott Williams & Wilkins, pp 478–500.

第95章 非去极化神经肌肉阻滞

Mohammad El-Orbany

病例概要

患者，女性，52 岁，既往有慢性肾功能不全病史，在神经肌肉松弛全身麻醉术后苏醒并气管拔管后产生了呼吸困难，胸壁和腹部反常运动以及间歇性上呼吸道梗阻。

问题分析

定义

据估计，拔管后神经肌肉阻滞残余（residual neuromuscular block，RNMB）（肌松药残余）的发生率高于 40%。如果不能正确识别和妥善管理，可能会因此导致严重的术后呼吸系统并发症。由于在拔管时肌松药未能充分逆转或长时间的神经肌肉阻滞超过了预期的作用持续时间，会致使患者术后长期肌无力。目前普遍认可，气管拔管时四个成串刺激（train-of-four，TOF）低于 0.9 时容易产生此并发症。残余肌无力可引起各种各样的症状，轻者会感觉不适、复视和吞咽困难，严重者则导致误吸和呼吸完全停止（框 95.1）。

在理想状态下，每种神经肌肉阻滞药物（neuromuscular blocking drug，NMBDs）均基于其药物代谢动力学特征以其可预测的速率进行代谢和清除。然而在临床实际应用中，同样要重视识别患者并存的疾病、术中事件和一些同时使用的药物治疗可能会延长 NMBDs 的作用持续时间并使其不易被拮抗。

框 95.1 肌松药残余的并发症

- 咽部协调能力和收缩力受损
- 吞咽功能障碍
- 食管上段括约肌张力减少
- 误吸风险增加
- 吸气流速下降
- 上呼吸道梗阻
- 低氧通气驱动受损和术后低氧血症风险增加
- 肌无力症状（视力障碍、面部无力、说话与饮水困难、全身无力）
- PACU 中发生严重呼吸事件的风险较高
- PACU 出室延迟
- 术后通气支持延长、插管次数增加
- 术后肺部并发症（肺不张或肺炎）的风险增高

PACU，麻醉后恢复室

识别

可以使用以下措施评估肌松药残余 / 肌肉力量的程度：

- **临床试验**：抬头 5 s，持续握手，伸舌试验；
- **主观监测指标（简单神经刺激器）**：视觉或触觉评价以评估 TOF、双短强直刺激或强直刺激的衰减；
- **客观监测指标（定性）**：加速肌电图、机械肌电图、肌电图和运动肌电图，以定性评估阻滞 / 肌肉力量的确切程度。

使用多种评估方式可能更准确地估计 RNMB 的恢复程度，并提示可以在无肌松残余作用下安全拔管的最佳时间。因此，如果在给予拮抗药后，患者仍然无法维持抬头 5 s；对 50-Hz 强直刺激、TOF 或双短强直刺激的反应衰减；TOF<0.9，则提示此时患者仍然存在一定程度的 RNMB，如果此时进行气管拔管，患者将极有可能产生与 RNMB 相关的并发症。在这种情况下最安全的做法是等待至患者在气管拔管前（TOF ≥ 0.9）恢复足够的肌肉力量，同时考虑以下可能会延长神经肌肉恢复的因素：

- 可能影响 NMBD 消除或代谢的共存疾病或病情；
- 与给药剂量和给药时机相关的预期恢复时间（表 95.1）。

使用常规神经肌肉监测（使用简单的神经刺激器或最好使用客观监测指标），根据手术要求和监测

表 95.1 不同非去极化神经肌肉阻滞药物的近似恢复时间

	剂量范围（mg/kg）	低剂量恢复时间（min）[a]	高剂量恢复时间（min）[a]
长效 NDMR			
泮库溴胺	0.1		40 ~ 60
多库氯铵	0.05 ~ 0.08	50 ~ 130（平均 91）	74 ~ 268（平均 177）
中长效 NDMR			
维库溴铵	0.10		25 ~ 45
罗库溴铵	0.6 ~ 1.2	15 ~ 85（平均 31）	38 ~ 160（平均 67）
阿曲库铵[b]	0.5		20 ~ 45
顺阿曲库铵[c]	0.15 ~ 0.20	28 ~ 65（平均 46）	31 ~ 103（平均 59）
短效 NDMR			
美维库铵[b]	0.25	11 ~ 29（平均 19）	

NDMR，非去极化肌肉松弛剂

[a] 基于包装插页和变异性，由生产商给出的可变性的近似恢复时间。除非另有说明，否则给出的值是恢复至肌颤搐幅度的 25%；

[b] 从高剂量恢复的时间是指需要给第一次维持剂量之前的时间；

[c] 恢复到颤搐高峰的 5%

结果，滴定 NMBDs 剂量和给药时机，并在肌松恢复到一定程度后给予适当剂量的拮抗药（TOF 刺激至少有 3 次反应），RNMB 的发病率可以显著降低。

风险评估

无论是已知的、未知的还是假定的机制，以下所有情况均可加强 NMBDs 的作用并增加拮抗的难度：

- 药物相互作用：抗生素（尤其是氨基糖苷类药物）、袢利尿剂（如呋塞米）、硫酸镁、锂盐、钙通道阻滞剂、奎尼丁或普鲁卡因胺；
- 肾或肝功能不全或衰竭，改变了依赖这些器官进行代谢及消除的药物作用时间，包括神经肌肉阻滞药物（表 95.2）；
- 低体温；
- 酸碱失衡。

启示

长时间阻滞会增加患者在手术室的时间，特别是某些门诊手术中心，要求患者必须拔管后方可转入麻醉后恢复室（postanesthesia care unit，PACU）。当在气管拔管前诊断出 RNMB 时，在 PACU 可能需要一段时间的术后机械通气支持，直到完全恢复。如果是这样，患者必须使用镇静剂以避免随后因部分或完全麻痹而引起的不良事件的回忆。

表 95.2 非去极化神经肌肉阻滞药物的代谢途径或消除途径

药物	肾	肝	酯酶水解	霍夫曼消除
泮库溴铵	主要	部分	无	无
多库氯铵	主要	主要	无	无
维库溴铵	少	主要	无	无
罗库溴铵	少	主要	无	无
阿曲库铵	无	无	主要	主要
顺式阿曲库铵	少	少	无	主要
美维库铵	少	少	主要	无

如果 RNMB 未被识别且气管导管被拔出，如前所述，患者可能会出现进一步的并发症，其中一些可能会很严重甚至会危及生命。患者可能没有足够的力量来保护气道，肺误吸的风险增加。这也可能导致呼吸功能不全，引起高碳酸血症和低氧血症。总的来说，这些情况可能会导致血流动力学不稳定、心律失常或呼吸停止。

管理

早期识别和及时治疗是降低可能与 RNMB 相关的发病率和死亡率的关键。如果在单次初始插管 NMBDs 剂量后时使用足够剂量的逆转药物且未达到所需的恢复水平，如可能，应寻求并纠正药物消除减少或增强的原因。

如果在手术结束时但在气管拔管之前未检测到神经肌肉阻滞延长，则安置患者在 PACU 中进行术后通气支持，患者保持镇静状态。神经肌肉恢复不足的证据包括以下内容：

- 无法维持抬头至少 5 s；
- TOF、50 Hz 强直刺激或双短强直刺激后衰减；
- 客观监测指标显示 TOF<90%。

在 PACU 期间，患者应保持镇静状态，直至头部抬高或周围神经刺激的结果表明其肌力充分恢复。

在病例概要中描述了一个不幸的事件。在未确保神经肌肉功能得到充分恢复的情况下拔除了气管导管。显然，在拔管前没有对患者进行充分评估，因而临床医师面临的窘境是患者在 PACU 发生了呼吸困难。在这种情况下，需要及时识别并立即采取措施，以确保充分的氧合和通气。这可以通过面罩通气、双水平正压通气或置入喉罩来实现，同时准备再次插管。后者通常需要实施，应经常评估患者以确保其在气管拔管前恢复足够的肌力。若未顾及到 RNMB 的影响，患者可发生严重的并发症，包括误吸或完全呼吸停止和（或）阻塞。

预防

通过遵守一些简单的规则，RNMB 将是一种可预防的并发症。首先，在不需要肌肉松弛时避免使用神经肌肉阻滞药（如在一些四肢手术中）。当有使用指征时，NMBDs 的选择应基于对以下情况的了解：可能影响肝或肾消除的并存疾病，同时使用的药物治疗以及可能影响肌肉松弛药临床持续时间的其他因素。

使用神经肌肉阻滞药时，应该常规用周围神经刺激仪（主观监测）或定量（客观）监测仪对神经肌肉阻滞的程度进行监测。这些监测可以指导临床医师正确选择诱导后气管插管的时机，确保术中保持适当的手术松弛程度，并在达到所需的阻滞恢复程度时提示安全拔管的时机。任何避免直接肌肉刺激产生误导效应的监测部位均可以接受，但应该记住不同肌群的恢复时间略有不同。神经肌肉监测最常见的部位是腕部尺神经、面神经或胫后神经，因为它们均较表浅，易于刺激。

尽管 TOF 反应的视觉或触觉评估在诱导和维持期间可能有用，但它们很难预测 NMBDs 是否充分恢复。当 TOF 比值高于 0.4 时，即使有经验的临床医生在使用视觉或触觉评估时也无法检测到对 TOF 刺激的衰减反应。选择双强直刺激或 5 s，50-Hz 强直刺激，结合临床症状，其检测 RNMB 的灵敏度更高，但仍不足以消除并发症。为避免 RNMB，气管拔管时 T_4/T_1 比应至少为 0.9，这只能通过使用客观监测指标来确定。预防 RNMB 的最后一项建议是，只要使用 NMBDs 时，就常规使用拮抗药物，且在肌肉松弛自然恢复到一定程度时使用（TOF 至少出现 3 个波，4 个最好）。必须指出的是，即使使用抗胆碱酯酶药物，完全恢复时间仍取决于 NMBD 的完全代谢和消除。此外，可能存在导致阻滞延长的活性代谢物。如果这些代谢物或母体药物代谢或消除缓慢，则恢复时间更为延迟，气管拔管应该推迟直至肌肉松弛充分恢复。

（杜兆宁　译　赵珍珍　校）

延伸阅读

Asai T, Isono S: Residual neuromuscular blockade after anesthesia: a possible cause of postoperative aspiration-induced pneumonia, *Anesthesiology* 120:260–262, 2014.

Cedborg AI, Sundman E, Bodén K, et al.: Pharyngeal function and breathing pattern during partial neuromuscular block in the elderly: effects on airway protection, *Anesthesiology* 120:312–325, 2014.

Debaene B, Plaud B, Dilly MP, et al.: Residual paralysis in the PACU after a single intubating dose of nondepolarizing muscle relaxant with an intermediate duration of action, *Anesthesiology* 98:1042–1048, 2003.

El-Orbany M, Ali HH, Baraka A, et al.: Residual neuromuscular block should, and can, be a "never event," *Anesth Analg* 118:691, 2014.

Eriksson LI: Evidence-based practice and neuromuscular monitoring: it's time for routine quantitative assessment, *Anesthesiology* 98: 1037–1039, 2003.

Fortier LP, McKeen D, Turner K, et al.: The RECITE study: a Canadian prospective, multicenter study of the incidence and severity of residual neuromuscular blockade, *Anesth Analg* 121:366–372, 2015.

Lien CA, Kopman AF: Current recommendations for monitoring depth of neuromuscular blockade, *Curr Opin Anaesthesiol* 27:616–622, 2014.

Murphy GS, Brull SJ: Residual neuromuscular block: lessons unlearned. Part I: definitions, incidence, and adverse physiologic effects of residual neuromuscular block, *Anesth Analg* 111:120–128, 2010.

Murphy GS, Szokol JW, Avram MJ, et al.: Postoperative residual neuromuscular blockade is associated with impaired clinical recovery, *Anesth Analg* 117:133–141, 2013.

Murphy GS, Szokol JW, Marymont JH, et al.: Intraoperative acceleromyographic monitoring reduces the risk of residual neuromuscular blockade and adverse respiratory events in the postanesthesia care unit, *Anesthesiology* 109:389–398, 2008.

Murphy GS, Szokol JW, Marymont JH, et al.: Residual neuromuscular blockade and critical respiratory events in the postanesthesia care unit, *Anesth Analg* 107:130–137, 2008.

Murphy GS, Szokol JW, Marymont JH, et al.: Residual paralysis at the time of tracheal extubation, *Anesth Analg* 100:1840–1845, 2005.

Plaud B: Neuromuscular monitoring, residual blockade, and reversal: time for re-evaluation of our clinical practice, *Can J Anaesth* 60(7): 634–640, 2013.

Todd MM, Hindman BJ: The implementation of quantitative electromyographic neuromuscular monitoring in an academic anesthesia department: follow-up observations, *Anesth Analg* 121:836–838, 2015.

围术期液体管理

第 96 章

Donald S. Prough, Christer H. Svenseén

病例概要

病例 1

患者，男性，72 岁，因非梗阻性结肠癌择期行横结肠切除和一期再吻合术治疗。患者既往有高血压病史，服用利尿剂控制良好，其他方面健康。

病例 2

患者，女性，35 岁，因胆石症择期行腹腔镜胆囊切除术治疗。患者除了轻度肥胖（术前体重 88 kg）外，其他方面健康。

问题分析

定义

输注液体可能是手术中最普遍的治疗措施。尽管经过数十年的研究，但该主题仍备受争议，在给予液体治疗的时间、输液量以及输液速度等问题仍无确定答案。不足或过度的液体治疗会导致相关并发症的发生，其程度从相对轻微到危及生命。最近研究表明，过去对围术期液体治疗的相关并发症的发生率和重要性估计不足。然而，在过去的十年中，已经实施了目标导向液体治疗方案，虽然对于重症患者的证据很不足，但对于择期外科手术患者而言已有更具说服力的证据。

液体治疗不足引起的危及生命的并发症，是由低灌注和相关的重要器官系统并发症所致。急性肾衰竭和多系统器官衰竭的预后最差。不太严重的并发症包括术后口渴、头晕、恶心、呕吐、疲劳和嗜睡。不足的液体治疗还可能短暂损伤术后运动耐量和肺功能。

过度液体治疗最令人担忧的并发症是原发性或继发性肺水肿。原发性肺水肿时，静脉回流和右心室前负荷增加，导致右心室流出和肺动脉流出增加，并最终导致肺毛细血管静水压升高。若压力迅速、持续增加，会导致肺泡毛细血管渗漏和肺泡积水。该机制类似于纳洛酮对阿片类药物的过度逆转作用。继发性肺水肿是由于左心室负荷过重和“前向”（心源性）衰竭所致。这在一些左心室功能受损的患者中更容易发生。与过度液体治疗相关的轻度并发症，发生较晚但不容忽视，包括外周性水肿、眶周水肿和胃肠功能受损或伤口愈合困难。这些症状常发生在离开麻醉恢复室后或在重症加强治疗病房中，因此较不易于被麻醉科医师所发现。

历史回顾

首次将液体输入循环中的尝试是为逆转霍乱患者腹泻或呕吐引起的脱水。20 世纪初至 20 世纪 60 年代中期，限制液体是围术期液体管理的主要策略。胶体液最初被使用是在 20 世纪中期、在二战期间，作为白蛋白的血管内替代物。在 20 世纪 60 年代，Shires 及其同事强调了在出血或大手术期间，细胞外液体积减少并需要用晶体液补充的概念，被称为“第三间隙”液体，这一个概念现已被广泛放弃。在越南战争期间，由于该项研究，输注大量的晶体液成了伤员治疗的标准。结果导致间质液体蓄积和外周水肿 [特别是急性呼吸窘迫综合征（acute respiratory distress syndrome，ARDS）]，但该方法也使得肾衰竭的发生率明显降低，随后被应用于平民外科手术患者的围术期管理。

尽管过度液体复苏与 ARDS 之间尚未建立明确的因果关系，但这种可能的联系一直困扰着临床医师。1999 年，Ariffe 报道了 13 例发生术后肺水肿的患者，其中 10 例康复，3 例发生严重的合并症。总体而言，在术中和术后 24 h 内，该组的净液体贮留量为 67 ml/kg。

在 2003 年一项具有里程碑意义的多中心研究中，Brandstrup 及其同事指出了在结直肠手术中限制性液体治疗的重要性。虽然这仅是一种胶体液-晶体液的使用方案，但明显的结果显示，该方案的优势是体重增加较少，而以往的研究结果发现体重增加与并发症发生率较高有关。接受短小手术的健康受试者，似乎可受益于输注中等量的晶体液，可防止术后恶心。而接受结直肠手术的患者，可受益于使用“限制性”目标导向方案模式的零平衡方案，即使其总输液量由于手术时间长超过了日间手术方案中的输液量。

近年来，随着加速康复外科（enhanced recovery after surgery，ERAS）方案的发展，以及用于评估液体治疗反应性的有创和无创设备的增加，围术期液体的输入量显著减少。这些方案包括对结肠、盆腔/直肠和胰腺手术的建议，目标是减少患者住院时间和恢复正常活动的时间，并通过遵循更积极的禁食原则，改进常规肠道准备、术前碳水化合物摄入以及早期活动来提高生存率（参见 Lobo et al.，2002）。

识别与评估

临床医师须充分认识液体治疗不足或过度的后果。低血压、心动过速和少尿是低血容量时明显而非特异性的表现；肺水肿是高血容量时明显而非特异性的表现。识别轻微的低血容量或高血容量通常更加困难。液体治疗被广泛认可的理论依据是其可改善心排血量和器官灌注，从而限制器官功能障碍的发生。

对血液和细胞外容量的临床评估，从肠梗阻、长期使用利尿剂、脓毒症、烧伤和创伤等相关容量欠缺疾病的认识开始。提示低血容量的体征包括少尿、仰卧位低血压和倾斜试验阳性。尽管少尿提示低血容量，但低血容量患者并不一定少尿，正常血容量患者可能由于肾衰竭或应激引起的内分泌反应而表现为少尿。仰卧位低血压提示血容量不足超过 30%，而正常的动脉血压对于老年或慢性高血压患者而言可能是相对的低血压。倾斜试验阳性是指患者直立时心率至少每分钟增加 20 次，收缩压降低至少 20 mmHg。年轻健康的患者可以耐受 20% 血容量的急性丢失，而仅表现出体位性心动过速；相比之下，20% ～ 30% 的老年患者尽管血容量正常却仍可能发生体位性低血压。

提示低血容量或细胞外容量减少的实验室证据，包括氮质血症、低尿钠、代谢性碱中毒（轻微低血容量）和乳酸酸中毒（严重低血容量）。急性出血几乎不会改变血细胞比容，直到输注液体或液体从间质转移到血管内。血尿素氮（blood urea nitrogen，BUN）正常值为 8 ～ 20 mg/dl，常因低血容量、高蛋白质摄入、胃肠道出血或加速分解代谢而升高，却因严重肝功能不全而降低。血清肌酐（serum creatinine，SCr）是肌肉分解代谢的产物，在老年人、女性、虚弱或营养不良的患者中含量常偏低，但在肌肉或急性分解代谢的患者中，它可能超过正常范围（0.5 ～ 1.5 mg/dl）。BUN/SCr 的比值超过正常范围（10 ～ 20）时表明患者脱水。肾前性少尿时，钠重吸收增加可使尿钠离子减少至 20 mEq/L 或更低；增强水重吸收应提高尿液浓度（尿液渗透压 >400，尿-血浆肌酐比值 >40：1）。然而，这些泌尿系统方面的指标，其变量的敏感性和特异性都不高。

评估术中液体复苏的充分性需综合多个临床变量，包括钠浓度、术中预估失血量以及对心率、血压、尿量、动脉氧合、pH 和中心静脉压的监测，但以上参数并非完全有帮助。众所周知，肉眼估计的术中失血量并不准确。此外，心动过速是一种不敏感的、非特异性的低血容量指标，中心静脉压同样如此。在严重低血容量时，间接血压测量值可能低于直接动脉压。直接监测动脉压的另一个优点可能是在伴血容量不足的正压通气的患者中，可以识别到收缩压的变异度增加。中至重度的低血容量时，尿量常急剧减少。因此，在无糖尿或未给予利尿剂的情况下，麻醉期间尿量为 0.5 ～ 1.0 ml/(kg·h) 时表明肾灌注充足。只有当组织灌注严重不足时，动脉血 pH 才会降低。尽管局部血流严重减少，心排血量仍可能保持正常。乳酸可以反映组织灌注，混合静脉血氧饱和度（mixed venous oxygen saturation，SvO_2）是全身组织和重要脏器灌注不良的特异性指标；但它们反映了多个器官的平均灌注情况，且需要放置肺动脉导管。其他替代参数如中心静脉血氧饱和度（central venous oxygen saturation，$ScvO_2$），需要放置中心静脉导管。这两种方法都不能预测特定器官的灌注不良。新技术正在开发中，如用于监测外周的旁流探头（图 96.1）。

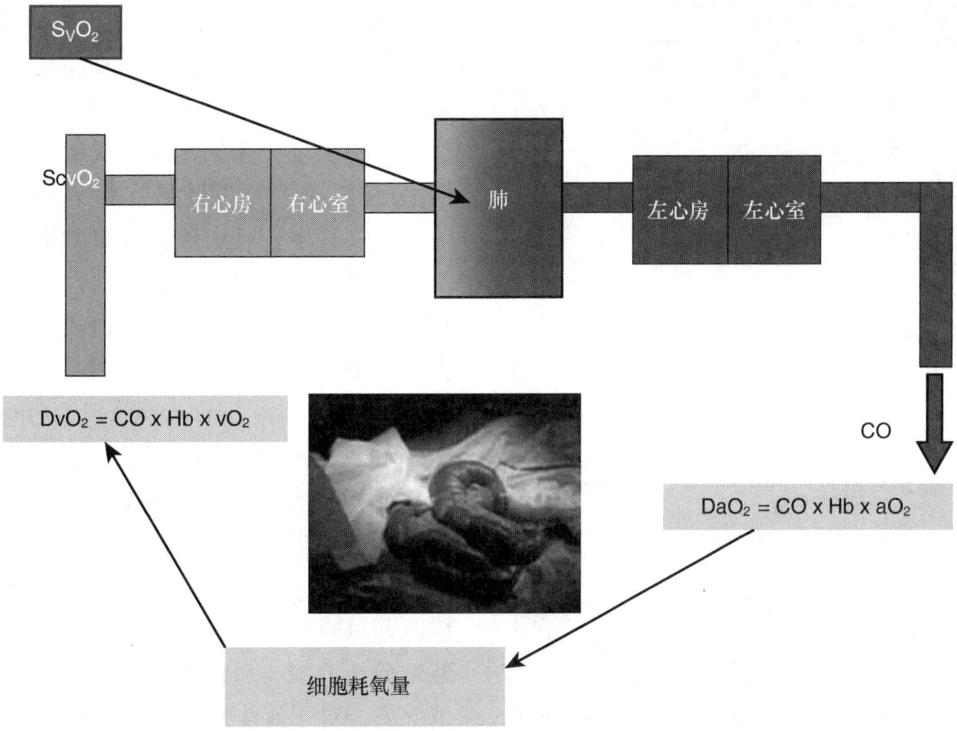

图 96.1 组织饱和度。CO，心排血量；DaO_2，动脉氧输送；Hb，血红蛋白；aO_2，动脉氧合；DvO_2，静脉氧输送；vO_2，静脉氧合；$ScvO_2$，中心静脉血氧饱和度；SvO_2，混合静脉血氧饱和度

个体化目标导向治疗

液体治疗更合理的方法是确定患者的**容量反应性**，通常需要通过监测患者血流动力学参数和确定每搏输出量（stroke volume，SV）的显著增加来判断。个体化目标导向治疗包括输注液体或使用正性肌力药物。患者在静脉快速补液（250 ～ 500 ml）后，SV 增加 10% ～ 15% 的被认为是**容量反应阳性**。容量反应性符合 Frank-Starling 原理，即随着前负荷的增加，SV 增加，直至达到最理想的前负荷时 SV 保持不变。如果增加液体负荷不再引起 SV 增加，则继续大量静脉补液可能并无益处。继续补液会增加心房压力，增加静脉和动脉的静水压，导致液体进入间质，造成组织水肿。组织水肿会进一步改变组织结构、影响氧交换、损伤毛细血管血流和淋巴回流。随着静脉压（平均循环充盈压）的升高，心房压的增加会向后传导，从而影响微循环。

每搏量变异度（stroke volume variation，SVV）和脉压变异度等功能性血流动力学参数可用于指导液体治疗，这两个参数都依赖于心脏和肺之间的相互作用（脉搏轮廓分析）。自主呼吸的患者，吸气时会降低胸腔内压力，从而增加静脉回流和前负荷，进而增加每搏输出量。而在机械通气患者中，则持续存在相反的情况，临床上可以通过研究机械通气时的动脉波形并观察曲线的移动情况来识别该现象。曲线的移动可实际反映低血容量的程度。针对 Frank-Starling 曲线的变化，如果变化发生在曲线的低位上升部分则可能导致较大改变，但如果发生在平台期，则仅会发生微小的改变（图 96.2）。因此，主要目的是达到足够的循环容量和较好的心血管功能。然而，在手术条件、体温变化和不同的麻醉条件下，可能会发生实质性的变化。

目标导向治疗的倡导者认为，鉴于患者不可避免的存在差异，有必要减少医务人员的变异性，特别是在高危患者和非 ERAS 计划中的患者。

不同监测系统

有创血流动力学监测设备，如 PiCCO（德国，慕尼黑，Pulsion Medical Systems），它可以通过股动脉或腋动脉置管以及中心静脉导管持续监测血流动力学。PiCCO 采用专利算法，假设主动脉压力波形曲线下的面积相当于每搏量曲线，将经脉搏轮廓分析的实时连续监测与经肺的间歇热稀释测量法相结合。该装置能够测量出经肺心排血量、胸内血容量、血管外肺水和心功能，心功能的参数需要从中心静脉导管注射冰盐水测得。该系统需要重新校准，特

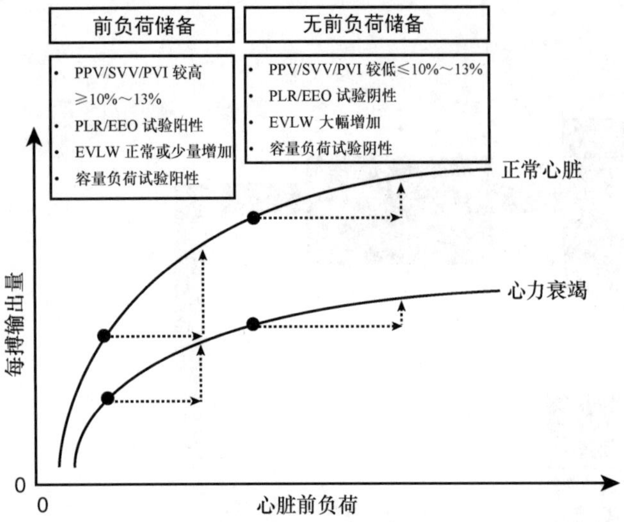

图 96.2 Frank-Starling 曲线描述了舒张期心肌张力（前负荷）与心脏收缩功能的关系。当心室功能处于曲线的上升支时，存在前负荷储备。该部分脉压变异度（PPV）、每搏量变异度（SVV）、脉搏血氧饱和度波形容积变异指数（PVI）较高，呼气末阻断试验（EEO）和被动抬腿试验（PLR）阳性。当心室功能在曲线平台期时，无前负荷储备（From Aditianingsih et al.: Guiding principles of fluid and volume therapy. *Best Pract Res Clin Anaesthesiol* 28[3]：249-260，2014.）

别是在发生快速变化时。

LiDCO（英国，伦敦，LiDCO 公司）是另一种脉搏轮廓分析法（或脉冲功率法），其在血管顺应性或阻力未发生重大变化的前提下，表示血管系统中净功率和净流量之间的线性关系。LiDCO 技术是通过锂稀释，在满足上述限制条件的情况下，对心排血量和每搏量进行可靠评估。LiDCO rapid 版不需要校准，仅用于监测心排血量和每搏量与基线的偏差。

FloTrac 或 Vigileo（加利福尼亚州，尔湾，Edwards 公司）系统需要连接到动脉线路上的传感器。该系统连续监测心排血量和 SVV，这与 Frank-Starling 有关。对于 Vigileo 系统，脉压的标准差与基于基础数据库的正常每搏量相关。主动脉阻抗也是根据既往数据得出，但实际的血管顺应性和阻力是通过动脉压力波形分析确定的。该装置不需要校准，操作简单，但由于使用血管活性药物时可靠性较低，使其应用受阻。当使用普通的升压药如去氧肾上腺素时，即使是最新的 3.0 软件版本其结果也不准确。此外，有效心排血量的测量需要获得最佳的动脉信号。SVV 测量也受到机械通气要求的限制，潮气量至少为 8 ml/kg。将 SVV 系统与血氧测定导管相结合从而提供中心静脉血氧饱和度（$ScvO_2$）测量的设备包，可提供更多血流动力学和容量数据。该装置的使用已经得到美国食品药品监督管理局的批准。所有这些装置都需要获得最佳的动脉信号，且当患者出现心律失常或正在接受主动脉内球囊反搏治疗时，所得到的监测结果均不可靠。

经食管多普勒引导治疗技术采用多普勒超声技术分析降主动脉血流。将一次性的探头插入食管并定位，用以测量每次心跳的血流量。然后将波形与生物特征数据进行比较，得出心脏的每搏量和校正血流时间（flow time corrected for heartbeat，FTc）。由于导管插入在食管下部，大约 70% 的循环血流量被计算在内。使用不同的算法，可为测量容量反应性提供机会。大多数算法使用少量胶体或晶体（2 ～ 3 ml/kg），主要目标是根据 Frank-Starling 曲线改善每搏量。增加前负荷会导致心排血量的增加。通过分析曲线，可以看出在不同心血管参数表现的情况下，对于液体疗法，哪些患者是“有反应”，哪些患者是“无反应”。逐步输液，直到认为患者对液体无反应为止。通常当每搏量或心排血量偏差小于 10% 时会出现这种情况。这已通过标准治疗方案验证，并显示能降低病残率和减少住院时间。在高危和行结直肠手术患者中，已使用经食管多普勒引导治疗技术。但最近的研究表明，在相对健康的患者或腹腔镜手术的患者中，采用经食管多普勒引导治疗和固定的治疗方案之间没有差异。

无创设备已经出现，如连续无创动脉压装置，将每次动脉搏动显示为可视化的波形。目前，尽管这些设备在临床上可能有助于跟踪压力趋势，但它们不够精确，不满足现有标准。脉搏血氧饱和度波形分析可用于评估液体反应性，已开发出了脉搏血氧饱和度容积描记（pulse oximetric plethysmographic，POP）波形振幅（δ POP）和脉搏灌注变异指数（plethysmographic variability index，PVI，其中灌注指数定义为外周毛细血管床中非搏动性血流与脉动性血流的比值）。

不同液体

液体的基本需求包括蒸发、水分和电解质通过汗液和尿液流失。钠离子对细胞外液容量有重要影响。麻醉和手术期间，抗利尿激素水平升高，减少了水的排出。如果给患者使用低渗溶液，血清钠

（serum natrium，S-NA）会降低，伴有潜在的低钠血症危险，这可能对脑细胞产生有害影响，特别是幼儿。

葡萄糖溶液

纯葡萄糖溶液分布至所有流体间隔室。葡萄糖溶液提供基本的热量，多数情况下有助于预防低血糖。添加醋酸根离子会降低氯离子含量。当氯离子供应减少、醋酸分解形成碳酸氢盐时，这种类型的溶液产生一定的缓冲能力，这就是“缓冲葡萄糖”的名称的由来。依据患者的营养状态，使用的葡萄糖含量不一（2.5% 或 5%，即 25 或 50 mg/ml）。葡萄糖和醋酸代谢过程中释放一定量的水，对总的水平衡起到了积极的作用。

等渗氯化钠溶液

等渗氯化钠溶液（9 mg/ml，单位体积内 0.9% 氯化钠）通常被描述为“正常”或“生理性”溶液，表明它与血浆和间质的渗透压类似。它由溶解在无菌水中的普通盐制成。该溶液提供的氯化物含量高于血浆，因此，等渗氯化钠可引起过量的氯离子，并可能导致高氯性酸中毒的发生，这是因为强离子差 [SID=（钠 + 钾 + 镁）-（氯离子 + 乳酸根离子）] 决定了细胞外液（extracellular fluid，ECF）的 pH 值。ECF 中的 SID 通常为 +40，但等渗氯化钠中的 SID 值为 0。因此，补充等渗氯化钠溶液会降低 SID 并导致酸中毒。在动物和健康志愿者中，已经证明氯化物会引起血管收缩，降低肾小球滤过率。因此，输注 0.9% 盐水会导致高氯血症，这与心脏收缩力减弱、肾灌注减少、胃血流量减少和肠道运动功能受损有关。尽管如此，等渗盐水仍然是世界上最常用的晶体溶液之一，它既便宜又与血液的相容性较好。

平衡液

平衡液模拟人体血浆的组成，其重要的特征还有等渗性，且氯离子浓度接近人体血浆。

可代谢的阴离子包含醋酸盐（醋酸）、乳酸盐（乳酸）、葡萄糖酸盐（葡萄糖酸）、苹果酸盐（苹果酸）或柠檬酸盐（柠檬酸）。这些阴离子消耗氢离子和氧气，在肝（主要是乳酸盐）或肌肉（主要是醋酸盐和苹果酸盐）中代谢以取代碳酸氢根离子。乳酸盐取代氯离子可降低总氯离子负荷，当乳酸在肝中代谢时，钠离子被释放并与其他阴离子相结合。故而平衡液的氯离子水平通常为 110 mmol/L，而等渗盐水中为 154 mmol/L。

世界各地几乎都在使用乳酸林格氏液（在英国被称为 Hartmann 溶液）。斯堪的纳维亚研究人员发现，乳酸的分解首先依赖于肝，且在一定程度上也依赖于肾。当外源提供乳酸时，糖异生是乳酸产生的主要途径，这可能对围术期管理有影响。美国国家科学院在 20 世纪 90 年代末发表的一份报告建议，乳酸林格氏液应该加以特别修饰改进，因为大多数制剂中的 D- 乳酸成分对危重患者有不良影响。

另一方面，醋酸盐可以被体内的大多数细胞代谢，表明它更适合于危重患者。与乳酸盐相比，醋酸盐更快地产生 HCO_3^-，消耗中等程度的氧，对呼吸商的影响更低，在糖尿病患者中无明显变化，可以作为缺氧标志物。与乳酸林格液一样，醋酸林格氏液中的钠含量比血浆中低很多。但最近的研究表明，当输注大量低钠液体时，存在发生术后低钠血症的风险，这在小儿人群中尤为明显，被认为是林格氏液的一个缺点，因此，在复方电解质液（Ringerfundin）中已经增加钠含量以解决这一问题。但与醋酸林格氏液（110 mmol/L）相比，这种液体含有的氯离子浓度更高（127 mmol/L）。

复方电解质注射液（Plasma-Lyte，勃脉力）

复方电解质注射液是一种渗透压和电解质含量更接近于血浆的溶液。缓冲能力由葡萄糖酸盐组成，葡萄糖酸盐是一种缓慢作用的弱缓冲液。许多人认为它是“理想的”晶体。目前，澳大利亚和新西兰的一项大型临床试验表明，对比使用缓冲晶体和等渗盐水，两组对危重患者的急性肾损伤或死亡率的影响没有差异。

胶体液

理想的胶体液中的大分子应能增加血浆容量，从而使产生的胶体渗透压接近于血浆渗透压。与晶体液相比，胶体液在血管内液体中保留的时间更长，意味着所需要的量更少。因此，理想情况下，胶体液取得积极效果的速度比使用相同体积的晶体液更快。此外，间质液体空间扩张的可能更小，从而减少水肿程度，改善微循环，也为组织的充足供氧提供了更好的条件。这适用于多糖蛋白复合物和内皮屏障完整的患者。

胶体液分为天然胶体和人工胶体两类。多年来，人们一直在争论使用哪种胶体液，并讨论胶体液与晶体液的优点。然而，研究结果并未表明一种溶液比另一种溶液有任何普遍的优势。

血浆

血浆输注使血管内液体扩张的空间略小于输注血浆的体积。与注入等量的右旋糖酐、羟乙基淀粉或白蛋白溶液相比，血浆在容量扩张方面效果稍差，因为血浆中含有增加毛细血管通透性的成分。输注血浆会引起炎症反应的激活，且级联系统也可被激活。因此，只有主要目的是为了提供凝血因子或凝血抑制剂时，才应给予输注血浆。

白蛋白

白蛋白是一种天然胶体，是人体血浆中的主要蛋白质。生理盐水中加入 4% ～ 5% 的人白蛋白时可作为一种用于容量复苏的胶体。白蛋白占血液中胶体渗透压的 60% ～ 80%。正常的毛细血管渗漏率为每小时 5% ～ 10%。白蛋白通过淋巴系统返回血液中。在创伤或脓毒症的情况下，毛细血管渗漏可能会增加，这会导致白蛋白的重新分布，使其大部分最终进入组织间隙（“白蛋白捕获”）。由于白蛋白与液体结合造成血管外水肿，进而阻碍微循环并损伤组织氧合。生理盐水与白蛋白的液体评估（Saline versus Albumin Fluid Evaluation，SAFE）研究显示，对危重患者随机分配液体后，28 天的死亡率没有显著差异。然而，在预先确定的亚组中进行的其他研究显示，白蛋白可增加创伤性脑损伤患者的死亡风险，但对脓毒症患者略有益处，尽管该作用在后续的研究中尚未完全确定。

人工胶体

右旋糖酐

右旋糖酐是由葡萄糖制成的多糖组成，一部分通过肾排出，其余部分在血浆中分解成二氧化碳和水。最常见的制剂是 6% 右旋糖酐 70、3% 右旋糖酐 60 和 10% 右旋糖酐 40。其扩张血浆容量的能力从略小于输入量（3% 右旋糖酐 60）到大于输入量（10% 右旋糖酐 40）不等，且 6% 右旋糖酐 70 的作用持续时间最长。推荐的最大使用剂量为每 24 h 1.5 g/kg。为了降低过敏反应发生的风险，使用低分子右旋糖酐 -1（半抗原）以结合针对右旋糖酐的任何抗体上的反应点。抗体可能是在早期使用右旋糖酐时产生的，也可能是胃肠系统中天然存在的。

右旋糖酐抑制血小板聚集，降低凝血因子Ⅷ / von Willebrand 的水平，并降低白细胞黏附。因此，右旋糖酐已不再被广泛使用。

明胶

明胶是由牛明胶制成的多肽组成，平均分子量为 30 ～ 35 kDa。明胶对凝血系统和器官完整性方面无损害作用，但可能引起肾功能障碍。

羟乙基淀粉

羟乙基淀粉（hydroxyethyl starch，HES）是一种人工聚合物，由玉米或马铃薯中提取的支链淀粉经羟乙基取代而成。现有的几种 HES 溶液（6% 或 10%）可根据分子量（70 ～ 450 kDa）、摩尔取代级和 C2/C6 比值进行区分。低分子量溶液（130 kDa）至今被使用得最多。

淀粉一部分被淀粉酶分解，然后通过肾分泌，其余积聚在网状内皮组织中，引起瘙痒。围术期可使用的制剂是低分子 HES 130/0.4（玉米淀粉）和 HES 130/0.42（马铃薯淀粉）。马铃薯淀粉是与平衡液（Tetraspan）混合而成，玉米淀粉溶液是与普通盐溶液（Voluven）或平衡液（Voluyte）混合而成。

在 21 世纪初期，研究者猜测分子量较大（>200 kDa）的 HES 会导致肾问题。虽然认为是分子大小本身的原因，但现在已证实，在危重病环境中，低分子量的制剂也会出现肾毒性问题。其中一些研究因设计不当而受到批评。有关围术期的研究存在相互矛盾的数据和综述。目前，HES 受到广泛的限制，截至本文撰写时，该产品已被世界各地的许多监管机构回收封存。也有人认为，在术中输血阈值前，仍存在一个可使用 HES 来代替失血的安全区域。

管理

对于 72 岁的横结肠切除术的男性患者来说，合理的选择是按照 ERAS 理念管理液体。若采用该方法，患者在术前给予碳水化合物，无预负荷，在诱导期间最小化晶体液输注。监测内容可以通过置入食管多普勒导管来评估 SV 和 FTc。如果出现诱导后低血压，在等待手术刺激开始的同时，使用血管升压药治疗。小剂量（100 ～ 200 ml）的晶体液或胶体液均可增加 SV 并降低 FTc。胸段硬膜外麻醉是最佳选择。维持液由晶体液（乳酸林格液或复方电解质注射液，3 ml/h）组成。所有失血一般都用胶体代替，按 1∶1 的比例将液体负荷降至最低，除非失血量超过 1500 ml 时，将酌情给予输注血液成分。

对于接受腹腔镜胆囊切除术的 35 岁女性患者而言，液体策略会有所不同。在整个过程中注入 1 ～ 2 L 晶体可能就足够。现有证据表明，该方法与改善术后症状有关。

（金培培　译　熊源长　校）

延伸阅读

Aditianingsih D, George YW: Guiding principles of fluid and volume therapy, *Best Pract Res Clin Anaesthesiol* 28(3):249–260, 2014.

Annane D, Siami S, Jaber S, et al.: Effects of fluid resuscitation with colloids vs crystalloids on mortality in critically ill patients presenting with hypovolemic shock: the CRISTAL randomized trial, *JAMA* 310(17):1809–1817, 2013.

Arieff AI: Fatal postoperative pulmonary edema: pathogenesis and literature review, *Chest* 115(5):1371–1377, 1999.

Brandstrup B, Svensen C, Engquist A: Hemorrhage and surgery cause a contraction of the extracellular space needing replacement"—evidence and implications, *Surgery* 139:419–432, 2006.

Brandstrup B, Svendsen PE, Rasmussen M, et al.: Which goal for fluid therapy during colorectal surgery is followed by the best outcome: near-maximal stroke volume or zero fluid balance? *Br J Anaesth* 109(2): 191–199, 2012.

Brandstrup B, Tønnesen H, Beier-Holgersen R, et al.: Effects of intravenous fluid restriction on postoperative complications: comparison of two perioperative fluid regimens, *Ann Surg* 238:641–648, 2003.

Caironi P, Tognoni G, Masson S, et al.: Albumin replacement in patients with severe sepsis or septic shock, *N Engl J Med* 370(15):1412–1421, 2014.

Carrico CJ, Coln CD, Lightfoot SA, et al.: Extracellular fluid volume replacement in hemorrhagic shock, *Surg Forum* 14:10–12, 1963.

De Hert S, De Baerdemaeker L: Why hydroxyethyl starch solutions should NOT be banned from the operating room, *Anaesthesiol Intensive Ther* 46(5):336–341, 2014.

Finfer S, Norton R, Bellomo R, et al.: The SAFE study: saline vs. albumin for fluid resuscitation in the critically ill, *Vox Sang* 87(Suppl 2):123–131, 2004.

Hamilton MA, Cecconi M, Rhodes A: A systematic review and meta-analysis on the use of preemptive hemodynamic intervention to improve postoperative outcomes in moderate and high-risk surgical patients, *Anesth Analg* 112(6):1392–1402, 2011.

Jacob M, Chappell D, Rehm M: The "third space"—fact or fiction? *Best Pract Res Clin Anaesthesiol* 23(2):145–157, 2009.

Kancir ASP, Johansen JK, Ekeloef NP, et al.: The effect of 6% hydroxyethyl starch 130/0.4 on renal function, arterial blood pressure, and vasoactive hormones during radical prostatectomy: a randomized controlled trial, *Anesth Analg* 120(3):608–618, 2015.

Lobo DN, Bostock KA, Neal KR, et al.: Effect of salt and water balance on recovery of gastrointestinal function after elective colonic resection: a randomized controlled trial, *Lancet* 359:1812–1818, 2002.

Lowell JA, Schifferdecker C, Driscoll DF, et al.: Postoperative fluid overload: not a benign problem, *Crit Care Med* 18:728–733, 1990.

Manoach S, Weingart SD, Charchaflieh J: The evolution and current use of invasive hemodynamic monitoring for predicting volume responsiveness during resuscitation, perioperative, and critical care, *J Clin Anesth* 24(3):242–250, 2012.

Marik P, Bellomo R: A rational approach to fluid therapy in sepsis, *Br J Anaesth* 116(3):339–349, 2016.

Moore FD, Shires GT: Moderation. *Ann Surg* 166:300–301, 1967.

Moritz ML, Ayus JC: Maintenance intravenous fluids in acutely ill patients, *N Engl J Med* 374(3):290–291, 2016.

Mouncey PR, Osborn TM, Power GS, et al.: Protocolised Management In Sepsis (ProMISe): a multicentre randomised controlled trial of the clinical effectiveness and cost-effectiveness of early, goal-directed, protocolised resuscitation for emerging septic shock, *Health Technol Assess* 19(97):i–xxv, 1–150, 2015.

Myburgh JA, Finfer S, Bellomo R, et al.: Hydroxyethyl starch or saline for fluid resuscitation in intensive care, *N Engl J Med* 367:1901–1911, 2012.

Peak SL, Delaney A, Bailey M, et al.: Goal-directed resuscitation for patients with early septic shock, *N Engl J Med* 371(16):1496–1506, 2014.

Pearse RM, Harrison DA, MacDonald N, et al.: Effect of a perioperative, cardiac output-guided hemodynamic therapy algorithm on outcomes following major gastrointestinal surgery: a randomized clinical trial and systematic review, *JAMA* 311(21):2181–2190, 2014.

Perner A, Haase N, Guttormsen AB, et al.: Hydroxyethyl starch 130/0.4 versus Ringer's acetate in severe sepsis, *N Engl J Med* 367:124–134, 2012.

Shires GT, Williams J, Brown F: Acute changes in extracellular fluid associated with major surgical procedures, *Ann Surg* 154:803–810, 1961.

Sinclair S, James SA, Singer M: Intraoperative intravascular volume optimisation and length of hospital stay after repair of proximal femur fracture: randomised controlled trial, *BMJ* 315:909–912, 1997.

Vallet B, Blanloeil Y, Cholley B, et al.: Guidelines for perioperative haemodynamic optimization, *Ann Fr Anesth Reanim* 32(10):e151–e158, 2013.

Van Der Linden P, James M, Mythen M, et al.: Safety of modern starches used during surgery, *Anesth Analg* 116(1):35–48, 2013.

Wakeling HG, McFall MR, Jenkins CS, et al.: Intraoperative oesophageal Doppler guided fluid management shortens postoperative hospital stay after major bowel surgery, *Br J Anaesth* 95:634–642, 2005.

Yealy DM, Kellum JA, Huang DT, et al.: A randomized trial of protocol-based care for early septic shock, *N Engl J Med* 370(18):1683–1693, 2014.

Young P, Bailey M, Beasley R, et al.: Effect of a buffered crystalloid solution vs saline on acute kidney injury among patients in the intensive care unit: the SPLIT randomized clinical trial, *JAMA* 314(16):1701–1710, 2015.

第 97 章 拮抗剂：纳洛酮、氟马西尼和舒更葡糖

William J. Sauer，Juliana Barr

纳洛酮

病例概要

患者，男性，65 岁，体重 80 kg，既往体健，行冠状动脉旁路移植术，手术历时 3 h，芬太尼总用量 2 mg。术后患者带气管导管转运至 ICU 病房，生命体征平稳。外科医师选择早期拔除气管导管，但此时患者仍处于深镇静状态，对疼痛刺激无反应，并且机械通气时无明显自主呼吸，随即给予纳洛酮 2 mg 静脉注射，5 min 后患者出现严重低氧血症，肺部听诊有啰音并出现泡沫样分泌物。胸部 X 线片提示急性肺水肿。心电图显示室性心律失常。

问题分析

定义

纳洛酮是非选择性阿片类受体拮抗剂，具有极高的亲和力，主要适应证为：①阿片类药物引起的呼吸抑制（即术后使用或新生儿受其母体中用药影响而致的呼吸抑制）；②急性阿片类药物过量；③阿片类药物引起的瘙痒（超适应证用药）。其化学结构与吗啡和氢吗啡酮类似，可竞争性抑制阿片类激动剂对所有阿片类受体的作用（μ> κ = δ），临床上主要用于拮抗阿片类药物的呼吸抑制作用和逆转镇静（μ 受体拮抗剂）。纳洛酮能同时逆转阿片类药物的镇痛作用，引起患者疼痛和（或）急性阿片类药物戒断样症状，所以使用时须滴定使用（表 97.1）。不同剂量的纳洛酮带来的不良反应也不同，可表现为显著的心肺功能不稳定（高血压、心律失常、肺水肿和心脏停搏等）、躁动和癫痫发作，尽管这些不良反应很少见，但大剂量应用纳洛酮仍时有发生。

常用给药途径有静脉、肌内、气管内，但以静脉注射为首选。由于生物利用度低和肝首过效应高（95%），使得纳洛酮口服无效。纳洛酮起效快（< 2 min），其持续作用时间取决于给药剂量（30 ～ 240 min），见表 97.2。其主要在肝内代谢，并由肾排出无活性代谢产物。大多数阿片类激动药物的半衰期比纳洛酮要长，必要时重复给药以预防出现再次进入麻醉状态。

识别

静脉注射纳洛酮尤其大剂量（0.4 ～ 2 mg）注射时，心血管并发症会在几分钟内迅速发生。通常认为，这是由于继发于交感神经兴奋，大量儿茶酚胺释放，引起高血压、心律失常、肺血管和全身性

表 97.1 术后镇静和呼吸抑制的拮抗药物剂量

药物	间歇给药 [a]	持续静脉输注 [a]
纳洛酮	静脉给药：20 ～ 40 μg 每 1 ～ 2 min（5 ～ 20 μg 每 1 ～ 2 min）	4 ～ 8 μg/（kg·h）[4 ～ 8 μg/（kg·h）]
氟马西尼	静脉给药：0.2 mg 每 2 ～ 5 min，最多 1.0 mg；重复给药每 20 min；最大剂量 =3.0 mg/h（4 ～ 20 μg/kg）	0.5 ～ 1.0 μg/（kg·min），最多 3 mg/h 总剂量 [0.5 ～ 1 μg/（kg·min）]

括号内为儿童剂量

表 97.2 拮抗药物的临床药理学

药物	起效（min）	峰值效应（min）	持续时间（min）	清除半衰期（min）
纳洛酮	1 ～ 2	5 ～ 15	60 ～ 240	40 ～ 60[b]
氟马西尼	1 ～ 2	2 ～ 10	45 ～ 90	50[c]

[a] 时间仅代表静脉注射所需时间；纳洛酮也可以静脉注射、肌内注射、皮下注射或气管内注射。不同患者之间的起效时间、达峰时间、持续时间和效应程度可能有很大差异。

[b] 新生儿的清除半衰期加倍。

[c] 药物的清除半衰期在新生儿中减半，在肝病患者中延长。

血管收缩、肺水肿和癫痫所致。如果纳洛酮消除快于残余阿片类药物，则可能会再次出现镇静和呼吸抑制（再次麻醉），因此需始终对患者进行监护，必要时重复给予纳洛酮。

风险评估

纳洛酮给药后并发症的确切发生率尚不明确，术后不良事件极少发生，尤其小剂量滴定给药时。长期使用阿片类药物 / 滥用、患有癫痫病史以及其他原因导致出现戒断症状（如恶心、呕吐、出汗、激动）的患者更容易出现不良事件。另外 ICU 患者中不良事件也较常见，可能跟 ICU 患者大剂量使用阿片类药物有关（如心脏大手术或非心脏手术、阿片类药物过量入院等）。最后，生理应激可能在纳洛酮的毒性中发挥一定的作用，因为据所有的个案报道，纳洛酮的毒性易发生于遭受事件时出现剧痛和应激的患者中。

在过去的十年里，与阿片类药物过量相关的死亡率逐年飙升，全球范围内大约 69 000 人因此丧命。世界卫生组织呼吁扩大纳洛酮药物的社区普及范围来降低死亡人数。既往前瞻性研究表明，对阿片类药物过量的患者紧急静脉注射纳洛酮（中位剂量 0.2 mg），其不良反应发生率为 1.3%，即使此因果关系并未得到证实。动物实验表明，纳洛酮使用前避免显著的高碳酸血症（面罩通气）可减少该药对心肺系统的不良反应。

启示

虽然最初推荐纳洛酮的给药方式为大剂量快速静脉注射，但现在更主张从小剂量谨慎开始，并间歇给药（见表 97.1），以降低发生心血管和神经系统并发症的可能性。心血管监护应持续至给药数小时后，以防止再次麻醉。

管理

如果出现并发症，应立即停止使用纳洛酮。支持患者氧供并行机械通气（球囊面罩、喉罩或气管内导管）、监测和治疗心血管并发症，同时安排患者转入 ICU 进一步治疗。

预防

避免纳洛酮大剂量注射，仔细滴定并严密监测血流动力学。小剂量（低至 20 ～ 40 μg）静脉推注或持续输注 [4 ～ 8 μg/（kg·h）] 即可拮抗阿片类药物的呼吸抑制和镇静，而不拮抗阿片类药物的镇痛效果，也不会诱发心血管不稳定。静脉注射纳洛酮比其他途径更具预测性，应尽可能使用该途径给药。纳洛酮能通过胎盘屏障，可导致新生儿和阿片类药物依赖的母体出现急性戒断症状或癫痫发作。

氟马西尼

病例概要

患者，男性，42 岁。因在家中昏迷被紧急送入院。既往有抑郁症和焦虑症。患者被发现时，旁边有阿米替林和地西泮的空瓶。入院后心率 95 次 / 分，呼吸频率 10 次 / 分。对疼痛刺激无回避反应，且无咽反射。遂予氟马西尼 1 mg 静脉注射，数分钟后患者出现癫痫大发作。予其静脉注射劳拉西泮后仍无反应。遂对其行紧急气管插管以保护气道，并收治入 ICU。

问题分析

定义

氟马西尼是一种 1,4- 咪唑并苯二氮䓬衍生物，可通过影响 γ - 氨基丁酸 A（γ -aminobutyric acid A，$GABA_A$）受体来发挥临床作用，具有非选择性、高亲和力以及竞争性的特点，主要用于：①逆转苯二氮䓬类药物的镇静作用；②苯二氮䓬类药物中毒时的解毒剂。氟马西尼可用于逆转苯二氮䓬类药物引起的镇静、遗忘、定向力障碍和低通气。因为氟马西尼仅与 $GABA_A$ 受体结合（苯二氮䓬类药物结合位点），所以它对阿片类或其他 GABA 能物质（如巴比妥类、乙醇、丙泊酚或其他全身麻醉药）没有影响（图 97.1）。由于长期使用 / 滥用苯二氮䓬类药物的患者有癫痫发作的风险，目前过量服用的现象已经极其少见（风险大于益处）。

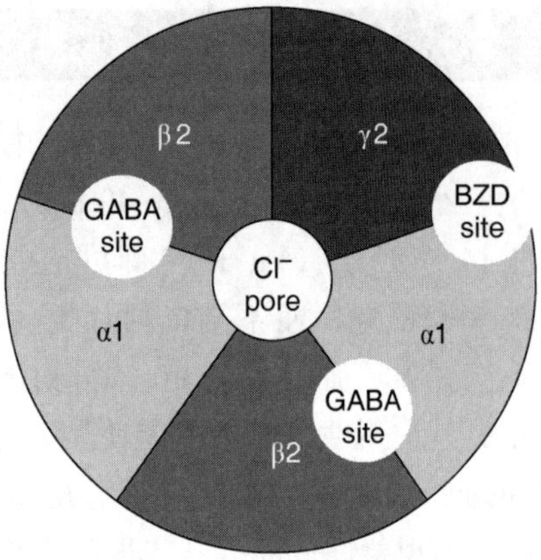

图 97.1 GABA$_A$ 受体（From Wikipedia.org. At https://en.wikipedia.org/wiki/GABAA_receptor#cite_note-pmid22446838-1.）

氟马西尼单次静脉注射后，数分钟内见效快（表 97.2）。其他给药途径有肌内注射、口服或直肠给药，这些非静脉途径通常用于长期应用氟马西尼的患者。氟马西尼经肝快速清除，因此作用时间短，其代谢产物无活性、无毒性。在严重肝病患者中，由于肝清除速度减慢，氟马西尼的代谢时间可能延长。与纳洛酮类似，氟马西尼的效应持续时间通常短于苯二氮䓬类药物（特别是在 ICU 中使用），一旦氟马西尼的作用消退会导致患者再次镇静。

识别

氟马西尼能诱发癫痫和药物戒断的其他症状，主要发生于长期服用苯二氮䓬类药物的患者、正在经历苯二氮䓬类药物戒断的患者或同时服用或过量应用三环类抗抑郁药（或其他抗惊厥类药物）的患者。这就导致了“黑框”警告和氟马西尼应用的减少。然而，那些长期应用苯二氮䓬类药物实施镇静的 ICU 患者，并未出现氟马西尼使用后诱发癫痫的报道。

虽然氟马西尼起效很快，但要完全且持续拮抗苯二氮䓬类药物的不良反应，所需氟马西尼的总剂量因使用的苯二氮䓬类药物的效力和残留血浆浓度不同而异。即使使用最大剂量的氟马西尼，患者的呼吸抑制作用仍可能不能被完全逆转。和纳洛酮相似，应用氟马西尼时进入镇静状态较为常见，需对患者进行严密监测。

风险评估

如果在麻醉或镇静中应用了小剂量苯二氮䓬类药物，氟马西尼可以有效逆转其残留的镇静和呼吸抑制作用。由于氟马西尼作用持续时间短，长期或大量使用苯二氮䓬类药物的 ICU 患者应用氟马西尼后，一旦其拮抗作用消退，可能会出现再次镇静和呼吸抑制现象。因此，这类患者不应使用氟马西尼来加快苯二氮䓬类药效的结束。然而，危重患者停用苯二氮䓬类药物后在合理的时间框内仍不能苏醒时，可试验性使用氟马西尼来帮助诊断。如果给予最大剂量的氟马西尼仍未清醒（即在 1 h 分 3 mg 氟马西尼静脉注射），应考虑导致持续镇静或呼吸抑制等其他因素。对氟马西尼有反应的患者，最后一次给药后应仔细观察 2 h，以确定是否有镇静或呼吸抑制复发的征象。

启示

很多专家认为，氟马西尼除了用于拮抗小剂量苯二氮䓬类药物的镇静，当其作为解毒剂时导致癫痫发作 / 不良事件的风险大于其潜在益处。大多数急性苯二氮䓬类药物过量患者的呼吸抑制程度低于阿片类药物过量的患者，必要时可提供机械通气和心血管支持，直至过量药物作用消退。如果氟马西尼用于治疗苯二氮䓬类药物过量，这些患者应收至 ICU 密切监测。

管理

与纳洛酮类似，如果出现并发症，立即停止给予氟马西尼。癫痫发作时，进行抗癫痫药物治疗，需要了解的是，如果之前用过氟马西尼，那么癫痫发作时，小剂量的苯二氮䓬药物无效。

预防

氟马西尼能逆转苯二氮䓬类药物引起的短期镇静和呼吸抑制，且安全有效，但不适于长期依赖的患者。氟马西尼应小剂量分次给药，给药后必须仔细观察患者有无再次镇静和呼吸抑制现象，持续至少 2 h。氟马西尼用药需小剂量（0.2 mg）重复静脉推注或小剂量持续静脉滴注 [0.5 ～ 1 μ/（kg · min），可达 3 mg/h]，通过滴定以达到目标镇静和通气水平。这种给药方式能可靠地避免患者术后出现再镇静现象，亦可避免突然或完全逆转抗焦虑作用。最后，应避免对长期依赖苯二氮䓬类药物或疑似三环类抗抑郁药过量的患者使用氟马西尼。

舒更葡糖

病例概要

患者，男性，87 岁，拟急诊行腹腔镜胆囊切除术。给予罗库溴铵（1.2 mg/kg）快速序贯诱导后完成气管插管。手术用时 1 h，术中未再追加罗库溴铵，手术结束时，四个成串刺激（train-of-four，TOF）显示为 0/4。给患者注射舒更葡糖，2 min 后其神经肌肉阻滞被完全逆转（TOF=4/4，肌颤搐不衰减）。但随后患者出现急性心动过缓（30 次 / 分）。立即静脉注射格隆溴铵 0.2 mg，恢复窦性心律（74 次 / 分）。

问题分析

定义

舒更葡糖（布瑞亭）是一种 γ-环糊精，可以选择性结合甾体类神经肌肉阻滞药（neuromuscular blocking agent，NMBA），因此，成为首个选择性神经肌肉阻滞拮抗剂。国际上舒更葡糖已用于临床很多年，而最近美国食品药品管理局（Food and Drug Administration，FDA）批准其在美国境内使用的适应证为：①常规拮抗罗库溴铵和维库溴铵引起的神经肌肉阻滞；②紧急拮抗罗库溴铵引起的神经肌肉阻滞。后一种适应证可能改变麻醉科医师对罗库溴铵诱导后“不能插管，不能通气”患者的处置方式。以往，医生一般选择胆碱酯酶抑制剂（如新斯的明、依酚氯铵）拮抗非去极化肌肉松弛药作为传统的标准处理方式。与此不同的是，舒更葡糖可以封被甾体类 NMBA，减少罗库溴铵或维库溴铵与烟碱受体的相互作用（一种真正的拮抗剂，而不仅仅是通过增加神经肌肉接头处乙酰胆碱的量来与剩余的 NMBA 竞争）（图 97.2）。

由于对高敏反应和心动过缓等方面的顾虑，FDA 曾三次拒绝批准舒更葡糖上市。但是全世界超过 900 万的患者使用过这种药物，而且后续的重复剂量试验表明，使用舒更葡糖后，严重的不良事件极其罕见（不到 1%）。如果舒更葡糖的注射剂量不足，神经肌肉阻滞可再次发生。其他方面的顾虑还包括凝血功能障碍患者的部分凝血活酶时间（partial thromboplastin time，PTT）延长，还可能会降低体内雌激素和（或）孕激素用以避孕的浓度。舒更葡糖亦有报道可能会延长 QT 间期。常见的副作用包括头痛、恶心、头晕和呕吐。

在使用与神经肌肉阻滞程度相匹配的合理剂量时，舒更葡糖在静脉注射后可迅速起效（<3 min）（表 97.3）。由于其不经过肝代谢，所以肝功能障碍

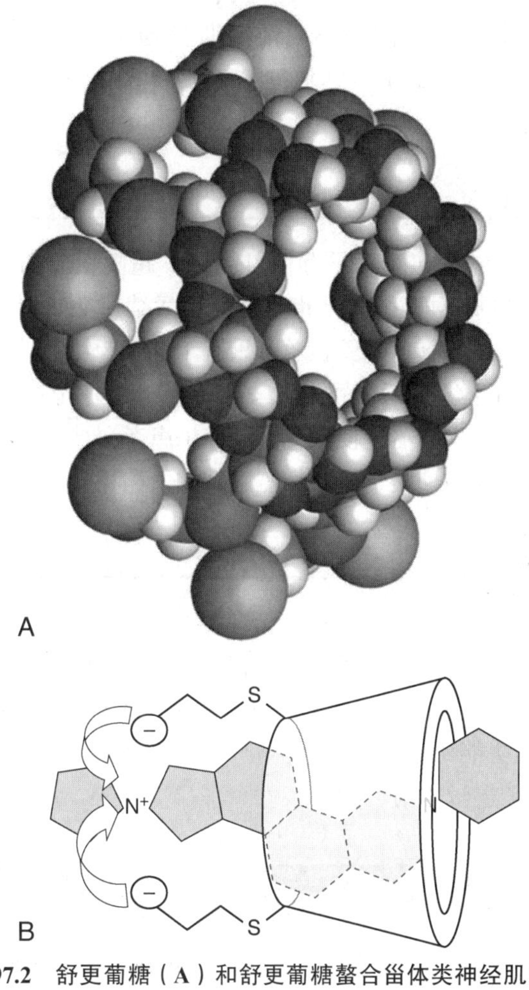

图 97.2 舒更葡糖（A）和舒更葡糖螯合甾体类神经肌肉阻滞药罗库溴铵的图示（B）（From Wikiwand. Available ai http://www.wikiwand.com/en/Sugammadex.）

表 97.3 舒更葡糖（甾体类神经肌肉阻滞药拮抗剂）剂量

TOF>2	TOF<2	即刻（TOF<0）[a]
2 mg/kg	4 mg/kg	16 mg/kg

[a] 给予罗库溴铵后立即拮抗的剂量（不包括维库溴铵）

TOF，四个成串刺激。

并不影响舒更葡糖的给药剂量；但需考虑患者有无凝血功能异常。舒更葡糖几乎全部经肾排泄，其半衰期约为 2 h（严重肾功能损伤的患者可达 19 h）。

识别

严重的不良反应（如超敏、心动过缓）通常在舒更葡糖用药后 5 min 内即可发生，因此在给药后应即刻严密监测。抗胆碱能药物和经典的抗过敏药物应备好随时可用。应进行神经肌肉监测以确保 NMBA 完全逆转。神经肌肉阻滞的复发问题（舒更葡糖剂量不足时）在既往研究中已有描述。如果患者在舒更葡糖给药后需要再次进行神经肌肉阻滞，那么应该使用不同类型肌松药（即非甾体类 NMBA），因为舒更葡糖对非甾体类 NMBA 没有影响。

风险评估

虽然最初对舒更葡糖可能引发超敏反应的顾虑导致 FDA 对其批准上市延迟。但后续对 299 例患者进行的重复剂量试验显示，只有 1 例患者发生过敏反应。由于舒更葡糖可延长 PTT，因此有明显凝血异常的患者应该避免使用此药。如果患者深神经肌肉阻滞程度已被逆转，应密切监测其肌力和呼吸力度。

启示

舒更葡糖比胆碱酯酶抑制剂起效快，且更有效地逆转神经肌肉阻滞，因此未来临床使用可能更为频繁。无论使用哪种拮抗剂，都应密切监测患者心肺功能（ASA 标准监测）和神经肌肉恢复状态（TOF 定量监测）。

管理

如果患者出现心动过缓，应迅速给予抗胆碱能药物（如格隆溴铵）。因超敏反应出现支气管痉挛或低血压时应立即进行妥善的药物治疗。

预防

在可能发生过敏反应的患者中，应避免使用舒更葡糖（有反应史）。如果患者存在凝血异常，应谨慎使用。正在使用雌激素和（或）孕激素避孕的患者应告知其舒更葡糖对这些药物疗效有干扰作用。

（王家强 译 李晓菲 校）

延伸阅读

Abrishami A, Ho J, Wong J, et al.: Sugammadex, a selective reversal medication for preventing postoperative residual neuromuscular blockade, *Cochrane Database Syst Rev* (4):CD007362, 2009.

Barnett V, Twycross R, Mihalyo M, et al.: Opioid antagonists, *J Pain Symptom Manage* 47(2):341–352, 2014.

Dahan A, Aarts L, Smith TW: Incidence, reversal, and prevention of opioid-induced respiratory depression, *Anesthesiology* 112:226–238, 2010.

Ledowski T: Sugammadex: what do we know and what do we still need to know? A review of the recent (2013 to 2014) literature, *Anaesth Intensive Care* 43(1):14–22, 2015.

Ngo AS, Anthony CR, Samuel M, et al.: Should a benzodiazepine antagonist be used in unconscious patients presenting to the emergency department? *Resuscitation* 74(1):27–37, 2007.

Osterwalder JJ: Naloxone—for intoxications with intravenous heroin and heroin mixtures—harmless or hazardous? *J Toxicol Clin Toxicol* 34:409–416, 1996.

Rosow CE, Dershwitz M: Clinical pharmacology of opioids. In Evers A, Maze M, Kharasch E, editors: *Anesthetic pharmacology: basic principles and clinical practice*, ed 2, Cambridge, 2011, Cambridge UP, pp 531–547.

Rudolph U, Davies MF, Barr J: Benzodiazepines. In Evers A, Maze M, Kharasch E, editors: *Anesthetic pharmacology: basic principles and clinical practice*, ed 2, Cambridge, 2011, Cambridge UP, pp 466–477.

Stoelting RK, Hillier SC, editors: *Pharmacology and physiology in anesthetic practice*, ed 4, Philadelphia, 2005, Lippincott Williams & Wilkins.

World Health Organization: Community management of opioid overdose. 2014 Available at www.who.int/substance_abuse/publications/management_opioid_overdose/en/. Accessed August 27, 2017.

琥珀胆碱

第 98 章

Eugene B. Freid

病例概要

患者，女性，52 岁，因患双相抑郁症接受其首次电休克治疗（electroconvulsive therapy，ECT）。既往病史包括婴儿期脑膜炎导致的偏瘫、停滞性脑病和高血压，其余正常。目前主要治疗药物包括拉莫三嗪、鲁拉西酮和赖诺普利。该病患者接受的单侧 ECT 疗法麻醉诱导采用 80 mg 美索比妥和 60 mg 琥珀胆碱，过程顺利，患者接受单侧 ECT 治疗。手术结束 15 min 后患者仍无呼吸，且无 TOF 反应。患者予以镇静、插管和机械通气。60 min 后，患者较为虚弱，4 个抽搐减弱，TOF 中度衰减，接受 ECT 治疗后 2 h 拔除气管导管。检测结果表明，丁酰胆碱酯酶活性为 55%，辛可卡因值为 25，与丁酰胆碱酯酶的非典型变异相一致。

问题分析

定义

50 年来，琥珀胆碱因起效迅速，作用时间短，比其他神经肌肉阻滞药具有独特的优势。然而，琥珀胆碱也具有多种众所周知的并发症，主要与其作用机制或药物代射动力学有关，或作为特异质效应发生（框 98.1）。最严重的反应是高钾血症、非预期的肌肉松弛延长和恶性高热（见第 195 章）。存在易发生乙酰胆碱受体上调或横纹肌溶解病情的患者可能在使用琥珀胆碱后不久出现高钾血症诱导的心脏停搏（框 98.2）。

琥珀胆碱应用后，出现Ⅱ相阻滞或代谢下降时，可能会发生长时间肌肉松弛。单次大剂量、重复给药或长时间持续输注琥珀胆碱，接头后受体可能会不能对乙酰胆碱产生正常反应，即使受体-通道再极化后，受体也可能会对乙酰胆碱产生耐药性，这被称之为**Ⅱ相阻滞**。

正常情况下，琥珀胆碱的短效作用是丁酰胆碱酯酶（butyrylcholinesterase，BChE）对其快速水解的结果，BChE 也称为**假性胆碱酯酶**或**血浆胆碱酯酶**。90% 的琥珀胆碱静脉注射后被 BChE 迅速水解成一种几乎无活性的代谢物。当琥珀胆碱从终板扩散到细胞外液后其神经肌肉阻滞作用终止，BChE 通过控制水解速率影响药物的起效和持续时间。当正常 BChE 的数量显著减少或 BChE 的突变体存在时，琥珀胆碱的持续时间可能会延长。

框 98.1 琥珀胆碱用药并发症

- 心血管系统
  - 心动过速（神经节刺激）
  - 心动过缓、窦性停搏、交界性心律（心脏毒蕈碱样）
- 高钾血症、钾离子过度释放
- 肌束震颤；肌痛[a]
- 肌红蛋白尿，血浆肌酸磷酸激酶升高
- 肌肉持续收缩（强直性肌营养不良、先天性肌强直）
- 恶性高热
- 咬肌强直
- 肌松作用延长
  - Ⅱ度阻滞
  - 假性胆碱酯酶活性不足
- 眼内压增高
- 颅内压增高
- 胃内压升高
- 组胺释放
- 变态 / 过敏样反应

[a] 琥珀胆碱预处理可能会减轻（去肌颤）

识别

琥珀胆碱给药后不久出现 T 波升高、QRS 波群

框 98.2 琥珀胆碱诱发钾过度释放的情况

热损伤
上运动神经元或下运动神经元缺陷
  脊髓损伤
  轻偏瘫，下运动神经元病变
  多发性硬化
  脑卒中
  Guillain-Barré 病
  脑炎伴运动神经受累
  中枢神经系统创伤
肌病，肌营养不良
严重创伤
废用性萎缩，长期化学性去神经支配
严重感染，破伤风

宽大和正弦曲线的 QRS 波形（见第 87 章）以及心搏停止或心室纤颤，这是钾释放过多和高钾血症患者的心电图（electrocardiogram，ECG）上观察到的特征性改变。血清钾离子浓度测定可证实是否存在高钾血症。但如果 ECG 异常，在确定血清钾离子浓度之前即应先进行治疗。

既往体健的患者在接受正常剂量的琥珀胆碱时，通常只有在全身麻醉苏醒失败和肌无力延长时，才发现异常 BChE 的存在。极低水平的正常 BChE 或异常形式的 BChE 会导致不同程度的神经肌肉阻滞延长（表 98.1）。这些异常情况并不少见。最近在瑞士进行的一项观察性研究中，16% 的患者接受 1 mg/kg 琥珀胆碱快速序贯诱导的阻滞持续时间超过 10 min。可通过周围神经刺激的特征性发现来进行诊断，包括四个成串刺激比值（T4/T1）小于 30%、衰减现象及强直后易化，这种典型的Ⅱ相阻滞，是由于神经肌肉接头处未代谢的琥珀胆碱浓度升高所致。

风险评估

钾释放

在正常情况下，骨骼肌的去极化发生在运动终板的乙酰胆碱受体（acetylcholine receptor，AChR），琥珀胆碱作用于 AChR 后，可使血清 K^+ 浓度升高达 0.5 mEq/dl。然而，在一些病理条件下，使用琥珀胆碱后钾离子过量释放会导致血清钾离子浓度过高（见框 98.2）。在易感患者中，不成熟的 AChR 上调，α-7AChR 遍及整个肌膜。实际上，整个肌膜发挥运动终板的作用。上调的突触外 AChR 对琥珀胆碱更敏感，代谢更慢，导致肌细胞持续去极化和钾离子向胞外过度外流。用非去极化松弛剂预处理不能可靠地消除高血钾反应。

琥珀胆碱引起的钾离子过度释放发生的时机取决于损伤的性质，并发生于 AChR 超敏形成的时机之后。通常在热损伤或创伤后 5 ～ 15 天开始，20 ～ 60 天达到高峰，并持续长达 3 个月。患有上或下运动神经元疾病的患者始于第 7 天，并持续约 6 个月，甚至偶有持续数年的病例。相反，患有停滞性脑病（例如脑性瘫痪）的患者在琥珀胆碱给药后通常不出现过度的 K 离子释放，因为其神经系统损伤发生久远且已状态稳定。

在使用琥珀胆碱后，患有肌病的患者可能发生横纹肌溶解，可引发危及生命的高钾血症。在婴儿和儿童中，肌病临床症状不明显，仅在琥珀胆碱引起的高钾性心脏停搏出现后才得以诊断。

Ⅱ相阻滞

临床中无论重复给药或连续输注，琥珀胆碱总剂量低至 4 mg/kg 时Ⅱ相阻滞可能会发生。快速耐受的发生通常与临床相关的Ⅱ相阻滞同时发生。

假性胆碱酯酶

新生儿、老年人、妊娠、肝病、营养不良、恶性肿瘤、热损伤以及使用某些药物或长期接触有机磷杀虫剂的患者血浆 BChE 活性下降。在行血浆置换后 BChE 水平可能会急剧下降（框 98.3）。正常 BChE 的含量降低一般不会导致影响临床症状的琥珀胆碱阻滞作用延长，只有正常 BChE 的活性降低 75% 时才可能出现（正常活性 4.9 ～ 12 IU/ml）。相反，在遗传异常的 BChE 患者中，恢复正常的神经肌肉功能的延迟时间可能从 10 ～ 15 min（轻度）到 2 ～ 4 h（重度），这取决于 BChE 突变体。BChE 由染色体 3q26 上的单个基因位点转录。目前已发现 50 多个 BChE 基因突变位点，其中某一个氨基酸的改变会导致酶功能异常，另一些位点突变会抑制 BChE 的产生。一个 BChE 基因可能携带多个突变位点。许多但不是全部 BChE 的表型差异能通过标准化实验条件下测定化合物（如地布卡因、氟化物）抑制 BChE 对苯甲酰胆碱的水解能力来确定。地布卡因对正常（Eu Eu）患者的苯甲酰胆碱水解有 80% 的抑制作用。

最常见的突变体是 Kalow 突变体（K）和 Ea

框 98.3 诱发丁酰胆碱酯酶活性降低的病情

生理性（新生儿、妊娠和老年人）
肝病、营养不良
恶性肿瘤（尤其是肺、胃肠道和泌尿生殖系统）
热损伤
药物治疗（糖皮质激素、甲氧氯普胺、雌激素、环硫磷、班布特罗、苯乙肼和环磷酰胺）
有机磷杀虫剂
血浆置换

地布卡因耐药突变体（非典型）（表 98.1）。在非典型突变体中，地布卡因抑制的苯甲酰胆碱水解降低至不到 30%。其他 BChE 质的变异包括 2 个对氟化物耐药的突变体和几个沉默突变体，其点突变导致 BChE 活性极低，且既不显示地布卡因也不显示氟化物诱导的抑制作用。也有三种 BChE 量的突变体，为 J、K 和 H，BChE 水平下降。k- 多态性突变体本身只会使琥珀胆碱作用时间稍微延长，但可能合并其他突变，显著延长神经肌肉阻滞。表 98.1 总结了正常和遗传异常 BChE 突变体的特征。

启示

琥珀胆碱引起的高钾血症的后果包括心律失常和心脏停搏。琥珀胆碱引起的肌肉松弛延长需要气道管理和机械通气（需镇静），直到神经肌肉无力症状消退。携带异常 BChE 突变体患者也显示米库氯铵和酯类局部麻醉药持续时间延长。由于 BChE 不参与艾司洛尔和瑞芬太尼的代谢，在非典型或异常 BChE 患者中，它们的代谢未受影响。

管理

高血钾

心脏停搏和心室纤颤采用标准高级心血管生命支持（advanced cardiovascular life support，ACLS）方案治疗。此外，必须以钙剂（氯化物或葡萄糖酸盐）稳定心肌，积极采取过度通气以及碳酸氢钠和 β- 激动剂治疗高钾血症。目前心脏停搏和心室纤颤的治疗方案不再将钙离子和碳酸氢钠纳入初始治疗中，因此早期识别高血钾症至关重要。钙离子可减轻心脏高钾对细胞的影响。过度通气、碳酸氢盐和 β- 肾上腺素能受体激动剂（肾上腺素）有助于钾离子内流。较轻度高钾血症可使用过度通气、钙、碳酸氢钠和胃肠外或吸入 β- 肾上腺素能受体兴奋剂

表 98.1 正常、非典型和异常的丁酰胆碱酯酶

基因型	表型（通用名）	阻滞延长（90% T1，min）	地布卡因值	氟值	酶活性	频率
Eu Eu	野生型（通常）	正常 9.3（4 ~ 16）	70 ~ 80	60	100%	96%
Kalow（k）多态性	（K-variant）	最少 11.6（7 ~ 14）	80	60	67%	Eu/K：1/4 KK：1/63
Eu Ea		轻微 15（9 ~ 38）	60	50	77%	1/25
Eu Ef		轻微 15（11 ~ 23）	75	50	86%	1/200
Eu Es		轻微	80	60	50%	1/190
Ea Ef		中度 29（23 ~ 36）	50	50	59%	1/20 000
Ef Es		中度	65	35	37%	1/15 000
Ef Ef	耐氟化物 F1、F2	中度	65	35	74%	0.002 1/154 000
Ea Ea	地布卡因耐药（非典型）	显著 130（90 ~ 180）	20	20	43%	0.018 1/2000
Es Es	静默型 S1、S2、S3	显著	—	—	0 ~微量	1/100 000
Ea Es		显著	20	20	22%	1/29 000

Data from Pantuck EJ，Pantuck CB：Prolonged apnea following succinylcholine administration. In Azar I，editor：*Muscle relaxants*. New York，Marcel Dekker，1987，pp 206-229；Whittaker M：Plasma cholinesterase variants and the anaesthetist. *Anaesthesia* 35（2）：174-197，1980；Bretlau C，S?renson MK，Vedersoe AL，et al.：Response to succinylcholine in patients carrying the K-variant of the butyrylcholinesterase gene. *Anesth Analg* 116(3)：596-601，2013.

（沙丁胺醇或特布他林）进行治疗。葡萄糖和胰岛素也可使用，但由于它们的起效较慢，所以一般不考虑作为一线治疗药物使用。对于高钾导致心脏停搏的患儿，应对潜在的肌肉疾病进行术后评估。

阻滞延长

由于发现有遗传异常的 BChE 患者在麻醉肌肉松弛期间知晓的情况仍有报道，肌肉松弛延长的治疗不仅包括保证气道通畅和气体交换，还包括镇静/镇痛，直至Ⅱ期阻滞消退和肌力恢复。单纯Ⅱ相阻滞可应用抗胆碱酯酶药逆转。然而，琥珀胆碱过量或非典型或异常的假胆碱酯酶所致的阻滞属于混合阻滞（Ⅰ相和Ⅱ相），抗胆碱酯酶治疗可延长Ⅰ相阻滞的时间。大多数医生只是继续通气支持，直到阻滞消退，肌肉力量恢复到其正常水平。尽管库存血液和血浆中含有活性 BChE 成分，但输血的相关风险大于逆转长时间阻滞的获益。怀疑有非典型或异常 BChE 的患者应检测 BChE 活性、地布卡因数值和遗传检测（如可行），并告知其病情。在患者的病历中应有提示，注明患者对琥珀胆碱“过敏”，而且患者应该佩戴医疗警示手环。

预防

预防琥珀胆碱并发症的最好方法是完全避免使用该药，除非有明显的适应证或使用优势。对于幼儿，特别是患有临床症状不明显的肌病的男性，这似乎更有必要。在许多国家，舒更葡糖钠的获批应用使得在大多数情况下用罗库溴铵替代琥珀胆碱成为可能。数项研究已表明，大剂量罗库溴铵和舒更葡糖钠的起效和恢复速度已经能够与琥珀胆碱持平甚至更快。

如果反复使用琥珀胆碱，则应将琥珀胆碱的总剂量控制在 5 ～ 6 mg/kg 以下，以减少Ⅱ相阻滞的发生。在术前评估过程中，应询问患者是否有长期肌无力或麻醉苏醒延迟的家族史。由于 BChE 的遗传性，某些地区的遗传异常更为常见，在这些地区，术前实验室筛查 BChE 活性可能会有一定的作用。

（袁　炜　译　陈　玲　校）

延伸阅读

Dell-Kuster S, Levano S, Burkhart CS, et al.: Predictors of the variability in neuromuscular block duration following succinylcholine: a prospective observational study, *Eur J Anaesthesiol* 32:687–696, 2015.

Gronert GA: Cardiac arrest after succinylcholine, *Anesthesiology* 94:523–629, 2001.

Jensen FS, Viby-Mogensen J: Plasma cholinesterase and abnormal reaction to succinylcholine: twenty years' experience with the Danish Cholinesterase Research Unit, *Acta Anaesthiol Scand* 39:150–156, 1995.

Larach MG, Rosenberg H, Gronert GA, et al.: Hyperkalemic cardiac arrest during anesthesia in infants and children with occult myopathies, *Am J Anesth* 24:241–247, 1997.

Levano S, Ginz H, Siegemund M, et al.: Genotyping the butyrylcholinesterase in patients with prolonged neuromuscular block after succinylcholine, *Anesthesiology* 102:531–535, 2005.

Martyn Jr JA, White DA, Gronert GA, et al.: Up-and-down regulation of skeletal muscle acetylcholine receptors, *Anesthesiology* 76:822–843, 1992.

Martyn JA, Richtsfeld M: Succinylcholine-induced hyperkalemia in acquired pathologic states: etiologic factors and molecular mechanisms, *Anesthesiology* 104:158–169, 2006.

Pantuck EJ: Plasma cholinesterase: gene and variations, *Anesth Analg* 77:380–386, 1993.

Pantuck EJ, Pantuck CB: Prolonged apnea following succinylcholine administration. In Azar I, editor: *Muscle relaxants*, New York, 1987, Marcel Dekker, pp 206–229.

Sørensen MK, Bretlau C, Gätke MR, et al.: Rapid sequence induction and intubation with rocuronium-sugammadex compared with succinylcholine: a randomized trial, *Br J Anaesth* 108:682–689, 2012.

Thomsen JL, Nielsen CV, Eskildsen KZ, et al.: Awareness during emergence from anaesthesia: significance of neuromuscular monitoring in patients with butyrylcholinesterase deficiency, *Br J Anaesth* 115(Suppl 1):i78–i88, 2015.

Viby-Mogensen J: Correlation of succinylcholine duration of action with plasma cholinesterase activity in subjects with the genotypically normal enzyme, *Anesthesiology* 53:517–520, 1980.

挥发性麻醉药：器官毒性

第 99 章

Evan D. Kharasch

病例概要

患者，女性，53 岁，在氟烷麻醉下保留自主呼吸行声带乳头状瘤激光切除术。患者之前接受过数次手术，最近的一次为 1 个月前，均使用氟烷麻醉且顺利。然而，此次术后 1 周，患者出现发热、恶心及萎靡，同时伴有严重的黄疸和血清转氨酶浓度明显升高。

问题分析

定义

挥发性麻醉药引起的器官毒性是从麻醉药用药至麻醉药消除之后细胞结构或功能持续改变的结果。对于挥发性麻醉药最令人关注的是其肝毒性和肾毒性。

本文未做讨论但值得提及的是，挥发性吸入麻醉药与干燥的二氧化碳吸收剂相互作用可能形成潜在的有毒化合物，如一氧化碳和化合物 A。可能发生肺和肾毒性，也有发生火灾和爆炸的报道（有关更多详情，请参阅“推荐阅读”中列出的 Baum 和 Woehlck 的文献。）

肝毒性

肝毒性最常见于氟烷用药后，恩氟烷、异氟烷、七氟烷和地氟烷用药后也可发生肝毒性但概率较低。氟烷可导致两种类型的肝损伤：

- 暴发性肝坏死（“氟烷性肝炎”）；
- 轻度亚临床肝毒性。

暴发性肝坏死的临床特征是发热和黄疸，血清转氨酶水平明显升高。肝活检显示大量小叶中央型坏死。目前，暴发性肝坏死被认为是一种由氟烷氧化代谢为中间产物引起的免疫现象。随后中间产物与肝蛋白质结合并诱导三氟乙酰化，使蛋白质具有抗原性。这些抗原刺激抗体的形成，当再次暴露于氟烷（或恩氟烷、异氟烷或地氟烷）时，引发免疫介导的肝坏死。这种坏死是罕见的，氟烷用药后每 6 000 ～ 35 000 人中有 1 例发生；恩氟烷用药后每 100 万人中则有 2 例发生；异氟烷用药后有一些病例报道；地氟烷用药后有 1 例确诊病例。也有报道七氟烷用药后发生肝功能障碍，但认为不是由免疫介导的坏死，其与麻醉的关系尚不清楚。

氟烷用药后通常发生轻度肝毒性（约占 25%），但其他挥发性麻醉药用药后不发生。其特点是血清转氨酶和谷胱甘肽 -S- 转移酶浓度轻度短暂升高及术后药物代谢改变。然而，临床上显著的肝细胞疾病并不是轻度肝毒性的特征，这种轻度肝毒性是由于氟烷还原（无氧）代谢，其活性代谢产物引起脂质过氧化并与细胞色素 P-450 结合。这两种形式的麻醉药物肝毒性被认为是不相关的。

急性肾衰竭

急性肾衰竭是围术期常见问题，但它极少是使用挥发性麻醉剂的直接后果。有几个术语需要定义：

- **肾衰竭**是可导致血清生化发生改变的肾功能减退，可表现为少尿、非少尿或多尿；
- **肾功能不全**是血清生化正常的较轻的肾功能减退；
- **少尿**指尿量少于 20 ml/h（70 kg 成人），意味着肾衰竭；
- **非少尿性肾衰竭**比少尿性肾衰竭更常见，被认为是较轻微的肾损伤；

- **多尿**指尿量大于 100 ml/h（70 kg 成人）。

少尿和非少尿性肾衰竭可能是肾后性（梗阻性）、肾前性（由于低血容量、低血压、肾血流减少或心血管手术引起的肾灌注不足）或肾性（由肾毒素如氨基糖苷类抗生素、肌红蛋白、血红蛋白、造影剂或非甾体抗炎药引起）。多尿性肾衰竭，即肾浓缩能力下降，是由中枢性尿崩（抗利尿激素分泌不足，通常是由于垂体功能障碍）或是由肾性尿崩（肾对抗利尿激素无反应）引起。

麻醉相关性肾功能不全通常是肾前性的，由低血压或肾灌注改变引起。它受麻醉时间限制，且为可逆性。由麻醉药引起的肾衰竭仅在使用甲氧氟烷时观察到，可引起血管加压素抵抗性多尿、高钠血症、高渗透压和脱水；它还能增加血尿素氮（blood urea nitrogen，BUN）和肌酐水平。甲氧氟烷的肾毒性与甲氧氟烷的代谢呈剂量相关性。与毒性相关的血浆氟化物浓度范围 50 ～ 80 μM 不等。长期使用恩氟烷后可出现轻微但可逆的浓缩功能障碍。恩氟烷、异氟烷、地氟烷或七氟烷均未观察到直接肾毒性，即使全身氟化物浓度远超过 50 μM。全身的氟浓度作为肾毒性的作用因素已经被忽视。

识别

临床上暴发性肝坏死表现为术后 3 ～ 6 天出现发热、恶心、食欲缺乏、寒战、萎靡和皮疹，紧接着术后 6 ～ 10 天出现严重黄疸。实验室检查表现包括血清转氨酶水平明显升高、高胆红素血症和凝血酶原时间延长，但这些并不是其特异性表现。病理检查结果包括小叶中心和中央带坏死，但同样，这些表现也非特异性的。临床上氟烷用药后的轻微肝毒性通常是无症状的，实验室检查只有轻微的、可逆的肝酶增加（天冬氨酸氨基转移酶、丙氨酸转氨酶、γ- 谷酰基转移酶和谷胱甘肽 -S- 转移酶）。它们在术后 1 ～ 2 天升高，通常在几天内消退。然而，该水平可能持续升高最多 2 周。

麻醉相关性肝炎的特异性诊断是非常困难的，其临床表现和形态学特征与病毒性肝炎非常相似。事实上，围术期隐匿性肝炎（病毒性、感染性、酒精性）的发病率为 1/700，其中 30% 的病例术后出现黄疸，这远远高于麻醉相关的暴发性肝炎的发病率。甲、乙、丙、丁型肝炎或其他感染性疾病（如巨细胞病毒、EB 病毒）的血清标志物阳性可能有助于排除麻醉是术后肝炎发生的病因，但血清标志物阴性时也不能排除，尤其是近期存在感染的情况下。少数实验室可以检测血清中抗三氟乙酰化蛋白抗体，这有助于麻醉相关性肝炎的诊断。然而，该试验缺乏足够的特异性，不能常规使用。丙肝是术后肝炎最常见的病因，但也应排除肝脏缺血、其他药物、输血和胆汁淤积。

肾功能不全和急性肾衰竭的临床表现前面已经列出。根据肾对脱水和抗利尿激素的反应来鉴别中枢性和肾性尿崩症。少尿性肾衰竭是由血尿素氮-肌酐比值、尿钠和渗透压、尿-血浆渗透压、尿-血浆肌酐、钠排泄分数和对液体冲击的反应性来确定。在甲氧氟烷后的时代，对挥发性麻醉药引起肾衰竭的特异性诊断极为罕见。

风险评估

暴发性肝坏死的临床危险因素包括：

- 多次接触氟烷；
- 既往有麻醉后发热或黄疸史；
- 肥胖；
- 女性；
- 中年。

氟烷通过细胞色素 P-450 2E1 氧化代谢。因此，酶诱导（酒精、异烟肼、肥胖）增加了抗原形成及风险，而酶抑制（双硫仑）则降低代谢。短时间内（<6 周）多次反复接触氟烷是氟烷性肝炎的最大危险因素。

由于未知原因，即使反复接触氟烷，儿童的患病风险也大大降低。肝病本身不是氟烷性肝炎的危险因素。轻度肝毒性的临床危险因素是指那些增加氟烷还原代谢的因素。通过 P-450 3A4 和 2A6 对氟烷进行无氧还原代谢，因此，酶的诱导（如巴比妥类药物、苯妥英钠、丙戊酸）可以促进代谢，减少肝血流量。后者被氟烷进一步还原。虽然恩氟烷、异氟烷和地氟烷也会导致新抗原的形成，但其程度远小于氟烷，因此在氟烷致敏的患者中使用这些药物患肝炎的风险要小得多。

术后肾衰竭唯一明确的临床危险因素如下：

- 术前肾功能差（BUN 或肌酐水平升高）；
- 高龄；
- 心力衰竭。

通常，治疗和预防低血容量和术前补液的主要目标是减轻挥发性麻醉药对心血管和肾血流影响。机械通气和呼气末气道正压是与挥发性麻醉药相关的降低肾功能的其他次要因素。虽然与麻醉无关，但某些药物的代谢产物（巴比妥类药物、异烟肼、乙醇）则增加甲氧氟烷的代谢和毒性。

启示

氟烷引起的暴发性肝坏死几乎有一半具致命性。目前尚不清楚轻度肝毒性的临床意义。围术期急性肾衰竭占所有需要急性透析患者的一半，死亡率达到 50%。这种情况数十年来一直没有得到改变。

治疗

对于暴发性肝坏死或轻度肝毒性均无特异性治疗方法。轻度肝毒性不需要治疗，而肝坏死只有支持治疗和原位肝移植。急性肾功能不全的治疗包括恢复正常血容量和肾血流量；甘露醇、髓袢利尿剂（有争议）、多巴胺和非诺多泮（试验性）的使用和透析治疗。

预防

没有必要采取措施预防轻度肝毒性。预防暴发性肝坏死的唯一安全可靠的方法是对于先前接触过氟烷的患者完全避免使用氟烷、恩氟烷、异氟烷和地氟烷。仅接触一次氟烷的成年人和儿童出现肝炎较为罕见。保守的方法是在有已知暴发性坏死危险因素的患者中避免使用氟烷，尤其是近期接受氟烷麻醉的患者。最保守的方法是完全避免氟烷接触。

预防术后肾衰竭唯一最有效的措施是维持肾灌注，尽量减少肾缺血。充分的水化至关至要。甘露醇可能是一种有效的预防药物。

（时 鹏 译 韩 烨 校）

延伸阅读

Baden JM, Mazze RI: Polyuria. In Gravenstein N, Kirby RR, editors: *Complications in anesthesiology*, ed 2, Philadelphia, 1996, Lippincott-Raven, pp 493–498.

Baum JA, Woehlck HJ: Interaction of inhalational anaesthetics with CO_2 absorbents, *Best Pract Res Clin Anaesthesiol* 17:63–76, 2003.

Brown BR: Inhalation anesthesia and hepatic injury. In Gravenstein N, Kirby RR, editors: *Complications in anesthesiology*, ed 2, Philadelphia, 1996, Lippincott-Raven, pp 701–710.

Dooley JR, Mazze RI: Oliguria. In Gravenstein N, Kirby RR, editors: *Complications in anesthesiology*, ed 2, Philadelphia, 1996, Lippincott-Raven, pp 479–491.

Gut J, Christen V, Frey N, et al.: Molecular mimicry in halothane hepatitis: biochemical and structural characterization of lipoylated autoantigens, *Toxicology* 97:199–224, 1995.

Novis BK, Roizen MF, Aronson S, et al.: Association of preoperative risk factors with postoperative acute renal failure, *Anesth Analg* 78:143–149, 1994.

Pearson JD, Gelman S: Liver complications after anesthesia. In Benumof JL, Saidman LJ, editors: *Anesthesia and perioperative complications*, St. Louis, 1992, Mosby–Year Book, pp 413–433.

Prough DS, Zaloga G: Hypovolemia and renal dysfunction. In Benumof JL, Saidman LJ, editors: *Anesthesia and perioperative complications*, St. Louis, 1992, Mosby–Year Book, pp 434–465.

Ray DC, Drummond GB: Halothane hepatitis, *Br J Anaesth* 67:84–99, 1991.

Woehlck HJ: Sleeping with uncertainty: anesthetics and desiccated absorbent, *Anesthesiology* 101:276–278, 2004.

第 100 章 血液和血液制品感染

Jason A. Ochroch, Gaurav Malhotra

病例概要

患者，男性，70 岁，既往冠状动脉疾病史，诊断为腹主动脉瘤，拟行腹主动脉瘤开腹修补术。麻醉科医师在术前等候区对其进行术前评估。患者血红蛋白为 10 g/dl，麻醉科医师决定获得患者对可能输注血液制品的知情同意。在谈话的过程中，患者表现出明显不安。通过进一步的询问，得知患者非常担心“会从血液中传染某些东西”，并希望了解更多信息。

问题分析

定义

血源性感染是患者、家属和医务人员共同关心的问题。患者可能因输注库存的血液制品而被感染。此外，输注同种异体血行为本身就可能诱发受血者免疫调节进而增加感染的风险。作为血液制品的最大使用者，麻醉科医师了解感染的风险及处理流程尤为重要。

输血传播感染性疾病（transfusion-transmitted infectious disease，TTID）被发现已有数十年的历史，自 20 世纪 80 年代开始不断有新进展，并且发现了血液相关的人类免疫缺陷病毒（human immunodeficiency virus，HIV）。血液制品可以传播病毒、细菌和寄生虫。在整个献血过程中，多项机制的建立包括献血者筛选和检测可减少这些风险。

识别

血液筛查过程从询问病史开始，以识别当前有感染症状和有潜在感染风险的患者。然后，通过抗体和核酸检测，对捐献的血液进行病毒和寄生虫病原体的检测（框 100.1）。此外，供者血小板在捐献后 24 h 进行自动培养，以排查细菌污染。典型传染性疾病如变异克-雅病、疟疾、登革热和巴贝斯虫病虽不检测，但在献血时询问病史可筛查出来。

框 100.1 捐献血液制品中的传染源检测

- 人类免疫缺陷病毒 1 型和 2 型
- 人类嗜 T 细胞病毒 1 型和 2 型
- 乙型肝炎病毒（HBV）
- 丙型肝炎病毒（HCV）
- 西尼罗病毒
- 巨细胞病毒
- 梅毒（梅毒螺旋体）
- 恰加斯病（克鲁兹锥虫）——仅适用于首次捐献者

Adapted from Goodnough LT：Blood management：transfusion medicine comes of age. *Lancet* 381（9880）：1791-1792，2013.

细菌感染

输血传播细菌感染（transfusion-transmitted bacterial infection，TTBI）常见于输注血小板，因为其为室温储存。采血过程包括供者血液、静脉采血和后续处理的污染导致一系列的生物感染引起 TTBT。革兰氏阳性菌和革兰氏阴性菌均可在血小板中生长，最常见的病原体是小肠结肠炎耶尔森菌。

输血相关性免疫调节

输血相关性免疫调节（transfusion-related immunomodulation，TRIM）是另一种输血并发症，可引起受血者感染性损伤。以往认为，同种异体输血可以提高肾移植受者的生存率。然而，人们也发现输血导致与输注成分无关的术后细菌感染率增加、内源性 HIV 和巨细胞病毒的激活、恶性肿瘤切除术后的复发率和术后短期内（3 个月）总死亡率增加。TRIM 的病理生理学目前尚不清楚，其机制可能涉及包括供体白细胞、可溶性白细胞衍生介质和人类白细胞抗原肽在内的免疫抑制和促炎反应。减白细胞技术可改善但无法完全解决这个问题。

风险评估

尽管 TTID 的风险随着血液储存技术的进步而显著减少，但并非零风险。目前最常见的 3 种病毒性 TTID 感染风险如下：

- HIV：1∶2 000 000 次输血；
- HBV：1∶500 000 次输血；
- HCV：1∶2 000 000 次输血。

其他病毒和寄生虫感染的发生率很难准确报告。值得注意的是，在制备诸如静脉注射免疫球蛋白和白蛋白等血液衍生产品时，HIV、HBV 和 HCV 已失活，不具有传染性。目前认为 TTID 可能通过 3 种途径传染：献血者处于感染的“窗口期”，无法检测出；筛选分析中无法避免的假阴性；以及血液储存流程中工作人员的失误。

血小板的细菌感染率为 0.04% ～ 10%，输血感染率为 1∶10 000，输血导致脓毒症的死亡率为 1∶500 000。风险与剂量相关，因此多供体输血比单供体输血的感染风险高。研究发现，脓毒症相关的死亡率是输血死亡的第三大原因，仅次于输血相关急性肺损伤（transfusion-related acute lung injury，TRALI）和急性溶血性输血反应（acute hemolytic transfusion reaction，AHTR）（见第 101 章）。

职业暴露

血液污染性伤害（如针刺伤）属于可能导致感染的职业健康风险。被 HIV 或 HCV 污染的血液针刺伤后感染概率分别为 0.3% 和 1.8%；被 HBV 污染的血液针刺伤后，感染风险在 23% ～ 62%，取决于患者 HBeAg 的水平。由于职业暴露很少被报道，其真实发生率尚不清楚。

启示

输血或其他形式的血液接触后，TTID 可导致深远的影响。尽管这些疾病仅能追溯到患者输血史或职业接触史，但对症状的识别和合适的转诊仍极其重要。

HIV 或肝炎的诊断取决于检测指标，以及暴露后数周至数月病毒引起症状的发展。尽管约半数患者感染 6 周内会出现病毒感染症状（如发热、咽炎、肌痛、淋巴结肿大），但 HIV 感染初期通常无明显症状。随后的抗体和核酸检测可证实 HIV 感染。同样，HBV 或 HCV 感染初期也可能是无症状或在暴露数周甚至数月后出现流感症状。其中不到 1/3 的患者会出现临床黄疸。血液暴露数周后若出现肝炎症状（如萎靡、黄疸），应立即转诊进行适当的血液学检查。新确诊的患者应及时进行药物和心理治疗。

管理

细菌感染

TTBI 相关性脓毒症因感染的病菌接种量、病菌毒力和受体免疫状态而表现不同，但从输血结束到出现症状的时间中位数为 30 min（从 0 ～ 5 h）。临床上无法根据症状出现的时间与 AHTR 相鉴别（见第 101 章）。

发生严重的输血反应时，初始治疗应包括立即停止输血，支持治疗和复苏，重新采血（从对侧手臂采血）进行血型鉴定、交叉配血试验、检测直接抗球蛋白、血浆游离血红蛋白和血培养，通知血库并检查是否存在人为错误。如果高度怀疑感染（即输注血小板），可考虑经验性使用广谱抗生素。

职业暴露

若发生职业暴露，请务必遵循所在医院的处理流程。应将暴露情况报告给相应的办公室，以便记录、咨询和管理。通常，应立即用肥皂和清水清洗受伤的区域，受累的黏膜可用清水或适当的盐溶液冲洗。

若感染源为 HIV 患者，暴露后的 24 ～ 36 h 内使用抗逆转录病毒药物进行化学预防可能降低感染风险。HBV 暴露后预防措施包括检查以前的疫苗接种史、必要时接种疫苗和给予乙型肝炎免疫球蛋白进行被动免疫。HCV 尚无公认的暴露后预防措施，通常是血清学随访。

预防

有很多方法可以预防 TTID。如前所述，大多数病毒和寄生虫感染可通过献血过程中的询问病史和相关检测被筛查出来。TTBI 可以通过适当的供体筛选、无菌样本采集、储存期间振荡血小板、减少白细胞、改进培养方法和时机以及杀菌处理进行预防。

知情同意和备选方案

鉴于 TTID 风险可对患者情绪产生影响，在术前访视时必须以合适的视角向患者阐述这一问题。任何可能涉及术中大量失血的手术前均应征得患者的输血同意。虽然每家医院都有自己的输血同意书，但其内容都应该包括输血的潜在风险和益处、替代输血的方案和患者有机会提出疑问。

血液制品不应作为一般性扩充血容量使用，而应用于特定的指征，如增加携氧能力或增加凝血因子或血小板水平。术前采集自体血液、使用等容血液稀释和术中血液回收技术可能有助于避免接触同种异体血液制品。然而，术前采集自体血液仍然可能因血库工作人员的失误以及采集和储存不当而导致感染。此外，尽管理论上使用限制性输血策略可以降低感染风险，但研究表明仅能略微改善。

职业暴露

预防职业暴露主要是正确使用标准预防措施（框 100.2），包括隔离预防措施、避免锐器伤和手卫生。二级预防包括暴露前预防，如必要时接种疫苗。尽管目前尚无 HIV 或 HCV 疫苗，但建议感染风险高的包括麻醉科医师在内的医疗从业人员应接种 HBV 疫苗。

框 100.2 标准预防措施要点

对所有患者进行隔离预防措施，防止血液和体液接触

接触血液或体液或破损的皮肤黏膜时戴手套（不要清洗或消毒手套，因为消毒剂会导致手套破损）

如果进行喷洒操作，应使用隔离衣、面具、眼镜防护

避免锐器伤

锐器应放入特定容器，并及时处理

避免回套针帽

摘除手套后或任何血液或体液接触后及时洗手

心肺复苏置入人工气道设备后及时洗手

Data from Siegel JD，Rhinehart E，Jackson M，et al.：2007 guideline for isolation precautions：preventing transmission of infectious agents in health care settings. *Am J Infect Control* 35（10 Suppl 2）：S65-S164，2007.

（袁宁平 译 盛 颖 校）

延伸阅读

Beekmann SE, Henderson DK: Protection of healthcare workers from blood-borne pathogens, *Curr Opin Infect Dis* 18:331–336, 2005.

Carson JL, Carless PA, Hebert PC: Transfusion thresholds and other strategies for guiding allogeneic red blood cell transfusion, *Cochrane Database Syst Rev* (4):CD002042, 2012.

Centers for Disease Control and Prevention: Updated US Public Health Service guidelines for the management of occupational exposures to HBV, HCV, and HIV and recommendations for postexposure prophylaxis, *MMWR Morb Mortal Wkly Rep* 50:1–54, 2001.

Dienstag JL: Acute viral hepatitis. In Kasper D, Fauci A, Hauser S, et al.: *Harrison's principles of internal medicine*, ed 19, New York, 2015, McGraw-Hill.

Fauci AS, Lane C: Human immunodeficiency virus disease: AIDS and related disorders. In Kasper D, Fauci A, Hauser S, et al.: *Harrison's principles of internal medicine*, ed 19, New York, 2015, McGraw-Hill.

Goodnough LT: Autologous blood donation, *Crit Care* 8(Suppl 2):S49–S52, 2004.

Goodnough LT: Blood management: transfusion medicine comes of age, *Lancet* 381:1791–1792, 2013.

Goodnough LT, Shander A: Patient blood management, *Anesthesiology* 116:1367–1376, 2012.

Hart S, Cserti-Gazdewich CM, McCluskey SA: Red cell transfusion and the immune system, *Anaesthesia* 70(Suppl 1):38–45, e13–e16, 2015.

Perez P, Salmi LR, Follea G, et al.: Determinants of transfusion-associated bacterial contamination: results of the French BACTHEM case-control study, *Transfusion* 41:862–872, 2001.

Perkins HA, Busch MP: Transfusion-associated infections: 50 years of relentless challenges and remarkable progress, *Transfusion* 50:2080–2099, 2010.

Rohde JM, Dimcheff DE, Blumberg N, et al.: Health care-associated infection after red blood cell transfusion: a systematic review and meta-analysis, *JAMA* 311:1317–1326, 2014.

Siegel JD, Rhinehart E, Jackson M, et al.: 2007 guideline for isolation precautions: preventing transmission of infectious agents in health care settings, *Am J Infect Control* 35(10 Suppl 2):S65–S164, 2007.

Vamvakas EC, Blajchman MA: Transfusion-related immunomodulation (TRIM): an update, *Blood Rev* 21:327–348, 2007.

Welsby IJ, Hathaway JA: Blood and blood component therapy. In Longnecker DE, Brown DL, Newman MF, et al.: *Anesthesiology*, ed 2, New York, 2012, McGraw-Hill, pp 1438–1452.

血液和血液制品：输血反应和并发症

第 101 章

Seth Perelman

病例概要

患者，女性，33 岁，G3P2002，孕 34 周，既往有前置胎盘病史，对胎盘增生进行超声检查。患者在硬膜外麻醉下成功实施剖宫产术，但需要同种异体输血，包括 6 单位红细胞悬液（packed red blood cell，PRBC）、2 单位新鲜冰冻血浆（fresh frozen plasma，FFP）和 6 单位血小板。患者在手术结束时血流动力学稳定；但术后 5 h 在麻醉后恢复室后出现发热、急性呼吸窘迫和低血压，需要机械通气。

问题分析

定义

输血反应是对输注同种异体血液成分所产生的任何不良反应。输血反应可为急性，也可能延迟发生，可能临床无危害性，也可能是危及生命的反应。本文重点结合所呈现的临床病例，讨论各种输血反应及其处置。

识别

同种异体输血和不良反应之间存在一定的时间关系，即意味着输血反应的发生。这些反应可能包括一系列的体征和症状，包括发热、寒战、皮疹、腰痛、血流动力学不稳定、支气管痉挛、凝血功能障碍、血红蛋白尿和呼吸困难。该特异性反应可能提示一种正在发生的输血反应，并可能有助于描述该反应的类型；然而，接受输血的患者往往有基础并存疾病，可能会出现类似输血反应的症状。在手术室难以将这些症状归因于输血，可能会使病情进一步复杂化，因为全身麻醉可能会掩盖或混淆这些症状。因此，必须迅速评估可疑的反应，以尽量减少其影响。

输血反应类型（表 101.1）

急性反应

异体输血（allogeneic blood transfusion，ABT）反应可分为急性和迟发性、免疫介导性和非免疫介导性。本节将讨论具体的诊断和管理策略，以及减

表 101.1　输血反应的发生率

输血反应类型	发生率（每 100 000 单位输血）
变态性输血反应	112.2
输血过敏反应	8
急性溶血性输血反应	2.5 ～ 7.9
延迟溶血性输血反应	40
延迟血清学输血反应	48.9 ～ 75.7
发热性非溶血性输血反应	1000 ～ 3000
高溶血性输血反应	未知
低血压输血反应	1.8 ～ 9.0
大量输血相关反应（柠檬酸，钾，冷毒性）	未知
输血后紫癜	未知
脓毒性输血反应	0.03 ～ 3.3（取决于输血制品）
输血相关性循环超负荷	10.9
输血相关性移植物抗宿主疾病	使用辐射或病原体灭活方法极为罕见（接近 0%）
输血相关性坏死性小肠结肠炎	未知
输血相关性急性肺损伤	0.4 ～ 1.0（因成分和风险缓解策略实施的不同而不同）

少输血相关的病残率和死亡率的策略（表 101.2）。

急性溶血性输血反应

急性溶血性输血反应（acute hemolytic transfusion reaction，AHTR）是由于供体红细胞抗原与受体抗体结合形成免疫复合物造成的急性血管内溶血导致危及生命的反应。这些反应通常是由于输血错误（输血成分不正确）引起的。这些 Ag-Ab 免疫复合物引起补体固定、白细胞活化、血管内溶血和血红蛋白尿，并诱导细胞因子的形成，导致血流动力学不稳定、腰痛、发热、寒战和弥散性血管内凝血（disseminated intravascular coagulation，DIC）。 严重的反应通常是 ABO 血型不合的结果，或者可能是由于之前的同种异体免疫导致的其他红细胞（red blood cell，RBC）抗体的反应。输血反应的严重程度取决于受体的 Ab 滴度、输液量和输液速度。大多数死亡病例与输血量大于 200 ml 有关，输血量大于 1000 ml，死亡率接近 44%。改进的管理系统减少了 ABO 血型不合引起的 AHTR 的发生率，美国食品药物管理局报告称，1976—1985 年因 ABO 血型不合 AHTR 死亡共有 131 例，而 2010—2014 年的死亡人数为 13 例。实验室发现包括血红蛋白血症、血红蛋白尿、直接抗体试验（direct Ab test，DAT）阳性和 DIC（凝血酶原时间延长 / 部分凝血活酶时间延长、血小板减少、低纤维蛋白原血症）。尽管存在超过 250 种红细胞抗原，AHTR 通常是 ABO 或 RHD 组不相容导致的。

表 101.2　输血反应类型

急性输血反应	延迟输血反应
溶血	溶血
非溶血	血小板减少
• 发热	移植物抗宿主病
• 荨麻疹	传染性传播-病毒，细菌，寄生虫，朊病毒
• 变态反应-瘙痒，荨麻疹和发热	输血相关性免疫调节
• IgA 介导的过敏反应	铁超载
• 输血相关性肺损伤	
• 输血相关性脓毒症	
• 输血相关性循环超负荷	
• 凝血功能障碍	

IgA，免疫球蛋白 A

Modified from Proctor LT：Blood and blood products：transfusion reaction. In Atlee JL：*Complications in anesthesia*，2nd ed. Philadelphia，Saunders，2006，pp. 202-203.

发热性非溶血性输血反应

发热性非溶血性输血反应（febrile nonhemolytic transfusion reactions，FNTR）是一种常见的以发热为特征的反应，可能与输液过程中或输液后数小时出现的寒战、僵直和不适有关。它们通常是由受体抗体对供体白细胞抗原反应，释放补体介导的内源性致热原 [白细胞介素 -1（interleukin-1，IL-1）、IL-6、肿瘤坏死因子 - α] 形成抗原-抗体复合物引起的。治疗通常给予解热药物对症处理，但 FNTR 是排除的诊断，因为发热反应也可能同时伴发更严重的反应，如 AHTR、输血相关性急性肺损伤和脓毒症。在大多数情况下，临床可以减少输血的比例但不可能不输血。在普遍应用去白细胞血制品的国家，FNTR 有所减少。

变态反应

变态反应较为常见，通常症状轻微，表现为荨麻疹、瘙痒以及可能的发热。大多数是由抗体-抗原对供体血浆中血清蛋白的反应所致，其通过免疫球蛋白 E（immunoglobulin E，IgE）介导。出现荨麻疹输血反应（urticarial transfusion reaction，UTR）并不意味着必须放弃输血。可以停止输血，使用抗组胺剂，当症状减轻时，可以恢复输血。

过敏性输血反应很少见，但在遗传性免疫球蛋白 A（immunoglobulin A，IgA）缺乏，且输液产品中含有 IgA 抗体或其他供体血浆成分抗体的患者中，往往发生严重的过敏性输血反应。这种抗 IgA 免疫复合物的相互作用立即发生，与剂量无关。除了 UTR 中出现的荨麻疹外，临床特征还包括血管性水肿、支气管痉挛和低血压。治疗方法与其他原因引起的过敏性反应相同，取决于反应的严重程度，包括液体复苏、肾上腺素、抗组胺药和皮质类固醇。

输血相关性急性肺损伤（框 101.1）

在发达国家，输血相关性急性肺损伤（transfusion-related acute lung injury，TRALI）被认为是导致输血相关疾病和死亡的主要原因之一。输血相关性急性肺损伤在输血后 6 h 内表现为急性呼吸窘迫综合征，它的发病率因国家不同而异，而且由于 2004 年以前缺乏一致的定义，很可能被低估。临床排除诊断

框 101.1 输血相关性急性肺损伤的定义（TRALI）

疑似 TRALI
- 输血后 6 h 内急性发作
- PaO_2/FiO_2 小于 300 mm Hg，或 P：F 比例恶化
- 胸部 X 线片的双侧浸润性改变
- 无肺水肿迹象（肺动脉楔压≤ 18 mmHg 或中心静脉压≤ 15 mmHg）
- 没有其他急性肺损伤的危险因素

可能的 TRALI
- 与疑似 TRALI 相同，但是急性肺损伤的另一个危险因素

延迟的 TRALI
- 与（可能的）TRALI 相同，并在输血后 6 ～ 72 h 内发病

From Vlaar AP，Juffermans NP：Transfusion-related acute lung injury：a clinical review. *Lancet* 382（9896）：984-994，2013

法和不同的报告方法（主动和被动的输血监测）是其被低估的主要因素。最近的综述指出，每单位输血的发生率高达 1.12%，高危受体每单位输血的发生率为 8%，相应的报告也有所增加。TRALI 是指在输血结束后 6 h 内，在没有其他急性肺血管超负荷危险因素的情况下，出现急性肺损伤（acute lung injury，ALI）的新发症状。临床特征包括低氧血症、呼吸困难、发绀和心动过速，可伴有发热和低血压。区分 TRALI 和其他形式的 ALI 非常重要，包括循环超负荷和心肌或瓣膜性心脏病。急性低氧血症的定义是 PaO_2/FiO_2 小于 300 mmHg，伴双侧肺浸润的胸部 X 线片表现，无心源性肺水肿征象。由于接受 ABT 治疗的同时并存肺部疾病的患者将被排除在 TRALI 的诊断之外，加拿大共识小组在 2004 年将“可能的 TRALI”的定义包括在输血后出现 ALI 恶化的一个或多个危险因素的患者中。在这一高危人群中，“延迟 TRALI”的发生在输血后 72 h 内也有描述，并与高死亡率有关。

据报道，TRALI 可发生于所有类型的血液成分中。然而，大多数的反应都发生在含有 50 ml 以上血浆的产品中，而传统的 FFP 是最常涉及的成分。降低风险的策略包括延迟使用经产妇供体血浆和使用单采血小板，可降低 FFP 相关 TRALI 的发生率。目前，与其他血液成分相比，红细胞相关的 TRALI 因血浆供体延迟使用和红细胞输注量，使其导致的 TRALI 相关死亡发生率最高。

最初提出的 TRALI 病理生理机制归因于抗体介导的模型，其中供体血浆的白细胞（white blood cell，WBC）抗体[人类白细胞抗原（human leukocyte antigen，HLA）Ⅰ和Ⅲ类或特异性中性粒细胞]针对受体 WBC 抗原在受体肺的微循环中相互作用引起直接或间接的中性粒细胞活化。该抗体滴度和含 Ab 血浆的体积是可能的风险改变因素，这可能表明在特定的风险亚组和低风险受体中可能需要不同的阈值来形成 TRALI。在 65% ～ 90% 的 TRALI 病例中，已在供体血浆中鉴定出 Ab，多胎妇女和近期有过输血史供者发生 HLA 抗原异体免疫的风险较高。然而，并不是所有的 TRALI 病例都是 Ab 介导的，也不是所有输注含有 HLA Ab 的血制品都会引起 TRALI。这就引出了另一种假设，即所谓的二次打击模型。

在“第一次打击”中，患者潜在的危险因素所引起的肺内皮细胞活化导致细胞因子的释放和黏附分子的表达，从而动员多形核白细胞（polymorphonuclear leukocyte，PMN）扣压于肺内皮细胞内。由于受体的危险因素，PMN 的动员通常发生在输血前。危重患者发生 TRALI 的风险最高，但各种研究都揭示了特定的受体风险因素：APACHE 评分高、休克、大量输血、液体正平衡、吸烟、高气道峰压的机械通气、脓毒症、紧急心脏手术、肝病、慢性酒精滥用和近期手术。“第二次打击”涉及 PMN 与白细胞抗体和（或）血浆中存在的生物反应调节剂（biologic response modifier，BRM）的相互作用，BRM 中含有随贮存而积累的血液成分（生物活性脂质和其他可溶性因子）。Ab 或 BRM 与 PMN 的相互作用导致细胞因子、氧化酶、蛋白酶和活性氧的释放，破坏肺毛细血管内皮，导致渗漏和随后的非心源性肺水肿。TRALI 的治疗以支持为主，包括积极的呼吸支持，补充氧气，必要时以足够低的压力和潮气量进行机械通气，以避免气压伤。

输血相关性循环超负荷

输血相关性循环超负荷（transfusion-associated circulatory overload，TACO）是另一种导致呼吸功能不全的输血相关性病因，但继发于容量超负荷。它通常发生在老年人和婴儿中，或在短时间间隔内接受血液成分治疗的有基础心肌疾病的患者中。它经常被漏报和漏诊，是向 FDA 报告的输血相关死亡的第二大常见原因。最近的一项前瞻性分析发现，血小板相关 TACO 的发生率为 1：167，远高于目前被

动上报的发生率。通过对TACO相关危险因素和输液治疗的回顾性分析，发现患者有充血性心力衰竭、肾功能不全和年龄大于70岁的病史，常常采用不适当的输液治疗和次优的液体管理策略。鉴别TACO和TRALI颇具挑战，尤其是当两者可以共存时，但TRALI通常与发热、低血压和渗出性肺浸润有关，而TACO则与循环超负荷、N-proBNP升高和（或）心肌功能障碍有关，通常对利尿剂治疗有反应。

输血相关性脓毒症

输血相关性脓毒症（transfusion-associated sepsis，TAS）是由输注被细菌污染的血液成分所引起。最初的症状可能包括发热、寒战、低血压和心血管衰竭，通常发生在输血后4 h内。污染通常是由供体静脉穿刺处的皮肤菌群所引起，较少见的污染来源于无症状的供体菌血症，或极少的污染发生在血液处理过程中。血库的储存温度导致出现不同种类细菌感染的倾向。红细胞储存在4℃下，更容易受到革兰氏阴性菌（如小肠结肠炎耶尔森菌和假单胞菌）的污染和增殖。血小板在室温（22℃）下储存，更容易受到革兰氏阳性菌（如表皮葡萄球菌、金黄色葡萄球菌和芽孢杆菌）的污染。2004年，自动细菌检测单采血成分（单供者）的应用大大降低了TAS的发生率，并从全血制品多采血小板转变为单供体灭活血小板，但在输血相关死亡病例中，TAS仍然排在第三位。血小板仍然占总死亡数的70%，因为在4℃下储存可导致细菌呈指数性增殖和许多受体免疫功能受损。尽管最佳的采集技术和被动的血液预警，但在静脉穿刺时，少量的细菌进入血液成分，许多脓毒症反应并非由输血引起，而是由于患者原有的感染。因此，TAS的真实发生率可能被低估。在最近的一项研究中，Hong及其同事确定了细菌性血小板污染单位的发病率为1：2572。在高度怀疑出现TAS时才需要治疗，包括应用广谱抗生素以及血流动力学支持。尽管血小板病原灭活系统目前还没有广泛使用，但其与脓毒症事件发生率降低有关。

凝血功能障碍

红细胞缺乏凝血因子、纤维蛋白原和血小板，因此大量输入红细胞可能导致稀释性凝血病。稀释性凝血病或复苏相关的凝血病也可能是由于出血时输注大量的晶体液或不平衡的血液成分所引起。这种凝血功能障碍还可能是创伤所导致的凝血功能障碍，即灌注延迟或灌注不足导致的凝血因子的激活和消耗，此外还可能是继发于低温、酸中毒和长时间休克引起的凝血功能障碍。创伤相关性凝血病导致了固定比例血液成分治疗方案的发展，也被称为“损伤控制”疗法，该疗法基于对大量创伤患者的临床观察研究，通过固定比例血液成分治疗提高了患者的生存率。对于大量输血的患者，在进行成分治疗时，稀释性凝血障碍应通过实验室凝血试验或黏滞弹性试验进行确诊。

延迟反应

延迟溶血性输血反应

延迟溶血性输血反应（delayed hemolytic transfusion reaction，DHTR）是由于在以前的输血、妊娠或移植过程中发生的异源融合的遗忘反应而引起的免疫介导的输血反应。受体抗体，通常是Kidd或Rh，由于Ab滴度低，常常无法识别，但再次暴露时，通常在输血后3～30天对供体抗原引起Ab非介导的反应。DHTR的发生率为1：2500，但在镰状细胞病的患者中发生率升高至11%。暴露后，Ab滴度迅速升高，常发生延迟溶血反应。血管外溶血呈渐进性，不像急性反应那么严重，血红蛋白意外降低，患者出现黄疸或直接抗球蛋白试验阳性。最常见的临床特征是黄疸和血红蛋白尿，其次是发热、背痛、呼吸困难、寒战和高血压。通常不需要治疗，但应通知血库进一步鉴别抗原，以避免将来发生类似的反应。

输血相关移植物抗宿主病

输血相关移植物抗宿主病（transfusion-associated graft-versus-host disease，TA-GVHD）是一种罕见的异种异体输血并发症，它发生于当供者来源的T淋巴细胞发起的抗宿主组织的免疫应答时。在大多数输血中，在供者淋巴细胞对宿主产生免疫反应之前，这些淋巴细胞会被受者的强大的免疫系统破坏。在免疫功能受损或供者与受者之间存在部分HLA匹配的患者中，免疫应答不能产生，供体淋巴细胞可对宿主产生应答。临床特征包括黄斑丘疹、腹痛、腹泻、肝功能异常和供体淋巴细胞破坏宿主骨髓导致的全血细胞减少。TA-GVHD通常在输血后4～30天内发生，并且普遍致命，因此预防尤其重要。在免疫功能低下的患者中，接受来自家庭供体的血液成分的患者，或接受过造血细胞移植的患者，可通过

γ 射线放射来实现输入淋巴细胞的失活从而达到预防作用。

输血后紫癜

输血后紫癜（posttransfusion purpura，PTP）是一种罕见的免疫介导的延迟输血反应，在输血后 5 ～ 10 天内，任何含有血小板（RBC、血小板）的血液成分都会发生这种反应。PTP 主要发生于女性，它涉及抗体介导的对供者血小板的人类血小板抗原 1a（the human platelet antigen 1a，HPA-1a）的反应。HPA-1a 阴性的妇女（<2% 的白种人）因怀孕而致敏，男性和女性都可能因先前的输血而致敏。虽然机制未明，但免疫复合物介导的反应可能导致输注者血小板的破坏。通过检测血小板特异性同种抗体可以确诊 PTP。治疗包括静脉注射免疫球蛋白，虽然亦有报道称其对类固醇激素有反应。

输血传播感染

自 20 世纪 80 年代人类免疫缺陷病毒（human immunodeficiency virus，HIV）流行达到顶峰以来，人们对输血传播感染（transfusion-transmitted infection，TTI）的认识已有实质性地提高，输血传播感染的风险已大大降低。用于减轻输血感染风险的策略包括供血延期使用、供者筛查、抗体检测、核酸检测、去白细胞和病原体灭活。尽管实施了这些保障措施，但我们仍然面临着这些检测的固有局限性，感染性病原体和未经检测的病原体的不同窗口期，以及新出现感染的持续威胁。随着每一个新出现的传染威胁，我们在识别输血相关病原体和开发适当的筛查和检测方法之间都存在着延迟。尽管从认识到 HIV 威胁到实施供者检测仅用了 3 年时间，仍发生了大约 12 000 例输血相关 HIV 感染病例。1970—1990 年间，对丙型肝炎病毒（hepatitis C virus，HCV）的识别和检测间隔较长，导致 480 万输血相关的 HCV 感染。任何具有无症状血源相关的感染性病原体都有可能发生输血相关传播。病原体必须能够在收集的输血成分中存活，并通过静脉途径引起感染。HIV 和 HCV 的感染期较长，但西尼罗河病毒和登革热病毒的潜伏期短得多。2009 年，一个共识小组确认了对美国血液供应具有威胁的 68 种新出现的传染病，其中，人类变异克-雅病、登革热病毒和巴贝西亚物种威胁最大。自该共识发布以来，该名单中又增加了六种病原，包括黄热病病毒、虫媒病毒、异向性鼠白血病相关病毒、人细小病毒 / 博卡病毒，最近又增加了中东呼吸综合征冠状病毒（the Middle East respiratory syndrome coronavirus，MERS-COV）。在巴西有记录的输血传播病例中，寨卡病毒是对我们血液供应的最新威胁。无症状感染的高发生率限制了供体延期使用的有效性，高流行地区正在进行血液试验。虽然在发达国家，TTI 的一般风险仍然很低，但零风险的血液供应仍然难以实现，TTI 仍然是“输血医学的一个固定和不可避免的特性”。

输血相关性免疫调节

人们意识到同种异体输血的免疫抑制作用已有 40 多年，对提高输血受者的肾移植存活率具有益处。自 20 世纪 80 年代以来，输血相关免疫调节（transfusion-related immunomodulation，TRIM）的不良影响，细菌感染、癌症复发和潜伏感染激活等风险的增加一直受到争议。TRIM 的发病机制被认为与大量引入多种抗原有关，尤其是在白细胞上，在 ABT 期间提呈给受体，导致免疫异常，产生临床不良反应。尽管 TRIM 是一个真实的生物学事件，但经 T 辅助细胞、自然杀伤细胞、单核细胞和巨噬细胞功能的实验室免疫异常以及细胞因子产生减少证实，其临床效果仍存在争议。虽然观察性证据对 ABT 相关的术后感染具有说服力，但并非绝对证据，观察性研究容易受到混杂因素的影响从而难以解释。ABT 可能是其他可导致不良临床结局的不良预后因素的替代标志物。心脏手术人群可能比较独特，因为有更一致的随机临床试验证据支持短期风险的增加与含白细胞的 ABT 有关。尽管与输血治疗相关的医源性和医院获得性感染并非通过输血传播引起，但它们与输血相关，并对临床结局产生了主要影响。尽管 TRIM 与同种异体白细胞输注有关，但目前实施普遍的去白细胞方法以特异性降低 TRIM 的影响还为时过早。

输血性铁超载

尚无生理性机制可以有效地清除多余的铁，因此全身铁主要受铁吸收和铁流失的调节，多余的铁可能有剧毒性。一个健康的个体每天吸收大约 1 ～ 2 mg，而 300 ml 的血液含有大约 200 mg 的血红素铁。输血性铁超载（transfusional iron overload，TIO）主要是输血依赖性贫血的慢性输血治疗引起。当输血铁超过转铁蛋白的结合能力时，非转铁蛋白结合的铁沉积在组织中，实质性铁超载将导致终末器官功能障碍，特别是肝、心脏、胰腺和其他内分泌器官。沉积的游离铁可参与氧化反应，导致活性氧物质生成并产生相关毒性。此外，TIO 还与胰岛素抵抗、肿瘤和感染有关（图 101.1）。治疗 TIO 的主要方法是使用铁螯合物，铁超载应怀疑血清铁蛋白水平大于 1000 ng/ml，这一水平可能在 80 kg 成人中使用 20 单位 PRBC 后出现。虽然 TIO 的风险通常表现在慢性输血依赖人群中，但由于铁依赖性细菌生长引起的感染风险仅输入几个单位后即可发生。

管理

围术期输血反应的管理因所涉及的反应类型而异，尽管围术期可能发生的反应具有紧急性质，但必须了解急性和延迟反应的频率和影响。与急性反应相关的死亡率非常罕见，估计约为 200 万分之一，但通常轻微反应的症状可能是更严重反应的迹象，而且许多症状和体征可能在全身麻醉下被掩盖。TRALI、TACO、AHTR、脓毒症和过敏反应是最可能与主要病残率和死亡率相关的急性反应。图 101.2 给出了处理各种输血反应的流程。

当怀疑有急性输血反应时，应立即采取某些措施。输血应该立即终止，并联系输血机构。患者静脉输液通道应保持通畅，并开始支持治疗和对症治疗。继续输血或停止输血将取决于输血反应的病因和其他症状的关系。发热可能仅是 AHTR、TRALI、脓毒症、不太严重的 FNTR 或患者的部分基础疾病的体征。此时，应确认计划中的血制品已提供给正确的患者。应重新评估患者是否有其他症状和体征，如发热、呼吸窘迫、心血管稳定性、血管性水肿、荨麻疹、血红蛋白尿、支气管痉挛和凝血障碍。若患者清醒，我们需要注意患者的其他症状和体征包括寒战、背痛、胸痛和瘙痒。根据一系列的体征、症状和其他支持性数据，临床医师也许能够确定该反应是否危及生命，以及当时必须采取哪些复苏措施。如果反应被视为危及生命，应将剩余的血液制品或管道保留，并将其送至血库，另外还应进行其他输血部门推荐的实验室检测 [DAT、全血细胞计数、尿分析、乳酸脱氢酶（lactate dehydrogenase，LDH）]。额外的输血通常需推迟到初步评估完成，除非需要额外的血液制品来治疗潜在的疾病，如出血。

输血相关性临床病史的初步评价

发热 / 寒战

发热和寒战是由 FNTR 引起的最常见的临床

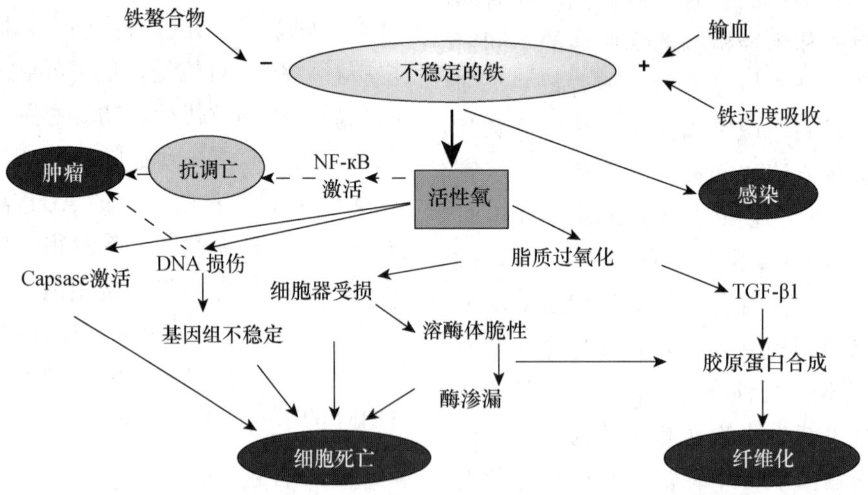

图 101.1 铁超负荷的病理机制和临床结局。由于反复输血或长期铁吸收增加而导致的铁超载中，未与转铁蛋白或铁蛋白等天然分子或治疗性铁螯合物结合的铁，会产生各种活性氧（ROS），多数为羟基自由基。这发生在储存铁蓄积的细胞中（特别是肝、内分泌组织和心肌），从而增加储存和不稳定细胞铁的水平。ROS 增加脂质过氧化和细胞器受损，导致由转化生长因子（TGF）-β1 介导的细胞死亡和纤维化。ROS 还会使 DNA 损伤，可能导致基因组不稳定、突变、细胞死亡或瘤变。ROS 直接激活 Caspase，从而加速细胞凋亡。矛盾的是，ROS 也可能通过激活 NF-kB（虚线）而具有抗细胞凋亡作用，这可能有助于骨髓增生异常综合征转化和铁介导的瘤变，如肝癌（From Porter JB，Garbowski M：The pathophysiology of transfusional iron overload. *Hematol Oncol Clin North Am* 28[4]：683-701，2014. Adapted from Porter JB：Pathophysiology of iron overhead. *Hematol Oncol Clin North Am* 19[Suppl 1]：7-12，2005.）

当患者发生输血反应时必须停止所有输血，并由医师评估
提供支持性治疗以支持重要器官功能（心脏，肺，肾）
有关输血反应诊断或治疗的问题，请致电输血部门或其他相应的医师

体温升高

反应	症状	干预
可能发热的非溶血反应	基线以上增加<1℃，且无其他新症状	• 密切观察，连续监测生命体征 • 如果稳定且无其他新症状，则继续输血
可能的细菌污染 可能的溶血	基线以上增加≥1℃，或增加<1℃但出现以下任何新症状（寒战或僵直，低血压，恶心或呕吐）	• 停止输血，保持静脉通路开放，评估患者，检查患者ID和血液制品ID以及一致性 • 退热药 • 考虑血培养（患者）;如果中性粒细胞减少则经验性给予抗生素 • 不要恢复输血 • 如果温度升高2℃或临床高度怀疑脓毒症，则强烈建议血液制品培养 • 通知输血实验室：退回血液制品（连同管理配套装置），输血后的患者血样送至输血实验室

对于由于潜在疾病或治疗而持续发热的患者，如果可能：
- 如果患者的体温升高，则避免开始输血
- 在开始输血前用退热药物治疗发热
- 如果温度逐渐升高到基线以上≥1℃，按上述方法治疗（停止并且不要恢复输血，如果有指征则进行培养）
- 通知输血实验室，退回血液制品（连同输注装置），输血后患者的血样亦送至输血实验室

变态反应症状

反应	症状	干预
荨麻疹	轻度荨麻疹，皮疹或仅皮肤瘙痒	• 停止输血，保持静脉通路开放，并评估患者 • 抗组胺药 • 通知患者临床医师和输血实验室；不需要样品 • 如果症状消失，则可以恢复输血 • 如果症状没有改善或恶化或复发，则停止输血；退回血液制品（连同输血装置）至输血实验室
可能的过敏反应	荨麻疹、皮疹、瘙痒和（或）任何其他新症状（喉部、眼睛和舌头肿胀等）	• 停止输血，保持静脉注射线开放，评估患者，检查患者ID和血液制品ID以及一致性 • 抗组胺药 • 不要恢复输血 • 通知输血实验室：退回血液制品（连同输血装置），输血后患者血样送至输血实验室

呼吸系统症状

反应	症状	干预
可能的过敏反应，输血相关性循环超负荷，脓毒性输血反应或输血相关性急性肺损伤	支气管痉挛，呼吸困难，呼吸急促和低氧血症，大量泡沫粉红色液体（来自气管导管）	• 停止输血，保持静脉通道开放，评估患者，检查患者ID和血液制品ID以及患者一致性 • 有指征时对症治疗（肾上腺素，抗组胺药，类固醇；氧气和呼吸支持，利尿剂；液体，血压和肾支持） • 若提示存在输血相关性急性肺损伤，行胸部X线检查是否存在双侧间质性浸润 • 血液培养（患者和血液制品），如果临床怀疑脓毒症 • 不要恢复输血 • 通知输血实验室：退回血液制品（连同输血装置）和输血后患者血样。对相关血制品进行检疫隔离

所有其他症状

反应	症状	干预
可能的过敏反应，溶血性输血反应，液体过量或输血相关性急性肺损伤	寒战，僵直，低血压，恶心或呕吐，濒死感、背部或胸痛，静脉输注部位疼痛，咳嗽，呼吸困难，缺氧	• 停止输血，保持静脉通路开放，评估输血单位，检查患者ID和血液制品ID以及患者一致性 • 有指征时对症治疗（肾上腺素，抗组胺药，类固醇;氧气和呼吸支持，利尿剂；液体，血压和肾支持） • 血液培养（患者和血液制品），如果高度临床怀疑脓毒症 • 不要恢复输血 • 通知输血实验室：退回血液制品（连同输血装置）和输血后患者血样。对相关血制品进行检疫隔离

图 101.2 输血反应处理流程（From Delaney M，Wendel S，Bercovitz RS，et al.：Transfusion reactions：prevention，diagnosis，and treatment. *Lancet* pii：S0140-6736（15）01313-6，2016. [Epub before print.]）

表现。但是，首先必须排除潜在的致命反应，如AHTR、脓毒症和TRALI。如果怀疑存在AHTR，则需要对输血者输注的血液制品确认是否正确，并且应下医嘱进行实验室检测，以排除存在免疫介导的溶血反应（DAT、重复交叉匹配、凝血试验、LDH、未结合胆红素、血清结合珠蛋白、系列血红蛋白）。脓毒症会伴有血流动力学不稳定，应检查血液制品是否变色和是否存在气泡。如果怀疑有脓毒症，应对患者和供体的血液制品进行培养。TRALI可能伴有发热或寒战，但需要存在呼吸相关的表现。FNTR是一种不太严重的反应，但它是一种排除诊断，不伴有任何全身性的参与，通常涉及非去白细胞的血液制品。

呼吸困难

呼吸窘迫可能由TRALI、过敏反应或TACO引起。过敏反应可能伴有支气管痉挛、荨麻疹和血管性水肿，起病迅速是其突出的特征。TRALI和TACO可能很难区分，特别是因为两者可能同时发生。区别特征可能包括较大的输注量、既往心脏病史和证实TACO患者心源性肺水肿的支持性检查。TRALI可能与短暂性白细胞减少有关，常伴有发热。

荨麻疹

单独的荨麻疹发作通常并无危害，只要它们不出现提示过敏反应的症状。它们通常发生在输血后4 h，最常与血小板输注有关。一旦发生荨麻疹，应暂停输血，服用抗组胺药，若不出现其他症状，可恢复输血。不需要实验室检测。

低血压

围术期低血压可能由低血容量引起，若低血压不是由手术出血所致，且与输血存在临时相关性，则应怀疑是输血反应。低血压可能继发于过敏反应、AHTR、TRALI和脓毒症。过敏反应的症状除了低血压，通常还伴有急性血管性水肿、皮疹和支气管痉挛。TRALI的主要特征是呼吸窘迫，而脓毒症除了发热和感染病因的实验室证据外，可能还伴随着休克的其他发现。除血流动力学不稳定外，AHTR通常包括溶血、发热和凝血障碍。另一个不常见的低血压原因是通过激活内源性凝血级联激活途径——缓激肽（或其代谢物）介导的低血压。这种不常见的表现更可能发生在接受血管紧张素转换酶抑制剂（angiotensin-converting enzyme inhibitors，ACEI）治疗的高血压患者中。ACEI降低缓激肽的代谢，通过带负电荷的去白细胞过滤器接收血液制品。低血压通常比较短暂，但可能需要辅助治疗，应排除其他低血压原因。许多这种过滤器市场上已不再售用，但在鉴别诊断中应考虑到这种不常见的低血压原因。

预防

同种异体输血是围术期患者治疗的重要组成部分，在某些人群中可以挽救生命，但这与已知和未知的重大风险以及社会成本有关。彻底了解输血风险、管理和预防是患者最佳治疗的必要组成部分。尽管已有不少降低风险的成功策略，但仍不能实现零风险血液供应，而且随着全球化的不断发展，新出现的威胁，特别是传染性威胁的风险将继续威胁我们的血液供应。所有这些都将增加社会成本，并将继续扩大发达国家和发展中国家之间的差距。尽管输血可以挽救生命，但不应想当然地认为它是安全的，益处就一定会大于其风险。减少同种异体暴露是减少输血治疗相关风险的有效方法，虽然效果并不总是明显。许多观察性研究证实，在相似的临床环境中输血治疗的巨大差异提示这些机构存在许多没有适应证的输血。美国血库协会（American Association of Blood Banks）在《理智选择运动》发布了作为输血的第一条推荐声明“不是绝对需要，不要输入过多单位的血液”。患者血液管理策略依赖于血液成分的循证使用，包括优化红细胞生成、减少失血和治疗贫血，以及实验室检查指导的输血流程，这些流程已被证明可以减少同种异体血接触、降低输血风险和改善临床结局。减少输血反应的风险需要使用全方位措施，从供者选择到储存期，解决血液供应的安全问题，并通过供者选择和供血推迟、筛查、减少和灭活病原体，将风险降至最低。在输血期间，医疗团队有责任随时对任何不良反应保持高度警觉，对其进行识别，并在输血部门或血库的参与下治疗并发症。无论是免疫介导的还是感染性的延迟反应都需要识别。这种反应可能是输血介导的，可能需要回顾输血计划来识别和跟踪供者血液单位。

（谢　芳　译　朱科明　校）

延伸阅读

Alter HJ: Pathogen reduction: a precautionary principle paradigm, *Transfus Med Rev* 22(2):97–102, 2008.

Andreu G, Morel P, Forestier F, et al.: Hemovigilance network in France: organization and analysis of immediate transfusion incident reports from 1994 to 1998, *Transfusion* 42(10):1356–1364, 2002.

Borgman MA, Spinella PC, Perkins JG, et al.: The ratio of blood products transfused affects mortality in patients receiving massive transfusions at a combat support hospital, *J Trauma* 63(4):805–813, 2007.

Callum JL, Waters JH, Shaz BH, et al.: The AABB recommendations for the Choosing Wisely campaign of the American Board of Internal Medicine, *Transfusion* 54(9):2344–2352, 2014.

Centers for Disease Control and Prevention, National Center for Emerging and Zoonotic Infectious Diseases (NCEZID), Division of Vector-Borne Diseases (DVBD): Zika and blood transfusion. August 31, 2016. Available at http://www.cdc.gov/zika/transmission/blood-transfusion.html. Accessed September 22, 2016.

Cotton BA, Au BK, Nunez TC, et al.: Predefined massive transfusion protocols are associated with a reduction in organ failure and postinjury complications, *J Trauma* 66(1):41–48, 2009.

Delaney M, Wendel S, Bercovitz RS, et al.: Transfusion reactions: prevention, diagnosis, and treatment, *Lancet*, 2016. pii:S0140–6736(15)01313-6 [epub ahead of print].

El Kenz H: Van der Linden P: Transfusion-related acute lung injury, *Eur J Anaesthesiol* 31(7):345–350, 2014.

Gajic O, Rana R, Winters JL, et al.: Transfusion-related acute lung injury in the critically ill: prospective nested case-control study, *Am J Respir Crit Care Med* 176(9):886–891, 2007.

Goodnough LT, Shander A: Patient blood management, *Anesthesiology* 116(6):1367–1375, 2012.

Holcomb JB, Wade CE, Michalek JE, et al.: Increased plasma and platelet to red blood cell ratios improves outcome in 466 massively transfused civilian trauma patients, *Ann Surg* 248(3):447–458, 2008.

Hong H, Xiao W, Lazarus HM, et al.: Detection of septic transfusion reactions to platelet transfusions by active and passive surveillance, *Blood* 127(4):496–502, 2016.

Lieberman L, Maskens C, Cserti-Gazdewich C, et al.: A retrospective review of patient factors, transfusion practices, and outcomes in patients with transfusion-associated circulatory overload, *Transfus Med Rev* 27(4): 206–212, 2013.

Marik PE, Corwin HL: Acute lung injury following blood transfusion: expanding the definition, *Crit Care Med* 36(11):3080–3084, 2008.

Maxwell MJ, Wilson MJ: Complications of blood transfusion, *Contin Educ Anaesth Crit Care Pain* 6:225–229, 2006.

Mendler MH, Turlin B, Moirand R, et al.: Insulin resistance-associated hepatic iron overload, *Gastroenterology* 117(5):1155–1163, 1999.

Murphy W: Managing threats rather than risks in blood transfusion: robust design for a complex system, *Transfusion* 46(11):2011–2013, 2006.

Opelz G, Sengar DP, Mickey MR, et al.: Effect of blood transfusions on subsequent kidney transplants, *Transplant Proc* 5(1):253–259, 1973.

Porter JB, Garbowski M: The pathophysiology of transfusional iron overload, *Hematol Oncol Clin North Am* 28(4):683–701, 2014.

Raval JS, Mazepa MA, Russell SL, et al.: Passive reporting greatly underestimates the rate of transfusion-associated circulatory overload after platelet transfusion, *Vox Sang* 108:387–392, 2015.

Sayah DM, Looney MR, Toy P: Transfusion reactions: newer concepts on the pathophysiology, incidence, treatment and prevention of transfusion related acute lung injury (TRALI), *Crit Care Clin* 28(3):363–372, 2012.

Sazama K: Reports of 355 transfusion-associated deaths: 1976 through 1985, *Transfusion* 30(7):583–590, 1990.

Shander A, Lobel GP, Javidroozi M: Transfusion practices and infectious risks, *Expert Rev Hematol* 9(6):597–605, 2016.

Shander A, Sazama K: Clinical consequences of iron overload from chronic red blood cell transfusions, its diagnosis, and its management by chelation therapy, *Transfusion* 50(5):1144–1155, 2010.

Sharma RR, Marwaha N: Leukoreduced blood components: advantages and strategies for its implementation in developing countries, *Asian J Transfus Sci* 4(1):3–8, 2010.

Silvergleid AJ: Approach to the patient with a suspected acute transfusion reaction. In Kleinman S, Tirnauer JS, editors: UpToDate, Waltham, MA. Accessed September 22, 2016.

Skeate RC, Eastlund T: Distinguishing between transfusion related acute lung injury and transfusion associated circulatory overload, *Curr Opin Hematol* 14(6):682–687, 2007.

Stramer SL: Current perspectives in transfusion-transmitted infectious diseases: emerging and re-emerging infections, *ISBT Sci Ser* 9(1):30–36, 2014.

Stramer SL, Hollinger FB, Katz LM, et al.: Emerging infectious disease agents and their potential threat to transfusion safety, *Transfusion* 49(Suppl 2): 1S–29S, 2009.

Stramer SL, Musso D: Zika virus: a new challenge for blood transfusion, *Lancet* 387(10032):1993–1994, 2016.

Toy P, Bacchetti P, Grimes B, et al.: Recipient clinical risk factors predominate in possible transfusion-related acute lung injury, *Transfusion* 55(5):947–952, 2015.

U.S. Food and Drug Administration: Fatalities reported to FDA following blood collection and transfusion: annual summary for fiscal year 2011. Available at http://www.fda.gov/BiologicsBloodVaccines/SafetyAvailability/ReportaProblem/TransfusionDonationFatalities/ucm302847.htm. Accessed September 22, 2016.

U.S. Food and Drug Administration/Center for Biologics Evaluation and Research: Fatalities reported to FDA following blood collection and transfusion: annual summary for fiscal year 2014. Available at http://www.fda.gov/downloads/BiologicsBloodVaccines/SafetyAvailability/ReportaProblem/TransfusionDonationFatalities/UCM459461.pdf. Accessed September 22, 2016.

Vamvakas EC: WBC-containing allogeneic blood transfusion and mortality: a meta-analysis of randomized controlled trials, *Transfusion* 43(7):963–973, 2003.

Vamvakas EC, Blajchman MA: Blood still kills: six strategies to further reduce allogeneic blood transfusion-related mortality, *Transfus Med Rev* 24(2): 77–124, 2010.

Vamvakas EC, Blajchman MA: Transfusion-related immunomodulation (TRIM): an update, *Blood Rev* 21(6):327–348, 2007.

Vamvakas EC, Blajchman MA: Transfusion-related mortality: the ongoing risks of allogeneic blood transfusion and the available strategies for their prevention, *Blood* 113(15):3406–3417, 2009.

Vamvakas EC, Pineda AA, Moore SB: Incidence of delayed hemolytic transfusion reactions, *Vox Sang* 69(1):86, 1995.

Vlaar AP, Binnekade JM, Prins D: Risk factors and outcome of transfusion-related acute lung injury in the critically ill: a nested case-control study, *Crit Care Med* 38(3):771–778, 2010.

Vlaar AP, Juffermans NP: Transfusion-related acute lung injury: a clinical review, *Lancet* 382(9896):984–994, 2013.

Vogelsang G, Kickler TS, Bell WR: Post-transfusion purpura: a report of five patients and a review of the pathogenesis and management, *Am J Hematol* 21(3):259–267, 1986.

第102章 硬膜外麻醉：意外鞘内注射

Tomas McCutchen，J.C. Gerancher

病例概要

患者，虚弱女性，79岁，55 kg，在一家骨科专科手术中心安排为当天第一台手术行择期全髋关节置换术。考虑到术中麻醉和术后镇痛，麻醉方式选用硬膜外麻醉。患者坐在手术台上，导管置入顺利。15 ml局部麻醉药（2%利多卡因和5 μg/ml肾上腺素）分3次，每次5 ml，每次间隔3 min以上通过硬膜外导管注入。髋关节炎性疼痛随即缓解，患者的下肢变得没有感觉。5 min后，患者主诉无力感和呼吸困难，紧接着出现呼吸暂停，意识丧失，继而出现低血压和血氧饱和度下降。在给予面罩通气后行气管插管。予以麻黄碱和静脉输液维持血压。

问题分析

定义

当通常用于硬膜外镇痛或麻醉剂量的局部麻醉药意外进入蛛网膜下腔（鞘内）时，患者可能由于高位脊椎麻醉而出现病残甚至死亡。这种情况可见于穿刺针或鞘管部分或完全穿透硬脊膜和蛛网膜后给予局部麻醉药时。

识别

意外鞘内注射的临床结局取决于进入脑脊液（cerebrospinal fluid，CSF）的局部麻醉药的剂量。低剂量导致下肢麻木；大剂量导致广泛扩散，甚至出现可能引发由于脑干麻醉所导致的意识丧失和呼吸停止。

风险评估：解剖学因素

硬膜外腔位于硬脊膜外，脑膜坚韧的外层与枕骨大孔的骨膜相融合。硬膜外腔横向外侧延伸至脊神经根，在椎间孔中与神经外膜融合，向尾部延伸至骶尾韧带，由前至后分别是后纵韧带、黄韧带和椎板。硬膜外腔隙通过椎间孔与椎旁间隙相通。硬膜外腔的后部和侧部的内容物主要是脂肪，硬膜外腔的外侧和前侧主要为瓣膜静脉。

蛛网膜是一层纤薄的膜，紧靠硬脊膜的内表面。它由多层扁平细胞组成，在层与层之间由结缔组织纤维穿行其中。细胞通过紧密连接相连，这可能解释了蛛网膜是药物从硬膜外腔向鞘内扩散的主要生理屏障的事实。在有椎间孔的区域，脊神经根穿过蛛网膜和硬脊膜，蛛网膜通过硬脊膜疝出形成颗粒。脊髓和颅内蛛网膜颗粒均被看作是CSF的门户，其成分为中枢神经系统的出口。

软脑膜是脑膜更为纤薄的层，黏附于脊髓上。鞘内腔隙是位于蛛网膜和软脑膜之间的空间，其中充满了CSF。脊髓内的CSF直接与颅内CSF联通。

启示

由于大多数硬脊膜与椎管壁紧密相连，硬膜外腔实际上是一个潜在的间隙。它也是一系列不连续的隔间，只有在注入液体或空气时才会变得连续。与蛛网膜下腔麻醉相比，硬膜外麻醉或镇痛需要更大剂量的局部麻醉药。这一解剖结构也解释了硬膜外麻醉时给药平面形成的带状阻滞区，其进一步扩散与注射的局部麻醉药体积直接相关。相对而言，当局部麻醉药注入鞘内通过 CSF 直接作用于脊髓时，它可以产生远高于和低于注射平面的阻滞。麻醉平面扩散的效果不仅与药物的量和浓度相关，还与患者的体位以及溶液的比重相关。如果溶液是等比重的，麻醉平面扩散的效果主要由药物的浓度和容量决定，而低比重和高比重溶液的扩散更依赖于患者的体位。

硬膜外麻醉时大容量的局部麻醉药可能会麻痹 C3 ～ C5 神经根，由于膈神经发自 C3 ～ C5 神经，因此双侧膈神经麻痹可能导致清醒状态的呼吸麻痹。此外，由于颅内和脊髓周围 CSF 的连续性，局部麻醉药可到达脑干并使之麻醉。

治疗

尽早发现意外的鞘内注射对于防止更多的给药和减少可能的并发症至关重要。如果有疼痛症状的患者（例如，产程活跃的产科患者）正在经硬膜外注射药物，意外鞘内注射的第一个征兆可能是给予试验量后几乎所有的疼痛立即消失。患者随后可能出现运动和感觉障碍，麻醉平面的扩散远比硬膜外注射后迅速和广泛。

意外鞘内注射的治疗主要为支持治疗，包括确保呼吸道通畅、给氧和通气，以及用液体和血管升压药（如果需要）维持血压，直到阻滞平面消退。在任何实施椎管内麻醉的场所，必须配备基本的气道设备随时待用，并准备好处理意识丧失、呼吸暂停甚至可能的完全性循环衰竭的预案。

预防

在硬膜外针穿刺和导管放置过程中，需要保持高度的怀疑，在注入预定的硬膜外麻醉剂量前，必须仔细抽吸，并先行给予试验剂量。在定位硬膜外腔隙的过程中，如果穿刺针或者导管有明显的 CSF 回流，则不可注入硬膜外阻滞剂量和体积的局部麻醉药。通常，导管或穿刺针意外进入鞘内并不明显。例如，在硬膜外穿刺过程中，穿刺针尖可能会撕裂硬膜，但若针尖大部分位于硬膜外腔隙内，可能不会出现 CSF 回流，但硬膜外留置导管可能会通过硬膜撕裂口进入蛛网膜下腔。在这种情况下，在注射药物之前缓慢、谨慎的回抽导管可能会发现 CSF。

如果使用生理盐水判断落空感，或者是重置硬膜外导管前给予了一定剂量的硬膜外药物，则可能难以确定回抽液体的性质是生理盐水，或是预先注入的局部麻醉药，还是脑脊液。为了区分 CSF 和其他液体，可以通过以下操作来实施，包括测量液体的 pH、温度或葡萄糖含量。然而尚无一种方法得到广泛的临床应用。如果在回抽的过程中伴有气泡，且可回抽的清亮液体总量小于 3 ～ 5 ml，那么导管在鞘内的可能性就**非常小**。然而，多孔导管的某一个孔可能是处在鞘内的。这种情况下，应当重置导管，或者在充分的测试之前不应按硬膜外剂量给药。

硬膜外试验剂量由少量局部麻醉药组成。原因是这种剂量的局部麻醉药注入鞘内，容易产生明显的运动和感觉障碍，但不会造成高平面的脊椎麻醉；如果硬膜外注射相同的试验剂量，它应该产生很小或不明显的效果。常规的试验剂量是 40 ～ 60 mg 的利多卡因。这个剂量的药物如果注射至鞘内，将很快产生相对低平面脊髓阻滞的体征和症状。但需要注意的是，如果进行腰-硬联合麻醉，在给予足以手术的蛛网膜下腔阻滞剂量后，试验剂量可能会引起高平面的脊椎麻醉。

在每一位患者中，通过同一硬膜外导管重复给药的量均应逐次增加。这个病例中已经注意到导管意外移入鞘内。在追加药物时，需要有适当的时间间隔来评估鞘内注射的可能性，以及时发现导管的意外移位。鞘内留置导管应予以标注，以防硬膜外麻醉的药物意外注入蛛网膜下腔。

硬膜外麻醉期间使用的药物不仅仅是局部麻醉药。作为一种临床常识，大多数临床麻醉科医师在硬膜外麻醉时都会避免使用若误注入鞘内会导致脊髓损伤的药物。事实上，有几种药物，例如芬太尼、肾上腺素和不含有葡萄糖成分的局部麻醉药，虽然没有标注用于脊椎麻醉，但是在临床实践中，这些药物用于椎管内麻醉是安全的。但是两种药物是例外，对此尚有很多争议，即局部麻醉药氯普鲁卡因和含有防腐剂偏亚硫酸钠的制剂。虽然不在本文探讨的范围内，但如果原本用于硬膜外腔的大量药物，意外进入鞘内，则发生的脊髓神经毒性可能与此相关。

硬膜外自体血充填的操作过程中，血液同样进入硬膜外腔。尽管血液进入蛛网膜下腔的后果仍不清楚，但是在一些病例报告中，仍然将其当作并发症之一。目前推测症状和体征是由于误入蛛网膜下腔的血液对脊髓刺激，引起的蛛网膜炎甚至是脑膜炎所导致的。症状范围从无痛到永久性疼痛甚至包括神经系统病损。症状的分布和严重程度可能与意外注入蛛网膜下腔的血液量和扩散程度有关。文献中的病例报告表明大多数此类患者背部、腿部以及臀部疼痛逐渐发作，除止痛药外无需其他干预即可逐渐好转。在硬膜外自体血填充的操作过程中，在注入自体血前，麻醉科医师必须非常谨慎地确定穿刺针位于硬膜外腔而不是位于蛛网膜下腔。这些操作包括轻柔地抽吸，反复地确认，仔细地观察是否有 CSF 从穿刺针中溢出。并时刻牢记针尖误入蛛网膜下腔的发生率仍然未知。在穿刺寻求落空感的过程中，借助空气而不是生理盐水可有助于麻醉科医师辨别回流液体是否是 CSF。在一些情况下，硬膜外自体血填充前，建议预先给予试验剂量的局部麻醉药来确认针尖位置。如果怀疑血液意外注入蛛网膜下腔，须积极处理。磁共振成像可以排除明显的蛛网膜下腔血肿。与患者讨论可能会发生的体征和症状，使用镇痛药治疗疼痛，监测患者的神经状态。

（李 岩 译 文平山 校）

延伸阅读

Bernards CM: Epidural and spinal anesthesia. In Barash PG, Cullen BF, Stoelting RK, editors: *Clinical anesthesia*, ed 4, Philadelphia, 2001, Lippincott Williams & Wilkins, pp 689–713.

Bernards CM, Hill H: The spinal nerve root sleeve is not a preferred route for redistribution of drugs from the epidural space to the spinal cord, *Anesthesiology* 75:827, 1991.

Calimaran AL, Strauss-Hoder TP, Wang WY, et al.: The effect of epidural test dose on motor function after a combined spinal-epidural technique for labor analgesia, *Anesth Analg* 96:167–172, 1996.

Drasner K: Chloroprocaine spinal anesthesia: back to the future? *Anesth Analg* 100(2):549–552, 2005.

Hogan Q: Epidural catheter tip position and distribution of injectate evaluated by computed tomography, *Anesthesiology* 90:964–970, 1994.

Kalina P, Craigo P, Weingarten T: Intrathecal injection of epidural blood patch: a case report and review of the literature, *Emerg Radiol* 11:56–59, 2004.

Liu S, Pollock JE, Mulroy MF, et al.: Comparison of 5% with dextrose, 1.5% with dextrose, and 1.5% dextrose-free lidocaine solutions for spinal anesthesia in human volunteers, *Anesth Analg* 81(4):697–702, 1995.

Poblete B, Van Gessel EF, Gaggero G, et al.: Efficacy of three test doses to detect epidural catheter misplacement, *Can J Anaesth* 46:34–39, 1999.

Reisner LS: Epidural test solution or spinal fluid? *Anesthesiology* 44: 451, 1976.

Tessler MJ, Wiesel S, Wahba RM, et al.: A comparison of simple identification tests to distinguish cerebrospinal fluid from local anaesthetic solution, *Anaesthesia* 49:821–822, 1994.

Visser WA: Delayed subarachnoid migration of an epidural catheter, *Anesthesiology* 88:1414–1415, 1998.

Waters JH, Rizzo VL, Ramanathan S: A re-evaluation of the ability of thiopental to identify cerebrospinal fluid in epidural catheter aspirate, *J Clin Anesth* 7:224–227, 1995.

局部麻醉药全身毒性 第103章

Craig E. Cummings

病例概要

患者，男性，76岁（身高184 cm，体重58 kg，ASA Ⅲ级），拟行全肩关节置换术。其内科病史是冠状动脉疾病远端金属裸支架置入术后和心房纤颤。术后拟行连续肌间沟阻滞镇痛。患者经静脉注射咪达唑仑和芬太尼镇静后，在超声引导下行臂丛神经周围置管。经导管负压抽吸后，逐步加量注入0.5%布比卡因与肾上腺素5 μg/ml（20 ml），持续约1 min。注射完成后，患者出现肌肉抽搐和室性心动过速的心电图改变。

问题分析

定义

局部麻醉药（局麻药）通过阻断电压门控钠通道，抑制兴奋性组织中电冲动的产生和传导。局麻药与通道内孔 α 亚基的特定区域相互作用，可阻止通道激活的构象变化并导致通道的物理闭塞。这就阻碍了通常与膜去极化有关的钠离子内流。局麻药不同于经肠外或肠内给药的药物，因为它们被积聚在预定的作用部位附近，并通过全身吸收进入循环而被清除。局麻药可直接注射到神经周围组织或关节间隙，渗透到皮下组织，或局部应用于皮肤和黏膜表面，提供麻醉和镇痛作用。静脉注射可以产生局部麻醉，减少插管时颅内压升高，治疗心律失常。

从1884年可卡因引入临床使用以来，就有对局麻药的毒性作用的描述，而寻找安全性更高的化合物对这类药物的发展产生了重大影响。局麻药的不良反应可以是局部的，也可以是全身性的。局麻药引起的肌肉毒性和神经毒性将不予讨论。局麻药全身毒性（local anesthetic systemic toxicity，LAST）是局麻药血浆浓度过高所致，主要累及中枢神经系统（central nervous system，CNS）和心血管系统（cardiovascular system，CVS）。潜在的毒性与局麻药本身的麻醉强度相当，效力越强、脂溶性越强的化合物风险越大。蛋白结合力的降低和药物清除的减少也增加了潜在的毒性。LAST的临床表现变异极大，其范围从给药部位吸收局麻药至全身引起的轻微症状到意外血管内注射后的致命性心血管性虚脱（cardiovascular collapse，CC）。较少见的全身毒性包括变态反应和高铁血红蛋白血症。

识别

中枢神经系统毒性

中枢神经系统比心血管系统更容易受到局麻药的毒性影响。局麻药很容易穿过血脑屏障，以剂量依赖的方式产生典型的症状模式（图103.1）。随着局麻药血浆浓度的上升，主要症状从口周麻木、耳鸣、头晕和视觉障碍进展到精神状态的改变、震颤和强直性阵挛发作。这种最初的中枢神经系统兴奋被认为与大脑皮质中抑制性神经元的早期阻滞有关，使易化神经元的活性未遇到阻抗。随着局麻药血浆和中枢神经系统浓度的进一步升高，神经元活动受到无差异的抑制。导致全部中枢神经系统抑制，表现为意识不清和呼吸停止。

虽然局麻药的全身毒性作用与剂量相关，但血浆水平的变化速率也是一个重要因素。缓慢静脉注射或全身吸收局麻药引起的毒性更容易出现中枢神经系统的先兆症状，并以常规方式缓慢进展。意外血管内注射大量局麻药继发的毒性可能进展迅速，并且在无先兆症状的情况下，早期可能就表现为全身强直性阵挛发作或心血管系统毒性。

外部因素对中枢神经系统的毒性潜在影响也

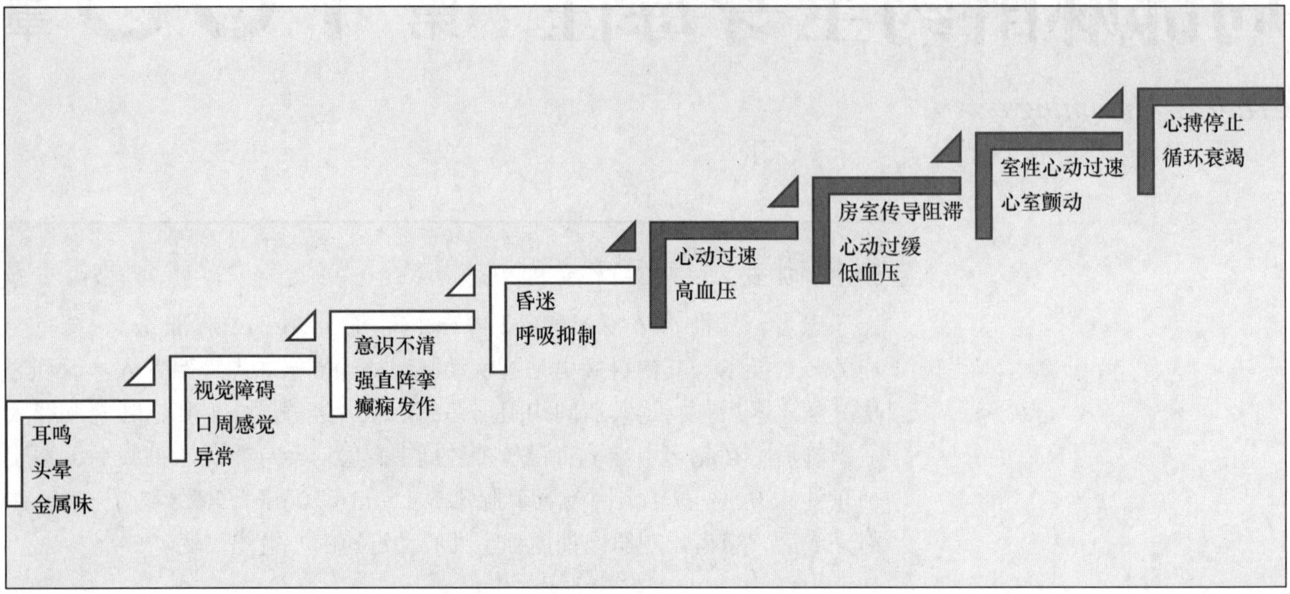

图 103.1 局麻药全身毒性（LAST）临床症状和体征的典型进展，与缓慢的静脉注射或从给药部位逐渐全身吸收局麻药有关

很大。酸中毒通过降低蛋白质结合，增加游离药物跨过细胞膜的比例而加剧毒性。动脉二氧化碳分压（arterial carbon dioxide tension，$PaCO_2$）升高使脑血管扩张，增加脑血流量，增加局麻药向大脑的输送。局麻药溶液中加入肾上腺素，可通过增加脑灌注和局麻药药理活性成分的比例，增加中枢神经系统的毒性。服用苯二氮䓬类药物可以提高惊厥发作的阈值，但过量镇静会导致通气不足、高碳酸血症和缺氧。镇静药物引起的精神状态改变也可能减轻毒性的先兆症状。

心血管系统毒性

局麻药的心血管毒性是由直接心脏效应和神经机制共同作用的结果。局麻药通过阻断心脏钠通道、钙通道和线粒体代谢直接干扰心脏的正常电生理和收缩功能。心脏毒性的最初症状和体征包括心动过速和高血压，往往与中枢神经系统毒性的早期兴奋同时发生。局麻药血浆浓度升高导致以下情况：

- 房室传导阻滞；
- 心动过缓；
- 左心室抑制；
- 致死性心律失常，如室性心动过速和心室颤动。

直接的心脏抑制作用可与外周血管舒张作用同时发生，因为高水平的局麻药可使平滑肌松弛。局麻药血浆浓度的升高，通过抑制自主神经血管收缩和其他中枢神经系统介导的血管调节机制，导致低血压的发生。

诱发心血管虚脱所需要的布比卡因的血浆浓度仅为诱发惊厥所需要的浓度（CC/CNS 比值）的 3 倍，导致其安全范围窄，布比卡因血浆浓度达到中毒水平时迅速从中枢神经系统毒性发展到心血管毒性。这种比例在常用的局麻药中并不相同，在利多卡因和甲哌卡因等效力较弱的局麻药中，CC/CNS 比值增加提供了更大的安全范围。与利多卡因相比，布比卡因对静息和失活心脏钠通道具有更强的结合亲和力，并在舒张期间与这些通道紧密结合。布比卡因从钠通道缓慢解离降低心室传导速度，延长不应期，通过诱发折返性室性心律失常，增加心脏毒性。在全身麻醉期间，或服用苯二氮䓬类药物或其他提高惊厥发作阈值的药物的深度镇静患者，心律失常或循环衰竭是 LAST 常见的表现体征。此外，布比卡因容易诱发恶性室性心律失常，当患者静脉注射大剂量布比卡因静脉时，其主要毒性症状表现为无前驱症状的心血管性虚脱。

变态反应

对无防腐剂酰胺类局麻药极少产生真正的免疫介导反应。局麻药的不良反应通常与意外的血管内注射或局麻药的全身吸收有关，从而导致轻微的毒性症状。肾上腺素等添加剂的全身效应亦常被报道为局麻药过敏。由免疫球蛋白 G（immunoglobulin G，IgG）或 IgE 抗体介导的真正变态反应主要由酯类局麻药引起，主要与代谢物对氨基苯甲酸（para-aminobenzoic acid，PABA）有关，这是已知的化妆品中一种常见的过敏原。市场上销售的多种酰胺类局麻药，经常含有防腐剂对羟基苯甲酸甲酯，其化学结构与 PABA 相似，也可引起免疫介导反应。

高铁血红蛋白血症

血红蛋白的亚铁形式（Fe^{2+}）被氧化成正铁形式（Fe^{3+}），正铁形式无法结合或运输氧气，导致高铁血红蛋白血症。苯佐卡因和丙胺卡因的代谢物邻甲苯胺，可以作为氧化物导致形成高铁血红蛋白。临床可将 2.5% 丙胺卡因和 2.5% 利多卡因制成混合物即丙胺卡因乳剂（EMLA 乳剂）。但与成人相比，儿童患者还原酶途径不成熟，更易患高铁血红蛋白血症，因此 EMLA 乳剂常作为表面麻醉药使用。在支气管镜、内镜和经食管超声心动图检查前，临床上也使用苯佐卡因作为黏膜表面麻醉剂。高铁血红蛋白血症的特点是对氧疗无效的难治性中枢性发绀，通常在高铁血红蛋白水平超过 15% 时发生。症状的严重程度从焦虑、呼吸困难、头痛和恶心到精神状态改变和血流动力学不稳定。症状的严重程度与血液中高铁血红蛋白的水平成正比。高铁血红蛋白水平超过 50% ～ 70% 则十分严重，通常会危及生命。当存在巧克力色的血液，以及脉搏血氧仪和动脉血气分析的血氧饱和度出现差异时，临床诊断需要警惕高铁血红蛋白血症。通过碳氧血红蛋白监测技术定量测定高铁血红蛋白可以确诊。治疗症状性高铁血红蛋白血症的方法是静脉注射亚甲蓝（1 ～ 2 mg/kg）。

风险评估

许多因素会影响局麻药全身毒性的发生，包括患者个体特征（框 103.1）和区域麻醉技术。严重肝病的患者蛋白质合成减少以及肝降解能力降低，因此在使用酰胺局麻药时更容易发生局麻药全身毒性。存在缺血性心脏病或心脏传导异常的患者对局麻药的心脏毒性更敏感。酸碱状态在局麻药全身毒性的发生中起重要作用，因为代谢紊乱导致 $PaCO_2$ 升高或 pH 降低可降低惊厥发作阈值，同时增加脑血流。酸中毒状态的最终结果是向中枢神经系统运输更多的局麻药。

框 103.1 增加 LAST 发生可能的患者个体特征和并存疾病

极端年龄（<4 个月或 >70 岁）
心脏传导缺陷
缺血性心脏病
肝病
线粒体疾病
酸中毒

局麻药通过给药部位吸收和分布进入体循环。在没有意外血管内注射的情况下，局麻药的血浆水平取决于以下因素：

- 注射部位的组织血流；
- 局麻药的总剂量；
- 单个局麻药的理化性质；
- 血管收缩剂的联合使用。

已经证实，局麻药的全身吸收与注射部位的组织灌注呈正相关。肋间神经阻滞后，局麻药的血浆峰值浓度最高，从骶管间隙、臂丛、坐骨沟及皮下组织浓度逐渐降低。局麻药总剂量的增加（体积浓度）导致全身吸收增加和血浆浓度峰值升高，而在硬膜外麻醉和周围神经阻滞期间，加用肾上腺素可降低血浆峰值水平。当肾上腺素添加到具有内在血管舒张特性的局麻药如利多卡因中时，血管收缩的有益作用最为显著。

管理

尽管我们尽了最大的努力，局麻药全身毒性仍可能发生，毒性的严重程度取决于监测的及时性和治疗的充分程度。局麻药全身毒性的临床表现与发病时机、初始表现和持续时间不一致。诊断除需要临床警惕外，还需要了解这些变异性。在接受可能产生毒性剂量局麻药的患者中出现不典型的体征和症状时，应怀疑是否发生局麻药全身毒性。及时的识别和治疗可以阻止心血管性虚脱的毒性进展，并有利于复苏。

布比卡因诱发的恶性心律失常后的心肺复苏尤具挑战性，而且往往对标准的高级心脏生命支持药物治疗和技术无效。然而，动物研究和人类病例报告均表明，静脉注射脂肪乳剂与高质量的基本生命支持结合时，复苏策略显示出可重复性的成功。在局麻药全身毒性的疑似病例中，应强调气道管理的首要地位。缺氧和酸中毒会加重局麻药全身毒性，并可能降低脂肪乳剂治疗的效果，因此必须确保最佳的氧合和通气。苯二氮䓬类药物可迅速消除惊厥发作。丙泊酚或巴比妥类药物只能在没有苯二氮䓬类药物的情况下使用，且在血流动力学不稳定的情况下慎用。小剂量的琥珀胆碱可用于消除肌肉活动和预防因长期强直性阵挛发作引起的代谢性酸中毒。

在局麻药全身毒性情况下，对心脏骤停应进行标准的高级心脏生命支持，并实施以下改进后的药物治疗方案：

- 动物模型中已证实，大剂量使用肾上腺素会导致肺水肿和延迟性血流动力学损害，因此在需要血流动力学支持时，应减少肾上腺素的标准复苏剂量，仅使用小于 1 μg/kg 的重复剂量。
- 在中毒性心肌病的情况下，应避免使用强效的缩血管药物（如血管升压素）提高外周血管的阻力，因为会进一步影响心排血量从而阻碍复苏。
- 胺碘酮是治疗室性心律失常的首选抗心律失常药物，利多卡因和普鲁卡因胺可进一步增加局麻药全身毒性。
- 应避免使用 β-受体阻滞剂、钙通道阻滞剂和其他降低收缩力的药物。
- 当出现严重局麻药全身毒性的症状，应考虑静脉脂肪乳剂治疗。

在局麻药全身毒性情况下，脂肪乳剂给药的最佳时机仍存在争议，但推荐的 20% 脂肪乳剂初始治疗应包括以下内容：

- 初始给药量 1.5 ml/kg，继而以 0.25 ml/kg/min 持续给药，循环稳定后至少持续 10 min。
- 可重复初始给药量，持续性心血管虚脱时输注速度加倍至 0.5 ml/（kg·min）。
- 最初 30 min 最大剂量约为 10 ～ 12 ml/kg。

丙泊酚脂质含量低（10%），且具有直接心脏抑制作用，因此不应将其作为脂肪乳剂治疗的替代品。对于局麻药全身毒性严重，经脂肪乳剂输注和血管升压治疗无效的患者，应考虑体外循环。

严重的冠状动脉疾病可能会降低静脉脂肪乳剂的疗效，因为要快速从心脏组织中消除局麻药，必须将其送入冠状动脉血管床。局麻药在血液中被分割成脂质室或“脂质库”，可部分恢复心血管指标。脂肪乳剂还可以增加血管内容积和直接正性肌力作用，通过脂质代谢和线粒体加工，产生强心作用。心排血量的增加加速了局麻药的肝脏代谢。骨骼肌内局麻药浓度亦观察到短暂升高。局麻药的沉积物会随着时间的推移重新分布到循环中，因此推荐所有发生 LAST 的患者，在事件发生后应严密观察至少 12 h。

尽管越来越多的病例报告描述了脂肪乳剂治疗的有效性，但脂肪乳剂在局麻药全身毒性治疗中的解毒作用和其他亲脂药物过量并非不会产生意外后果。在实验中已证实静脉注射脂肪乳剂与胰腺炎、急性呼吸窘迫综合征和脂血干扰实验室检查结果有关，但迄今尚未证实存在因果关系。虽然标准的长链甘油三酯乳剂和混合中长链甘油三酯乳剂的配方均已成功使用，但用于逆转 LAST 的静脉脂乳剂的最佳配方尚未确定。

预防

尽管局麻药引起严重不良事件的情况很罕见，但严重的 LAST 确实有可能导致显著的病死率。最近 ASA 对 1990 年以后发生的周围神经阻滞相关的并发症已结案索赔进行分析，其中 5% 的索赔涉及意外的血管内注射或局麻药的吸收。此外，近 1/4 与死亡或脑损伤有关的索赔涉及 LAST。

虽然没有单一干预措施能够可靠地消除 LAST 的风险，但应强调预防在降低毒性发生率和严重程度方面的重要性。使用术前检查清单，可以避免在给药前忽略患者的重要特征，并确保复苏设备和药物的立即可用。患者在局部麻醉期间和之后都应使用 ASA 标准监护仪进行监测，因为有报道显示存在迟发性 LAST。在进行区域麻醉时，应考虑使用最小或不使用镇静药物。苯二氮䓬类镇静药会提高惊厥发作的阈值，但会降低患者表达中枢神经系统毒性主观症状的能力。

最佳临床实践应包括尽量减少意外血管内注射的可能性和限制从给药部位全身吸收过量局麻药的技术（框 103.2）。根据动物模型、临床经验和中毒病例报告的推断，应谨慎使用最大推荐剂量的局麻

框 103.2 预防局部麻醉的全身毒性麻醉临床实践的改进

术前检查清单
ASA 标准监护仪
最小或不使用术中镇静
血管内标记物或“试验剂量”
针或导管反复抽吸
局麻药小剂量增量注射
使用最小有效剂量
超声引导

药。临床医师应该关注达到预期结果所需的最低有效剂量。对于易发生 LAST 患者的病情或疾病状态应进一步调整给药方案（见框 103.1）。效力较低的替代品左旋对映体，如罗哌卡因，也可降低心脏毒性。局麻药的注射应以少量、分次的方式进行，每次注射的时间间隔应一个循环时间以上。每次注射前都应对针或导管进行抽吸，并在注射过程中也经常抽吸，以评估血管内放置情况。在无禁忌证的情况下，建议在给予潜在毒性剂量的局麻药时，使用血管内标记物，如肾上腺素。肾上腺素以 1：200 000（5 μg/ml）的浓度加入局麻药溶液，有助于识别血管内注射，并通过收缩局部血管减少全身吸收进入循环。使用这项技术的操作者应该熟悉肾上腺素测试阳性剂量的各种标准，并了解其不同临床情况中的局限性。

超声引导的应用对 LAST 的发生率有显著影响。2013 年发表的一项大型多中心试验中，20 021 例患者接受了 25 336 次周围神经阻滞，证实了 LAST 是一种罕见的事件，总发病率为 0.87/1000。该研究还表明，超声引导可降低 LAST 风险（优势比 0.19：0.28），使用超声引导可提高患者的安全性，与周围神经阻滞后 LAST 风险降低有关。超声引导可降低意外血管穿刺的风险，减少用于周围神经阻滞的局麻药剂量，理论上都可降低 LAST 的风险。

致谢

感谢 Francis V. Salinas 博士对本章上一版的贡献。

（陈 君 译 王 薇 校）

延伸阅读

Abrahams MS, Aziz MF, Fu RF, et al.: Ultrasound guidance compared with electrical neurostimulation for peripheral nerve block: a systematic review and meta-analysis of randomized controlled trials, *Br J Anaesth* 102: 408–417, 2009.

Barrington MJ, Kluger R: Ultrasound guidance reduces the risk of local anesthetic systemic toxicity following peripheral nerve blockade, *Reg Anesth Pain Med* 38:289–299, 2013.

Berde CB, Strichartz GR: Local anesthetics. In Miller RD, editor: *Miller's anesthesia*, ed 8, Philadelphia, 2015, Elsevier, pp 1028–1053.

Boren E, Teuber SS, Naguwa SM, et al.: A critical review of local anesthetic sensitivity, *Clin Rev Allergy Immunol* 32:119–128, 2007.

Butterworth JF, Mackey DC, Wasnick JD: Local anesthetics. In Butterworth JF, Mackey DC, Wasnick JD, editors: *Morgan and Mikhail's clinical anesthesiology*, ed 5, New York, 2013, McGraw-Hill, pp 263–276.

Casati A, Baciarello M, DiCianni S, et al.: Effects of ultrasound guidance on the minimum effective anaesthetic volume required to block the femoral nerve, *Br J Anaesth* 98:823–827, 2007.

DiGregorio G, Neal JM, Rosenquist RW, et al.: Clinical presentation of local anesthetic systemic toxicity a review of published cases 1979 to 2009, *Reg Anesth Pain Med* 35:181–187, 2010.

Evans JA, Wallis SC, Dulhunty JM, et al.: Binding of local anaesthetics to the lipid emulsion Clinoleic™ 20%, *Anaesth Intensive Care* 41:618–622, 2013.

Fettiplace MR, Akpa BS, Ripper R, et al.: Resuscitation with lipid emulsion dose-dependent recovery from cardiac pharmacotoxicity requires a cardiotonic effect, *Anesthesiology* 120:915–925, 2014.

Fettiplace MR, Lis K, Ripper R, et al.: Multi-modal contributions to detoxification of acute pharmacotoxicity by a triglyceride micro-emulsion, *J Control Release* 198:62–70, 2015.

Guay J: The epidural test dose: a review, *Anesth Analg* 102:921–929, 2006.

Heavner JE: Local anesthetics, *Curr Opin Anaesthesiol* 20:336–342, 2007.

Hiller DB, Gregorio GD, Ripper R, et al.: Epinephrine impairs lipid resuscitation from bupivacaine overdose: a threshold effect, *Anesthesiology* 111: 498–505, 2009.

Jamaty C, Bailey B, Larocque A, et al.: Lipid emulsions in the treatment of acute poisoning: a systematic review of human and animal studies, *Clin Toxicol* 48:1–27, 2010.

Lee LA, Posner KL, Kent CD, et al.: Complications associated with peripheral nerve blocks: lessons from the ASA closed claims project, *Int Anesthesiol Clin* 49:56–67, 2011.

Levine M, Skolnik AB, Ruha AM, et al.: Complications following antidotal use of intravenous lipid emulsion therapy, *J Med Toxicol* 10:10–14, 2014.

Mazoit JX, LeGuen R, Beloeil H, et al.: Binding of long-lasting local anesthetics to lipid emulsions, *Anesthesiology* 110:380–386, 2009.

McEvoy MD, Hand WR, Stoll WD, et al.: Adherence to the guidelines for the management of local anesthetic systemic toxicity is improved by an electronic decision support tool and designated "reader," *Reg Anesth Pain Med* 39:299–305, 2014.

Mulroy MF, Weller RS, Liguori GA: A checklist for performing regional nerve blocks, *Reg Anesth Pain Med* 39:195–199, 2014.

Neal JM, Bernards CM, Butterworth JF, et al.: ASRA practice advisory on local anesthetic systemic toxicity, *Reg Anesth Pain Med* 35:152–161, 2010.

Neal JM, Hsiung RL, Mulroy MF, et al.: ASRA checklist improves trainee performance during a simulated episode of local anesthetic systemic toxicity, *Reg Anesth Pain Med* 37:8–15, 2012.

Rosenberg PH, Veering BT, Urmey WF: Maximum recommended doses of local anesthetics: a multifactorial concept, *Reg Anesth Pain Med* 29: 564–575, 2004.

Ruan W, French D, Wong A, et al.: A mixed (long- and medium-chain) triglyceride lipid emulsion extracts local anesthetic from human serum in vitro more effectively than a long-chain emulsion, *Anesthesiology* 116:334–339, 2012.

Salinas FV: Local anesthetic systemic toxicity. In Atley JL, editor: *Complications in anesthesia*, ed 2, Philadelphia, 2006, Saunders, pp 230–234.

Salinas FV, Auyong DB: Essential drugs in anesthetic practice: local anesthetics. In Evers AS, editor: *Anesthetic pharmacology: basic principles and clinical practice*, ed 2, New York, 2011, Cambridge University Press, pp 574–588.

Sites BD, Taenzer AH, Herrick MD, et al.: Incidence of local anesthetic systemic toxicity and postoperative neurologic symptoms associated with 12,668 ultrasound-guided nerve blocks, *Reg Anesth Pain Med* 37:478–482, 2012.

Takahashi R, Oda Y, Tanaka K, et al.: Epinephrine increases the extracellular lidocaine concentration in the brain: a possible mechanism for increased central nervous system toxicity, *Anesthesiology* 105:984–989, 2006.

Weinberg GL: Lipid emulsion infusion: resuscitation for local anesthetic and other drug overdose, *Anesthesiology* 117:180–187, 2012.

第104章 脊椎麻醉后呼吸抑制

Perumal Tamilselvan，Joanna David

病例概要

病例 1

患者，男性，75 岁，在脊椎麻醉下接受全膝关节置换术，脊椎麻醉用药为局部麻醉药、300 μg 二乙酰吗啡或 100 μg 吗啡。当天晚上，患者严重嗜睡，在鼻导管吸氧下氧饱和度 94%。

病例 2

患者，女性，60 岁，在脊椎麻醉下接受经阴道全子宫切除术，脊椎麻醉用药为局部麻醉药和 300 μg 二乙酰吗啡。在恢复室里，患者主诉严重的瘙痒和恶心呕吐。吸空气下氧饱和度为 98%。

问题分析

定义

硬膜外和鞘内给予阿片类药物已应用于临床数十年。椎管内应用阿片类药物产生深度节段性抗伤害作用的剂量远小于全身给药所需要的剂量。在脊椎麻醉中加入芬太尼可以延长感觉阻滞的时间，但不延长出院时间，是门诊手术常用的麻醉方法。鞘内给予阿片类药物行分娩镇痛可降低局部麻醉药的用量，因此接受硬膜外麻醉的产妇可以行走（可行走的硬膜外麻醉）。

识别

鞘内和硬膜外使用阿片类药物的副作用列于框 104.1。最常见的有：

- 呼吸抑制；
- 镇静；
- 瘙痒；
- 恶心和呕吐。

总的来说，椎管内使用阿片类药物相关的副作用与静脉、肌内或口服阿片类药物类似。然而，由于阿片类药物与其在脊髓和大脑中的受体之间的相互作用，其严重程度、发生率和发生时机差异很大。最严重的并发症是呼吸抑制，可为早期或迟延性发作。

框 104.1　椎管内麻醉的并发症

呼吸抑制
镇静
瘙痒
恶心和呕吐
尿潴留
胃肠功能障碍
过敏反应
痛觉超敏
行为问题
头晕或低血压
体温调节功能障碍

风险评估

呼吸抑制

阿片类药物在脑脊液中向喙侧扩散的程度和速度决定了呼吸抑制副作用的发生特征。脑脊液的自然循环可使残留的药物直接接触到位于第四脑室底的大脑呼吸中枢。一般来说，腰段脑脊液到达大脑需要 4 ～ 6 h。因此，决定药物到达喙侧脑脊液量的因素包括给药位置（鞘内 vs. 硬膜外；胸椎 vs. 腰椎）、剂量和脂溶性。当鞘内给予高亲脂药物芬太尼或舒芬太尼时，其可迅速穿透脊髓组织直接作用于背角神经元。脑脊液中药物残留浓度低，因此该类药物具有更强的节段性镇痛作用。相比之下，吗啡的亲脂性不高，其经脊髓吸收和从脑脊液中流出（通过蛛网膜颗粒）较慢。因此，高浓度的药物在脑脊液中停留的时间更长。因此，与芬太尼或舒芬太尼相比，吗啡更有可能到达大脑的呼吸中枢从而导致延迟性呼吸抑制。

如果硬膜外给予阿片类药物，它可以有脊髓或脊髓外（全身）的作用，从而有双重抑制呼吸。其可表现为早期呼吸抑制（<2 h），其原因为血管摄取和再分配，类似于肌内注射后发生的情况；或晚期呼吸抑制（6 ～ 12 h），其原因为药物在脑脊液向喙侧迁移。脊髓效应和脊髓外效应的比例取决于有多少药物被吸收至硬膜外静脉丛，有多少沉积在硬膜外脂肪中，有多少穿透脑脊膜进入脑脊液。药物的脂溶性、分子量和形状在很大程度上决定其硬脑膜的穿透性和在脑脊液中停留足够长时间以使其能够向喙侧扩散的药物量。这就解释了为什么亲水性吗啡或氢吗啡酮比高亲脂性药物（如芬太尼或舒芬太尼）具有更强的硬膜穿透力（脊髓作用）。基于同样的原因，当吗啡或氢吗啡酮用于高位胸段或颈段硬膜外时，呼吸抑制的风险更大。

被认为呼吸抑制风险增加的患者包括老年人和体弱者，有严重肺部疾病（包括睡眠呼吸暂停）的患者，以及同时服用阿片类药物或中枢神经系统抑制剂的患者。长期应用阿片类药物治疗的患者可出现耐药，因此这些患者较少出现中枢介导、椎管内阿片类药物导致的呼吸抑制。产后患者也较少发生呼吸抑制，可能是由于她们比较年轻，同时妊娠增加了通气驱动。最后，报道的椎管内应用阿片类药物的严重呼吸抑制（需要治疗）的总发生率为 0.2% ～ 2%，这与更传统的使用方法（约 1%）差别不大。框 104.2 列出呼吸抑制的危险因素。

镇静

镇静与呼吸抑制相关，原因有二：首先，阿片类药物可经由脑脊液向喙侧扩散从而直接作用于丘脑、边缘系统或大脑皮质；其次，如果确实发生了严重的呼吸抑制，由此引起的高碳酸血症可能会产生二氧化碳麻醉。在此之前，当患者在椎管内使用阿片类药物后变得越来越嗜睡时，即使呼吸频率和氧合在可接受的限度内，也应仔细考虑间歇性低通气和呼吸抑制。

框 104.2 增加呼吸抑制风险的因素

阿片类药物的特征
- 剂量较大
- 鞘内注射
- 亲水性吗啡或氢吗啡酮
- 重复给药和连续输注

患者的特征
- 老年
- 体弱
- 严重肺部疾病
- 睡眠呼吸暂停
- 初次使用阿片类药物
- 正在使用阿片类药物或中枢神经系统抑制剂

瘙痒

椎管内使用阿片类药物最常见的副作用是瘙痒。可以是全身性的，但更常见于面部、颈部或上胸部。发生率差异很大，从 0% ～ 100%，通常只有在直接询问之后才被发现。严重的瘙痒较罕见，仅约 1% 的患者发生。阿片类药物的剂量越高，瘙痒的风险越大。由于雌激素与阿片类受体发生相互作用，因此产科患者更为常见。所有的阿片类药物都能引起瘙痒，而芬太尼和吗啡则更为常见。瘙痒的可能机制是由于阿片类药物通过脑脊液的喙侧扩散与位于髓质的三叉神经核（瘙痒中心）的阿片类药物受体相互作用。这也许可以解释为何瘙痒在面部区域更常见。组胺释放不是瘙痒的原因；但与之相反，抗组胺剂可以缓解症状。

恶心与呕吐

鞘内和硬膜外阿片给药后恶心呕吐发生率约为 30%。虽然其潜在机制与药物的全身吸收无关，但与静脉注射阿片类药物后恶心呕吐的发生率是相同的。通常在注射后 4 h 内出现恶心，随后出现呕吐。其发生率与阿片类药物的剂量可能有关，也可能无关，但鞘内注射吗啡的发生率更高。女性比男性更容易发生恶心呕吐。鞘内和硬膜外使用阿片类药物可能导致药物在脑脊液中向头侧迁移，并随后与位于该区域的阿片类受体相互作用。对运动敏感的前庭系统和阿片类药物导致的胃排空减少也可能在鞘内和硬膜外应用阿片类药物引起的恶心和呕吐中发挥作用。

尿潴留

鞘内和硬膜外应用阿片类药物后尿潴留的发生

率差异很大，从 0% 到 80% 不等，最常见于年轻男性志愿者，其发生率与阿片类药物的使用剂量无关，而鞘内应用吗啡的发生率可能更高，其潜在机制与药物的全身吸收无关。鞘内和硬膜外使用阿片类药物后发生尿潴留比静脉或肌肉注射等量阿片类药物后发生尿潴留更为常见。鞘内和硬膜外应用阿片类药物引起的尿潴留可能与位于骶髓的阿片类药物受体的相互作用有关。这种相互作用抑制了骶副交感神经系统的放电，从而导致逼尿肌松弛和最大膀胱容量的增加，从而导致尿潴留。在人体中，硬膜外注射吗啡在 15 min 内即可导致明显的逼尿肌松弛，可持续 16 h，且易被纳洛酮逆转。内源性阿片类药物可能在膀胱功能的正常控制中发挥重要作用。

胃肠功能障碍

众所周知，静脉和肌内注射阿片类药物可改变胃肠道运动。鞘内和硬膜外阿片类药物也可导致胃排空延迟和肠道转运时间延长。鞘内或硬膜外阿片类药物给药后胃肠动力下降的原因与药物的全身吸收无关，似乎是与位于脊髓的阿片类受体相互作用所致。在人类志愿者中，硬膜外使用吗啡可以延缓胃排空。在小鼠中，鞘内注射吗啡可引起剂量依赖性胃肠功能障碍和纳洛酮可逆转的小肠转运时间延长。接受鞘内或硬膜外阿片类药物治疗的患者可出现肠梗阻的体征和症状，进而导致恶心和呕吐。

启示

患者的合理选择和小心谨慎可以减少椎管内应用阿片类药物的严重不良反应，尤其是中枢性呼吸抑制。谨慎的术后管理很有必要，因为使用亲水性药物（吗啡、氢吗啡酮）可导致延迟发作的和较长时间的呼吸抑制。椎管内使用吗啡或氢吗啡酮后需要监测至少 24 h。过度嗜睡可能是首发症状，这就是为何在术后观察时应该进行精神状态评估。应避免同时使用其他麻醉性镇痛药物或中枢神经系统抑制剂，尤其是对于首次使用阿片类药物的患者。

小剂量的亲脂药物，如芬太尼，可在门诊手术环境中安全使用。研究表明，即使对于老年患者，鞘内使用芬太尼的剂量小于 25 μg 时呼吸抑制的风险可降至最低。对于术后接受硬膜外镇痛的患者，如果芬太尼的使用剂量合理，即使使用胸段硬膜外导管，也不需要特别监测。

诸如瘙痒、恶心呕吐和尿潴留等副作用可能被视为麻烦但轻微的并发症，但即便如此，也可能产生不良后果。如果严重到一定程度，可能会出现非计划入院或延迟出院，治疗药物所导致的不愉悦的副作用，或不必要的操作，如由于无法排尿而留置膀胱导管。

在分娩过程中鞘内应用麻醉性镇痛药越来越普遍。已有并发症被报道，如延长早期产程和严重胎儿心动过缓，但其因果关系在产科文献中仍存争论。胎儿心率异常，尤其是心动过缓的发生率可能与剂量相关。推测原因可能为快速镇痛后循环儿茶酚胺不平衡导致子宫过度活跃。应当强调的是，这种心率异常对传统治疗措施有反应，且与新生儿不良结局无关。

管理

对于严重的副作用，包括呼吸抑制，最好的拮抗剂是纯阿片拮抗剂，如纳洛酮。虽然静脉使用纳洛酮的起效速度很快，但单次注射的持续时间可能不足，因此经常需要静脉输注。对于不太严重的副作用（如瘙痒），纳洛酮可能很难滴定至起效且不拮抗部分镇痛作用。基于此，像纳布啡这样的混合激动拮抗剂可能更合适。研究表明，在不改变疼痛控制水平的情况下，纳布啡可以有效地治疗瘙痒、恶心或呕吐。

已用于治疗椎管内阿片类药物副作用的其他药物见表 104.1。血清素 5-HT_3 拮抗剂（如昂丹司琼）是治疗瘙痒和恶心的有效药物。弱血清素拮抗剂氟哌利多可能有助于治疗瘙痒，但对恶心和呕吐更有效。丙泊酚抑制背角信号传递，能有效治疗恶心和瘙痒；然而，用于此目的的丙泊酚输注的管理和成本可能会超过它的益处。尽管组胺释放不是阿片类药物引起瘙痒的机制，但抗组胺药物如苯海拉明的镇静作用可能通过打破瘙痒–抓痒循环而产生益处，但它们不能直接减轻瘙痒。

这些药物可在不影响镇痛的情况下减轻瘙痒、术后恶心呕吐等副作用。由于呼吸抑制是一种中枢介导的作用，因此不太可能使用这些药物进行治疗。

表 104.1 椎管内使用阿片类药物并发症的处理

并发症	处理
呼吸抑制	• 呼吸频率小于 8 次 / 分或难以唤醒
	• 给氧 6 ～ 8 L/min
	• 每 2 ～ 3 min 静脉注射纳洛酮 100 ～ 200 μg 直至呼吸速率大于 8 次 / 分；由于纳洛酮持续时间短，将需要重复给药；或者采用输注纳洛酮 50 ～ 100 μg/h
镇静	• 如果嗜睡但可被唤醒，则通过鼻导管给氧
	• 检查呼吸频率和氧饱和度
	• 如果无法唤醒，请寻求帮助
瘙痒	• 昂丹司琼 [4 mg 静脉注射（IV）]
	• 小剂量丙泊酚（每次 10 ～ 20 mg，IV）
	• 氯苯那敏（可能有效，但因镇静作用而增加呼吸抑制的风险，不应作为一线治疗用药）
	• 低剂量纳洛酮（100 μg 皮下注射或静脉注射）；每 30 min 重复一次
恶心和呕吐	• 按处方给予止吐药（通常是昂丹司琼、丙氯哌嗪或甲氧氯普胺）
	• 如果常规止吐药不能缓解，考虑给予低剂量纳洛酮（100 μg/h）
尿潴留	• 导尿管

预防

限制椎管内阿片类药物的剂量可以减少不良反应的发生率。因此，多模式的术后镇痛方法可能是最佳预防方案。非甾体抗炎药可以降低阿片类药物的需求，提供镇痛，甚至可能通过抑制前列腺素的合成而有预防瘙痒的作用。地塞米松也是一种有效的预防恶心呕吐的药物，如果剂量较高，可能会增强镇痛效果。氟哌利多可减少术后恶心呕吐。预防性应用昂丹司琼已被证明可以减少恶心、呕吐和瘙痒。然而，纳布啡可能是治疗优于预防的药物。术中注射丙泊酚不能预防术后瘙痒或恶心。持续硬膜外镇痛时加入低浓度的局麻药可通过协同作用减少阿片类药物的用量。

（杨迪迪 译 孟 岩 校）

延伸阅读

Chaney MA: Side effects of intrathecal and epidural opioids, *Can J Anaesth* 42:891–903, 1995.

Etches RC, Sandler AN, Daley MD: Respiratory depression and spinal opioids, *Can J Anaesth* 36:165–185, 1989.

Szarvas S, Harmon D, Murphy D: Neuraxial opioid-induced pruritus: a review, *J Clin Anesth* 15:234–239, 2003.

Van de Velde M, Teunkens A, Hanssens M, et al.: Intrathecal sufentanil and fetal heart rate abnormalities: a double-blind, double placebo-controlled trial comparing two forms of combined spinal epidural analgesia with epidural analgesia in labor, *Anesth Analg* 98:1153–1159, 2004.

第四部分

设备相关并发症

第 105 章 麻醉回路

Michael R. Mathis，*Satya Krishna Ramachandran*

病例概要

患者，女性，57 岁，重度吸烟史，在麻醉诱导期间发生气管插管困难。面罩通气亦有困难，部分原因是需要较高的吸入压力，另一部分原因是面罩贴合不佳导致面罩和面部之间的漏气较多。首次和随后的气管插管尝试时，均出现呼吸球囊下难以通气，且未见 CO_2 波形；每次均试探性判断为食管插管，并迅速移除导管。每次插管后，面罩通气都更加困难。在此期间，患者间歇性地出现低血压。诱导后约 30 min，观察者注意到麻醉呼吸系统的呼气单向阀在整个呼吸周期中都保持静止。更换阀门后该问题得以解决；患者能够通气，且成功插管，"不能通气，不能插管"的情况出现意外转折。

问题分析

定义

麻醉呼吸系统（anesthetic breathing system，ABS）曾由美国测试和材料协会在设备标准中定义为"与患者直接相连，出现呼吸压力时供气流通过的气体通道；该通道往往配有单向阀；特定混合成分的气体通过它进行传输"。ABS 的特殊组件之一 CO_2 吸收器，将在第 106 章讨论。

几乎每一件医疗设备都存在操作错误或故障的风险。麻醉呼吸系统有多重机械部件和连接，且因生产厂商和设计而异，容易引发严重事故导致患者受伤。在美国最受欢迎的 ABS 是回路系统；框 105.1 列出了该系统的组件，并将故障模式列在框 105.2 中。

涉及 ABS 的严重事故可以被大致归类为操作者错误或设备故障。美国麻醉科医师协会（American Society of Anesthesiologists，ASA）主张使用以下定义对各 ABS 相关问题索赔结案分析和精确限定。**操作者错误**是指"设备准备、维护或使用相关的故障或人为错误"，而**设备故障**指的是"虽经过日常维护且曾正常使用的设备出现意外的故障"。ABS 中的单向阀突然无法打开就是设备故障的一种。**断开**被定义为最初以功能性和常规方式配置的呼吸回路中接合部件连续性丧失。错误连接被定义为呼吸回路部件或附件的无功能和非常规配置。

框 105.1 回路系统的组件
新鲜气体流入口
吸气管路
呼气管路
呼吸单向阀
CO_2 吸收剂
Y 形连接管
呼吸机 / 储气球囊
可调限压（"弹出"）阀
麻醉气体清除系统

该患者发生的通气困难，是 ABS 相关的许多潜在致命或伤害性并发症之一。尽管麻醉机设计和麻醉监测的进步已使过去 20 年里 ABS 引起全身麻醉索赔的频率得以降低，但涉及 ABS 的严重事故仍可能威胁生命。在 1990 年后的全身麻醉结案索赔中，20% 被确认为由 ABS 引起，其中一半导致不可逆转的脑损伤或死亡。卡住的单向阀——就像本病例概要中患者所发生的——代表了多数的 ABS 结案索赔。这种事件可能是进展最迅速的破坏性麻醉事件；在封闭呼气系统中，气体进入肺部无法排出，

框 105.2 麻醉呼吸回路故障

断开
可能的断开的部位，请参见框 105.1

堵塞（气道压力升高）
机械压缩 / 变形
电路内异物
加热软管
清除系统连接不当
水冷凝
缓慢进展的微生物过滤器堵塞

泄漏（降低气道压力）
吸气管路
呼气管路
任何其他管道或小接头

阀门故障
阻塞
失能
逆流 / 复呼吸

CO_2 吸收剂失效
钠石灰耗尽
CO 生成
钠石灰干燥
过热
未去除包装
吸收罐破裂

污染
微生物、病毒
颗粒物质

气道压力迅速上升到一定水平可能会导致肺部破裂。其他索赔包括错误连接，以及机械通气故障时未能使用自动充气手控通气装置（self-infating manual ventilation device，SIMVD）。

识别

众所周知，识别 ABS 问题很困难，如所示案例概要。它们似乎与麻醉科医师完成的任何事情（例如转动刻度盘、注射药物或插入气管导管）都没有关系，这些事件往往难以预估且具有灾难性。除非高度怀疑，否则麻醉科医师可能会专注于更常见的原因——比如该病例中的食管插管。目前的监护本身可能对判断 ABS 问题帮助不大；然而，麻醉机检查仍然是最有价值的预防方法之一。结案的索赔分析评论者认为，对于大多数呼吸回路索赔，通过麻醉前机器检查可以避免相关损伤（75%）。最重要的监护是警觉的麻醉科医师，他们监测呼吸音和胸廓运动，并持续观察监视器。

风险评估

任何接受全身麻醉的患者易受 ABS 相关并发症风险的影响。更高的潮气量、呼吸频率、新鲜气流增加了风险，尤其是对于较小的患者。肺部疾病病患者，尤其是肺大泡患者，特别容易被增高的气道压力所损伤（**气压伤**）。麻醉状态降低了心血管保护性反应机制，并进一步导致正压通气下心血管损害。正如病例概要中所述，血容量或心功能降低的患者会有更大的风险。快速上升的气道压力迅速阻碍静脉回流，进而使每搏量减少、动脉压降低，即使在健康患者中也是如此。

导致或促成 ABS 发生问题的原因包括磨损、部件损坏、设计缺陷、疏于或不当维护、装配不当、粗心以及使用前未检查麻醉工作站。在 20 世纪 80 和 90 年代，使用前未进行设备检查是大部分重大事件中的一个常见原因。在 Cooper 及同事的调查中，20.5% 的事件涉及“未进行检查”。在澳大利亚的一项调查中，“未进行设备检查”在所有事故中占 11.8%。此后，澳大利亚进一步对 1000 例严重麻醉事故进行调查，发现 395 例由设备问题造成，因未能执行麻醉机检查而导致的事故比例有所降低（2.5%）。尽管如此，ABS 故障引起的严重事故不仅威胁生命，而且在大多数情况下是可预防的，因此应当继续努力改善 ABS 设计和安全检查。

在 Cooper 及同事的开创性报告中，与 ABS 相关的严重事件排在榜单前列：机械通气时呼吸回路断开（5.2%）、呼吸回路泄漏（1.7%）、呼吸回路连接错误（1.7%）和呼吸回路控制差错（1.4%）。呼吸回路相关的严重事件占所有严重事件的 10%。澳大利亚对严重事件的最新调查也显示了类似结果；395 例与设备问题有关的严重事件中，61 例（15%）源自通气故障或泄漏，21 例（5.3%）由于电路断开，8（2.0%）来自单向阀故障，7（1.8%）由错误连接造成。

在最新的 ASA 结案索赔分析中，气体输送装置相关索赔自 1990 年以来逐步降低；然而，根据专家判断，其中许多索赔仍可避免。在分析中，85% 的气体输送装置索赔涉及麻醉科医师过失，其中 41%

被认为是可通过麻醉机器检查预防的。最常被引用的事件涉及卡住的吸气/呼气阀；其他事件包括来自回路的塑料阻塞了回路内腔，呼气末正压阀连接到错误的（吸气）回路分支，以及储气球囊的错误安放。

启示

呼吸回路并发症能够造成严重后果。过去几十年里发表了一些关于麻醉结局的大规模调查结果，其中涉及气体输送装置引起的严重损伤。这些研究中约 5% ～ 23% 的麻醉相关死亡和脑损伤是由气体输送装置故障引起的。在 ASA 完结索赔项目最新资料中，自 1990 年以来共有 6022 例索赔涉及全身麻醉，其中 40 例（0.7%）为呼吸回路并发症所致。在与呼吸回路并发症相关的索赔中，15 例（38%）死亡或出现了严重脑损伤。

由于呼吸回路并发症所带来的危及生命的后果，人们近 20 年来一直在努力减少事件的发生。事实上，1990 年以来与气体输送装置相关的索赔数量和损伤严重程度均得以降低。麻醉给药系统的改进——专注于更安全的机器、呼吸机和回路设计，同时改进了安全检查工具并加强了算法触发预警，为索赔发生率及严重程度的降低提供了合理的解释。与先前结案索赔分析有所不同，现在已没有回路断开相关的索赔，回路连接错误相关索赔比例也得以降低。尽管有了上述改进，患者安全仍需由警觉的、训练有素的麻醉科医师来保障，绝大多数（86%）气体输送索赔仍然与可避免的麻醉科医师过失相关。

总之，人为错误在 ABS 并发症的发生中起着重要作用。ABS 并发症对患者造成的伤害往往具有严重程度高且医疗花费大的特征。过去 20 年中，安全核查的实施和 ABS 设计的改进使 ABS 相关并发症的发生率得以降低，但索赔持续存在，其中一半索赔由吸气或呼气单向阀卡住引起。

管理

处置方式通常很简单，尤其是当 ABS 相关状况识别相对较早时。偶尔需要使用备用麻醉机替代故障机器；这是一件既非琐碎也不容易的事情。当这种情况发生或诊断确认后，应该使用另一种方法来保证供氧和通气。在这方面，重要的是认识到，快速使用带有麻醉呼吸系统故障排除流程中的 SIMVD 的作用。在更新的 ASA 完结索赔分析中，三个低严重程度的索赔中成功地使用了 SIMVD；相比之下，另两例索赔中出现死亡或严重脑损伤，虽然 SIMVD 可用，但没有进行尝试；还有一例中 SIMVD 不可用，另一例在通气不足时确认了心脏停搏后才使用 SIMVD，错过了最佳时间。有趣的是，尽管涉及 SIMVD 使用不当导致的完结索赔反复出现，但研究表明确认 SIMVD 可用是 ASA 2008 麻醉前检查中最常被忽略的步骤。

预防

防止大多数 ABS 相关事件的最佳方法已使用了数十年，也就是麻醉工作站检查。正式的检查清单由美国 FDA 自 1986 年制定并生效。此外，ASA 于 1993 年制定了一份检查建议清单，并于 2008 年更

框 105.3　FDA 推荐 ABS 相关的麻醉工作站检查

呼吸系统的初始状态：
将选择开关设置在“气囊”模式
检查**呼吸回路**是否完整、完好、通畅
验证 CO_2 吸收剂是否足够。
安装呼吸回路**附件设备**［例如加湿器、呼气末正压（PEEP）阀］。
呼吸系统泄漏检查：
将所有气体流量设置为零（或最小）
关闭**可调压力限制（APL；“弹出”）阀**并堵住 Y 型连接管
将氧气呼吸系统的压力维持在 30 cmH_2O
打开 APL 阀，确保压力降低
通气系统和单向阀：
将第二个呼吸球囊与 Y 型连接管相连
为下一位患者设置合适的呼吸机参数
切换到自动通气（呼吸机）模式
用 O_2 充满**风箱**和第二个呼吸球囊，然后打开呼吸机
将 O_2 流量设置为最小，其他气体流量设置为零
确保在吸气时风箱能提供合适的潮气量，且呼气时风箱能完全充满
将新鲜气体流量设定为约 5 L/min
确认呼吸机风箱和模拟肺能够适当充满和排空，且呼气结束时没有持续的压力
检查**单向阀**是否动作正常
确保**呼吸回路附件**功能正常
关闭呼吸机，并切换到手动通气（气囊/APL）模式
手动通气，确保人工肺能够充气和放气，且感觉到合适的系统阻力和顺应性
取下第二个呼吸球囊

新。检查方案通常需要四项基本活动：核查备用设备和用品（例如加压气瓶），检查设备配置（例如呼吸回路连接），检查设备机械力学（例如单向阀的正确动作），以及监护仪准备（例如校准、功能验证和警报激活）。ASA 的结案索赔分析显示，更好地选择和使用监护仪可以防止气体输送系统索赔中的绝大多数并发症。

我们无法展示整个 FDA 检查流程，与 ABS 相关的部分见框 105.3。ASA 制定的麻醉前检查步骤详见表 105.1。在本章开头的场景中，简单地在麻醉前从 ABS 吸气和呼气管道上拆除 Y 型连接管，并分别使用两根管道完成吸入和呼出，这种方法可以明显降低发生灾难的可能性。

由于高气道压力会带来严重并发症，装置标准应考虑到警报本身可能无法给临床医师足够时间来识别警报、诊断问题，并实施补救行为。因此，每

表 105.1　ASA2008 关于麻醉前检查程序的推荐

	每天、移动机器或更换挥发罐后完成	
待完成项目		**责任方**
项目 #1	确认辅助氧气瓶和手动通气装置（加压给氧气囊）可用且功能正常	麻醉科医师和技术员
项目 #2	确认患者吸引装置足以清理气道	麻醉科医师和技术员
项目 #3	打开麻醉输送系统，并确认 AC 电源可用	麻醉科医师或技术员
项目 #4	确认所需监护的可用性，包括警报	麻醉科医师或技术员
项目 #5	确认安装在麻醉机上的备用氧气瓶压力足够	麻醉科医师和技术员
项目 #6	确认管道气体压力≥ 50 psig	麻醉科医师和技术员
项目 #7	确认挥发罐是已充分填充；若是，则填充口应紧密关闭	麻醉科医师或技术员
项目 #8	确认流量计和公共气体出口之间的供气管线没有泄漏	麻醉科医师或技术员
项目 #9	测试气体清除系统功能	麻醉科医师或技术员
项目 #10	校准或确认氧气检测的校准，并检查低氧警报	麻醉科医师或技术员
项目 #11	确认二氧化碳吸收剂新鲜且未耗尽	麻醉科医师或技术员
项目 #12	执行呼吸系统压力和泄漏测试	麻醉科医师和技术员
项目 #13	确认吸气和呼气过程中气体能够正确地流经呼吸回路	麻醉科医师和技术员
项目 #14	记录检查流程的完成情况	麻醉科医师和技术员
项目 #15	确认呼吸机设置，并评估提供麻醉护理的准备情况（ANESTHESIA TIME-OUT）	麻醉科医师
	每次使用前完成	
两个病例之间需要完成的项目亚组		**责任方**
项目 #2	确认患者吸引装置足以清理气道	麻醉科医师和技术员
项目 #4	确认所需监护的可用性，包括警报	麻醉科医师或技术员
项目 #7	确认挥发罐是已充分填充；若是，则填充口应紧密关闭	麻醉科医师
项目 #11	确认二氧化碳吸收剂新鲜且未耗尽	麻醉科医师或技术员
项目 #12	执行呼吸系统压力和泄漏测试	麻醉科医师和技术员
项目 #13	确认吸气和呼气过程中气体能够正确地流经呼吸回路	麻醉科医师和技术员
项目 #14	记录检查流程的完成情况	麻醉科医师和技术员
项目 #15	确认呼吸机设置，并评估提供麻醉护理的准备情况（ANESTHESIA TIME-OUT）	麻醉科医师

From American Society of Anesthesiologists：ASA Library of Anesthesia Workstation Checkout Procedures（checkout procedure submission template），2008. Available at http://www.asahq.org/resources/clinical-information/2008-asa-recommendations-for-pre-anesthesia-checkout/sample-procedures. Accessed August 19，2016.

种麻醉工作站必须有固定的呼吸压力限制保护模块，其最大压力不能超过 125 cmH_2O（12.5 kPa）。此外，如果**固定**呼吸压力限制保护模块为 80 cmH_2O 或更大，现代麻醉工作站需要具备可调呼吸压力限制保护模块。如果没有呼吸机，或麻醉工作站在手动或自主呼吸模式下，储气球囊袋可被视为气道压力限制保护模块。保护模块在本病例中提供的保护程度有限，这是由呼气阀阻塞导致呼出气体无法到达储气球囊袋或呼吸机。

总之，怀疑、观察和强制能使 ABS 相关并发症得以预防、识别和处理。麻醉科医师的座右铭"警惕"无比重要，对 ABS 并发症而言更需要持续保持警惕。在麻醉过程中，气道压力的急剧增加或由泄漏导致的潮气量完全丧失是真正的紧急情况，致命或致残损伤可能在几秒钟内发生。

（刘洪伟 译 汪 惠 校）

延伸阅读

American Society of Anesthesiologists: 2008 recommendations for preanesthesia checkout, 2008. Available at http://www.asahq.org/resources/clinical-information/2008-asa-recommendations-for-pre-anesthesia-checkout. Accessed August 19, 2016.

ASTM F1208 (Anesthesia Breathing Systems). In *Medical devices. Emergency medical services*, vol. 13.01. West Conshohocken, PA, 1994, American Society for Testing and Materials.

Cooper JB, Newbower RS, Kitz RJ: An analysis of major errors and equipment failures in anesthesia management: considerations for prevention and detection, *Anesthesiology* 60:34–42, 1984.

DeMaria Jr S, Blasius K, Neustein SM: Missed steps in the preanesthetic set-up, *Anesth Analg* 113:84–88, 2011.

James RH: 1000 anaesthetic incidents: experience to date, *Anaesthesia* 58: 856–863, 2003.

Kusmaphanyo C, Charluluxananan S, Sriramatr D, et al.: The Thai Anesthesia Incident Monitor Study (Thai AIMS) of anesthetic equipment failure/malfunction: an analysis of 1996 incident reports, *J Med Assoc Thai* 92: 1442–1449, 2009.

Mehta SP, Eisenkraft JB, Posner KL, et al.: Patient injuries from anesthesia gas delivery equipment a closed claims update, *Anesthesiology* 119:788–795, 2013.

Russell WJ, Webb RK, Van der Walt JH, et al.: Problems with ventilation: an analysis of 2000 incident reports, *Anaesth Intensive Care* 21:617–620, 1993.

CO_2 吸收器

第 106 章

Marc Sherwin，James B. Eisenkraft

病例概要

患者，女性，75 岁，因憩室炎穿孔在全身麻醉下接受腹腔镜部分结肠切除术。患者腹部被吹入 CO_2，压力在 15 ～ 20 mmHg，持续 45 min。在此期间，呼气末 CO_2 在未对分钟通气量进行任何调节的情况下升至 50 mmHg。最后 15 min 时，最终的呼气末 CO_2 甚至增至 55 mmHg，吸入 CO_2 值本应该为零，此时却上升到 6 mmHg。经检查发现，CO_2 吸收器中吸收剂的颜色并未发生变化。

问题分析

定义

在紧闭和半紧闭的呼吸回路中，CO_2 吸收剂对消除 CO_2 是必不可少的。吸收剂与 CO_2 的化学反应允许使用新鲜低流量气体且不会引起复吸入。患者呼出的气体通过装有吸收剂颗粒的储罐，根据吸收剂的组成产生不同程度的碳酸盐、水和热量。

当前的麻醉系统中最常用的吸收剂包括 Sodasorb、Medisorb、Drägersorb 800 Plus、Amsorb Plus、Litholyme 和 Spiralith。吸收剂的成分都不相同，如氢氧化钙含量、催化剂（NaOH 或 KOH）、含水量和指示物（表 106.1）。

Sodasorb、Medisorb 和 Drägersorb 800 Plus 都使用不同剂量的活性剂与碳酸（H_2CO_3）反应生成碳酸盐（CO_3）。当患者呼出的 CO_2 与吸收剂中的 H_2O 发生反应时，首先会产生碳酸；生成的碳酸盐随后与氢氧化钙 [$Ca(OH)_2$] 反应生成不溶性碳酸钙（$CaCO_3$）沉淀；氢氧化钠（NaOH）和氢氧化钾（KOH）在最后的反应中再生，当所有的氢氧化物都变成碳酸盐时，吸收剂被耗尽。吸收剂均含有乙基紫，乙基紫随 pH 降低颜色发生变化，当吸收剂耗尽时乙基紫会变成紫色。其化学公式如下：

1. $CO_2+H_2O=H_2CO_3$
2. $H_2CO_3+2NaOH$（或 KOH）$=Na_2CO_3$（或 K_2CO_3）$+2H_2O+$ 热量
3. Na_2CO_3（或 K_2CO_3）$+Ca(OH)_2=CaCO_3+2NaOH$（或 KOH）+ 热量

Amsorb Plus 与其他吸收剂的不同之处在于，其未使用碱性氢氧化物（NaOH 和 KOH）。碱性氢氧化物是很强的一价碱性物质，它能将强效吸入麻醉

表 106.1　吸收成分的比较

成分	Sodasorb	Medisorb	Drägersorb 800 Plus	Amsorb Plus	Litholyme	Spiralith
$Ca(OH)_2$	76.5%	81%	82%	>75 %	>75%	0%
NaOH	2.25%	1% ～ 2%	2%	0%	0%	0%
KOH	2.25%	0.003%	0.003%	0%	0%	0%
LiOH	0%	0%	0%	0%	0%	95%
LiCI	0%	0%	0%	0%	<3%	0%
水	18.9%	18%	16%	14.5%	12% ～ 19%	化学结合
指示剂	是	是	是	是	是	否

Data from Materials Safety Data Sheets，Occupational Safety and Health Administration，U.S. Department of Labor.

剂分解成有害物质，包括氟甲基-2-2-二氟1-（三氟甲基）乙烯醚（化合物A）和一氧化碳（CO）。Amsorb成分包括氢氧化钙、水，用于保持水分的氯化钙、硫酸钙以及提高硬度和孔隙度的聚乙烯吡咯烷酮。其化学公式如下：

1. $CO_2+H_2O=H_2CO_3$

2. $H_2CO_3+Ca(OH)_2=CaCO_3+2H_2O+$ 热量

Litholyme和Spiralith是最新型的吸收剂，它同样也不使用催化剂，从而避免形成化合物A和CO。Litholyme采用了不与吸入麻醉剂发生化学反应的氯化锂作为催化剂，以实现CO_2的吸收。由于没有NaOH或KOH，故不会导致NaOH或KOH的再生，pH指示剂也不会反复变色。此外，使用氢氧化锂还可降低放热反应，减少火灾风险，改善经济/环境影响。Epstein等发现，由于七氟烷的消耗减少，用Litholyme代替钠石灰可以使麻醉科医师在七氟烷麻醉时使用更低的新鲜气体流量（<2 L/min）。节省的费用基本可抵消了Litholyme增加的成本。

Spiralith与Litholyme在许多不同之处。与其他所有先与水发生反应的吸收剂不同，Spiralith将无水氢氧化锂（LiOH）粉末部分溶解在一种非颗粒状聚合物基质中。这产生了更大的反应面积、更低的温度、更长的使用时间以及成本效益。环境影响也是选择吸收剂时因素之一，制造商声称这是Spiralith的一个亮点，因为其将粉末包裹于可回收聚合物板上。Spiralith在耗尽时没有pH指示剂警示。因此，必须定期更换吸收剂并须严格监测患者呼吸回路中吸入CO_2浓度。氢氧化锂（LiOH）与CO_2的化学反应如下所示：

$$2LiOH*H_2O+CO_2=Li_2CO_2+3H_2O-\text{热量}$$

（$*H_2O$是指水合LiOH）

识别

吸收剂耗尽的迹象包括呼气末CO_2和吸入CO_2增加，以及吸收罐内产生过多热量。如果在CO_2监测仪上设置适当的CO_2过低或过高报警值，一旦超过限值就会报警。$PaCO_2$升高可能引起高血压和心动过速，也可作为吸收剂耗尽的临床指征。急性高碳酸血症会引起脑血流量增加和颅内压升高，在神经外科手术中可以通过手术部位的出血量来监测。$PaCO_2$升高会增强呼吸驱动，可能也会观察到呼吸机的“过度呼吸”现象。

在开始麻醉前，请务必先确认好吸收剂是否已耗尽。吸收器被设计成透明即为便于检查吸收剂乙基紫pH指示剂的颜色变化。当患者呼出的气体通过吸收器时，上层吸收颗粒首先出现颜色变化。现代麻醉工作站预装一次性吸收剂的“快速更换”吸收罐。呼吸回路中有自密封的吸收器支架，在拆卸吸收器时应避免泄漏，这在更换吸收剂时非常重要。在以前的设计中，更换吸收剂时必须打开呼吸回路中的吸收器，打开的呼吸回路会造成麻醉剂泄漏，直至吸收剂更换完成，吸收器被关闭。Seif和Olympio曾报道，当麻醉科医师更换GE Aestiva/5麻醉机Medisorb吸收剂时，一名全麻患者的气道无法连接到复苏气囊上。开放式吸收器中产生的巨大泄漏，导致持续正压通气以及呼吸环路失效。在这种情况下，呼气支管路与主设备断开连接并直接连接到可以通过呼气支进行通气的复苏气囊上。

乙基紫是吸收剂中的pH指示剂。当pH从13.5降至10.3时，指示剂随着氢氧离子的消失而由无色变为紫色。当吸收剂未及时更换时会出现异常，由于NaOH和KOH会在耗尽的容器中再生，pH逐渐升高，一旦超过变色阈值，就会出现即使吸收剂已耗尽，但颜色不再呈现为紫色。此外，还有其他方法使乙基紫失效导致颜色不再变化。Andrews等发现，Sodasorb暴露在荧光灯8 h后pH指示剂浓度下降50%，即使在黑暗环境中，只要暴露在荧光灯下乙基紫就会失效。较新的吸收剂如Litholyme和Spiralith不存在催化剂再生的问题。Litholyme中没有NaOH和KOH化合物，指示剂可保持紫色。Spiralith由100%氢氧化锂组成，所以无pH指示剂。由于无法观测到颜色变化，麻醉科医师需持续监测$FiCO_2$，以定期更换吸收剂。

风险评估

在麻醉过程中，耗尽的CO_2吸收剂很可能会出现高碳酸血症的迹象或警示，但须鉴别其他导致高碳酸血症的原因。如果患者处于持续通气状态，高碳酸血症可能是由CO_2产生（或注入）量增加或CO_2排出量减少导致。CO_2产生量增加见于高代谢状态（如脓毒症、发烧、患者体温过高）、腹腔镜下注入的CO_2扩散、浅麻醉所致的儿茶酚胺释放、与

H^+ 反应产生 H_2O 和 CO_2 的碳酸氢盐治疗、甲状腺危象和恶性高热。高碳酸血症也可能是医源性的，如部分机器被设计成能够输送 CO_2，而这种输送可能在无意中发生。其他潜在原因还包括跨过 CO_2 吸收器或将其从回路中移除；或者如 Ellett 等所报道的，一次错误的连接 / 交叉管道导致 CO_2 通过 N_2O 输送系统输出，而 N_2O 软管连接到 CO_2 出口。CO_2 排出减少的最常见原因是通气不足，可能由分钟通气量不足或自主呼吸的患者由药物引起的呼吸抑制。CO_2 复吸入会导致高碳酸血症，无论是通过吸收性差、功能不全或单向阀缺失的气流通道，还是吸收剂耗尽合并新鲜气体流量不足，无法通过废气清除系统清除 CO_2。

启示

耗尽的吸收剂除导致高碳酸血症外，还会导致许多危险的并发症。其中之一是由于干性吸收剂生成的化合物 A 和 CO。在新鲜低流量（<2 L/min）、氢氧化钡石灰、高浓度七氟烷、高温和干燥的吸收剂等条件下，化合物 A 可致大鼠中毒性肾损害，该结论是否适用于人类尚不清楚。事实上，Yamakage 等研究发现，与 Drägersorb 800 Pus（2% KOH）相比，七氟烷在新鲜气体流 1 L/min 下与 Medisorb 或 Amsorb[分别包含最小（0.003%）KOH 和不含 KOH] 混合 4 h 后，化合物 A 的浓度并没有增加或仅微量增加。Epstein 等还建议，当使用惰性 LiOH 时，更低流量下使用七氟烷可能更安全、更经济。尽管如此，我们仍建议吸入麻醉下新鲜气体流量应大于 2 L/min，且肾功能不全患者应避免使用七氟烷。

干性吸收剂与强挥发性麻醉药，特别是地氟烷反应造成的一氧化碳中毒，则更为罕见。Stabernack 等在 2000 年的研究表明，锂吸收剂和 Amsorb 都缺乏 NaOH 和 KOH，从而降低了 CO 产生量，而氢氧化钡石灰（Baralyme）的 CO 含量最高。上述案例的场景如下：在周末，忘记关闭的环路中高气流使吸收剂变干，周一早上的第一例患者使用了该环路。每日手术麻醉结束后关闭机器和使用不包含 NaOH 和 KOH 的干燥剂，可以降低 CO 产生的风险。

另一罕见但幸运的病例是 CO_2 吸收器过多产热而引起火灾和爆炸。当 CO_2 升高并伴有体温升高时，还必须考虑恶性高热。如前所述，由于放热反应，CO_2 的中和反应产生水和热。该反应产生的热量随吸收剂的组成而变化。曾经被广泛使用的干燥剂 Baralyme 由于与几起火灾有关，于 2005 年被撤出美国市场。Laster 和 Eger 报告称碳酸钙可与不同浓度的挥发性麻醉剂反应，与七氟烷反应甚至会导致温度高达 90℃，然而并没有火灾发生。如果感觉吸收器明显发热，建议断开患者呼吸回路，并更换吸收剂。

管理

在 CO_2 吸收剂耗尽和潜在并发症处理中，最重要的措施是确保患者有足够的氧气和通气。必要时可能需更换通气方式（如呼吸气囊和氧气）。如果是吸收剂耗竭所致，增加新鲜气体并建立无复吸系统会有效清除回路中 CO_2，同时尽量减少有害降解产物。尽管如此，最有效的管理措施依旧是及时更换吸收剂，即使在没有可见的颜色变化下。更换吸收器最好在使用呼吸机间歇期，以免出现无法更换吸收器的情况。

当发现 CO_2 增加时，重要的是还应考虑吸收剂耗竭以外的其他原因（如表 106.2 所示）。时刻留意患者体温是否有过热或发烧的迹象，减少外部加热可能帮助。需牢记的是，腹腔镜下操作也是导致 CO_2 增加的一个重要因素，还应注意恶性高热，通常可通过其他相应临床体征鉴别诊断。应意识到，分钟通气量和任何变化都会造成 CO_2 增加，适当增加潮气量或呼吸频率可以清除 CO_2。最后，检查麻醉机吸、呼气单向阀有无失灵或吸收剂耗尽，用新的吸收剂替代即将失效的吸收剂，有助于判断是否为相应原因导致的 CO_2 增加。

表 106.2 二氧化碳升高的原因

与吸入相关	与呼出相关
吸收剂耗尽	发热 / 脓毒症
通路	恶性高热
单向阀不工作	给予碳酸氢盐
通过环路吸入二氧化碳	通气不足
管道开关	腹腔镜下操作
	浅麻醉

预防

麻醉工作站使用前，麻醉科医师应检查是否有吸收剂，吸收剂是否耗尽，同时需要对换向阀的装配是否正确、功能是否正常也进行检查。目前，这些检查还不能实现自动化，因此必须由麻醉科医师执行。为防止使用干性吸收剂，建议建立定期更换吸收器的制度。正如前面所讨论的，NaOH 和 KOH 可以再生并使乙基紫还原为无色，所以 pH 指示剂并不能可靠地指导是否应该更换吸收剂，而 Spiralith 不含 pH 指示剂。CO_2 吸收剂耗尽的最常见结果是高碳酸血症，对 CO_2 升高的临床症状保持警惕至关重要。$FiCO_2$ 浓度是一个非常重要的指标，当麻醉工作站 /CO_2 监测仪监测的 $FiCO_2$ 值超过 2 ~ 3 mmHg 时应及时更换吸收剂。

2005 年，麻醉患者安全基金会发表了相关建议。如果遵循以下建议，将有效降低 CO_2 吸收剂引起并发症的风险。建议如下：

- 当暴露于挥发性吸入麻醉药时，所使用吸收剂不会发生降解；
- 制定防止干燥和干燥发生时的管理策略，如在机器不使用时应关闭气流；
- 定期更换吸收剂，尤其在周一早上第一个病例前；
- 当颜色变化表示用尽或不确定是否用尽时，应更换吸收剂；
- 使用多分配盒系统时，更换所有吸收剂。

（周　艳　译　文平山　校）

延伸阅读

Andrews JJ, Johnston Jr RV, Bee DE, et al.: Photodeactivation of ethyl violet: a potential hazard of Sodasorb, *Anesthesiology* 72(1):59–64, 1990.

Ellett AE, Shields JC, Ifune C, et al.: A near miss: a nitrous oxide-carbon dioxide mix-up despite current safety standards, *Anesthesiology* 110(6):1429–1431, 2009.

Epstein RH, Dexter F, Maguire DP, et al.: Economic and environmental considerations during low fresh gas flow volatile agent administration after change to a nonreactive carbon dioxide absorbent, *Anesth Analg* 122(4):996–1006, 2016.

Laster MJ, Eger 2nd EI: Temperatures in soda lime during degradation of desflurane, isoflurane, and sevoflurane by desiccated soda lime, *Anesth Analg* 101(3):753–757, 2005.

Levy RJ: Anesthesia-related carbon monoxide exposure: toxicity and potential therapy, *Anesth Analg* 123(3):670–681, 2016.

Mazze RI: Novel CO_2 absorbents and low-flow sevoflurane, *Anesth Analg* 91(6):1562–1563, 2000.

Olympio MA: Carbon dioxide absorbent desiccation safety conference convened by APSF, *Anesthesia Patient Safety Foundation Newsletter* 20(2):25–44, 2005.

Pond D, Jaffe RA, Brock-Utne JG: Failure to detect CO_2-absorbent exhaustion: seeing and believing, *Anesthesiology* 92(4):1196–1198, 2000.

Rose G, McLarney JT: Carbon dioxide absorber. In Rose G, McLarney JT, editors: *Anesthesia equipment simplified*, New York, 2014, McGraw-Hill Education, pp 93–101.

Seif DM, Olympio MA: Expiratory limb ventilation during unique failure of the anesthesia machine breathing circuit, *Anesthesiology* 118(3):751–753, 2013.

Stabernack CR, Brown R, Laster MJ, et al.: Absorbents differ enormously in their capacity to produce compound A and carbon monoxide, *Anesth Analg* 90(6):1428–1435, 2000.

Walker SG, Smith TC, Sheplock G, et al.: Breathing circuits. In Ehrenwerth J, Eisenkraft JB, Berry JM, editors: *Anesthesia equipment: principles and applications*, ed 2, Philadelphia, 2013, Elsevier, pp 95–125.

Wissing H, Kuhn I, Warnken U, et al.: Carbon monoxide production from desflurane, enflurane, halothane, isoflurane, and sevoflurane with dry soda lime, *Anesthesiology* 95(5):1205–1212, 2001.

Yamakage M, Yamada S, Chen X, et al.: Carbon dioxide absorbents containing potassium hydroxide produce much larger concentrations of compound A from sevoflurane in clinical practice, *Anesth Analg* 91(1):220–224, 2000.

中心静脉压监测

第 107 章

John T. Lemm，Jonathan B. Mark

病例概要

患者，男性，65 岁，被送往手术室进行冠状动脉搭桥术。麻醉诱导后右颈内静脉置入三腔中心静脉导管（central venous catheter，CVC）。手术过程中没有并发症，结束后患者被送往重症加强治疗病房。患者手术恢复后，由于难以建立外周静脉（intravenous，IV）通路，治疗团队决定保留他的 CVC。术后第 4 天患者出现发热、寒战，随后出现心动过速和低血压。

问题分析

定义

使用 Sven-Ivar Seldinger 首创的技术置入 CVC 革命性地改变了医学领域。CVC 的置入已经成为一种相对简单和安全的操作，仅在美国，每年记录的 CVC 日就超过 1500 万。虽然 CVC 置入的并发症并不常见，但机智的临床医师应尽可能了解其潜在的风险，因为如果不能识别这些风险，许多会导致严重的损伤。并发症通常分为两类：与 CVC 置入相关的突发问题，以及由于长期留置导管导致的问题。这些并发症分别列于表 107.1 和 107.2。诸如对缺乏经验的操作者进行强制性监督和使用超声引导等策略已被广泛采用，并可能减少突发的不良事件，如动脉穿刺和气胸。即使采取了这些预防措施，临床医师也应在 CVC 置入过程中始终密切监测患者，因为心律失常、低血压、精神状态改变或氧饱和度下降都是潜在问题的征兆。

中心静脉置管的一个特别可怕的并发症是导管相关性血流感染（catheter-related bloodstream infection，CRBSI）。发热、血流动力学不稳定、置管部位炎症和精神状态改变均提示 CVC 相关脓毒症，尤其是当没有其他明确的感染源时。CRBSI 的诊断始于临床怀疑，其次是微生物学诊断。CRBSI 最严格地定义为对于一个没有其他明确感染源的患者，从导管尖端和外周血样本或者从导管接口和外周血样本中分离出相同的生物体。

识别

以下情况可以识别 CRBSI：

- 留置静脉导管或者 CVC 的患者发热；
- 静脉导管或中心静脉导管置入部位的炎症或化脓；
- 导管培养和外周血培养结果阳性；
- 无其他明确的感染源。

CRBSI 最敏感的特征是发热，任何留置静脉导管的患者发热的鉴别诊断必须包括 CRBSI，直到找到其他原因。然后采用系统性的方法排除其他感染源，包括痰培养和尿培养，手术伤口和皮肤完整性检查，以及全面的体格检查。最后，应检查所有导管置入部位是否有炎症和化脓。

为了获得导管的培养样品，必须拔除 CVC 或外周静脉导管。拔除 CVC 时，患者可能仍然需要中心静脉通路。如果是这种情况，最好将新的 CVC 放置在不同的部位，而不是通过导丝更换导管，因为使用这种技术会大大增加血流感染的风险，特别是当 CVC 留置时间超过 3 天时。当然，如果存在明显的局部感染迹象，则绝不应该尝试进行“导丝”更换。培养用血样本应在 CVC 或 IV 导管更换前后或当时从外周部位获取，以便与导管尖端培养结果进行比较。从导管样本和外周血培养物中分离出相同的病原体可证实 CRBSI 的诊断。

半定量和定量的导管培养比传统培养基培养对感染的诊断具有更高的特异性；然而，我们必须认识到，不是每个阳性培养结果都意味着 CRBSI。在无感染迹象的情况下，血培养阳性仅仅代表导管定

表 107.1　中心静脉压力监测置管时的并发症

并发症	预防	识别	治疗
空气栓塞	置管时使用 Trendelenburg 体位	呼吸困难	给予 100%O_2
		氧饱和度下降	必要时心血管支持
	自主呼吸患者中堵塞开放式针头和导管接头处	低血压	
气胸	常见于锁骨下入路	置管时咳嗽	胸腔闭式引流
		氧饱和度下降	<15% 可继续观察
		呼吸困难	
	使用小针进行“探路”	低血压	给予 O_2
	针插入时持续抽吸注射器	胸部影像学检查	必要时心血管支持
	正压通气更常见	呼吸音减弱	
心律失常	避免导丝插入 >15 cm	心电图表现	拔出导丝
		可听见的脉搏规律性的改变	罕见、抗心律失常药物或体外电复律
动脉穿刺	注意定位标志	血液呈鲜红色	拔针，直接按压≥ 10 min
	触摸动脉搏动	搏动性血流	使用扩张器或导引器放置，血管外科医师会诊
	使用小针“探路”	扩展性血肿	
	使用压力计（延长管）或压力传感器确认静脉通路	气道受损（颈动脉穿刺）	气道支持，必要时气管插管
	使用便携式超声引导		
心脏压塞	避免暴力操作导管的导丝和扩张器	心血管失代偿	手术清除
	胸片证实导管放置正确	与导管放置的时间关联	
		超声心动图	

表 107.2　中心静脉压力监测留置时的并发症

并发症	预防	识别	治疗
血管侵蚀	胸部 X 线片确认导管尖端位置正确（上腔静脉与右心房交界处）	胸腔积液	外科手术修复
	多见于左侧锁骨下和颈内静脉，多于右侧	心血管失代偿（血胸、压塞）	
		呼吸功能不全	
血栓形成	有肝素保护层的导管可能降低风险	可能是“无症状”	考虑使用溶栓药物或肝素
	仅在有绝对指征情况下使用导管	上肢或肩部水肿或压痛	严重时外科血栓清除
		可能发生肺栓塞	
感染	严格无菌操作技术	无其他感染源的发热	拔除感染的导管
	最大防护措施	局部红肿、压痛、化脓	抗生素治疗
	仅在有绝对指征情况下使用导管	导管和外周血培养出同一种微生物	
	考虑使用抗菌导管		
	每日检查置管部位		
误读	传感器正确的“调零”和“调平”	与临床状态的相关性	
	宣教和培训	传感器经常性的“调零”和“调平”	

植而不是 CRBSI，尽管导管定植被认为是向明显感染发展的主要步骤。当使用半定量培养技术时，从外周血培养的同一微生物在导管样本生长超过 15 个菌落形成单位支持导管定植的诊断。当患者出现感染迹象时，可诊断为 CRBSI。定量培养是诊断导管相关性感染更为敏感的方法。导管样本中超过 10 000 个菌落形成单位的生长表明导管定植。同样的结果合并全身感染的迹象构成 CRBSI 的诊断。

在某些临床情况下，比如建立血管通路困难的患者，在明确 CRSBI 诊断之前拔除导管可能并非明智之举。在此类情况下，定量血培养和差异报警时间（differential time to positivity，DTP）技术是可行的诊断替代方法。定量培养依赖于从 CVC 导管和外周静脉穿刺部位获得的成对血样的比较。从导管获得的菌落计数比从外周血培养获得的菌落计数高 3 倍可支持 CRBSI 的诊断。当无条件进行定量培养时，就像许多实验室一样，DTP 是一种有用的替代方法。DTP 指从导管样本比外周血样本中至少提前 2 h 检测出微生物生长。与定量培养一样，DTP 对诊断 CRBSI 具有高度的敏感性和特异性。

风险评估

据估计，医院内血流感染的发生率约为每年 25 万例，大多数感染与使用留置血管内装置有关。CVC 约占所有 CRBSI 的 90%。尤其令人不安的是，无论是住院患者还是门诊患者，需要这些导管作为长期血管通路的患者的数量正在稳步上升。自 20 世纪 90 年代初以来，CRBSI 的发生率稳步下降，主要是由于宣教的改善，无菌技术的依从性以及导管管理的改进。许多机构曾报告，在过去每 1000 导管日血流感染率高达 8.5，新近的数据表明，这些机构已很容易实现每 1000 导管日血流感染率低至 0.73。然而，由于许多因素影响感染率，包括医院规模、高危患者人群、导管使用频率和 CRBSI 诊断方案等，感染率出现差异较为常见。

文献反复证实 CRBSI 的风险随着中心静脉置管时间的延长而增加。有了这些知识，许多机构采用了常规的 CVC 更换方案，认为其能降低感染率。Cobb 及其同事 1992 年进行的一项随机对照试验表明这种做法并无效果。除了不增加感染风险外，常规导管更换会增加机械性并发症的风险，导致了患者的不适，并极大地占用了医护人员时间。

任何 CVC 患者均有感染的风险。但有几个宿主因素会显著增加 CRBSI 的风险，包括严重烧伤或其他皮肤完整性缺失的患者、骨髓移植受者、中性粒细胞减少患者、接受全肠外营养的患者以及既往有 CRBSI 的患者。最常见的感染源是定植在穿刺点皮肤上的微生物，而重度皮肤定植患者和 CRBSI 之间有很强的相关性。这些生物体沿着导管伤口的经皮通道从皮肤迁移，最终定植于导管的内外侧。

启示

CRBSI 和死亡率在 12% ～ 25% 之间、显著的发病、住院时间延长、额外医疗费用高达 16 500 美元相关。在假体植入这类患者（如心脏瓣膜、血管移植物）中，这些感染尤其具有破坏性。假体材料一旦暴露于血流细菌中就很容易受到损害，一旦感染通常需要冒风险取出材料并随后更换这些材料。

治疗

一旦怀疑有 CRBSI，治疗的第一步就是立刻拔除感染的导管。如果患者仍旧需要血管通路，最好在新的位置放置新的静脉导管。只有在仔细分析后，新置入导管造成的机械性损伤的风险明显超过此类交换的感染风险（例如，具有挑战性的血管通路患者），那么才只考虑使用导丝辅助更换受感染的导管。一旦取出，应将旧的导管尖端和皮内节段进行半定量或定量培养。同时，两组血培养物的数量应进行比较分析，理想的血培养物应来自不同的外周部位。

早期进行广谱抗菌治疗是治疗 CRBSI 的主要手段，但应在获得交换导管和血培养结果后使用。抗生素应选择覆盖革兰氏阳性和革兰氏阴性的药物，特别高危患者还应包含抗真菌药物。一旦获得了培养结果并且了解其药物敏感性，必须针对特定微生物使用抗生素以免抗生素耐药性的发生。

图 107.1 和图 107.2 分别提供了诊断疑似非隧道式 CVC 感染患者急性发热的流程图，以及处理非隧道式 CVC 相关血流感染患者的方法。

预防

严格遵守疾病预防控制中心（the Centers for

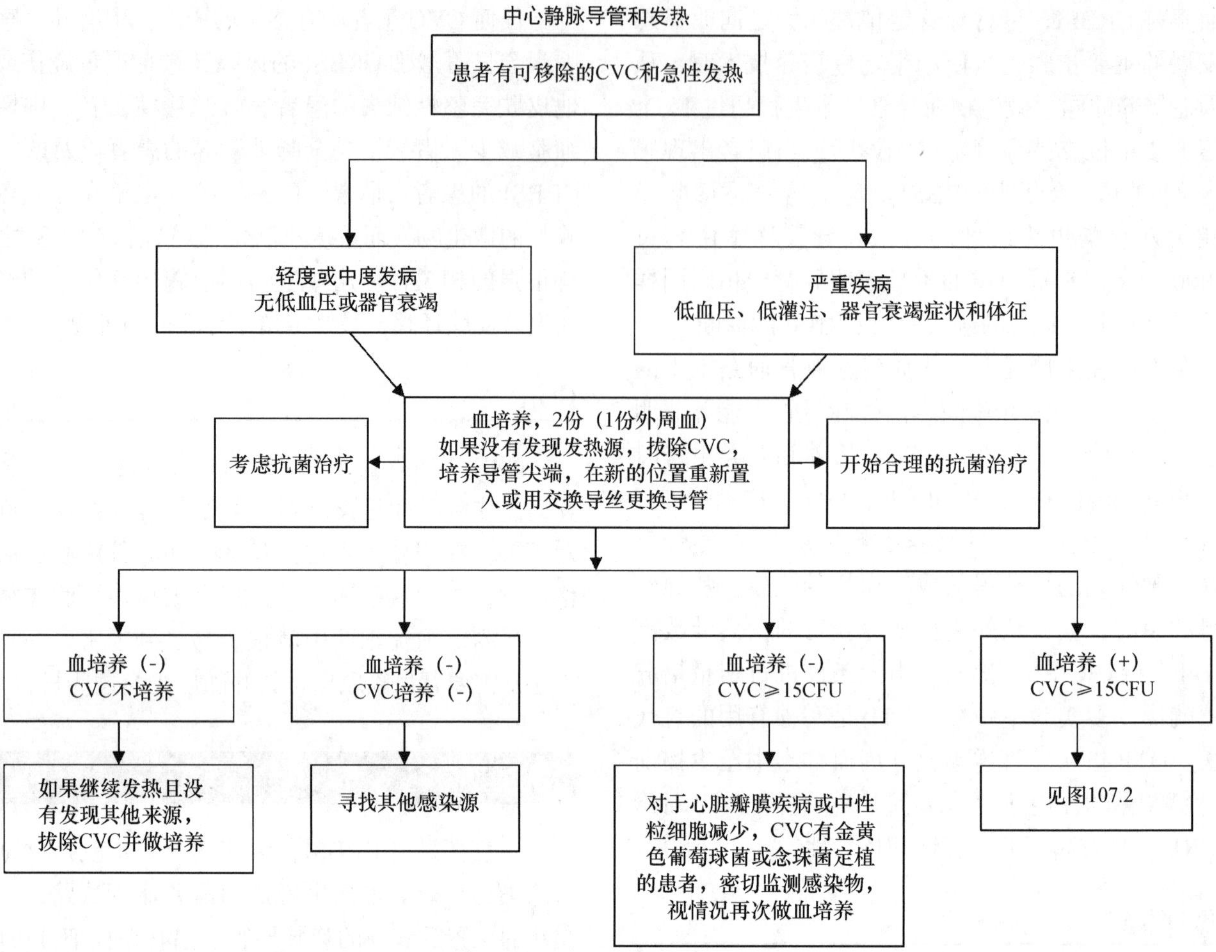

图 107.1 疑似非隧道式中心静脉导管（CVC）感染的急性发热患者的诊断。CFU，菌落形成单位（Adapted from Mermel LA，Farr BM，Sheretz RJ，et al.：Guidelines for the management of intravascular catheter-related infections. *Clin Infect Dis* 32[9]：1249-1272，2001.）

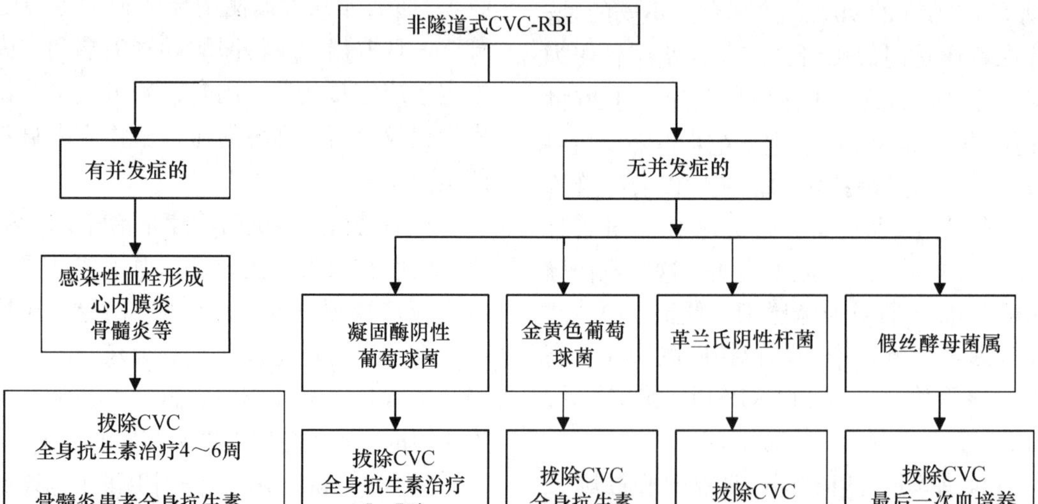

图 107.2 非隧道式中心静脉导管血流感染（CVC-RBI）患者的处理。TEE，经食管超声心动图（Adapted from Mermel LA，Farr BM，Sheretz RJ，et al.：Guidelines for the management of intravascular catheter-related infections. *Clin Infect Dis* 32[9]：1249-1272，2001.）

Disease Control and Prevention，CDC）制定的预防血管内导管相关感染的指南是预防 CRBSI 的关键。

这些推荐的要点包括：

- 只有在确实需要时才使用 CVC，一旦不需要立刻拔除；
- 对置入和管理 CVC 者进行宣教和培训；
- 在放置 CVC 时严格遵守洗手和最大限度的无菌屏障预防措施；
- 使用 2% 氯己定制剂进行皮肤消毒；
- 避免常规更换 CVC 作为预防感染的策略；
- 使用无菌的或者抗生素浸渍的 CVC 装置。

任何血管内装置都为微生物进入血液提供了入口（图 107.3）。患者的皮肤和导管的置入者是最可能的感染微生物来源。如前所述，置入部位的重度皮肤定植似乎是 CVC 感染风险增加的预测因素。严格遵守洗手和皮肤消毒是减少 CRBSI 的基础。与 10% 聚维酮碘或 70% 酒精相比，使用 2% 氯己定进行皮肤消毒与 CVC 相关的局部感染和 CVC 相关菌血症的发生率较低相关，因此 2% 氯己定被 CDC 推荐用于皮肤准备。导管位置也会影响 CVC 感染的风险。应尽可能避免股静脉置管，因为与锁骨下或颈内静脉置管相比，股静脉置管的感染率明显较高。与颈内静脉相比，锁骨下静脉可能具有较低的感染风险，但必须权衡这些益处与放置过程中患者机械性损伤的风险，尤其是对于缺乏经验的操作者。

与不太严格的预防措施（无菌手套和小的手术单）相比，最大限度的无菌屏障预防措施（包括使用长袖手术衣、手术口罩和大的手术单）可显著降低 CRBSI 的风险。事实上，Raad 及其同事证明，当这些最大的屏障预防措施得到实施时导管相关性脓毒血症的发生率降低了 6 倍。鉴于绝大多数数据支持使用最大限度的无菌屏障预防措施来预防 CRBSI，CDC 建议对所有中心静脉导管的置入采取最大限度的屏障预防措施，但紧急情况除外。

所有血管内装置的置入部位必须每日进行检查和触诊，因为早期识别局部导管相关感染可能有助于防止进展为血流感染。敷料护理是 CVC 维护的一个有争议的方面。尽管出于患者舒适和方便的原因，大多数机构使用透明 CVC 敷料，但与纱布敷料相比，研究一再证明使用透明敷料时定植率和感染率更高。近来，使用葡萄糖酸氯己定浸渍海绵附着的透明敷料已变得普遍，虽然目前只有微弱的数据表明它们能显著降低了感染率。目前的指南建议每 2 天更换一次纱布 CVC 敷料，每 7 天更换一次透

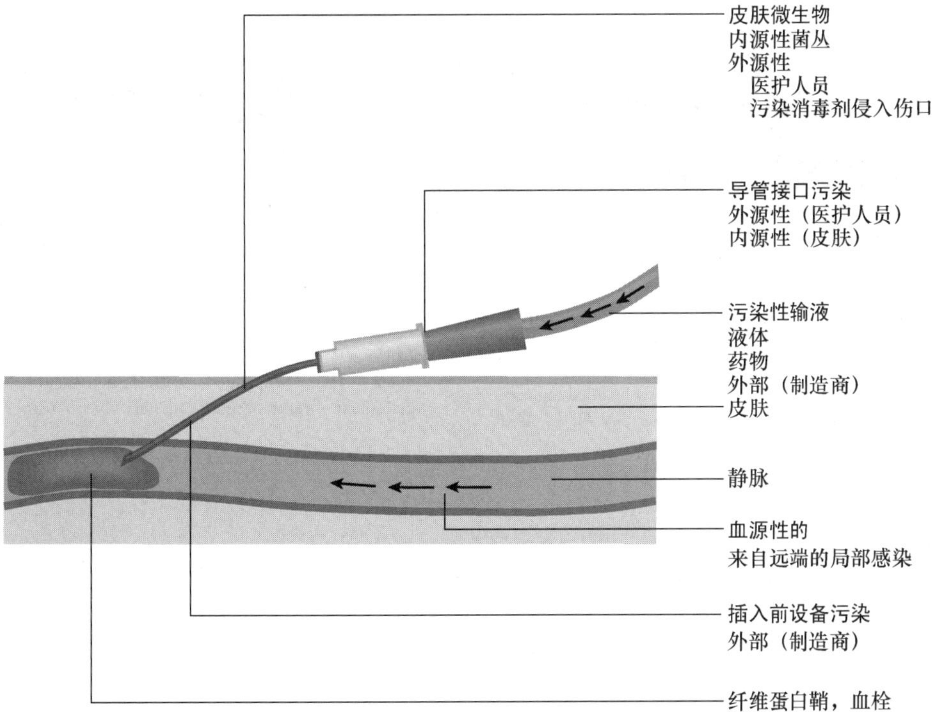

图 107.3 血管内套管感染的来源。主要来源是皮肤菌群，导管接口的污染，输液的污染，以及血管内装置及其纤维连接蛋白-纤维蛋白鞘的血源性定植和医护人员（From Maki DG：Infections due to infusion therapy. In Bennett JV，Brachman PS，editors：*Hospital infections*，3rd ed. Boston，Little，Brown，1992，pp 849-898.）

明敷料，以有效减少定植和 CRBSI。

抗菌药物浸渍导管的使用已被证明可显著降低 CRBSI 的风险。目前，这些抗菌导管主要有两种类型：氯己定-磺胺嘧啶银涂层导管和米诺环素-利福平涂层导管。最大的 meta 分析回顾了 11 项研究，共 2611 例 CVC，与无涂层 CVC 相比，导管定植和导管相关感染的总优势比分别为 0.44 和 0.56。尽管与传统的无涂层导管相比，这两类药物均能明显减少 CRBSI，尽管证据仍然薄弱，米诺环素-利福平涂层导管比氯己定-磺胺嘧啶银涂层导管可以提供更好的抗菌效果。

随着 CVC 使用率的不断上升，临床医生将继续看到置管的并发症。正确处理包括 CRBSI 在内的中心静脉导管的并发症至关重要，机构必须将关注重点放在风险预防上。坚持培训导管的置入者和日常管理者是有效降低风险的基石。诸如中心静脉固定等方案有效地限制了包括感染在内的不良事件，但总依从性仍然难以确定。机制的临床医师必须认识到自满的风险，并努力每天观察这些重要的质量指标。

致谢

感谢 Peter J. Lee 博士和 James G. Ramsay 博士对本章上一版的贡献。

（成天华 译 陆 军 校）

延伸阅读

Bowdle A: Vascular complications of central venous catheter placement: evidence-based methods for prevention and treatment, *J Cardiothorac Vasc Anesth* 28(2):358–368, 2014.

Casey AL, Mermel LA, Nightingale P, et al.: Antimicrobial central venous catheters in adults: a systematic review and meta-analysis, *Lancet Infect Dis* 8(12):763–776, 2008.

Cobb DK, High KP, Sawyer RG, et al.: A controlled trial of scheduled replacement of central venous and pulmonary artery catheters, *N Engl J Med* 327(15):1062–1068, 1992.

Domino KB, Bowdle TA, Posner KL, et al.: Injuries and liability related to central vascular catheters: a closed claims analysis, *Anesthesiology* 100(6):1411–1418, 2004.

Eyer S, Brummitt C, Crossley K, et al.: Catheter-related sepsis: prospective, randomized study of three different methods of long-term catheter maintenance, *Crit Care Med* 8(10):1073–1079, 1990.

Ezaru CS, Mangione MP, Oravitz TM, et al.: Eliminating arterial injury during central venous catheterization using manometry, *Anesth Analg* 109(1):130–134, 2009.

Keenan SP: Use of ultrasound to place central lines, *J Crit Care* 17(2):126–137, 2002.

Kluger DM, Maki DG: *The relative risk of intravascular device related bloodstream infections in adults. In Abstracts of the 39th Interscience Conference on Antimicrobial Agents and Chemotherapy*, San Francisco, 1999, American Society for Microbiology, p 514.

Maki DG, Weise CE, Sarafin HW: A semiquantitative culture method for identifying intravenous-catheter-related infection, *N Engl J Med* 296(23):1305–1309, 1977.

Mermel LA, Maki DG: Infectious complications of Swan-Ganz pulmonary artery catheters, *Am J Respir Crit Care Med* 149(4 Pt 1):1020–1036, 1994.

Mermel LA, McCormick RD, Springman SR, et al.: The pathogenesis and epidemiology of catheter-related infection with pulmonary artery Swan-Ganz catheters: a prospective study utilizing molecular subtyping, *Am J Med* 91(Suppl 3B):197S–205S, 1991.

O'Grady NP, Alexander M, Burns LA, et al.: Guidelines for the prevention of intravascular catheter-related infections, *Clin Infect Dis* 52(9):e162–e193, 2011.

Pronovost P, Needham D, Berenholtz S, et al.: An intervention to decrease catheter-related bloodstream infections in the ICU, *N Engl J Med* 355(26):2725–2732, 2006.

Pronovost PJ, Goeschel CA, Colantuoni E, et al.: Sustaining reductions in catheter related bloodstream infections in Michigan intensive care units: observational study, *BMJ* 340:c309, 2010.

Raad II, Hohn DC, Gilbreath BJ, et al.: Prevention of central venous catheter-related infections by using maximal sterile barrier precautions during insertion, *Infect Control Hosp Epidemiol* 15(4 Pt 1):231–238, 1994.

Ramsay J, Nolte F, Schwartzman S: Incidence of catheter colonization and catheter related infection with an antiseptic impregnated triple lumen catheter, *Crit Care Med* 22:A115, 1994.

Ruesch S, Walder B, Tramer M, et al.: Complications of central venous catheters: internal jugular versus subclavian access—a systematic review, *Crit Care Med* 30(2):454–460, 2002.

Rupp SM, Apfelbaum JL, Blitt C, et al.: Practice guidelines for central venous access: a report by the American Society of Anesthesiologists Task Force on Central Venous Access, *Anesthesiology* 116(3):539–573, 2012.

Seldinger SI: Catheter replacement of the needle in percutaneous arteriography; a new technique, *Acta Radiol* 39(5):368–376, 1953.

Timsit JF, Schwebel C, Bouadma L, et al.: Chlorhexidine-impregnated sponges and less frequent dressing changes for prevention of catheter-related infections in critically ill adults: a randomized controlled trial, *JAMA* 301(12):1231–1241, 2009.

Vannucci A, Jeffcoat A, Ifune C, et al.: Retained guidewires after intraoperative placement of central venous catheters, *Anesth Analg* 117(1):102–108, 2013.

电气安全

第108章

Jeffrey J. Schwartz，*Jan Ehrenwerth*

病例概要

强电击

患者，男性，50岁，平素体健，在全身麻醉下行腹腔镜胆囊切除术。在手术过程中，麻醉科医师感到刺痛，患者发生心室纤颤。立即复苏及除颤后患者恢复正常窦性心律。将正在使用的故障监护仪移除后，手术继续顺利进行。

微电击

在相邻手术间，一名植入临时起搏器的60岁男性患者，正在进行下肢血管旁路术。麻醉科医师调整起搏器导线时，患者发生心室纤颤。立即复苏及除颤后患者恢复正常窦性心律。

问题分析

定义

当人体成为一条电路的部分或全部，就会发生电击伤。要成为电路的一部分，患者必须在具有不同电压的两点上发生接触。这种接触不需要一定是电线。盐水浸湿的洞巾可导电，金属底座由于电路故障而导电，泄漏的电流可在任意两个导体间传递。

电击的机制可分为两类：

- **强电击**是指大量电流通过完整的皮肤表面：5毫安（mA）被认为是人体最高安全电流阈值；10～20 mA可引起持续的肌肉收缩；100～300 mA可导致心室纤颤。
- **微电击**是指相对较小电流直接作用于心肌。电流密度高，仅100微安（μA）即可导致心室纤颤。由于电流太小，手术者不会感到刺痛感。

识别

对电气问题的认识不仅包括能够意识电击的发生，而且能准确评估可能发生的电击。在手术室（operating room，OR）内经常发生的电击伤常表现为，患者突发性心室纤颤（ventricular fibrillation，VF）或室性心动过速（ventricular tachycardia，VT）。麻醉科医师通常认为心室纤颤或室性心动过速是由心源性因素造成，但同时应始终记住存在发生电击的可能。任何不明原因的刺痛感都可能提示存在电击危险，应立即进行排查。微电击的产生通常没有先兆，仅在恰当的临床环境中被识别。

风险评估

暴露于电气设备环境中的所有患者和工作人员，都存在强电击的风险。生理盐水的常规使用及电气设备的频繁使用，使手术室成为一个电击高风险环境。患者携有与心脏相连的导电性植入物，如含有生理盐水的中心静脉导管或起搏器导线，发生微电击的风险都会增加。

强电击最常见的原因是电气设备损坏和电路故障。电力公司提供的电压（110～220 V）使用绝缘电线来隔绝电流。但绝缘层会发生磨损，电流可通过金属物品传递或直接传递到患者。一次电击的发生意味着大量安全防护措施（见下文）的疏漏，如防护措施无效、被忽略，甚至没有使用。

启示

电击的产生取决于以下各点：

- 电流量；

- 电流频率；
- 电流持续时间；
- 电流是否直接作用于心肌。

大多数手术室电气设备使用的额定电压为 110 V 或 220 V。根据欧姆定律，在 120 V 电压下，流经的电流量（安培）=120 V ÷ 以欧姆（Ω）为单位的电阻。在同等电压下，干燥皮肤的电阻约为 120 000 Ω，只传递 1 mA 电流。而潮湿皮肤的电阻大约为 1200 Ω，可传递 100 mA 电流，这是一个潜在致命的电流。美国的电流频率是 60 Hz，恰巧也是最危险的电流频率。

电流作用人体后影响电兴奋组织。电流流经神经和肌肉时可引起疼痛和收缩，就像周围神经刺激器的电刺激一样。当电流流经心脏时，则可引起心室纤颤或室性心动过速，甚至死亡。

管理

电击发生后的处理由恰当的复苏组成，包括心肺复苏和除颤。如果能够及时识别电击，则必须迅速移除电源和故障设备。然而，电击通常被排除在诊断之外。

线路隔离监视仪

在使用隔离电源（即线路隔离电路）的手术室中，线路隔离监视仪（line isolation monitor，LIM）可监测隔离的完整性。如果线路隔离监视仪发生报警，则说明电路不再隔离，在发生电力故障事件时则会产生电流。此时，手术室仍处于安全状态，电气设备正常运行。监视仪报警通常是故障设备插入了电源插座。应将非必要的电气设备电源依次与插座分离，直到故障设备被识别出来。不太常见的是，许多正常运行的设备也存在较小的泄漏电流，可能会同时连接至同一电路中。由于对错误报警较为敏感，线路隔离监视仪的报警阈值已从 2 mA 变为 5 mA。

接地故障电流漏电保护器

在使用接地故障电流漏电保护器（ground fault circuit interrupter，GFCI）的手术室中，故障设备会导致 GFCI 切断由它提供服务的所有设备电源。断路器有一个复位按钮来恢复电流，前提是故障设备必须已被识别并移除，否则断路器会再次触发断开电源。

预防

由于麻醉科医师、设备制造商以及手术室建筑工程师采取了各种各样的安全防护措施，电击是一种极为罕见的并发症。

接地

手术室的大多数电气设备是接地的。这意味着设备底座、金属外壳和其他内部组件，可通过三叉插头连接地线插槽与地面连接。这种连接可将故障电流安全地分流到地面，而不传递给与设备接触的人员（图 108.1）。

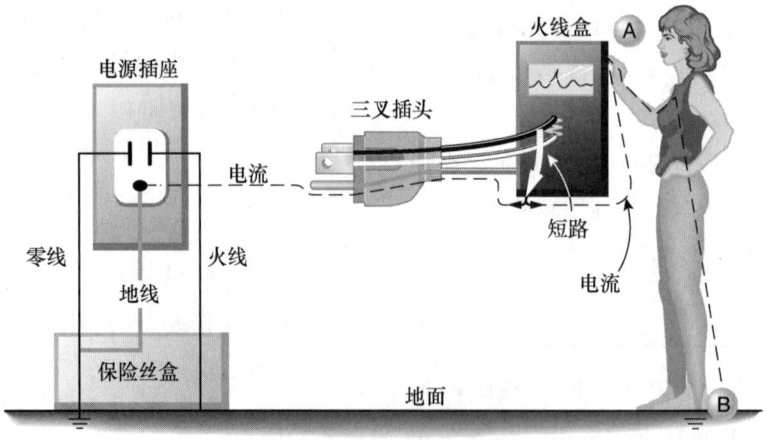

图 108.1 当带地线插座的故障设备与接地插座正确连接时，电流（虚线）优先流向低电阻地线。一个人站在地面上（B 点），触碰箱子（A 点），会形成完整的电流回路；然而，只有一小部分的电流会通过人体（From Ehrenwerth J，Seifert HA：Electrical and fre safety. In Barash PG，Cullen BF，Stoelting RK，et al.，editors：*Clinical anesthesia*，ed 7. Philadelphia，Wolters Kluwer，2013，pp 189-218.）

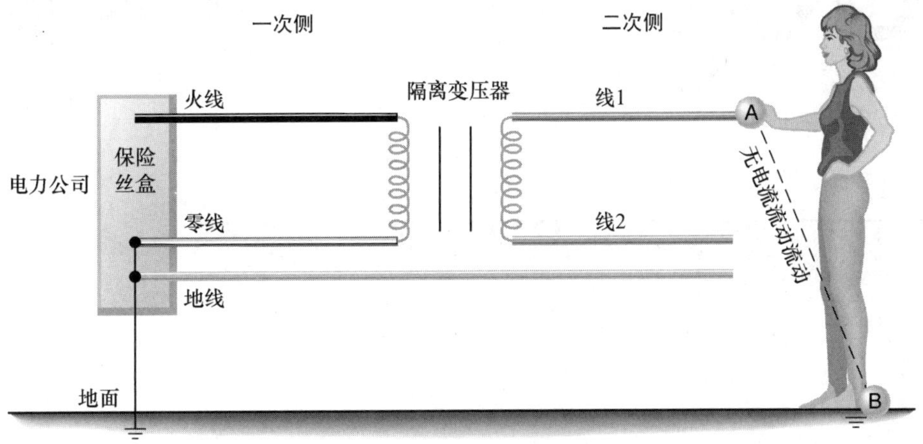

图 108.2 隔离电力系统（IPS）的安全特性。当人体与 IPS 的一侧（A 点）接触，同时站在地面（B 点）时，不会受到电击。在这种情况下，因为人体没有连接电路的两点，所以没有形成回路。点 A 是 IPS 的一部分，点 B 是电路的一次侧或接地侧（From Ehrenwerth J，Seifert HA：Electrical and fre safety. In Barash PG，Cullen BF，Stoelting RK，et al.，editors：*Clinical anesthesia*，ed 7. Philadelphia，Wolters Kluwer，2013，pp 189-218.）

电源隔离

许多手术室中使用电源隔离以降低电击风险。电力公司提供接地电源，即其中一条输送电力的电线同时也与一根埋藏在地下的大导电杆相连。这为手术室电源供应提供了额外安全保障。然而，这也意味着，在某种程度上，所有患者都已经直接连接到电流回路的一部分。由于电路故障，只要一个额外的接触，患者必然会形成电流回路。隔离变压器可以把设备接地线转换成与地面无直接连接的隔离线路（图 108.2）。因此，故障设备的两个接触点之间就不太可能发生电击。

线路隔离监视仪

如果使用了隔离电源，必须监测隔离的完整性，否则系统故障电流意外地接地分流，不会有任何警报。线路隔离监视仪可持续监测手术室电路与地面之间的阻抗。阻抗应该是（接近）无穷大。如果监测到阻抗降低和电张不再绝缘，则发出警报。

接地故障电流漏电保护器

一些手术室安装了 GFCI 以降低风险。GFCI 持续监测设备电流输入和输出的电流差。如果差值超过一定阈值（常规设置为 5 mA），断路器会提前切断电源防止事故发生。如果断路器安装在一个所谓的菊花链插座，一台设备发生故障将中断其他几个正常运行的设备电源。这对于手术室运作具有潜在的危险。因此，最新的 NFPA-99（美国消防协会制定的医疗设备规范）标准，将要求任何手术室的 GFCIs 只控制一个插座，禁止类似菊花链插座的使用。

中心静脉导管与起搏器导线使用注意事项

中心静脉导管和起搏器导线必须在佩戴手套的情况下进行操作，同时不接触其他物品，以减少泄漏弱电流形成传递的可能性。

检查

必须定期由生物医学工程部门或仪器设备科对设备进行检查和测试，以便在电击事故发生前检测出故障电路、设备接地线破损或电流泄漏过大。

（饶苗苗 译 张丽君 校）

延伸阅读

Bruner JMR, Leonard PF: *Electricity, safety and the patient*, Chicago, 1989, Year Book Medical Publishers.

Ehrenwerth J: Electrical and fire safety. In Barash PB, Cullen BF, Stoelting RK, et al., editors: *Clinical anesthesia*, ed 8. Philadelphia, Lippincott Williams & Wilkins, 2017, pp 109–140.

Litt L, Ehrenwerth J: Electrical safety in the operating room: important old wine, disguised new bottles, *Anesth Analg* 78(3):417–419, 1994.

National Fire Protection Association: *NFPA-99: Health care facilities code, 2015 edition*, 2015. Quincy, MA.

Schwartz JJ, Ehrenwerth J: Electrical safety. In Lake CK, editor: *Clinical monitoring for anesthesia and critical care*. Philadelphia, WB Saunders, 1994, pp 35–42.

Schwartz JJ, Ehrenwerth J: A case-oriented approach to electrical safety. In Morell RC, Eichhorn JH, editors: *Patient safety in anesthetic practice*, New York, 1996, Churchill Livingstone, pp 55–70.

Wills JH, Ehrenwerth J, Rogers D: Electrical injury to a nurse due to conductive fluid in an operating room designated as a dry location, *Anesth Analg* 110(6):1647–1649, 2010.

第109章 手术室着火

Herodotos Ellinas

病例概要

患者，男性，35岁，因脸部枪伤出现面部和颈部血肿，被送往手术室行紧急清醒气管切开术。使用葡萄糖酸氯已定作为消毒剂，给予患者纯氧吸入的同时，铺盖手术单。

问题分析

定义

火是一种可燃物质（燃料）快速、持续、放热的氧化反应，可以释放热能和光能，通常伴有火焰。手术着火属于罕见事件，每年发生550～650起，是指实施手术患者的体表或体内物质的燃烧。这与手术室火灾不同，手术室火灾是指手术室内发生的火灾，不一定涉及患者。患者体内发生火灾的例子包括气道火灾，如激光引燃气管导管，以及火花引燃肠道气体引起腹腔内火灾。患者体表火灾的例子包括用外科电气设备引燃手术单、海绵或其他燃料。大约62%的手术火灾发生在呼吸道或面部，24%发生在患者体表，14%发生在患者体内。虽然外科手术引起的火灾罕见，但可造成严重损伤或死亡，而且在大多数情况下可以预防。

即使使用不易燃的麻醉药，手术室仍然可能发生火灾。火灾由“着火三要素”（引火源、氧化剂和燃料）引起（图109.1）。造成火灾的原因包括无效沟通、缺乏培训、误解和不正确使用医疗器械。常见的引火源有外科电气设备（59%）、激光（32%）和电凝、热丝烧灼、光纤光源、除颤仪和高速牙钻等热源。氧化剂是助于燃料燃烧的物质，有助于火燃烧得更旺。虽然空气、氧气和笑气不具有爆炸性，但它们是手术室内常见的氧化剂。在手术室有许多潜在的燃料，包括手术单、手术衣、海绵、气管导管、皮肤消毒液、头发和皮肤。有些燃料比其他燃料更易燃，而有些燃料只有在氧化剂存在时才会燃烧。

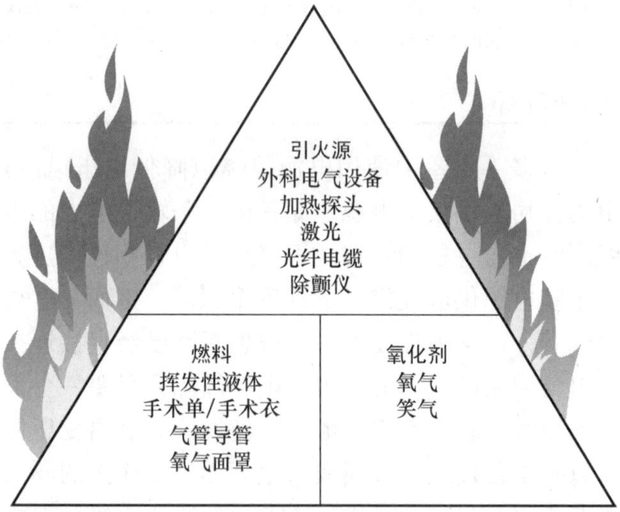

图109.1 着火三要素

手术室内发生的火灾通常与实施气道的激光手术有关。它们通常是在保护不充分的气管导管内着火（图109.2），或放置在气道内的任何易燃物（如湿棉絮）被激光束直接、过长时间照射引起。这种火灾的发生率为0.5%～1%。大多数火灾开始只发生在气管导管的外表面；如果未及时发现，则在到达管腔时可能产生类似喷灯样火焰，而导管内富含的氧气会增强其燃烧过程。

根据一项结案的索赔分析发现，90%的火灾索赔与电凝有关；监测麻醉下的手术区域富氧环境，如头、颈和上胸部手术，是发生火灾的主要原因。头、颈部和气道手术中发生火灾的风险增加，其原因为手术单下或口咽腔内氧气和笑气的聚集。取决于不同的手术，富含氧气的气体可直接靠近或包围操作部位。有几种可能导致氧气增多的情况。在局部麻醉下行头、颈部手术时，面罩、鼻导管或其他

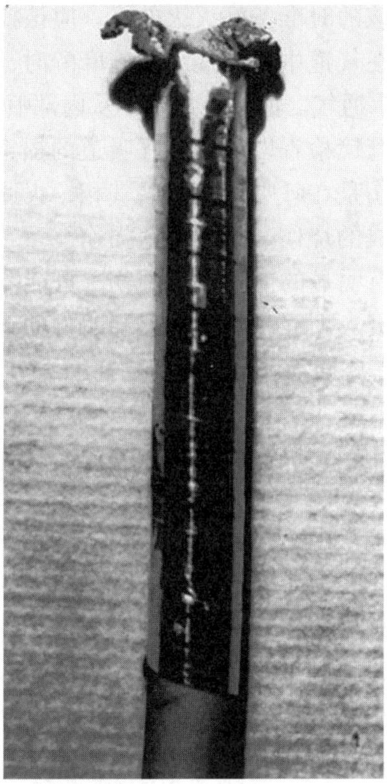

图 109.2 激光引发气道着火后的气管导管（密歇根大学医学中心 Allan Brown 博士提供）

开放呼吸系统可将氧气泄漏到患者的口、鼻或气道附近，并在手术单下聚集。在扁桃体及类似手术中，套囊充气不足的气管导管泄漏的氧气会聚集于口咽部。电凝设备在富含氧气的气道内使用，占了着火三要素中两项，而气管导管的套囊成为三要素中最后一要素。

火灾也可能是由激光误射或（通过金属表面）反射到任何不稳定的易燃材料引起，如覆盖患者的手术单。手术室内的许多液体（如皮肤消毒液、酊剂、脱脂剂、缝合包溶液）都含易燃、易挥发的有机化学物质。皮肤消毒液可能含有酒精或丙酮，在液体蒸发前都具有易燃性。如果使用不当，可能会导致溶液渗入患者的头发，聚集于患者的皮肤上或身体下面，渗透床单。如果患者在溶液完全干燥前盖好手术单，蒸汽就会被截留并输送和暴露于含有热源和引火源的手术区域。同样，外科透热法也可能引燃肠道气体。肠道气体含有不同浓度的氮气、二氧化碳、氢气、甲烷和氧气，在一定比例下可以燃烧。此外，笑气及其放热分解成分、氧气和氮气会使这些气体更加易燃。

静电、易燃易爆性麻醉气体（如乙醚、环丙烷），这些引火源相互作用而引起的火灾和爆炸在过去较为关注。而如今，含有干燥的二氧化碳吸附剂与强效吸入麻醉药的相互作用，可产生一氧化碳、高温、烟雾，引起火灾和爆炸（框 109.1）。

识别

火花、爆裂声和闪光预示有可能发生了着火、燃烧或爆炸。大多数手术室明火是通过火焰和烟雾发现。麻醉科医师应监测二氧化碳吸收器是否有过热迹象，并监测七氟烷吸入浓度与挥发罐设置的关系。与挥发罐设置相比，吸入七氟烷浓度的异常延迟上升或意外下降可能预示放热七氟烷的降解（框 109.3）。

风险评估

无论何时，只要存在高能量的引火源（如电刀或激光）、潜在的易燃材料（如气管导管、含酒精的皮肤消毒液、手术单）和氧化剂（氧气、笑气或二者兼有），就存在着燃烧的可能性。氧化剂的浓度越高，火灾的风险越大。因此，建议将吸入氧浓度尽可能降至最低。

无论是否使用激光，任何接受气道手术的患者都有发生气道着火的危险。Silverstein 火灾风险评估量表可用于确定手术中发生火灾的风险，并利于更好的沟通，以防止不可预见的后果。该评估基于三个因素（1 ～ 3 分）进行评分，即手术部位、开放的氧源和存在的引燃物。当激光手术或使用电凝的气道手术（如扁桃体切除术、气管切开术）实施麻醉时，任何时候都应保持高度警惕。使用开放呼吸系统（如鼻导管、面罩）在局部麻醉下实施头颈部手术时，发生火灾的风险也很高。

当吸附剂干燥时，二氧化碳吸附剂与七氟烷之间的放热反应最有可能发生。大多数吸附剂引起的火灾发生于麻醉机不使用后间隔一段时间，如，周一上午的第一台手术。

框 109.1 引起手术室着火和爆炸的原因

- 清醒吸氧患者实施头、颈和上胸部手术时使用电凝
- 在气管导管内特别是在气管造口术中使用电凝或激光
- 食管或气管的激光手术
- 易燃的皮肤消毒液或肠道气体
- 强效吸入麻醉药（如七氟烷）与干燥的二氧化碳吸附剂（钡石灰）之间的放热反应

启示

大多数外科手术引起的火灾，如果处理得当，不会对患者造成影响，或者伤害很少。然而，不适当的处理可能造成灾难性的后果，包括死亡，在ICU由于肺水肿长期期行机械通气、脓毒症或多器官衰竭综合征。气道火灾的一个晚期并发症是气管狭窄。

管理

手术室工作人员应开展关于手术火灾性质、预防和扑灭方面的宣教。采用培训、模拟和演习的形式，让工作人员熟悉手术火灾的反应和应对方法。综合训练包括在大型火灾的救援、警报、控制和疏散（rescue，alert，containment，and evacuation，RACE）反应方面的指导。推荐使用二氧化碳灭火器，并应放置在手术室方便取用之处。工作人员应熟悉此类消防设备、医疗气体供应切断阀、便携式电池供电的照明系统、通风系统、建筑物警报和电路系统的位置和操作方法。

小火通常可以通过戴手套的手或毛巾轻拍火焰，从而安全、简单地熄灭。并且应仔细检查该区域，以确保所有燃烧的物质都已熄灭。手术小组成员应评估导致火灾的原因，并努力防止再次发生。

需要立即采取行动扑灭发生在患者身上的大火，保护患者不受（额外的）热损伤，如果患者受伤并给予治疗。全面的应对措施需要麻醉科医师、外科医师和手术室护士的通力合作。麻醉科医师应该关闭氧流量，换成空气继续给患者通气。外科医师或护士应从患者身上移除燃烧的物品并将其扑灭。尤为重要的是，由于纸制手术单不透水，用水洒在此类手术单并不能扑灭其下面的火。同样重要的是，即使已燃材料已经熄灭，也要从患者身上取下，防止余热造成进一步烫伤。外科医师应对患者伤势进行评估和治疗。如果火势过猛，高温和浓烟可能会迫使手术团队撤离该区域。医疗队应该设法营救和疏散患者，然而这种可能性比较低。

在发生气道火灾或爆炸时，麻醉科医师、外科医师和护士必须迅速果断地采取行动，从而减少对患者的伤害。应立即从患者体内取出气管导管或其他点火源或火源，并必须停止供氧以防氧气接触火焰。气管导管灭火必须使用桶中的水，所以在激光手术中应该随时准备好灭火的水。应该检查是否有东西遗留在气道中。当继续实施麻醉时，患者应使用纯氧面罩通气。如果火灾属于从内部喷出的类型，应行支气管镜检查以评估下呼吸道的损害情况。下呼吸道损伤是在呼吸周期的吸气相，火通过气管导管腔内造成的烧伤。如呼吸道损伤严重，应重新插管。如果有明显的上呼吸道损伤，可能需要实施气管切开。吸入烟雾和热损伤引起明显的下呼吸道损伤，可能需要插管进行长时间的通气维持。

预防

美国麻醉科医师协会制定的手术室火灾处理流程图（图 109.3），概述了预防手术室火灾的四种措施：

- 避免引燃物靠近氧化剂；
- 策略性地放置手术单，从而有效避免氧气聚集；
- 使用易燃皮肤消毒液需要给予充足的待干时间；
- 在引燃物附近备好湿润的海绵和纱布。

在实施监护麻醉过程中，尤其在头颈部手术，麻醉科医师和其他医护人员必须考虑给予氧气的风险效益比。根据患者术前呼吸空气条件下氧饱和度的情况，考虑是否需要术中给氧。当需要较高浓度的氧气来维持氧饱和度时，手术团队应做好随时发生着火的准备。在靠近患者头颈部或气道使用引火源前，至少需要停止 1 min 供氧。

不同种类皮肤消毒液的酒精含量各不相同，最新指南推荐使用含有 70% 异丙醇的葡萄糖酸氯己定，它具有抗菌覆盖广的优势，但其属于一种高度易燃的物质。在择期手术中充足的待干时间（每一种产品均需要——无毛皮肤超过 3 min，湿的毛发长达 1 h）必须强制执行。急诊手术中应使用替代产品（如氯己定、必妥碘）。此外，避免消毒液聚集的改进铺单技术，小心放置呼气软管，并使用主动净化系统，这些措施可以保障高风险的手术。

手术中激光导致气道火灾的风险，可以通过避免激光在手术区域内外的误射，以及避免意外照射到手术单或患者脸部进行控制（框 109.2）。患者的眼睛应该用湿纱布垫覆盖，不要用胶布贴闭双眼，因为胶布具有可燃性。在激光气道手术中，应使用带套囊的激光气管导管。尽管市面上有许多可用于激光手术的气管导管，但尚无一种可完全防燃。

手术火灾需要所有相关人员的警觉和深思熟虑

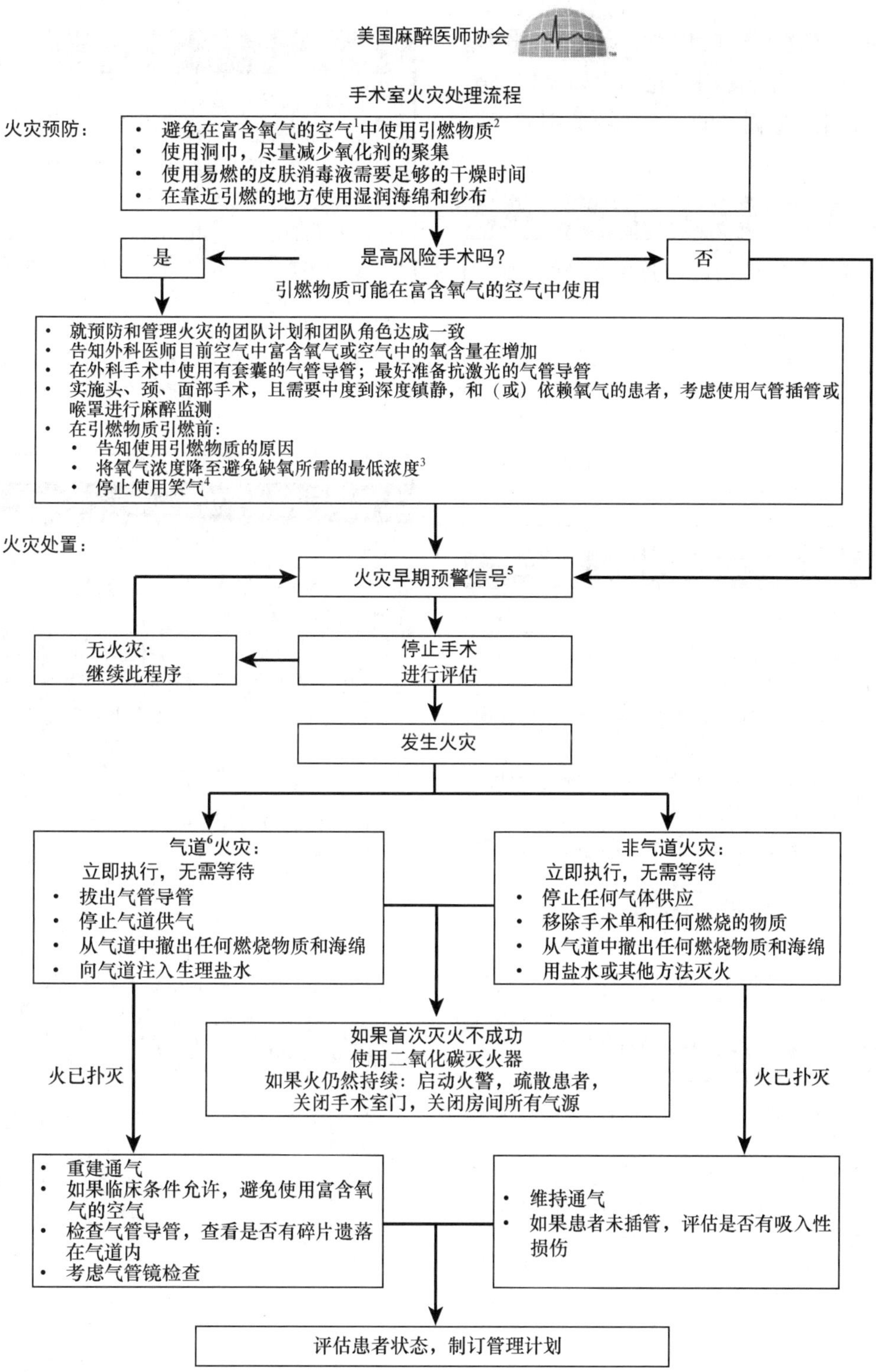

1.点火源包括但不仅限于电刀、电凝和激光。
2.当室内空气上方的氧浓度增加，和（或）存在任何浓度的笑气时，就会产生富含氧化剂的空气。
3.在尽量减少供氧量，等待一段时间（如1～3min）后再使用引火源。对于依赖氧的患者，将供氧量减少到避免缺氧的最低限度。监测脉搏氧饱和度，如果可行，监测吸入、呼出和（或）输送的氧气浓度。
4.停止输送笑气后，等待一段时间（如1～3 min）后再使用引火源。
5.意外的闪光、火焰、烟雾或热，不寻常的声音（如“砰”“啪”）或气味、手术单的意外移动、手术单或呼吸回路的变色、患者的不正常体动或主诉。
6.在该流程中，气道着火是指气道或呼吸回路的着火。
7.如有必要，可在患者身上使用二氧化碳灭火器。

图 109.3 ASA 手术室火灾处理流程（From Apfelbaum JL，Caplan RA，Barker SJ，et al.：Practice advisory for the prevention and management of operating room fires. An updated report by the American Society of Anesthesiologists Task Force on Operating Room Fires. *Anesthesiology* 118[2]：271-290，2013.）

的准备。表 109.1 概述了关于使用引火源（如电刀、电凝）的注意事项。关于使用氧化剂（如氧气、笑气）、燃料和二氧化碳吸附剂的注意事项分别列于框 109.3、表 109.2 和框 109.4。

框 109.2 手术室内避免激光引发火灾的推荐

- 在高风险手术暂停核查时，讨论处理火灾预防的计划
- 使用最低的吸入氧浓度（<0.3），避免使用笑气
- 在高风险手术中使用抗激光气管导管
- 口咽手术（如扁桃体切除术）时，气管导管的套囊应尽量置于气管远端
- 在套囊注入染色盐水，可及早发现气管导管套囊破裂
- 在气管导管套囊上方使用湿的脱脂棉，其中不能有金属丝
- 使用喷射通气或间歇性呼吸暂停

表 109.1 手术室引火源使用的注意事项

引火源种类	管理指南
电刀 / 电凝	使用双极电凝限制点火电位 尽量降低供氧浓度 当不使用电刀时，应将其探头放置在皮套内或者远离患者和手术单 在氧气浓度升高的手术部位（咽喉、口腔）使用电刀时要格外小心 选择恰当的电刀模式进行切割，避免使用电弧凝固模式 在靠近烧灼处使用盐水浸泡纱布 避免电极尖端有焦痂，必要时进行清除
手术激光	激光输出功率降至最低可接受范围，并限制脉冲持续时间 在安全表面上做激光着火测试 不使用时，将激光器置于待机模式 只有当激光的尖端完全在外科医师的直视下方可激活 只有使用激光的工作人员才可以将其激活 在将激光从手术部位撤离前，将其停用并置于待机模式 在进行内镜激光手术时，将激光纤维置于内镜中，然后引导进入患者体内 在上呼吸道手术中选择合适的抗激光导管
光纤电缆和光源	在激活光源前，确保光纤连接完成 在将镜子与光电缆断开之前，请先关闭光源
除颤仪	根据产品说明书使用 避免在富含氧气的空气中放电 培训操作人员如何正确使用除颤仪 尽可能使用一次性除颤器胶粘片，取代非一次性电极板 最大限度地让患者与胶粘片或电极板的表面接触 当使用电极板时，选择合适的导电胶

框 109.3 氧化剂（氧气和笑气）使用的注意事项

- 在开放式呼吸系统中，使用空气或吸入氧浓度低于 30%
- 识别和改善富氧气的环境
- 当在开放式呼吸系统中给患者供氧时，用手术单覆盖于患者的头部和颈部
- 在头颈部附近使用电刀前停止供氧 1 min
- 行口咽部手术时，如果气管导管套囊未充分堵住气道，可以使用湿纱布或海绵以减少氧气进入口咽部
- 当不使用时关闭氧气
- 避免使用笑气；笑气和氧气混合物的危险性并不比纯氧低；笑气扩散进入肠道气体，产生了额外的氧化剂，从而助燃氢气和甲烷

表 109.2 手术室可燃物的使用注意事项

燃料种类	管理指南
可燃性皮肤消毒液（脱脂剂、丙酮、酒精）和软膏（胶棉、凡士林、苯甲酸酊、气溶胶、石蜡）	尽量减少使用酒精含量高的皮肤消毒液 小心使用皮肤消毒液；不要让消毒液渗入头发或床单中；避免消毒液聚集在患者身上或身下 等待皮肤消毒液完全干燥后再进行铺单
床单、手术单、手术衣、口罩、面罩、帽子	所列举的均具有易燃性，即使贴上“防燃”的标签也不例外 在靠近激光位置使用湿手术单和毛巾 使用洞巾将手术区域与燃料和氧化剂隔开 尽可能使用湿的纱布海绵
麻醉相关物品（气管导管、面罩、鼻导管、胶布、血压计袖带）	尽可能使用带有套囊的气管导管 上呼吸道激光手术使用抗激光导管 气道激光手术使用亚甲基蓝染色盐水注入套囊内（用来提示套囊破裂） 在气道激光手术中使用湿脱脂棉保护套囊
患者头发	用无菌手术水凝胶涂抹于手术部位附近的头发，防止其点燃
肠道气体	避免使用笑气 避免使用含甘露醇的肠道准备液 如果需要，可以用惰性气体稀释肠道气体

框 109.4 手术室二氧化碳吸附剂、卤代麻醉剂的使用注意事项

- 提醒麻醉相关人员，包括技术人员和麻醉科医师，注意这种危险的性质
- 制定麻醉机的设置和维护规程，确保吸附剂不会干燥并定期更换

框 109.4 手术室二氧化碳吸附剂、卤代麻醉剂的使用注意事项（续）

- 在两次使用之间应减少或消除流经吸附剂的气体，并在一天结束时关闭麻醉机，以避免干燥
- 如果吸附剂的水化状态出现问题，应更换吸附剂
- 定期监测二氧化碳吸收罐的温度
- 与挥发罐设置相比，吸入七氟烷浓度异常延迟上升或意外下降，可能预示放热七氟烷的降解
- 考虑使用不含强碱化合物的替代吸附剂（如 Amsorb）

致谢

感谢 Paul E. Kazanjian 博士和 Anthony R. Doyle 博士对本章上一版的贡献。

（钱晓春　译　薄禄龙　校）

延伸阅读

Bruley ME: Surgical fires: perioperative communication is essential to prevent this rare but devastating complication, *Qual Saf Health Care* 13:467–471, 2004.

ECRI Institute: New clinical guide to surgical fire prevention. Patients can catch fire—here's how to keep them safer, *Health Devices* 38:314–332, 2009.

Kaye AD, Kolinsky D, Urman RD: Management of a fire in the operating room, *J Anesth* 28:279–287, 2014.

Macdonald AG: A short history of fires and explosions caused by anaesthetic agents, *Br J Anaesth* 72:710–722, 1994.

Mathias JM: Scoring fire risk for surgical patients, *OR Manager* 22:19–20, 2006.

Mehta SP, Bhananker SM, Posner KL, et al.: Operating room fires: a closed claims analysis, *Anesthesiology* 118:1133–1139, 2013.

Rampil IJ: Anesthetic considerations for laser surgery, *Anesth Analg* 74:424–435, 1992.

Rinder CS: Fire safety in the operating room, *Curr Opin Anaesthesiol* 21:790–795, 2008.

Scheinbein DS: Laser surgery and fire hazards in ear, nose, and throat surgeries, *Anesth Clin* 28:485–496, 2010.

Smith LP, Roy S: Operating room fires in otolaryngology: risk factors and prevention, *Am J Otolaryngol* 32:109–114, 2011.

Stoelting RK, et al.: Preventing on-patient fires in the operating room, *Anesthesia Patient Safety Foundation Newsletter* 26:41, 2012.

Van Der Spek AFL, Spargo PM, Norton ML: The physics of lasers and implications for their use during airway surgery, *Br J Anaesth* 60:709–729, 1988.

Watson DS: New recommendations for prevention of surgical fires, *AORN J* 91:463–469, 2010.

第 110 章 流量计

Robert G. Loeb

病例概要

患者，男性，20 岁，平素体健，刚完成麻醉诱导，正在接受腹股沟疝修补术。气体流量设置为氧气（O_2）1 L/min 和笑气（N_2O）2 L/min。当氧气分析仪报警时，氧饱和度开始下降（图 110.1）。启动氧气冲洗阀暂时解决了该问题。

问题分析

定义

流量计故障是麻醉机故障的一个罕见原因，因为现代麻醉机正是为防止许多流量计问题而设计的。尽管最后一次流量计事故是在 2004 年公布的，但流量计故障仍偶尔会报告至美国食品和药品管理局。

曾有患者因流量计错误设置而死于吸入低氧混合气体。流量计设计不当有时是一个影响因素，因为过去的麻醉机被设计为两个并联流量计组件，分别连接两种气体。如今改进的流量计设计，减少了用户出错的可能性。此外，自 20 世纪 80 年代起，所有麻醉机都配备了一个比例装置，可限制 O_2 和 N_2O 相对流速，以防止错误地使用低氧混合气体（见第 117 章）。例如，Dräger 生产的麻醉机配备了 O_2 比例调节器，GE Healthcare 生产的麻醉机则安装了名为 Link-25 的机械联动装置。两者通常都是可靠的，但有报告称 Link-25 偶尔会出现故障。

流量计组件由带有相关流量计的流量控制阀组成（图 110.2）。**传统**流量计组件由一个机械流量控制阀和一个或两个串联连接的玻璃流量计管组成，分别用于对应的压缩气体。**电子**流量计系统具有电子控制阀和用于每种气体的电子流量计，用户通过计算机界面控制气体流量。在具有混合流量计的麻醉机中，每种气体都有一个机械流量控制阀和一个电子流量计。

机械流量控制阀是可变阻力针阀。逆时针方向转动阀门可以减小阀门上的阻力，从而增加气体流量。合成流量取决于阀门阻力和阀门入口与出口之间的压差；因此，上游或下游的压力波动将导致流量变化。根据相关流量计读数可手动调节流量。

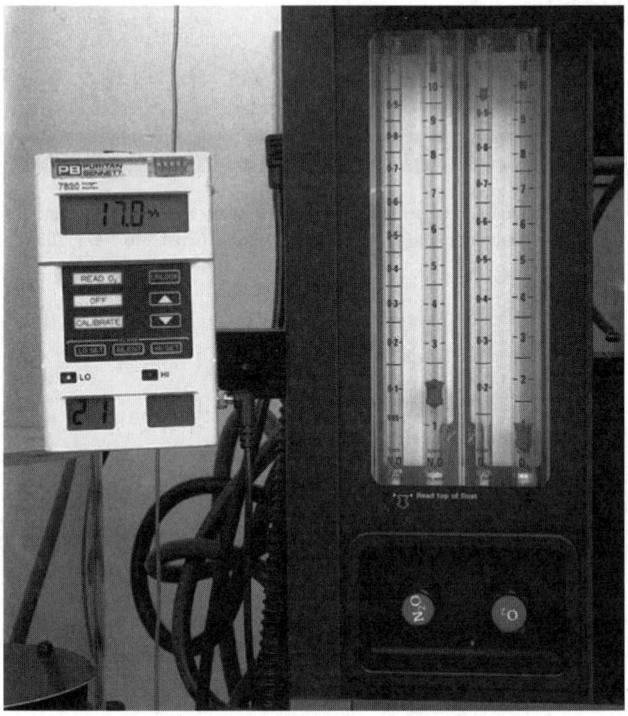

图 110.1　吸入的氧浓度非常低，与流量计设置不一致

电子流量控制阀是电子调节阻力阀，由电力驱动。用户按顺时针方向转动电子旋钮，或使用屏幕控制来增加所需的气体流速。然后电子微处理器降低阀门阻力，不断调整阀门，使得测量流量和设定流量之间的差值为零。某些系统可以控制总流量并设置 O_2 浓度。

曾有患者死于流量计直接连接到气管导管而没有气体的出口通路。在对一项与设备相关的已结案

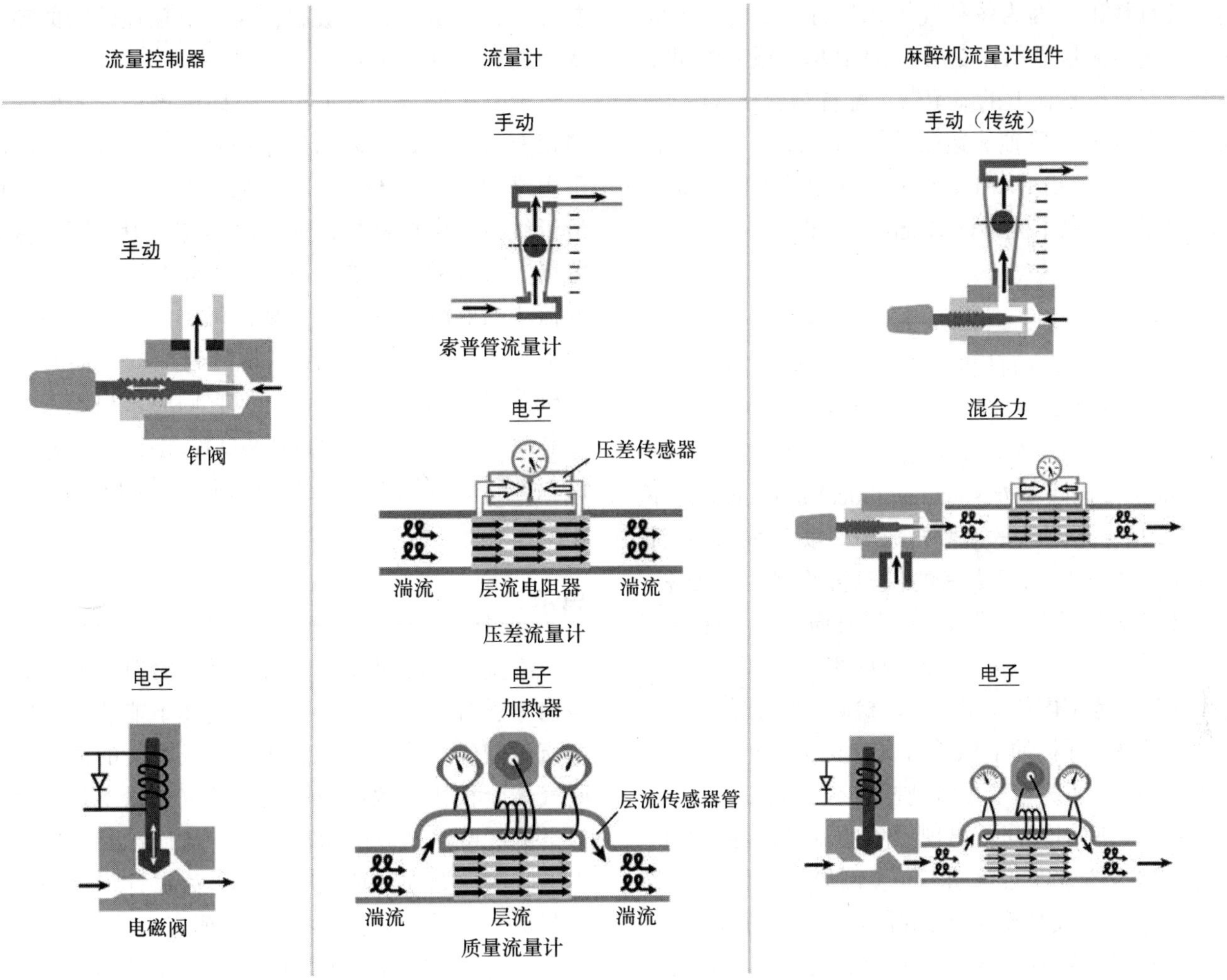

图 110.2　三种类型的麻醉机流量计组件：传统（手动）、混合和电子。传统的流量计组件包括手动针阀和下游 Thorpe 管流量计。一些新的麻醉机全部为电子流量计组件，每个组件包括电动和电子控制阀以及电子流量计。其他现代麻醉机具有混合流量计组件，其中气体流量通过手动针阀控制，但以电子方式测量和显示流量。有各种类型的电子气体流量计，例如压差流量计，其测量气体通过流量电阻器时的压降和测量气体的对流传热的质量流量计

索赔进行分析时，滥用手术室外传输管道的给氧占 40 例中的 9 例，每例都导致患者气胸。例如，如果氧气传输管道直接连接到气管导管，有意或无意地阻塞了 T 形出口，则可能发生这种情况。至关重要的是，所有临床医师都应了解流量计的最大出口压力应等于其入口压力，标称值为 50 PSI。该数字看起来很小，但应务必记住。1 PSI 约等于 70 cmH_2O，故 50 PSI 相当于 3500 cmH_2O。

麻醉机玻璃流量计管和壁挂式氧气或空气流量计，由锥形玻璃管及里面的浮标组成，其内径顶部大，底部小。准确地说，流量计管必须处于垂直位置，并且浮标的运动不得受到静电、水或管内污垢的干扰。流量计被校准为与之匹配的管道和浮标；更换任一组件都可能导致严重误差。现代玻璃流量计为永久密封，以防止在维护期间匹配管道和浮标时出错。每个流量计都针对特定气体进行校准，测量任何其他气体的流量都不准确。为防止在机器维修期间出现错误，现代流量计只能安装在相应气体的外壳中。为保护流量计管免受破损，它们安装在塑料保护罩后面。

麻醉机越来越多地使用电子流量计而非玻璃流量管。电子流量计的优点包括可靠性提高和维护减少，低流量下的精准度提高，以及将流量数据转换成电子记录和自动控制气流的能力。多种技术可用于电子测量流量，包括质量流量和压差。质量流量传感器根据热扩散原理运行，测量在气流通道中维持加热元件温度所需的能量。

每个传感器都针对特定气体进行校准，每种气体都有不同的特定热指数。压差流量计测量固定流量电阻器上的压差。同样，每个传感器都针对特定

气体进行校准，因为每种气体都具有不同的密度和黏度。气体流量显示在专用LED显示屏或麻醉机屏幕上。麻醉机平板上的显示器可配置为数字或图形，也可配置为显示单独流速或计算的总流速，并设置为 O_2 浓度。除由RAM电池故障导致校准因子缺失外，没有关于电子流量计出现问题的报告。

识别

麻醉机使用前的检测期间，最容易检测到流量计故障。美国麻醉科医师协会（American Society of Anesthesiologists，ASA）开发了一个检测程序（可以从http://asahq.org/resources/clinical-information/下载），以检测最严重的麻醉机故障。**项目8：确认流量计和公共气体出口之间的供气管路是否有泄漏，可检测流量计缺失、泄漏、破裂或损坏。**目视检查流量管可能会发现流量计破裂或损坏。通过调节所有气体在整个范围内的流量，可以检测到粘于管中的浮标，同时检查浮标的平稳滑动。应该注意的是，ASA麻醉设备检查不太可能检测到校准不当的流量计。

在术中使用期间，出现故障的流量计导致呼吸回路中的气体浓度与预期不同（例如，O_2 浓度高或低于设置值）或从麻醉机到呼吸回路的意外流速。尽管没有源自麻醉机的气体流量监测，但在极端情况下，医师可能会注意到储气囊或呼吸机风箱未能充气。Y形连接处呼吸气体分析仪和呼吸回路中的 O_2 分析仪，是针对来自麻醉机的气体浓度的流量阀后最近的监测仪。由于复吸入，监视器上的读数很少与麻醉机设置相匹配。在低流量期间，浓度表盘数据与呼吸回路气体浓度之间的差异尤为明显。如果怀疑存在流量计问题，麻醉科医师可从新鲜气体软管中取样气体，检查从麻醉机流出的气体成分；如不能实施上述操作，可以在高流速下检查呼吸回路中的气体浓度。

风险评估

麻醉机故障是导致危急事件的罕见原因。例如，在澳大利亚事故监测研究中报告的前2000起事件中，只有4起涉及麻醉机故障。然而，其中2起由流量计问题引起，并被认为可能危及生命。美国FDA医疗器械报告数据库中偶尔有流量计故障的报告，其中大部分包括流量计和气体出口之间的管道断开，或流量计管道破裂，通常出现在较旧的独立或辅助氧气流量计中。

麻醉机的定期维护对于预防因磨损而引发的故障很有必要。具有讽刺意味的是，一些麻醉机故障是由维护过程中出现的错误造成的。因此，当使用最近维修过的机器时，临床医师应对设备问题保持警惕。旧麻醉机可能造成最大的安全隐患。一项对爱荷华州麻醉机的调查发现，机器的工作年限范围为1～28年（平均8年）。尽管较旧的机器并未比新机器更频繁地发生故障，但它们通常缺乏安全功能和必要的监控（例如 O_2/N_2O 流量报警、O_2 分析仪）。因此，临床医师应该对没有这些功能的旧机器保持警惕。

启示

流量计故障可能表现为呼吸回路泄漏或呼吸回路内不适合的气体成分。尽管气体不能从呼吸回路逆流至破碎的流量计，但从破裂或缺失的流量计泄漏气体会很快导致呼吸回路中的气体量不足，表现为空的呼吸囊或呼吸机风箱，并被误诊断为更常发生的呼吸回路泄漏或断开故障。流量计组件的大量泄漏是一个严重问题，因其会妨碍患者的有效通气。

流量计不准确或破裂 O_2 流量计的小泄漏，可能会导致麻醉机将低氧气体混合物分配到呼吸回路中，而 O_2 分析仪旨在检测这种情况。其他流量计问题不容易导致患者受伤。其他气体的泄漏不同于 O_2，不会导致低氧混合物，因为流量计的设置是为了防止在这种情况下优先损失 O_2。

管理

一次 O_2 冲洗可暂时纠正因流量计问题导致的呼吸回路中容量损失或缺氧。O_2 冲洗绕过麻醉机的许多内部组件，包括流量计组件。此外，大多数麻醉机上的单向阀（或包含单向阀的挥发罐）可防止冲洗后 O_2 的逆行泄漏。

当在手术中检测到严重的流量计故障时，应使用替代方法，例如使用加压给氧气囊对患者进行通气。应该移除有缺陷的机器，直至它由经过培训的技术人员进行维修和彻底检查。

预防

大多数流量计故障都是预先存在的。因此，对麻醉机进行彻底预检可防止流量计故障引起的相关事件。使用 ASA 推荐的麻醉机检查程序可检测到许多问题，包括流量缺失、泄漏、破裂或损坏的流量计。但在此检查程序中，并未对流量计校准进行验证。

通过常规预检可避免许多与设备相关的故障。令人关注的是，麻醉从业者不擅长检测麻醉设备故障。例如，麻醉科医师和注册麻醉护士在一次会议展览中平均只检测到 44% 的预设麻醉机故障。只有 15% 的参与者发现 O_2 流量计被错误校准为仅能提供 10% 的指示流量。核查清单的使用并未明显提高检出率。麻醉科医师使用自己的检测方法只能检测到 26% 的麻醉机故障，在使用 FDA 检查程序（1986 年版）时可检测出 29% 的故障。但是，他们在使用 FDA 核查清单时未得到使用指导，而强化指导可以提高仪器检测的准确率。

（薛孜孜 译 张丽君 校）

延伸阅读

Buffington CW, Ramanathan S, Turndorf H: Detection of anesthesia machine faults, *Anesth Analg* 63:79–82, 1984.

Chandradeva K: A serious incident with the Blease Frontline Genius anaesthetic machine, *Anaesthesia* 59:627, 2004.

Cooper M, Ali D: Oxygen flowmeter dislocation [letter], *Anaesth Intensive Care* 17:109–110, 1989.

Eger II EI, Hylton RR, Irwin RH, et al.: Anesthetic flow meter sequence—a cause for hypoxia, *Anesthesiology* 24:396–397, 1963.

Eng TS, Durieux ME: Automated machine checkout leaves an internal gas leak undetected: the need for complete checkout procedures, *Anesth Analg* 114:144–146, 2012.

Feldman JM, Olympio MA, Martin D, et al.: New guidelines available for pre-anesthesia checkout. APSF Newsletter 23:6-7, 2008. Available at http://www.apsf.org/newsletters/html/2008/spring/05_new_guidelines.htm. Accessed February 1, 2016.

Hay H: Delivery of an hypoxic gas mixture due to a defective rubber seal of a flowmeter control tube, *Eur J Anaesthesiol* 17:456–458, 2000.

Kumar V, Hintze MS, Jacob AM: A random survey of anesthesia machines and ancillary monitors in 45 hospitals, *Anesth Analg* 67:644–649, 1988.

March MG, Crowley JJ: An evaluation of anesthesiologists' present checkout methods and the validity of the FDA checklist, *Anesthesiology* 75:724–729, 1991.

McHale S: A critical incident with the Ohmeda Excel 410 machine [letter], *Anaesthesia* 46:150, 1991.

Mehta SP, Eisenkraft JB, Posner KL, et al.: Patient injuries from anesthesia gas delivery equipment: a closed claims update, *Anesthesiology* 119:788–795, 2013.

Olympio MA, Goldstein MM, Mathes DD: Instructional review improves performance of anesthesia apparatus checkout procedures, *Anesth Analg* 83:618–622, 1996.

Singh S, Loeb RG: Fatal connection: death caused by direct connection of oxygen tubing into a tracheal tube connector, *Anesth Analg* 99:1164–1165, 2004.

Webb RK, Russell WJ, Klepper I, et al.: The Australian Incident Monitoring Study. Equipment failure: an analysis of 2000 incident reports, *Anaesth Intensive Care* 21:673–677, 1993.

第 111 章 颅内压监测

Adrian Pichurko，Paul Smythe

病例概要

患者，男性，18 岁，因机动车事故造成开放性长骨骨折和重型颅脑损伤。格拉斯哥昏迷量表评分为 6 分，头颅计算机断层扫描显示弥漫性脑水肿。监测脑室内压力为 30 mmHg。已对升高的颅内压启动治疗，并转至手术室治疗长骨骨折。

问题分析

定义

颅内压（intracranial pressure，ICP）是由颅内容物对硬质颅腔壁所产生的压力。正常成人中，颅内容物由 80% 的脑组织、10% 的血液和 10% 的脑脊液（intracranial pressure，CSF）组成。

正常的 ICP 约为 5 ～ 13 mmHg（7 ～ 18 cmH_2O）。无颅内病变的患者颅内容物具有正常的弹性，这意味着颅内容积的微小增加不会导致 ICP 升高。根据 Monro-Kellie 假设，某一腔室体积增加时，另一腔室的体积减小相等的量，使总体积保持不变。这种类型的补偿是必要的，因为三种颅内容物几乎是不可压缩的。当颅内容积接近颅腔容积时，弹性降低。在这种情况下，颅内容积的小幅度增加就会导致严重的、危及生命的 ICP 升高。

在过去的 5 年里，ICP 监测的诊断和治疗性使用没有明显的变化。大多数中心认为正常的 ICP 上限是 20 mmHg，而有些中心以 15 mmHg 为标准。ICP 高于 15 ～ 20 mmHg 被认为是颅内高压（intracranial hypertension，ICH，见第 150 章）。ICH 的治疗通常开始于 20 ～ 25 mmHg。ICH 患者治疗时应考虑脑灌注压（cerebral perfusion pressure，CPP）。CPP 被定义为平均动脉压减去 ICP，是反映驱动脑血流的压力梯度、氧供和代谢产物的生理变量，因此与脑缺血密切相关。CPP 的最佳水平尚不清楚，但几项临床研究表明维持 CPP 高于 70 mmHg 能显著降低死亡率和提高生存质量。此外，还可增加严重创伤性脑损伤（severe traumatic brain injury，TBI）后的缺血性脑灌注。在大多数 TBI 中，机体通过调节血管内容量或诱发全身高血压来调控 CPP。

识别

ICP 监测有助于诊断和治疗 ICH。所有的 ICP 监测从连接的物理部件到监测的系统都有一些共同的特点。ICP 监测仪和颅内腔之间的连接要求由水密封接口、与弹性膜连接的硬质管组成。监测 ICP 时必须确保腔室密闭。任何漏出都表明存在严重的潜在病理问题，病情可能从脑脊液漏（最好的情况）到脑疝（最坏的情况）。在无漏出时时，ICP 的任何变化都会导致与腔室相连的弹性膜发生一定程度的变形。

结构

变形的弹性膜与传感器相连接。连接介质（即硬质管）的作用是要准确地传输每一个 ICP 脉冲引发的弹性膜变形。传感器将这些连接的或发射的脉冲信号转换为电信号，电信号被放大后显示出来。显示器本质上是一个电压表，连接到示波器或触针记录器，以显示 ICP 波形和压力变化。ICP 监测系统的不同主要由变形弹性膜和传感器之间的连接方式及每个系统放置的解剖位置决定。

归零

所有的 ICP 监控装置必须将 ICP 转换成电压并显示出来。该关系以方程 $y=mx+b$ 表示，其中 y 为电压，x 为压力，m 为 ICP 曲线斜率。传感器的特点是电压和压力之间存在线性关系，即 m（在“校准”一节进一步讨论）。当施加在传感器上的压力等于零时，监控装置取值为零电压是最佳的。调整方程式中的 b 为 0，使关系变为 $y=mx$，从而实现归零。归零意味着，如果传感器在被测压力为零时产生电压，则必须通过反向的内部施加电压进行平衡或补偿。生物压力监测系统的零压力始终是环境大气压。调零是通过打开传感器上的三通或阀门来检测环境或室内空气压力为零来实现的。现代系统需要按下调零按钮，该设置会自动记忆。传感器调零（ICP 或其他任何压力传感器）很重要，此步骤的错误会影响后续压力读数。

传感器位置

ICP 监测装置的传感器既可以位于外部，也可以位于颅内导管尖端。位于外部的 ICP 监测装置，可随时重新调零外部传感器。位于颅内导管尖端的必须在将导管放入颅内之前将传感器调零。除了新型的气囊转换技术，大多数导管尖端压力传感器一旦放置就不能重新调零。

校准

校准是通过调整公式 $y=mx+b$ 的 m 项或斜率来完成的。在可调整式的 ICP 监测系统上的控制键标记为“校准”“增益”“放大系数”或“斜率”。当前大多数传感器都内置了一个可预先校准的小型微处理器。它们产生一个与压缩程度成比例的小恒定电压，称为**校准系数**。最常见的校准系数是 200。在 200 mmHg 时意味着传感器在额定压力下输出的电压可能大于或小于它应该输出的电压。可通过向传感器施加已知压力并调整监视器显示以读取与施加的已知压力相同的读数来检查校准。建议定期交叉检查所有传感器的校准。

漂移

零点和增益设置随时间发生变化，称之为**漂移**。由于没有完美的传感器，所有的传感器放大器都会有一定程度的漂移。

传感器类型

现代 ICP 监测仪使用两种不同类型的传感器。一类是**应变式传感器**，它由一个物理连接在磁铁上的薄膜组成，磁铁在一系列线圈内随脉冲运动。当线圈中的磁通量发生变化时，就会产生与磁运动的程度和频率成比例的电流。该电流与施加在应变式传感器上的压力成正比。然而，最常用的应变式传感器是高度专业化**压电式传感器**。这是一种在施加压力时产生电压的高标准化陶瓷晶体。在大多数压电系统中，传感器中类似于变形弹性膜的结构是晶体本身。预设的校准系数一般为 200。

第二类传感器是**光纤传感器**。它使用激光束将膜片运动与传感器的电子元件耦合起来。这种系统仍然依赖于随 ICP 变化而变化的膜片。膜片的传感器侧具有反射性（镜像），激光束指向膜片的这一侧。当膜片产生移动时，就会将激光束以不同的角度反射出去。该反射光信号与入射光信号有关，从而对由 ICP 变化引起的膜片变形进行定量估计。产生的信号需放大，并与膜的运动成正比。

误差源

外部传感器精确且可以重新校准。它们必须放置在相对于患者头部的固定参考点，以避免测量误差。内部传感器（导管尖端应变式或光纤式传感器）在置入颅内前应进行校准，一旦放置（即没有单独的脑室内导管）则无法重新校准。如果设备测量漂移，尤其是在 ICP 监测仪使用数天的情况下则可能出现 ICP 测量不准确。

脑室 ICP 监测

最常监测的颅内腔是脑室内、实质内、蛛网膜下腔、硬膜下和硬膜外（表 111.1）。脑室内 ICP 监测被认为是比其他 ICP 监测更精确的金标准，还具有引流脑脊液治疗 ICH 的作用。ICP 监测设备已根据其准确度、稳定性和引流脑脊液的能力进行了排名。连接到外部传感器或导管尖端压力传感器的脑室内导管是监测 ICP 最准确和最可靠的方法，可用于脑脊液引流。导管尖端压力传感器测量实质内 ICP 与直接测量脑室内 ICP 压力相似。蛛网膜下腔或硬膜下液体耦合装置和硬膜外 ICP 监测装置的精确度较低。

持续 ICP 监测

通过连续的 ICP 监测，可以观察到三种波形：A、B 和 C。B 波和 C 波分别与呼吸和动脉血压的变化有关，临床意义有限。A 波，称为高原波，具有临床意义。A 波是由升高的 ICP 产生，可达 50 ～ 120 mmHg，持续 2 ～ 20 min。此种波型是对

表 111.1 用于监测颅内压的颅内空间

颅内空间	压力传导方法	脑脊液引流	再校准
脑室内	颅外流体耦合应变式	+	+
	导管尖端流体耦合应变式	+	+
	导管尖端流体耦合光纤式	+	+
脑实质	导管尖端应变式	-	-
蛛网膜下腔	颅外流体耦合应变式	-	+
硬膜下腔	导管尖端应变式	-	-
	导管尖端光纤式	-	-
	颅外流体耦合应变式	-	+
硬膜外腔	颅外流体耦合应变式	-	+
	气动式	-	+

+ 可能需要或必要，- 不需要或不必要

脑血容量的增加而引起 CPP 波动的反应，只出现在血管床整体自我调节完好时。A 波意味着 ICP 容量补偿机制已到极限。

不同的无创监测 ICP 方法具有不同的准确性。形态学检查包括磁共振成像、CT、超声和眼底检查，以检测颅内顺应性降低的征象。除了其他体征外，还可以通过对比视神经直径和视神经鞘直径来评估。生理学评估方式包括经颅和经眼多普勒、鼓室声导抗和近红外光谱，以及神经生理学工具，如脑电图和视觉诱发电位。这些模式都不足以单独用于 ICP 的评估。

风险评估

ICP 监测在 TBI 患者中应用最为广泛（见第 150 章），可达到以下作用：

- 有助于早期发现颅内占位性病变；
- 限制可能有害的控制 ICP 的治疗方法的滥用；
- 通过脑脊液引流降低 ICP，从而改善脑灌注；
- 有助于判断预后；
- 改善预后。

脑外伤昏迷患者（格拉斯哥昏迷量表评分 3～8 分）、CT 结果异常时应进行 ICP 监测。CT 结果正常的昏迷患者如果有以下两种或两种以上的危险因素，也应进行 ICP 监测：

- 40 岁以上；
- 单侧或双侧异常姿势；
- 收缩压低于 90 mmHg。

对于格拉斯哥昏迷量表评分大于 9 分且有大面积病变的 TBI 患者和不能配合检查来连续监测的小儿患者，也需要进行 ICP 监测。

轻度或中度颅脑损伤患者不需要常规监测 ICP。当颅内病变患者出现意识障碍且不能执行指令性动作时，与 ICH 相关的死亡率增加了 2～10 倍。在以下情况，包括蛛网膜下腔出血（伴或不伴脑积水）、脑出血、脑积水、脑炎、脑膜炎、静脉窦血栓形成、缺血性梗死伴肿胀和肝性脑病时，建议进行 ICP 监测。表 111.2 按设备位置列出了各种 ICP 监测的优缺点。

启示

在高危患者中常规监测 ICP 的证据并不完全清楚。研究显示结果不确定，包括无影响甚至增加死亡率。尽管如此，依据中度强度证据，目前的共识指南还是推荐将其作为高危患者治疗方案的一部分。更多高级证据显示推荐使用 ICP 和 CPP 来监测危及生命的脑疝。

ICP 监测并发症包括感染、出血、神经损伤、意外注射、发生故障、阻塞和位置不当。因为在大型前瞻性研究中尚未报告与 ICP 监测相关的有临床意义的颅内感染，所以细菌定植是比感染更准确的表述。ICP 监测装置植入 5 天后细菌定植显著增加。液体耦合式 ICP 监测器的冲洗显著增加了细菌定植。无论是导管尖端传感器还是光纤传感器，脑室、蛛网膜下腔、硬膜下腔和脑实质的细菌定植率分别为 5%、5%、4% 和 14%。然而，临床上严重颅内感染并不常见。与 ICP 装置相关性血肿的总发病率为 1.4%。据报道，液体耦合式监测器脑室导管、蛛网膜下腔或硬膜下导管的故障或阻塞发生率分别为 6.3%、16% 和 10.5%。当 ICP 测量值大于 50 mmHg 时，会发生信号和波形的阻塞和丢失。脑实质和脑室内压力光纤导管尖端式传感器装置的故障率为 9%～40%，这需要重新插入新的光纤设备。

在患者体位改变时，由于设备断开或调零不当，脑室外引流也会造成脑脊液过度流失的风险。这可能导致动脉瘤的再出血、桥静脉破裂引起的硬膜下出血以及反向脑疝。于 2017 年麻醉与重症神经科学

表 111.2 ICP 监测设备放置位置的优缺点

设备位置	优点	缺点	波形质量
脑室内	金标准	导管可能被血液或组织阻塞	极好
	准确测量 ICP	感染或出血风险	
	可进行 CSF 引流或取样	可能需要频繁调零	
	可使药物或染色剂直接注入 CSF		
	确定 $\delta P/\delta V$		
脑实质	脑室通路不可取时可用	可能发生明显漂移	好
	精确	光纤电缆断裂	
	只需要归零一次	放置后无法重新校准	
	无需将传感器调整到患者位置	无法行 CSF 取样	
蛛网膜下腔	脑实质不受干扰	管腔可能被血液或组织阻塞	差
	快速插入	易出现衰减波形	
	脑室通路不可取时可用	高 ICP 时精准度较低	
		必须经常调零	
		存在脑脊液漏的顾虑	
硬膜下腔	开颅术后有益	存在衰减的风险	较差
	易于放置	过高时 ICP 值被低估	
	当 ICP 相对较低时精准度最佳		
硬膜外腔	不穿透硬脑膜	传感膜必须与硬脑膜保持共面	较差
	感染风险低	存在错误或误导性读数的风险	
	易于置入	对 ICP 监测仪不敏感	

CSF，脑脊液；ICP，颅内压 $\delta P/\delta V$，压力的变化随容积变化的函数
Modified from Guidelines for the Management of Severe Head Injury. Brain Trauma Foundation，1995.

学会发布的指南推荐，若设备意外断开，应立即夹闭脑室外引流并更换所有污染的部件。同时还推荐在患者体位变动前夹紧脑室外引流。然而，当患者转运时间过长（如院间转运）时，这一决定应个体化以避免 ICH 的风险。

管理

当 ICP ≥ 20 mmHg 或者有明显的脑水肿时，推荐进行 ICH 治疗（另见第 150 章）。治疗方案通常根据需治疗的颅内容物进行分类，包括以下内容：

- 脑组织容积；
- 脑脊液量；
- 脑血容量；
- 肿块病变。

脑组织含水量为 75% ～ 80%，治疗旨在通过减少脑组织含水量以减少脑组织容积。使用高渗剂如甘露醇的目的就在于此。甘露醇使脑血和脑组织之间产生渗透梯度，有利于水从组织中进入到血管。甘露醇也可以通过降低继发于自由水运动的血液黏度来降低脑血容量。血液黏度降低可使脑血流增加，从而促使具有正常调节功能的脑组织区域的血管收缩。这样就会减少脑血容量，降低 ICP。甘露醇的有效剂量为 0.25 ～ 1 g/kg 体重。注意维持血容量，且血浆渗透压不宜超过 320 mOsm。呋塞米和其他利尿剂可通过增加血液渗透压来降低脑组织含水量，有利于水从脑组织进入脑血管。据报道，当血管源性水肿是导致脑组织水含量增加的主要原因时，皮质类固醇可降低脑组织含水量；然而在治疗其他类型的脑水肿或血管源性水肿和其他类型水肿并存的情况下，皮质类固醇的效果甚微。急性颅脑损伤时，不建议使用皮质类固醇治疗 ICP 增高，因为其相关

的不良反应可能会使结果更差。不良反应包括脑组织以外部位的免疫反应降低、内源性类固醇产生抑制和高血糖。

脑脊液量的减少可直接改善升高的ICP，提高脑水肿区脑组织水的清除。降低脑脊液量的最直接方法是脑脊液引流，通常是在脑室内或腰椎蛛网膜下腔放置导管。由于存在急性脑疝的风险，ICH患者建议谨慎使用后者。将头高位有利于脑脊液从颅内转移到脊髓蛛网膜下腔，从而减少颅内脑脊液量。

降低脑血容量的方法包括：过度通气、使用已知的脑血管收缩剂以及限制使用损害脑自动调节的药物、头部抬高至心脏水平以上、抑制脑代谢、通过控制气道或机械通气将升高的胸腔内压力降至最低。过度通气下的低碳酸血症通过收缩脑血管来减少脑血流量，后者是由血管周围pH的快速升高所介导。然而，低碳酸血症可能会因脑血管收缩而致脑灌注不足，特别是TBI患者。在不升高ICP的前提下，TBI患者应避免进行长期的过度通气治疗（动脉二氧化碳分压为25 mmHg）。此外，在TBI后的前24 h内应避免预防性过度通气，因为此时本已减少的脑血流的进一步下降会加重脑灌注不足。如果ICH对镇静、肌肉松弛、脑脊液引流和渗透性利尿剂不敏感，则在急性神经功能恶化时可能需要短期或延期的过度通气治疗。镇静催眠药（如巴比妥类药物、依托咪酯、丙泊酚）可收缩脑血管并降低ICP。极端情况下，需要巴比妥类药物诱导昏迷来控制ICP。

损害脑自动调节的药物可以增加脑血容量和ICP，包括吸入麻醉剂和直接性血管扩张剂（如硝普钠、硝酸甘油、钙通道阻滞剂、前列环素、腺苷）。用间接性血管扩张剂（如拉贝洛尔、曲美他嗪）控制血压可防止脑血容量和ICP的增加。头部抬高至心脏水平以上可增加颅内静脉回流从而减少脑血容量。也可通过低温和巴比妥类药物诱导昏迷来抑制脑代谢。

颅内占位性病变增加了总脑容量，从而增加了ICP。其治疗包括肿瘤切除、化疗或放疗，还可为正常颅内容物创造额外空间如减压或颅骨切除术。

预防

尚无可以确切预防ICP升高的措施，这也不属于上一节所述的ICP管理部分。对于未手术治疗（例如颅内出血、肿瘤体积增大或脑积水）的患者，通过干预颅内三大内容物（即脑组织容积、脑脊液量和脑血容量）可以防止ICP升高。归纳如下：

- 脑组织容积：
  - 利尿剂（甘露醇）；
  - 皮质类固醇（用于血管源性水肿）。
- 脑脊液容量：
  - 脑室引流术；
  - 腰椎引流。
- 脑血流量：
  - 过度通气；
  - 头高位；
  - 停止吸入麻醉剂（和其他脑血管收缩剂）；
  - 巴比妥类药物；
  - 镇静剂和肌肉松弛剂。

（吴 玮 译 盛 颖 校）

延伸阅读

Albin MS, editor: *Textbook of neuroanesthesia with neurosurgical and neuroscience perspectives*, New York, 1997, McGraw-Hill, pp 61–117. 1137–1177.

Chesnut RM, Temkin N, Carney N, et al.: A trial of intracranial-pressure monitoring in traumatic brain injury, *N Engl J Med* 367:2471–2481, 2012.

Fahy BG, Sivaraman V: Current concepts in neurocritical care, *Anesth Clin North Am* 20:441–462, 2002.

Le Roux P, Menon DK, Citerio G, et al.: The International Multidisciplinary Consensus Conference on Multimodality Monitoring in Neurocritical Care: a list of recommendations and additional conclusions: a statement for healthcare professionals from the Neurocritical Care Society and the European Society of Intensive Care Medicine, *Neurocrit Care* 21(Suppl 2): S282–S296, 2014.

Lele AV, Hoefnagel AL, Schloemerkemper N, et al.: Perioperative management of adult patients with external ventricular and lumbar drains: guidelines from the Society for Neuroscience in Anesthesia and Critical Care, *J Neurosurg Anesthesiol* 29(3):191–210, 2017.

Marik PE, Varon J, Trask T: Management of head trauma, *Chest* 122:699–711, 2002.

Robba C, Bacigaluppi S, Cardim D, et al.: Non-invasive assessment of intracranial pressure, *Acta Neurol Scand* 134(1):4–21, 2015.

Shafi S, Diaz-Arrastia R, Madden C, et al.: Intracranial pressure monitoring in brain-injured patients is associated with worsening of survival, *J Trauma* 64:335–340, 2008.

静脉给药系统

第 112 章

Rajamani Sethuraman

病例概要

患者，男性，35 岁，体重 90 kg，拟行下颌骨骨折修复术。在吸入氧气和空气下，患者接受丙泊酚和瑞芬太尼持续泵注的静脉麻醉 4 h。手术结束前 20 min，患者心率 130 次 / 分，血压 170/100 mmHg。手术结束后，患者苏醒时烦躁不安，给予吗啡 15 mg 缓解疼痛后逐渐平静。患者主诉术中意识清楚，可回忆起手术室内谈话。在手术结束撤除洞巾时，发现丙泊酚输注管路漏液。

问题分析

定义

该病例描述的患者苏醒时疼痛明显，是由瑞芬太尼和丙泊酚的再分布和清除所致。这两个因素在药物血药浓度下降中起重要作用，而血药浓度下降又受输注时间影响。由于丙泊酚输液管道漏液，患者主诉在手术麻醉中发生知晓。瑞芬太尼能快速被血浆酯酶消除，故瑞芬太尼的再分布并不特别重要。在开始输注前需单次推注一定剂量以产生给定药物血浆浓度，该单次剂量通过以下公式计算：

$$单次剂量 = Ct \times VD$$

其中，Ct 是目标浓度，VD 是给定药物的分布容积。VD 是表观分布容积，包括中央室和外周室的药物分布。随着输注时间延长，药物在两室之间达到稳态浓度，呈稳态分布容积。根据初始 VD 计算，则单次剂量会偏低，而使用最终 VD 计算则会剂量偏高。因此，此处引入药物峰值效应的 VD 这一概念，在达到峰值效应时血浆和效应部位的药物浓度相似。维持输注速度（maintenance infusion rate，MIR）计算如下：

$$MIR = Ct \times Cls$$

其中，Ct 是目标浓度，Cls 是清除率。

时量相关半衰期（context-sensitive half-time）是指维持血浆恒定浓度的连续输注停止后，药物血浆浓度降低 50% 所需的时间。当连续输注具有多室动力学的麻醉药时，需了解时量相关半衰期这一概念。此时，药物进出外周室的净分布因输注持续时间而变化。此处，“时量”是指输注时间（图 112.1）。在某些情况下，药物血浆浓度降低 50% 以上，可能更具临床意义。一个更通用的术语，时量相关递减时间，适用于这种情况。此处效应部位药物浓度的降低，正如血浆浓度下降所示，推测其可模拟效应部位浓度的降低。时量相关递减时间提供了一个有效的临床理论框架，便于理解药物输注时间和患者苏醒所需时间的关系（图 112.2）。

根据实际的给药方案，自动给药系统可精确预测血浆（或效应部位）药物浓度变化所需的时间。这

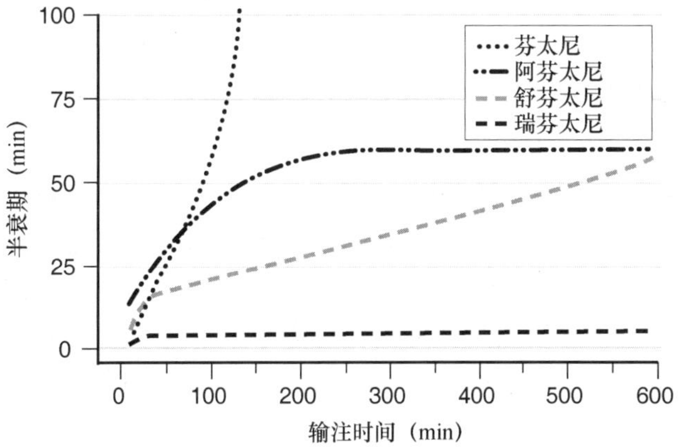

图 112.1 在模拟的药代动力学模型中，时量相关半衰期作为输注时间的函数（From Glass PA，Shafer SL，Reves JG：Intravenous drug delivery systems. In Miller RD，editor：*Anesthesia*，5th ed. New York，Churchill Livingstone，2000.）

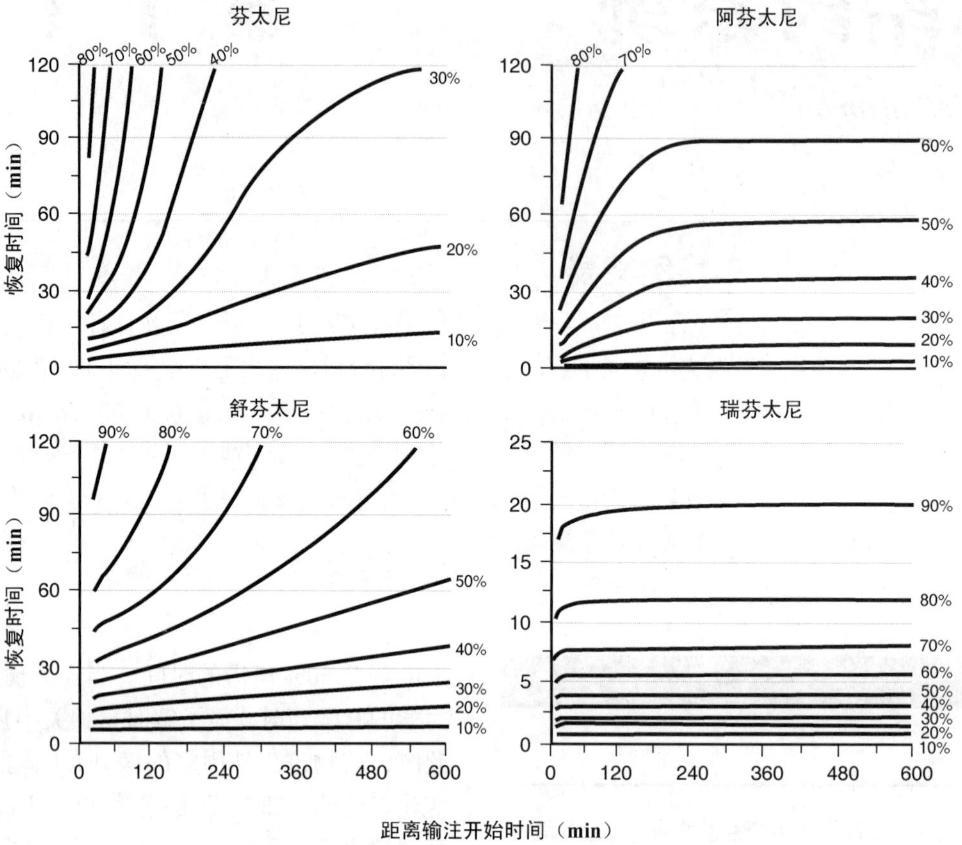

图 112.2 芬太尼、阿芬太尼、舒芬太尼和瑞芬太尼的恢复（递减时间）曲线显示，输注结束后术中效应部位浓度，从维持值下降到给定百分比（为每条曲线标记）所需的时间。给予负荷剂量后，需给予高输注速度应对再分布，然后再调整到最低的输注速度，以维持足够的麻醉或镇静深度。负荷剂量给予超过 5 ～ 10 min 可达到镇静效果，并根据患者反应进行调整。可联合应用咪达唑仑和阿片类药物，以达到麻醉效果（From Glass PA，Shafer SL，Reves JG：Intravenous drug delivery systems. In Miller RD，editor：*Anesthesia*，5th ed. New York，Churchill Livingstone，2000.）

些预测可帮助临床医师在合适的时间终止输注药物。不过，药物输注后动力学与消除半衰期无关。瑞芬太尼持续输注即为一个例证。即使在输注 3 h 后，瑞芬太尼的时量相关半衰期也短于其终末半衰期。据此我们可认为，瑞芬太尼是一种非时量相关的药物。

识别

阿片类药物使用过量可引起呼吸缓慢、心动过缓和瞳孔针尖样缩小。随着短效阿片类药物（如瑞芬太尼）的出现，如果过早终止输注，且未及时进行进一步镇痛，则可能出现相反的反应，就像本例患者。

了解所用药物的药代动力学很重要，但也不应该忽视系统设置中的实际错误。最常见的问题如下：

- 静脉管路断开；
- 静脉管路中存在空气；
- 管路闭塞；
- 注射泵电量过低；
- 注射器或药盒脱离；
- 管路断裂；
- 液体滴空。

另一可能影响麻醉起效和随后剂量调整的因素是输注管道距离患者的长度。当输液以背驮方式连接时，药物到达血液循环的速度与静脉流速直接相关，与输注连接点和静脉穿刺点之间的管道死腔容积量呈反比。因此，药物连接点应尽可能靠近静脉导管，以尽量减少静脉输液速度对药物输注的影响。鉴于上述问题，对静脉给药装置保持警觉非常重要。此外，较新型的输液泵还安装了发声警报器，当泵处于闲置状态、电池故障、空注射器及注射器变空前 3 min 时，会出现报警提示。

风险评估

时量相关半衰期和时量相关递减时间，在维持静脉药物输注的安全方面发挥着重要的作用。对大多数静脉麻醉药，患者在恢复清醒状态前需要降低 50% 浓度，门诊患者在安全离院前需要降低 80%～90% 浓度。药物消除半衰期通常一致性较好，时量相关半衰期和时量相关递减时间却并非如此。正如本病例概要所示，与其他阿片类药物相比，瑞芬太尼的代谢速度更快，且很少分布到外周室，故其时量相关递减时间更短。

与静脉给药系统使用相关的并发症，通常由人为过失导致。如果遵循常规检查清单，可将此类错误降至最低（表 112.1）。使用交流电源，使用专用的静脉管道，清除管道和注射器中的所有空气，并时刻保持警觉，可防止泵注中断。

表 112.1 静脉给药系统常见问题及推荐预防措施

问题	原因	预防措施
输注泵设置错误	浓度或速度错误	双人核对 使用预充式注射器或输液袋
	抽药或泵设置错误	复核单位及速度（如 mg/h 或 ml/h）
输注不足	设备故障	检查设备保修日期 检查注射器卡夹和输送机械运动是否平稳
	机械松弛导致启动延迟	正常情况下，开机时报警声响，进行自检
	输注管道有空气	冲洗并重启管路
	管路闭塞	检查静脉通路 检查是否需要增加堵塞压的上限
输注过量	设备故障	见上文
	虹吸作用	检查注射器是否破裂，注射器筒和柱塞是否紧密贴合 将输注泵放置在与患者相同的高度 应用抗虹吸阀
	闭塞后推注	在解除阻塞前，先释放管道压力 在第二管道中增加一个防回流阀
	推注药物治疗	输注泵与患者保持同一水平面 当注射器从输注泵上取出时，断开输液管
沟通	标签缺失或错误	使用正确的标签，颜色编码
	记录缺失或错误	检查注射量是否与注射剂量和持续时间相匹配
	在患者转移或移交治疗期间，信息缺失或不正确	在转移治疗前，提供完整及准确的患者病程资料

Modified from Keay S，Callander C：The safe use of infusion devices. *BJA Contin Educ Anaesth Crit Care Pain* 3：81-85，2004.

启示

目前已有商用靶控输注系统。靶控输注系统是全凭静脉麻醉系统，可设定所输药物的目标血浆和效应部位浓度。临床医师可根据患者人口数据（包括年龄、理想体重、身高和性别）来设置其所需目标浓度。一旦输液终止，该系统还可预测恢复时间。

较新的闭环输注系统可根据听觉诱发电位和脑电双频指数的反馈调整输液速度。在不久的将来，这些系统将成为日常麻醉实践的一部分。这些输注泵根据药代动力学模型的软件算法驱动，多种不同药物的药代动力学参数可在系统内编程。图 112.3 示意了旨在预防术中知晓的药代动力学药物输注系统的潜在错误来源。

不管使用何种药物，理解药代动力学十分重要，尤其是静脉输注药物。例如，与芬太尼、阿芬太尼和舒芬太尼相比，瑞芬太尼有完全不同的消除模式。在本文的病例概要中，由于未考虑到这种差异，患者苏醒时镇痛效果不佳。药物意外中断还导致患者术中知晓。

管理

药物输注失败时，可从以下几个方面寻找原因：

- 输注泵是否工作？
- 输注泵中药物是否减少？
- 输注的液体是否通畅？
- 连接是否紧密且无泄露？
- 血管通路是否通畅？

如不能迅速识别和纠正故障原因，就应改用另一种麻醉技术，以尽量降低患者术中知晓的风险。如果患者因过早停止输注而出现疼痛，应酌情进行追加镇痛和麻醉。贴牌和预充式注射器的使用，避免了与商用靶控输注系统的不兼容性。靶控输注系统用于不同患者时需重新设置；否则，输注泵将使用错误的患者信息。全凭静脉麻醉输注泵的绝对性能误差（过度输注或输注不足）适中。使用全凭静脉麻醉时必须维持足够的麻醉深度，尤其当患者处于肌松状态时。使用麻醉深度监测仪如脑电双频指数、听觉诱发电位，熵指数合临床指标变化，可以

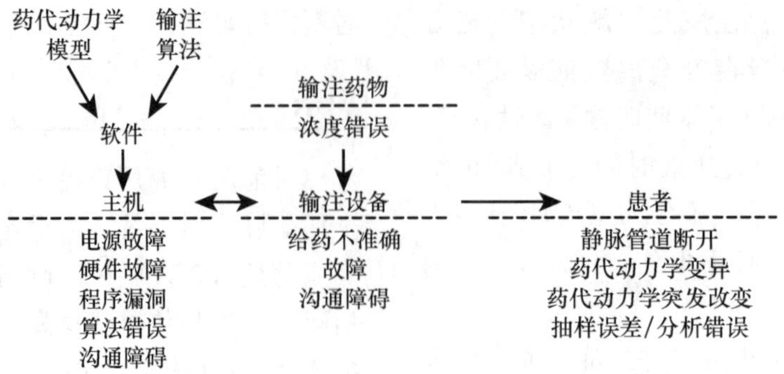

图 112.3 商用的靶控输液系统将计算机功能集成到设备中。图中示意了基于药代动力学模型的药物输注系统的潜在错误来源（From Glass PA，Shafer SL，Reves JG：Intravenous drug delivery systems. In Miller RD，editor：*Anesthesia*，5th ed. New York，Churchill Livingstone，2000.）

避免麻醉知晓。表 112.1 中列出了潜在问题和相关知识，有助于避免大部分错误。

预防

如果根据初始分布容积计算负荷剂量，给予的剂量可能不准确。计算输注速度时，应将其他隔室平衡和清除考虑在内。滴定剂量和输注速度，应根据临床需求进行调整。随着时间推移，当外周室与血浆浓度平衡时，必须降低输注速度，以维持效应部位的所需浓度。了解药物和患者的药代动力学和动态特征，通过滴定输注达到特定效应，可以实现这一目标，这与使用吸入麻醉药呼气末浓度分析仪类似。与后者不同的是，目前尚无血浆药物浓度实时分析仪。对输液管道、注射器、输液泵和临床参数保持持续的警觉，有助于避免给药过量或不足的问题。表 112.2 列举了部分给药方案。熟悉静脉药物输注系统，将避免在药物浓度的峰值和谷值间歇性给药，有助于最终改善患者血流动力学的稳定性和复苏时间，减少静脉药物用量并提高患者满意度。

（王树欣 译 张丽君 校）

延伸阅读

Eyres R: Update on TIVA, *Pediatr Anesth* 14:374–379, 2004.

Glass PSA, Shafer SL, Reves JG: Intravenous drug delivery systems. In Miller RD, editor: *Anesthesia*, ed 5, New York, 2000, Churchill Livingstone.

Kapila A, Glass PSA, Jacobs J, et al.: Measured context sensitive half-times of remifentanil and alfentanil, *Anesthesiology* 83:968–975, 1995.

Keay S, Callander C: The safe use of infusion devices, *BJA Contin Educ Anaesth Crit Care Pain* 3:81–85, 2004.

Leslie K, Absalom A, Kenny GNC: Closed loop control of sedation for colonoscopy using the bispectral index, *Anaesthesia* 57:693–697, 2002.

Milne SE, Kenny GNC: Future applications for TCI anaesthesia, *Anaesthesia* 53:56–60, 1998.

表 112.2 吸入 66%N_2O 和 O_2 时的人工输注方案

	麻醉		镇静或镇痛	
药物	负荷剂量（μg/kg）	维持剂量 [μg/（kg · min）]	负荷剂量（μg/kg）	维持剂量 [μg/（kg · min）]
阿芬太尼	50 ～ 150	0.5 ～ 3	10 ～ 25	0.25 ～ 1
芬太尼	5 ～ 15	0.03 ～ 0.1	1 ～ 3	0.01 ～ 0.03
舒芬太尼	0.25 ～ 2	0.01 ～ 0.05	0.1 ～ 0.5	0.005 ～ 0.01
瑞芬太尼	0.5 ～ 1	0.1 ～ 0.4	[a]	0.025 ～ 0.1
氯胺酮	1500 ～ 2500	25 ～ 75	500 ～ 1000	10 ～ 20
丙泊酚	1000 ～ 2000	50 ～ 150	250 ～ 1000	10 ～ 50
咪达唑仑	50 ～ 150	0.25 ～ 1.5	25 ～ 100	0.25 ～ 1
美索比妥	1000 ～ 1500	50 ～ 150	250 ～ 1000	10 ～ 50

[a] 静脉镇静时无负荷剂量

激光并发症

第113章

Arul Prakash Pandian James

病例概要

患者，男性，75岁，因转移性非小细胞肺癌，在全身麻醉下使用激光行支气管镜下肿瘤消融术。患者临床表现为慢性无痰咳嗽，计算机断层扫描显示肿瘤侵犯右侧支气管。

问题分析

定义

过去10年间，由于激光技术的改进、可靠性的提高以及成本的降低，医疗激光的应用越来越多。激光是通过激发原子发射光子以一束连续的单色光束的形式提供无菌的、强烈的能量。医疗激光对患者和手术室（operating room，OR）人员也存在某些危害，包括空气污染、组织结构或血管意外穿孔、点燃易燃材料和栓塞。

对于医疗激光，虽然没有联邦安全要求，但有国家安全标准。国家安全标准的制定是为了减少和防止激光事故。激光危害从无风险到重大风险，分为四个风险等级。医疗激光属于最高风险等级，必须由经过专业培训的人员，在有防护设备的前提下进行正确操作。

识别

医疗激光有好几种类型。其差异在于所用媒介和产生的波长不同（表113.1）。激光除共有的危害外，不同类型的激光有其独特风险。例如，二氧化碳（CO_2）激光的波长处于远红外线范围，可被其遇到的第一表面吸收，故需要对患者和手术室人员进行眼睛保护以防角膜损伤。

氩、KTP：YAG和Nd：YAG在可见光和近红外线范围内可以通过透明材料传输，并被色素组织吸收，在穿透角膜后可损伤视网膜组织。

激光危害可分为光束相关和非光束相关的危害。非光束相关的危害包括电击和激光产生的空气污染。与光束相关的危害包括血管穿孔、气管插管的套囊

表113.1　常用激光及其相关风险

媒介	波长（nm）	颜色	特性	潜在风险
CO_2	10600	远红外线	易被所有生物组织吸收；非常精确、表面穿透力强；非光纤传输	角膜损伤
钬：YAG	2060 2140（脉冲）	红外线	精确切割；热能扩散少；止血好；光纤传输	角膜损伤；可穿透金属
Nd；YAG	1064	近红外线	可光纤传输；采用光凝加热；组织穿透力强	晚期并发症发生率高；脑水肿；组织脱落；视网膜损伤
红宝石	694	红	可被色素吸收（血红蛋白除外）	视网膜损伤
氦-氖	632	红	可用作 CO_2 和Nd：YAG激光的瞄准光束	无害，除非直射眼睛
KTP：Nd：YAG	532	绿	光纤传输；分散及坏死（小于Nd：YAG）	类似于Nd：YAG（较少的视网膜损伤和组织穿透）
氩	488，514	蓝/绿	光纤传输；可被血红蛋白和色素组织吸收	视网膜损伤

破裂和热损伤。使用某些激光后可能会出现延迟的并发症。尤其是 Nd：YAG 激光，当穿透深度超过预期，在激光照射后几小时至几天内，组织坏死和水肿达到最大程度时，就会出现出血或穿孔。

风险评估

在使用激光束时，必须保护患者和手术室人员免受激光危害。反射光束可以照射到非目标区域，造成眼睛损伤、易燃材料着火或烧伤。

在气道手术中使用激光时，气道燃烧是最常见的严重并发症，导致严重病残甚至死亡。激光与易燃的气管导管接触会发生燃烧，在富含氧气的气道环境中，点燃的烟雾可导致更巨大的破坏。吸入 1 g 组织蒸发产生的烟雾相当于吸食 6 支未经过滤的香烟。这种烟雾或“激光烟雾”可能是病毒传播的一种载体，但目前尚无医务人员因此感染疾病的文献支持。

启示

激光的临床应用在过去数年大幅增加。成本低和可靠性强使医疗激光在各类手术应用中具有吸引力。除了切除肿瘤，激光还用于治疗良性前列腺增生、黄斑变性、冠状动脉成形术，以及治疗各种皮肤病和眼科疾病。然而，医疗激光使用的增加导致并发症随之增加。激光需要训练有素的高技能人员操作。他们必须时刻保持警惕，能够预测相关风险并采取措施保护患者和其他医务人员。如果及时并妥善处理，并发症通常轻微且可治疗。

管理

气道燃烧是激光治疗的最严重并发症。为尽量减少此类并发症，手术室团队必须行动迅速、协调一致，采取以下措施：

- 断开氧源，移除燃烧的气管导管和其他物品；
- 使用生理盐水灭火；
- 在纯氧条件下行面罩通气继续麻醉；
- 使用诊断性喉镜或硬支气管镜检查气道损伤程度；
- 去除一切杂物；
- 如果出现气道损伤，重新气管插管；
- 如果损伤严重或再插管失败，考虑气管切开；
- 必要时行机械通气；
- 必要时采用激素治疗；
- 拍摄胸部 X 线片。

手术巾单具有防火性，但如果被点燃则很难熄灭，因为它们也具有防水性。使用手术巾单时，应配备灭火器。任何手术室人员受伤，必须采取适当的治疗措施并生成事件报告。同时应调查此类事件发生的原因以杜绝再次发生。

预防

预防取决于需要避免哪些特定的并发症。只有受过专业培训，获得激光使用证书，具备安全防护措施的人员才能操作激光。在使用过程中，应保护手术室人员免受已知的激光危害。

眼睛防护

由于眼睛最容易受伤，所有人员都必须戴上合适的护目镜。建议使用带侧护板的环绕式护目镜，而标准眼镜不能挡住侧面的反射光束，隐形眼镜几乎没有保护作用。护目镜片必须能够吸收所使用的特定激光波长。透明镜片适用于 CO_2 激光，但对于其他激光，镜片必须着色。

患者的眼睛必须受到保护。清醒的患者应佩戴激光防护眼镜。如果不是手术部位，必须使麻醉后的患者的眼睛闭合，并用盐水浸湿的纱布或非闪耀金属护罩覆盖。

除 CO_2 激光以外的所有激光都能穿透透明玻璃，所以手术室窗户必须采取防护。在所有手术室入口处的显著位置应放置警示标志以提醒正在使用激光，并且所有入口处都应配备护目镜。

穿孔风险

当不指向目标组织时，应将激光束关闭或设置为待机模式。错误定向的激光束可能导致空腔脏器的意外穿孔。

在激光血管成形术期间，可导致冠状动脉穿孔，造成严重并发症（如心脏压塞、急性心肌梗死、紧急的冠状动脉旁路手术）。目前，这种穿孔发生的风险接近 1%。

穿孔并发症有可能在术后数天才发生。也有报道使用激光后导致空气栓塞及严重并发症。

皮肤损伤

避免激光长时间对非目标区域皮肤照射。手术部位附近的皮肤应采用湿润的巾单保护。与角膜相比，皮肤有一层角质细胞可减少激光损伤。

环境危害

激光烟雾（如前所述）会产生难闻的气味，可导致流泪或支气管刺激，也可能会成为病毒载体。通过使用高效烟雾排出器和使用特殊的激光防护口罩，可以最大限度地减少这种烟雾的吸入。然而，这种口罩在潮湿时需要定期更换。此外，对于由激光产生的空气中的碎片，一些激光防护口罩可能也无法提供全面的保护。

气道燃烧

目前尚无预防措施可以保证不发生气道燃烧。如果可能，可将吹气技术或喷射通气用于气道手术，但必须密切监测患者以防发生气压伤和胃扩张。

通过使用防激光气管插管，即在传统气管导管上包裹金属箔，或者商用金属导管，都可降低气管导管的可燃性。金属箔包裹的导管边缘比较粗糙，易磨损气管组织，还可能存在缝隙，暴露可燃部分。金属导管的套囊具有易燃性。金属导管弹性较差，内径较小，通气相对困难，且价格昂贵。当导管套囊破裂时，应注入染色的生理盐水进行标识。气管导管周围放置湿润的棉絮也可预防燃烧。

在维持患者足够的血氧饱和度的条件下，尽量降低吸入氧浓度。应禁止使用笑气，因其具有助燃作用。

致谢

感谢 Pattricia Klarr 博士对本章上一版的贡献。

（郑　敏　译　张丽君　校）

延伸阅读

Brown SG: Science, medicine, and the future: new techniques in laser therapy, *BMJ* 316:754–757, 1998.

Kestenbaum A: New revision of ANSI Z136.1 (laser safety standards), *LIA Today* 8(3), May 8, 2000. Available at http://hps.org/hpspublications/articles/ansiz136.1.html. Accessed September 23, 2016.

Koster R, Kahler J, Brockhoff C, et al.: Laser coronary angioplasty: history, present and future, *Am J Cardiovasc Drugs* 2:197–207, 2002.

Laser Institute of America: Laser safety information bulletin. Available at https://www.lia.org/subscriptions/safety_bulletin/laser_safety_info/. Accessed September 23, 2016.

Rampil IJ: Anesthesia for laser surgery. In Miller RD, editor: *Anesthesia*, ed 5, New York, 2000, Churchill Livingstone, pp 2199–2212.

第 114 章 机械通气设备

Brian J. Woodcock

病例概要

患者，男，68 岁，100 kg，行全麻气管插管，确认过双侧呼吸音。呼吸机设定参数为：潮气量 600 ml，通气频率为 10 次 / 分，吸呼比 1∶2。2 min 后，脉搏血氧仪音调降低警示麻醉科医师发现患者无胸廓起伏。通气设备似运转正常，麻醉科医师拿起听诊器，准备调节切换阀为手控，但发现阀门已处于手控位置。

问题分析

定义

手控通气一段时间后，未将呼吸机从手控通气切换到机控通气，是大量机械通气设备并发症的根源，可能对患者造成严重影响。在美国麻醉科医师协会（American Society of Anesthesiologists，ASA）关于已结案的麻醉不良事件索赔案的分析中，错误使用通气设备或操作者失误引起麻醉不良事件是设备故障的 3 倍。

通气设备误用或操作者失误的示例如下：

- 手控通气一段时间后未打开机控呼吸；
- 按患者体型设定的呼吸频率或潮气量不合适；
- 对于患者体型，最大压力限制设置得太高；
- 最大压力限制设置得太低，导致潮气量低；
- 不适当的吸-呼比；
- 气体流量高导致潮气量增加；
- 在通气设备吸气期间快速充氧；
- 操作者关闭压力、容量或吸入氧浓度（fraction of inspired oxygen，FiO_2）报警，以致察觉故障延迟。

设备故障或组装不正确可能包括以下原因：

- 风箱破损；
- 风箱安装不正确，使风箱和套管之间不密封；
- 电气或机械故障，机器停止运转；
- 无压力、呼吸暂停或 FiO_2 的故障报警。

呼吸机故障的其他原因还出现在麻醉机方面。这些并发症在其他章节有详细介绍，包括：气体驱动压力失效（见第 116 章），呼吸环路断开、通气活瓣粘连和呼吸环路管道的错误连接（见第 105 章）以及清除系统方面的错误（见第 120 章）。

识别

未能识别并及时纠正通气设备问题可能会产生灾难性后果。在 ASA 已结案的索赔分析中，12 例与通气设备问题有关，7 例导致死亡，5 例导致脑损伤。在通气设备工作异常后可供发现并纠正的时间窗很短，如不能在此窗口期及时发现并纠正，很快会产生不良生理事件。

打开呼吸机

实际上不能打开呼吸机较为常见，这通常发生于快速诱导后，可能持续数分钟都不会被注意到。

如果机控-手控开关尚未切换到机控位置，则会出现以下征象：

- 呼气末二氧化碳（end-tidal carbon dioxide，$ETCO_2$）波形消失；
- 激活 $ETCO_2$ 呼吸暂停报警；
- 如果关闭 APL 阀，储气球囊会膨胀、气道压上升。

如果呼吸机尚未打开但机控-手控开关已切换到机控位置，则显示如下：

- 无 $ETCO_2$ 波形；
- 无气道压力显示；
- 激活呼吸暂停压力报警和 $ETCO_2$ 报警。

呼吸机频率和潮气量的设定

潮气量或呼吸频率设置不当可能导致过度通气或通气不足，从而导致 $ETCO_2$ 下降或上升。对于儿童或体型较小成人，由于潮气量和胸膜腔内压增加导致的静脉回流减少可导致低血压。也可能发生气压伤，伴有气胸或皮下气肿。若成人患者按儿童的通气参数设置，最显著的特征是通气不足，包括气道峰压低，如果通气严重不足，则引起 $ETCO_2$ 升高和氧饱和度下降。

压力限制

高压限制设置不当可能会导致过大的潮气量和压力，导致气压伤。低压限制设置可能导致潮气量不足和高碳酸血症。

吸-呼比

当呼吸机频率异常时，可能会产生不合适的吸-呼比。例如，在手术结束时，设置较低的通气频率可使患者 $PaCO_2$ 升高。通气频率较低时，1∶2 的吸-呼比可能导致吸气时间过度延长。

新鲜气流

在患者插管后未能将新鲜气体流量设置降低可能导致患者过度通气。在吸气期间，设定的风箱潮气量还会加入回路的新鲜气体。例如，当新鲜气体流量为 10 L/min，呼吸率为 10 次 / 分，吸-呼比为 1∶2，每次潮气量会比预设值大 333 mL 以上。如果最大压力限制设置得太高，可能会导致小体型患者出现严重的过度通气或气压伤。

在吸气期间按下快速充氧按钮会导致大量气体进入患者，造成的气压伤可导致气胸形成。

呼吸机报警

呼吸机有两个报警设置，**呼吸机报警**和**压力阈值报警限值**（threshold pressure alarm limit，TPAL）报警。呼吸机报警有两个按钮，“报警静音”按钮和“报警关闭”按钮。在手控通气期间，按“静音报警”按钮可以防止呼吸暂停一段时间后呼吸机报警发出声音。当使用手控通气或在有限时间内暂停通气时，应按下“报警静音”按钮以取消该报警 60 s 或 120 s。如果操作者按下呼吸机“报警关闭”按钮，该按钮会无限期地停止呼吸机报警，若操作者未能重新激活，则消除呼吸机报警自动恢复的功能。

TPAL 报警显示了吸气时气道压力水平。但这是可调整的，它应设置低于吸气峰压（≤ 5 cmH_2O）。这样系统泄漏导致吸气峰压降低时就会触发报警，而不是要等到波形完全丧失时才报警（图 114.1）。当为

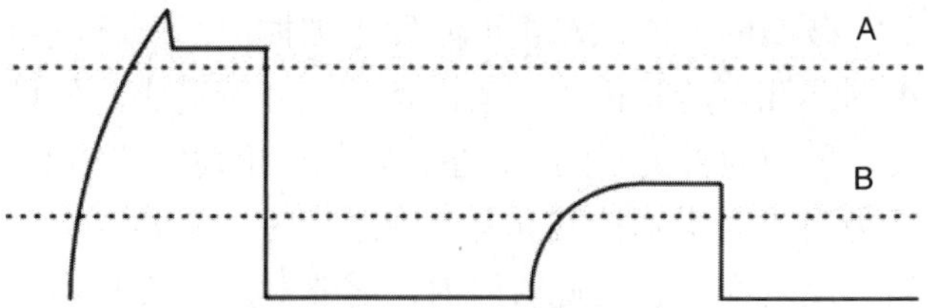

图 114.1 压力阈值报警限值（TPAL；虚线）描绘了吸气时所检测到的气道压力水平。当 TPAL 可调节时，应将其数值设置在比吸气峰压下低于 5 cmH_2O（设定 A）的范围内。在 TPAL 设置正确的情形下，如同在气道呼吸环路系统漏气（第二次呼吸）时发生的一样，系统将会检测到气道峰压降低的呼吸，视其为没有呼吸，如果情况继续会触发呼吸暂停警报。但是，如果 TPAL 过低（设置 B），系统会检测到呼吸减少，但呼吸机不会警报声音。当系统中的泄漏导致吸气峰压下降时，适当高的 TPAL 设置可允许触发警报，即使有气道压力波形的情况下也可触发

当前压力峰值设置的压力报警过低时，Narkomed 2B 麻醉机会发出（无声的）建议性通知。

呼吸机报警应被视为手术室中最重要的报警。一旦报警响起，警惕的麻醉科医师应会有不适感。即使报警的原因是已知的和可预料的（例如，在手术结束时，拮抗肌松后切换到自主通气），也不应允许持续报警而无人顾及。应纠正任何呼吸机报警状况，或将报警重置为患者当前最新状况的合适水平。同样，当手术结束患者离开手术室时，也不能任由机器持续报警。

呼吸机风箱

风箱中出现泄露口可以通过以下方式识别：

- 吸入麻醉气体的浓度降低；
- 如果驱动气体为 O_2，则 FiO_2 升高；
- 如果驱动气体是空气或空氧混合物，则 FiO_2 下降；
- 过度通气或通气不足。

如果风箱安装不当或风箱中有漏口，则用于给风箱提供驱动力的 O_2 直接与回路气体相通。由于驱动气体有较高压力，它进入风箱并与回路气体混合。因此，它会稀释回路中的麻醉气体并升高 FiO_2；如果使用空气作为驱动气体，在这种情况下 FiO_2 会下降（见第 116 章）。风箱泄漏的主要结果是在使用快速充氧阀后无法保持正常容积。尽管这种故障可能导致通气不足，但更可能的是，驱动气体会导致患者过度通气。发生这种情况是因为风箱运动不足以操控感应机制，导致呼吸机持续输送大量气体。此外，如果呼吸环路断开或泄漏，风箱可能在呼气期间掺杂室内空气。

破旧的老式风箱更可能发生破损泄漏。新风箱中的漏孔可能是由于厂家检查不充分所造成。如果安装风箱的人员不熟悉设备，可能会出现安装错误。因为当成人手术接在儿科手术之后时，需要改变风箱，反之亦然，在此时间内，需要对风箱安装的相关问题保持警惕。

呼吸机故障

呼吸机控制组件出现电气或机械问题是导致呼吸机故障的主要原因。总电路故障容易识别，但由于内部泄漏或阀门通气活瓣故障导致的部分机械问题可能更难以识别。

风险评估

某些情况与呼吸机问题的风险增加有关。在下列情况下，可能会出现设置呼吸机开关或转换阀错误：

- 诱导后不久；
- 经过一段时间的手控通气后；
- 当麻醉科医师分心时；
- 当存在多个麻醉管理人员时。

最大风险的时期是在诱导结束且听诊确认双肺呼吸音之后，麻醉科医师因放置其他监测装置或患者的血流动力学不稳定而分散注意力。因为长时间未使用呼吸机，冠状动脉搭桥术后恢复通气是另一个高风险期。“麻醉科医师反比率”表明，给予患者的监护程度与麻醉科医师数量成反比。当存在多名麻醉人员时，每个人都可能认为其他人已经打开了呼吸机。

不适当的呼吸机设置通常发生在成人手术后开始儿科手术或在儿科手术后开始成人手术时。潮气量或通气频率的错误设置会导致不适合该患者的分钟通气量。体型非常小的儿科患者采用成年人的呼吸机设置时会出现高度风险。患儿发生气压伤的风险非常高，继发于高吸气压和过度通气。相反，成年人采用儿童通气参数模式有严重通气不足的风险。

启示

这里讨论的大多数问题最终导致通气异常，如高碳酸血症或低碳酸血症。长期无通气可能导致缺氧。缺氧发生之前的时间长短不一，这取决于呼吸暂停前的 FiO_2 和患者的呼吸状态。其他并发症包括由于静脉回流减少导致的严重低血压和过度充气引起的显著的气压伤。

管理

对任何与机械通气相关问题的第一反应是立即

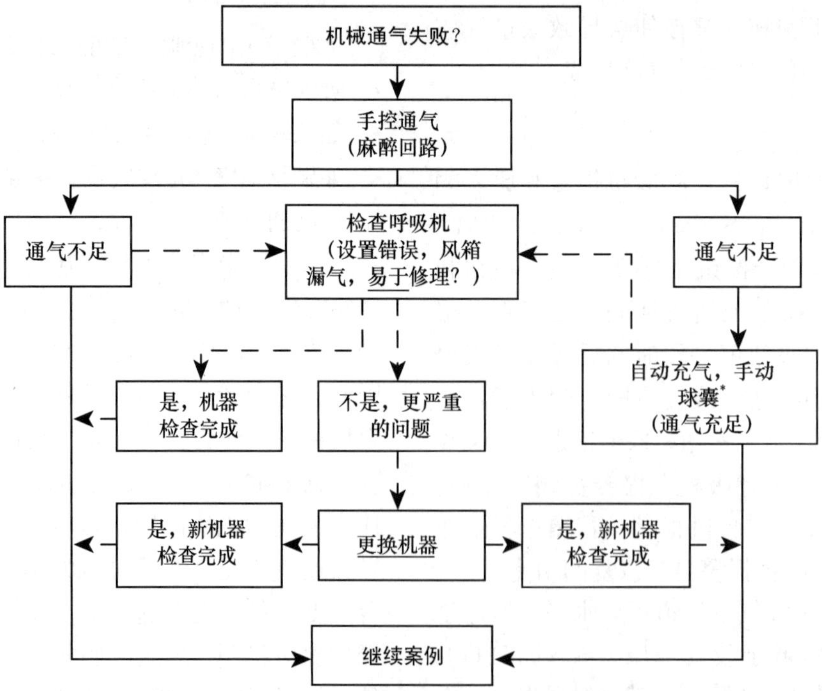

图 114.2 对于机械通气问题而建议的操作规程示意图。* 如果不能立即使用手控球囊通气，则经口对气管导管通气。实线，立即行动；虚线，补救行动。不可修理在使用中的机器

切换到手控通气（图 114.2）。

首先，这是使用麻醉回路完成的。如果患者仍然没有充分通气，则使用自充气手控复苏球囊或经口对气管导管进行通气。一旦建立了手控通气，就可以对呼吸机全面检查故障原因。应该确认对该患者的呼吸机设置是否正确；如果不正确，应该重置。如果风箱中有漏孔，应立即更换风箱，或更换麻醉机。在手术室修理正在使用的机器永远是不妥的行为。

预防

预防与机械通气设备有关的问题取决于以下方面：

- 操作者（麻醉科医师）的警惕性；
- 监测气道压力和呼气量，并正确设置报警；
- 熟练操作日常维护；
- 按照美国食品药品管理局指南，在每个手术之前执行彻底的检查程序：
  - 如果存在切换阀，请分别在手控和机控模式下检测其功能；
  - 必要时关闭 APL 阀（airway pressure leak，气道压力泄漏），并在患者端阻塞系统；
  - 通过适当的呼吸周期进行漏气和压力释放试验（具体流程因呼吸机的类型而异）；
  - 在环路的面罩端上连接储气球囊，将气体注满系统，然后让呼吸机进行周期性工作，确保球囊正常膨胀和排空。

（阮林星 译 马 宇 校）

延伸阅读

Brockwell RC, Andrews JJ: Complications of inhaled anesthesia delivery systems, *Anesthesiol Clin North Am* 20:539–554, 2002.

Brockwell RC, Andrews JJ: Inhaled anesthetic delivery systems. In Miller RD, editor: *Miller's anesthesia*, ed 6, Philadelphia, 2005, Churchill Livingstone, pp 298–303.

Caplan RA, Vistica MF, Posner KL, et al.: Adverse anesthetic outcomes arising from gas delivery equipment: a closed claims analysis, *Anesthesiology* 87:741–748, 1997.

Dorsch JA, Dorsch SE: *Understanding anesthesia equipment*, Philadelphia, 1999, Lippincott Williams & Wilkins.

Ehrenwerth J, Eisenkraft J: *Anesthesia equipment: principles and applications*, St. Louis, 2004, Mosby–Year Book.

第115章 患者加温系统

Michael P. Eaton

病例概要

患者，男性，76岁，因右侧回肠动脉损伤急诊入手术室行开腹修复术。术中，患者身下置入加温毯，其与功能正常的强制通风加热系统相连，并设置为最高温度（43℃）。术后，医护人员发现患者右下肢后内侧发生部分和全层烧伤。

问题分析

定义

众所周知，围术期低体温与病残率显著增加相关。因此预防低体温是麻醉管理的重要目标之一，但低体温防护装置在使用过程中并非没有风险。此类装置导致的主要并发症是组织烧伤，其他并发症包括体温过高、体温过低（与设备设定错误或设备运行故障有关）、触电和潜在感染。

患者加温装置可分为两大类：①装置本身的设计并非用于给患者加温，却被用来为患者加温；②装置本身为预防和处理低体温专门设计和制造。美国麻醉科医师协会（American Society of Anesthesiologists，ASA）关于患者加温装置所致损伤的结案索赔分析指出，大多数索赔都属于第一类产品。这类产品包括以下：

- 加热的静脉注射液袋；
- 加热的冲洗瓶或其他液体；
- 重复使用的“热袋”。

专门设计和制造用于预防和处理体温过低的设备，包括：

- 循环水毯；
- 电阻加热垫/毯；
- 强制通风加热毯；
- 辐射加热器；
- 普通或反光毯；
- 呼吸回路加热加湿器；
- 静脉输液加温器。

最后一个设备即静脉输液加温器，将在第119章中讨论。表115.1列出了部分加热装置导致损伤的发病机制、风险因素和预防措施等。

识别

连续监测核心温度可以识别患者术中是否发生体温过低和体温过高。按照现有的ASA标准，预计出现体温不稳定的患者应按要求进行体温监测。

遗憾的是，手术患者的烧伤通常在术后才会被识别，这对预防损伤来说为时已晚。通常，患者会主诉烧伤部位的疼痛。由于术后患者常需镇痛药物治疗手术相关疼痛，因此会掩盖与烧伤相关的疼痛并延误诊断。一旦使用加温装置，手术结束时医护人员都应对患者背部或其他接触部位进行检查。该检查通常由手术室护士在患者转运时完成，但团队所有成员都应认识到此项工作的重要性。早期识别有利于采取积极治疗，从而预防可能危及患者生命的潜在感染。

风险评估

不同患者群体使用这两类加温装置的风险不尽相同。近期，通过对加热静脉注射溶液袋相关烧伤的结案索赔分析，发现患者通常是女性、年龄38岁左右、术前并未预料到患者术中可能发生明显的低体温。导致风险的主要因素是使用了那些并非用于患者加温的装置。这些溶液袋通常保存在温度调节不佳的加热毯或烘箱中，或是由不能进行温度控制的微波炉加热所致。一项关于医院使用加热静脉注

表 115.1 与患者加温装置相关的损伤

设备	损伤机制	风险因素	预防措施
加热静脉注射溶液袋	传导传热	过度加热的液体	不使用
电阻加热垫	传导传热触电	温度设置过高 设备故障	仅限于清醒警觉患者 设置为最低有效温度
导电织物毯 / 垫循环水毯	传导传热	设备磨损 / 维护不当 患者组织灌注不足	每次使用前检查 做好日常维护
导电织物毯	传导传热	机器热量输出过高 机器故障	覆盖在患者身上，而非垫于身下（减少压力性损伤） 设置为最低有效温度 每次使用前检查 做好日常维护
加热灯	辐射传热	离患者过近 改装灯具	按照设备说明书维持患者与设备之间的距离 使用厂方推荐的扩散器或灯泡
强制通风加温装置	对流传热	未使用毯子或使用错误的毯子 PACU 使用机器或设置温度过高 患者组织灌注不良	仅使用同一厂家或制造商的毯子 仅使用已经获批在手术室内使用的装置并设置为最低有效温度 对血管功能不全的患者设置较低的温度 不在止血带或阻断的远端使用

射溶液袋的围术期调查发现，有数家机构允许将这些液体袋加热至 50℃以上。有两家医院将袋子保存在高于 70℃环境下，而机体暴露在这一温度几秒钟内即可导致烧伤（图 115.1）。

患者加温装置导致的损伤，更可能与患者自身或设备故障或误用有关。先前针对美国食品药品管理局的制造商和用户设施设备经验（Manufacturer and User-Facility Device Experience，MAUDE） 数据库进行的一次检索表明，使用某公司强制通风加温设备造成的损伤中，在 30 起案件中有 24 起可以确定损伤的原因是，在设备使用期间未使用加热毯（仅有软管）或使用时违反了制造商的推荐。

常见的与损伤相关的患者因素是，与加温装置接触部位的局部组织灌注不良。这类伤害通常以骨性突出区域（压力点）最为严重。对行血管手术（如该病例患者）、糖尿病及心肺转流术的患者，发生与加热设备相关的热损伤风险会有所增加。这些患者往往因疾病状态、手术或体外循环导致相应区域组织灌注较差，而血流不足又可影响到施加热量的重新分布，最终导致部分区域温度达到损伤程度。加温装置接触皮肤部位的压力也会影响该处灌注并增加受伤可能性。在水循环系统引起的伤害报告中，接触点的压力也是影响因素。

极端年龄患者发生热损伤风险的可能性增加，

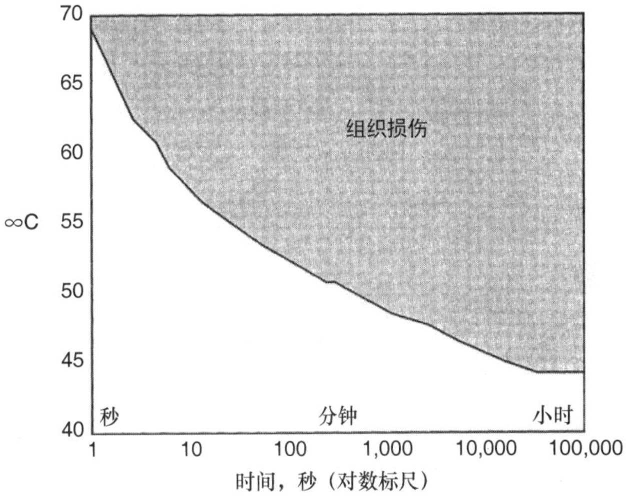

图 115.1 在不同温度下接触物体导致烧伤所需的时间（Data from Moritz AR，Henriques FC Jr：Studies of thermal injury. II. The relative importance of time and surface temperature in the causation of cutaneous burns. *Am J Pathol* 23[5]：695-720，1947.）

主要与该类患者术中发生低体温的风险增加，以及因此导致的使用加温装置的可能性增加。另外，还因为该类患者也存在发生组织灌注不足的问题。

设备日常维护不当或没有按照厂房说明书使用设备，则设备故障可能会给患者造成伤害。如果设备允许的偏差超过组织安全吸收和转移热量的能力，则即使设备得到正确使用和维护也可能会产生伤害。此类损伤尤其可能发生在当加温装置和患者存在高温度梯度时。部分常用的循环水毯即使经过相应的校准和维护，其允许的水温也高达48℃。而当温度超过45℃时，就可能引起热损伤，其损伤程度取决于暴露时间（见图115.1）。

患者加温系统需要高压电流，当设备维护不良或被液体污染时可能导致设备过热并引起火灾，对医护人员和患者都会构成危险。虽然隔离电力系统触电的可能性较小，但触电仍是电气设备故障的另一风险。

最近有许多报告称，强制通风加温装置（forced-air warming，FAW）会增加感染风险，特别是对于关节置换手术。目前所有34份关于某FAW制造商的MAUDE数据库报告中，均有手术部位感染（surgical site infection，SSI），由此导致了对设备制造商的诉讼。尽管有医疗事故律师和一些竞争产品制造商的证词，但FAW和SSI之间的联系尚未得到证实。使用FAW可能会破坏手术室内清洁高效微粒空气过滤的层流效果，但最近的两篇回顾指出，尚无足够证据可以证明FAW和SSI之间存在联系。由此得出的两大重要结论是：①该领域相关研究的质量较差；②目前FAW是维持体温的最常用方法，该方法已经被证明可降低SSI发生率，因此不能因为担心伤口污染而简单地弃用FAW。

启示

施行血管大手术或涉及心肺转流术的患者通常心血管储备功能下降，因此严重烧伤可能成为致命并发症。不太严重的烧伤也可能导致严重病残。出于好意但加温方式错误也会给患者带来永久性毁容瘢痕，使医护人员面临严重的法律诉讼风险。

高热在导致患者心脏和呼吸做功和氧耗增加，对患者有限的生理储备造成过度应激。血管扩张和出汗可能引起相对或绝对血容量不足和酸中毒，代谢亢进状态可能引起低血糖。医源性高热可能被误诊为恶性高热，导致一系列的非必需治疗。极度高热可能导致中枢神经系统损伤和死亡。

手术部位感染是围术期发病率和死亡率的主要因素。发生SSI的患者住院时间显著延长，医疗成本大幅增加。据估计，美国在手术部位感染所花的医疗保险总费用为34亿至100亿美元。

管理

识别出患者发生烧伤后，立即将患者转诊至擅长烧伤治疗的医师非常重要。烧伤的正确处理在许多教科书都有介绍，这里不做进一步讨论。

高热的处理包括关闭或移除加温装置并将患者充分暴露于环境之中。除非过度加热是温度骤然升高的唯一原因，否则极少需要给予主动降温；另外，许多温度管理设备具备主动冷却与加热双重功能。如果患者温度骤升严重或对被动冷却无反应，则应寻找其他原因，如感染、脓毒症或恶性高热。

预防

患者加温装置相关损伤的最佳管理策略是预防。ASA对此类损伤的结案索赔分析发现，在28起案件中，除1例使用加热的静脉注射溶液袋导致烧伤外，其他17起案件都被认为是护理不符合标准。以下设备绝对不应使用：设计目的并不是用于患者加温的装置、无效的设备，可能会给患者带来不可接受的损伤高风险的设备。

经批准使用的患者加温装置造成的伤害更难预防，关注下述重要细节可能会减少伤害的发生：

- 所有设备应该按照制造商的推荐做好设备维护。
- 任何在日常维护中未通过安全检测的设备都应该立即停用。
- 负责患者管理的麻醉人员应该亲自检查所用设备的设置。
- 使用人员应该熟悉并遵守制造商提供的设备使用推荐。除非经制造商批准，否则不得对设备进行任何改装。
- 手术期间必须始终保持警惕，以确保加热装置中不能直接接触患者的部分，如水毯的管道或强制通风床垫的软管等部位不会接触患者。
- 如果可能，应在患者身体的上方而非下方使用水毯装置。一方面，这可以使灌注不良的组织与装置接触的风险最小化；另一方面，这也提高了装置的功效，因为患者的热量主要散失在手术间，而手术台床垫已经提供了足够的隔热。事实上，加温装置通常是通过减少或消除患者自身的代谢热量而不是通过外在加热起效的。
- 不得将压力（如来自体位辅助设备）施加在与导

热设备接触的身体部位。换言之，在患者按照计划的程序正确摆放体位之前，不应使用水毯或电阻毯。

- 不应将加温装置放置在止血带或血管阻断远端的身体任何部位，否则可能会产生较大的温度梯度而造成伤害。

致谢

感谢 Stewart Lustik 博士对本章上一版的贡献。

（张　婉　译　韩文军　校）

延伸阅读

Chaney FW, Posner KL, Caplan RA, et al.: Burns from warming devices in anesthesia: a closed claims analysis, *Anesthesiology* 80:806–810, 1994.

Crino MH, Nagel EL: Thermal burns caused by warming blankets in the operating room, *Anesthesiology* 29:149–150, 1968.

Moritz AR, Henriques Jr FC: Studies of thermal injury. II. The relative importance of time and surface temperature in the causation of cutaneous burns, *Am J Pathol* 23:695–720, 1947.

Raphael DT, Ayoub N: Storage of plastic intravenous solution bags in operating room warmers, *Anesth Analg* 84:S203, 1997.

Sessler DI: Perioperative thermoregulation and heat balance, *Lancet*, January 7, 2016. [epub ahead of print].

U.S. Food and Drug Administration: Manufacturer and User Facility Device Experience database (MAUDE). Available at http://www.accessdata.fda.gov/scripts/cdrh/cfdocs/cfMAUDE/search.cfm?searchoptions=1. Accessed August 29, 2017.

Wood AM, Moss C, Keenan A, et al.: Infection control hazards associated with the use of forced-air warming in operating theatres, *J Hosp Infect* 88:132–140, 2014.

第116章 管道源性故障

James F. Szocik

病例概要

这是医院新门诊手术室运营的第一天。麻醉科医师到岗上班，期待一整天的病例都是ASA Ⅰ级的门诊轻症患者。然而，在第一台手术过程中，他就听到微弱的啁啾声并伴有氧气供应不足的报警。几秒钟后，麻醉科医师注意到呼吸机风箱并没有充气，麻醉呼吸机周期性运行的声音消失，随即响起刺耳的报警声，包括呼吸暂停压力和容量报警以及分钟通气量报警。

问题分析

定义

管道故障通常有两种类型，定量问题主要表现为管道内压力过低或过高，定性问题则是管道内存在污染物（框116.1）。极端情况下，替换下的管道内完全被污染的气体占据。管道由大量部件组成（图116.1），任何一个部件都可能发生故障。

识别

管道气源供应中的定量故障可以通过压力传感器检测出来。按照美国食品药物管理局推荐的指南进行机器检测，可以检测出管道压力不足或压力过高。现代麻醉机都配有低氧压力报警装置，在手术过程中，当发生氧气供应故障时麻醉机会发出低氧警报声提醒手术医师和麻醉科医师。笑气（N_2O）管道故障时，麻醉机不发出警报。其他气体的供气管道可能有中央压力报警系统。

定性错误则较难通过检测被发现。使用氧气传感器可检测到氧气气源的污染，氧气传感器在正常室内空气中的校准数值为21%，供应纯氧时氧气传感器示数应大于90%。当管道中的氧气混入任何一种其他气体时，经正确校准后的氧气传感器都会有所变化。目前，还没有监测仪或分析仪能确定管道系统中所有的潜在污染源（如一氧化碳、三烯类、溶剂类），尤其当污染源的浓度很低时。通过嗅觉也许会检测到一些污染气源，但会使工作人员暴露在潜在的危险污染源中。

框116.1 管道问题列表

A. 定量问题

Ⅰ. 管道压力低
1. 与机器连接的软管扭结
2. 与机器连接的软管泄漏
3. 与机器连接的双软管泄漏
4. 管道阻塞
5. 通道阀门关闭
6. 管道泄漏
7. 氧气无供应
8. 储备气体无法激活供应
9. 调节器冻结在关闭位置

Ⅱ. 管道压力高
1. 调节阀冻结在开启位置
2. 管道内液相气体在膨胀

B. 定性问题

Ⅰ. 管道污染
1. 允许交叉连接的索引安全系统错误
2. 管道交叉
3. 管道内有其他异物
4. 管道内有清洗液

Ⅱ. 气源污染
1. 储气罐内气体错误
2. 储气罐内有清洗液
3. 气源连接错误

风险评估

患者接受室内空气以外的气体治疗都存在风险。多数管道故障都涉及压力过高或过低的定量问

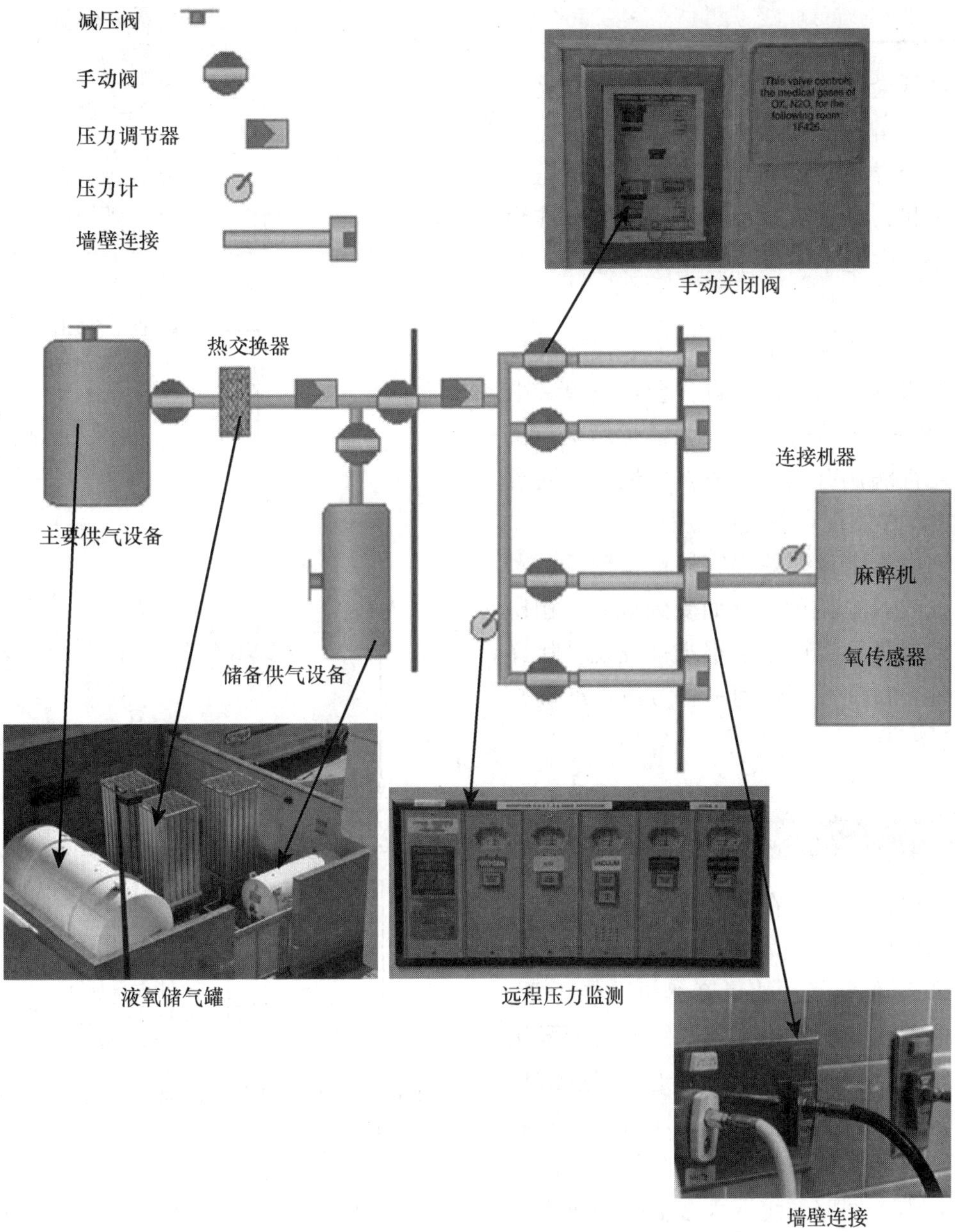

图 116.1 管道气体传输系统示意图。主要供气设备可为大型液体储气罐，或床旁压缩机。麻醉科医师应检测发生在麻醉机的管道问题（压力计或氧传感器），它们是组成管道供气系统的大量组件的最后共同道路

题。2004 年的 1 例涉及三重冗余系统（即主要供气装置、次级供气装置和备用储气钢瓶）的个案报道，强调了这种系统的弹性特征。由于连接失败引起大量液态氧气泄漏，导致主要供气装置和次级供气装置的关闭，但备用氧气瓶仍能满足多个手术室和 ICU 病床的需求。一项针对 200 多个医学院附属麻醉科的调查中，上报的 76 例麻醉事故中有 37 例与氧气管道压力低有关。氧气管道压力可在标准麻醉机正常检测时发现。更为严重的是供应管道交叉错误（管道接口接错），这可能导致缺氧。使用管道气体作为标准麻醉机检查的一部分，当涉及氧气源交叉故障的管道供应交叉错误（管道接口接错）时，可以通过氧气传感器示数大于 90% 予以发现和证实。与氧气源交叉故障相比，气体污染则更加危险。污染源可能发生在气体制造或精炼过程中，也可能发生在管道清洗液使用不当或焊接技术不当的情况下。对患者端气体的详细分析，是检测此类故障的唯一方法。许多故障和污染实例与管道系统的构造和改造有关。无论何时，在对管道问题进行检修处理时，都应提高警惕。

启示

管道压力过低会导致患者供气不足。比如笑气供应不足会出现麻醉过浅和术中觉醒。氧气供应不足则更为严重，会导致缺氧和器官损伤。管道压力过高会损坏麻醉机，导致流量计损坏、读值不准确或内部组件破裂。一旦术中发生管道压力过高，必须立即更换麻醉机。

若管道中一种不能维持生命的气体取代氧气导致患者窒息；如果混入的气体有毒，会导致患者中毒。根据 Moss 和 Evans 的报告，三氯乙烯污染与德克萨斯州 4 例死亡病例有关。医务人员最初是注意到氧气气味异常，才发现有毒气体污染。

综上所述，由于定量误差很容易被检测，患者不应该因为氧气或 N_2O 浓度不足而受到危害。相比之下，除管道接错外，定性错误很难被发现。除详细的气体分析外，目前没有任何一种方法可准确检测到管道气体的污染。

管理

处理包括管道源性污染在内所有管道故障的应对策略，见图 116.2。在管道发生问题时，必须为患者提供足够的氧气和通气。如果麻醉机功能正常，通过断开墙壁氧气供应，替换为氧气钢瓶为麻醉机供氧，可以很容易地保证患者氧气和通气。麻醉机优先选择墙壁氧气源，当发生故障时应首先断开麻醉机连接管路，再断开墙壁氧气，预防管道内的其他污染气源进入整个回路系统。大多数呼吸机由氧气供应的压力驱动，在紧急情况下改用人工手控通气可以节约氧气。如果麻醉机已受到高压损坏，或管道供气和钢瓶供气都已发生故障或怀疑受到污染，此时需要使用简易呼吸器（加压给氧气囊）维持患者最低有效通气，直到备用设备可用为止。此时，使用全凭静脉麻醉可以维持麻醉需要。排除故障和修复可能损坏的麻醉机不应浪费过多宝贵的时间。最后，将故障信息迅速传达到其他患者治疗区域，以便合理的处理和应对更大范围的故障和污染源。

医院生物医学工程部门有责任确定故障组件的来源和特性。与低压策略类似，可以通过确定整个系统或系统的一部分是否受到影响来确定故障组件（最有可能是调节器）的来源。

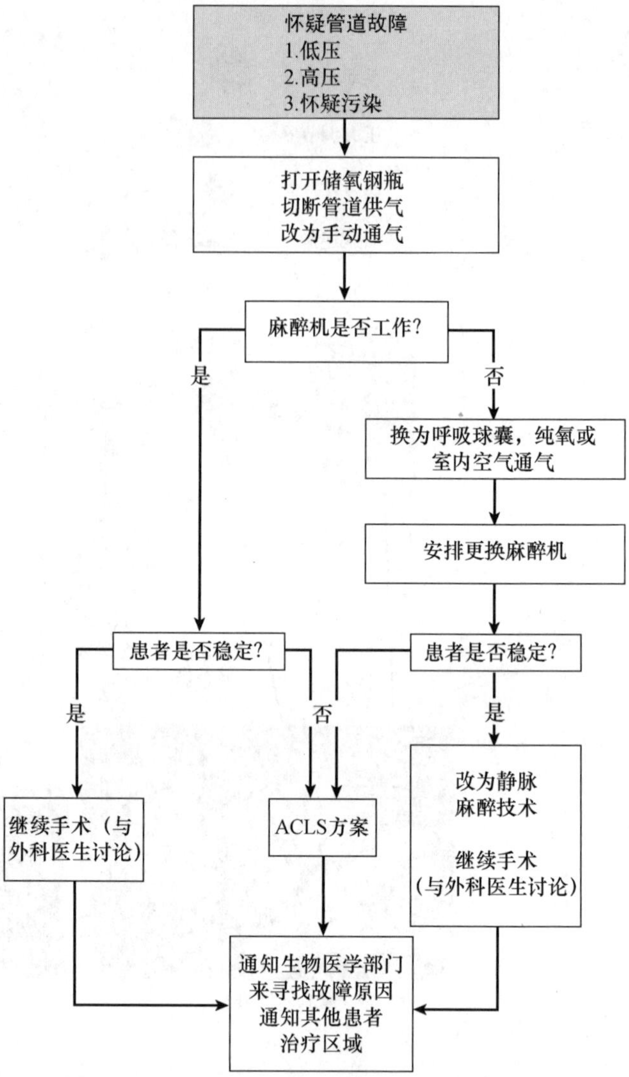

图 116.2 处理管道故障的简易流程图。ACLS，高级心血管生命支持

如果怀疑有污染物，应启动钢瓶供气装置，切断麻醉机与气源的连接，并通知生物医学工程师采集气体样本进行分析。此外，对管道的改造和维护保养记录有助于确定操作和维护的具体时间。

预防

管道故障所致灾祸的预防既有机械因素，也有人为因素。管道气体供应是机械结构，而所有机械结构均有一定的发生故障率。如果长时间使用，阀门、调节器或其他管道部件都有故障可能。此时自动激活储备装置和次级供气装置、激活减压阀和其他机械安全装置，有助于预防患者损伤。专业人员适当的检查和合理维修有助于预防机械故障。然而，计算机控制的系统在没有警告时可能出现严重问题。此时，人为因素变得至关重要。

预防患者损伤涉及之前提及的所有的机械保护装置，并加上更为重要的人为因素。由于所有机械保护装置都可能失灵，此时需依赖警觉性较高的麻醉科医师发现故障并激活适当的次级供气系统，这就要求每一台手术都需要一台经过正确检查过的麻醉机。

（吴 巧 译 陈元杰 校）

延伸阅读

Anderson WR, Brock-Utne JG: Oxygen pipeline supply failure: a coping strategy, *J Clin Monit* 7:39–41, 1991.

Dorsch JA, Dorsch SE: *Understanding anesthetic equipment*, ed 5, Baltimore, 2008, Lippincott Williams & Wilkins, pp 1–50.

Ehrenwerth J, Eisenkraft JB, Berry J: *Anesthesia equipment: principles and applications*, ed 2, Philadelphia, 2013, Elsevier, pp 3–24.

Feeley TW, Hedley-Whyte J: Bulk oxygen and nitrous oxide delivery systems: design and dangers, *Anesthesiology* 44:301–305, 1976.

Gilmour IJ, McComb RC, Palahniuk RJ: Contamination of a hospital oxygen supply, *Anesth Analg* 71:302–304, 1990.

Johner J, Rise G: Loss of pipeline oxygen supply, *Internet J Anesthesiol* 16(2):1–3, 2007. Available at http://ispub.com/IJA/16/2/5985. Accessed June 6, 2016.

Mehta SP, Eisenkraft JB, Posner KL, et al.: Patient injuries from anesthesia gas delivery equipment, a closed claims update, *Anesthesiology* 119:788–795, 2013.

Moss E, Evans F: Hospital deaths reportedly due to contaminated O_2, *Anesth Patient Safety Foundation Newslett* 11:13–24, 1996.

Schumacher SD, Brockwell RC, Andrews JJ, et al.: Bulk liquid oxygen supply failure, *Anesthesiology* 100:186–189, 2004.

Weller J, Merry A, Warman G, et al.: Anaesthetist's management of oxygen pipeline failure: room for improvement, *Anaesthesia* 62:122–126, 2007.

第 117 章 配比供给系统

Stewart J. Lustik，*Keith M. Franklin*

病例概要

患者，女性，45 岁，既往体健，在全身麻醉下行经腹全子宫切除术。纯氧给氧去氮后，丙泊酚麻醉诱导。琥珀胆碱肌肉松弛后气管插管顺利。氧化亚氮（N_2O）和异氟烷吸入。尽管呼气末二氧化监测正常，双侧呼吸音清，血压正常，但患者很快出现 SpO_2 下降。O_2 分析仪读数为 14%。流量计显示 5 L/min 的 N_2O 和 0.8 L/min 的 O_2。

问题分析

定义

由于配比供给系统缺陷，低氧混合气体被输送至该患者。配比供给系统（proportioning system）是被设计用来阻止低氧混合气体输送给患者的若干安全设置之一。一个正常运转的配比供给系统允许传送不超过 75%N_2O 和 25%O_2 的混合气体。

先前生产的 Modulus、Modulus Ⅱ和 Excel 系列麻醉机，已运用 Link-25 配比供给系统，GE 医疗生产的 Aestiva 和 Aespire 麻醉机也配备了此款控制系统。通过联锁齿轮机制和调节气体入口压力相结合，阻止传送超过 3∶1 以上的 N_2O 和 O_2。N_2O 控制阀有一个 24 齿链轮，通过链条连接到 O_2 控制阀的 48 齿链自由滑动轮（图 117.1）。N_2O 和 O_2 控制阀可独立移动，以提供高达 75% 的 N_2O；当 N_2O 和 O_2 比例上升到 3∶1 时，O_2 齿轮的进气标签与 O_2 控制旋钮上的止动螺钉接合。因此，N_2O 和 O_2 控制阀连接在一起。任何 N_2O 的进一步增加都会按比例增加 O_2 流量，以防止超过 3∶1。同样，尝试减少 O_2 流量将按比例减少 N_2O 流量至保持在 3∶1 的比例。当 N_2O 和 O_2 控制阀连接时，由于调节进气口压力，2∶1 链

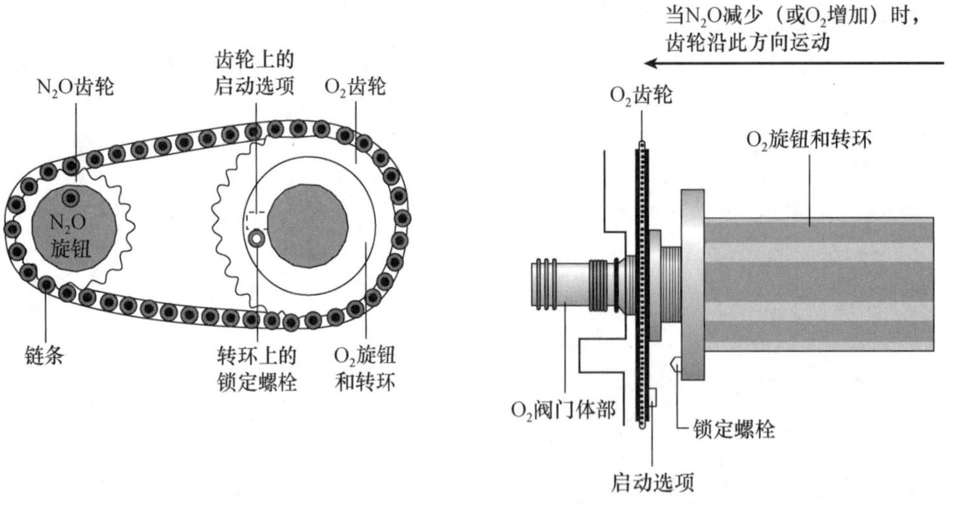

图 117.1 Ohmeda Link-25 配比供给系统。随着 N_2O∶O_2 的增加，O_2 齿轮向 O_2 旋钮移动。当 N_2O∶O_2 比例达到 3∶1 时，O_2 齿轮与 O_2 旋钮连接，O_2 旋钮与 N_2O 旋钮相关联

轮比导致最终输出的气体比例为 3∶1。第二级 N_2O 调节器将入口压力降低至 38±0.5 磅 / 平方英寸表压，O_2 调节器调节至 20.75±3.75 磅 / 平方英寸表压。

先前由北美 Dräger 公司制造的麻醉机配比供给系统，被称为敏感氧比例控制器（S-ORC）（图 117.2）。O_2 和 N_2O 通过各自的电阻器进行调控，在上隔膜（O_2）和下隔膜（N_2O）上施加反向压力发挥作用。这种反向压力，与上下弹簧的不同弹簧常数，导致连接在配比阀上的活塞运动。当 N_2O 流量增加 >72%～78% 时，活塞就会移动，配比阀限制 N_2O 流量进一步提高。例如，如将 O_2 流量计设置为 1 L/min，S-ORC 将不允许超过 3 L/min 的 N_2O。如果转动 N_2O 控制旋钮，使流量增加到 3 L/min 以上，N_2O 隔膜上的压力将移动活塞，防止 N_2O 流量进一步增加。同样，如将 O_2 流减少到 22%～28% 以下，则将按比例减少 N_2O 流量，以保持所需的 O_2 百分比。

许多最新设计的麻醉机，如 GE Healthcare Aisys CS2、Dräger Perseus 500 和 Mindray A7（图 117.3），均采用电子配比供给系统，O_2 和 N_2O 流量通过电子技术进行测量。如 N_2O 流量太高，电流驱动配比阀会限制 N_2O 流量并允许至少 25% 或 26% 的氧气。配比阀必须每 12 个月检查校准一次。这些机器还允许用户通过数字输入，设置所需的新鲜气体流量和 O_2∶N_2O 比例。

识别

诊断配比供给系统故障需要识别的机械性故障的征象，输送低氧混合物，接收低氧混合物，或以上均有：

- 机械性故障：
  - 当 N_2O 流量增加导致其在混合物中超过 75%，Link-25 系统缺乏可听见和感知的叮当声。

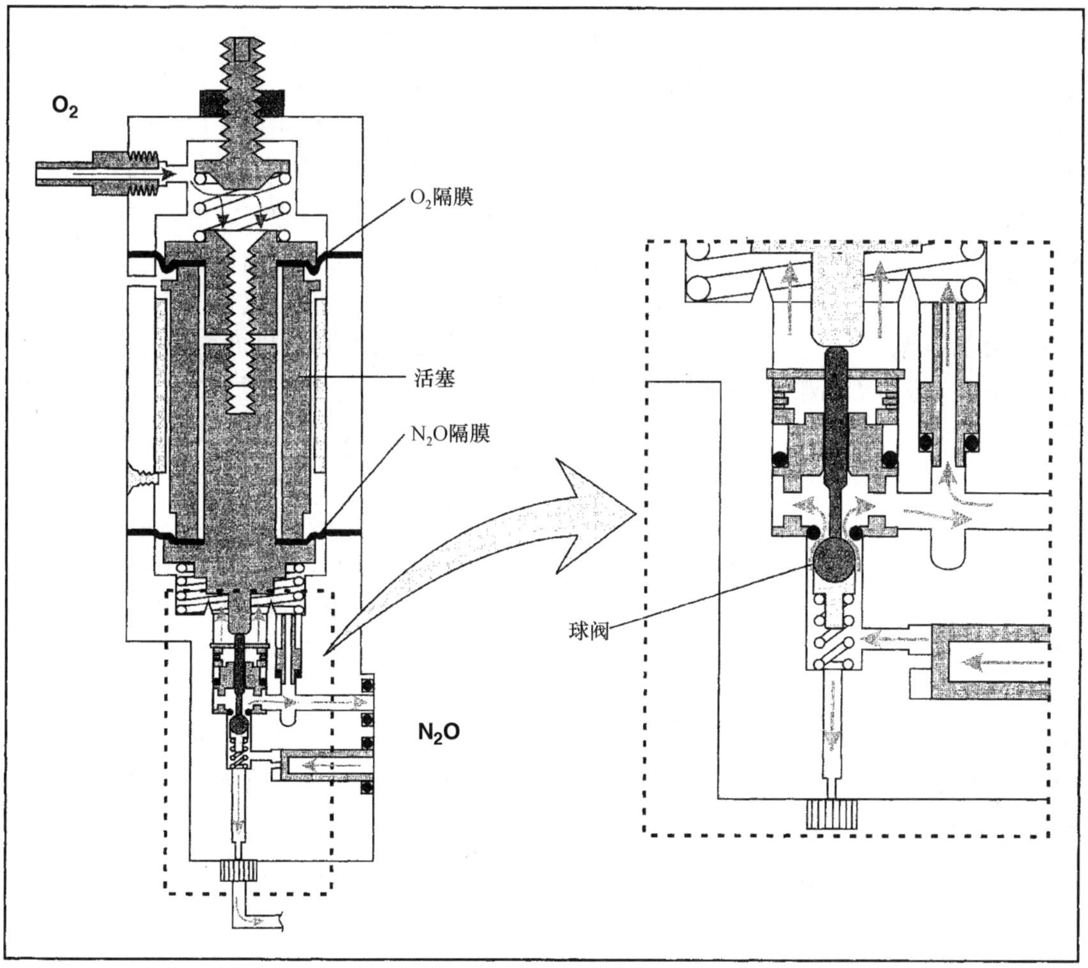

图 117.2 Narkomed 氧比例控制器。当 O_2 流量降低到 25%±3% 以下时，上部滚动隔膜上的 O_2 压力小于下部滚动隔膜片上的 N_2O 压力，活塞向上运动。这使得球阀下方的弹簧迫使球阀向上运动，部分阻挡 N_2O 的流量，直到达到新的平衡状态。增加氧气流量直到超过 25%±3% 时，氧气会将活塞和球阀向下推，减少对 N_2O 流量的阻碍

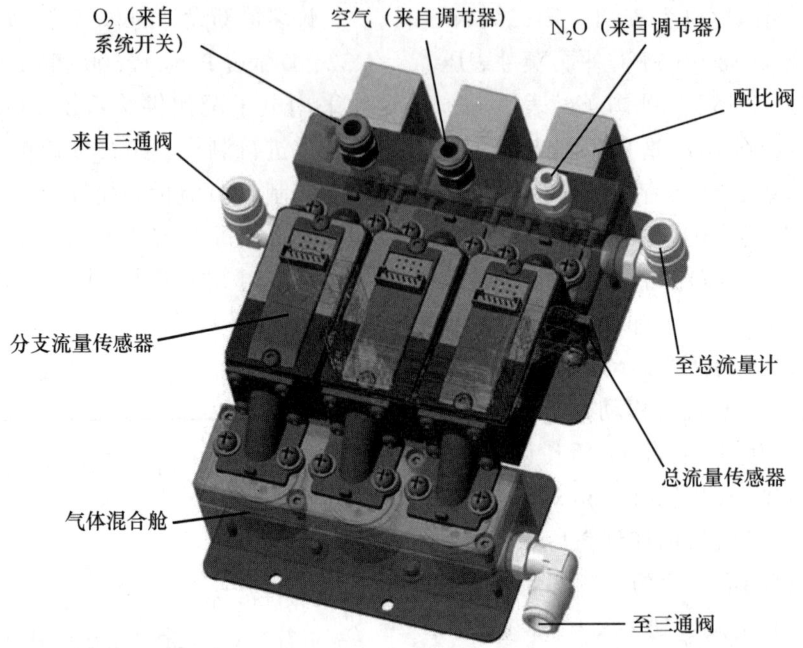

图 117.3 Mindray A7 电子流量控制系统。三个电子流量传感器将信号反馈给配比阀；这些阀门控制 O_2、空气以及 N_2O 的新鲜气体流量。当使用 N_2O 时，O_2 浓度不能设置低于 26%

- N_2O 和 O_2 流量计管或柱状图的高度标识比值 >3：1。流量计管被卡住也可能是原因之一。
- 输送低氧混合物：
  - 氧气分析仪显示低读数。
- 接收低氧混合物：
  - 缺氧会增加肾上腺素能张力，导致心动过速和高血压。如不纠正，最终会导致心动过缓、低血压和心脏停搏。
  - 外周血红蛋白氧饱和度的测定采用脉冲血氧仪。
  - 患者出现发绀。

风险评估

由配比供给系统损坏导致输送低氧混合物较为罕见，以下是配比供给系统故障的几个潜在原因。首先，配比供给系统的机械缺陷可能导致低氧混合物的输送。已有关于 Ohmeda 麻醉机上 Link-25 配比供给系统故障的案例报告。在一例故障中，链轮之间的连接链断裂使 N_2O 增加到缺氧浓度。在后来的模型中，链条由塑料改为不锈钢制成，增加了其抗拉强度。然而，在后来的情况中这并没有阻止链条从 O_2 旋钮上脱落。另一案例中，螺柱上 O_2 控制旋钮位置不正确，尽管仍输送了 100% 的 N_2O，但旋钮无法与螺柱接合。此外，目前已发现至少 3 起事件是由氧气控制旋钮上的止动螺钉松动，引起机器产生缺氧混合物。此外，Link-25 系统另一故障涉及链轮从旋钮脱离的情况。目前为止没有任何电子配比供给系统故障的报告，但阀门故障也可能导致麻醉机输送低氧混合物。尽管 S-ORC 组件（如隔膜、弹簧、活塞、调节螺钉、电阻器）的任何缺陷都可能导致低氧混合物的输送，目前北美 Dräger 麻醉机出现问题的报告仍不多见。

第二，GE 麻醉机的气动元件可能会失灵。如果 Ohmeda 麻醉机上的二级 O_2 或 N_2O 调节器失去校准，可能会导致 75% 以上的 N_2O 输送。Dräger 麻醉机不使用二级调节器，因此不存在以上隐患。

第三，目前所使用的现代麻醉机配比供给系统（Aisys CS_2、Perseus、Mindray A7）的电子元件可能会失效。当给予患者的总气体流量大于 N_2O+O_2 的设定流量时，系统会将 N_2O 的输送自动关闭，但仍存在潜在风险。

第四，尽管配比供给系统功能正常，在以下几种情况中，低氧混合物或意外的 N_2O 可能被输送给患者：

- 配比供给系统只控制 O_2 和 N_2O 比例，如向混合物中加入另一种气体（如氦气），会导致低氧气体的产生。即使使用了 Aisys 麻醉系统，当将空气混合地氟烷使用时，也可能会使混合气体的 O_2 浓度低于 21%。

- 当有 O_2 以外的气体存在于气体管道或气缸中时。
- 配比供给系统下游有泄漏，包括 O_2 流量计。
- S-ORC（North American Dräger）可能导致 N_2O 意外输送。当 N_2O 以 3∶1 输送时，如果 O_2 流量减少，N_2O 也会按比例减少。如果之后需要增加 O_2 浓度，增加 O_2 流量会导致 N_2O 流量也以 3∶1 上升，直到达到初始 N_2O 流量。

启示

低氧混合物的输送若不及时纠正，可能导致动脉血氧饱和度降低，器官缺血，循环衰竭甚至最终死亡。

管理

若低氧混合物输送由配比供给系统故障所致，应立即切断 N_2O 控制按钮。通过快速充氧阀或单独的氧气瓶经由旁路绕过配比供给系统。如果必要，麻醉机应该停止使用，直到服务商代表检查和替换配比供给系统。

预防

实施麻醉前，检查麻醉机时应当常规检查配比配给系统。美国食品和药物管理局麻醉设备检查指南推荐："浓度建立低氧性 O_2/N_2O 混合物，并确认气流和（或）报警是否得到正确的纠正"。在 Ohmeda 麻醉机中，尝试增加 N_2O 气流使 N_2O∶O_2 超过 3∶1 时会相应增加 O_2 流量；尝试减少 O_2 流量使 O_2∶N_2O 低于 1∶3 时会相应减少 N_2O 流量。在 Dräger 麻醉机和新一代 GE 麻醉机中，则不可能使 N_2O∶O_2 气流比例的增加超过 3∶1，而减少 O_2 流量至低于 1∶3 时会相应地减少 N_2O 流量。

美国麻醉科医师协会指南要求麻醉期间监测 O_2 浓度。实施麻醉前 O_2 分析仪必须校准，这是侦测低氧混合物输送最为可靠的方法。必须在术前对 Dräger 麻醉机行正压漏气测试，对 Ohmeda 麻醉机行负压漏气测试，以检测配比供给系统的下游是否泄漏，不然可能会导致低氧混合物的输送。

（栾延敏 译 陈 玲 校）

延伸阅读

Abraham ZA, Basagoitia J: A potentially lethal anesthesia machine failure, *Anesthesiology* 6:589–590, 1987.

Cheng CJ, Garewal D: A failure of the chain-link mechanism on the Ohmeda Excel 210 anesthesia machine, *Anesth Analg* 92:913–914, 2001.

Eisendraft JB: The anesthesia machine. In Ehrenwerth J, Eisenkraft JB, editors: *Anesthesia equipment: principles and applications*, St. Louis, 1993, Mosby–Year Book, pp 43–45.

Gordon PC, James MF, Lapham H, et al.: Failure of the proportioning system to prevent hypoxic mixture on a Modulus II Plus anesthesia machine, *Anesthesiology* 82:598–599, 1995.

Mindray North America: *A7 anesthesia system service manual*, Mahwah, NJ, 2015, Mindray, Inc. Available at http://www.mindraynorthamerica.com/cmsAdmin/uploads/h-046-006272-00-a7-service-manual-4-0.pdf, Accessed August 19, 2016.

Modulus II anesthesia system operation and maintenance manual, Madison, WI, Ohmeda, 1985, BOC Group, Inc.

Narkomed Service Group: *Operating principles of Narkomed anesthesia systems*, ed 2, Telford, PA, 1997, WE Andrews.

Rice J, Kolek B: *Explore the anesthesia system*, Madison, WI, 1996, Ohmeda, pp 43–44.

Richards C: Failure of a nitrous oxide-oxygen proportioning device, *Anesthesiology* 71:997–998, 1989.

U.S. Food and Drug Administration: *Anesthesia apparatus checkout recommendations*, Rockville, MD, 1986, Food and Drug Administration.

第 118 章 肺动脉压力监测

Yuriy S.Bronshtey，*Jonathan B.Mark*

病例概要

患者，女性，73 岁，重度二尖瓣反流，并安装永久性心脏起搏器，因尿脓毒症和难治性低血压被送入外科重症监护室。由于患者血流动力学对液体治疗没有反应，遂经右颈内静脉置入肺动脉导管（pulmonary artery catheter，PAC），深度 53 cm。肺动脉（pulmonary artery，PA）压力显示为 90/30 mmHg。次日清晨，肺动脉压为 76/20 mmHg，波形显示见图 118.1。重症医师给 PAC 气囊充气以记录肺动脉楔压值。数秒内患者出现焦躁、呼吸急促、咳出鲜红色血。怀疑咯血由肺动脉破裂引起，重症医师决定行气管插管。胸部 X 线证实 PAC 尖端位于右肺动脉远端，右肺出现新的浸润影。在透视引导下将支气管封堵器置入右主支气管隔离右肺，行左肺单侧通气。由于持续低氧血症，后行动静脉血体外膜肺氧合，患者气体交换和血压有所改善。次日患者成功接受右肺动脉近端分支弹簧圈栓塞术。

问题分析

定义

麻醉科医师和重症医师通常使用 PAC 指导循环休克患者的血流动力学管理，并监测患有严重肺动脉高压和（或）严重心室功能障碍的手术患者。放置 PAC 时需将引导鞘插入颈内静脉、锁骨下静脉或股静脉等大静脉，也可通过腋静脉置入。然后将 PAC 通过鞘管置入静脉腔内，对球囊充气，在血流助推下导管通过右心房（right atrium，RA）、右心室（right ventricle，RV）和 PA 近端。使用连续压力监测指导 PAC 推进，以确定导管尖端位置并确认适当的位置。透视引导也可用来辅助 PAC 放置。最近，经食管超声心动图引导下肺动脉置管技术已有介绍。

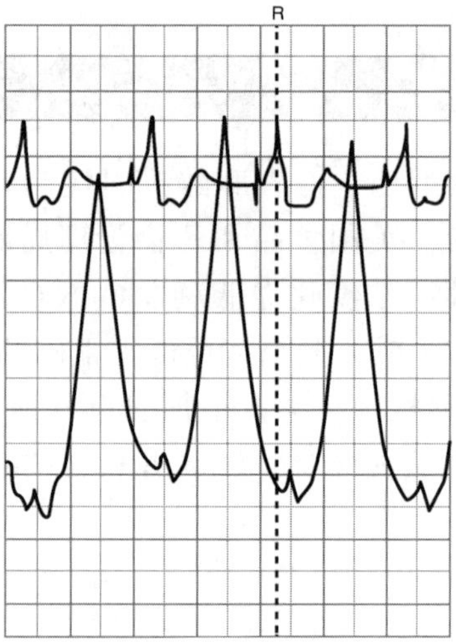

图 118.1 患者肺动脉导管在球囊充气前的波形。监护显示器记录的压力为 76/20 mmHg。注意，心电图显示心室起搏，R 波以虚线垂直线突出显示（Modified from Mark JB: *Atlas of cardiovascular monitoring*. New York，1998，Churchill Livingstone.）

PAC 监测的并发症可能发生在置管过程中或置管后。与置管相关的并发症包括所有中心静脉置管期间发生的并发症，但用于 PAC 的扩张器和鞘管可能导致更严重的血管损伤（与中心静脉置管相关的并发症参见第 105 章）。除中心血管损伤外，在 PAC 置入和监测过程中出现的其他机械性损伤包括心律失常、三尖瓣或肺动脉瓣损伤和肺动脉穿孔。除机械性损伤并发症外，PAC 监测还可能导致中心血管血液感染、感染性心内膜炎和肺血栓栓塞。最后，也可能是最重要的一点是，肺动脉导管滥用和监测数据的误读，也许是最常见的临床并发症。

心律失常或束支传导阻滞

当 PAC 通过 RA 和 RV 时，最常发生房性和室性心律失常，如房性或室性异位搏动和非持续性室性心动过速发生（在所有 PAC 放置中估计占 13% ～ 70%）。心室异位搏动也可发生在已放置好 PAC 的患者和拔除导管期间。大多数由导管操作引起的房性心律失常和室性心律失常是良性和自限性的。然而，部分患者发生室上性心动过速（如心房颤动）可能会引起需要治疗的严重低血压。血流动力学影响显著的持续性室性心动过速或心室颤动非常罕见，但也可能发生并且需要将 PAC 从心脏完全退出方可终止。

多达 5% 的患者在 PAC 插入期间或之后不久，可新发右束支传导阻滞（right bundle branch block，RBBB）。既往存在左束支传导阻滞（left bundle branch block，LBBB）的患者几乎不受影响。在这些患者中，可能发生完全性心脏传导阻滞，导致严重的血流动力学不稳定，需要紧急心脏起搏或其他标准的严重心动过缓或心搏停止的相应治疗。研究表明，这种情况并不常见，发生率 <1%。

导管尖端错位

从 PAC 获得准确的血流动力学数据，取决于导管尖端在肺动脉主干或近端肺动脉（距肺动脉瓣 3 ～ 5 cm）的位置。导管尖端位置不当会产生错误的数据，导致血管损伤。当 PAC 尖端无意中位于 RV 而非 PA 时，显示的“舒张压”出现错误（RV 舒张压与 PA 舒张压相反）（图 118.2），心排血量和混合静脉血氧饱和度的测量也不准确。

PAC 在最初置入后，由于导管变软，血流推动其进入更远端和更小的肺动脉分支，导管尖端可能向远端漂移。导管尖端持久位于“楔住”位置可导致肺梗死或肺动脉破裂，特别是试图在此位置将球囊充气。另外，将“楔压”误认为肺动脉收缩压可能导致不适当的治疗。值得注意的是，存在显著的二尖瓣反流患者中，两种压力描记很难区分（图 118.3）。

肺血栓栓塞

尸检研究显示，PAC 患者中导管相关血栓的发生率极高（约 60%）。血栓通常附着在导管引导鞘的插入部位或附近。血栓也发生在内皮或心内膜表面，这些内皮或心内膜表面因 PAC 放置或留存时受到创伤。血栓通常较小，但也可能是大块的，并导致临床上严重的肺栓塞。此外，血栓可以通过阻塞 RA 和 PA 中的导管测量端口和用于测量心排血量的导管尖端热敏电阻来改变血流动力学测量的准确性。

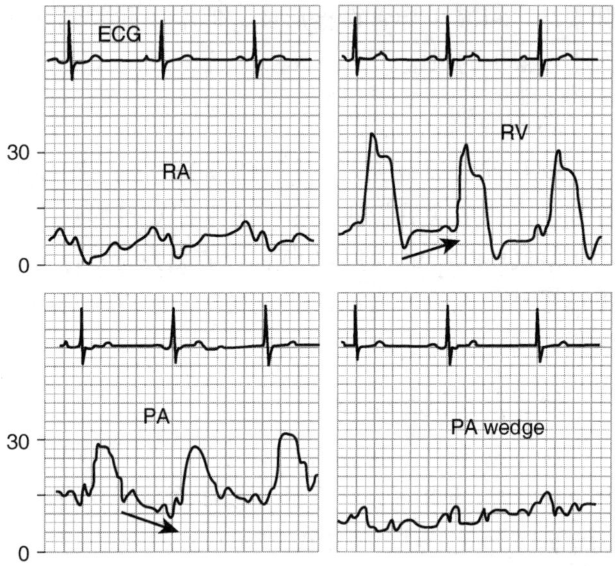

图 118.2 左上图，右心房（RA）描记显示正常的中心静脉或 RA 压力波形。右上图，右心室（RV）描记显示较 RA 升高的收缩压。左下图，肺动脉（PA）描记显示较 RV 描记升高的舒张压。右下图，PA 楔压描记显示类似于 RA 描记图的静脉压力波形，但表示的是左心房下游压力的间接测量值。注意，在本例中，RV 和 PA 压力的绝对值相似（大约 30/10 mm Hg），可能无法通过检查显示器上显示的数字识别。然而，RV 和 PA 波形明显不同。舒张期 RV 压力因 RV 充盈而升高，而舒张期 PA 压力因 PA 流向肺和左侧心脏（箭头）而降低（Modified from Mark JB：*Atlas of cardiovascular monitoring*. New York，1998，Churchill Livingstone.）

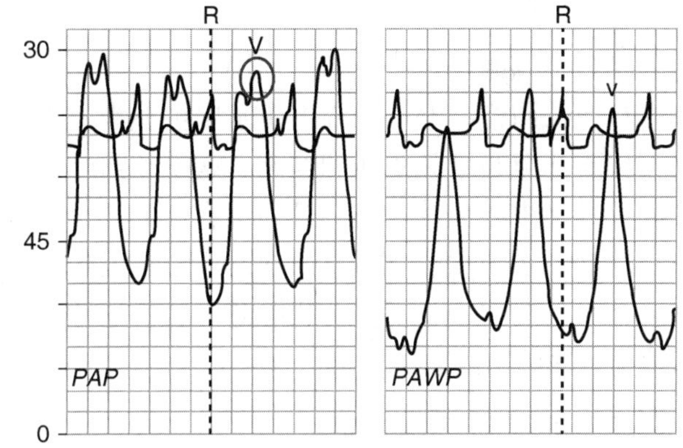

图 118.3 左图，严重二尖瓣反流患者的肺动脉压（PAP）描记图。注意，初始压力峰值在心电图（ECG）T 波前出现。右图，同一患者的肺动脉楔压（PAWP）描记图。注意，在心电图 T 波后有一个压力峰值的反流性高 V 波。同样的反流 V 波可能会使 PAP 描记波形变形，使其出现缺口或裂痕。如图 118.2 所示，监视器的数字显示值可能不能清楚地区分 PAP 和 PAWP（Modified from Mark JB：*Atlas of cardiovascular monitoring*. New York，1998，Churchill Livingstone.）

肝素结合可减少导管血栓形成，但增加肝素诱导的血小板减少的风险。

球囊破裂

PAC 球囊反复充气 / 放气以及通过引导鞘及其外部止血阀多次重新插入均可损坏 PAC 球囊。当试图用空气（1.5 ml）将其充气而没有阻力时，以及缓慢抽吸球囊腔返回血液而非空气时，就能识别球囊破裂。

肺动脉穿孔或破裂

肺动脉损伤，包括假性动脉瘤、穿孔或破裂，是 PAC 最严重和危及生命的并发症之一。其确切发病率尚不清楚，估计在 0.03% ～ 0.2%，死亡率估计为 41% ～ 70%。Barash 等根据离体全肺的尸检研究，提出了 PAC 相关穿孔或破裂的可能机制：

- PAC 推进过远导致尖端可能刺穿血管；
- 球囊偏心充气可推动导管尖端穿过血管壁；
- 球囊过度膨胀可导致球囊内压力达到 250 mmHg，压力部分或全部传导至肺动脉壁，导致过度膨胀和破裂。

另外，尝试给已经位于楔住位置的导管气囊充气，可能导致血管损伤和穿孔（见病例概要）。

导管打结或缠绕

PAC 可以缠绕在心脏结构周围，也可以在患者体内打结。同样，PAC 在心内手术中可能被心脏缝线夹住，并与心脏乳头肌和腱索、起搏和除颤器导线以及其他中心血管通路导管纠缠在一起。打结或缠绕的 PAC 常在尝试拔除或推进导管时被发现。有许多技术可在非手术下安全拔除导管，但通常需介入放射科医师协助。

导管细菌定植和脓毒症

约 1% ～ 2% 的 PAC 会发生血流感染。此外，PAC 本身可损伤三尖瓣和肺动脉瓣的心内膜表面，容易引起感染性心内膜炎，尤其是人工心脏瓣膜的患者。因此，放置 PAC 时应采用严格的无菌技术和全屏障隔离措施。

不当使用和数据误读

PAC 是一种诊断工具，需要恰当的解读数据以指导相应的治疗。20 世纪 90 年代，欧洲和美国进行的相关研究表明，重症医师和护士在 PAC 数据解读的基本知识上存在多重差距。大约一半医师无法做到下述几点：

- 根据清晰的波形描记来确定肺动脉“楔”压（见图 118.2）；
- 确定氧输送的决定因素；
- 识别与动脉置管相一致的血气结果。

值得注意的是，上述知识都是安全和有效使用 PAC 的基础。

识别

表 118.1 总结了与 PAC 特异性并发症相关的体征和症状。图 118.2 总结了 RV、PA 和楔压描记图的形态差异。

风险评估

在 PAC 置管期间或之后发生心律失常的危险因素包括：

- PAC 通过 RA 和 RV 所需的总时间；
- 既往有心肌梗死或缺血，特别是 RV 缺血或 LBBB（完全性心脏传导阻滞的风险）；
- 存在低氧血症或酸中毒；

表 118.1 PAC 并发症的体征和症状

并发症	相关症状和体征
导管缠绕或打结	1. 导管推进或拔出时有阻力 2. 初始 RV 压力波形出现时，导管向前推进超过 20 cm 或右颈内静脉绝对插入深度 60 cm 时，持续存在 RV 波形 3. 胸部 X 线确诊
PAC 感染	插入部位出现红斑或脓液，伴有全身感染症状（发热、白细胞增多等）
PAC 尖端在 RV	舒张期压力描记显示压力增加，而不是降低（见图 118.2）
PAC 尖端意外处于楔住位置	1. PA 描记显示球囊未充气时的楔压波形（见图 118.2） 2. 胸部 X 线显示 PAC 尖端在中线右侧或左侧 >5 cm 3. 从 PAC 尖端采集的血液显示典型的动脉血氧饱和度（≥ 85%）和 PaO_2（≥ 55 mmHg）值，而非典型的混合静脉值（<80% 和 <50 mmHg）
PA 破裂	焦虑、呼吸困难、咯血、血胸、低血压、低氧血症

PA，肺动脉；PAC，肺动脉导管；RV，右心室

- 电解质失衡（尤其是低钾或低镁血症）。

框 118.1 列出了与 PA 破裂、梗死或假性动脉瘤风险增加的有关因素。在心脏手术中，当右心腔在体外循环期间被排空时，对心脏操作或冷硬的 PAC 尖端远端迁移易导致 PA 穿孔。随着导管留置时间的延长，PAC 相关感染的风险增加。血栓形成的发生率随着导管留置时间的延长和病情严重程度而增加。

启示

与所有侵入性操作一样，PAC 也有相关风险和益处。严重并发症的发生率估计为 0.1% ～ 5%。这种风险必须与迅速识别和管理血流动力学紊乱的潜在益处进行权衡。最近一项 Cochrane 综述的结论认为，危重患者放置 PAC 不会增加死亡率、重症监护病房或住院时间、费用。作者也承认 PAC 可能有益于特定情况下的部分患者，但具体未知。

美国麻醉科医师协会肺动脉导管工作组建议，在决定是否适合放置 PAC 时，应考虑患者、手术操作和操作环境。最近的大量回顾性研究表明，PAC 的使用可以改善老年和（或）严重创伤患者预后，并减少心脏手术患者输血需求。临床医师目前依靠 PAC 指导复杂心力衰竭患者的治疗，包括接受心脏手术的患者和需要体外循环支持的患者。最后，在医师和护士有足够培训水平和熟悉其使用的情况下，PAC 更有可能使患者受益。

管理

PAC 并发症的处理建议见表 118.2。Addante 等提出了一种处理 PAC 所致肺动脉破裂的流程。框 118.2 中介绍了该处理流程的修改版本。动静脉体外膜肺氧合不仅能稳定气体交换，而且能引导血流远离肺出血部位。其他可能的治疗方法包括：

- 肺动脉弹簧圈栓塞术；
- PA 直视手术修补术；
- 肺动脉结扎联合（或不联合）肺切除术。

框 118.1 肺动脉破裂的危险因素

年龄 >60 岁
肺动脉高压
肺动脉导管远端移位
心肺转流术
抗凝
低体温
肺动脉导管球囊过度充气

表 118.2 PAC 并发症的推荐处理策略

并发症	处理策略
房性或室性心律失常	导管进入肺动脉或退出上下腔静脉
完全性心脏传导阻滞	经皮或经静脉起搏
导管扭结	在透视或不使用透视下，小心重新放置导管
导管打结	1. 胸部 X 线和（或）超声心动图确诊 2. 通过放射介入和（或）手术移除
导管相关感染	拔除导管并全身使用抗生素
导管相关血栓	抗凝及考虑早期拔除导管
球囊破裂	小心拔除 PAC

PAC，肺动脉导管

框 118.2 PAC 相关肺动脉破裂的处理流程

第 1 步：重新调整靠近出血部位的 PAC 尖端，重新对 PAC 球囊充气
第 2 步：单腔或双腔气管插管保护气道
第 3 步：确定出血的偏向侧（例如，使用胸部 X 线或经食管超声心动图检查 PAC 的偏向侧）；如果可行，将患者置于侧卧位，使出血侧朝下
第 4 步：使用以下任何一种方法实现肺隔离：
1. 使用双腔气管导管
   a. 给两个套囊充气，未受影响的肺通气
   b. 考虑将 PEEP 应用于受影响的肺
2. 使用单腔气管导管（SLET）
   a. 右侧肺动脉破裂：插入支气管封堵器，用透视或支气管镜确认在右主支气管的位置
   b. 左侧肺动脉破裂：插入 SLET，用透视或支气管镜确认其位置在右主支气管
第 5 步：启动动静脉体外膜肺氧合

PAC，肺动脉导管；PEEP，呼气末正压

预防

PAC 并发症的预防首先要仔细考虑患者风险、潜在益处和替代方案。值得注意的是，PAC 置入术是一种择期有创操作，其临床价值仍有争议。例如，对于严重三尖瓣反流患者，热稀释方法可能高估或低估心排血量，限制 PAC 作为血流动力学监测工具

的价值。应始终考虑PAC的替代方案，特别是在PAC相关并发症高风险的患者中（参见本章的风险评估）。例如，也可通过超声心动图评价心功能，或者利用动脉脉搏轮廓或胸部生物电阻抗和生物反应原理的心排血量监测来评估。

只有避免PAC放置，才能完全预防PAC并发症，但遵循安全原则可降低PAC相关的部分风险。在扩张目标血管前，常规使用超声引导静脉穿刺和压力传感器以确认其在静脉血管内，可减少PAC血管通路相关并发症。在需要PAC的LBBB患者中，如果在PAC放置期间发生完全性传导阻滞，临床医师可立即行快速经皮起搏。然而，这一预防措施仍存在争议，因为即使在接受PAC置入术的LBBB患者中，完全性心脏阻滞的发生率也很低。通过限制球囊充气次数，可以降低球囊破裂的风险。

预防肺动脉破裂需要在PAC置入、操作、快速拔除导管的过程中保持谨慎，初始置入时一旦获得PA楔压波形，应将球囊放气，导管后退2～3 cm，同时仍记录PA压力波形。理想情况下，PAC的尖端应在距肺动脉瓣3～5 cm处。通常右颈内静脉置管时，其置入深度为40～50 cm，但深度因置入部位和患者身高不同而有很大差异。此外，测量“楔压”①可能增加肺动脉穿孔的风险，②可根据肺动脉舒张压（重度肺动脉高压和肺血管阻力增加的患者除外）来估算，③常规液体治疗指导不需要PA。只要有可能，应通过X线或超声心动图确认PAC处于适当位置。常规胸部X线片可能会提醒操作者注意PAC尖端意外移位或操作相关并发症。例如，在胸部X线片上，PAC尖端距肺门不应超过2 cm，距中线不应超过5 cm。任何放置PAC的操作者都应考牢记肺动脉破裂的处理预案（见框118.2）。此外，任何在原位使用PAC的患者至少每天都需要重新评估导管，以鼓励及时拔除不必要的PAC。

此外，任何放置PAC的患者至少应每天都重新评估导管，以鼓励及时移除不必要的PAC。

医师必须具备放置和解读PAC数据的能力。这需要对右心导管和PAC置入术进行正规培训。确保有PAC放置操作能力的最低操作次数尚有争议，但必需进行持续的技能训练。鉴于过去20年来PAC的使用有所减少，此类培训部分可能需在模拟环境中进行。

致谢

感谢 Matthew D. Caldwell 和 Paul E. Kazanjian 博士对本章上一版的贡献。

（封莉莉 译 杨宇光 校）

延伸阅读

Addante RA, Chen J, Goswami S: Successful management of a patient with pulmonary artery rupture in a catheterization suite, *J Cardiothorac Vasc Anesth* S1053-S0770(16):4–5, 2016.

American Society of Anesthesiologists Task Force on Pulmonary Artery Catheterization: Practice guidelines for pulmonary artery catheterization: an updated report by the American Society of Anesthesiologists Task Force on Pulmonary Artery Catheterization, *Anesthesiology* 99(4):988–1014, 2003.

Balik M, Pachl J, Hendl J: Effect of the degree of tricuspid regurgitation on cardiac output measurements by thermodilution, *Intensive Care Med* 28(8):1117–1121, 2002.

Barash PG, Nardi D, Hammond G, et al.: Catheter-induced pulmonary artery perforation. Mechanisms, management, and modifications, *J Thorac Cardiovasc Surg* 82(1):5–12, 1981.

Brovman EY, Gabriel RA, Dutton RP, Urman RD: Pulmonary artery catheter use during cardiac surgery in the United States, 2010 to 2014, *J Cardiothorac Vasc Anesth* 30(3):579–584, 2016.

Connors Jr AF, Castele RJ, Farhat NZ, et al.: Complications of right heart catheterization. A prospective autopsy study, *Chest* 88(4):567–572, 1985.

Connors Jr AF, Speroff T, Dawson NV, et al.: The effectiveness of right heart catheterization in the initial care of critically ill patients. SUPPORT Investigators, *JAMA* 276(11):889–897, 1996.

Cronin B, Robbins R, Maus T: Pulmonary artery catheter placement using transesophageal echocardiography, *J Cardiothorac Vasc Anesth* S1053-S0770(16): 30276–30272, 2016.

Damen J, Bolton D: A prospective analysis of 1,400 pulmonary artery catheterizations in patients undergoing cardiac surgery, *Acta Anaesthesiol Scand* 30(5):386–392, 1986.

Domino KB, Bowdle TA, Psoner KL, et al.: Injuries and liability related to central vascular catheters: a closed claims analysis, *Anesthesiology* 100(6):1411–1418, 2004.

Evans DC, Doraiswamy VA, Prosciak MP, et al.: Complications associated with pulmonary artery catheters: a comprehensive clinical review, *Scand J Surg* 98(4):199–208, 2009.

Friese RS, Shafi S, Gentilello LM: Pulmonary artery catheter use is associated with reduced mortality in severely injured patients: a National Trauma Data Bank analysis of 53,312 patients, *Crit Care Med* 34(6):1597–1601, 2006.

Godoy MC, Leitman BS, de Groot PM, et al.: Chest radiography in the ICU: part 2. Evaluation of cardiovascular lines and other devices, *AJR Am J Roentgenol* 198(3):572–581, 2012.

Heerdt PM, Blessios GA, Beach ML, et al.: Flow dependency of error in thermodilution measurement of cardiac output during acute tricuspid regurgitation, *J Cardiothorac Vasc Anesth* 15(2):183–187, 2001.

Marik PE: Obituary: pulmonary artery catheter 1970 to 2013, *Ann Intensive Care* 3(1):38, 2013.

Martin C, Auffray JP, Saux P, et al.: The axillary vein: an alternative approach for percutaneous pulmonary artery catheterization, *Chest* 90(5):694–697, 1986.

Mermel LA, McCormick RD, Springman SR, Maki DG: The pathogenesis and epidemiology of catheter-related infection with pulmonary artery Swan-Ganz catheters: a prospective study utilizing molecular subtyping, *Am J Med* 91(3b):197s–205s, 1991.

Morris D, Mulvihill D, Lew WY: Risk of developing complete heart block during bedside pulmonary artery catheterization in patients with left bundle-branch block, *Arch Intern Med* 147(11):2005–2010, 1987.

Murthi SB, Hess JR, Hess A, et al.: Focused rapid echocardiographic evaluation versus vascular catheter-based assessment of cardiac output and function in critically ill trauma patients, *J Trauma Acute Care Surg* 72(5):1158–1164, 2012.

Narasimhan M, Koenig SJ, Mayo PH: Advanced echocardiography for the critical care physician: part 1, *Chest* 145(1):129–134, 2014.

Ramsingh D, Alexander B, Cannesson M: Clinical review: does it matter which hemodynamic monitoring system is used? *Crit Care* 17(2):208, 2013.

Rosen KR, Sinz EH: Simulation case library: the case of the coiled cardiac catheter, *J Educ Perioper Med* 4(2):E022, 2002.

Shah KB, Rao TL, Laughlin S, El-Etr AA: A review of pulmonary artery catheterization in 6,245 patients, *Anesthesiology* 61(3):271–275, 1984.

Swan HJ, Ganz W, Forrester J, et al.: Catheterization of the heart in man with use of a flow-directed balloon-tipped catheter, *N Engl J Med* 283(9):447–451, 1970.

第119章 液体和血液快速输注系统

S. Devi Chiravuri，L. Kareen Porter

病例概要

患者，男性，65岁，因腹主动脉瘤破裂被送入手术室进行急诊修复。患者行气管插管，存在低体温（34.5℃）和低血压（血压85/60 mmHg）。随即进行加压输液行容量复苏，输注液体采用1H-1200级静脉输液加温器加温。患者切皮前，患者血压降至60/30 mmHg，呼气末二氧化碳（$ETCO_2$）从35 mmHg急剧下降至10 mmHg，提示大量静脉空气栓塞。

问题分析

定义

当静脉内液体或血液必须以大于自由流动速度甚至输液加压袋装置所能达到的速率输注时，通常使用快速液体和血液输注（rapid fluid and blood delivery，RFBD）装置。现在的RFBD设备允许流量为1000 ml/min，具有“按刻度输入”流量的能力。除此之外，它还可以选择或设置输液的温度。

高压力提供高流量。RFBD的加压可以通过两种方法实现：外部气动加压和封闭式滚筒泵。而它的加热由水浴传导热交换或磁感应加热器提供。

除了可以提高流量和输液加温外，RFBD装置还必须能够检测或排放空气。空气收集器能够抽取小体积的夹带空气，但过多的空气有可能超出收集器的能力范围。很多市售RFBD设备都包含有安全保险机制，通过在检测到空气时关闭输液来防止空气被输送到患者体内。

与设备使用或故障相关的潜在并发症包括：

- 空气栓塞；
- 容量过多或输液过量（输血相关性循环超负荷）；
- 液体过度加热；
- 低体温；
- 溶血；
- 电击伤。

识别

静脉空气栓塞

静脉空气栓塞是麻醉中已经被详细阐述的并发症之一（见第127和186章）。无论是通过手术部位的夹带，或是通过静脉导管不慎进入，当大量空气进入静脉通路时都会发生这种情况；与外周静脉相比，中心静脉更易发生。空气进入心脏，会显著减少心排血量。它还可以通过卵圆孔未闭到达左心[反常空气栓塞（paradoxic air embolism，PAE）]，并可能导致冠状动脉缺血或脑缺血。麻醉科医师可以通过超声心动图、心前区多普勒或$ETCO_2$的突然下降来判断空气栓塞。空气栓塞的临床表现包括：

- 体循环低血压；
- 中心静脉或肺动脉压力升高；
- 心律失常；
- 低氧血症；
- $ETCO_2$急剧下降；
- 肺顺应性降低；
- 心血管衰竭。

高血容量

高血容量最初可导致高血压，但随着左心室前负荷和舒张末期容积的增加而最终脱离 Frank-Starling 曲线（前向左心室衰竭），随后可出现低血压。如果有中心静脉监测，则可见肺动脉压和肺毛细血管楔压升高。

低体温或高体温

如果输液时体温监测不当或加热装置出现故障，患者患者可能会发生低体温，可导致凝血障碍、心律失常、周围血管收缩和神经肌肉阻滞延长。

体温过高和体温过低一样有害，应通过温度监测检测高温。中心体温监测比皮肤温度监测更为准确。体温过高可引起血红蛋白等分子变性，引起血红蛋白血症和溶血反应。临床上表现为出汗、血管扩张、酸中毒和血红蛋白尿。

电击伤

电击伤并非 RFBD 设备所独有，任何与患者接触的电气设备都可能发生这种情况。电击可能导致疼痛、肌强直、热损伤或短暂性心律失常。

风险评估和影响

保持警惕性是医师必不可少的素质，特别是使用任何医疗设备期间。机器故障或操作错误都可能导致致命的并发症。

治疗

静脉空气栓塞的管理包括防止进一步空气进入和治疗空气栓塞。过去麻醉科医师所学到的方法是通过采用呼气末正压或 Valsalva 动作来降低右心房与左心房压力梯度来预防 PAE。然而，这些方法已被证明会增加 PAE 的风险，且由于颈静脉压迫操作效果更好，因此传统方法已在实践中被放弃。

如果怀疑发生静脉空气栓塞：

- 如果手术部位有空气进入，应立即提醒外科医师；
- 停止快速输液装置；
- 降低患者头部，并将患者置于左侧卧位（如可能）。进行颈静脉压迫；
- 停止氧化亚氮的使用；给患者吸入 100%FiO_2；
- 如果有中心静脉导管，尝试抽吸空气；
- 必要时，予以血流动力学支持，包括血管升压药物和实施胸外按压。

如果患者出现低体温，可通过提高室温、使用加热床垫和空气加温毯以及加温静脉输液来恢复正常体温（见第 115 章）。如果患者出现体温过高，通过关闭所有加热装置，并暴露皮肤或强制空气对流进行主动降温。

溶血反应常见的原因有：超压输液产生的剪切应力，血液和血液制品过热，输血反应或血型不匹配。治疗原则如下：

- 停止输血；
- 通知血库，重新检查血型交叉配对；
- 维持尿量；
- 碱化尿液；
- 监测有无弥散性血管内凝血的征象；
- 治疗高钾血症。

血容量过多可表现为肺或循环衰竭。治疗原则包括：

- 循环支持；
- 利尿；
- 扩血管治疗；
- 辅助通气或正压通气；
- 在极端情况下，施行放血治疗。

预防

提高警惕性是降低手术室麻醉风险的关键。在连接静脉输液管路和输液设备之前进行充分的排气是非常重要的步骤。仔细监测 $ETCO_2$ 是必要的预防措施。

通过积极治疗和中心体温监测可以预防体温过低和体温过高。皮肤温度监测有时会提供虚假信息，尤其是血管处于收缩状态时。

密切关注患者的容量状态也非常重要。尿量、中心静脉压、脉压变异度和经食管超声心动图也可提供有用的信息。

提高工作警惕性和正确维护手术室中的所有电气设备，可以将电击伤风险降至最低。可以从绝缘和接地故障检测报警器的快速检查开始着手。

最后，对于熟悉并正确使用和维护 RFBD 设备的重要性无论怎么强调都不过分。应该优先制订与此类设备相关的工作培训计划，保持设备的正常工作状态。使用者必须熟悉这些设备在不同情况下的能力和局限性，例如使用电池时和使用交流电源时的不同。为了避免不相容和凝血的风险，不应通过RFBD装置进行药物输注。应按照制造商的建议定期维护RFBD装置，以防止水浴加热装置出现故障或污染。RFBD系统可在需要大容量复苏的手术中发挥关键作用（例如重大创伤、心血管手术、肝移植），但只有在具有良好判断力的麻醉科医师正确使用的情况下才能发挥作用。

（孙媛媛 译 孟 岩 校）

延伸阅读

Bedford RF: Air embolism. In Gravenstein N, Kirby RR, editors: *Complications in anesthesiology*, Philadelphia, 1996, Lippincott-Raven, pp 271–280.

Comunale ME: A laboratory evaluation of the Level 1 Rapid Infuser (H1025) and the Belmont Instrument Fluid Management System (FMS 2000) for rapid transfusion, *Anesth Analg* 97:1064–1069, 2003.

Grady MS, Bedford RF, Park TS: Changes in superior sagittal sinus pressure in children with head elevation, jugular venous compression and PEEP, *J Neurosurg* 65:199–202, 1986.

McLellan E, Clark B, Townsend R: Mechanical failure of a Level 1 Rapid Infuser as a potential source of septicaemia, *J Hosp Infect* 66(4):399–401, 2007.

Poder TG, Nonkani WG: Tsakeu Leponkouo É: blood warming and hemolysis: a systematic review with meta-analysis, *Transfus Med Rev* 29:172–180, 2015.

Smith CE: Principles of fluid warming in trauma, *Semin Anesth Periop Med Pain* 20:51–59, 2001.

废气清除系统

第 120 章

Marc Sherwin，*James B. Eisenkraft*

病例概要

患者，男性，25 岁。无特殊既往史，行扁桃体切除术。麻醉诱导气管插管后，新鲜气体流量（fresh gas flow，FGF）6 L/min，以 O_2、N_2O 和异氟烷混合气体维持麻醉，患者通过循环呼吸系统保持自主呼吸。在外科医师要求下将麻醉机移动位置后，呼吸回路的储气囊开始逐渐膨胀。将可调节压力限制阀（APL 或 "popoff"）完全开放，也无法降低储气囊内的压力。呼吸回路需间断从麻醉机断开，才能减轻压力。当 FGF 降低到 2 L/min 时，才不再需要经常断开呼吸回路来减压。从关闭的废气清除系统接口处可听到嘶嘶声，储气囊此时完全空瘪。

问题分析

定义

新鲜气体从麻醉机持续流入循环呼吸系统；因此，必须留出相同容量的空间以避免呼吸回路压力的增加。废气清除系统是被设计用于患者自主呼吸时，收集呼吸回路中呼气末通过 APL 阀的废气，或在机械通气时收集通过压力释放阀（pressure relief valve，PRV）的废气，并排出手术室。该系统旨在减少呼吸回路中混合的麻醉气体对手术室环境的污染。

废气清除系统的基本组成是废气收集组件、输送管道、净化接口、废气排出管路和废气清除组件（图 120.1）。通过 APL 阀和呼吸机 PRV 排放的废气经输送软管送至净化接口端。经过净化后，废气进入气体排出管路，排出管道通常是一个单独的医院负压系统，使用紫色软管将其与医院主负压系统使用的白色软管区分开来。

净化端口设计既可以是具有正 PRV 和负 PRV 的**封闭**容器，或是一个提供评估系统功能的储气袋，也可以是与大气相通的**开放**容器。

在封闭容器设计中，正压释放阀的开启压力为 5 cmH_2O（一些新设备的开启压力为 10 cmH_2O），压力超过阈值时废气将被排放到室内（图 120.2）。如果负压流速不足（如紫色真空管未连接）或处理系统下游管路堵塞，则可能出现这种情况。在本病例中，正压 5 cmH_2O（或 10 cmH_2O）被反馈至呼吸系统，并形成呼气末正压（positive end-expiratory pressure，PEEP）出现在呼吸系统的压力监测器上。负 PRV 在 -0.5 cmH_2O（和 -1.8 cmH_2O）开放。这种情况发生在负压流速大于废气流量进入封闭容器的速度时。房间内的空气被负 PRV 抽吸时可能会产生嘶嘶声。在开放系统中，容器内的空气可由固定端口进入或排出，取决于端口内的压力大小。

清除装置可以分为主动系统和被动系统。主动系统包括应用吸力（真空负压）将废气从端口清除，而被动系统则允许气体通过管道被动流到手术室的排气格栅。主动系统的负压应能吸入 25 L/min 的气体，以便应对麻醉诱导和其他紧急情况下的 FGF 增高。气体排出管路和输送管路一样，应设计成防堵塞、不贴地面走线，以尽量减少受压或堵塞的可能性。

识别

废气清除系统的故障可能会将患者置于危险处境。呼吸系统压力增加超过设定限度将引起警报发声。压力监测系统在峰值压力过高、PEEP 过高、持续高压、压力过低和出现负压时会警报。如果患者自主呼吸，储气囊状态提供了评估压力的简单方法。如果呼吸回路压力增加，表明气体进入速度快于排

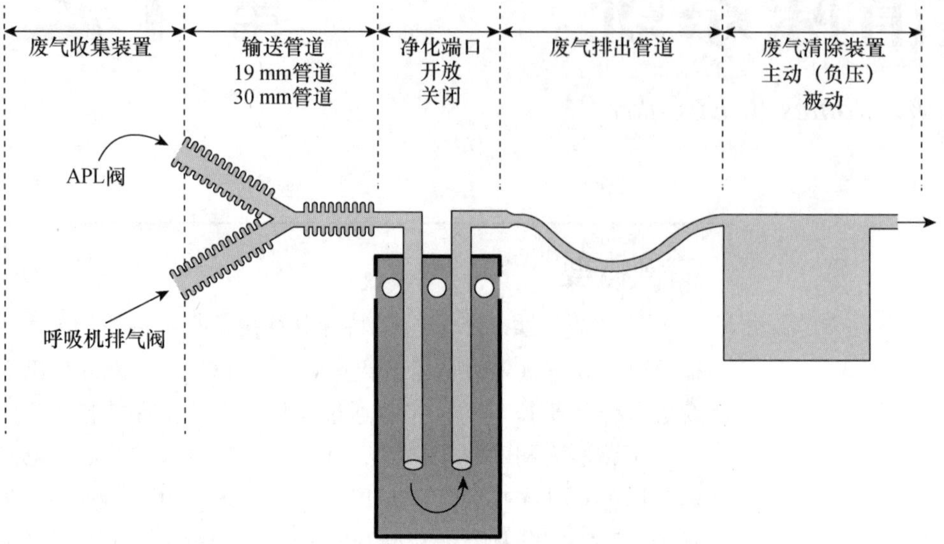

图 120.1　麻醉废气清除系统的组成部分。图中显示的接口为开放储存设计。当负压抽吸气体的速度超过从输送管流入的气体速度时，开放的端口允许空气进入接口

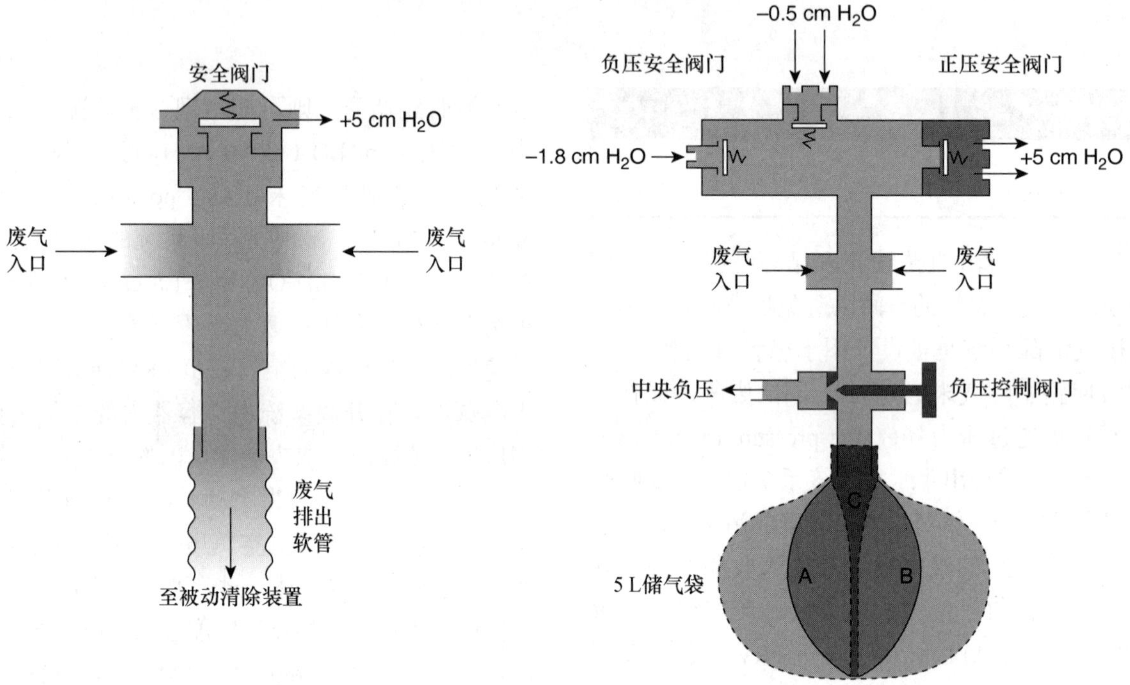

图 120.2　封闭的储存净化端口。左图：与被动处理系统连接的端口。右图：与主动系统连接的端口

出速度，必须从上游到下游检查气流路径，以确定受压或阻塞位置。如果气体收集装置部件（APL 阀和呼吸机 PRV）工作正常，气体将被释放到输送管路中，再到净化端口。如果输送管道堵塞，则废气不能流入净化端口。在评估端口时，识别所使用的系统类型（封闭容器和开放容器）十分重要。在有活性处理组件的封闭界面中，应检查储气袋是否膨胀过度或不足。压瘪的袋子表明气体排出量超过流入量。如果输送管路被堵塞（例如移动麻醉工作站时，管路被轮子压过），就会发生这种情况。由于没有气体到达端口，来自医院真空负压接口的持续负压抽吸导致房间空气通过 PRV 进入端口，造成嘶嘶声。

风险评估

由于麻醉科医师的不当操作或设备故障，可能会造成手术室空气被麻醉废气污染。增加污染的操作例子包括以下：

- 在将呼吸回路连接到患者前，打开麻醉气体；
- 在麻醉气体流出时，断开患者呼吸回路；
- 使用无气囊的气管导管或气管导管的气囊未充气；
- 在麻醉诱导或维持过程中，麻醉气体从面罩泄漏；
- 向挥发罐内加药时，液体麻醉气体溅出；
- 冲洗呼吸回路时。

除麻醉科医师失误外，机械性问题也会导致手术室污染。麻醉机、循环系统和废气系统的泄漏都可以污染空气。

废气收集装置回收通过 APL 阀或麻醉机 PRV 排出的麻醉气体，并通过两个独立管道将其汇入输送管道。如果废气收集装置或输送管路的任何部位有堵塞，导致气体不能进入净化端口，呼吸回路内的压力就会增大。高压可导致气压伤，甚至可能导致张力性气胸。

如果阀门系统出现故障，废气净化端口也可能出现问题导致危害。在封闭系统中，如果压力释放阀发生故障，清除系统中的负压或正压将传递到呼吸回路。接口压力释放阀可能堵塞，特别是负压释放阀。在开放系统中，如果端口意外堵塞，气体无法通过处理系统排出，产生的压力将被传输到呼吸回路。

启示

清除系统的问题对患者有潜在危险。极端负压会限制通气，引起肺泡塌陷，甚至可能引起负压性肺水肿。正压可能干扰通气，引起气压伤和张力性气胸。在大多数情况下，PRV 可防止清除系统的并发症，但无论阀门功能如何，进入的废气流速、负压流速和储气囊大小都会影响封闭储气系统。

通常认为，手术室内废气污染对麻醉科医师和手术室工作人员有害。1977 年，美国职业安全与健康研究所发表了每 8 h 内（时间加权平均值）空气中麻醉气体的最大允许值建议。这些建议从未颁布成法律，因此职业安全与健康管理局尚无法采取强制措施。目前为止，还没有研究最终证明手术室空气中微量的麻醉废气对人体健康有危害。

Allen 和 Lees 报告了一起工程设备室着火的案例，该设备室是一家医院负压泵的处理场所。被处理的废气通常含有极易燃浓度的氧气，如果直接输送到条件适宜的环境，就会导致危险的火灾发生。

表 120.1 国家职业安全与健康研究所建议的微量气体水平

麻醉气体	最大时间加权平均浓度（百万分之一）
只含卤化剂：	2
只含氧化亚氮：	25
卤化剂与氧化亚氮的混合气体：	
卤化剂：	0.5
氧化亚氮：	25
牙科设备（只含氧化亚氮）：	50

From U.S. Department of Health，Education and Welfare：*Criteria for a recommended standard*：*occupational exposure to waste anesthetic gases and vapors*. Washington，DC，U.S. Department of Health，Education and Welfare，1977.

管理

如果怀疑废气清除系统出现故障，应将患者与麻醉呼吸系统断开。患者可使用简易呼吸球囊进行通气，如果需要继续麻醉，应使用静脉麻醉药物维持。检查系统是否出现明显异常的迹象十分重要，如管路堵塞或阀门堵塞。如不能确定故障原因，应立即更换设备。如果患者出现负压损伤，如肺不张或肺水肿，应给予正压通气和纯氧治疗。如果正压导致张力性气胸，应置入胸管并进行妥善治疗。

预防

当使用 N_2O 和高浓度吸入麻醉药物时，麻醉机应配备功能正常的废气清除系统。麻醉工作站的使用前检查应包括废气清除系统。传输管道的直径应为 30 mm 或 22 mm，30 mm 管道以黄色标记，以区别于 22 mm 传输管道。为防止堵塞，传输管道应尽可能短而质硬，因这部分系统靠近净化端口的 PRV，在扭曲时会导致危险情况的发生。应检查是否存在可能干扰阀门或端口的松散物件。管路应在高处，如果在地面上，则不应将设备置于管道上，以防意外堵塞。废气必须从医院排放到不能再循环的地方。

为防止泄漏，避免对手术室空气的污染，麻醉设备应定期进行检查，包括气瓶阀门开启时检查 O_2 和 N_2O 供应是否有泄漏。还应进行适当的泄漏测试。如果使用无气囊的气管导管，手术室污染的风险更高。

（罗金华　译　陈元杰　校）

延伸阅读

Allen M, Lees DE: Fires in medical vacuum pumps: do you need to be concerned? *ASA Newsletter* 68:22, 2004.

ASTM: *Standard specification for anesthetic gas scavenging systems: transfer and receiving systems (ASTM F1343-02)*, Conshohocken, PA, 2005, ASTM International.

Barwise JA, Lancaster LJ, Michaels D, et al.: Technical communication: an initial evaluation of a novel anesthetic scavenging interface, *Anesth Analg* 113:1064–1067, 2011.

Carvalho B: Hidden hazards of scavenging, *Br J Anaesth* 83:532–533, 1999.

Eisenkraft JB, McGregor DG: Waste anesthetic gases and scavenging systems. In Ehrenwerth J, Eisenkraft JB, Berry JM, editors: *Anesthesia equipment: principles and applications*, ed 2, New York, 2013, Elsevier, pp 125–147.

Elakkumanan LB, Vasudevan A, Krishnappa S, et al.: Obstruction to scavenging system tubing, *J Anaesthesiol Clin Pharmacol* 28:270–271, 2012.

Joyal JJ, Vannucci A, Kangrga I: High end-expiratory airway pressures caused by internal obstruction of the Dräger Apollo® scavenger system that is not detected by the workstation self-test and visual inspection, *Anesthesiology* 116:1162–1164, 2012.

Kanmura Y, Sakai J, Yoshinaka H, et al.: Causes of nitrous oxide contamination in operating rooms, *Anesthesiology* 90:693–696, 1999.

McGregor DG: *Waste anesthetic gases: information for management in anesthetizing areas and the postanesthesia care unit (PACU)*, Park Ridge, IL, 1999, ASA Task Force on Trace Anesthetic Gases, American Society of Anesthesiologists.

Miller MG, Cullen BF: The cost of scavenging: is it worth it? *Anesth Analg* 58:265–266, 1979.

Mychaskiw G, Morris S: Dangerous design flaw in the Ohmeda Aespire anesthesia system, *Anesth Analg* 100:1543–1544, 2005.

Oliver Jr WC, Abenstein JP, Nuttall GA: Ventilator alarm failure due to modification of the scavenging system, *Anesthesiology* 93:1351–1352, 2000.

Panni KM, Corn SB: The use of a uniquely designed anesthetic scavenging hood to reduce operating room anesthetic gas contamination during general anesthesia, *Anesth Analg* 95:656–660, 2002.

Patel KD, Dalal FY: A potential hazard of the Dräger scavenging interface for wall suction, *Anesth Analg* 58:327–328, 1979.

Tavakoli M, Habeeb A: Two hazards of gas scavenging, *Anesth Analg* 57:286–287, 1978.

U.S. Department of Health, Education and Welfare: *Criteria for a recommended standard: occupational exposure to waste anesthetic gases and vapors*, Washington, DC, 1977, U.S. Department of Health, Education and Welfare.

外科电灼设备

第 121 章

Jeffrey J. Schwartz，Jan Ehrenwerth

病例概要

患者，男性，59 岁，行右侧结肠癌切除术。由于之前手术造成的粘连，术野暴露较为困难。外科医师数次抱怨术中所用的电外科设备（electrosurgical unit，ESU）工作状态不良，须增加能量。巡回护士按其要求，更换了一套新的 ESU 设备，但是仍未解决设备工作状态欠佳的问题。手术耗时 3 小时，术后患者被转运至麻醉恢复室（postanesthesia care unit，PACU）。PACU 护士在更换心电图（electrocardiogram，ECG）电极时发现患者与两个电极片接触的皮肤出现了 2 度烧伤。

问题分析

定义

外科手术使用电外科设备（也称为 ESU 或 Bovie）凝固血管或切割组织，为 500 000 ～ 1 000 000 赫兹（周期每秒）的高频交流电能。在该频率下的电流不会刺激心脏组织，而且当其穿过组织时不会产生电休克或心室颤动。

外科医师使用的手持设备是接触面积很小的电极，能在小范围内集中了较高的电流密度，达到切割或凝固组织的作用。而电流回路是通过一个较大的表面区域凝胶电极完成，称为负极板或分散电极，将其放至于患者体表并连接到 ESU 主机。分散电极具有表面积广，电流密度低，可安全传导能量的特点（图 121.1）。应注意，该分散电极常常被称为接地板。但这种理解绝对不正确，因为患者永远不会在手术室（operating room，OR）有意“接地”，因为这会增加电休克的风险。

如果分散电极没有正确地连接于患者，例如凝胶已干燥或使用不当，高频电流将寻找另一条回路。最常见的是 ECG 电极。然而，由于 ECG 电极的接触面积与分散电极相比小得多，电流密度较高，因此患者粘贴 ECG 电极的皮肤或接触放置不当的分散电极的皮肤会频繁出现烫伤（图 121.2）。温度探头和脑电双频指数监测电极也可能作为是回路电流的路径并造成烧伤。金属首饰如果与手术床接触，也可成为电流替代路径并导致烧伤。

识别

术中发现 ESU 的问题可能非常困难。由于 ESU 的工作频率很高，所以即使没有正确使用负极板，电流回路也很容易形成。甚至在很多情况下，ESU 似乎运行正常。新一代的设备具有提醒用户注意某些安全问题的功能。例如，如果来自负极板的电线未连接主机，主机会发出报警声。

ESU 出现问题也可能表现为，外科医师多次要求增加功率，术中难以切割或止血，以及清醒的患者有热感或烧灼感。

ESU 的使用还涉及其他几个问题。其中一个主要问题是电磁干扰（electromagnetic interference，EMI）。EMI 可干扰心脏起搏器，引起心律失常；干扰监控设备；在植入自动转复除颤仪（automated implantable cardioverter-defibrillator，AICD）的患者中模拟室颤的发生。

植入心脏起搏器的患者可能会出现快速型心律失常或抑制心率抑制。监测问题主要被视为电气干扰或电噪声。ESU 干扰可能导致植入 AICD 的窦性心律患者发生休克，并导致心室颤动。

其他 ESU 问题包括使各种化学品或病毒颗粒蒸发。此外，ESU 已被认为是大多数手术室火灾中的热源。

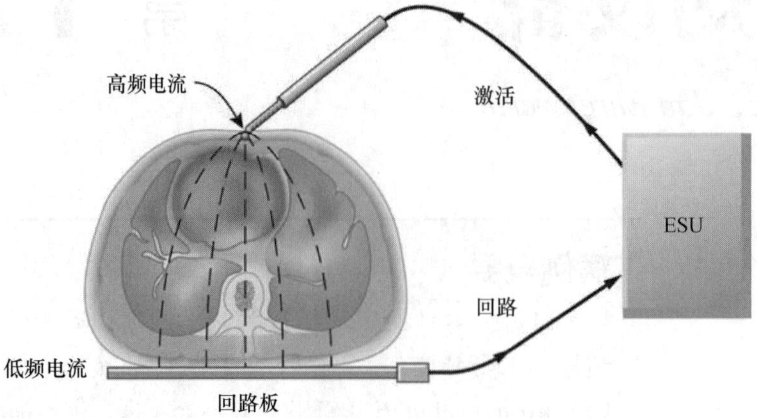

图 121.1 电外科设备负极板的正确使用。其电流较低，不会对患者造成危害（From Ehrenwerth J，Seifert HA：Electrical and fre safety. In Barash PG，Cullen BF，Stoelting RK，et al.，editors：*Clinical anesthesia*，7th ed. Philadelphia，Wolters Kluwer，2013，pp 189-218.）

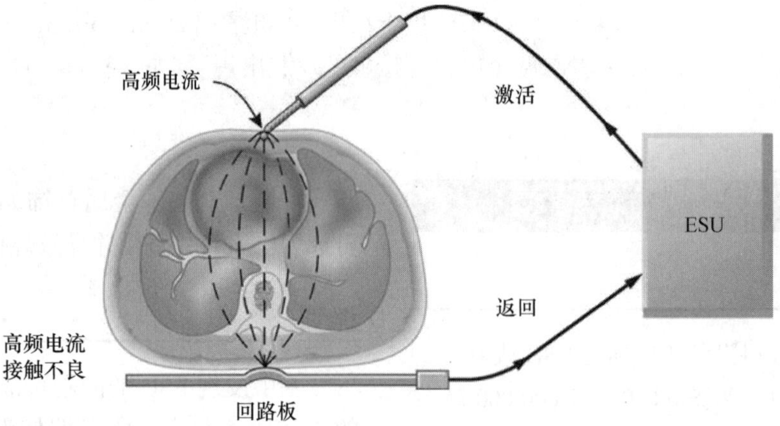

图 121.2 电外科设备负极板使用不正确。其接触不良时可引起高能电流甚至导致患者烫伤 / 烧伤（From Ehrenwerth J，Seifert HA：Electrical and fre safety. In Barash PG，Cullen BF，Stoelting RK，et al.，editors：*Clinical anesthesia*，7th ed. Philadelphia，Wolters Kluwer，2013，pp 189-218.）

风险评估

评估 ESU 使用的风险取决于 ESU 的类型和使用年限。较新的型号内置了安全防护系统，可以在出现问题时发出警报。大多数 ESU 问题涉及普通的单极 ESU，为外科医师手持能量电极，并通过大表面积的返回电极形成回路。双极 ESU 是电线钳，钳子的两头分别是正极和负极。不需要负极板，功率相对较低，因此风险较低。

另一种风险较小的设备是电烙器。这是一种电池供电的手持设备，用于凝固组织或止血，可用于眼科或其他小手术病例。

管理与预防

安全须知

确保 ESU 及其所有组件在使用前正常运行，可以防止 ESU 发生故障导致的烧伤。虽然通常是由手术间巡回护士负责检查 ESU 的安全性；但麻醉科医师、外科医师和所有手术团队成员都有责任。

围术期注册护士协会（the Association of peri-Operative Registered Nurses，AORN）发布了关于 ESU 使用的实践建议。该建议包括以下内容：

- 检查分散电极的有效期，在使用前立即打开包装，检查分散电极是否损坏。尤其是导电凝胶表面不应该干燥。
- 分散电极的导电侧应放置在清洁、干燥、无毛发的皮肤上，尽可能靠近手术部位，覆盖血管良好的肌肉块。如果可以避免，分散电极不应放置在植入的金属假体上，更不应放置于文身处，因为这些电极会将电流汇集在一起从而导致局部加热。分散电极不应放置在骨性隆起处，因为其不规则表面可能导致凝胶和皮肤之间不能完全接触。分散电极不应放置在止血带的远端或疤痕组织上，因为它们不能很好地导电。如果在术中改变患者的体位，则应重新检查分散电极的位置。

新一代的 ESU 可监视整个电路的阻抗，并且在分离电极环路被阻断或不良应用中发现电阻抗增加时，则可以发出警报或禁用。但这不是万无一失的。如前所述，如果出现活动性电极处温度增高，或外科医师频繁要求提高功率，此时应立即对电极板及连接回路做出评价。

腹腔镜手术存在 ESU 灼伤的额外风险，其与分散电极的不当放置无关。对于腹部手术来说，活动性电极周围的绝缘层的损坏可能导致杂散电能进入目标以外的部位。即使具有完整的绝缘，也可以在活动性电极的手柄和非目标组织之间具有电容耦合。

如果确实发生烧伤，患者应该接受烧伤治疗。损坏的绝缘层应该由生物医学工程师将 ESU 移除等待测试，尽管分散电极的故障可能性更大。范围较小的一度烧伤通常只需要用芦荟或其他保湿剂进行局部治疗。更严重的烧伤则需要会诊是否需要做整形手术或进行植皮手术。因为热量来源于身部内部，所以可能存在比表面上可见的更多的组织损伤。

其他电外科手术风险

对于心脏植入式电子设备（cardiac implantable electronic device，CIED）的患者，应将分散电极尽可能远离植入设备，以尽量减少对其的电子干扰。当需要在 CIED 15 cm 范围内使用活动性电极时，应考虑在手术期间改变 CIED 的功能。针对这种情况已经制定了各项管理指南。总之，最安全的策略是植入 AICD 的患者应该在手术期间暂停抗心动过速功能。具有心脏起搏器依赖的患者应该将起搏器切换到非同步模式。

为防止 ESU 引起火灾，所有基于酒精的制备溶液应在制造商建议的时间内（通常为 3 min）彻底干燥，然后再进行铺单。在气道未安全固定的头颈部手术中，必须注意限制使用供氧，因为富氧环境将显著增加所有手术室材料的可燃性。

（李盼盼　译　王晓琳　校）

延伸阅读

American Society of Anesthesiologists: Practice advisory for the perioperative management of patients with cardiac implantable electronic devices: pacemakers and implantable cardioverter-defibrillators: an updated report by the American Society of Anesthesiologists Task Force on Perioperative Management of Patients with Cardiac Implantable Electronic Devices, *Anesthesiology* 114(2):247–261, 2011.

Crossley GH, Poole JE, Rozner MA, et al.: The Heart Rhythm Society (HRS)/American Society of Anesthesiologists (ASA) Expert Consensus Statement on the perioperative management of patients with implantable defibrillators, pacemakers and arrhythmia monitors: facilities and patient management: executive summary, *Heart Rhythm* 8(7):e1–e18, 2011.

Ehrenwerth J: Electrical and fire safety. In Barash PB, Cullen BF, Stoelting RK, et al., editors: *Clinical anesthesia*, ed 8. Philadelphia, Lippincott Williams & Wilkins, 2017, pp 109–140.

RP Summary: Recommended practices for electrosurgery, *AORN J* 95:388–390, 2012.

Spruce L, Braswell ML: Implementing AORN recommended practices for electrosurgery, *AORN J* 95(3):373–384, 2012.

第122章 经食管超声心动图

Jack S. Shanewise

病例概要

患者，女性，75岁，诊断为不稳定性心绞痛，因血管介入治疗时缺乏合适导管导致血管重建不全而紧急行冠状动脉旁路移植术。心肺转流术期间发现置入经食管超声心动图（transesophageal echocardiography，TEE）超声探头困难。几次尝试后探头突然前移，随即发现探头尖端突破咽部后进入了心脏前方的手术区域。随后与家属沟通得知，患者有20年的吞咽困难史。

问题分析

定义

由于常需应用TEE，麻醉科医师需要了解其潜在的并发症及其预防方法。大多数TEE并发症较轻微，多为置入探头所导致的口咽部创伤。在极少数情况下会出现更严重的问题，如咽部穿孔、食管穿孔和胃肠道出血。

伴有声带功能障碍的喉部损伤是手术室特有的TEE并发症。这可能发生在坐位开颅手术期间进行TEE监测且长时间颈部过度屈曲的患者中。TEE探头的放置和操作可以压迫支气管或引起气管插管移位，特别是在儿童手术中。另外，TEE探头可能无意中插入未插管患者的气管而不是食管。同时，TEE探头的尖端有时会在食管中弯曲反折，造成退出操作困难而发生危险。

尽管由于探头过热造成食管灼伤在理论上存在可能性，但这种并发症尚未见报道。当探头温度超过安全水平时，大多数TEE系统会自动关闭。在TEE监测期间，麻醉科医师可能会因为分心于TEE而忽略更急更重要的生命体征变化。此外，如果缺乏正确的培训和知识，TEE监测可能被误读而导致错误的管理决策。

识别

口咽部损伤直接肉眼可见，或表现为口腔出血。而胃肠道出血可能是隐匿性的，甚至表现为低血容量性休克或不明原因的贫血。若置入胃管可以明确诊断。食管穿孔可在术野发现，也可能表现为随后出现的脓毒症，清醒患者可自诉有严重的胸痛。TEE后食管穿孔的诊断常被延误，特别是伴有其他并发症的患者，所以对心脏术后情况不佳的患者我们应该考虑到这一点。探头尖端弯曲可导致探头退出困难，常伴有异常成像（方向倒置）和控制旋钮活动度降低。

风险评估

在插入TEE探头之前，应尽量了解患者的所有食管症状和既往疾病，询问以下三个问题：

1. 您的食管有无问题？
2. 您是否存在吞咽困难？
3. 您有没有呕过血？

如果患者的回答均为“否”，则可继续进行操作。当患者无法交流时，应询问其家属。医生至少应检查医疗记录中的食管相关问题。

框122.1列出了TEE的禁忌证。然而，如果TEE能提供重要信息但患者有食管疾病史，可考虑使用纤维食管镜进行术前胃肠道评估。插入TEE探头前应评估患者口腔、牙齿松动情况并规避可预见性的损伤。另外，TEE探头转向线缆过紧或过松时均可能导致探头在食管中弯曲反折，应在使用前进行修复。

框 122.1 经食管超声心动图的禁忌证

绝对禁忌证
- 食管梗阻
  - 缩窄
  - 肿瘤
- 食管上括约肌或下括约肌肥厚
- 食管损伤
- 穿孔
- 近期食管手术
- 食管瘘
- 食管憩室
- 颈椎不稳定

相对禁忌证
- 未明确诊断的吞咽困难
- 食管静脉曲张
- 上消化道出血

大多数使用术中 TEE 时，会有其他监测和介入设备占据与 TEE 探头相同或临近的途径。这些装置包括气管导管、温度监测装置、胃肠引流管和鼻饲管。考虑到 TEE 探头的尺寸和硬度，这些装置中任何一个均有可能发生移位。装置移位的潜在并发症包括轻微影响（如胃管不在位）到可能危及生命的情况（如气管导管移位至主支气管造成通气异常）。

启示

TEE 的并发症虽然罕见，但可能是致命的。与所有医疗操作一样，在进行 TEE 检查前必须进行风险-获益分析。然而，大量的经验表明在合理筛查患者且操作得当时，风险是非常小的。

管理

经 TEE 检查后发现口腔出血时，应迅速、仔细地检查口咽部，以确定损伤的部位和程度。通常情况下，口咽部的轻微创伤不需要特殊治疗，但对于更广泛的损伤，可能需要使用抗生素。值得注意的是，对于 TEE 检查后出现的持续性胃肠道出血，应实施内镜检查。除了探查出血部位之外，也可提供治疗，如电灼和（或）血管收缩剂浸润治疗。疑似食管穿孔的患者，可口服水溶性造影剂进行 X 线诊断。穿孔通常被视为外科急诊。咽部穿孔可通过直视检查进行诊断，如果严重，需要紧急通知耳鼻喉科医师会诊实施外科引流。气道通畅始终优先于 TEE 监测，如果出现气道问题，应立即取出探头。如果 TEE 探头的末端在食管中反折，则应将其进至胃部，以获取更大空间使探头伸直以便取出。

预防

术前食管疾病的评估和探头置入与操作仔细而轻柔是预防 TEE 并发症的两个基石。置入和撤出 TEE 探头时，需关注与其占用相同路径的其他装置。遇到明显阻碍时绝不能使用暴力通过。不要长时间将探头锁定在弯曲位置，并且当探头手柄锁定时，探头不应向前或向后移动。

胃病患者可以安全地进行 TEE 检查，但操作者不得让 TEE 探头超出食管以外，以避免插入胃引起潜在问题。对 TEE 设备的损坏虽然并非严格意义上的并发症，但产生这种后果是极不可取的。通常情况下，TEE 设备是最昂贵的手术室设备之一，并且维修成本极高。同时，考虑到这些复杂电子设备的脆弱性，应特别强调轻柔操作 TEE 探头的必要性。

致谢

感谢 Patrick Benedict 博士对本章上一版的贡献。

（王 晓 译 王嘉锋 校）

延伸阅读

Augoustides JGT, Hosalkar HH, Milas BL, et al.: Upper gastrointestinal injuries related to perioperative transesophageal echocardiography: index case, literature review, classification proposal, and call for a registry, *J Cardiothoracic Vasc Anesth* 20:379–384, 2006.

Disibeyaz S, Parlak E, Koksal AS, et al.: What to do if a transesophageal echocardiography probe buckled in esophagus? *Echocardiography* 29:E85–E86, 2012.

Hilberath JN, Oakes DA, MD, Shernan SK, et al.: Safety of transesophageal echocardiography, *J Am Soc Echocardiogr* 23:1115–1127, 2010.

Kallmeyer IJ, Collard CD, Fox JA, et al.: The safety of intraoperative transesophageal echocardiography: a case series of 7200 cardiac surgical patients, *Anesth Analg* 92:1126–1130, 2001.

O'Shea JP, Southern JF, D'Ambra MN, et al.: Effects of prolonged transesophageal echocardiographic imaging and probe manipulation on the esophagus—an echocardiographic-pathologic study, *J Am Coll Cardiol* 17:1426–1429, 1991.

Piercy M, McNicol L, Dinh DT, et al.: Major complications related to the use of transesophageal echocardiography in cardiac surgery, *J Cardiothoracic Vasc Anesth* 23:62–65, 2009.

Spahn DR, Schmid S, Carrel T, et al.: Hypopharynx perforation by a transesophageal echocardiography probe, *Anesthesiology* 82:581–583, 1995.

第123章 挥发罐

Christopher J. Curatolo，James B. Eisenkraft

病例概要

患者，男性，54岁，美国麻醉科医师协会（American Society of Anesthe-siologists，ASA）分级Ⅱ级，全身麻醉下行腹腔镜腹壁疝修补术。患者基础血压为120/70 mmHg。顺利完成静脉诱导和气管插管后，将七氟烷挥发罐浓度刻度盘设置为以6 L/min的新鲜气流量输送3%浓度的七氟烷。开始机械通气后，再次测量患者血压为50/30 mmHg，而呼吸回路气体分析仪显示吸入浓度为4.4 vols%异氟烷。

问题分析

定义

假设分析仪的读数正确，患者接受的是异氟烷而非预期的七氟烷，而且浓度比挥发罐浓度刻度表盘上的设定值大得多。麻醉剂的不同可能是无意或故意将不同的麻醉剂（本病例为异氟烷）加注于特定药剂的七氟烷挥发罐所致。而导致麻醉气体输送浓度增加的因素，包括挥发罐注错药物、故障、倾倒、过多注药和通过挥发罐的气体逆流。

识别

这些情况的最终结果是麻醉剂和（或）浓度与预期不同，导致患者出现一些麻醉剂过量相关的临床症状和血流动力学表现，包括本病例所发生的严重低血压。鉴别药剂错误并测量其在呼吸回路中的浓度，对做出正确诊断至关重要。在尝试排除过量和不正确药剂的原因前，临床医师应立即停止使用有问题的挥发罐，并用氧气清除呼吸系统以快速降低麻醉剂浓度。同时注意纠正心血管抑制。麻醉科医师也可以考虑将患者与麻醉机的呼吸回路断开，并采用替代系统进行肺部通气，比如自动充气的手控通气装置（如简易呼吸气囊）或用不同的麻醉回路（如Bain）连接氧气源。

此外，还需做一些调查工作来确定麻醉剂过量是由挥发罐还是呼吸回路所致。由于现代强效挥发性吸入麻醉剂通过机装、校准，指定吸入麻醉剂的挥发罐输送，将挥发罐浓度刻度盘设为某一数值（例如1%），并会对从麻醉机的共同气体出口（common gas outlet，CGO）流出的气体中的药剂浓度进行取样和分析。CGO是麻醉机流量计和挥发罐产生的气体混合物离开机器进入呼吸系统的新鲜气体入口处。因此，CGO是输送系统中最靠近挥发罐出口的取样位置。校准完成的挥发罐其新鲜气体流量设置为5 L/min时（Dräger挥发罐的校准载气为空气，GE、Datex-Ohmeda和Penlon挥发罐的校准载气为氧气），浓度刻度盘设置为1%，使用校准的麻醉剂分析仪测量从CGO流出气体的药剂浓度。挥发罐在校准状态下（根据厂商说明），测量到的浓度应在挥发罐设定浓度的10%～15%（例如，若刻度盘设置为1%，则测量到的浓度应该在0.85%～1.15%）。

如检测到不同的麻醉剂，说明特定药剂的挥发罐并未含有它所标记的药剂，这种挥发罐应立即停用（必要时还应停用麻醉机），直到在非临床环境中对其进行检查和测试。如果检测浓度高于预期浓度，则可能是挥发罐而非呼吸回路出现问题。如果测得的药剂浓度与稀释浓度一致，则很可能是麻醉回路中有液体药剂。如果使用独立式挥发罐[例如，安装在新鲜气源和呼吸回路之间（以及灌注师在体外循环中使用的挥发罐）]，则应检查以确保新鲜气流经过挥发罐的方向正确（即新鲜气体通过挥发罐流入端进入，而非流出端进入）。

风险评估

挥发罐故障

除地氟烷外，目前大多数麻醉机挥发罐都采用可变旁路设计。新鲜气体被分成两条通道进入。大部分气体通过旁路，不接触麻醉剂蒸汽；少量气体进入蒸汽室并在饱和蒸汽浓度下与麻醉剂一起流出。当两路气流在挥发罐出气口混合时，旁路气流与挥发罐流出物混合以产生预期（设定的）浓度。虽然少见，但挥发罐本身也会出错。例如，挥发罐药液水平指示器可能失效，但并不表示挥发罐中没有吸入麻醉剂，这一情况很难被发现，除非使用者能警惕地察觉到麻醉剂呼气末浓度远低于挥发罐浓度表盘设定值。部分麻醉机，除高浓度报警外也有低浓度报警，有利于发现上述问题。已结案索赔案例的分析发现，因吸入麻醉剂不足导致的术中知晓时有发生。

特定药剂挥发罐的错误灌注

有数种情形下可能会出现挥发罐被灌注错误的麻醉剂。在某种实际情况下，排空挥发罐以保存液体麻醉剂，也可合理保管好一段时间内不会使用的挥发罐。在排空挥发罐时，可能出现药剂不匹配（即将一种药剂排放到标有不同药剂的空瓶中）。在世界的某些地区，只有一到两种挥发罐，无法与现有吸入麻醉剂罐相匹配。Adler 等描述了如何在执行医疗任务时尽可能安全地做到这一点，并根据挥发罐和麻醉剂不匹配时探索了挥发罐输出的数学和实验模型。尽管在灌注设计上取得进展（例如，密匙灌注和便捷灌注转换器），但仍有报告称，有使用者逾越了这些安全特性，并对挥发罐进行了错误填注。图 123.1 为挥发罐的填注系统。

过度填注和倾倒

挥发罐的过度灌注或倾倒可能导致来自挥发罐（或药槽）的液体药剂进入旁路，而该旁路设计仅用于气体（如氧气、氧化亚氮、空气）。引入旁路的极少量液体制剂可能导致潜在致死浓度的麻醉剂被输送入患者回路。这是因为，吸入麻醉剂（在 20℃和 1 个大气压下）的饱和蒸汽浓度范围从七氟烷的 21 vols% 到地氟烷的 88 vols%。在此条件下，1 ml 液体试剂蒸发可产生约 200 ml 蒸汽（表 123.1）。如果循环呼吸回路的容积约为 5 L，则进入该回路的 1 ml 液体药剂在完全混合的情况下可能导致约 [（200/5000）× 100]=4% 的浓度；在不完全混合的情况下，则可能导致更高的浓度。

在美国，挥发罐的灌注结构可能有不同设计（例如，漏斗式填注、密匙填注）。漏斗式填注挥发罐缺少特定的药剂填注系统（见图 123.1）。在填注过程中必须仔细检查，以确保药槽中的液位不超过

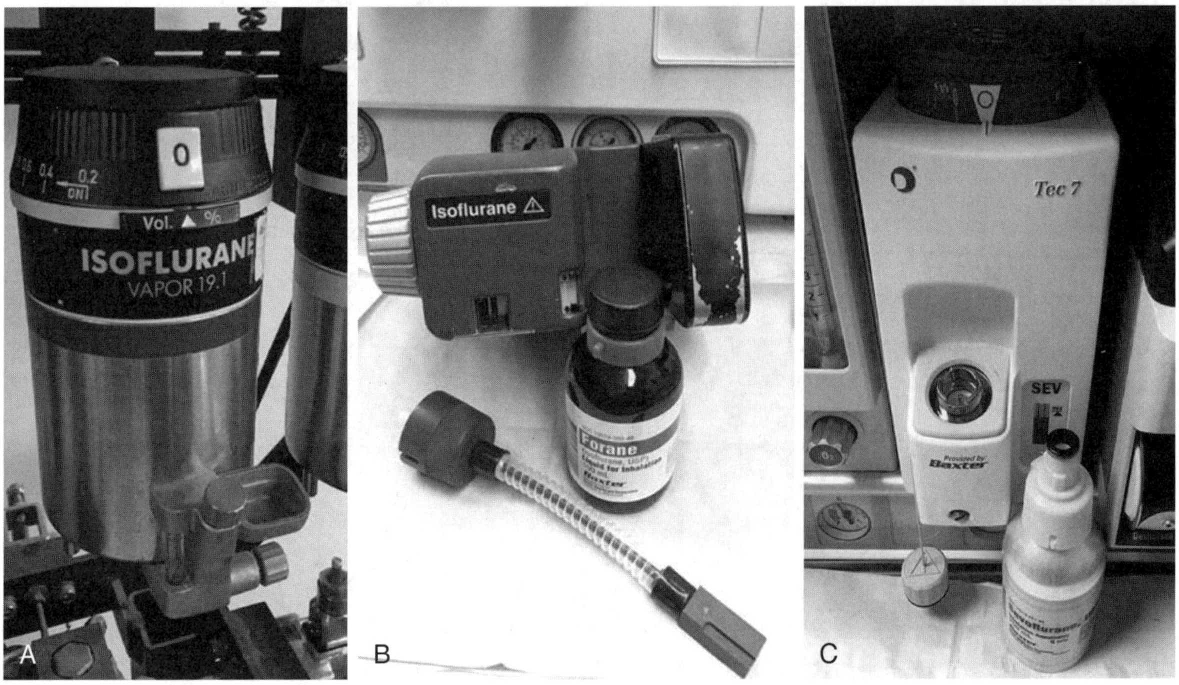

图 123.1　特定麻醉剂蒸发器的填注系统。图 A. 漏斗式填注；图 B. 密匙填注；图 C. 便捷填注

观察窗上指示的最高填注线。密匙填注挥发罐的过度填注已被广泛描述。密匙填注系统被设计为装有麻醉剂液体的瓶子和匹配挥发罐间有一个密封接头，而挥发罐刻度盘转到关闭位置。正确应用以下两种机制可防止发生过度填注。首先，当填注达到挥发罐中液体最大安全水平时，麻醉剂瓶内的空气吸入中断；其次，当挥发罐处于关闭位置时，挥发罐顶部的空气空间被密封，从而防止过度填注。密匙填注挥发罐的填注速度较慢，导致使用者会采取不当做法来加快填注。这种做法包括松开密匙填注装置和挥发罐之间的密封件，从而允许室内空气直接进入瓶子，并将浓度表盘旋转到接通位置。这种双重故障状态会允许过量的空气进入药剂瓶，由此允许过量的液体药剂进入挥发罐。这种挥发罐的过度填注会导致麻醉剂过量和神经损伤。

许多挥发罐有倾倒可能。如果将挥发罐从麻醉机中取出并倾斜在一边，则挥发罐药槽中的液体药剂可能会进入挥发罐的气体进出通道。Dräger Vapor 2000 和 3000 系列的挥发罐装有旋转装置（通过将试剂刻度盘浓度转至“T”来选择），可将挥发罐从麻醉机的安装架上移除，并隔离液体药剂室，从而防止其倾倒。GE Aladin 蒸发系统使用的是特定药剂的卡盒设计，此设计使得倾倒对挥发罐输出没有影响（图 123.1B）

独立式挥发罐和逆流

现代输送系统使用的挥发罐均安全安装在麻醉机的一个集合管上，但在兽医机构和实验室的体外循环机上仍在继续使用独立式挥发罐。独立式挥发罐更容易发生倾倒，因此特别危险。与浓度刻度盘设置相比，独立式挥发罐的浓度输出可能显著增加。此外，通过可变旁路、浓度校准或特定药剂的挥发罐，气体流动方向的逆转可严重影响其性能，这具体取决于模型。图 123.2 为安装在体外循环机上的独立挥发罐。请注意制造商对流出连接（outflow connection，OUT）的明确标记，以预防逆流事故的发生。据报道，此类逆流事件会导致吸入麻醉剂浓度过高的风险。最后，未经授权擅自改动麻醉机，可能导致挥发罐集合管的气流连接被接反。

启示

麻醉剂浓度超过挥发罐浓度刻度盘设定数值时，可能导致一系列并发症，从轻度的血流动力学不稳定到完全的心血管衰竭等。所有的吸入药物都是心肌抑制剂和外周血管扩张剂。准备使用七氟烷却错误地使用了过量的异氟烷，可能造成灾难性后果。异氟烷（20℃时为 238 mmHg）的饱和蒸汽压（saturated vapor pressure，SVP）高于七氟烷（20℃

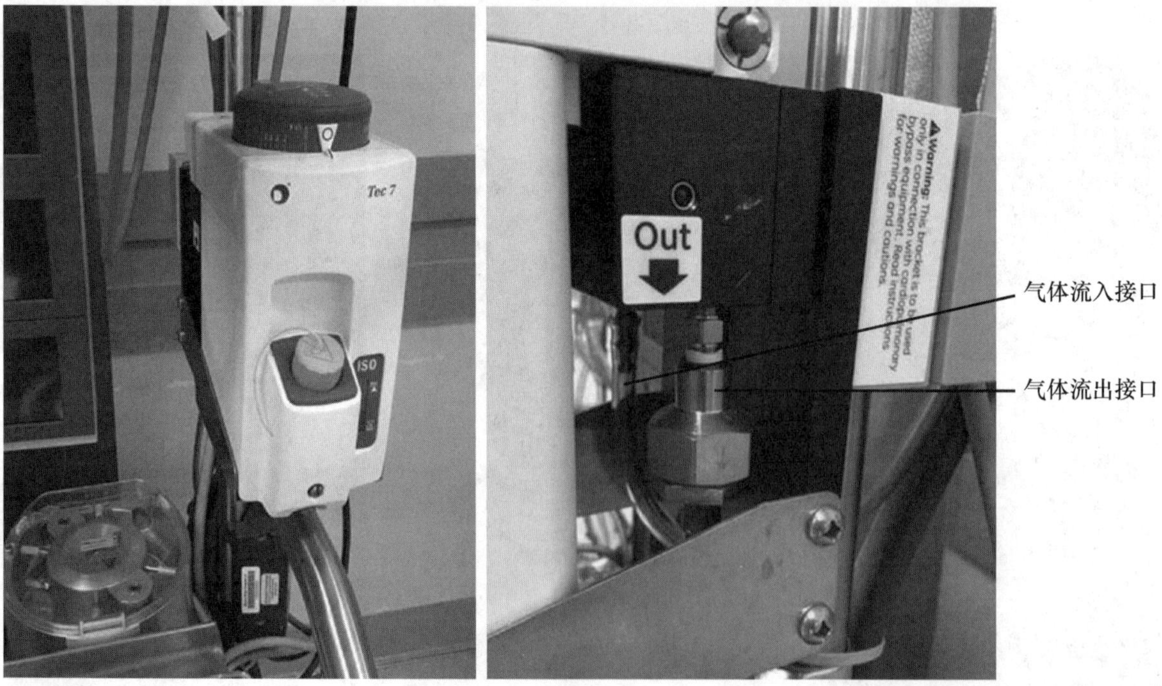

图 123.2 **图 A.** 安装在体外循环机上的独立挥发罐；**图 B.** 侧视图显示了入口和出口软管，如果装反可能导致麻醉气体浓度增加的风险

时为 160 mmHg），因此会产生更高的蒸汽输出浓度。再加上异氟烷 [最低肺泡有效浓度（minimum alveolar concentration, MAC）1.2%] 比七氟烷（MAC 2%）更有效，这一错误的影响是双重的，挥发罐效能（MAC 当量）更为显著。本病例概要中的患者，挥发罐输出的并非预期浓度为 3%（1.5 MAC）七氟烷，因为错误灌注，挥发罐提供的是浓度为 4.4%（3.7 MAC）的异氟烷。

对于特定药剂的可变旁路挥发罐，通过调节旁路和挥发罐输出的气体流量比例来产生所需的麻醉剂浓度。该比例取决于麻醉剂的物理性质、温度和稀释浓度。由于各种药剂的挥发特性存在区别，其饱和蒸汽压与温度呈曲线关系（表 123.1）。为达到所需的稀释浓度，表 123.2 为可变旁路的特定药剂挥发罐产生的旁路流量与蒸发室流出量的比值。在本病例中，七氟烷在 20℃时的饱和蒸汽压为 160 mmHg；因此，在一个大气压下，七氟烷将代表挥发罐中大气压的 21%（SVP/P_{atm}=160/760=21%）。如果从挥发罐中排出 100 ml/min 气体，就有 21 ml 气体为七氟烷蒸汽。为产生 1% 的浓度，必须将 21 ml 七氟烷稀释至 2100 ml 总体积。当总体积为 2100 ml 时，进入挥发罐的 2079 ml/min 流量会发生分流，使 79 ml 气体进入挥发罐，2000 ml 流入旁路（2100-79-21）。

表 123.1 20℃时每毫升液体麻醉剂的麻醉蒸汽体积	
麻醉剂	蒸汽 / 液体（ml/ml）
地氟烷	182
恩氟烷	195
氟烷	226
异氟烷	196
七氟烷	182

From Eisenkraft JB：Anesthesia vaporizers. In Ehrenwerth J，Eisenkraft JB，Berry JM，editors：*Anesthesia equipment*：*principles and applications*，2nd ed. Philadelphia，Elsevier，2013，p 67.

表 123.2 20℃时经旁路流至挥发罐的流出稀释比			
浓度	氟烷	异氟烷	七氟烷
1%	32：1	30：1	20：1
2%	10.6：1	14.5：1	9.5：1
3%	7：1	9.3：1	6：1

Adapted from Eisenkraft JB：Anesthesia vaporizers. In Ehrenwerth J，Eisenkraft JB，Berry JM，editors：*Anesthesia equipment*：*principles and applications*，2nd ed. Philadelphia，Elsevier，2013，p 67.

最后，流出稀释比是旁路流量与挥发罐流出量的比值。在本病例中，比例为 2000：100 或 20：1。

如果稀释为 3% 七氟烷（以达到 1.5 MAC 当量），则旁路气流和挥发罐流出气流之间将产生 6：1 的流出气流稀释比 [因为 21/（100+600）=3%]。当设置为 3% 的七氟烷挥发罐被错误灌注为异氟烷（20℃时 SVP 为 238 mmHg）时，挥发罐中则变为浓度为 31%(238/760）的异氟烷蒸汽。此时，当气体以 100 ml/min 从挥发罐流出时，31 ml 异氟烷蒸汽被稀释到 700 ml（100 + 600）的总体积中，导致异氟烷浓度为 31/700=4.4%（或 3.7 MAC 当量）。

表 123.3 为异氟烷错误填注至七氟烷挥发罐时导致的预测药物浓度和麻醉效能（MAC 当量）。

ASA 已结案的索赔项目，为识别麻醉相关不良后果提供了许多有价值的参考。1997 年，Caplan 等报告一项由气体输送设备引起麻醉不良后果的分析。分析显示，挥发罐是麻醉设备中仅次于呼吸回路引起不良后果的最常见原因。在 Mehta 等更新的（2013 年）类似分析中，自 1990 年以来，挥发罐问题（剂量不足和过量）是麻醉气体输送设备索赔的最常见原因。尽管很少发生并发症，但其中许多事件出现了灾难性的后果，患者病残率和死亡率高。

表 123.3 错误填注的挥发罐的预测蒸汽浓度和效能					
挥发罐	挥发罐内药剂	表盘浓度设置（%）	稀释比例	输出（%）	输出 MAC
异氟烷	异氟烷	1	30：1	1.00	0.83
	七氟烷	1		0.68	0.34
	异氟烷	2	14.5：1	2.00	1.67
	七氟烷	2		1.35	0.68
	异氟烷	3	9.3：1	3.01	2.51
	七氟烷	3		2.04	1.02
七氟烷	七氟烷	1	20：1	1.00	0.50
	异氟烷	1		1.48	1.23
	七氟烷	2	9.5：1	2.00	1.00
	异氟烷	2		2.95	2.46
	七氟烷	3	6：1	3.00	1.50
	异氟烷	3		4.43	3.69

管理

麻醉剂分析仪应设置合适的高浓度报警限值，这并非ASA麻醉基本监测的标准，却至关重要。这是检测浓度过高或不同药剂意外输送的最敏感方法，正如本病例概要所述。尽管许多麻醉从业人员依赖于单个挥发罐的精确校准，但若缺乏麻醉剂分析仪，则会大幅增加吸入麻醉剂过量或不足的可能，且不能预防不同药剂的意外输送。包括心电图和血压在内的标准监护仪，对检测潜在过量用药对血流动力学的影响至关重要。如果患者有自主呼吸，可能出现呼吸模式的改变。当蒸汽浓度大大超过浓度刻度盘设定值时，应立即给患者提供一种可替代的肺部通气方法（参见1993年美国食品药品管理局、2008年ASA的推荐）。如上所述，应对过量麻醉剂的来源或发生机制进行调查。

预防

灌注挥发罐时不应超过观察窗中的最大填注线以避免过度灌注；对密匙填注挥发罐，应遵循厂家说明（例如，将挥发罐刻度盘设置到"off"位置，并确保密匙填注喷嘴和挥发罐之间的密封性），此方法可以避免挥发罐的过度填注。

如果挥发罐已经倾倒或倾斜过大，则应采用来自机器流量计（不用绕过挥发罐的氧气冲洗）的高流量新鲜气体清洗挥发罐，同时将挥发罐浓度刻度盘设置为最大浓度，直到检测不到该药剂为止。该设置可最大限度地增加通过挥发罐入口和出口通道以及通过旁路的流量。然后重新填注挥发罐，并在挥发罐重新使用前，按照前述重新进行检查校准。

独立式挥发罐可能比安装在机器上的挥发罐的潜在危险更大。GE Ohmeda挥发罐可以用专门设计的支架安装在体外循环机上。使用这种独立式挥发罐时，在运输和使用过程中应注意避免倾倒。应该检查新鲜气体入口和出口与挥发罐之间的连接，确保没有接反——一旦接反则可能导致蒸汽浓度输出增加。

应该按照制造商的建议每天对麻醉机进行相应检查，在每个病例开始前还应行简化检查。低浓度和高浓度麻醉剂报警有助于检测药物剂量不足和过量。通过对结案的索赔案例分析发现，这两种情况都是导致不良结果的原因。正确地使用挥发罐可能有助于降低意外剂量甚至麻醉剂类型错误的可能性。如果发生此类故障，应立即对呼吸回路中的气体进行分析，然后迅速识别并采取适当措施，以防止对患者造成伤害。总之，一名警惕性高的麻醉科医师应懂得如何化险为夷，避免患者因此病残或死亡。

（凡丽华　译　韩文军　校）

延伸阅读

Adler AC, Connelly NR, Ankam A, et al.: Technical communication: inhaled anesthetic agent-vaporizer mismatch: management in settings with limited resources: don't try this at home, *Anesth Analg* 116:1272–1275, 2013.

Aisys anesthesia machine technical reference manual, Madison, WI, 2005, Datex-Ohmeda.

Andrews JJ, Johnston Jr RV, Kramer GC: Consequences of misfilling contemporary vaporizers with desflurane, *Can J Anaesth* 40:71–76, 1993.

Caplan RA, Vistica MF, Posner KL, et al.: Adverse anesthetic outcomes arising from gas delivery equipment: a closed claims analysis, *Anesthesiology* 87(4):741–748, 1997.

Dräger Vapor 19.1 operating instructions, Lübeck, Germany, 1992, Drägerwerk AG.

Dräger Vapor 2000 Anaesthetic Vaporizer: instructions for use, ed 2, Lübeck, Germany, 1998, Dräger Medical.

Eisenkraft JB: Anesthesia vaporizers. In Ehrenwerth J, Eisenkraft JB, Berry JM, editors: *Anesthesia equipment principles and applications*, ed 2, Philadelphia, 2013, Elsevier.

Eisenkraft JB: A commentary on anesthesia gas delivery equipment and adverse outcomes, *Anesthesiology* 87:731–733, 1997.

Found P, Forrest AP: Vaporizer level obstruction detected by anesthetic vapor analysis, *Anesth Analg* 88:469, 1999.

Hardy J-F: Vaporizer overfilling [Editorial], *Can J Anaesth* 40:1–2, 1993.

Martin ST: Hazards of agent-specific vaporizers. A case report of successful resuscitation after massive isoflurane overdose, *Anesthesiology* 62:830–831, 1985.

Mehta SP, Eisenkraft JB, Posner KL, et al.: Patient injuries from anesthesia gas delivery equipment: a closed claims update, *Anesthesiology* 119:788–795, 2013.

Ohmeda Tec 5 continuous flow vaporizer: operation and maintenance manual, Madison, WI, 1989, Ohmeda.

Sinclair A, Van Bergen J: Vaporizer overfilling, *Can J Anaesth* 40:77–78, 1993.

Tobias JD: Administration of sevoflurane using other agent-specific vaporizers, *Am J Therap* 5:383–385, 1998.

第五部分

围术期事件

第124章 神经后遗症：中枢神经损伤

Rebecca M. Gerlach，Mark A. Chaney

病例概要

患者，男性，68岁，合并胰岛素依赖型糖尿病和高血压，有吸烟史80包年，拟行4支冠状动脉旁路移植术（coronary artery bypass grafting，CABG）。麻醉平稳诱导后，经食管超声心动图发现主动脉弓处有严重的主动脉粥样硬化，遂在主动脉置管前进行了主动脉周围超声扫描，以确定最佳置管位置。心肺转流术（体外循环）期间患者体温维持在32℃，平均动脉压为50～60 mmHg。在未输注血制品的情况下，血红蛋白维持在7 mg/dl以上。尽管手术操作成功，但患者术后出现了明显的短期记忆丧失和手灵活性下降。出院后患者先入住了一家专业的康复护理机构，最后入住了一家辅助生活中心（assisted-living home）。

问题分析

定义

许多患者，尤其是老年和大手术患者，术后会出现神经功能整体下降，其原因既非间断的缺血性事件（卒中），也非急性疾病或药物作用（谵妄）。这种功能下降可能是暂时的，也可能持续数周至数月，甚至可能导致永久性残疾和功能改变。术后中枢神经功能损伤综合征的诊断，可通过术后神经心理学测试的认知能力与患者术前基线水平相比较来诊断。然而，神经心理学测试费时费力，并非术前常规检查，因此许多患者术后即使临床上怀疑，也未被正式诊断为术后认知功能障碍（postoperative cognitive dysfunction，POCD）。与谵妄的诊断不同，POCD既没有DSM-V的明确诊断标准，也没有明确的神经心理学测试的下降程度的诊断标准。麻醉后中枢神经功能障碍的范围很广，本章将重点讨论POCD；术后谵妄（见第166章）、苏醒延迟（见第137章）、苏醒期躁动（见第189章）和血栓栓塞并发症（见第183章）将在本书其他章节详细讨论。

识别

患者出现神经功能障碍的首发症状可能是患者自诉“感觉不对”，或是家属注意到患者“行动迟缓”或健忘加重。过去，由于此种功能下降最常见于心脏手术后，因此被认为完全与体外循环有关（如“pump head”）。现在认识到，虽然这种现象仍最常见于心脏手术后，但它可发生在任何大手术后。非心脏大手术和心脏手术后患者在出院时的POCD发病率高得惊人，两类手术的POCD发病率分别为30%～40%和>50%。这一比例在青年和中年非心脏大手术患者出院3个月后降至约5%，老年患者仍超过12%。心脏手术后患者即使出院数月后，患病率仍接近30%。

用于诊断POCD的神经认知功能测试可评估认知功能的几个方面，包括总体功能、执行功能、学习和记忆能力、视觉空间功能和（或）精神运动功能（表124.1）。简易精神状态检查（Mini Mental Status Examination，MMSE）是一种床旁问卷形式的评估量表，方便用于评估患者的整体神经认知功能，并涵盖了诸多认知功能相关的领域（表124.2）。虽然MMSE原本是设计用于痴呆筛查的工具，但也

表 124.1 用于术后认知功能障碍诊断的神经认知测试

核心领域	认知过程	测量	所需时间
整体功能	多重的	蒙特利尔认知评估（MoCA）	约 15 min
执行能力	简单注意力	韦氏成人智力量表中的顺序数字广度测试—第 3 版修订版（WAIS- Ⅲ）	约 5 min ～ 10 min
	复杂的记忆力（工作记忆）	逆序数字记忆广度测试（WAIS- Ⅲ）	约 5 min ～ 10 min
	反应抑制	斯特鲁普色词测试	3 min ～ 4 min
	思维灵活性	特雷尔 A/B 测试	每个子测验约 5 min
	语言流畅性	对照口语词汇联想测试（COWA）	3 min
学习和记忆	听觉-语言的学习和记忆	霍普金斯语言学习测试-修订版（HVLT-R）	35 min
	视觉的学习和记忆	简化视觉空间学习测试-修订版	45 min
视觉空间功能	视觉运动整合	数字符号编码测试（WAIS- Ⅲ）	5 min
	复杂的视觉空间感知	霍伯视觉组织测试（HVOT）	约 10 min ～ 12 min
精神运动功能	手动灵活性和运动速度	拉斐特槽钉板实验	约 5 min

Modified from Berger M，Nadler JW，Browndyke J，et al.：Postoperative cognitive dysfunction：minding the gaps in our knowledge of a common postoperative complication in the elderly. *Anesthesiol Clin* 33（3）：517-550，2015.

表 124.2 简易精神状态检查（MMSE）中的认知能力测试

认知能力	评分	测试
定向力	10	报告时间和地点准确
重合度	3	复述物品的名称
注意力和计算能力	5	执行简单的运算和拼写
回忆	3	回忆之前指定的物品
语言	9	说出某物品名称、重复一个简单的短语遵循一个三个步骤的命令和一个简单的书面命令，写简单的一句话，复制一张简单的绘画

可用于患者术后认知改变及其随时间而改善的情况的筛查。该测试需耗时 5 ～ 10 min，需对 30 分的总分值进行评分。该测试要求患者具备基本的读写能力，并且随着测试时间的推移容易受到学习效应的影响，可能会对结果的准确性造成干扰。与进行更广泛的神经认知功能测试相比，MMSE 难以区分功能障碍的特定领域。

测试中应该涵盖的认知领域的数量仍是未知的，但推荐至少应涵盖四个方面。即使进行了一整套测试，诊断 POCD 的阈值也尚未确定。仅有某一领域评分显著下降的意义也不明确。测试通常在手术的急性期影响消退后进行（一般在手术 1 周后）。

风险评估

POCD 的确切机制尚不清楚，它可能是由多种途径共同作用的结果，包括脑微栓子和手术或麻醉所致的中枢神经炎症反应。已经识别出多种相关的特殊危险因素，它们既与患者因素相关，也与操作因素有关，但其中多种危险因素是不可调控的。高龄一直被认为是 POCD 的危险因素，随着手术人群年龄的持续增长，寻找可调控的危险因素变得更加重要。

不可调控的危险因素：

- 高龄；
- 神经认知储备的基础水平（教育水平、遗传风险、海马体积）；
- 既往有卒中史；
- 原有神经系统疾病；
- 术后谵妄。

有调控可能的危险因素：

- 吸烟；
- 术后感染；
- 术后呼吸系统并发症或肺部基础疾病；
- 麻醉、手术或住院时间；
- 周围血管疾病；
- 糖尿病；

- 高血压，尤其是入院时收缩压大于 180 mmHg；
- 过量饮酒；
- 全身麻醉相对于局部麻醉（有争议）；
- 麻醉相对过量（有争议）。

值得注意的是，尽管数据存在争议，仍有数项研究提示，全身麻醉药的过度暴露可能会导致 POCD，而以脑电双频指数（bispectral index，BIS）监测指导滴定麻醉药用量可能将这种风险降到最低。但仍需要进行深入研究以确定两者之间的关系。

心脏手术特有的危险因素：

- 近端主动脉粥样硬化或既往 CABG 术史；
- 术后心房颤动；
- 体外循环期间灌注压低；
- 体外循环期间血液稀释；
- 高血糖；
- 从低体温状态下快速复温；
- 体外循环下（on-pump）[与非体外循环下（off-pump）相比]行 CABG。

外科医师的某些技术操作增加了大脑微栓塞的风险，这与 POCD 的发生有关，包括置管过程中对主动脉的操作，如钳夹阻断、侧壁钳夹、松开钳夹或提起心脏等。体外循环回路相关的操作和体循环时间过长，由于增加了发生空气栓塞和微血栓栓塞的风险，也被认为是发生中枢神经系统损伤的危险因素。

启示

围术期中枢神经系统损伤作为一种灾难性的并发症，可严重影响患者的生活质量，并占用大量的医疗资源。对于神经认知功能储备有限的患者，即使是轻微的神经认知改变也往往意味着严重的后果，患者难以恢复至原有的基础功能状态和生活自理。丹麦的一项前瞻性研究显示，POCD 持续 3 个月的患者死亡率显著增加[经性别、年龄及是否是癌症患者等因素校正后的危害比为 1.63（1.11 ～ 2.38）]。POCD 持续 1 周的患者，更容易因残疾或提前退休而永远地离开劳动力市场[经性别和年龄校正后的危害比为 2.26（1.24 ～ 4.12）]，而且在更长的时间段内，患者需要的社会转移支付也显著增加（60% vs. 41.2%）。由于手术患者年龄一直在持续增长，因而如何预防和治疗 POCD 已成为一个重要的公共健康问题。

处理

有关 POCD 的病因、危险因素和处理等方面仍存在许多未能解答的问题（表 124.3）。患者一旦发生 POCD，除了进行认知功能康复的支持治疗外，对理想的治疗方案仍知之甚少。由于许多患者会自行康复，因此这方面的研究也很少。既然术后谵妄和炎症状态是 POCD 的危险因素，因此对这些方面进行优化治疗应该是前景可期的，包括对危重症或感染的治疗，以及避免患者出现长时间的未经治疗的术后疼痛。

预防

尽管人们对围术期认知功能下降的药物预防有相当大的兴趣，但尚无较好的给药方案或治疗共识。有几种药物对早期认知功能的改善有帮助，被认为是与这些药物的抗炎作用有关。一项 51 例患者的随机研究显示，麻醉诱导时单次静脉注射氯胺酮（0.5 mg/kg）可改善心脏手术后 1 周内患者的认知功能。同样，其他两项随机试验也显示，硫酸镁可改善心脏或血管手术后数日内患者的认知功能。然而，这些药物的疗效持续时间短，临床效果有限。有关硫喷妥钠、丙泊酚、尼莫地平、谷氨酰胺 / 天冬氨酸、来昔帕

表 124.3 术后认知功能障碍（POCD）相关的未解答的问题

因素	问题
年龄	衰老是如何影响 POCD 风险的?
麻醉方式	对何种患者麻醉方式（全身麻醉 vs. 区域麻醉）可能影响 POCD 的风险?
痴呆	POCD 是否长期伴有痴呆风险的增加?
共存的退行性疾病	退行性疾病如何导致与 POCD 有关的中枢神经炎性病变，如阿尔茨海默病?
风险评估	是否存在 POCD 的 CSF 生物标志物?
SSRI 的作用	SSRI 是预防 POCD 的有效治疗选择还是过程中的改进?
缺血预处理	缺血预处理是否可以预防 POCD ?
预先锻炼	身体或认知功能的术前预先锻炼是否能有效降低 POCD 的严重程度?

CSF，脑脊液；SSRI，选择性 5- 羟色胺再摄取抑制剂

Adapted from Berger M，Nadler JW，Browndyke J，et al.：Postoperative cognitive dysfunction：minding the gaps in our knowledge of a common postoperative complication in the elderly. *Anesthesiol Clin* 33（3）：517-550，2015.

泛（lexipafant）、利斯的明、氙气、促红细胞生成素和瑞马酰胺等进行的随机研究均未能证实对降低 POCD 发生率有益。

在过去的十年中，优化心脏手术后患者的脑功能预后一直是很多临床研究关注的主题。目前，使用能探测脑灌注不良的监测有望能改善患者认知功能的结局［例如，近红外光谱（near-infrared spectroscopy，NIRS）监测］。脑氧饱和度监测常用于心脏手术中监测患者脑血流的氧饱和度。迄今为止，在氧饱和度较基线值下降 20% 时即采取干预措施以优化脑的氧合的方法并未能降低 POCD 的发病率，但长时间脑氧去饱和大于 50% 则与出现神经认知功能下降的风险之间存在明确的关系。针对高危患者采用的多模式监测策略，包括血流动力学监测、体温监测、NIRS，甚至 BIS 监测，是改善大手术后患者认知状况最有前景的策略。但仍须确定的是，何种患者、何时和如何进行这些监测，以及哪些干预措施最为有效。

致谢

感谢 David Muzic 博士对本章上一版的贡献。

（王树欣 译 倪 文 校）

延伸阅读

Berger M, Nadler JW, Browndyke J, et al.: Postoperative cognitive dysfunction: minding the gaps in our knowledge of a common postoperative complication in the elderly, *Anesthesiol Clin* 33:517–550, 2015.

Bilotta F, Gelb AW, Stazi E, et al.: Pharmacological perioperative brain neuroprotection: a qualitative review of randomized clinical trials, *Br J Anaesth* 110(Suppl 1):i113–i120, 2013.

Chan MT, Cheng BC, Lee TM, et al.: BIS-guided anesthesia decreases postoperative delirium and cognitive decline, *J Neurosurg Anesthesiol* 25:33–42, 2013.

Fedorow C, Grocott HP: Cerebral monitoring to optimize outcomes after cardiac surgery, *Curr Opin Anaesthesiol* 23:89–94, 2010.

Fines DP, Severn AM: Anaesthesia and cognitive disturbance in the elderly, *Contin Educ Anaesth Crit Care Pain* 6:37–40, 2006.

Folstein MF, Folstein SE, McHugh PR: Mini-Mental State: a practical method for grading the cognitive state of patients for the clinician, *J Psychiatr Res* 12:189–198, 1975.

Grigore AM, Grocott HP, Mathew JP, et al.: The rewarming rate and increased peak temperature alter neurocognitive outcome after cardiac surgery, *Anesth Analg* 94:4–10, 2002.

Hudetz JA, Iqbal Z, Gandhi SD, et al.: Ketamine attenuates post-operative cognitive dysfunction after cardiac surgery, *Acta Anaesthesiol Scand* 53:864–872, 2009.

Monk TG, Weldon BC, Garvan CW, et al.: Predictors of cognitive dysfunction after major noncardiac surgery, *Anesthesiology* 108:18–30, 2008.

Newman MF, Kirchner JL, Phillips-Bute B, et al.: Longitudinal assessment of neurocognitive function after coronary-artery bypass surgery, *N Engl J Med* 344:395–402, 2001.

Stanley TO, Mackensen GB, Grocott HP, et al.: The impact of postoperative atrial fibrillation on neurocognitive outcome after coronary artery bypass graft surgery, *Anesth Analg* 94:290–295, 2002.

Steinmetz J, Christensen KB, Lund T, et al.: Long-term consequences of postoperative cognitive dysfunction, *Anesthesiology* 110:548–555, 2009.

第125章 神经系统不良后遗症：周围神经损伤

Elizabeth Healy，Mohammed M. Minhaj

病例概要

患者，男性，62岁，接受冠状动脉旁路移植手术。该手术通过胸骨正中切口进行，术中取内乳动脉用来移植。在例行术后访视中，患者主诉左手无名指和小指有“刺痛”感。体格检查发现手指感觉减退，尺神经支配区出现轻微肌力下降。神经科会诊后，患者被诊断为臂丛神经损伤。

问题分析

定义

周围神经损伤（peripheral nerve injury，PNI）是围术期一种较常见且被充分认识的麻醉并发症。损伤通常较为短暂，却涉及大多数诉讼案件。美国麻醉科医师协会（American Society of Anesthesiologists，ASA）最新的完结索赔分析中，PNI占16%。这一比例在10年间保持稳定（以前为15%），这意味着我们对PNI病理生理学缺乏认识，当前预防策略未达到理想效果。尺神经损伤是PNI最常见损伤类型，其次为臂丛神经损伤、腰骶神经根损伤和脊髓损伤。近年来，尺神经损伤的索赔比例一直在下降，但脊髓损伤的索赔不断增加。

在66%的相关病例中，人们认为麻醉并无差错，进一步表明对该并发症的认识不够充分，该并发症可能是多因素所致。通常认为，造成PNI的机制包括：

- 直接创伤/撕裂（即颈内静脉置管、第一肋骨骨折穿透神经丛）；
- 压缩/拉伸（导致传导阻滞或缺血的机械性压迫）；
- 毒素（即直接注射局部麻醉药物）；
- 双重损伤——预先存在的神经损伤（糖尿病或类风湿性关节炎）会使同一区域或附近神经更易受到损伤。

事实证明，PNI真实发病率很难确定，部分原因是许多研究为回顾性研究，漏报率较高。据报道，PNI总发病率为0.03%～0.14%。在心脏手术中，PNI发病率为0.2%～38%。尽管PNI在心脏手术中的发病率最高，其在不同专科中都有报道，包括神经外科、骨科、普外科、结直肠外科、产科和妇科。事实上，一项逾10年超过380 000例患者的研究发现，PNI在神经外科、心脏外科、普外科和骨科发生最多。许多文献报道了臂丛神经损伤，也有腓神经、膈神经和交感神经损伤等报道。该研究还指出，与外周神经阻滞、监护下麻醉和腰麻相比，PNI与硬膜外麻醉和全身麻醉具有相关性。椎管内麻醉通常更多与下肢神经损伤相关。

识别

大多数PNI在术后即刻被发现。少数病例在术后几天到几周内才被发现。从外科手术到症状出现的过程存在较大差异，提示术后可能存在特定的触发事件。也有观点认为，先前存在的外周神经病变可能在此时表现出来。

PNI可出现感觉障碍、运动障碍或两者兼有。一些作者认为，在臂丛神经损伤时，功能障碍的出现是疾病进展的一个过程——感觉和运动神经细胞死亡的时机不同。对接受正中胸骨切开术的患者，有人认为低位神经根损伤更易出现感觉丧失，高位及中位神经根损伤更易表现出运动功能丧失。心脏手术后，臂丛损伤更易出现在较低位的神经根，表现为感觉缺失。非心脏手术相关的损伤倾向于发生在高位或中位神经干。

术中使用躯体感觉诱发电位（somatosensory evoked potential，SSEP）检测 PNI 尚存在争议。使用 SSEP 监测潜在神经损伤在神经外科文献中已有报道。Hickey 等试图将其应用于心脏手术。其研究指出，当放置胸骨撑开器时，SSEP 波形明显变化，但这些变化与术后神经病变并不相关，使其术中预测 PNI 的能力受到质疑。手术结束时检测到的 SSEP 变化，可能能够更好地预测周围神经病变。

继发于体位摆放的神经损伤通常为单侧，且仅影响单根神经。应当将其与其他原因导致的神经功能障碍区分，如颈椎损伤、肌肉骨骼损伤、自身免疫性神经系统疾病或急性臂丛神经炎（Parsonage-Turner 综合征）。急性臂丛神经炎（每年 1.6/100 000）以快速发作的剧烈双肩疼痛并向上臂辐射为特征。疼痛通常不会伴随神经根分布，最终演变为肌肉无力或肌肉萎缩。臂丛神经炎由手术所致压力反应引起，可能伴随手术而出现，通常与 PNI 高风险因素有所区别。臂丛神经炎以支持治疗为主，通常在几个月内自行缓解。

风险评估

文献证实，某些神经在麻醉期间受到损伤的风险更大。目前普遍认为，出现损伤最多的是尺神经和臂丛神经，这可能与其解剖位置有关。尺神经从髁突上绕过时位置表浅，易在髁间沟受压。臂丛神经近端出椎管处和远端腋筋膜处极易受损伤。多个骨性凸起也增加了神经丛对压迫性损伤的易感性，如锁骨、第一肋骨、肱骨头和喙突。

如上所述的解剖关系，被认为是正中胸骨切开术造成神经损伤的重要原因。Vander Sal 等在一项尸体研究中发现，正中胸骨切开术增加了第一肋骨骨折的发生率。其描述 15 例中有 11 例肋骨移位到神经丛中。在另外 15 具尸体中，胸骨撑开器放置更靠近尾侧，则没有发现肋骨骨折。该作者随后也注意到，肋骨骨折和臂丛神经损伤并不相关，但当撑开器靠近尾侧时，对臂丛损伤的发生率具有明显影响。

胸骨撑开器已多次被证实会导致神经损伤，但其机制尚未明确。可能机制是第一肋骨向头侧和后侧旋转导致神经丛受压或缺血。Lederman 等认为，颈内静脉置管可能通过直接针刺伤或随后形成的血肿导致神经损伤。

心脏手术中冠状动脉旁路移植术（coronary artery bypass graft，CABG）需要不对称的胸骨牵开，这被认为是 PNI 主要的风险因素。需要取内乳动脉（internal mammary artery，IMA） 进 行 CABG 时，PNI 发生率接近 10%；其他情况下 PNI 发生率接近 1%。Jellish 等利用 SSEP 对该结果进行验证，发现使用不对称胸骨撑开器时双臂波幅均明显降低。一些作者假设，“举手”姿势有助于缓解臂丛张力，减少神经损伤。Jellish 等也证实，与手臂放在两侧相比，举手姿势下 SSEP 改变更小，但分析认为所观察到的变化更可能是尺神经受影响所致，举手姿势并未明显减少臂丛神经损伤。

许多作者试图确定增加 PNI 风险的患者或手术室特征。被引用较多的危险因素包括超重、男性（尤其是尺神经病变）、糖尿病或周围血管病等先前即存在的神经病变（框 125.1）。心脏手术中，PNI 显著危险因素包括体温过低、不对称胸骨撑开及获取 IMA 进行 CABG（框 125.2）。

启示

大多数 PNI 约 1 个月后自行缓解。其最好预后是轻微损伤导致的机能性麻痹，仅因神经传导受阻导致暂时性功能丧失。较之更重的损伤是轴突断裂，其预后亦较理想。这种损伤只造成轴突和周围髓鞘损伤，尚完好的间质框架为再生提供了支持。神经离断是最严重的损伤形式，会导致完全性功能丧失，且通常难以恢复至术前水平。糖尿病等基础疾病与 PNI 恢复期延长相关。

框 125.1　围术期神经损伤的解剖学和病理生理危险因素

- 糖尿病
- 神经病变
- 酗酒
- 带状疱疹
- 结节性多动脉炎
- 外周血管疾病
- 凝血因子缺乏
- 高血压
- 甲状腺功能减退
- 颈肋骨
- 肩部畸形或臂丛神经起源畸形

框 125.2 心脏手术围术期神经损伤的危险因素

胸骨撑开
　放置胸骨撑开器
　不对称胸骨撑开
获取内乳动脉
手术持续时间
体外循环持续时间
低体温
胸骨切开术中第一肋骨骨折导致的穿透损伤
颈内静脉置管时的损伤
　直接与针刺相关的伤害
　血肿形成导致臂丛神经受压

治疗

当怀疑出现 PNI 时，处理的第一步是细致的神经学检查。如果检测到损伤，则应进行神经科会诊。可以考虑术后即刻进行肌电图（electromyography，EMG）检测，尤其是对怀疑先前即有神经功能障碍的患者。该检查可发现感觉和运动神经传导速度的改变。大部分神经损伤后 2 ～ 3 周才出现 EMG 改变。术后即刻检查的任何阳性发现，都提示患者先前即有神经病变。若症状持续，应于 3 ～ 4 周后再次进行检查，以确认是否发生神经性改变。

PNI 的治疗为支持治疗，很大程度上取决于病变严重程度。在急性期可能很有必要使用镇痛药如阿片类药物或神经病理性治疗药物（如加巴喷丁）。物理疗法是治疗运动功能损伤的基石。根据运动受限程度，可能需要考虑使用夹板以防止进一步损伤，且有助于日常活动。对难以痊愈的严重损伤，应当考虑外科治疗。外科干预通常限于涉及解剖异常的情况，如胸廓出口综合征、第一肋骨骨折或骨性凸起压迫。一些作者认为早期手术干预可以提高神经的再生能力。

预防

由于 PNI 的多因素性及对其认识的不充分性，使得预防变得尤为困难。充分了解臂丛和其他常见受损神经的解剖，对确保正确定位至关重要。在这些案例中，几乎没有证据可以指导麻醉管理。2011 年，ASA PNI 预防工作组提出了一个主要基于共识观点的建议。该建议主要关注患者的适当体位，框 125.3 中对其进行了总结。ASA 还主张对患者术后神经功能进行评估，以提高 PNI 早期发现率。

框 125.3 ASA 周围神经损伤预防工作组推荐

术前检查患者耐受预期手术体位的能力
仰卧时将手臂外展限制在 90° 以内
保持前臂的中立位（无论是内收还是外展）
旋后可能有助于减轻尺骨槽上的压力
对术中所需体位保持警觉
四肢的适当衬垫（衬垫过紧可能增加神经病变风险）
侧卧位患者使用胸部绑带可能降低周围神经损伤的风险
在头低脚高位手术中不恰当放置肩部支架可能会增加风险

如前所述，心脏手术具有臂丛神经损伤的特异性危险因素。除前面提到的步骤外，大多数医师还有如下建议：

- 尽量减小胸骨撑开，尤其在获取 IMA 时；
- 胸骨撑开器靠近尾端放置；
- 保持头部在中立位，使臂丛的牵张力最小化；
- 正中胸骨切开术（避免不对称胸骨撑开）。

（刘洪伟　译　李　黛　校）

延伸阅读

Alvine FG, Schurrer ME: Postoperative ulnar-nerve palsy: are there predisposing factors? *J Bone Joint Surg Am* 69:255–259, 1987.
Ben-David B, Stahl S: Prognosis of intraoperative brachial plexus injury: a review of 22 cases, *Br J Anaesth* 79:440–445, 1997.
Burnett MG, Zager EL: Pathophysiology of peripheral nerve injury: a brief review, *Neurosurg Focus* 16:1–7, 2004.
Cheney FW, Domino KB, Caplan RA, et al.: Nerve injury associated with anesthesia: a closed claims analysis, *Anesthesiology* 90:1062–1069, 1999.
Eggers KA, Asai T: Postoperative brachial plexus neuropathy after total knee replacement under spinal anaesthesia, *Br J Anaesth* 75:642–644, 1995.
Hanson MR, Breuer AC, Furlan AJ, et al.: Mechanism and frequency of brachial plexus injury in open-heart surgery: a prospective analysis, *Ann Thorac Surg* 36:675–679, 1983.
Hickey C, Gugino LD, Aglio LS, et al.: Intraoperative somatosensory evoked potential monitoring predicts peripheral nerve injury during cardiac surgery, *Anesthesiology* 78:29–35, 1993.
Healey S, O'Neill BO, Bilal H, et al.: Does retraction of the sternum during median sternotomy result in brachial plexus injuries? *Inter Cardiovasc Thorac Surg* 17:151–158, 2013.
Jellish WS, Martucci J, Blakeman B, et al.: Somatosensory evoked potential monitoring of the brachial plexus to predict nerve injury during internal mammary artery harvest: intraoperative comparisons of the Rultract and Pittman sternal retractors, *J Cardiothorac Vasc Anesth* 8:398–403, 1994.
Kroll DA, Caplan RA, Posner K, et al.: Nerve injury associated with anesthesia, *Anesthesiology* 73:202–207, 1990.
Lalkhen AG, Bhatia K: Perioperative peripheral nerve injuries, *Contin Educ Anaesth Crit Care Pain* 12:38–42, 2012.
Lederman RJ, Breuer AC, Hanson MR, et al.: Peripheral nervous system complications of coronary artery bypass graft surgery, *Ann Neurol* 12:297–301, 1982.

Mahla ME, Long DM, McKennett J, et al.: Detection of brachial plexus dysfunction by somatosensory evoked potential monitoring—a report of two cases, *Anesthesiology* 60:248–252, 1984.

Practice advisory for the prevention of perioperative peripheral neuropathies, *Anesthesiology* 114:1–14, 2011.

Tomlinson DL, Hirsch IA, Kodali SV, et al.: Protecting the brachial plexus during median sternotomy, *J Thorac Cardiovasc Surg* 94:297–301, 1987.

Unlu Y, Velioglu Y, Kocak H, et al.: Brachial plexus injury following median sternotomy, *Inter Cardiovasc Thorac Surg* 6:235–237, 2007.

Vahl CF, Carl I, Muller-Vahl H, et al.: Brachial plexus injury after cardiac surgery: the role of internal mammary artery preparation: a prospective study on 1000 consecutive patients, *J Thorac Cardiovasc Surg* 102:724–729, 1991.

Vander Salm TJ, Cereda JM: Cutler BS: Brachial plexus injury following median sternotomy, *J Thorac Cardiovasc Surg* 80:447–452, 1980.

Vander Salm TJ, Cutler BS, Okike ON: Brachial plexus injury following median sternotomy. Part II, *J Thorac Cardiovasc Surg* 83:914–917, 1982.

Warner MA: Perioperative neuropathies, *Mayo Clinic Proc* 73:567–574, 1998.

Welch MB, Brummett CM, Welch TD, et al.: Perioperative peripheral nerve injuries, *Anesthesiology* 111:490–497, 2009.

第 126 章 不良事件和意外结局：全面披露

Scott A. Falk，Dale W. Lanks

病例概要

患者，女性，38 岁，高血压和肥胖（体重指数为 32），拟行腹腔镜胆囊切除术治疗慢性复发性胆囊炎。患者术前评估时告知麻醉科医师其对青霉素过敏。进一步追问病史后，患者解释道，她母亲说她在童年曾发生过一次过敏，具体情况已记不清楚。

患者入手术室后常规全身麻醉诱导，经口气管插管顺利。麻醉科医师同外科医师讨论抗生素选择后认为，头孢唑啉预防术后手术部位感染的效果最佳。负责给药的麻醉科医师认为，该患者既往对青霉素反应可能很小，且头孢菌素和青霉素之间的过敏原交叉反应性很低。

给予头孢唑啉后 3 min，患者通气困难且血压极低。遂启动复苏和抗过敏，患者稳定后，但仍需肾上腺素输注。麻醉科医师和外科医师决定推迟手术并将患者带气管导管送至重症监护病房（ICU）。

引言

不幸的是，在医疗服务过程中不良事件和意外结局时有发生。高达 13.5% 的医保受益患者在接受诊疗时曾经历不良事件。然而，不良事件并不完全意味着临床医师犯错、疏忽或偏离医疗原则。不管何种原因，不良事件意味着某些事情没有按预期或计划进行。无论何时发生不良事件或意外结局，患者及家属都希望知晓治疗过程中发生的事情，并获悉全面解释及原因。因此，了解如何有效地披露不良事件或意外结局，可对最终发生的不良结果产生重要而有益的影响，有助于维护医患信任关系，减少任何潜在的职业责任风险。不良事件或意外结局，再加上医患关系不佳，将造成更大的职业责任风险。

临床麻醉实践一直致力于提高患者安全，但也可能面对发生不良事件或意外结局等特殊挑战。患者在医院或门诊可选择特定的外科医师实施手术，但在大多数情况下，患者通常在手术前不久才会接触到麻醉科医师，无法选择特定的麻醉科医师为自己实施麻醉。换言之，麻醉科医师与患者基本上未建立融洽或信任关系。但是，麻醉科医师必须积极参与披露麻醉相关事件，并且要制订可供遵循的处理方案，对明事理与闹事患者给予不同处理措施。

国际医院认证联会委员会（Joint Commission，JCI）自 2001 年起就要求，除做正确和道德上允许的事情外，还应充分披露不良事件或意外结局。任何对患者有临床影响的非预见事件，不管是暂时还是永久的，均需要披露。全国质量论坛等组织也鼓励充分披露，认为全面披露是保障医疗安全的举措之一。此外，披露也是美国多个州的法定要求。

为何需要披露？

- JCI 要求披露；
- 部分州的相关法要求披露；
- 披露是患者的期望；
- 能提供致歉和缓和愤怒的机会；
- 披露可改善医患信任度；
- 促进患者安全和质量改进；
- 披露为早期干预奠定了基础；

- 有助于将潜在职业责任风险降至最低；
- 无论如何，披露是正确的做法。

准备披露

当事件未能正确或按计划进行，即使未偏离治疗标准且未造成永久伤害，也应进行全面公开的披露。及时披露是必要的，但须经过深思熟虑并组织协调好，以合适的方式进行。每个机构都应积极推动披露文化，以便达到最佳的临床实践水平。做好披露准备是重要的第一步，不仅涉及相关临床医师，更关系到整个团队。团队可能包括不参与实际披露但在必要的听证会中帮助解释或澄清事件的人员。应确定披露内容、负责披露人员、披露时间及披露后预期的行动方案。披露准备团队的所有成员，包括主持披露的临床医师，应当是与患者和家属保持联系的负责人，需要知道并理解所披露的信息。上述过程有助于保证信息传递的持续性和一致性。

披露

在大多数情况下，即使事件的全部事实和具体情况尚不清楚，也应尽快进行披露。公开披露最好能与患者和（或）家庭/替代决策者面对面进行。只应披露已知的事实和客观信息。谨记，永远都不应肆意推测、指责、批评其他临床医师，或就有关事件具体情况或尚未确定的事实发表意见。及时披露有助于避免患者和家属质疑为何需等待这么长时间，有助于消除试图隐藏或隐瞒信息才告知事件已发生的误解。初次披露通常不能达到完全披露的目的，这可能是一个持续过程。初次披露时至少给予初步事实很重要，但没必要回答全部问题，且不可能预测患者和（或）家庭成员可能要问的问题。必须让患者及家属知晓，当有更多信息和事实时，将进行更多披露。在披露过程中，当被询问的问题尚无答案时，应该说："我不知道，但我会找到更多信息，回来与您探讨。"

如情况合适且必要，披露应由包括涉事麻醉科医师在内的小型披露团队执行，这也是团队的责任与义务。在大多数情况下，特别是患者事先未见过涉事麻醉科医师时，让外科医师或初级保健医师同时出席亦有帮助。这既让患者不感到陌生，还因其与他们已建立持续信任的医患关系，也最有资格回答患者的问题（例如，"这对我的健康意味着什么？"或"这会改变我的预后吗？"）。此外，所披露的信息可能使患者不知所措，而临床医师仍会参与患者后续治疗，故其参与有助于能精确回忆所披露内容和讨论过程。

披露团队的另一个关键成员是，患者事件发生前后在手术间的主管护士。参与披露讨论的主管护士要确保患者和家属对告知信息已清楚，并知晓其对披露信息的反应。主管护士可与该手术间护理人员分享这些信息。护理人员应与患者和家属进行更多的持续和频繁接触，回答其反复询问的一连串问题。重要的是，护理人员应了解该事件，并知道应向谁报告患者和家属可能提出的问题。作为披露团队的成员，主管护士不仅可作为患者和家属的联系人，同时也是护理人员的联系人。

同样，尽可能让家庭成员出席披露非常重要，这有助于在场其他人员能听到并记住事实，还能为患者提供情感支持。但也要意识到，家属可能受信息影响，在披露不良事件后照顾患者和家属同等重要。可能需患者和家属服务、教牧关怀或社工服务等部门帮助，以提供支持并帮助患者和家属应对。

根据事件性质，医疗机构的医疗负责人或患者安全负责人出席披露可能有益。这有助于证明，不管事件情况如何，管理部门将认真对待，认真评估医疗工作，并在必要时为患者转院等。对患者及家属而言，医疗机构将充分学习并吸取不良事件或意外结局中的经验，努力防止未来再发生类似事件。

讨论可能的补偿

在初次披露讨论期间，若患者或家属突然提出补偿问题，最恰当的回应是告知对方：补偿问题将由院方相关管理部分处理，后续将有人员对此回应。决不应当对可能的赔偿做出任何承诺。也可能出现下述情况，不良事件或意外结局导致严重和（或）永久性损伤，确实与治疗标准有偏差。一旦如此，在披露预备会议期间，应与医院管理层和相关高级管理人员讨论这些情况，巧妙地向患者和家属保证医院/机构将会讨论采取补偿措施。尽管后续商讨中关于补偿的讨论会很多，但当前最好不讨论任何补偿。在满足患者急需的医疗需求后，再告诉患者

和家属最终会讨论补偿问题。既往有与麻醉药相关的诉讼案件中给予重大经济补偿的案例

表达悔意或致歉

长期以来，人们不愿对不良事件或意外结局表示遗憾或悔意，也不愿在适当时间道歉。临床医师经常担心，表达悔意或致歉会被认为是承认有错，让患者或家属愤怒，导致诉讼可能性增加。许多患者最初可能不会因不良事件或意外结局而生气，但若感到不被重视时才会生气，而挥之不去的愤怒是寻求法律诉讼解决的主要因素。目前，担心向患者表达悔意或道歉会增加诉讼是没有根据的。实际上，道歉和充分披露日渐降低了患者提请诉讼的概率。表达悔意或道歉可能是困难或尴尬的，但这样做会使披露更为人性化，并为所有相关人员（包括临床医师）提供巨大的情感支撑和益处。根据不良事件或意外结局的性质及所涉及的内容，确定道歉方式和由谁去进行道歉是披露准备的一部分（框 126.1）。

文书

文书与披露同等重要。这既包括对实际不良事件或意外结局的记录文书，还应包括公开讨论的文书。在医疗文书记录中，患者临床状态的记录应全面、明确和客观，关于披露讨论的文书记录也应如此。

披露文书应包括以下内容：

- 日期和时间；
- 披露内容；
- 披露出席人员；
- 患者和家属对披露的反应；
- 所提问题及回答；
- 后续计划。

如不确定如何记录，应向院方的风险管理部门寻求指导。

框 126.1 披露的要点

- 必须包括涉事的麻醉科医师
- 必须包括患者的外科医师或初级保健医师
- 必须包括护理管理人员
- 必须根据当时已知的事实，以实际、客观和非评判的方式，用非专业术语解释不良事件或意外结局的性质、严重程度和原因
- 必须描述事件对患者临床过程和预后的潜在影响
- 必须表示遗憾或悔意，并在适当时机致歉
- 必须留出提问时间
- 必须确定后续计划
- 必须确保所有联系渠道畅通无阻
- 绝不讨论任何与治疗标准相偏差可能情况
- 绝不讨论相关人员的临床能力
- 绝不对潜在赔偿要求做出承诺

随访

当患者和家属听到不良事件或意外结局的消息后，认为其会想到所有可能的问题或疑虑是不现实的。对刚收到的信息，患者和家属需要时间理解并做出反应。不良事件或意外结局对患者的影响程度，在披露时可能无法确定，在相当长的一段时间内可能也无法确知。因此，与患者和家属保持联系至关重要。要告知他们会保持随访，并解答未来可能遇到的任何问题。应提供联系信息，保持双方处于可联络状态。在此期间，医护团队不仅要为患者提供必要的医疗护理，还应为家属提供支持。这可能包括为家庭成员安排与患者一起住院或附近就医，报销酒店、餐饮和停车等费用。这一做法所带来的积极影响，有助于为不良事件和意外结局提供改善机会。应与风险管理或医疗部门合作，确定提供哪些医疗服务适当，包括可能针对特殊情况制定的干预措施。鉴于不可能知道患者家属的最迫切需求是什么，建议直接询问对方可以做些什么来满足相关需求。

病例概要分析

披露准备团队

- 涉事的麻醉科医师；
- 外科医师；
- 围术期主管护士；
- ICU 主管护士；
- 风险管理部门代表；
- 患者和医疗服务代表。

披露团队

- 涉事的麻醉科医师；
- 外科医师；

- ICU 主管护士。

披露信息

因患者在 ICU 内且气管插管，该事件最初向其丈夫披露。

- 在您妻子全身麻醉后，给她使用了一种名为头孢唑啉的抗生素，以帮助预防术后感染。
- 给予头孢唑啉后不久，她对这种药物出现明显的过敏反应。
- 当她病情稳定后，医师认为最好推迟手术时间，并将她转到 ICU。
- 她提及童年时对青霉素过敏，并与她就此讨论过。然而，她童年所经历的具体反应类型不清楚。
- 在与她的外科医师讨论后，决定使用头孢唑啉。该药是术后手术部位感染最有效的预防性抗生素。已知或潜在对青霉素发生过敏反应患者，对头孢唑啉的过敏反应发生率很低。
- 给予头孢唑啉后，她的血压显著降低，并需要持续输注肾上腺素来维持血压。
- 她将在 ICU 中接受密切监测，一旦清醒且血压不需要肾上腺素维持时，就能够拔除气管导管。
- 发生这样的事件，我们感到非常抱歉，一旦她脱离呼吸机恢复自主呼吸，我们会向她解释为何发生这种情况。在此期间，您有什么问题吗？我们能为您做些什么吗？

麻醉文书记录

2016 年 9 月 1 日上午 10：30

1 名 38 岁女性拟行腹腔镜胆囊切除术。术前评估时，其自述童年曾有青霉素（penicillins，PCN）过敏。她不记得所经历的过敏类型，只是听她母亲说过。在与外科 X 医师讨论后，考虑到患者童年有 PCN 过敏，遂决定给予头孢唑啉，因其能有效预防感染且与青霉素过敏原的交叉反应性低。平稳进行全麻诱导和气管插管后，给予头孢唑啉。3 min 后，患者发生通气困难和血压降低。随即开始复苏和抗过敏治疗。开始输注肾上腺素后，患者血压逐步稳定。手术取消并将患者带气管导管送至 ICU。与 X 医师和 ICU 主管护士一起，与患者丈夫会面并充分解释该事件，包括使用头孢唑啉前做出选择的决定过程。患者丈夫稍微有点不高兴，询问患者何时醒来以及机械通气多长时间的问题。已告诉对方，预计患者会逐渐醒来，一旦清醒并能足够的自主呼吸时即拔管。同时还告诉他，患者清醒后，将立刻将事件完整解释给本人。我向他解释说，我们都很遗憾发生了这件事，并告诉他将在今天下午晚些再来访视。我的联系信息也已提供给他。

随访计划

- 涉事的麻醉科医师和外科医师，将继续与患者及其丈夫保持联系。
- ICU 主管护士将成为患者及其丈夫的指定联系人，以便回答所有问题并满足其迫切需求。
- 根据患者及其丈夫最迫切的需求，应尽力为患者和家属提供服务以促进医疗服务工作的恢复，例如为患者丈夫安排住宿、提供餐券或停车券等。

讨论

发生麻醉相关不良事件或意外结局后，主动、负责、坦率和恳切地对待患者和家属，是降低责任风险最核心的步骤。虽然患者和（或）家属可能对事件感到愤怒，但若对方感受到尊重和善意对待，便不会因感觉到被规避或隐瞒真相而更加愤怒。

在医疗活动中，确保诊疗过程一切顺利是不可能的。当无法按预期发展时，掌控和管理方式将对不良事件和意外结局的发展产生重大影响。公开、坦诚、透明、及时、关怀和善解人意的全面披露，所带来的益处将在恢复信任中不可估量，且很大程度上减轻不良事件或意外结局对患者、家庭、涉事临床医师和医疗机构可能造成的影响。

（李盼盼　译　沈　锓　校）

延伸阅读

Agency for Healthcare Research and Quality: *Communication and Optimal Resolution (CANDOR)*, Rockville, MD, May 2016, AHRQ. Available at http://www.ahrq.gov/professionals/quality-patient-safety/patient-safety-resources/resources/candor/index.html. Accessed September 23, 2016.

Amori G: *Disclosure of unanticipated events in 2013*, American Society for Healthcare Risk Management, 2013. Available at http://www.ashrm.org-/pubs/files/white_papers/Disclosure-of-Unanticipated-Events-in-2013_Prologue.pdf. Accessed September 23, 2016.

ECRI Institute: *ECRI executive summary: incident reporting and management.* Available at www.ecri.org, 2012. Accessed September 23, 2016.

Heard GC, Sanderson PM, Thomas RD: Barriers to adverse event and error reporting in anesthesia, *Anesth Analg* 114(3):604–614, 2012.

Kain ZN: The National Practitioner Data Bank and anesthesia malpractice payments, *Anesth Analg* 103(3):646–649, 2006.

Levinson DR: *Adverse events in hospitals: national incidence among Medicare beneficiaries. Department of Health and Human Services*, Office of the Inspector General, 2010. Available at https://oig.hhs.gov/oei/reports/oei-06-09-00090.pdf. Accessed September 23, 2016.

Lipira LE, Gallagher TH: Disclosure of adverse events and errors in surgical care: challenges and strategies for improvement, *World J Surg* 38:1614–1621, 2014.

Moffatt-Bruce SD, Ferdinand FD, Fann JI: Patient safety: disclosure of medical errors and risk mitigation, *Ann Thorac Surg* 102(2):358–362, 2016.

National Quality Forum (NQF): *Serious reportable events in healthcare—2011 update: a consensus report*, Washington, DC, 2011, NQF.

Singh V, Cunningham CJ, Panda M, et al.: Disclosure and documentation of reported unanticipated medical events or outcomes: need for healthcare provider education, *J Healthc Risk Manag* 32(1):14–22, 2012.

Souter KJ, Gallagher T: The disclosure of unanticipated outcomes of care and medical errors: what does this mean for anesthesiologists? *Anesth Analg* 114:615–621, 2012.

Szypula K, Ashpole KJ, Bogod D, et al.: Litigation related to regional anaesthesia: an analysis of claims against the NHS in England 1995–2007, *Anaesthesia* 65(5):443–452, 2010.

Wagner TH, Taylor T, Cowgill E: Intended and unintended effects of large-scale adverse event disclosure: a controlled before-after analysis of five large-scale notifications, *BMJ Qual Saf* 24:295–302, 2015.

空气栓塞

第 127 章

Lisa Wise-Faberowski，*Michael I. Chen*

病例概要

患儿，8 周，行颅骨矢状缝早闭去骨瓣术。外科医师切开颅骨时，心前区多普勒超声出现声音变化，血压迅速下降（图 127.1）。

问题分析

定义

血管系统内的气泡被称为**气体栓子**或**空气栓子**。当静脉中的空气栓子进入动脉循环，被称为**反常空气栓子**。静脉空气栓子或反常空气栓子可通过**泡腾**方式进入血液，或通过外部**注入**进入血液。

溶解在液体中的气体量与温度和压力呈函数关系。温度突然升高，可导致气泡通过泡腾的方式从含有气体的溶液中释放。这一情况可发生在低温心肺转流后快速复温期间或快速加温冷的静脉液体或血制品时，也可发生于经历快速减压的潜水员（“减压病”）。

气体更常通过注入的方式进入血液（如腹腔镜、胸腔镜、关节镜期间）或通过加压系统输注液体和血制品。不易塌陷的静脉也可进入空气，如骨静脉窦、粗大且处于开放状态的中心静脉和高于心脏水平开放的静脉。当静脉开口位置高于心脏一定水平且超过中心静脉压时，可导致空气栓子的产生（如坐位开颅术）。静脉和反常空气栓塞可发生在仰卧位、俯卧位或侧卧位。自主呼吸期间的低静脉压或胸内负压会增加空气栓塞的风险。

儿童更易发生静脉空气栓塞。短时间内可出现明显快速的失血，少量失血即占儿童血容量的很大一部分。儿童的颅骨很薄，开颅手术期间尤需注意。儿童头部占身体比例相对较大，导致在仰卧或俯卧位开颅术期间，手术部位高于心脏水平。最后，由于心内分流（卵圆孔未闭）的普遍存在，虽然一定量的静脉空气栓塞对成人可能微不足道，但其导致的反常性空气栓塞对新生儿则是灾难性的。

识别

清醒患者可能因静脉空气栓塞出现呼吸困难和咳嗽。在麻醉期间，当出现大量空气栓塞后，生命体征才会产生变化。按灵敏度递减顺序，检测静脉

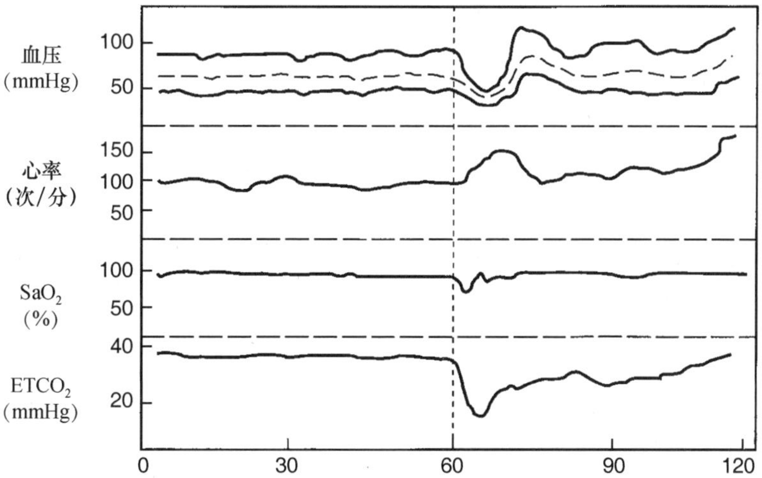

图 127.1　8 周龄婴儿颅骨矢状缝修复手术期间的血压、心率、氧饱和度（SaO_2）和呼气末二氧化碳（$ETCO_2$）浓度的趋势记录示意图。虚线处表示多普勒声音发生剧烈变化。注意血压和 $ETCO_2$ 突然降低，并伴有心动过速，但 SaO_2 几乎没有变化

空气栓塞的监测方法包括：
- 超声心动图或多普勒超声检查；
- 呼气末二氧化碳（end-tidal carbon dioxide，$ETCO_2$）降低或新出现呼气末氮气（end-tidal nitrogen，ETN_2）；
- 肺动脉压升高；
- 中心静脉压升高；
- 血压下降；
- 心电图（electrocardiogram，ECG）改变（例如，右心室劳损、缺血、心律失常）；
- 心脏听诊“磨轮样”杂音。

超声心动图和多普勒监测的灵敏度很高，它们甚至可检测出常规静脉注射的微小气泡和轻微夹带的空气。当超声心动图和多普勒监测到空气栓塞时，临床团队需引起重视，同时需考虑空气栓塞的严重程度（体积、持续时间和相关临床症状）和临床情况（例如，开颅术）。心电图的改变相对滞后，心脏听诊“磨轮样”杂音最不敏感；然而，当与超声心动图或多普勒监测到静脉空气栓塞的证据相符时，则考虑已出现大量空气栓塞。

超声心动图

经胸或经食管超声心动图（transesophageal echocardiography, TEE）能够识别分散和大量的（即暴雪模式的密度）气泡。此外，TEE 可定位左心或右心栓子，并可检测出心脏异常（室间隔缺损），这些异常可增加反常空气栓塞的风险。TEE 已应用于体重低至 2.5 kg 的新生儿。其广泛使用的局限性包括：
- 高成本；
- 麻醉和手术期间需要有一个单独的、训练有素的观察者；
- 咽、喉和食管有损伤风险；
- 可导致气管插管移位，尤其在婴儿气管插管期间操作。

因此，尽管 TEE 是检测静脉空气栓塞非常敏感的技术，目前在许多机构中并不实用，并且无需作为常规监测。

多普勒超声

心前区多普勒超声检查与 TEE 同样敏感，可用于检测静脉空气栓塞。它可对空气栓塞进行半定量评估，但不能定位空气栓塞位于左心或右心。婴儿心脏和胸壁之间的距离较小，从而提高了多普勒超声的敏感性。探头需放置在心脏的右侧，通常位于胸骨右侧乳头线上。轻微活动可使探头移位，因此应将其牢靠固定在胸部。通过静脉导管注入几毫升液体，当多普勒声音出现大的特征性变化时，可确认探头的位置正确。多普勒探头容易移位，并可导致患者俯卧位时局部皮肤压迫性坏死。通过将多普勒探头固定于患者背部，可避免婴儿出现这种情况。电刀和超声心动图会干扰多普勒超声检查。

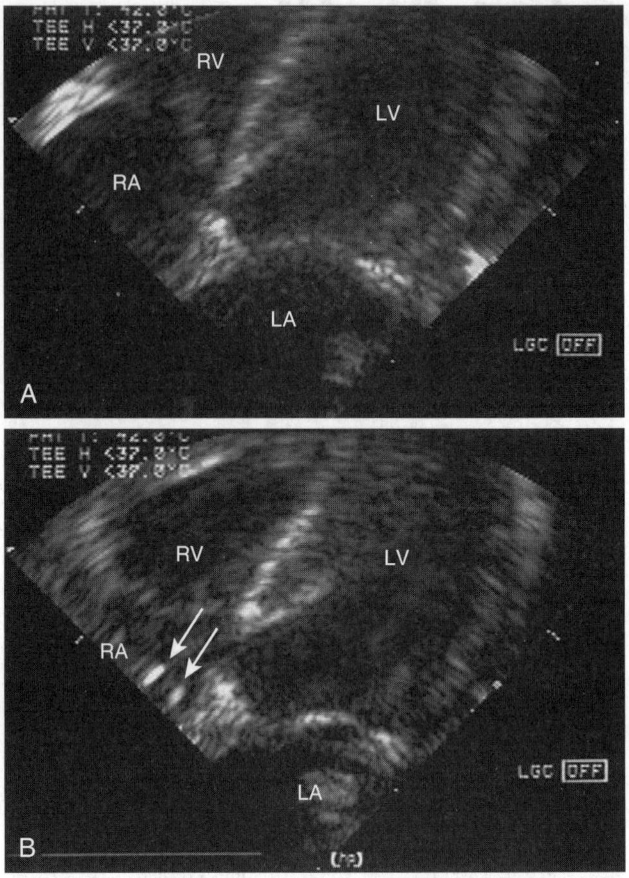

图 127.2　左心房（LA）、右心房（RA）、左心室（LV）和右心室（RV）经食管超声心动图四腔心视图。图 A，没有静脉空气栓塞（VAE）的心脏视图。**图 B，**箭头表示在 VAE 期间 RA 中的气泡产生的反射

呼气末二氧化碳

由于死腔通气增加，静脉空气栓塞显著降低 $ETCO_2$ 浓度。此外，肺血栓栓塞导致肺血流减少、突发的大量失血、静脉回流减少，或由于心功能不全、心动过缓或心律失常导致的心排血量减少均可导致 $ETCO_2$ 降低。除非在气管导管尖端附近采样，否则因为气体泄漏或无气囊的气管导管周围夹带的空气或小潮气量被新鲜气体所稀释，均可能导致虚假的低 $ETCO_2$。即使如此，之前基线稳定的 $ETCO_2$

突然发生的变化通常也较为明显。

呼出的氮气

除非在吸入气体中加入空气，否则呼吸气体中不会含有氮气（N_2）。N_2 再次出现表明静脉空气栓塞导致回路泄漏或肺泡扩散。如果没有漏气，突然出现 ETN_2 诊断静脉空气栓塞的特异度高，但灵敏度较差；大的静脉空气栓塞仅使 ETN_2 增加 1% ～ 2%。

肺动脉导管

当空气导致肺血管栓塞时，肺动脉导管显示肺动脉压升高。与低中心静脉压相似，低肺动脉楔压可能意味着静脉空气栓塞和反常空气栓塞。但大多数情况下，肺动脉导管对婴幼儿并不实用。

中心静脉导管

中心静脉置管对高危手术患者是合理的，如坐位开颅手术，即便小儿也应实施。当手术体位为平卧时，对健康的儿童而言，中心静脉置管几乎没有必要。如果难以开放外周静脉通路，中心静脉导管可用于补液和用药，并可监测中心静脉压。低中心静脉压可能表明患者需要补液以降低静脉空气栓塞风险；中心静脉压突然升高可能预示大静脉空气栓塞。有时可通过中心静脉导管吸出大静脉内的空气栓子，特别是当导管尖端有多个开口且靠近上腔静脉和右心房交界处。临床上可通过 X 线片或通过右心房 ECG 适配器记录单极 ECG 来确认空气栓塞的位置。为此，将导管导线替换为 V 导联，并观察导管前进到右心房时特征性的 P 波变化（P 波振幅升高，高尖的 P 波可能超过 R 波或 S 波振幅）。

动脉血压

动脉置管不仅可连续监测血压，还可进行动脉血气测定。动脉置管适用于任何具有出血或静脉空气栓塞风险的手术，尤其是小儿手术。

脉搏血氧测定

对明显的静脉空气栓塞，脉搏血氧测定可检测到氧饱和度的降低。动脉血气分析可显示高碳酸血症和动脉-肺泡氧分压差增加。

风险评估

在以下操作过程中，儿科患者静脉空气栓塞的风险将会增加：

- 任何外科手术，当其手术部位足够高于心脏，特别是突发大出血时；
- 开颅手术且行大面积颅骨切开术（例如，颅缝早闭修复术）；
- 开颅手术时直接在较大的硬脑膜静脉窦上进行操作（例如，后颅窝探查）；
- 颅脑手术（例如，额叶或中段前移）行骨切除和术中为减少出血而抬高头部；
- 某些骨科手术（例如，脊柱侧凸手术）；
- 进入大静脉结构（例如，肝静脉、下腔静脉）的高风险普外科手术（例如肝手术）；
- 肝移植手术；
- 任何心脏直视手术；
- 血管造影和心导管检查；
- 安装、使用和停用心肺转流或体外膜肺氧合装置；
- 血液透析、血浆置换或中心静脉导管置入；
- 正压通气期间的气压伤；
- 阻力消失法使用空气来确认硬膜外腔时。

启示

严重的肺空气栓塞可导致心排血量减少、肺动脉高压和循环衰竭，其病因如下：

- 气泡阻塞外周肺血管；
- 肺大血管或心脏中的气体栓子导致气体阻隔；
- 反射性肺血管收缩；
- 继发于肺动脉高压的右心室衰竭；
- 电机械分离或心律失常；
- 冠状动脉灌注压降低、冠状动脉反常空气栓塞以及低氧血症引起的心肌缺血。

肺功能受损导致二氧化碳潴留和动脉血氧饱和度下降，可由以下原因引起：

- 肺血管阻塞引起通气死腔量增加，通气-血流比例失衡；
- 反应性支气管收缩伴气道阻力增加；
- 间质性肺水肿。

气泡直接或通过心内交通进入动脉循环。大多数新生儿卵圆孔未闭，通常存在左向右分流。婴儿卵圆孔未闭的发生率为 25% ～ 50%，成人卵圆孔未闭发生率为 20% ～ 30%，但很少分流。然而，静脉空气栓塞导致的右心压力升高可能促进反常空气栓子通过未闭的卵圆孔。反常的空气栓塞可导致心肌或脑缺血。

管理

手术期间成功处理静脉空气栓塞的关键是，麻醉科医师和外科医师应密切沟通。此外，应考虑以下准则：

- 每个人都应该听到多普勒声音。在进行可能引起多普勒声音变化的静脉注射时要提前说明。
- 如果多普勒超声检查显示静脉空气栓塞与注射无关，外科医师应使用相关措施（例如，使用骨蜡，用生理盐水覆盖手术区，用蘸湿生理盐水的纱布覆盖）以减少空气进入。
- 当怀疑静脉空气栓塞时，寻找与 $ETCO_2$ 或血压下降相关的明显的静脉空气栓塞或失血。如果监测到 ETN_2 再现，则可确认静脉空气栓塞的诊断。
- N_2O 虽然并不禁忌用于这些手术，但当出现静脉空气栓塞时，应立即停用。随后，对患者进行纯氧通气，以避免进一步增大气泡，并治疗低氧血症。
- 调整手术床，尽量使手术部位低于心脏水平。同时确保患者牢固地固定在手术台上。
- 建议对颈静脉进行轻柔按压，以减少空气进入并暴露空气可能的进入部位，但必须避免颈动脉受压迫。
- 虽然空气可通过中心静脉或肺动脉导管吸出，但通常无法吸出进入的大量空气。
- 建议将患者置于左侧卧位以利于复苏，但在某些手术中可能不实用。
- 建议使用额外的静脉输液或正性肌力药（麻黄碱、肾上腺素）支持循环。临床上很少需要进行心肺复苏，特别是快速检测到栓子并采取适当措施后。

预防

仔细询问病史和体格检查，以及对手术计划的熟悉程度，对评估静脉空气栓塞或反常空气栓塞风险至关重要。建议使用心前区多普勒超声作为敏感且无创性检查，以尽早发现静脉空气栓塞。当预计有明显或快速的液体或血液置换时，考虑使用过滤器或除泡器。对高风险手术，需采取相应措施减少空气进入和静脉空气栓塞（例如体位、使用骨蜡、液体覆盖手术区域）。

（张　婉　译　吉　栋　校）

延伸阅读

Cucchiara RF, Bowers B: Air embolism in children undergoing suboccipital craniotomy, *Anesthesiology* 57:338–339, 1982.

Eldredge EA, Soriano SG, Rockoff MA: Pediatric neurosurgical anesthesia. In Coté CJ, Todres ID, Goudsouzian NG, et al.: *A practice of anesthesia for infants and children*, ed 3, Philadelphia, 2001, WB Saunders, pp 493–521.

Faberowski LW, Black S, Mickle JP: Incidence of venous air embolism during craniectomy for craniosynostosis repair, *Anesthesiology* 92:20–23, 2000.

Harris MM, Strafford MA, Rowe RW, et al.: Venous air embolism and cardiac arrest during craniectomy in a supine infant, *Anesthesiology* 65:547–550, 1986.

Harris MM, Yemen TA, Davidson A, et al.: Venous embolism during craniectomy in supine infants, *Anesthesiology* 67:816–819, 1987.

Markhorst DG, Rothuis E, Sobotka-Plojhar M, et al.: Transient foramen ovale incompetence in the normal newborn: an echocardiographic study, *Eur J Pediatr* 154:667–671, 1995.

Sethna NF, Berde CB: Venous air embolism during identification of the epidural space in children, *Anesth Analg* 76:925–927, 1993.

被控渎职行为

第 128 章

David S. Smith，*Mary Ellen Nepps*

病例概要

孕妇，23 岁，因胎儿心动过缓和胎盘早剥全身麻醉下急诊行剖宫产术。手术开始时，患者出现低血压（血压 70/30 mmHg）和心动过速（心率 150 次 / 分）。分娩后，胎儿 Apgar 评分较低，胎儿出现酸中毒（脐带血 pH 7.01）。术后，患者主诉术中知晓。婴儿成长期间出现脑瘫、癫痫和发育迟缓。2 年后，患方提出医疗事故诉讼，指控麻醉科医师渎职。

问题分析

医疗事故索赔的要素

诉讼是指为赔偿损害而要求经济补偿的民事案件。在该案例中，诉讼是基于职业过失的索赔。其他可构成职业责任诉讼基础的情形包括缺席（执业者有义务在现场但没有在场）或缺乏知情同意。为在渎职索赔中获胜，原告（即起诉人）必须明确以下几点：①被告对患者负有义务，②被告违反了该义务，③是造成伤害的原因，以及④损伤。原告有责任证明每一项要素。一般而言，在民事案件中举证责任由证据比重决定，而非像刑事案件那样证据必须确凿无疑。在大多数情况下，责任问题并无争议，因其以医患关系为基础。为证明被告违反了这一义务，原告必须提供有说服力的专家证词，证明被告（被起诉人）没有遵守医疗标准。不好的结果本身，并不是渎职的证据。陪审团面对的问题是，在相同或类似的情况下，执业人员是否行使了执业者通常行使的医疗和技能水平。对自称是专家的执业人员，对他的标准可能比普通执业者高一些。就因果关系而言，原告通常必须确定偏离照护标准是造成索赔损伤的直接原因。然而，在美国某些州，该标准在某些类型的案件中有所放宽，以允许原告通过确定这种偏离增加损害风险的程度来要求被告承担其责任。最后，原告必须证明所要求的伤害赔偿，通常包括经济损失（收入损失、医疗费用等）和非经济损失（疼痛和痛苦、丧失生活乐趣等）。根据各州情况，陪审团对非经济损害赔偿的金额的确定可能有上限，也可能没有。

潜在的索赔通知

麻醉科医师可通过几种方式察觉潜在的医疗事故诉讼，患者或家属对治疗工作的不满是引起诉讼的一个重要原因。因此，患者或家属对护士的抱怨可能是其提起诉讼的第一个征象；也可能是患者在急诊治疗期间或在术后门诊就诊期间向外科医师或其助手抱怨；另一种可能是，患者向医院管理人员正式投诉麻醉科医师的某一做法。通常情况下，当麻醉科医师接到诉讼通知时，患者或家属诉讼意图的第一个迹象早已出现。

诉讼始于正式向法院提交法律文件。在大多数情况下，最初的申请被称为投诉。在一些州，诉讼可通过传票提起，传票只是简单地通知你已经被提起诉讼，然后再提交一份包含更详细信息的诉状。在麻醉科医师收到投诉或传票前，不需要采取任何行动。诉状通常阐述诉讼的依据：原告是如何因所谓的不合格医疗和索赔依据的细节而受到伤害的。当收到此类投诉时，应立即通知医师或医疗事故责任人，并将收到的所有文件副本发送给他。特别是一旦接到诉讼通知，所有记录都必须保存好，并且不要销毁或变更记录或其他相关文件。如果被发现，试图修改或销毁文档会给人留下有过失的印象，并且会使辩护变得非常复杂，实际上还会损害辩护。

风险评估

近 20 年来，与麻醉相关的渎职诉讼的发生率有所下降。脉搏血氧监测和二氧化碳监测使用的增加，可能是气管插管误入食管、心搏骤停和脑损伤等以往容易被诉讼事件发生率降低的部分原因。框 128.1 列出了许多与麻醉相关渎职的原因。

大多数与麻醉有关的产科索赔涉及剖宫产，其中最常见的是产妇死亡（21%）和新生儿脑损伤（17%）。美国麻醉科医师协会（American Society of Anesthesiologists，ASA）从事此索赔项目的审查人员发现，在有关新生儿脑损伤的诉讼中，有近一半案件由不恰当的麻醉管理造成。在产科麻醉索赔中，有一半是针对轻伤（如头痛、背痛、手术时疼痛、精神损害）提出的。在 ASA 的所有诉讼中，尽管审查人员发现麻醉科医师采取了适当的麻醉管理，但仍有 40% 的项目给原告支付了赔偿。

准备辩护

提起医疗事故诉讼后，会发生一系列事件（框 128.2）。一旦正式提出投诉，就须在规定时间内做出答复。未能在最后期限做出答复，可能对辩护产生不利影响，并可能导致对医师的默认判决。专业责任的受托人可指派律师为麻醉科医师辩护，并准备对投诉做出回应。麻醉科医师可要求指定一名律师，只要该律师在医疗事故受托人批准的律师名单上，保险公司通常会向该律师提供担保。麻醉科医师也可以自费聘请私人律师，但通常没有必要，除非当诉讼可能导致执照问题或巨大经济困难。如果聘请私人律师，该律师应当与医疗事故保险公司指派的律师合作，指定律师将继续处理医师的诉讼辩护。

框 128.1 涉嫌渎职的部分原因

- 未能提供足够的氧合
  - 插管错误
  - 氧气供应失败
  - 呼吸道阻塞
- 未能维持充足的循环
  - 低血压
  - 心律失常
  - 心搏骤停
- 误吸
- 术中知晓
- 神经损伤
  - 外周神经损伤
  - 脊髓损伤
  - 硬膜外异物
- 牙齿损伤
- 角膜损伤
- 口咽部、杓状软骨、声带、气管的物理损伤
- 与体位有关的物理损伤，包括骨折、脱位、压疮、感染
- 术后视力丧失
- 误诊
- 未能与患者或治疗小组其他成员充分沟通

框 128.2 医疗事故诉讼的阶段

- 传票 / 投诉
- 对投诉做出回应
- 证据公开
- 专家报告 / 口供
- 提案
- 审前会议 / 调解会议 / 调解
- 和解或陪审团庭审

在早期的计划阶段，麻醉科医师必须对律师完全坦诚，并共享所有正面和负面信息。虽然处理医疗事故索赔的律师对医学比较熟悉，但麻醉科医师必须就案件的具体医学知识点对律师进行讲解，帮助律师准备辩护。提供关键文献、指导方针等会有助于准备强有力的辩护。保密是一个重要的考虑要素。律师和客户的交流通常是保密的，不受披露的限制。麻醉科医师与同事就病例实情进行讨论不可避免，且完全允许（在管理中探讨过程）。麻醉科医师在患者医疗记录中涉及的任何有关治疗问题的图表和事件记录均可以公开。因此，建议不要在医疗记录的文档之外创建有关问题的文档。电子邮件和短信也可以被公开。目前，原告律师通常可要求获得相关的电子通信资料，包括电子邮件、短信、社交媒体帖子和病历审计跟踪等。不同的电子供应商采取的备份方式不同，而电子邮件的保存期长得惊人。Face book 或 Twitter 等社交媒体是非临床的，不是讨论患者问题的场所，任何此类平台发布的内容都可以被公开。涉及医疗事故的文件应该被安全妥善保存。

诉讼程序

证据公开

这属于诉讼所有参与者之间的信息交流。原

告有权获得所有与患者治疗相关的非机密材料。表 128.1 列出了公开证据的主要方法。

证词可能是最常见的公开证据的方法。宣誓之后，被告会被问及其必须回答的问题。证词的格式与法庭采用的格式相似。双方的律师都在场，没有法官。有一名法庭记录员会把问题和答案用文字记录下来。麻醉科医师在证词中所说的话与他或她在法庭上所说的话同样重要。证词过程中的证词和审判过程中的证词若存在显著偏差，可以用来反对被告人。在提供证词过程中，专业的态度、外表和举止十分重要，原因有二。其一，证词通常是原告律师会见被告的最初机会。除问题答案提供的信息外，原告律师认为这次会面是评估麻醉科医师在陪审团面前是什么样的证人的一次机会；其次，对原告律师而言，将证词录下来，然后在法庭上回放部分证词已经成为一种越来越普遍的做法。因此，证词过程中所表现的行为举止，必须与审判时所表现的行为举止保持一致，这一点至关重要。

在宣誓作证前，麻醉科医师与其律师应该会面，讨论预期的情况和问题、如何回答具体问题以及如何表现。麻醉科医师应该听从律师建议。可使用下述指导策略：尊重流程和在场人员；回答要直接、实事求是；不主动提供任何信息；不要表现出愤怒、厌烦或沮丧；避免使用俚语、讽刺或幽默；必须避免对原告的轻蔑评论；在问题完整陈述前，不要开始回答；在回答前停顿 1 ～ 2 s，给辩护律师一个反对的机会；说话声音清晰，易于听懂；避免表述过快或过慢；避免过度使用医学术语。可以对原告所发生的事情表示同情，而不必承担责任。无论是在证词还是庭审作证过程中，目标都是让人们觉得自己是一名称职、有爱心的医师，已为患者尽了最大的努力。

表 128.1 证据公开过程

方法	描述
质问	由被告必须回答的一长串问题组成的书面要求
要求提供医疗信息	要求提供相关医疗记录的复印件；大多数医院都有专门的机构来确保涉及医疗事故行为的纸质和电子病历的安全
要求出示文件	这些文件可能涉及原告或被告认为对案件重要的任何文件（例如，原告可能要求一份董事会认证证书的复印件）；还可以要求提供信件、电子邮件、短信、电话交谈记录等
证人证词	经宣誓而作的证词，其格式与法庭上使用的格式相似

专家

如前所述，为确定医疗过失索赔，原告必须提供合格的医学专家鉴定，来证明麻醉科医师偏离了治疗标准，并且这种偏离是患者受伤的直接原因。通常，在诉讼过程中，原告需提供专家鉴定报告来支持索赔，而辩护律师将提供支持辩护的专家报告。在一些州，专家可能会在庭审前接受证词；在另一些州，庭审将是向专家证人询问其意见的第一次机会。

提案

提案是要求法院就案件中的某一特定问题作出命令的请求。其中，提案的类型包括：强制某些可以提出异议的公开证据的提案，阻止或限制某些类型证据公开的提案，以及限制或驳回某些权利要求或驳回某些当事人的提案。提案通常不需要医师出庭，律师将告知客户任何需要他或她参与的提案。

审前会议

在庭审开始前，所有参与案件的律师通常必须参加由法庭举行的听证会，麻醉科医师不参加此会议。在审前会议上，可以讨论诸如确定审讯日期、提交审前提案的截止日期和提交拟议的陪审团指示等事项。在一些司法管辖区，法院还会在案件开始时召开会议，确定完成审前询问的最后期限、专家证人的披露时间以及提交哪些类型的提案等。一些州有强制性的审前调解或强制和解会议，试图在庭审前解决案件。

庭审证词

庭审过程中的证词与供词中的证词相似，但也存在一定差异。由一名主审法官就所提出问题的实质和形式提及的反对意见作出裁决。有一个非专业的陪审团，其对医学的熟悉程度通常不如进行证词的律师。由于是由陪审团决定支持或反对被告，因此医师在陈述证词时应与陪审团联系，而不是聘请律师或法官，这一点非常重要。如前所述，证词应以缓慢、清晰的方式表述，尽量少用行话或复杂的医学术语，同时应注意避免对陪审团“居高临下”。陪审团可能不理解医学术语，也可能不清楚医疗过程的细节，但若确信被告是一个关心、尽责的医师，为患者已尽最大努力时，他们可能更倾向为被告辩护。庭审过程的简要概述见框 128.3。

证人通常在庭审过程中被传唤作证。这些证人大多了解所发生的事情，并且为其所看见、所听见的事作证。原告和被告几乎在所有案件中都会出庭作证。被告医师不仅可在辩护期间被传唤，也可在原告案件中被传唤，在此期间，被告医师可作为假设的敌对证人被讯问。还有一些“专家”证人，鉴于其具备专业知识，被允许就治疗标准、涉及的治疗是否符合相应治疗标准以及是否有任何违反治疗标准的行为而造成伤害等问题发表意见。法院决定是否接受证人作为专家，正方和反方的任何一方都可对专家作证的资格提出质疑。必要时，担保方通常也有权对专家意见的科学依据提出初步质疑。

虽然对诉讼程序进行了广泛讨论，但大多数医疗事故诉讼都在庭审前和解。造成这种情况的原因有很多。对任何一方而言，审判结果很难预计，无论哪一方胜诉，都可能导致长时间上诉；和解结果是确定性和终局性的；双方都要为庭审付出相当大的成本；有时人们担心索赔或辩护力度，或担心陪审团对案件某些方面的反应。

在决定是否进行庭审或和解时，保险范围也是重要的考虑因素。许多医师担心医疗事故赔偿金会超过他们保险单的限额。典型麻醉失误的保险限额为每次 100 万美元。在 ASA 索赔项目中，只有 4% 的付款超过该数额。自 ASA 开始收集数据以来，医疗事故赔偿额超过 100 万美元的案件比例并未增加。然而，由于案件所处的司法管辖区不同，超额裁决的风险可能有很大不同。医疗事故保险不补偿医师离开诊所的时间或与诉讼有关的收入损失。保险单通常有一个条款，即将那些故意不当行为排除在保险范围。大多数保单都有一个条款，要求医师与指定的律师和保险公司进行相应合作。医师如拒绝遵守公开证据请求、会见其律师、提供证词或出庭受审等，则可能损害其保险范围。

另一需要考虑的问题是，医疗事故的和解和赔偿应向国家执业人员数据库（National Practitioner Data Bank，NPDB）报告。美国国会于 1986 年成立 NPDB，其接收的报告包括：医疗事故赔偿（无论金额大小），不良行为（如拒绝或限制许可证、拒绝或限制医院权限、被排除在州或联邦卫生保健项目外、不利的专业社会行为等）以及与卫生保健相关的民事判决或刑事定罪。当医师申请或更新医院权限时，通常会查询此信息。可以理解的是，NPDB 条目可能会对其就业、许可或权限产生不利影响。州委员会和认证机构通常会关注鉴别那些以较为麻烦的方式支付的涉及临床问题以及代表医师支付的费用。少量的医疗事故报告通常不建议采用这种方式，也可能不会引起关注。涉及临床权限或许可证的不良行为报告可能更值得关注。

框 128.3 庭审过程

- 陪审团成员选择
- 双方律师的开场陈述
- 原告律师试图证明被告因疏忽大意而引起损伤。为促进目标的实现，原告团队将提出并审查证人（包括事实和专家），介绍证据等；辩护团队也可对任何证人进行交互讯问
- 被告律师使用上述相同技巧，试图证明被告对患者的照护是恰当和合适的，和（或）不会导致损伤
- 结束辩论，双方分别从各自的角度对本案进行总结陈述
- 审判长对陪审团的指示。法官解释适用于案件的法律，并就如何进行审议向陪审团提供指导
- 陪审团审议。陪审团讨论案件，审查证词，并审查证据，试图对被告作出支持或反对的决定
- 判决。陪审团裁决的公开声明，包括裁决的损害赔偿金额（如果有的话）

预防

医疗事故的预防首先应始终遵循相应的治疗标准。框 128.4 列出了几种有助于降低被起诉风险的行为策略。患者术前和术后访视非常重要，访视能加强与患者的交流并解决患者关心的问题。患者或家属对治疗的不满可能会增加诉讼的可能性。因此，与患者保持良好的关系不仅有助于临床麻醉，也有助于良好的风险管理。

近年来，人们努力打破“障碍”，改善不良事件后的沟通，允许医师表达同情、道歉或慰问，但不允许在后期诉讼中表现出这些姿态。支持者建议，这可能是患者和医师之间的润滑剂，并可能降低患者惩罚医师的欲望。现在，许多州都制定了法律，

框 128.4 有助于降低诉讼风险的行为

- 通过自学或参加讲座和课程进行持续的教育
- 与同事和机构合作，制订患者安全和质量持续改进的计划，识别并处理风险
- 制定术前患者访谈和回顾图表
- 就风险和备选方案进行明确解释；要友好、面带微笑、不要催促患者或家属
- 获得知情同意。确保患者和家属理解提出的建议、风险期望都是合理的
- 遵守 ASA 的监测建议
- 正确标识药物
- 保存准确、清晰的麻醉记录，记录不良事件或意外事件，并在发生任何不良事件后提供持续治疗
- 熟悉自己使用的麻醉和其他设备
- 适时请求协助，避免耽误援助请求
- 熟悉正在执行的操作流程
- 对麻醉患者进行体位护理
- 提供麻醉照护时避免分心
- 与外科医师、护士和其他人员保持良好的关系
- 亲自或电话进行术后随访

允许这些医师表达同情、道歉或慰问，而不用冒着后期在法庭上这些姿态可能会对医师不利的风险。虽然各州的保护范围各不相同，但在任何诉讼前最好做出这些姿态，但不应该包括承认过错。

被起诉似乎是所有医师面临的职业风险。Jena 及其同事表示，到 65 岁时，75% 的低风险专业医师和 99% 的高风险专业医师可能会在医疗事故索赔中被点名。在这一数据收集中，麻醉学被认为是一个低风险的专业。

被起诉的心理反应

诉讼过程中以及结案后被告方的心理反应在文献中尚未得到充分讨论或关注。根据 Charles 的简要总结，至少 95% 的医师在被起诉时都会经历一段时间的情绪困扰。在某些情况下，焦虑会导致严重的抑郁症、药物滥用或心房颤动之类的身体症状。认识到潜在的情感损失是建立适当应对机制的第一步。

致谢

感谢 Robert D. Kaye 和 Christophe M. D. Heard 博士对本章上一版的贡献。

（陈文颖　译　韩文军　校）

延伸阅读

Brenner IR: *How to survive a medical malpractice lawsuit*, Chichester, England, 2010, Wiley Blackwell, p 155.

Charles SC: Coping with a medical malpractice suit, *West J Med* 174:55–58, 2001.

Cheney FW, Posner K, Caplan RA, et al.: Standard of care and anesthesia liability, *JAMA* 261:1599–1603, 1989.

Davies JM, Posner KL, Lee LA, et al.: Liability associated with obstetric anesthesia, *Anesthesiology* 110:131–139, 2009.

Hickson GB, Federspiel CF, Pichert JW, et al.: Patient complaints and malpractice risk, *JAMA* 287:2951–2957, 2002.

Jena AB, Seabury S, Lakdawalla D, et al.: Malpractice risk according to physician specialty, *N Engl J Med* 365:629–636, 2011.

Ranum D, Ma H, Shapiro FE, et al.: Analysis of patient injury based on anesthesiology closed claims data from a major malpractice insurer, *J Healthc Risk Manag* 34(2):31–42, 2014.

Ross BK: ASA closed claims in obstetrics: lessons learned, *Anesthesiol Clin North Am* 21:183–197, 2003.

Saitta N, Hodge Jr SD: Efficacy of a physician's words of empathy: an overview of state apology laws, *J Am Osteopath Assoc* 112:302–306, 2012.

Satiani B: The National Practitioner Data Bank: structure and function, *J Am Coll Surg* 199:981–986, 2004.

U.S. Department of Health and Human Services: National Practitioner Data Bank—what you must report to the NPDB. Available at https://www.npdb.hrsa.gov/hcorg/whatYouMustReportToTheDataBank.jsp. Accessed November 30, 2016.

Watson-Dunham B: *Medical malpractice law and litigation*. West Legal Studies, Clifton Park, NY, 2006, Thomson Delmar Learning, p 354.

第129章 过敏和类过敏反应

Sylvia Y. Dolinski

病例概要

患者，女性，54岁，因卵巢肿瘤拟行子宫及卵巢切除术。给予丙泊酚、芬太尼和维库溴铵麻醉诱导，七氟烷维持，插管后不久给予2 g头孢替坦，随后20 min内，出现低血压，且对去氧肾上腺素和麻黄碱不敏感，呼吸末二氧化碳为22 mmHg。多次给予100 μg的肾上腺素以维持平均动脉压大于60 mmHg。随后手术被取消，患者转至重症监护病房。1周后再次手术。

问题分析

定义

患者在麻醉时接触大量静脉注射药物：麻醉药、抗生素、扩容液体、血液制品、镇痛药、消毒剂、染料和造影剂。因此，麻醉科医师很可能会在他们的职业生涯中遇到过敏反应患者。过敏反应是一种迅速发生的危及生命的全身性变态反应。然而，它只表现为单一的体征（支气管痉挛或低血压），与许多疾病表现相似，因此可能会误诊。在未经特殊治疗而恢复的轻度病例中，缺乏对过敏反应的认识可能导致再次暴露的致命后果。经典反应被描述为过敏反应[免疫球蛋白E（immunoglobulin E，IgE）介导]或类过敏反应（非IgE介导）。欧洲过敏与临床免疫学学会提出将临床反应定义为过敏反应及其亚型，并在实验室诊断确定机制后将其细分为变态反应或非变态反应。然而，美国过敏、哮喘与免疫学学会在2015年最新的指南中仍将该反应定义为过敏和类过敏反应。不管如何分类，对于麻醉科医师来说都不重要，因为无论病因如何，过敏反应的治疗都是一样的。麻醉过程中的大多数反应是由IgE介导的抗原，导致肥大细胞（组织）和嗜碱性细胞（血液）脱颗粒。高达50%的对神经肌肉阻滞药物（neuromuscular blocking drug，NMBD）发生I型超敏的患者否认曾接触过该药物。即使患者是第一次接触，也可能通过皮肤试验检测出NMBD特异性IgE。虽然这一理论尚未得到证实，但普遍认为之前接触过类似季铵盐基团的化合物会使患者致敏，从而形成特定的IgE分子。食品、化妆品、消毒剂和其他药物通常含有这种铵基。因此，当首次接触NMBD时，这些预先形成的IgE分子与NMBD的铵盐基团发生交叉反应。

识别

流行病学

在包括法国、英国、斯堪的纳维亚半岛在内的大部分欧洲国家，NMBD是引起围术期过敏反应最常见的麻醉药物（30%～50%）（图129.1和129.2）。在美国，只有一项针对38名患者的单中心研究，报道其发病率为11%。乳胶制品仍然排在第二位，由于加强了预防措施，美国可能有所减少。抗生素继续排在第三位，30多年来发病率有所上升，可能是由于抗生素预防的依从性增加。围术期麻醉期间过敏反应的发生率为1∶20 000～1∶3500，死亡率为1.4%～9%，高于非麻醉相关的过敏反应。尽管麻醉科医师迅速采取行动，但死亡率的增加与患者的基本情况、短时间静脉注射的巨大抗原负荷以及麻醉剂对心脏抑制作用有关，这种更为严重的过敏反应大多是IgE介导的。这种情况女性比男性高3倍。新出现的过敏原包括非甾体抗炎药（nonsteroidal antiinflammatory drugs，NSAIDs）、染料、放射造影剂和氯己定。

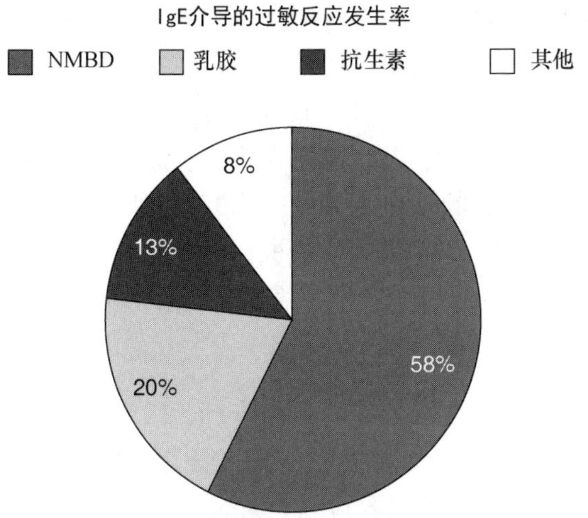

图 129.1 过敏反应最常见的原因（Data from Mertes PM，Alla F，Trechot P，et al.：Anaphylaxis during anesthesia in France：an 8-year national survey. *J Allergy Clin Immunol* 128[2]：366-373，2011.）

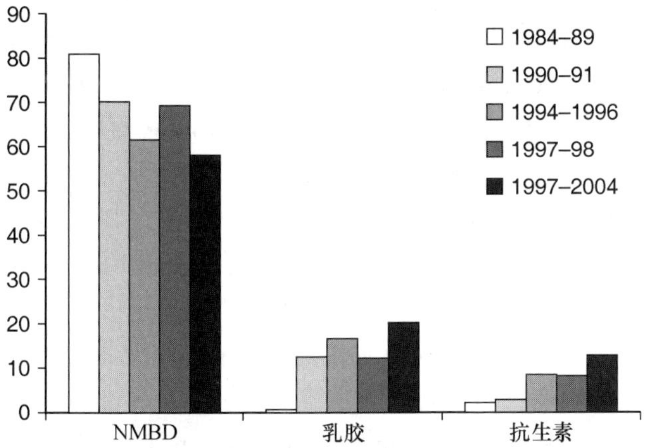

图 129.2 法国 30 年研究过敏反应发生率比较。（Data from Mertes PM，Laxenaire MC，Alla F，et al.：Anaphylactic and anaphylactoid reactions occurring during anesthesia in France in 1999-2000. *Anesthesiology* 99[3]：536-545，2003；and Mertes PM，Alla F，Trechot P，et al.：Anaphylaxis during anesthesia in France：an 8-year national survey. *J Allergy Clin Immunol* 128[2]：366-373，2011.）

发病机制

药物引起的过敏反应由 IgE 和非 IgE 依赖性通路介导。独立的通路包括补体和激肽释放酶的激活。典型的症状是单相的，反应在 3 h 内立即发生。双相过敏反应中，在 72 h 内重新启动前至少停止 1 h，且不与触发剂再次接触。在迁延性变异反应中，即时反应可持续数小时。

在 IgE 介导的通路中，先前存在的与肥大细胞和嗜碱性细胞结合的 IgE 抗体在暴露于抗原时发生交联反应。细胞激活伴随着大量的炎性介质（组胺、前列腺素 D2、白三烯 D4、血小板活化因子）的释放，这些介质促进血管扩张和平滑肌收缩。肥大细胞和嗜碱性细胞也可以通过补体（非 IgE 通路）直接激活。另一种机制是激活组织和血浆激肽释放酶（缓激肽和激肽）促进血管扩张、气道平滑肌收缩和增加血管通透性。虽然胰蛋白酶亦有释放，但尚不清楚它如何参与过敏进程。

Ring 和 Messmer（1977）制定了过敏反应围术期严重程度分级（框 129.1）。麻醉过程中，过敏反应通常表现为分布性休克和（或）支气管痉挛，甚至完全性心脏停搏。舌头和嘴唇会发生血管性水肿，如果患者已经插管，则可以避免窒息。心脏缺血不仅是严重的低血压的结果，也可能继发于冠状动脉本身肥大细胞激活（Kounis 综合征）。严重低血压时可能不出现荨麻疹，而血压恢复时可能出现。

风险评估

特异反应是乳胶引起过敏反应的危险因素，但它不是大多数药物引起过敏反应的危险因素。合并其他疾病如冠状动脉疾病、哮喘或肺气肿可能导致更严重的结果：①过敏反应所致的缺血（或肾上腺素治疗），或②严重的支气管痉挛（或呼吸困难）。使用 β- 受体阻滞剂或血管紧张素转换酶（angiotensinconverting enzyme，ACE）抑制剂的患者低血压可能更严重和难以治疗。

- 我们应充分认识到不同种类的 NMBD 之间存在 60% ～ 70% 的交叉反应。但 NMBD 皮肤测试阴性说明可以安全替代。
- 由于具有共同的 β- 内酰胺环，对青霉素或阿莫西林过敏的患者对第一代头孢菌素过敏发生率较高，但第二或第三代头孢菌素过敏发生率不高。

表 129.1 围术期高敏反应严重程度分级

分级	临床症状
Ⅰ 皮肤反应	红斑、荨麻疹、血管性水肿
Ⅱ 未危及生命的反应	皮肤反应 ± 低血压 ± 心动过速 ± 呼吸困难 ± 胃肠反应
Ⅲ 危及生命的反应，单器官或多器官	休克和（或）支气管痉挛
Ⅳ 心脏骤停	

From Dewachter P，Mouton-Faivre C，Emala CW：Anaphylaxis and anesthesia，*Anesthesiology* 111：1141-1150，2009.

- 蛋类和大豆过敏者不易对丙泊酚过敏。丙泊酚是一种含有大豆油和蛋黄中的卵磷脂的油水乳剂。这些化合物不是过敏原。蛋类过敏患者中，蛋清蛋白是过敏原。大豆过敏患者可以使用丙泊酚，因为在提炼过程中过敏性蛋白已被去除。丙泊酚的主要过敏原是异丙基和苯酚。
- 局麻药分为酯类和酰胺类。酯类引起的皮肤反应通常是由于对氨基苯甲酸（para-aminobenzoic acid，PABA）的代谢引起的。当使用肾上腺素以延长作用时间时，全身吸收可导致过敏症状：焦虑、震颤、心动过速和头痛。据报道，3000 名患者中，真正的 IgE 介导的过敏反应发生率为 0.97%。其中还包括局麻药中防腐剂对羟基苯甲酸甲酯的反应。

麻醉过程中的过敏原

- NSAIDs 越来越多地被用于多模式镇痛。如果需要进行疼痛治疗，皮肤测试以确定 NSAIDs 使用的安全性。
- 氯己定作为消毒剂在外科手术中的使用越来越多。它可以涂抹于中心静脉导管，如果出现长时间的过敏反应，不应忽视氯己定的致敏作用。
- 前哨淋巴结活检定位使用的异舒泛蓝等染料和术中使用的其他染料越来越多地导致过敏反应。亚甲蓝已被用于病毒灭活新鲜冷冻血浆（fresh frozen plasma，FFP）。
- 血液制品：具有 IgA 抗体的 IgA 缺陷的患者可对含有 IgA 抗原的 FFP 或血小板发生反应。除了与血液制品本身发生反应外，还必须考虑亚甲蓝。

过敏反应的临床表现

药物引起的过敏反应的表现包括皮肤反应（荨麻疹和血管水肿）、呼吸反应（支气管痉挛）和心血管反应（低血压和心动过速或心动过缓）。当严重低血容量的心室收缩时，Bezold-Jarisch 反射诱发心动过缓以改善心室充盈。面对这种心动过缓，使用阿托品可能立即发生心搏骤停。哮喘患者更容易发生严重的支气管痉挛，任何诱导后出现严重支气管痉挛并伴有低血压和需要肾上腺素治疗的患者，都应该检查胰蛋白酶水平。心脏病患者、服用 β- 受体阻滞剂或血管紧张素转换酶抑制剂的患者更容易出现严重的低血压。有多达 10% 的病例可见双相或长时间的表现。**假定的**诊断是根据**临床**基础和支持性**生物标志物**进行的围术期诊断，而最终诊断应依赖于变态反应学证据。如果不结合临床表现可能出现误诊或延迟诊断，因为低血压可能是由于多种麻醉药的不良反应、失血或并存疾病。胶体用于治疗其他原因引起的低血压（深度麻醉或硬膜外交感神经切除术）时，可能会被忽视。荨麻疹和血管性水肿也可能因为患者手术巾覆盖或插管而忽略。

诊断

组胺不是一个好的诊断指标，因为它短暂升高（半衰期为 10 ～ 20 min），在复苏期间就恢复到基线。但是它仍然需要检测。尿 N- 甲基组胺持续时间较长，可检测 6 h，但并非所有医院都可检测。胰蛋白酶浓度水平大于 25 μg/L 是高度敏感的标志。它在 60 min 左右达到峰值，半衰期为 2 h，当水平大于 11.4 μg/L 时，应考虑过敏性诊断。最近有研究表明，与过敏反应无关的心搏骤停或严重低血压的患者，组胺或胰蛋白酶水平没有升高。然而，尸检分析显示，其他死因可能导致胰蛋白酶水平超过 11.4 μg/L，这可能是因为血液溶血和嗜碱性粒细胞破坏。复苏（或死亡）后应尽快送检胰蛋白酶，1 h ～ 2 h、6 h、24 h 重复检测。所有指南都推荐检测胰蛋白酶水平。24 h 水平被视为基线水平，两倍于基础水平可以确诊。

通常在过敏反应发生后 4 ～ 6 周，应将患者转至过敏专科医师进行皮肤点刺试验（skin prick test，SPT）或皮内试验（intradermal test，IDT）以确定过敏药物。如果患者立即接受测试，肥大细胞可能会耗尽其储存的过敏介质。尽管如此，如果检测结果为阳性，立即（几天内）进行检测可能会有所帮助。如果手术很紧急，表 129.1 为推荐使用的方案。当风团直径等于阳性对照（如组胺）的一半，且大于阴性对照（生理盐水）至少 3 mm 时，SPT 为阳性。其他 NMBDs、阿片类药物和诱导剂也应进行评估，为今后手术时 IDT 提供选择。体外试验，如放射变应原吸附剂试验、酶联免疫吸附剂试验或荧光酶免疫试验，检测患者血清 IgE（serum IgE，sIgE）到假定的具有二级抗 IgE 的致敏剂抗体可检测 sIgE 结合量。这些测试通常是为寻找 NMBDs、乳胶、β- 内酰胺类、氯己定和环氧乙烷（手术器械用杀菌剂）的过敏。目前正在研究新的诊断试验，如嗜碱性粒细胞活化试验，它是用流式细胞术检测嗜碱性粒细胞暴露于特定过敏原后表达的嗜碱性粒细胞活化标记物。

框 129.1 需紧急手术的建议方案

1. 为过敏反应做准备：肾上腺素 10 ～ 20 μg/ml，2 根大直径静脉导管、动脉导管
2. 避免接触乳胶
3. 避免使用以前的抗生素，青霉素和第一代头孢菌素
4. 使用替代消毒剂：聚维酮 vs. 氯己定
5. 特异性血清 IgE（仅阳性试验有效）
6. 使用不同的方法：避免所有以前使用过的药物
   a. 区域阻滞技术
   b. 吸入麻醉药
7. 如果不可能采用替代技术，请尽早进行皮肤测试：
   a. 阳性：避免使用这些药物，并使用皮肤测试阴性药物
   b. 阴性：注意神经肌肉阻滞药物之间的高交叉反应性，抗组胺药和类固醇可以预防过敏反应

Adapted from Soetens F，Rose M，Fisher M：Timing of skin testing after a suspected anaphylactic reac-tion during anaesthesia. *Acta Anaesthesiol Scand* 56（8）：1042-1046，2012.

管理

由于 50% 的液体可迅速渗出导致低血压，因此应迅速给予 1 ～ 2 L 晶体液和（或）胶体液（除非认为其是过敏药物），并立即给予肾上腺素。因为肾上腺素能逆转血管扩张、支气管收缩和黏膜水肿。最初使用肾上腺素而不是去甲肾上腺素或抗利尿激素的关键原因是它能够增加 cAMP，从而直接抑制介质的进一步脱颗粒。了解患者的基本情况如冠状动脉疾病、高龄或卒中的风险十分重要，特别是在危急时刻，以免给患者使用过量的肾上腺素。肾上腺素的剂量应该从 10 ～ 50 μg 开始，最大增加到 100 ～ 300 μg。重复给药后应立即开始肾上腺素输注。将 1 mg（1∶1000）的肾上腺素加入到 250 ml 的液体内配置成 4 μg/ml 的肾上腺素，以 1 ～ 4 μg/min 的速度注入。当肾上腺素不能恢复血压时，应加用其他血管活性药物。抗组胺药物不能消除过敏反应且作用缓慢，但可以改善皮肤表现。需谨慎使用抗组胺药物，因为迅速注入 H_1 和 H_2 阻滞剂会引起低血压。类固醇可以预防双相性过敏反应。使用 β-受体阻滞剂的患者可考虑使用胰高血糖素。胰高血糖素可以直接激活腺苷酸环化酶，可减轻顽固性低血压和支气管痉挛。亚甲基蓝通过阻断一氧化氮诱导的血管扩张，有病例报告证实亚甲基蓝可以有效治疗儿茶酚胺和抗利尿激素难治性休克的患者。表 129.2 列举了过敏反应的治疗方案。

表 129.2 过敏反应的治疗

	理由
术中用药	
停止目前输注和之前给与的所有药物	
快速给与晶体 1 ～ 2 L	35% ～ 75% 的液体可在 15 min 内渗出
肾上腺素	阻断介质的释放
β_2 受体激动剂（沙丁胺醇）	对支气管痉挛治疗作用时间长于肾上腺素
100% 氧气类固醇	不建议立即使用，二级管理预防双相反应
抗组胺药	不建议立即使用，用于治疗荨麻疹、瘙痒、血管性水肿
诊断	
血清胰蛋白酶（直接）	含量 >11 ng/ml
血清组胺（直接）	可能继续提高到 1 h
尿组胺或 N- 甲基组胺	大多数医院可能无法提供
围术期	
血清胰蛋白酶（1、3、6、12 h）	诊断，检测峰值水平并返回基线
血清 IgE 特异性药物	琥珀胆碱、丙泊酚、抗生素、乳胶等
皮肤测试过敏咨询	识别致敏抗原

预防

预防麻醉期间过敏反应唯一方法是避免使用已知的致敏药物或麻醉前的可疑药物。除非不能避免使用同一类药物，否则在进一步麻醉前应对患者进行检测（包括皮肤测试）。麻醉科医师和过敏专科医师之间的合作对于确定过敏药物和使用安全麻醉剂替代至关重要。这种情况下，应该与外科医师讨论推迟手术。延迟并不理想，但在等待过敏测试的 4 ～ 6 周内可以进行化疗。但是，考虑到她是癌症患者，应认为其为紧急手术。进行麻醉时，避免使用所有可疑的药物和不使用 NMBD，胸腔硬膜外注射 1% 罗哌卡因可使肌肉充分松弛，七氟烷术中维持。患者手术很成功。事后看来，继续治疗的决定是明智的，因为卵巢肿瘤其实是阑尾癌，她可能接受了错误的化疗。此外，麻醉科医师和过敏专科医师还确定了以后手术的安全麻醉药物。事实上，她在数月

之后安全地接受了腹腔热灌注化疗手术。

（王靖云 译 王 薇 校）

延伸阅读

Dewachter P, Mouton-Faivre C, Castells MC, et al.: Anesthesia in the patient with multiple drug allergies: are all allergies the same? *Curr Opin Anesth* 24:320–325, 2011.

Dewachter P, Mouton-Faivre C, Emala CW: Anaphylaxis and anesthesia, *Anesthesiology* 111:1141–1150, 2009.

Hepner DL, Castells MC: Anaphylaxis during the perioperative period, *Anesth Analg* 97:1381–1395, 2003.

Joint Task Force on Practice Parameters, American Academy of Allergy, Asthma and Immunology and American College of Allergy: Asthma and Immunology: anaphylaxis—a practice parameter update 2015, *Ann Allergy Asthma Immunol* 115:341–384, 2015.

Kannan JA, Bernstein JA: Perioperative anaphylaxis. diagnosis, evaluation, and management, *Immunol Allergy Clin North Am* 35:321–334, 2015.

Laroche D, Gomis P, Gallimidi E, et al.: Diagnostic value of histamine and tryptase concentrations in severe anaphylaxis with shock or cardiac arrest during anesthesia, *Anesthesiology* 121:272–279, 2014.

Mertes PM, Alla F, Trechot P, et al.: Anaphylaxis during anesthesia in France: an 8-year national survey, *J Allergy Clin Immunol* 128(2):366–373, 2011.

Mertes PM, Tajima K, Regnier-Kimmoun MA, et al.: Perioperative anaphylaxis, *Med Clin North Am* 94:761–789, 2010.

Nell L, Eren E: Peri-operative anaphylaxis, *Br J Clin Pharmacol* 71(5):647–658, 2011.

Ring J, Messmer K: Incidence and severity of anaphylactoid reactions to colloid volume substitutes, *Lancet* 1:466–469, 1977.

Soetens F, Rose M, Fisher M: Timing of skin testing after a suspected anaphylactic reaction during anesthesia, *Acta Anaesthesiol Scand* 56:1042–1046, 2012.

Volcheck GW, Mertes PM: Local and general anesthetics immediate hypersensitivity reactions, *Immunol Allergy Clin North Am* 34:525–546, 2014.

血管性水肿和荨麻疹 第 130 章

Catherine Drexler

病例概要

患者，57 岁，非洲裔女性，患有高血压，最近开始使用血管紧张素转换酶（angiotensin-converting enzyme，ACE）抑制剂，在全身麻醉下接受腹腔镜胆囊切除术。患者入苏醒室 1 h 后，患者抱怨感觉舌头“发厚”。经检查，患者舌体剧烈肿胀并突出到口腔外，患者能够讲话且无呼吸困难或瘙痒，无荨麻疹或哮喘症状。患者对 15 min 前静脉给予的 25 mg 苯海拉明无反应。

问题分析

定义

血管性水肿和荨麻疹的病因复杂，包括免疫介导和非免疫介导的。二者常同时发生，症状从温和、自限性到危及生命，严重程度不一。

荨麻疹是指皮肤红斑，瘙痒性的皮肤水肿。血管性水肿的过程类似，但发生在真皮层、皮下和黏膜下层，弥漫性水肿较多。由于真皮层的作用，血管性水肿常不伴有瘙痒。

血管性水肿的部位包括面部、舌、喉部、四肢、生殖器和胃肠道。后者可能表现为急性腹腔内病变的症状。喉部受累可能导致危及生命的气道阻塞。

荨麻疹和血管性水肿可急性或慢性起病，病因通常不明。家族史可能包括遗传性血管性水肿（hereditary angioedema，HAE）和 C1 酯酶抑制剂（C1-INH）缺乏。C1-INH 缺乏引起的血管性水肿常发生于潜在的自身免疫性疾病或恶性疾病时。C1-INH 缺乏可激活补体级联反应，因其酯酶切割 C1，导致血管扩张和血管性水肿。

急性荨麻疹或血管性水肿是肥大细胞和嗜碱性粒细胞活化、脱颗粒或降解所致，可由免疫球蛋白 E（immunoglobulin E，IgE）或其他触发物（如补体介导或直接肥大细胞释放剂）介导。这些细胞释放或产生各种介质，导致血管扩张和血管通透性增加。这些介质包括组胺、组胺释放因子、前列腺素 D、白三烯 C4 和 D4、血小板活化因子、过敏毒素（C3a、C4a、C5a）、缓激肽、激肽释放酶、细胞因子如白细胞介素（interleukin，IL）-4 和 IL-5 以及干扰素 -γ。不管其分类和潜在原因如何，肥大细胞降解的临床特征均相似（框 130.1）。

识别

及时发现荨麻疹或血管性水肿对改善预后至关重要。

本病例较易识别，因相关症状由这名警醒的患者本人报告。然而，由于某些原因，术中诊断荨麻疹或血管性水肿可能很困难。手术单、保温毯和手术“准备”消毒液可能会阻碍和限制皮肤暴露，导致发现延迟。与组胺释放相关的支气管痉挛可能错误地归因于气道操作或哮喘。由全身反应引起的血管舒张导致的低血压可能被错误地推测为心肌抑制、麻醉药效应或血容量不足的表现。最后，短时间内可能给予多种具有免疫或非免疫肥大细胞激活和脱颗粒功能的药物，包括抗生素、神经肌肉阻滞剂及阿片类药物。因此，即使注意到一种反应，也可能难以辨别其原因，以及是否代表真正的“过敏性”（IgE 介导的）事件。

一旦发现荨麻疹或血管水肿，注意药物使用和反应开始之间的时间关系十分重要。反应可能延迟，导致对致病药物的错误结论。

框 130.1 血管性水肿的分类

特发性
免疫介导的血管性水肿
　免疫球蛋白 E 介导
　物理性荨麻疹
　接触反应

补体介导
C1 酯酶抑制剂（C1-INH）缺乏
　遗传性血管性水肿
　获得性 C1-INH 缺陷
免疫复合物型血清病
荨麻疹性血管炎
系统性红斑狼疮
输血反应

非免疫介导
直接肥大细胞或组胺释放
血管紧张素转换酶抑制剂相关

其他罕见综合征
肥大细胞增多症
C3b 灭活剂缺乏
感染
　驱虫药
　真菌
　病毒
系统性疾病
　甲状腺功能亢进症
　胶原血管病
恶性肿瘤（尤其是 B 细胞肿瘤）

风险评估

约 15% ～ 20% 人群在其一生中会经历一次血管性水肿或荨麻疹发作；血管性水肿在中年女性中更为普遍。与白种人相比，非洲裔美国人 ACE 抑制剂相关的血管性水肿发生率更高，可能与缓激肽裂解的其他（非 ACE）酶水平较低的遗传变异有关。没有既往史和家族史时，由于潜在原因的广泛性，难以前瞻性地识别有危险的患者。在这种情况下，患者服用 ACE 抑制剂被认为与血管性水肿相关。尽管通常在用药开始后数周至数月内发生，但在暴露多年后也可见到 ACE 抑制剂相关血管性水肿的报道。此外，也有在停用 ACE 抑制剂后血管性水肿继续发作的情况。气道操作（如气管内插管）和牙科操作已被视为血管性水肿的诱因。此外，患者围术期接受非甾体抗炎药（nonsteroidal antiinflammatory drugs，NSAIDs）也是常见诱因；与 NSAIDs 相关的荨麻疹和（或）血管性水肿的遗传易感多态性已被描述。

风险评估应从详尽的病史、体格检查及药物和治疗方法开始。正确诊断和治疗血管性水肿的关键是注意是否同时存在荨麻疹。荨麻疹和瘙痒症的存在表明该过程是“过敏性”或 IgE 介导，存在组胺释放。因此，抗组胺药物和肾上腺素治疗有效是可预计的。若无荨麻疹，缓激肽或补体等其他介质可能会诱发反应，而认识到这种区别对正确指导治疗十分必要。ACE 抑制剂相关的血管性水肿是非免疫性的，不太可能对抗组胺药、肾上腺素或皮质类固醇产生明显反应。

风险评估必须包括气道评估，要考虑喉部受累的可能性，这可由呼吸困难或声音变化提示。如需气管插管，纤维支气管镜检查可能是最佳选择。患者也可能需要气管切开术。发生血管性水肿的患者在气管拔管前也应检查气道。

启示

围术期荨麻疹或血管性水肿最主要的担忧是其可迅速发展为气道梗阻和（或）过敏反应，因此需要加强监测，并需有能力管理气道的医师在场。若出现血流动力学衰竭的全身反应，可能需要大量静脉输液。如果抗组胺药、肾上腺素和皮质类固醇无反应，应怀疑非组胺性血管性水肿，并采取不同的管理策略。在尝试大剂量（高达 4 倍常规剂量）抗组胺药后，应考虑抗组胺药无反应的情况。

管理

根据临床表现、病因（致病药物和化学介质）和治疗，血管性水肿大致分为组胺能性或非组胺能性。

在评估和管理气道和血流动力学状态后，应回顾患者所用药物并停用可能的致病药物。如出现血管内容量减少的症状，则应开始液体复苏。肾上腺素可用于循环衰竭、过敏反应或与支气管痉挛相关的严重呼吸衰竭。

有些反应是温和且自限性的，可在数小时至数天内解决。除适当加强监护外，不需要实验室检查（必要时）和消除致病因子以外的治疗。

对没有荨麻疹的急性血管性水肿，实验室检查包括促甲状腺激素和全血细胞计数。若存在荨麻疹，血清 IgE 和类胰蛋白酶水平常支持过敏这一机制。如怀疑遗传或获得性 C1-INH 缺乏或质量异常，可检测补体蛋白 C1-INH 和 C4。补体蛋白水平低支持 HAE 或 C1-INH 缺乏的诊断，在 ACE 抑制剂血管性水肿中可见正常值。根据最初测试的结果和潜在的系统性病因，可进行自身免疫行疾病或恶性肿瘤等其他疾病的进一步测试。

最近，许多药物被批准用于治疗急性非组胺能血管性水肿和 HAE 人群的长期治疗。鉴于美国最新的高血压治疗指南推荐使用 ACE 抑制剂，医师更可能遇到 ACE 抑制剂血管性水肿。已有较多成功使用这些药物治疗 ACE 抑制剂血管性水肿的报道。

血浆来源的 C1-INH（plasma-derived C1-INH，pdC1-INH，Berinert）于 2009 年被批准用于急性 HAE 发作。急性发作的治疗剂量为 20 IU/kg，静脉注射，HAE 患者在接受该药物使用培训后可自行使用。尽管缺乏大规模研究，与接受抗组胺药和类固醇标准治疗的历史对照相比，ACE 抑制剂诱导的血管性水肿患者应用血浆来源的 C1-INH 后，症状消退的时间缩短，插管或气管切开较少。

50 IU/kg 静脉用重组人 C1-INH（recombinant human C1-INH，rhC1-INH，Rhuconest）于 2014 年被批准用于 HAE。rhC1-INH 抑制 C1、血浆激肽释放酶、FX Ⅰ a 和 FX Ⅱ a 可被 C1-INH 抑制。与 pdC1-INH 一样，rhC1-INH 预计可用于治疗 ACE 抑制剂诱导的血管性水肿。rhC1-INH 的半衰期短于 pdC1-INH，但对其传播感染的关注较少。

艾替班特（Icatibant，Firazyr）是一种选择性缓激肽 B2 受体阻滞剂，于 2011 年批准用于成人急性 HAE 发作。最近一项涉及 ACE 抑制剂诱导的血管性水肿的随机试验报道，与抗组胺药和糖皮质激素的对症治疗相比，艾替班特更优，表现为起效更快，症状完全消退的时间更短。皮下注射 30 mg 后，起效时间为 2 h，完全代谢的时间为 8 h。

2009 年，美国批准激肽释放酶抑制剂艾卡拉肽（ecallantide，Kalbitor）用于急性 HAE 发作，皮下注射剂量为 30 mg。症状缓解时间为 2 h。与艾替班特不同的是，其过敏反应风险为 3%，未被批准用于自我给药。

上述特异性药物的缺点是成本高（每次治疗需要 5000 ～ 10 000 美元）和缺乏普遍可用性。

在新药批准前，新鲜冰冻血浆（fresh frozen plasma，FFP）（通常为 2 个单位）因含有激肽酶，可以分解过多的缓激肽，已被用于治疗 ACE 抑制剂诱导的血管性水肿。理论上，FFP 含有补体成分，用于补体介导的血管性水肿有加重症状的风险。这尽管比之前讨论的昂贵药物更具成本效益，但也存在感染传播、容量超负荷和其他输血相关并发症的潜在风险。

预防

在 ACE 抑制剂诱导的血管性水肿中，停药是唯一的预防方法。一些患者在服用血管紧张素受体阻滞剂时会出现血管性水肿，但发生率低于 ACE 抑制剂。

预防性治疗通常用于 HAE 人群，并分为术前预防和长期预防。牙科手术所致血管性水肿的风险特别高，需要进行术前预防。减毒雄激素对急性和长期预防有效，但有许多不良影响（特别是男性化），使其可能不适用于女性患者和儿童。血浆来源的 C1-INH 已被证明对急性预防有效，并可长期预防特定患者的发作。使用抗纤维蛋白溶解的氨甲环酸也有效，但前述其他药物效果更佳。

（罗金华　译　陈　玲　校）

延伸阅读

Baş M, Greve J, Stelter K, et al.: A randomized trial of icatibant in ACE-inhibitor–induced angioedema, *N Engl J Med* 372:418–425, 2015.

Bhardwaj N, Craig TJ: Treatment of hereditary angioedema: a review, *Transfusion* 54:2989–2996, 2014.

Blanca-López N, Barrionuevo E, Andreu I, et al.: Hypersensitivity reactions to nonsteroidal anti-inflammatory drugs: from phenotyping to genotyping, *Curr Opin Allergy Clin Immunol* 14:271–277, 2014.

Bork K: Angioedema, *Immunol Allergy Clin North Am* 34(1):23–31, 2014.

Busse PJ, Buckland MS: Non-histaminergic angioedema: focus on bradykinin-mediated angioedema, *Clin Exp Allergy* 43:385–394, 2012.

Caballero T, Farkas H, Bouillet L, et al.: International consensus and practical guidelines on the gynecologic and obstetric management of female patients with hereditary angioedema caused by C1 inhibitor deficiency, *J Allergy Clin Immunol* 129:308–320, 2012.

Cornejo-García JA, Flores C, Plaza-Serón MC, et al.: Variants of CEP68 gene are associated with acute urticaria/angioedema induced by multiple non-steroidal anti-inflammatory drugs, *PLoS One* 9(3):e90966, 2014.

Darlenski R, Kazandjieva J, Zuberbier T, et al.: Chronic urticaria as a systemic disease, *Clin Dermatol* 32(3):420–423, 2014.

Eli M, Joseph M, Kuznik B, Menachem S: Chronic idiopathic angioedema: a single center experience, *Int J Dermatol* 53:e421–e427, 2014.

Greve J, Bas M, Hoffmann TK, et al.: Effect of C1-esterase-inhibitor in angiotensin-converting enzyme inhibitor–induced angioedema, *Laryngoscope* 125:e198–e202, 2015.

Hsieh FH: Year in review: urticarial and angioedema, *Ann Allergy Asthma Immunol* 114:166–167, 2014.

Jensen NF, Weiler JM: C1 esterase inhibitor deficiency, airway compromise, and anesthesia, *Anesth Analg* 87:480–488, 1998.

Pedrosa M, Prieto-García A, Sala-Cunill A: Spanish Group for the Study of Bradykinin-Mediated Angioedema (SGBA) and the Spanish Committee of Cutaneous Allergy (CCA): management of angioedema without urticaria in the emergency department, *Ann Med* 46:607–618, 2014.

Riedl MA: Critical appraisal of androgen use in hereditary angioedema: a systematic review, *Ann Allergy Asthma Immunol* 114:281–288, 2015.

Sabroe R: Acute urticaria, *Immunol Allergy Clin North Am* 34(1):11–21, 2014.

Spyridonidou A, Iatrou C, Alexoudis A, et al.: Peri-operative management of a patient with hereditary angioedema undergoing laparoscopic cholecystectomy, *Anaesthesia* 65:74–77, 2010.

Stijiljkovic L: Renin-angiotensin system inhibitors and angioedema: anesthetic implications, *Anesthesiology* 25:356–362, 2012.

Vasekar M, Craig TJ: ACE inhibitor–induced angioedema, *Curr Allergy Asthma Rep* 12:72–78, 2012.

Zuberbier T: Methods report on the development of the 2013 revision and update of the EAACI/GA^{2}LEN/EDF/WAO guideline for the definition, classification, diagnosis and management of urticaria, *Allergy* 69:e1–e29, 2014.

自主神经反射障碍 第 131 章

David L.McDonagh，*Catherine B.Barden*

病例概要

患者，男性，35 岁，3 年前因车祸导致 T1 脊髓横断，拟行择期膀胱镜检查和膀胱取石术。患者在术前等候区感觉焦虑，有重击样头痛，颜面潮红，血压高（168/100 mmHg），而入院时血压 92/58 mmHg。

问题分析

定义

自主神经反射障碍（autonomic dysreflexia，AD）或反射亢进是脊髓损伤导致一系列自主神经活动过度的一种综合征，多见于完全性脊髓损伤，即损伤水平以下无感觉或运动功能。T6 或以上损伤（内脏交感传出神经以上）使患者有自主神经反射障碍的危险；T6 以下损伤很少引起该综合征。脊髓损伤水平以下的伤害性刺激可引起脊髓强烈的神经传入冲动和不受抑制的交感传出冲动。交感传出通常会被脊髓上（下行）抑制所抑制，但与大脑的联系已不存在。动物研究表明，长期失神经支配后，血管系统肾上腺素受体表达增加也可能参与自主神经反射障碍的病理生理过程。所导致的不受抑制的血管升压反应可引起高血压，甚至可导致终末器官损害。

识别

1860 年，Hilton 首次报道 1 例四肢瘫痪的自主神经反射障碍患者。症状包括焦虑、跳动性头痛、面部潮红、视力模糊、恶心和鼻塞，也可发生肌肉痉挛。体格检查的体征包括高血压和经常反射性心动过缓（框 131.1）。在脊髓损伤水平以下，交感传出占主导地位，皮肤表现为典型的冰凉感，并有毛发竖立。在副交感神经占优势的损伤水平以上，皮肤温暖、发红，大汗。患者一定会出现高血压，但不一定极高危。患者静息时血压可正常稍偏低（120/80 mmHg）。在受到伤害性刺激时，血压可升高至正常范围（>120/80 mmHg）或 1 期高血压（>140/90 mmHg，但 <160/110 mmHg），尽管可发生严重 2 期高血压（160/110 mmHg）（详见推荐阅读中 Chobanian 等的文献）。

框 131.1 自主神经反射障碍的体征和症状

- 高血压
- 心动过缓
- 心律失常
- 内脏和肌肉痉挛
- 毛发竖立
- 苍白或面色潮红
- 重度头痛
- 焦虑
- 抽搐
- 意识丧失
- 大汗
- 视力模糊
- 呼吸急促
- 恶心呕吐

风险评估

所有 T6 或以上的脊髓损伤患者，均应考虑有自主神经反射障碍的风险。其发病率大于 50%，男性较女性更常见，完全性脊髓损伤的风险最高。该综合征见于亚急性至慢性期脊髓损伤，即初始损伤致脊髓休克恢复后。对既往有自主神经反射障碍病史或有相应症状病史的患者，应高度警惕。近期出现相应症状时，应积极寻找诱发原因（框 131.2）。最常见原因是膀胱充盈、尿潴留和粪便阻塞。低于脊髓损伤水平（即感觉丧失区域）的各种有害刺激也可引起自主神经反射障碍，如分娩。值得谨记的

框 131.2 自主神经反射障碍的潜在诱发因素

膀胱充盈或尿潴留
粪便阻塞或直肠检查
脊髓损伤以下水平手术
子宫收缩、分娩
泌尿外科操作
肌内注射
褥疮溃疡
痔疮
急腹症
皮肤刺激或衣物束缚

是，任何外科手术或脊髓损伤以下的其他刺激都可能引发自主神经反射障碍，即使患者身体部位没有知觉。

启示

严重高血压是自主神经反射障碍的主要损害。如果不加控制，持续性高血压可导致终末器官损害，出现高血压急症。（注：高血压危象包括急症和亚急症，但都包括血压急性升高≥160/110 mmHg。高血压**亚急症**时，没有终末器官损害的证据，而高血压**急症**时有终末器官损害）。主要关注点包括癫痫发作、出血性卒中、隐匿性动脉瘤破裂引起的蛛网膜下腔出血、眼内出血、心律失常和导致心肌缺血的心肌劳损。在极少数情况下，自主神经反射障碍综合征可能是致命的（详见推荐阅读 Wan 和 Krassioukov 的文章）。

管理

麻醉管理包括以下内容：

- 寻找和治疗诱发原因（如留置尿管）；
- 直立或反向 Trendelenburg 体位；
- 麻醉选择（全身、椎管内、区域麻醉）；
- 合理的术中和术后监测；
- 血管扩张药（如硝酸甘油、尼卡地平、肼屈嗪）；
- 升压药和静脉内输液（治疗极度低血压）；
- 加深全身麻醉（如用丙泊酚、瑞芬太尼）；
- 如果血流动力学不能平稳控制，可以推迟择期手术。

尿潴留或粪便阻塞常诱发自主神经反射障碍。术中，低于脊髓损伤水平的手术刺激也可能是诱因。一定要考虑并排除类似的综合征，如产妇先兆子痫或子痫。让患者处于直立位引起的体位性低血压，是纠正高血压的最基本方法。潜在原因的初步治疗包括暂停外科手术、膀胱导尿（或冲洗留置导尿管），必要时清除粪便后行直肠检查。

麻醉方法的选择（区域麻醉或全身麻醉）应根据手术操作和患者需求决定。脊椎麻醉、硬膜外麻醉或区域麻醉对抑制导致自主神经反射障碍的传入神经活性非常有效，可适当使用（如分娩时硬膜外麻醉和脊椎麻醉）。值得注意的是，外周神经阻滞或皮肤浸润局麻药也存在诱发自主神经反射障碍的可能性。由于存在高血钾风险，脊髓损伤患者应避免使用琥珀胆碱。

对术中及术后监测，除标准监测外，可考虑动脉置管行有创血压监测或连续无创动脉压监测。应备好随时可用的血管扩张药。有多种药物可用于快速降压。静脉注射拉贝洛尔、尼卡地平、硝酸甘油和硝普钠均可使用，可通过推注给药或持续输注给药。此外，还应备好静脉输液和升压药，以治疗医源性低血压。如果使用全身麻醉药，应备好能够随时迅速加深麻醉。在一项针对经尿道碎石患者的研究中，除吸入麻醉药外，靶控输注瑞芬太尼是减少自主神经反射障碍的有效方法。在此情况下，静脉推注瑞芬太尼的应用尚未见报道，但在其他情况下已被证实可有效阻断自主神经对有害刺激的反应。最后，如患者术前自主神经反射障碍不能及时评估和治疗，应推迟择期手术。

预防

预防措施仅针对具体患者的诱发因素。对住院患者或门诊患者，常规导尿和使用泻药确保正常肠道活动较为重要。应教会患者认识其症状，尽可能纠正问题，必要时要求紧急医疗护理。应确定围术期高危患者，制订合适的麻醉方案（全身麻醉、椎管内麻醉和区域麻醉），考虑提前行膀胱导尿，并立即用药物（血管扩张药、推注麻醉药）控制急性高血压。

（成天华 译 周 懿 校）

延伸阅读

Chobanian AV, Bakris GL, Black HR, et al.: National Heart, Lung, and Blood Institute Joint National Committee on Prevention, Detection, Evaluation, and Treatment of High Blood Pressure. National High Blood Pressure Education Program Coordinating Committee. The Seventh Report of the Joint National Committee on Prevention, Detection, Evaluation, and Treatment of High Blood Pressure: the JNC 7 report, *JAMA* 289:2560–2572, 2003.

Krassioukov A, Warburton DE, Teasell R, et al.: Spinal Cord Injury Rehabilitation Evidence Research Team: a systematic review of the management of autonomic dysreflexia after spinal cord injury, *Arch Phys Med Rehabil* 90(4):682–695, 2009.

Kuczkowski KM: Peripartum anaesthetic management of a parturient with spinal cord injury and autonomic hyperreflexia, *Anaesthesia* 58:823–824, 2003.

Lee JS, Fang SY, Roan JN, et al.: Spinal cord injury enhances arterial expression and reactivity of α_1-adrenergic receptors—mechanistic investigation into autonomic dysreflexia, *Spine J* 16(1):65–71, 2016.

Stephenson RO: Autonomic dysreflexia in spinal cord injury, *eMedicine J*, 2015. Available at www.emedicine.medscape.com.

Wan D, Krassioukov AV: life-threatening outcomes associated with autonomic dysreflexia: a clinical review, *J Spinal Cord Med* 37(1):2–10, 2014.

Yoo KY, Jeong CW, Kim SJ, et al.: Remifentanil decreases sevoflurane requirements to block autonomic hyperreflexia during transurethral litholapaxy in patients with high complete spinal cord injury, *Anesth Analg* 112:191–197, 2011.

第 132 章 麻醉知晓

Jaideep J. Pandit

病例概要

“我以为我快要死了。（1 min 前）我被推到手术室进行一个相当常规的正畸手术。……突然，我意识到出了很大的问题。我能听到周围发生的事情，我惊恐地意识到我在手术中醒了过来，但我一动也不能动。……我躺在那里，疯狂地想我是不是要死了……就好像麻醉科医师把我的灵魂以外的一切都从我身上拿走了。”

—来自 NAP5 报告的一例患者经历

问题分析

定义

当患者在麻醉和手术中，本应处于无意识状态，但却在某个时刻出现知晓，称为全身麻醉期间的意外知晓（accidental awareness during general anesthesia，AAGA），可由患者自发报告。该定义取自英国第五国家审计项目（*5th National Audit Project*，NAP5），比一些较早的定义更能反映患者的经历。比方说，先前的定义仅关注手术期间 AAGA 的报告，但较新的定义包括了诱导期间（例如快速序贯诱导的诱导剂量可能不足但患者已经肌肉松弛）和苏醒期间（如麻醉药物已逐渐清除而神经肌肉阻滞尚未完全逆转，患者描述这种的随后意外发生的无力 / 瘫痪感为“意外知晓”）的患者体验。基于患者自发报告的 AAGA 总发病率约为 1∶19 000，但使用肌松药（约 1∶8000）与不使用肌松药（约 1∶136 000）之间存在显著差异。剖宫产的发病率极高（约 1∶670）。

除自发报告外，许多研究调查采用 Brice interview 问卷调查。该问卷针对患者设计了一些比较直接的问题，关键的一些问题是患者在“入睡”之前记得的最后一件事是什么以及患者醒来时记得的第一件事是什么。根据回答，询问者推测患者是否发生 AAGA（即使患者本人没有主动提及）。采用 Brice interview 得到的“阳性率”出乎意料地高达约 1∶600，但关于这是否是明确的 AAGA，或者仅仅是触发或提示诱导的内隐记忆，尚且存在争论。“知晓”的第三个方面是保留内隐记忆的可能性。外显记忆是对事物或事件的记忆；内隐记忆是指存在将无意识时可能遇到的事物或词语相关联的现象。著名的案例是“鲁滨逊·克鲁索”实验。很少有人会自发地把“星期五”和“鲁滨逊·克鲁索”联系在一起。除非他们在麻醉期间播放了一盘故事的磁带，那么大约 63% 的患者会将它们联系在一起。麻醉后此类内隐记忆的临床意义仍然不清楚。

识别、管理和预防

AAGA 的识别、处理和预防互有交叉重叠。NAP5 的结论极大地改变了我们对 AAGA 的实践方式。到目前为止，AAGA 最大规模的研究（其病例数超过了文献报道的总数），提供了 64 项临床实践推荐（以及 100 多项研究建议）。现在可以确定的是，未被发现的 AAGA 不会发生在没有肌松的患者身上——仅仅因为麻醉浅的患者可能会体动或者坐起来，但这肯定不会不被发现。NAP5 关键信息是指出神经肌肉阻滞是所有 AAGA 病例的主要危险因素。NAP5 还发现神经肌肉阻滞的监测率非常低，拮抗的使用率也很低。多数出现 AAGA 主要原因是神经肌肉阻滞剂使用不当、剂量过大和未监测剂量，而且在手术结束时没有拮抗。因此，主要推荐包括：①神经肌肉阻滞剂只在十分必要时使用并严格按照合适剂量给药；②使用时，应使用神经刺激仪监测；③应在手术结束时给予拮抗，然后再减浅麻醉，使患者苏醒。通过这种方式，肌肉松弛的程度被保持在一个足以手术的水平，如果患者偶然出现意外知晓的情况，也足以让患者移动。该指南现在是英国最低强制性要求。

令人惊讶的是，NAP5 并不建议大规模使用经过处理的脑电图（processed electroencephalogram，pEEG）监测，如脑电双频指数（Bispectral Index，BIS）或熵指数。这些监测的实用性仍存争议，一些临床试验（基于 Brice interview）表明它们可以降低 AAGA 的发生率，但其他试验未能重现这些结果。在更基本原则的层面上，pEEG 监测作为诊断工具的效用备受质疑，因其在相同的麻醉深度下它所显示的数值并不一致。已经确定的是，pEEG 读数与金标准“孤立前臂试验”无关，即使在完全清醒但肌松的志愿者中，pEEG 读数也非常低。虽然一些权威指南建议 pEEG 读数应小于 60 以避免 AAGA，但 NAP5 发现了一些病例报导，尽管数值低于 60，仍发生了创伤性 AAGA。更令人担忧的是，NAP5 发现了几例麻醉药浓度降至最低肺泡有效浓度（minimum alveolar concentration，MAC）只有 0.2 ～ 0.3 的情况，结果发生了 AAGA，原因是 pEEG 数值非常低（大约 40），错误地提示了麻醉过深。一些权威机构认为 MAC 应该保持在 0.7 以上并且设有合适的警报限值是合理的建议。

然而，当全凭静脉麻醉（total intravenous anesthesia，TIVA）与神经肌肉阻滞药一起使用时，NAP5 确实推荐使用 pEEG（或孤立前臂试验）监测。由于尚无其他办法来监测静脉注射剂是否真的输入体内，因此这是合乎逻辑的实用做法。有案例报道曾发生过几例由于没注意到静脉药管路断开而导致 AAGA 发生的事件。目前这一建议是英国所要求的最低限度的监测。

心理学意义

众所周知，AAGA 可导致创伤后应激障碍（posttraumatic stress disorder，PTSD）或无 PTSD 的严重症状。不良心理后遗症可能包括焦虑、抑郁、睡眠障碍伴梦魇、惊恐发作以及其他一些长期精神疾病。心理创伤因患者的怀疑而加剧，从而会延误治疗。NAP5 发现，比起疼痛而言，“瘫痪”的感觉更能导致心理创伤。NAP5 中阐述的 AAGA 心理支持方式为：首先向患者承认其经历可能是真实的并且在被认真对待。诚实的讨论（英国称之为医师的坦诚义务）应包括所有可能的原因，并将其作为调查的重点。应通过随访与患者保持接触，如果患者有任何心理障碍的迹象，请及早转诊寻求心理支持。

因果关系和法医学层面

AAGA 的发生并不总是表明麻醉科医师有过错。当然，某些情况可能非常难以解释：药物错误（例如，神经肌肉阻滞先于任何催眠药物使用，TIVA 管路断开，无法打开挥发性药物罐，未遵守现已公布的监测要求或神经肌肉阻滞药拮抗）。即使机器故障导致麻醉药物输送中断，也有人认为，根本原因是未能监测或未对呼气末挥发浓度下降做出反应（或 TIVA 中 pEEG 读数上升）。NAP5 的结果显示 AAGA 主要发生在诱导期和苏醒期而非麻醉维持期间，该结果有助于指导知情同意内容的调整，从而有助于管理患者的预期。在手术前提供详细的书面信息可以帮助解释关于 AAGA 的一些复杂的统计数据。在术前访视时，麻醉科医师应该解释，在诱导或苏醒期，对口腔中器械或导管的非常简短和模糊的感觉并不罕见，或者可能存在短暂的迅速消退的肌肉无力期。当遇到由于麻醉或神经肌肉阻滞药给药不平衡出现的罕见情况时，这可以帮助患者做好准备和消除顾虑。换句话说，由于 AAGA 可能会实际存在，我们并不能完全承诺会保证患者完全丧失意识（除非不使用神经肌肉阻滞药）。

然而，少数患者可能天生对麻醉药物产生抗药性。NAP5 发现，在大约 5% 的病例中，有家族麻醉史或重复的 AAGA 经历，提示患者有高于预期的麻醉药物需求。在大约 20% 的病例中，NAP5 审查小组可以发现麻醉剂的输送或所采用的剂量或监测策略没有缺陷。像所有其他药物一样，麻醉剂直接作用于特定的蛋白质受体和通道（而不是非特异性脂质膜），可能表现出自然变异（多态性）。因此，医务人员应当良好地遵守已发表的指南，特别是在管理神经肌肉阻滞药方面，但要意识到可能会存在耐药性。这些方面是驱动未来进一步研究的动力。

（杨心月　译　卞金俊　校）

延伸阅读

Andrade J, Deeprose C: Unconscious memory formation during anaesthesia, *Best Pract Res Clin Anaesthesiol* 21:385–401, 2007.

Avidan MS, Zhang L, Burnside BA, et al.: Anesthesia awareness and the bispectral index, *N Engl J Med* 358:1097–1108, 2008.

Avidan MS, Jacobsohn E, Glick D, et al.: Prevention of intraoperative awareness in a high-risk surgical population, *N Engl J Med* 365:591–600, 2011.

Checketts MR, Alladi R, Ferguson K, et al.: Recommendations for standards of monitoring during anaesthesia and recovery 2015, *Anaesthesia* 71:85–93, 2016.

Myles PS, Leslie K, McNeil J, et al.: Bispectral index monitoring to prevent awareness during anaesthesia: the B-Aware randomised controlled trial, *Lancet* 363:1757–1763, 2004.

Pandit JJ: Acceptably aware during general anaesthesia: "dysanaesthesia"—the uncoupling of perception from sensory inputs, *Conscious Cogn* 27C:194–212, 2014.

Pandit JJ: Isolated forearm—or isolated brain? Interpeting responses during anaesthesia—or dysanaesthesia, *Anaesthesia* 68:995–1009, 2013.

Pandit JJ: Monitoring (un)consciousness: the implications of a new definition of "anaesthesia," *Anaesthesia* 69:801–805, 2014.

Pandit JJ, Andrade J, Bogod DG, et al.: 5th National Audit Project (NAP5) on accidental awareness during general anaesthesia: summary of main findings and risk factors, *Anaesthesia* 69:1089–1101, 2014.

Pandit JJ, Cook TM: *NAP5: accidental awareness during general anaesthesia*, London, 2014, The Royal College of Anaesthetists and Association of Anaesthetists of Great Britain and Ireland.

Pandit JJ, Cook TM: National Institute for Clinical Excellence guidance on measuring depth of anaesthesia: limitations of EEG-based technology, *Br J Anaesth* 110:325–328, 2013.

Pandit JJ, Russell IF, Wang M: Interpretations of responses using the isolated forearm technique in general anaesthesia: a debate, *Br J Anaesth* 115(Suppl):i32–i45, 2015.

Schuller PJ, Newell S, Strickland PA, et al.: Response of bispectral index to neuromuscular block in awake volunteers, *Br J Anaesth* 115(Suppl 1):i95–i103, 2015.

缓慢性心律失常

第 133 章

Clare H. Ridley，Paul B. Zanaboni，Charles B. Hantler

病例概要

患者，男性，71 岁，在行开放性腹主动脉瘤修复术时，因急性失血导致严重低血压。平均动脉压为 40 mmHg，心电图（electrocardiogram，ECG）显示心率 35 次 / 分的宽 QRS 波形。患者术前 ECG 显示一度房室传导阻滞合并双束支传导阻滞。

问题分析

定义

缓慢性心律失常是指与缓慢的心室去极化率（<60 次 / 分）有关的心脏节律异常。当合并重要器官功能异常时，例如中枢神经系统损伤（晕厥、精神状态改变）、体位性低血压、心力衰竭或其他主要器官系统功能障碍（尤其是肾、肝或胃肠），这种节律紊乱具有临床意义。

缓慢性心律失常的病因包括冲动形成异常、冲动传导异常，或两者兼而有之（框 133.1）。图 133.1 描绘了参与心脏内冲动的产生和传导的解剖结构（即特殊传导系统）。

窦房结细胞的最大舒张电位在 −50 ～ −60 mV 之间。一旦达到最大舒张电位，窦房结细胞立即去极化。4 期自动去极化是由缓慢衰减的外向钾电流与缓慢恢复的内向钙电流不平衡所致。后者导致细胞内电位比细胞外的负值逐渐变小。只有当细胞内电位负值小于 −50 mV 时才会产生起搏电流。在窦房结细胞中，这种电流很可能通过 L 型钙通道形成。但在 4 期自动去极化（即正常自律性）的后半段，也可激活 T 型钙通道。窦房结细胞去极化至 +10 mV（最大动作电位超射值），最大幅度为 60 ～ 70 mV。一旦达到最大动作电位，窦房结细胞开始复极化。在早期复极化期间，特别是在心房肌、心室肌或浦肯野纤维（即“快反应”纤维）中，钠离子和钙离子内流，以及几种不同的钾离子复极化外流共同发挥了作用。[**注**：与窦房结或房室结细胞相比，“快反应”纤维的动作电位最大幅度更大，超射值更高，传导速度更快，早期快速（1 期）复极化也更明

框 133.1　缓慢性心律失常的病因

心肌内在原因
- 冲动形成异常
- 窦性心动过缓
  - 窦房结自律性降低
  - 窦房传导阻滞
- 颈动脉窦超敏
  - 神经心源性晕厥（交感神经传出减少）
- 冲动传导异常
- 房室结传导阻滞
  - 一度阻滞
  - 二度阻滞
    - Ⅰ型
    - Ⅱ型
  - 三度阻滞

外部因素
- 麻醉药
  - 高浓度吸入麻醉药（七氟烷，氟烷）
  - 镇静剂（阿片类，右美托咪定）
- 心脏加速纤维的局部阻滞（T1 ～ T4）
- 手术
  - 眼心反射
  - 腹膜刺激
  - 颈动脉体刺激
- 药物
  - β-受体阻滞剂，非二氢吡啶类钙通道阻滞剂，胺碘酮，地高辛
  - α-受体阻滞导致反射性心动过缓（去氧肾上腺素）

代谢性原因
- 低温
- 内分泌（甲状腺功能减退，艾迪生病）
- 电解质（高钾血症，高镁血症）

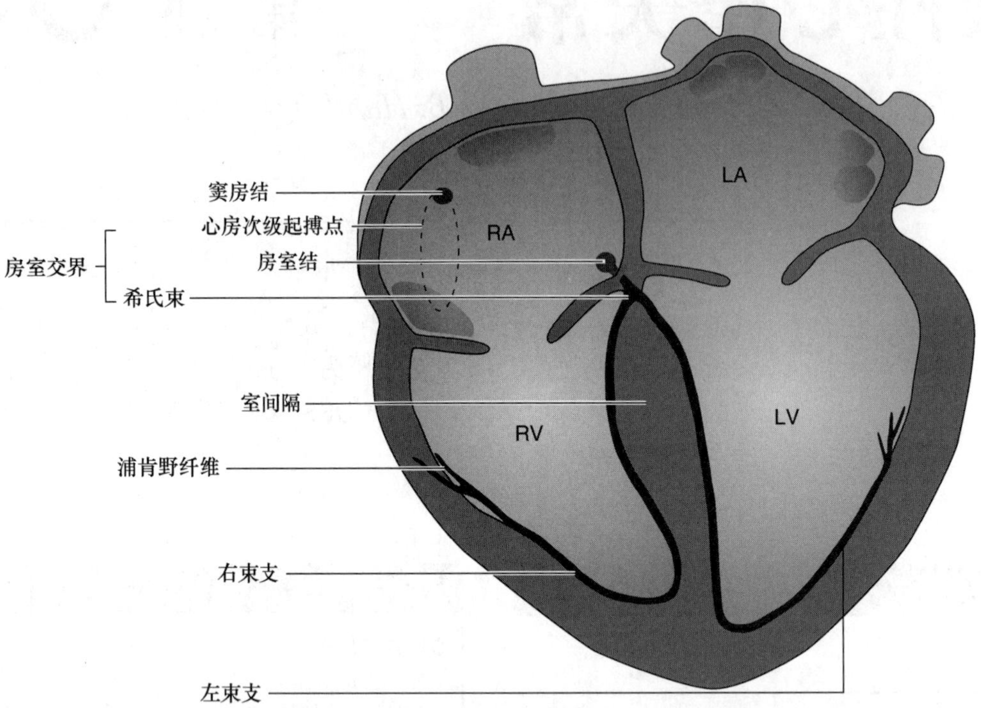

图 133.1　参与心脏内冲动的产生和传导的解剖结构（即特殊传导系统）。LA，左心房；LV，左心室；RA，右心房；RV，右心室

显]。总之，在所有类型的纤维中，复极化期间静电荷主要是以正电荷（主要是钾离子）外流为主，此外还有不同程度的钙离子和钠离子内流。去极化期间净电荷主要是以正电荷内流为主，也伴有减少的钾离子外流。

窦房结的正常起搏速率为 60 ～ 100 次 / 分。药物、神经冲动传入（交感神经和副交感神经）、体温和激素均可影响 4 期自动去极化的速率及产生可再生性（自给性）动作电位的阈值，进而改变窦房结去极化的速率。

除了窦性心动过缓（窦性心律，心率小于 60 次 / 分；图 133.2），当起源于低位起搏点时，还会出现缓慢的逸搏心律。这种逸搏心律（起源于房室结下方）通常与高度房室传导阻滞（二度）和三度房室传导阻滞有关。（高度房室传导阻滞定义为两个或多个连续 P 波阻滞，但有些 P 波可传导至心室。而三度房室传导阻滞时，无 P 波传导至心室。）

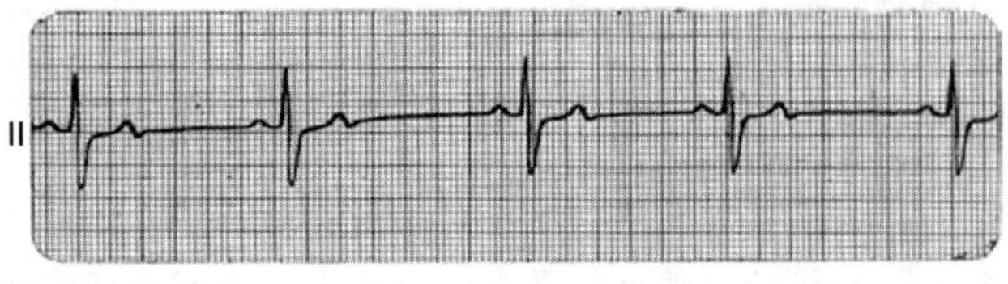

图 133.2　窦性心动过缓，P 波与 QRS 波关系正常，心率小于 60 次 / 分

心房次级起搏点

这些起搏点沿着界沟（界嵴）和冠状窦口分布。心房次级起搏点的特征是在正常直立的 P 波中（Ⅱ、Ⅲ和 aVF 导联）出现扁平，双向或负向（如游走性心房起搏点）的 P 波。心房次级起搏点的频率上下限与窦房结相似，P-R 间期与窦房结相同或略小（<0.1 s）。

房室交界起搏点

房室交界性心动过缓可能没有明显的 P 波，也可能与窦性心律中的正常直立 P 波相反。倒置（逆行）P 波多出现在 QRS 波群之前（P-R 间期小于 0.1 s），或者较少见地出现于 QRS 波群之后。

浦肯野纤维

典型的逸搏（如与高度或三度房室传导阻滞有关的逸搏心律），心率小于 50 次 / 分（成人可能更低），一般无相应的 P 波，可有孤立的直立 P 波。这些 P 波起源于窦房结或心房次级起搏点，因阻滞而无法下传，与 QRS 波群无关。然而，即使是高度或三度房室传导阻滞，逆行（心室–心房）传导也可能是完整的，因此可能产生相应的 P 波。这种 P 波的波形与正常 P 波相反。（**注：**在高度或三度房室传导阻滞期间，窦房结独立于心室搏动，速度比心室起搏点快。这是因为窦房结受自主控制，心室逸搏心律时血压偏低，并有压力反射介导的交感神经传出增加。）

心室肌纤维

心室肌纤维很少有自律性。只有静息膜电位缺失时才会出现。这种肌纤维部分去极化可能是疾病所致，通常与心肌缺血或梗死有关。心室率通常低于 40 次 / 分，罕有逆行 P 波。心房和心室各自搏动（房室分离）并不少见。

窦房结去极化后，冲动由心房特殊传导组织来传导。窦房传导阻滞是指冲动在心房内传导失败，其特征是 ECG 中无 P 波出现。当出现这种情况（或窦房结不能去极化）时，次级的起搏点必须承担起对心室的控制。最后，如前所述，窦房结最易受副交感或交感（自主神经）控制，这通常由压力感受器和心脏机械感受器来介导。

识别

本文已经讨论了窦性心动过缓和低位起搏的逸搏心律的 ECG 特征。此外，心动过缓也可能源于房室传导延迟或阻滞。一度房室传导阻滞仅表现为房室冲动传导延迟（P-R 间期 >0.12 s），心室搏动（QRS 波群）并未脱落。二度房室传导阻滞是指一些冲动在房室间传导受阻，进一步细分为莫氏Ⅰ型，莫氏Ⅱ型和高度（二度）房室传导阻滞。对于莫氏Ⅰ型（文氏）（图 133.3），一些但不是所有心房搏动被阻断，表现为 P-R 间期逐渐延长直至 QRS 波脱落。冲动传导和脱落的比率可以是固定的（如 3∶2，4∶3），也可以是变化的（如 4∶3 和 3∶2）。对于莫氏Ⅱ型，QRS 波群脱落之前无 P-R 间期逐渐延长，下传比例也是可变的（图 133.4）。高度（二度）房室传导阻滞会在两个传导的心跳之间有两个或两个以上的 QRS 波群脱落，同样，比例也是可变的。三度房室传导阻滞无心房搏动传导至心室（图 133.5）。心房和心室受不同的起搏点控制，QRS 波群可窄小（控制心室的起搏点位于希氏束分叉之上），也可宽大（位于分叉之下）。因此，在三度房室传导阻滞中，房室完全分离（心房和心室分别搏动）。

风险评估

缓慢性心律失常可由心肌内在原因或外部因素

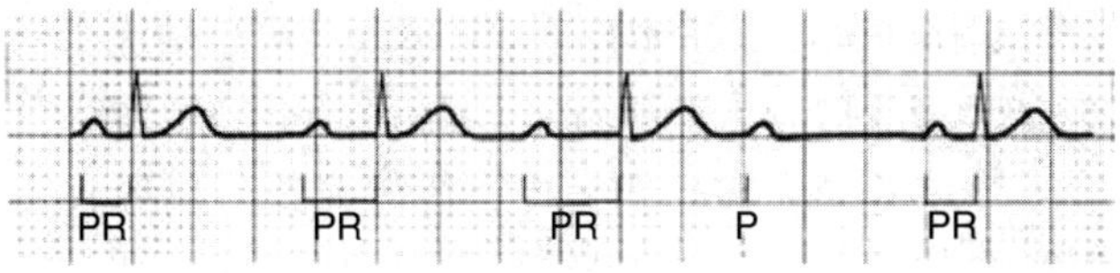

图 133.3 莫氏Ⅰ型（文氏）二度房室传导阻滞，P 波被阻断前（即第 4 个 P 波）P-R 间期逐渐延长。与一度房室传导阻滞相同，P-R 间期大于 0.12 s，但没有脱落的心室搏动。在本例中，如果下传的与未下传的心房搏动的比例发生变化（如 3∶2，4∶3），阻滞将是可变的（未显示），就像莫氏Ⅰ型二度房室传导阻滞通常发生的那样。阻滞通常发生在房室结点内或其边缘

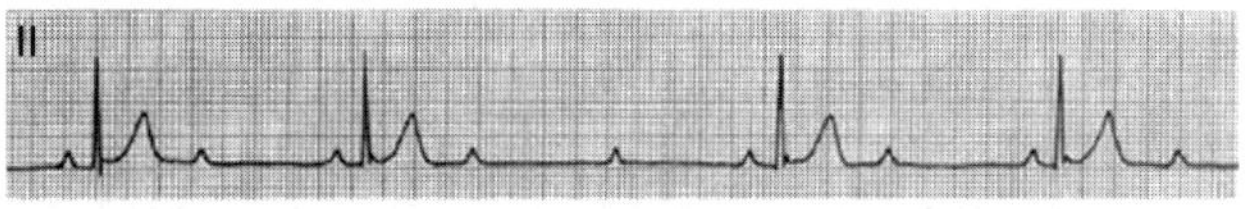

图 133.4 莫氏Ⅱ型二度房室传导阻滞，P-R 间期可能不发生改变（固定阻滞），阻滞也可能是可变的（如图所示）或间歇性的。如果是固定的，心房以某个固定的比例恒定下传搏动（如 2∶1，3∶1，4∶1）。如果是可变的，阻滞会重复变化（如 2∶1 和 3∶1）。如果阻滞是间歇性的，正常房室传导的周期会被偶尔下传的搏动打断，但不会重复发生。Ⅱ型二度房室传导阻滞最常发生在希氏束或其下方

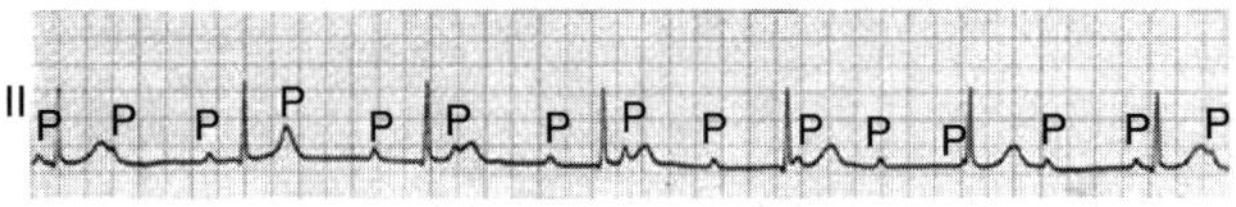

图 133.5 三度房室传导阻滞（几乎总是在希氏束或其下方），P 波独立于 QRS 波群（即完全房室分离，如同心室起源的缓慢性心律失常或快速性心律失常）。如果控制心室的起搏点位于希氏束分叉点内或其上方，QRS 波群窄小（如图所示），如果位于更远端，QRS 波群则宽大

引起，例如迷走张力增加或电解质紊乱。植入式人工心脏起搏器（见第 16 章）适用于有症状（如易疲劳、先兆晕厥或晕厥）且无法逆转的缓慢性心律失常患者。

全身麻醉和手术

全麻期间发生的缓慢性心律失常有多种原因。高浓度吸入麻醉药（尤其是早期挥发性麻醉药）和阿片类药物是麻醉期间发生严重心动过缓最为大家熟悉的原因。手术刺激可导致迷走张力相对增加，从而引起窦房结自律性、房室结传导或两者均变慢。最常见的例子是眼心反射、腹膜刺激和颈动脉体刺激。停止刺激后这些反应就会消失。尽管药物和手术引起的缓慢性心律失常通常对抗胆碱能药（阿托品、格隆溴铵）或拟交感药物（肾上腺素、异丙肾上腺素）有反应，但如果可以用起搏导线或经静脉

临时起搏（如心脏手术期间），那么起搏总是优于药物治疗。药物有可能引起心动过速，不易逆转，并可能导致心律失常。如果房室传导完整且可经食管或经静脉起搏，则优先采用起搏治疗窦性心动过缓和房室交界性心律。对有临床症状且药物治疗无效的严重缓慢性心律失常，通常采用外部（经皮）或内部（经静脉或心外膜）起搏来改善血流动力学。

椎管内麻醉

累及上胸段的椎管内麻醉可通过阻断源自上胸段脊髓的心脏加速纤维的交感神经传出而导致迷走神经占支配地位（心动过缓）。这种心动过缓通常对抗胆碱能药有很好的反应。

药物导致的心动过缓

许多接受手术的患者正在服用减慢窦性心率或房室传导的药物（如 β- 受体阻滞剂、非二氢吡啶类钙通道阻滞剂）。这些药物可与麻醉和手术共同导致严重的缓慢性心律失常。同样，抗胆碱能药或拟交感药物可逆转心动过缓。但使用时应谨慎，因为极度心动过速会使缺血性心脏病或心律失常患者面临更大的风险。对于择期手术，任何可能会引起意外的心率减慢或房室传导阻滞而导致严重心动过缓的药物均应减量。

代谢性原因

代谢状况可能导致术前或术中出现严重的缓慢性心律失常。包括低体温（普遍使用暖风加温毯后现在很少出现）、内分泌失调和电解质异常。严重低体温可导致窦性心动过缓或逸搏心律，伴或不伴 Osborne 波或 J 波（Osborne 波或 J 波是指 QRS 波群终末的突出切迹和伴 ST 段抬高）。甲状腺功能减退和艾迪生病患者通常会出现术前心动过缓，手术和麻醉期间可能因麻醉药的作用而加重临床症状。高钾血症（可使窦房结和房室结细胞超极化）也可引起严重的窦性心动过缓或房室结传导减慢。心电图显示缓慢、宽大 QRS 波。严重的高钾血症可导致房室传导阻滞或心脏停搏。高镁血症还可通过减少去极化期间钙离子内流引起窦性心动过缓。择期手术前应纠正高钾血症和高镁血症，以预防缓慢性心律失常。

启示

缓慢性心律失常通常导致心排血量降低，尤其当心房传输功能受损或丧失时（如慢心房颤动或逸搏心律），因此麻醉期间不易耐受心动过缓。此外，任何血管舒张、血容量不足或心肌抑制时，心脏更加不能耐受严重心动过缓。例如，如果不能增加心率或心排血量以维持组织灌注，急性低血压时则无法产生正常的生理反应。应牢记心排血量是心率和每搏量的乘积。每搏量除了受到心率增加的影响以外（阶梯效应或鲍迪奇效应除外，因为增加心率可增加心肌收缩力），还受心肌收缩力和前负荷的影响，心动过缓和缓慢性心律失常可减少心排血量，尤其当心房传输功能丧失时。心房适当、及时的收缩对心室舒张功能受损（舒张功能障碍）患者的左心室充盈至关重要，比如老年患者、慢性高血压、主动脉瓣狭窄或肥厚性心肌病患者。心室收缩功能受损的患者也难以耐受缓慢的心率。这种情况下，收缩末期容积增加导致每搏量减少，只能通过增加心率来促进血液向前流动。心率较慢会加重瓣膜反流，如二尖瓣关闭不全，这可能是由于二尖瓣瓣环变大所致。

管理

冲动形成异常

窦性心动过缓

有临床症状的窦性心动过缓应根据生理性损伤的严重程度来治疗。保守治疗包括停止或减少已知抑制窦房结的药物，或停止手术刺激（如眼心反射）等。如果上述治疗无效或不可能实现，则考虑使用抗胆碱能药（如阿托品）或拟交感药物（如麻黄碱、肾上腺素、异丙肾上腺素）。若仍无效果，或窦性心动过缓导致血流动力学严重紊乱，应进行人工起搏（经皮、经静脉或经食管）。

房室交界性逸搏心律

房室交界性心律，无论是心动过缓还是心动过速（>100 次 / 分），都可抑制心房传输，可能与三尖瓣或二尖瓣关闭不全有关。依赖心房传输的患者（严重舒张功能障碍的患者）极度需要恢复窦性心律。抗胆碱能药或拟交感药物通常无效，或仅增加房室交界性心律的速度。全麻期间使用 β- 受体阻滞剂（如艾司洛尔）可恢复窦房结的支配。然而，使用加重心动过缓的药物是有风险的，只有在房室交界性心律大于 60 次 / 分时才可尝试。其他措施还包括改用静脉麻醉药，与吸入麻醉药相比，静脉麻醉药对窦房结的影响较小。经食管心房起搏可恢复心房传输功能，并改善前负荷。

病态窦房结综合征

病态窦房结综合征包括窦性心动过缓，窦性停搏和变时性机能不全，也与室上性快速性心律失常（心动过缓–心动过速或“快慢”综合征）有关，其中最常见的是心房扑动或心房颤动。窦性心动过缓的治疗如前所述。第 161 章讨论了心动过速的治疗方法。始终要牢记的是，对于病窦综合征和有快速性心律失常病史的患者，任何积极的变时性治疗都可能导致极度心动过速或快速性心律失常的发生。有症状的病态窦房结综合征患者通常会植入双腔起搏器以及服用药物治疗，以预防快速性心律失常，减慢房室结传导。

冲动传导异常

一度房室传导阻滞

除非合并有症状或影响血流动力学的心动过缓或逸搏心律，一般不对一度房室传导阻滞进行治疗。但也有极少数例外，比如心脏手术，尤其是肥厚性心肌病修复术后，较短的 P-R 间期可改善舒张期充盈（前负荷）。因此，术中临时用起搏导线进行双腔顺序起搏可缩短 P-R 间期，改善心室充盈。如果是由于 P-R 间期延长导致血流动力学紊乱，则应考虑围术期和长期（如果有症状）双腔起搏。

二度房室传导阻滞

莫氏 Ⅰ 型房室传导阻滞通常源于房室结传导受损，很少进展为完全阻滞。只有影响到血流动力学或症状严重时，才考虑起搏（临时或永久）。莫氏Ⅱ型房室传导阻滞很可能源于希氏束内部或下部的疾病，且通常进展为二度或三度阻滞，如无术前症状，可保守治疗。如有症状或对血流动力学不利的心动过缓，可术中临时起搏。如症状持续，应永久起搏。

三度房室传导阻滞

先天性完全性房室传导阻滞的患儿如无症状，可推迟至青春期后再植入永久性起搏器。然而，对于所有三度房室传导阻滞的成年患者，除非病因可逆（如地高辛中毒、β - 受体阻滞剂过量），均应放置起搏器。

症状性心动过缓的治疗

2015 年高级心脏生命支持（advanced cardiac life support，ACLS）指南概述了有脉搏的症状性心动过缓的紧急处理方案（图 133.6）。值得注意的是，“症状性心动过缓”可直接导致晕厥或先兆晕厥、眩晕或脑灌注不足引起的意识混乱。如果患者的气道通畅且分钟通气量和氧合充足，治疗首选阿托品。如果无效，则启用输注 β - 受体激动剂（如肾上腺素或多巴胺）。若仍无效，则考虑经皮起搏。如果需要，应进行静脉起搏，因经皮起搏会引起患者不适，通常需要镇静。

预防

接受手术的患者放置永久起搏器的适应证与普通人群相似。美国心脏协会、美国心脏病学会以及北美起搏和心脏电生理学会（现在的心律协会）已经发布了有关植入永久起搏器的指南（见延伸阅读）。围术期临时起搏的指征尚不明确。然而，对于未植入心律管理装置的患者、衰弱综合征患者、具有不良心动过缓、逸搏心律或房室传导阻滞的患者，以及行中危或高危手术的患者，应强烈考虑临时起搏。

（孟庆元　译　卞金俊　校）

延伸阅读

Atlee JL: Perioperative cardiac arrhythmias: diagnosis and management, *Anesthesiology* 86:1397–1423, 1997.

Atlee JL, Pattison CZ, Mathews EL, et al.: Transesophageal atrial pacing for intraoperative sinus bradycardia or AV junctional rhythm: feasibility as prophylaxis in 200 anesthetized adults and hemodynamic effects of treatment, *J Cardiothorac Vasc Anesth* 7:436–441, 1993.

De Costa D, Brady WJ, Edhouse J: Bradycardias and atrioventricular conduction block, *BMJ* 324:535–538, 2002.

ECC Committee, Subcommittees and Task Forces of the American Heart Association: American Heart Association guidelines for cardiopulmonary resuscitation and emergency cardiovascular care: part 7.3: management of symptomatic bradycardia and tachycardia, *Circulation* 112(Suppl 24):IV67–IV77, 2005.

Epstein AE, DiMarco JP, Ellenbogen KA, et al.: ACC/AHA/HRS 2008 guidelines for device-based therapy of cardiac rhythm abnormalities, *Circulation* 117:e350–408, 2008.

Goodacre S, McLeod K: ABC of clinical electrocardiography, *BMJ* 324: 1382–1385, 2002.

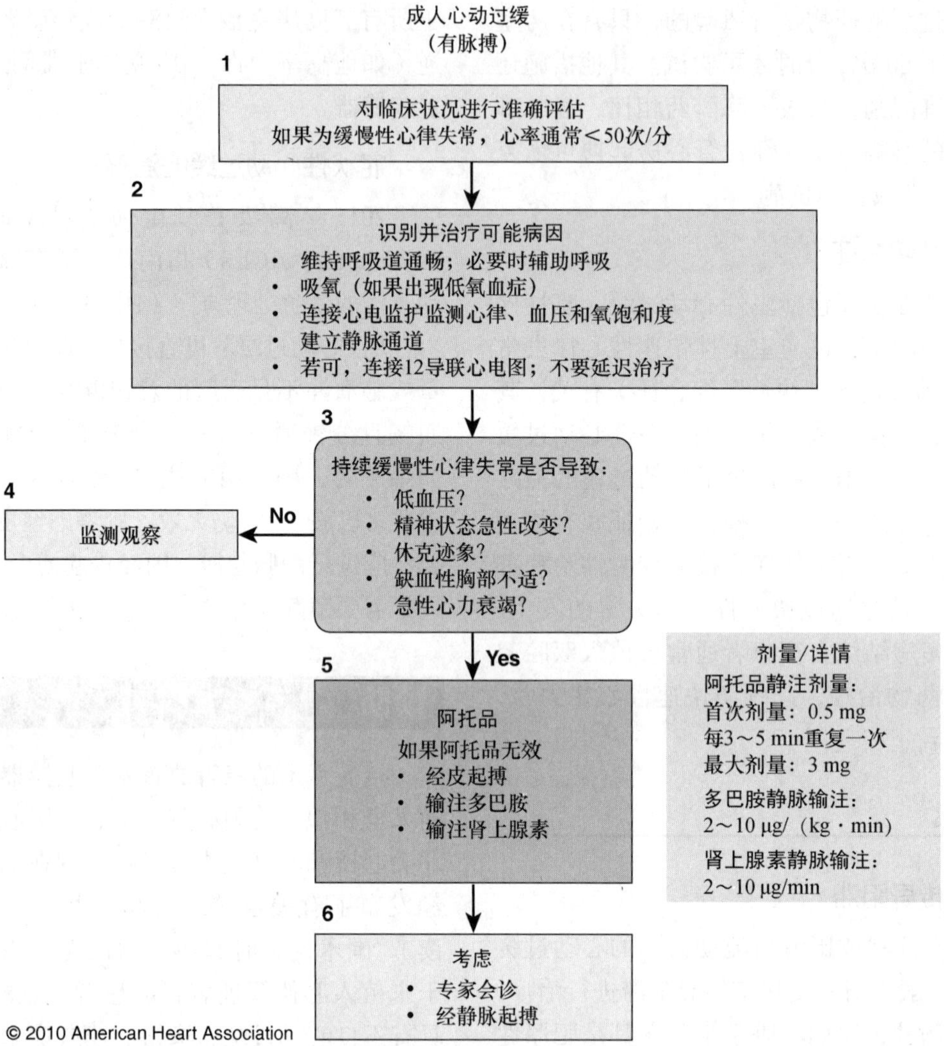

图 133.6 高级心脏生命支持（ACLS）对心动过缓的处理方案（Copyright by ACLS Training Center. This is current with respect to 2015 American Heart Association Guidelines for CPR and ECC. These guidelines are current until they are replaced in October 2020. After that date，please contact ACLS Training Center at support@acls.net for an updated document.）

Gregoratos G, Abrams J, Epstein AE, et al.: ACC/AHA/NASPE 2002 guideline update for implantation of cardiac pacemakers and antiarrhythmia devices: a report of the American College of Cardiology/American Heart Association Task Force on Practice Guidelines (ACC/AHA/NASPE Committee to Update the 1998 Pacemaker Guidelines), *Circulation* 106: 2145–2161, 2002.

Neumar RW, Otto CW, Link MS, et al.: Part 8: adult advanced cardiovascular life support: 2010 American Heart Association guidelines for cardiopulmonary resuscitation and emergency cardiovascular care, *Circulation* 122(18 Suppl 3):S729–S767, 2010.

Zimetbaum PJ, Josephson ME: Use of the electrocardiogram in acute myocardial infarction, *N Engl J Med* 348:933–940, 2003.

支气管痉挛

第134章

Joan Benca

病例概要

患儿，男性，6岁，有轻微间歇性哮喘病史，拟急诊行腹腔镜阑尾切除术。在预充氧和快速序贯诱导后，气管插管顺利，无误吸迹象。气管插管后，气道峰压由18 cmH_2O上升到35 cmH_2O，同时氧饱和度由100%下降至82%，血压由98/64 mmHg降低至68/34 mmHg，心率由80次/分升至130次/分。胸部听诊闻及双肺弥漫性呼气性喘鸣。监护仪显示呼气末二氧化碳曲线急剧上升。

问题分析

在哮喘患者中，支气管痉挛由支气管平滑肌痉挛性收缩引起。支气管痉挛是全身麻醉中的一种罕见现象，仅在1%～2%的全身麻醉药使用时发生。来自美国麻醉科医师协会（American Society of Anesthesiologists，ASA）的结案诉讼研究数据表明，支气管痉挛虽然不常见，但严重支气管痉挛可导致死亡或脑损伤。

支气管痉挛是一种排除性诊断，通常发生在麻醉诱导后、气管插管或拔管时。在麻醉诱导及气管插管时，引起支气管痉挛的原因众多。例如，所给药物可能导致组胺释放，气管插管时刺激副交感神经系统反射性引起支气管收缩等。无论是免疫球蛋白E（immunoglobulin E，IgE）介导的，还是非IgE介导的，药物均可能即刻诱发变态反应。

为判断患者发生了何种情况，应立即对患者行纯氧手动通气，以快速判断肺顺应性，同时听诊肺部以确认是否有喘鸣（框134.1）。如果气流非常低，呼吸音可能严重减弱或消失。此时立即确定气管导管位置及气管导管是否通畅至关重要。体格检查的主要目的在于排除肺水肿、黏液栓堵塞和张力性气胸等。此外，还应排除气管导管扭曲或堵塞的可能性。吸入异物或胃内容物、麻醉深度不足也可引起支气管痉挛的发生。

框134.1　患者麻醉中发生喘鸣的其他原因（除支气管痉挛外）

- 气管内导管或其他气道装置机械阻塞
- 张力性气胸
- 肺水肿
- 胃内容物误吸
- 肺栓塞
- 异物吸入（如牙齿）

管理

该患者表现出与支气管痉挛相一致的气道阻塞症状，包括喘鸣、呼气时间延长、呼吸音减弱、正压通气时气道压增加、氧饱和度降低及低血压等。呼气末二氧化碳曲线呈上升趋势，但仅此一项并非支气管痉挛的特异性现象；它只表明在呼吸环路过程中某个环节发生呼气障碍。在严重支气管痉挛时，尽管气流阻塞导致动脉血二氧化碳分压升高，但CO_2波形可能下降或消失。

一旦发生，应立即进行治疗。给予纯氧行手动通气，使用静脉麻醉药或吸入麻醉药加深麻醉，使用喷雾器通过气管导管给予短效选择性β_2-受体激动剂。当β_2-受体激动剂或加深麻醉无效时，此时应静脉注射肾上腺素0.1～1 μg/kg作为负荷量，随后以0.01 μg/（kg·min）的速度持续输注。吸入麻醉药七氟烷和异氟烷都是良好的支气管扩张剂，建议给予其中一种。地氟烷对气道有刺激作用，不建议用于支气管痉挛的治疗。另一种治疗急性严重支气管痉挛的方法是静脉注射镁剂（40 mg/kg）。

吸入镁剂在这种情况下未见益处。应考虑静脉注射大剂量类固醇，甲泼尼龙 2 mg/kg 为负荷剂量，以 0.5 ～ 1 mg/kg 持续输注 6 h。皮下注射特布他林（0.01 mg/kg，最高 0.3 mg），每 20 min 重复一次。在严重哮喘致支气管扩张剂或吸入麻醉药难以进入气道发挥作用时，特布他林可有一定的帮助。在紧急情况下，可能很难鉴别过敏反应与支气管痉挛，在发病 2 h 内可借助胰蛋白酶水平帮助诊断。如果需排除过敏反应，患者需在发生紧急情况 1 个月后寻求过敏专科医师的帮助，并进行皮肤针刺试验。大多数过敏反应患者会有皮疹或脸红表现。

如患者出现支气管痉挛和低血压的症状，应如前所述静脉注射肾上腺素。对不能耐受心动过速的患者，当发生支气管痉挛（如主动脉瓣狭窄患者）时，则可通过雾化器或定量吸入器给予抗胆碱能药物如异丙托溴铵。异丙托溴铵是一种季铵类药物，不会全身吸收，也没有全身副作用。在部分患者中，异丙托溴铵是继 β-受体激动剂之后的二线治疗药物。

预防

急性支气管痉挛并不局限于哮喘患者，但哮喘患者在围术期发生支气管痉挛的概率更大。在儿童患者中，发生支气管痉挛的危险因素还包括有湿疹或花粉热病史、湿疹家族史、吸烟史、年龄较小以及麻醉前 2 周内患有上呼吸道感染等。当儿童曾出现有夜间干咳、运动哮喘史或过去 12 个月发生 3 次以上哮喘，均提示该患儿围术期发生支气管痉挛风险增加。回顾既往麻醉记录和因哮喘发作住院治疗的病历记录，可能有助于制订麻醉计划。

术前对疾病严重程度及控制程度的评估应包括，患者呼吸道疾病或哮喘病史、目前症状控制情况、现在服用的药物、急救性药物使用的频率、以前是否有住院或气管插管治疗史，以及患者对麻醉和气管插管时的反应如何等。

确定患者存在围术期呼吸事件的风险后，做好术前准备改善患者病情非常重要。哮喘控制不佳的儿童麻醉前进行呼吸科会诊可有益处。吸入支气管扩张剂和吸入性糖皮质激素应使用至术日晨。对哮喘患者而言，良好的麻醉前准备意味着患者服药依从性好并处于稳定的呼吸状态，患有上呼吸道感染的患者手术应推迟至少 2 周，肺炎患者手术推迟 6 周。对急诊手术患者，麻醉前给予选择性 β_2-受体激动剂可能有益。

手术当日的术前体格检查应包括，肺部听诊、关注呼吸音类型和呼气相时长、检查胸廓起伏情况或辅助呼吸肌的参与情况、评估患者的生命体征、查看是否有呼吸频率的增加或氧饱和度下降等。对存在活动性喘鸣、呼吸做功增加、回缩、咳嗽、发烧或低动脉血氧饱和度等以上迹象的患者，都应推迟择期手术麻醉。

对此类患者，我们应严格制订麻醉计划，包括麻醉诱导剂的使用、气道管理以及肌松药和拮抗剂的使用等。

静脉诱导比吸入诱导更能降低支气管痉挛发生的危险。气道管理时建议选择面罩或喉罩，而非气管插管，以降低支气管痉挛的发生率。区域麻醉是另一可避免气管插管的方法，但对大多数儿童并不适用。与依托咪酯和苯巴比妥相比，丙泊酚和氯胺酮具有支气管扩张的作用，更能有效防止支气管痉挛出现。相比于地氟烷，七氟烷和异氟烷是较好的支气管扩张剂。气管插管前在声带上喷洒利多卡因可增加支气管痉挛的发生率，其可能原因是机械刺激所致。然而，与水溶性凝胶相比，放置喉罩前使用利多卡因凝胶润滑可减少支气管痉挛的发生率。静脉注射利多卡因目前存在争议，但比气管内使用利多卡因可能更有益。许多儿科麻醉科医师并不使用肌松药，因其是与即刻超敏反应最相关的药物。此外，肌松拮抗剂新斯的明可通过激活乙酰胆碱受体刺激气道反应。

抗胆碱能药物可引起支气管扩张，包括雾化异丙托溴铵、静脉注射格隆溴铵和静脉注射阿托品。静脉注射格隆溴铵和阿托品后支气管扩张起效至少需要 20 min，格隆溴铵较阿托品引起的支气管扩张时间更长。

尽管术前已充分准备，并合理选择麻醉方式，支气管痉挛仍可能发生（框 134.2）。麻醉患者术中发生支气管痉挛时的处理较为棘手。此时给予吸入麻醉药和（或）静脉注射丙泊酚、氯胺酮或右美托咪定，均为较好选择。然而，如果通气严重受限，将很难通过使用吸入麻醉药来加深麻醉。加深麻醉和治疗支气管痉挛的辅助措施还包括，静脉注射肾上腺素、皮下给予特布他林、静脉注射镁剂和抗胆碱能药物以及雾化吸入 β-受体激动剂。使用定量吸入器通过呼吸环路给予 β-受体激动剂处理支气管痉挛，不及使用喷雾器或强化雾化器有效。因此，建议使用定量吸入器时吸 8 ～ 10 次。当支气管痉挛导致严重通气障碍时，应给予肾上腺素，并同时使用静脉麻醉药物加深麻醉，直至能有效通气为止。框 134.3 列出了急性支气管痉挛的治疗步骤。

氯胺酮是一种具有良好支气管扩张作用的静脉麻醉药。糖皮质激素对急性支气管痉挛的治疗无法即刻发挥疗效。然而，急性支气管痉挛患者应当使用糖皮质激素，以帮助减少导致气道应激的持续炎症发生。如果喉罩通气患者表现为支气管痉挛，则应停止喉罩通气并尝试面罩通气。如果面罩通气不成功，建议气管插管。拔除气管导管是诱发支气管痉挛的另一个潜在诱因。如果患者在麻醉状态下接受过支气管痉挛的治疗，该患者应在深麻醉状态下拔管还是清醒状态下拔管，目前尚无统一意见。部分观点认为，清醒状态下气管拔管的理由是，如果患者在紧急情况下发生支气管痉挛，就需要气道来帮助治疗。另一部分观点则认为，选择深麻醉状态下拔管旨在避免出现气道刺激。最后，在气道操作或气管插管前以及手术过程中应维持足够的麻醉深度，这是预防全身麻醉期间支气管痉挛发生的最重要措施。确保足够的麻醉深度，并使其与外科医师或麻醉科医师操作时的刺激程度相匹配，这一点非常重要。

框 134.2　患者麻醉时发生支气管痉挛的原因

非特异性支气管高反应性
对药物、血液、乳胶的过敏或类过敏反应
琥珀胆碱、阿曲库铵、罗库溴铵
哮喘加重
药物：β-受体阻滞剂、前列腺素抑制剂、抗胆碱酯酶等
刺激副交感神经纤维、M2 和 M3 毒蕈碱受体
气管插管或拔管引起的气道刺激

框 134.3　急性支气管痉挛的治疗

使用强效吸入麻醉药（七氟烷、异氟烷）或静脉麻醉药（丙泊酚、氯胺酮、右美托咪定）增加麻醉深度
β 受体激动剂
通过雾化装置的沙丁胺醇定量吸入器（喷 2 次）
　麻醉回路雾化器（2.5 mg，3 ml 生理盐水中）
　通过套管接头定量吸入器（喷 8 ～ 10 次）
肾上腺素静脉注射 0.1 ～ 1 μg/kg 负荷量，随后以 0.01 μg/(kg·min) 输注
　气管给药 10 μg/kg
　肌内注射 10 μg/kg
特布他林皮下注射 0.01 μg/kg，最大剂量 0.3 μg
抗胆碱类
　异丙托溴铵定量剂吸入器（18 μg/ 喷）4 ～ 8 喷 q 20 min × 3 h
　异丙托溴铵喷雾器 250 ～ 500 μg q 20 min × 3 剂量
　格隆溴铵 4 μg/kg 静注
　阿托品 20 μg/kg 静注
类固醇激素
　甲泼尼龙 1 ～ 2 mg/kg，最大剂量 125 mg
　氢化可的松 2 mg/kg 静注
　地塞米松 0.1 ～ 0.5 mg/kg 静注，最大剂量 10 mg
硫酸镁
　40 mg/kg 每 20 min 静注

（解　健　译　陈　玲　校）

延伸阅读

Habre W, Petak F: Anaesthesia management of patients with airway susceptibilities: what have we learnt from animal models? *Eur J Anaesthesiol* 30:519–528, 2013.

Hamilton ND, Hegarty M, Calder A, et al.: Does topical lidocaine before tracheal intubation attenuate airway responses in children? An observational audit, *Paediatr Anaesth* 22:345–350, 2012.

Lauer R, Vadi M, Mason L: Anaesthetic management of the child with co-existing pulmonary disease, *Br J Anaesth* 109(51):i47–i59, 2012.

Liccardi G, Salzillo A, Sofia M, et al.: Bronchial asthma, *Curr Opin Anesthesiol* 25:30–37, 2012.

Luce V, Harkouk H, Brasher C, et al.: Supraglottic airway devices vs tracheal intubation in children: a quantitative meta-analysis of respiratory complications, *Paediatr Anaesth* 24:1088–1098, 2014.

Orestes M, Lander L, Verghese S, et al.: Incidence of laryngospasm and bronchospasm in pediatric adenotonsillectomy, *Laryngoscope* 122: 425–428, 2012.

Regli A, von Ungern-Sternberg B: Anesthesia and ventilation strategies in children with asthma: part I—preoperative assessment, *Curr Opin Anesthesiol* 27:288–294, 2014.

Regli A, von Ungern-Sternberg B: Anesthesia and ventilation strategies in children with asthma: part II—intraoperative management, *Curr Opin Anesthesiol* 27:295–302, 2014.

Schebesta K, Guloglu E, Chiari A, et al.: Topical lidocaine reduces the risk of perioperative airway complications in children with upper respiratory infections, *Can J Anesth* 57:745–750, 2010.

von Ungern-Sternberg BS, Boda K, Chambers NA, et al.: Risk assessment for respiratory complications in paediatric anaesthesia: a prospective cohort study, *Lancet* 376:773–783, 2010.

von Ungern-Sternberg BS, Boda K, Schwab C, et al.: Laryngeal mask airway is associated with an increased incidence of adverse respiratory events in children with recent upper respiratory tract infections, *Anesthesiology* 107(5):714–719, 2007.

von Ungern-Sternberg BS, Davies K, Hegarty M, et al.: The effect of deep vs. awake extubation on respiratory complications in high-risk children undergoing adenotonsillectomy, *Eur J Anaesthesiol* 30:529–536, 2013.

Woods BD, Sladen RN: Perioperative considerations for the patient with asthma and bronchospasm, *Br J Anaesth* 103:i57–i65, 2009.

第135章 腹腔神经丛阻滞的不良反应和并发症

Ignacio Badiola

病例概要

患者，男性，71岁，诊断为转移性胰腺癌，因继发性腹痛转诊到疼痛诊疗中心。该患者先前接受过腹腔神经丛局部麻醉药阻滞，腹痛减轻了80%。今日使用苯酚行神经丛毁损术。手术看似很顺利，但他被转移到苏醒室后主诉下肢麻木无力。

问题分析

定义

世界首例腹腔神经丛阻滞术于1914年进行，自那以后，发展出多种适应证和操作技术方法。并发症虽然罕见，但比较严重甚至是灾难性的。腹腔神经丛是支配从食管远端三分之一处到横结肠的神经结构，其还参与调节肾、肾上腺、脾、肝和胆道功能。腹腔神经丛阻滞术已成功用于包括胰腺癌和上消化道恶性肿瘤等在内的多种肿瘤患者的镇痛，以及慢性胰腺炎等非恶性疼痛疾病。在大多数情况下，先使用局部麻醉药行诊断性阻滞，然后使用苯酚或酒精行神经毁损术，从而获得长期镇痛效果。

腹腔神经丛主要是交感神经系统结构，用局部麻醉药阻断或用苯酚/酒精毁损交感神经后，可因副交感神经张力增加，从而产生症状。这会引起内脏循环血管扩张，静脉回流减少和心脏前负荷降低，导致血压下降。通常表现为直立性低血压。消化道副交感神经张力增加可致肠蠕动亢进和腹泻。

严重并发症罕见，然而，神经系统并发症可能是灾难性的。神经损伤、截瘫和主动脉夹层等并发症并不常见，但有可能发生。一项Meta分析报告了2%（13/628例）的严重不良事件。这些事件包括：下肢无力、感觉异常、硬膜外麻醉、腰椎穿刺、血尿、气胸和胸膜炎性胸痛。还可发生截瘫，特别是使用苯酚/酒精时，可能是由于Adamkiewicz动脉痉挛所致。

腹腔神经丛阻滞后可能发生的其他并发症包括肾损伤、腹膜后血肿、气胸、乳糜胸、穿透椎间盘、脓肿形成、疼痛加剧和射精障碍（框135.1）。

识别

直立性低血压通常发生在术后患者试图从仰卧位坐起来时。血压下降常伴有头晕、多汗，可能发生晕厥。恶性肿瘤患者可能表现更为显著，因为这些患者常因食水摄入减少而存在血容量不足。通过

框135.1 腹腔神经丛毁损并发症

- 局部疼痛
- 直立性低血压
- 腹泻
- 神经损伤
- 感觉异常
- 硬膜外麻醉
- 腰椎穿刺
- 肾损伤
- 血尿
- 气胸
- 腹膜后血肿
- 乳糜胸
- 射精障碍
- 疼痛加剧
- 椎间盘穿刺
- 感染

监测血压加上以上症状可以及时识别。应测量患者的基础血压、术中以及术后等时点血压，特别是当患者从俯卧位改为仰卧位，以及最后从仰卧位改为直立位时。患者应该逐渐而不是突然地恢复成坐位。

腹腔神经丛阻滞后发生肠蠕动亢进性腹泻比较常见。许多恶性肿瘤患者因服用阿片类药物而出现便秘，可认为此时的肠蠕动亢进有一定益处。应告知患者可能会发生腹泻，建议他们采取措施保持水分。

气胸是一种罕见的并发症。然而，因为胸膜向下反折可至 T12/L1 水平，如果患者腹腔神经丛阻滞后出现呼吸短促或低氧血症，则应考虑气胸并发症。

与感觉和运动变化相关的并发症通常在局部麻醉药或神经毁损剂注入后立即出现。识别包括在注入局部麻醉药或神经毁损剂之前进行多次检查确认。这包括影像引导 [计算机断层扫描（computed tomography，CT）或透视] 穿刺、注射前回抽有无血液或脑脊液、预先注射造影剂以帮助排除误入血管。在注入神经毁损剂前应注入少量局部麻醉药，以帮助排除不正确的穿刺针位置。注入试验剂量局部麻醉药后，如果出现无力或感觉变化，则表明穿刺针尖位于硬膜外 / 鞘内或神经根内，必须重新定位穿刺。

风险评估

与其他介入手术一样，治疗可获得的益处必须超过其风险。1995 年的一项 Meta 分析回顾了包括 1000 多名癌症患者（63% 胰腺癌，37% 非胰腺癌）的 24 项研究，结果显示，89% 的患者在神经毁损后的前 2 周内疼痛缓解可达良好至最好，且止痛效果可维持 3 个月。其他类型癌症的反应与胰腺癌患者类似。该研究者认为，腹腔神经丛毁损对多种消化道恶性肿瘤患者具有较长久的益处，常见不良事件包括局部疼痛（96%）、腹泻（44%）和低血压（38%），作用短暂且程度轻微。严重不良事件中，神经系统并发症（包括下肢无力、感觉异常、硬膜外麻醉和腰椎穿刺）占 1%。非神经系统并发症如气胸和血尿，发生率约为 1%。

启示

常见不良反应通常为自限性，并应该可以预料。手术前应与患者和护理人员沟通这些问题。肠蠕动亢进通常对癌症患者和严重疼痛患者有益，因为他们通常因服用阿片类药物而正忍受便秘痛苦。直立性低血压通常在血容量平衡后自行改善。

虽然多数气胸只需进行严密监护，但严重气胸可能需要有创性的胸腔闭式引流术和住院治疗。尽管不常见，但应在术前与患者沟通。

幸运的是，神经并发症如注入神经毁损剂导致截瘫并不常见。然而，发生这种情况的影响需要与患者强调，因为其可能造成永久伤害。

管理

治疗取决于所出现的并发症。发生直立性低血压时，应令患者保持仰卧位或头低足高位（Trendelenburg 体位）。由于其发生机制是血管扩张、静脉容量增加，因此可以经口或静脉补液。对于难治性病例，也可给予 α_1- 受体激动剂（如去氧肾上腺素）等药物进行治疗。

肠蠕动亢进最常见的原因是副交感神经活性过度，具有自限性，可以采用补液和拮抗剂（如洛哌丁胺）对症治疗。一篇文献报道了 2 例持续性腹泻患者的治疗经过（见文末推荐阅读中 Yang 等的研究），其中 1 例经奥曲肽治疗获得成功。

气胸的治疗取决于气胸的程度和临床症状。无症状的少量气胸通常可以严密观察，而有症状的大量气胸则需要行胸腔闭式引流术。

神经并发症的治疗更为复杂。如果注射试验剂量时即出现神经症状，应重新定位穿刺。如果在注射神经毁损剂过程中出现症状，应立即中止手术。可尝试回吸神经毁损剂，但可能不太有效。应立即咨询神经学 / 神经外科学专家和介入放射学专家，尽管逆转已出现损伤的方法目前仍十分有限。

预防

低血压和肠蠕动亢进是腹腔神经丛阻滞 / 毁损的常见不良反应。

通常认为，影像引导是预防并发症特别是神经并发症的重要方法。目前，常用的影像引导技术包括 CT、X 线透视检查和内镜超声。一项对 1145 例恶性肿瘤患者的 Meta 分析中，246 例（32%）神经阻滞未通过影像引导进行，214 例用 CT 引导，271

例用X线拍片引导，36例用X线荧光透视引导，7例用超声引导。基于影像学技术的结果分析表明，术中使用影像引导并未较非影像引导方法的不良反应发生率更低。然而，作者注意到大多数分析研究是回顾性研究。而且，1145例患者中只有7例使用了内镜超声引导，因此无法充分评估不良事件结局的差异。

一项包括了2730例腹腔神经丛阻滞的回顾性调查（给疼痛门诊发放问卷调查）显示，其中4例出现永久性截瘫，3例出现肛门和膀胱括约肌张力丧失。应注意，所有4例并发症都使用了造影剂进行影像学辅助。然而，没有具体说明使用了哪种影像学技术。

致谢

感谢Gilbert Y. Wong和David L. Brown博士对本章上一版的贡献。

（吴 玮 译 陈 辉 校）

延伸阅读

Davies DD: Incidence of major complications of neurolytic coeliac plexus block, *J R Soc Med* 86(5):264–266, 1993.

Eisenberg E, Carr DB, Chalmers TC: Neurolytic celiac plexus block for treatment of cancer pain: a meta-analysis, *Anesth Analg* 80(2):290–295, 1995.

Radpay B, Parsa T, Dabir S, et al.: Acute respiratory failure as a rare complication of celiac plexus block in a patient with adenocarcinoma of the ampulla of vater, *Tanaffos* 11(2):54–57, 2012.

Yang A, Brown J, Mak E: Persistent diarrhea after celiac plexus block in a pancreatic cancer patient: case report and literature review, *J Palliat Med* 19(1):83–86, 2015.

角膜损伤

第 136 章

Katharine H. Zentner，*Luis L. Llamas*，*Lois L. Bready*

病例概要

患者，女性，25 岁，在气管插管全身麻醉下行鼻息肉切除术后，在麻醉后恢复室（postanesthesia care unit, PACU）内主诉右眼疼痛及异物感。体格检查发现双眼周围残留有睫毛膏颗粒的油性软膏，右眼结膜红斑，明显流泪，畏光，视力减退。患者右手示指连接脉搏血氧饱和度探头。

问题分析

定义

角膜损伤（corneal injury，CI）在围术期并不常见，但会引起疼痛，降低患者满意度，并可能使 PACU 转出时间及出院时间延迟。围术期 CI 有 3 种类型：①角膜擦伤（corneal abrasions，CA），由机械性损伤引起；②暴露性角膜损伤，由麻醉过程中眼睑闭合不充分引起；③化学灼伤，通常由无意中接触皮肤消毒液引起。CA 是围术期最常见的眼科损伤，报道的发生率为 0.013% ～ 0.17%。其长期后遗症并不常见，但可能包括角膜溃疡或糜烂、视力丧失。化学灼伤通常会留下瘢痕。幸运的是，近年来与 CA 相关的麻醉索赔比例已显著下降（图 136.1）

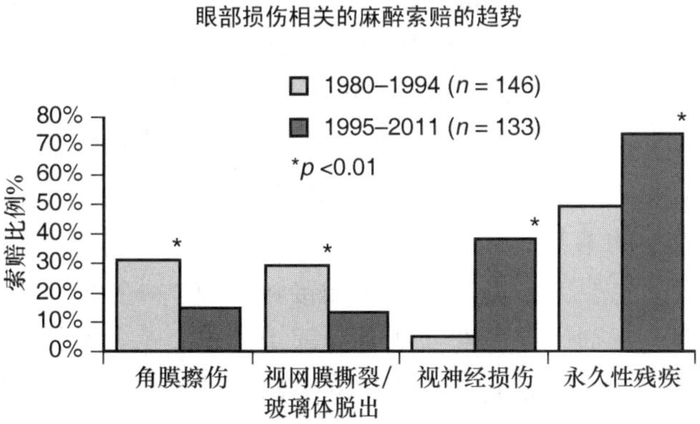

本分析不包括因眼部神经阻滞实施手术引发的索赔。随时间推移，由视神经永久性损伤引发的索赔率增加，由角膜擦伤、视网膜撕裂或玻璃体脱出引发的索赔率下降。

图 136.1　眼部损伤相关的麻醉索赔的趋势（From Posner KL, Lee LL：Anesthesia malpractice claims associated with eye surgery and eye injury：highlights from the anesthesia closed claims project data request service. *ASA Newsletter* 78[11]：28-30，2014.）

识别

角膜损伤的症状一般在麻醉结束后 1 ～ 3 h 内得以识别，可能表现为眼睛疼痛、流泪、异物感、畏光和视力减退。床旁检查可发现擦伤部位（图 136.2），尤其是斜向光检查时。擦伤可通过应用荧光素染料来观察，染料可填充角膜损伤处，并在钴蓝光下使其可见。

检查可发现与暴露区域相关的上下眼睑之间有一薄层角膜剥落（图 136.3A）或机械擦伤所致的线性缺损（图 136.3B）。化学性角膜毒性作用通常会导致结膜水肿（即球结膜明显水肿），伴有各种角膜上皮缺损，包括点状角膜炎（图 136.4）。

风险评估

眼部结构靠近气道和其他操作（图 136.5），有

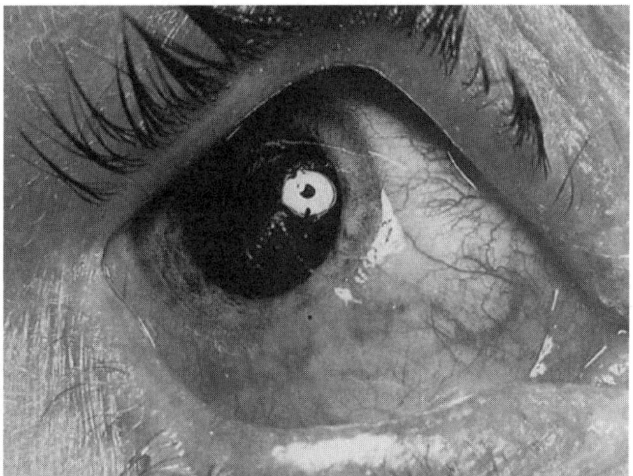

图 136.2　角膜磨损

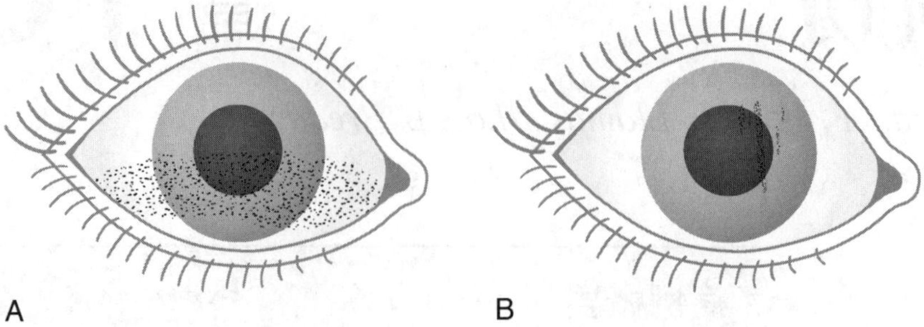

图 136.3 角膜及结膜染色类型。**图 A**，眼睑间擦伤（指眼睑闭合不完全而暴露）。**图 B**，线性缺损（提示机械擦伤）

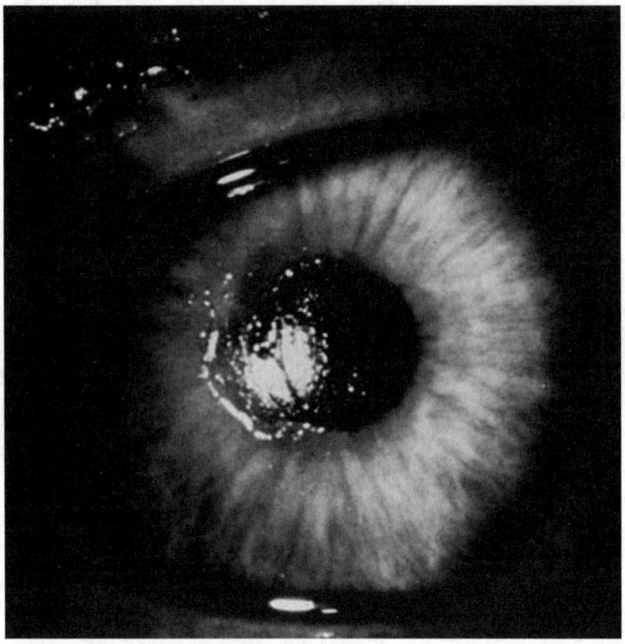

图 136.4 伴点状角膜炎的Ⅰ级化学灼伤（最轻微）

诸多可能导致角膜损伤的麻醉相关危险因素。角膜上皮脆弱，即使轻微碰触也可能造成创伤。高龄及全身麻醉是最常见的危险因素，但角膜损伤也可能发生在清醒镇静期间，患者镇静过度而无法对偶发性损伤或眼睑闭合不全做出反应。在全身麻醉期间，保护性角膜反射受到抑制，泪液生成减少，眨眼反射被抑制，抑制了润滑剂在眼球表面的重新分布。异物（即隐形眼镜、睫毛膏颗粒）可能存在。其他危险因素包括，患者转运/苏醒期间的吸氧及术中患者体位，特别是 Trendelenburg 体位。Trendelenburg 体位时，血管内、上巩膜静脉和眼内压升高，角膜厚度增加，导致眼球严重干燥及脱落和擦伤的风险增加。

化学灼伤

在对眼周皮肤进行消毒时（头颈部手术），消毒液可能会意外接触角膜。大多数皮肤消毒液有角

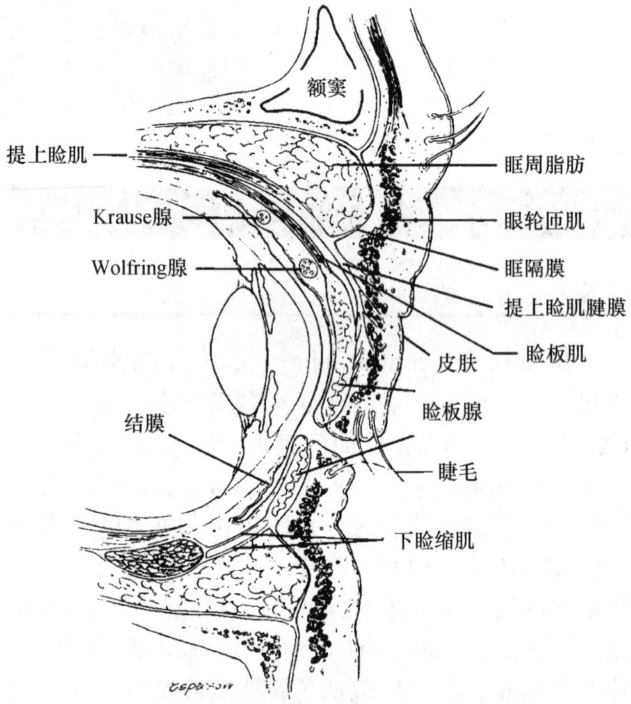

图 136.5 眼球及眶周横截面示意图

膜毒性，接触角膜可能导致化学灼伤，甚至可能导致失明（框 136.1）。如果消毒液不小心溅出或流进泪膜（即，头颈部手术术前准备），可能会产生强烈的毒性作用。据报道，洗必泰（4% 葡萄糖酸氯己定和清洁剂）可导致永久性角膜瘢痕。对角膜毒性最小的溶液是碘伏（10% 聚维酮碘）。影响角膜毒性的主要因素是溶液浓度和接触时间，一旦溅入化学消毒剂，妥善的做法是立即用盐水、平衡盐溶液或水冲洗结膜囊。已报道的大部分外科术前消毒液引起角膜损伤的病例，由非眼科医师在头颈部手术消毒时所致。这表明，未识别出溅入消毒液及冲洗不足可能是造成不良后果的原因之一。应注意，手术准备时消毒液可能从鼻腔通过鼻泪管逆行流入结膜囊。

接触酸性胃液也会导致角膜化学灼伤。如果发

框 136.1 皮肤消毒剂的角膜毒性

洗必泰（葡萄糖酸氯已定，清洁剂：4% 异丙醇）
pHisoHex（含 3% 六氯酚和清洁剂）
Lavacol（70% 乙醇）
Betadine 外科洗液（7.5% 聚维酮碘清洁剂）
碘酊（2% 碘，2.35% 碘酸钠，46% 乙醇）
含碘消毒液

From MacRae SM，Brown B，Edelhauser HF：The corneal toxicity of presurgical skin antiseptics. *Am J Ophthalmol* 97：221-232，1984.

现或怀疑这种暴露，仍建议冲洗结膜囊。

Manecke 等报告 1 例因使用含防腐剂的眼睛润滑剂引起双侧角膜严重损伤的病例。业已证实，防腐剂氯丁醇和苯扎氯铵可引起角膜上皮细胞脱落。如果使用眼用软膏，应选择无防腐剂的制剂。

角膜擦伤

面罩、头带、手臂、肘部、麻醉科医师或外科医师 ID 牌直接压迫眼球，或其他附近物体会擦伤角膜表面。角膜擦伤可能发生于以下时间：麻醉诱导期间，面罩或其他气道装置通气时，使用眼用润滑剂时（如果眼用润滑剂管的尖端接触角膜），手术中（外科医师或麻醉科医师的手、肘或器械对眼球的压迫），或苏醒期（原因与诱导期间相似，或患者擦拭眼部分泌物或润滑剂）。

管理

疼痛通常是角膜损伤患者的首要主诉。如前所述，使用荧光素染料进行床边检查可以早期诊断。应尽快进行眼科评估，但在等待眼科评估时，不应延迟治疗，以免导致患者疼痛不必要的延长。

新近报告指出，麻醉科医师主导围术期角膜擦伤的治疗方案取得成功。Segal 等建议，对所有术后眼部不适或疼痛的患者，PACU 麻醉工作人员及时予以眼用抗生素软膏进行治疗，同时进行眼科会诊。Chelly 等建议，2 ～ 3 h 内每 30 min 在患眼内滴入人工泪液，直到症状消失。如果症状持续超过 2 ～ 3 h，患眼每隔 6 h 应用 0.5% 红霉素眼药膏 1 次。如患者对红霉素过敏，可选择其他治疗方法，如环丙沙星、妥布霉素、杆菌肽。Chelly 的研究则指出，只有在次日晨症状还未好转时，才进行眼科会诊。

预防

充分认识眼损伤风险，对预防此类事件的发生至关重要。建立适当预案并准备，就有可能消除大多数对眼球有害的操作和潜在的破坏性物体。

使用胶带封闭眼睑可保护角膜免受外伤、化学损伤和脱水。除非实施快速气管插管，建议在气道管理前、眼睑反射消失后立即行水平方向粘贴胶带而不是垂直方向。术中应检查眼部以免胶带移位，导致眼球表面接触胶粘剂。麻醉结束时，胶带由上向下取下（以便取胶带时眼睑保持闭合），避免角膜上皮剥离和擦伤的危险。

非仰卧位或麻醉科医师无法观测眼部时，例如侧或俯卧位、头部或颈部手术覆盖头部、头部被包裹、上呼吸道手术，建议使用纱布护目垫或护目镜。虽然一些临床医师提倡常规使用护目镜，但因患者头部大小、瞳孔间距离等差异，其实施可能具有挑战性。

无防腐剂的眼用润滑剂可预防干眼，可降低角膜损伤的一种风险，但当患者擦拭眼睛以清除润滑剂时，可能带来另一种风险。

患者术晨不应使用睫毛膏，全麻诱导前应协助患者清除睫毛膏。必须摘除隐形眼镜，以免损伤角膜或隐形眼镜。最后，建议将脉搏血氧饱和度探头放置在示指以外的手指上（如第四或第五指），以防患者在麻醉苏醒过程中自行造成角膜擦伤。

致谢

感谢 Stacey Allen 博士对本章上一版的贡献。

（林安琪 译 樊玉花 校）

延伸阅读

A case report from the Anesthesia Incident Reporting System: Case 2014-11: Proper Eye Protection, *ASA Monitor* 78:44–56, 2014.

Chelly J, Marr L, Hudson M, et al.: A department-of-anesthesiology-based management protocol for perioperative corneal abrasions, *Clin Ophthalmol* 9:1689–1695, 2015.

Grixti A, Sadri M, Watts MT: Corneal protection during general anesthesia for nonocular surgery, *Ocul Surf* 11(2):109–118, 2013.

MacRae SM, Brown B, Edelauser HR: The corneal toxicity of presurgical skin antiseptics, *Am J Ophthalmol* 97:221–232, 1984.

Manecke GR, Tannenbaum DP, Mccoy BE: Severe bilateral corneal injury attributed to a preservative-containing eye lubricant, *Anesthesiology* 93(6):1545–1546, 2000.

Posner KL, Lee LL: Anesthesia malpractice claims associated with eye surgery and eye injury: highlights from the anesthesia closed claims project data request service, *ASA Newsletter* 78(11):28–30, 2014.

Segal KL, Fleischut PM, Kim C, et al.: Evaluation and treatment of perioperative corneal abrasions, *J Ophthalmol* 901:2014, 2014.

第137章 苏醒延迟

Somi R. Desikan

病例概要 1

患者，男性，65 岁，在全麻下行胫骨切开复位内固定术。既往有高血压和糖尿病病史，服用雷米普利和二甲双胍。使用咪达唑仑 2 mg、丙泊酚和瑞芬太尼诱导，置入 i-gel 喉罩行机械通气。至手术结束前共给予吗啡 20 mg。手术时间 150 min，在麻醉后苏醒室（PACU）拔除喉罩后 20 min，患者对语言刺激仍然无反应。

病例概要 2

患者，女性，80 岁，在全麻下行腹腔镜阑尾切除术。她的体重指数（body mass index，BMI）为 35（体重 95 kg），合并轻度慢性肾病（估计肾小球滤过率为 55）。使用芬太尼 100 μg、丙泊酚 200 mg、罗库溴铵 50 mg 行快速诱导，七氟烷吸入维持麻醉。手术 90 min 后，肌松恢复，拔除气管导管。随即患者出现意识模糊，呼吸浅快，氧饱和度下降。

病例概要 3

患者，女性，86 岁，在全麻复合髂筋膜阻滞下行股骨颈骨折切开复位内固定术。既往有高血压和房颤病史，服用氨氯地平和华法林。患者在家不慎摔倒，术前格拉斯哥昏迷量表评分（Glasgow Coma Scale，GCS）为 14 分。全身麻醉药物有丙泊酚 100 mg，芬太尼 75 μg，使用喉罩进行通气，术中使用七氟烷维持麻醉。45 min 后手术结束，送入 PACU 30 min 后，患者还未恢复知觉。

问题分析

定义

麻醉后苏醒延迟尚无明确的定义。在临床实践中，苏醒延迟是指在麻醉结束后 20 ～ 30 min 内患者未能恢复预期的意识水平。它还包括患者的一些异常表现，如严重的躁动。麻醉后意识恢复所需的时间受多种因素影响，如患者因素，麻醉药物的使用，手术时间以及围术期使用的各种药物之间相互作用等。在许多患者中可能为多种因素所致，但一般会有一个因素起主导作用。

麻醉恢复延迟的常见原因如下：

- 术前所用药物与麻醉药物的相互作用及增强作用；
- 镇静剂和麻醉药的绝对或相对过量；
- 同时使用苯二氮䓬类药物和阿片类药物；
- 患者对药物的敏感性（例如，初次使用阿片类药物的患者）。

不常见的原因包括：

- 代谢障碍；
- 电解质紊乱；
- 术后谵妄；

- 脓毒症。

罕见的原因包括：

- 血清素综合征；
- 中枢抗胆碱能综合征；
- 精神障碍；
- 脑卒中及其他神经并发症。

识别

对苏醒延迟的识别通常是通过简单的神经学评估如 AVPU[警觉（alert），只对口头刺激做出反应（responds only to verbal stimuli），只对疼痛做出反应（responds only to pain），没有反应（unresponsive）] 或 GCS 评分进行的。这是一种排除诊断，因此，麻醉科医师必须及时评估这些患者，以诊断和排除气道阻塞、呼吸衰竭和低血糖，区分苏醒延迟和虚假表现为苏醒延迟但威胁生命的问题。

应立即对患者进行生命体征评估，评估患者的气道（airway，A）、呼吸（breathing，B）、循环（circulation，C）（特别是自主呼吸的频率和特征以及血氧饱和度），并做好体格检查。应在苏醒延迟可能的整个过程中随时对 ABC 进行重新评估。图 137.1 概述了一种帮助评估和管理昏迷患者的方法。

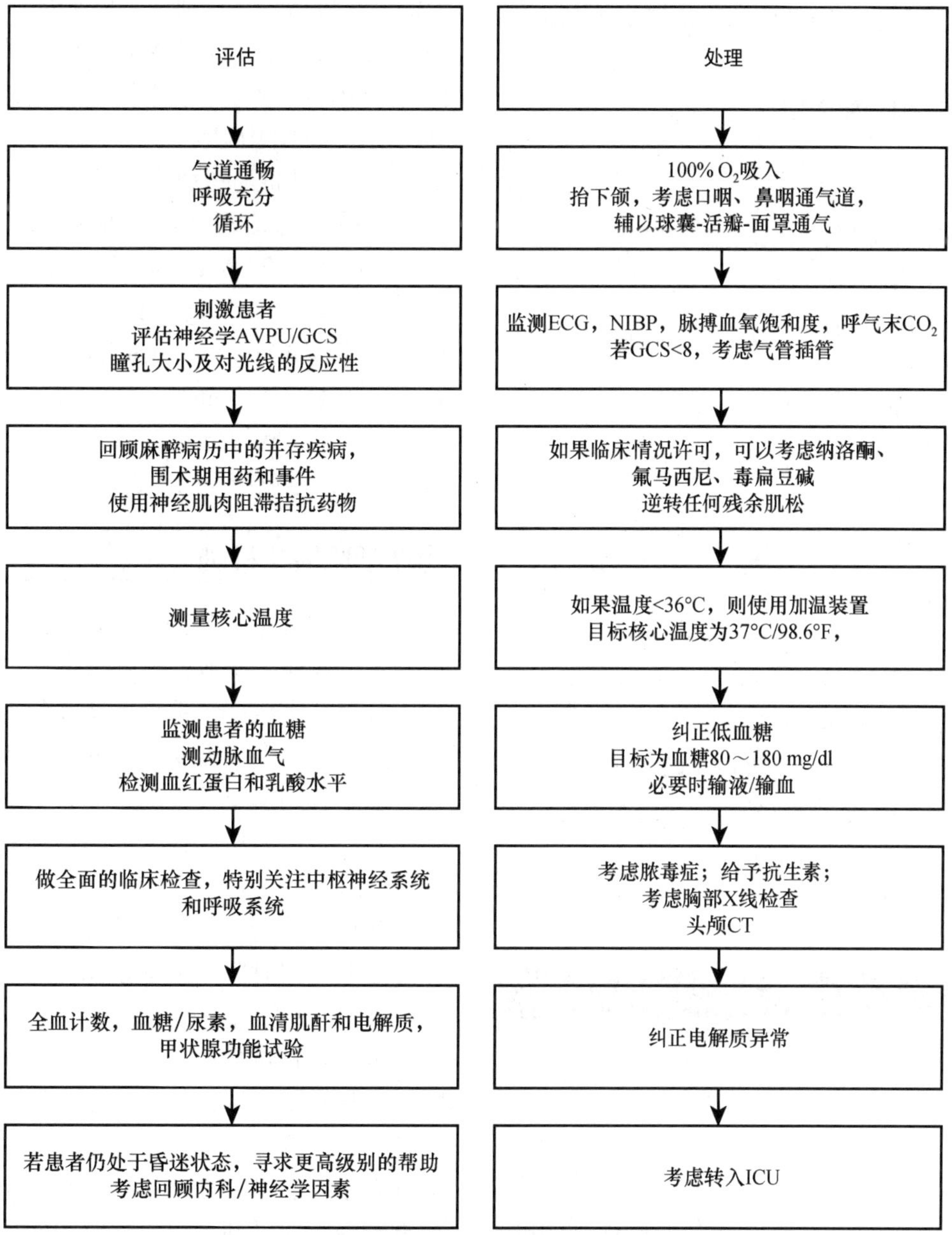

图 137.1 麻醉后苏醒延迟患者的评估与处理

风险评估

现代麻醉多使用短效麻醉药，大多数患者在手术后可以很快恢复，很多患者都可以在术后 1 h 内出 PACU。虽然苏醒延迟有很多原因，但到目前为止，它的可预见性和发生频率还没有得到很好的研究，因为大多数病例属于可疑病例，因此没有确切的发病率。虽然长效麻醉药的使用率可能会下降，但因为患者复杂的内科病情服用多种药物，使得大手术后苏醒延迟的实际发生率可能并不会下降。苏醒延迟的发生原因可能多样，例如老年痴呆症或肾功能损害的患者接受了长时间的全麻手术，第一个小时内出现苏醒延迟更可能是药理学原因；在第一个小时之后则更多的可能是代谢、神经学和其他罕见的原因。

苏醒延迟的风险因素包括：

- 高龄；
- 痴呆患者；
- 存在认知或精神障碍；
- 肝、肾损害患者；
- 手术时间和麻醉时间过长；
- 使用长效麻醉药；
- 麻醉药物绝对和相对过量；
- 服用镇静剂和抗精神病药物的患者；
- 中毒患者急诊手术；
- 术前休息不好的患者。

启示

大多数发生苏醒延迟的患者恢复良好。如果危及生命的问题能够得到迅速诊断和治疗，对大多数患者来说只需密切的观察和监测即已足够。有一些患者可能需要非计划入院或在重症监护室进行观察。极少数患者需要进行外科手术例如硬膜下血肿清除术，因为硬膜下血肿最初可能以苏醒延迟的形式出现。

管理

评估和调查

苏醒延迟是一种临床诊断，系统的方法（如图 137.1 所示）有助于及早发现治疗危及生命的问题。一旦排除了气道阻塞、呼吸衰竭和低血糖等问题，通常需要基于个体化的密切观察和监测管理。所有患者都应常规持续监测心电图、脉搏血氧饱和度、无创血压和体温。

无论是诊断还是排除具体的临床情况，均需要实施进一步的检查。在 PACU 中，确保随时可以实施血糖和神经肌肉监测，必要时还需行动脉血气（arterial blood gas，ABG）分析和放射学检查（如胸部 X 线或头部 CT 扫描）。应制定好使用这些检测的预案或转至其他机构进行这些检测的计划。

治疗

一旦排除了严重的问题，大多数患者会在密切监测下缓慢恢复，特别是药物原因引起的苏醒延迟。拮抗剂 [纳洛酮、氟马西尼、毒扁豆碱和新斯的明（舒更葡糖）] 可用于拮抗苯二氮䓬类、吸入麻醉剂和肌肉松弛剂的作用。

合理的拮抗药物剂量如下：

- 纳洛酮，每 2 min 静脉注射 40 μg，总量 200 μg；
- 氟马西尼，0.2 mg/min，静脉注射，总量 1.0 mg；
- 毒扁豆碱，1.25 mg 静脉注射；
- 新斯的明 50 μg/kg 和格隆溴铵 10 μg/kg；
- 舒更葡糖 2 ～ 4 mg/kg。

对于有症状的患者，应纠正电解质和代谢异常，但需谨慎以避免严重的不良反应。

药理学原因及机制

在恢复期的药物残留反应受到多重因素的影响，如剂量、代谢、排泄、患者易感性以及药物间相互作用等等。中枢神经系统敏感性的生物变异呈钟形曲线。一些患者只需要少量的诱导和维持药物，而另一些患者则需要较多的药物，当然，大多数人处于中间位置。到达大脑受体的药物浓度和受体对特定药物的敏感性决定了反应。

肝代谢下降常见于小儿、老年人、营养不良、体温过低和同时服用由肝微粒体酶解毒的几种药物（如乙醇、巴比妥酸盐）的患者。

虽然药物再分布是某些药物（如硫喷妥钠）作用时间较短的原因，但它也可能导致苏醒延迟，特别是在重复给药时。脂溶性药物，如吸入性麻醉药，会分布于脂肪中，其结果是脂肪储存库在麻醉结束后重新释放回循环系统。这对于使用长效麻醉药物的肥胖患者尤其如此。

苯二氮䓬类药物如咪达唑仑和地西泮常用于抗焦虑。较大剂量使用时，特别是与阿片类药物合用于老年患者时，往往容易造成苏醒延迟。阿片类药物有镇痛、镇静和呼吸抑制的作用，患者对阿片类药物的敏感性差别很大。阿片类药物还能剂量依赖性降低脑干化学感受器对 CO_2 的敏感性，这会导致高碳酸血症，而进一步降低患者的意识水平，有意识的患者使用神经肌肉阻滞可表现为无意识。

草药补充剂如卡瓦、圣约翰麦汁和缬草可能导致过度镇静和苏醒延迟。

静脉麻醉药意识障碍的持续时间受药物的时量相关半衰期、剂量、其他药物以及患者因素的影响。ICU 患者数天长期输注药物后，通常会出现苏醒延迟。吸入性麻醉的苏醒取决于药物的肺清除率和苏醒时最低肺泡有效浓度（MAC awake，即与按指令睁眼相关的呼气末药物浓度）。MAC awake 约等于 30%MAC。异氟烷和氟烷（相对于七氟烷或地氟烷）具有较高的气血溶解度，需要更长的时间才能从体内清除，可能导致苏醒延迟，尤其在肥胖患者长期手术后。

代谢原因及机制

低血糖可表现为混乱、行为异常、癫痫和昏迷。长期饥饿的患者和使用磺脲类和胰岛素的糖尿病患者特别容易发生低血糖。严重的高血糖也会使昏迷时间延长。低钠血症，特别是急性低钠血症，可导致嗜睡、苏醒延迟和癫痫发作。经尿道前列腺电切术（transurethral resection of the prostrate，TURP）使用大量低渗冲洗液时，尤其容易发生液体过量和低钠血症，导致 TURP 综合征。低钠血症、肺水肿和脑水肿会出现包括昏迷在内的不同的脑体征。用 ABG 测量电解质是确诊的最快方法。如果患者出现癫痫和昏迷，可能需要加强复苏和管理，包括插管、通气和心血管支持。在血清钠达到 130 mmol/L 之前，应缓慢调整使血清钠每小时升高不超过 2 mmol/L。在恢复期，也有可能出现高钠血症、尿毒症或昏迷加重。体温过低很常见，特别是在幼儿或老人以及长时间的手术之后。体温过低除了会减缓大脑活动外，还会减缓药物的代谢，导致药物作用时间延长，并在麻醉后发生苏醒延迟。许多患者低温和酸中毒会同时发生，这是由于酸中毒患者蛋白质结合减少而增强了芬太尼等药物的作用。多种原因造成的呼吸衰竭会导致低氧血症和高碳酸血症，导致无意识状态出现恶性循环，从而加剧呼吸衰竭。

术中心律失常、低血压或高血压都可导致颅内出血、血栓形成、脑梗死，尤其是脑血管病患者。局部麻醉药从硬膜外阻滞或星状神经节阻滞等部位扩散会导致意识丧失。

5.8% 的术后谵妄患者发生在冠状动脉旁路移植术后，而在接受急诊肿瘤手术的患者中发生率高达 28%。谵妄的表现多种多样，从抑制型到兴奋型不等。抑制型可能容易与麻醉药物的残余作用相混淆。

不常见原因

5- 羟色胺综合征通常发生在 2 种或 2 种以上的 5- 羟色胺能类药物同时给予时，表现为神经肌肉异常、自主神经活动亢进和精神状态改变三联征，临床表现可以是轻微到严重。抗帕金森药物（左旋多巴）和抗抑郁药例如选择性 5- 羟色胺再摄取抑制剂、选择性去甲肾上腺素再摄取抑制剂、三环抗抑郁药、单胺氧化酶抑制剂，都会增加 5- 羟色胺的水平。

中枢抗胆碱能综合征（central anticholinergic syndrome，CAS）虽然比过去发生少得多，但可能表现为脑刺激、躁动、木僵。阿托品、三环抗抑郁药（阿米替林）和抗精神病药（氯丙嗪）可诱发 CAS。一般对毒扁豆碱反应较好。

预防

对于出现苏醒延迟或声称以前有过苏醒延迟的患者的麻醉

- 询问患者的详细病史，包括患者是否需要非计划入院或入 ICU 治疗；
- 了解之前手术的麻醉和临床记录；
- 询问患者或查看患者相关的检查结果、专家意见；
- 回顾有无使用拮抗剂，如氟马西尼、纳洛酮或毒扁豆碱；
- 了解患者目前服用的药物的相互作用。

麻醉方案

- 对于拟行手术，如可能可考虑局部 / 区域麻醉；

- 避免术前应用镇静剂；
- 使用短效麻醉药；
- 根据年龄调整 MAC；
- 在病态肥胖患者中，使用调整后的公式，如理想体重（IBW）+40% 额外体重用于靶控输注丙泊酚。如有疑问，应滴定药物以达到效果并进行监测；
- 用 Broca 公式计算理想体重（IBW）：男性，（身高 cm−100）；女性，（身高 cm−105）。
- 使用麻醉深度监测，如脑电双频指数和熵。

关于病例的讨论

病例 1

该患者过去从未接受过全身麻醉，有保护性气道反射，呼吸频率为 8 ～ 10 次 / 分，对疼痛刺激有反应，瞳孔反应虽弱但有反应。患者血糖正常。对阿片类药物敏感是该患者苏醒延迟的原因。尽管考虑使用纳洛酮，但因为患者氧饱和度正常并且接受较为疼痛的大手术，所以决定未予注射纳洛酮。约在 PACU 停留 40 min 后，患者开始对语言刺激做出反应，但仍处于嗜睡状态约 1 h，2 h 后患者被送回病房。

病例 2

严格来说这并不是苏醒延迟，这个病例主要是 PACU 内由于肌松残余而导致的呼吸衰竭。该患者拔管后在给予纯氧，持续的气道正压和重复剂量的新斯的明后，情况继续恶化，正准备重新插管时，该患者被高度怀疑有肌松残余，所以决定给予舒更葡糖，此举迅速逆转肌松残余，改善了呼吸衰竭。

病例 3

在 PACU 的评估中，患者的 GCS 评分表明对疼痛刺激没有反应，右瞳孔扩张，对光反射消失，血糖正常，国际标准化比值为 1.4。对其进行气管插管和通气，其头颅 CT 显示急性慢性硬膜下血肿，患者随后被转移到神经外科中心进行硬膜下血肿清除术。

（张莹莹 译 刘 征 校）

延伸阅读

Brown DV, Heller F, Barkin R: Anticholinergic syndrome after anesthesia: a case report and review, *Am J Ther* 11:144–153, 2004.

Desikan SR, Khan M: Use of Sugammadex in post-extubation respiratory failure in a patient already reversed with neostigmine and glycopyrronium, *Acta Anaesthesiol Scand* 59(Suppl 121):47, 2015.

Krenk L, Rasmussen LS, Hansen TB, et al.: Delirium after fast tract hip and knee arthroplasty, *Br J Anaesth* 114:194–203, 2012.

Miller LG: Herbal medicinals. Selected clinical considerations focussing on known or potential drug-herb interactions, *Arch Intern Med* 158: 2200–2211, 1998.

Nakkahira J, Sawai T, Fujiwara A, et al.: Trans-urethral resection syndrome in elderly patients. A retrospective observational study, *BMC Anesthesiol* 14:30–35, 2014.

Raduege KM, Kleshinski JF, Ryckman JV, et al.: Anesthetic considerations of herbal kava, *J Clin Anesth* 16:305–311, 2004.

Sinclair RFC, Faleiro RJ: Delayed recovery of consciousness after anaesthesia, *Cont Educ Anaesth Crit Care Pain* 6:114–118, 2006.

Tzabaziz A, Miller C, Dobrow MF, et al.: Delayed emergence after anesthesia, *J Clin Anesth* 27:353–360, 2015.

Wilson L, Rooney T, Baugh RF, et al.: Recognition and management of perioperative serotonin syndrome, *Am J Otolaryngol* 33:319–321, 2012.

牙齿损伤

第 138 章

Myrna C. Newland

病例概要

患者，女性，54 岁，拟全身麻醉行腹腔镜下胆囊切除术。术前查体提示颈部较短，体重指数 32，麦氏评分（Mallampati score）Ⅲ级。牙科检查可见多处龋齿，磨牙多处牙冠修复，上切牙突出。患者被告之此前有“困难气管插管”史。全身麻醉下应用可视喉镜进行气管插管，插管成功且无牙齿损伤。

问题分析

定义

全身麻醉下气管插管导致的牙齿损伤，被认为是与麻醉相关的最常见并发症之一，也是医疗投诉的来源之一。患者牙列在围术期的任何（可能需要或不需要牙科干预治疗的）显著变化被称为**牙齿损伤**。1986 年，Lockhart 等对美国各麻醉培训项目负责人展开调研，评估麻醉过程中牙齿损伤情况。据估计，约 100 万例麻醉操作中，牙齿损伤发生率为 1/1000。1999 年，梅奥诊所 Warner 等研究发现，牙齿损伤在全身麻醉下气管插管患者中的发生率为 1/2805，而 285 000 例区域麻醉或麻醉监护病例中未发现牙齿损伤。

我们分析了内布拉斯加大学医学中心数据库 14 年共 161 687 例麻醉相关不良事件中所有围麻醉期牙齿损伤病例，发现 78 例牙齿损伤，发生率为 1/2073。2012 年，美国外科医师学会（American College of Surgeons，ACS）发布 2005—2008 年重大外科手术患者上呼吸道损伤流行病学调查，同年发布美国外科质量改进计划（National Surgical Quality Improvement Program，NSQIP）报告。一项前瞻性研究收集 251 家医院接受重大外科手术的全身麻醉患者数据，563 190 例患者中发生气道损伤 1202 例。气道损伤的独立危险因素为困难气道和高龄。最常见的气道损伤为唇部撕裂伤 / 血肿，其次为牙齿损伤。牙齿损伤可能发生在手术室外。2011 年，一项针对手术室外紧急气道控制的研究显示，3423 例急救患者有呼吸道相关并发症者共 144 例，其中牙齿损伤 6 例，发生率为 1/570；10% 的患者出现插管困难，出现插管并发症的预测因素包括，≥ 3 次尝试插管、急诊室插管、Ⅲ或Ⅳ级声门显露和普通病房插管。气管插管的主要原因为，患者出现呼吸窘迫或心搏骤停。

质控分析与结案索赔

Vallejo 等对一大型医学院附属研究机构（包括社区初级、专科三级和四级医疗中心）8 年共 816 690 例麻醉质量保险资料进行统计，发现牙齿损伤是患者投诉并需要医学鉴定的气道并发症中最常见原因，发生牙齿外伤 360 例。全身麻醉患者牙齿损伤发生率为 1/1754。儿童患者发生率低得多，为 1/7692。牙齿损伤的主要危险因素是对既往牙列不良患者进行全麻插管操作。

2007—2012 年期间，一家名为 Doctors Company 大型医疗事故保险公司对麻醉科患者术中伤害进行分析，发现共有 607 起索赔。最常见索赔原因为牙齿损伤（20.8%）和死亡（18.3%）。牙齿损伤多数与气管插管或拔管等操作有关。插管困难和牙齿状况差是牙齿损伤的常见原因。牙冠折断和种植牙脱落，牙齿贴面脱落，有时需要胃镜、气管镜等取出被吞咽或吸入的脱落牙齿、牙冠或牙桥。多数案例因术前没有对牙齿或口腔矫治状况进行评估与记录。此类案件对牙齿损伤的平均赔偿为 6174 美元。

识别

牙齿损伤可能发生在手术室、麻醉后（恢复室）苏醒室、重症监护病房或医院其他地方，可能由患者、护士或麻醉从业人员发现。牙齿损伤及其定义包括以下内容：

- 釉质断裂：牙釉质刮痕或缺口；
- 半脱位：牙齿支持结构损伤，伴有异常松动，但牙齿无移位；
- 脱臼：牙齿从牙槽中部分移位；
- 撕脱：牙齿从牙槽内完全移位；
- 牙折：牙冠单独折裂或牙冠和牙根同时折裂；
- 其他损伤：烤瓷牙、种植牙、人工牙冠、固定局部义齿（桥）损坏和贴片脱落。

牙齿损伤的危险因素有，全身麻醉下气管插管、牙列不良、喉镜检查与插管困难。最常受伤的牙齿是上颌切牙。乳牙易松动脱落，导致儿童牙齿损伤风险增加。Tan 等对一家三级儿科中心 80 811 例全身麻醉患儿病例的回顾性分析发现，过去 12 年间共发生 2 ～ 15 岁患儿牙齿损伤 42 例，其中 69% 损伤发生于 5 ～ 8 岁儿童。全身麻醉患儿牙齿损伤的发生率为 1/1924。62% 牙齿损伤发生于牙科病史不准确的患儿。2 名患儿需要多次麻醉下拔牙与牙齿修复。

管理

牙科损伤通常由麻醉从业人员在操作时发现。在研究中，82% 的病例存在牙列不良或牙齿重建的情况，86% 的牙齿损伤是麻醉从业人员在手术室（68%）或术后监护病房（14%）发现的。术前牙列不良或牙齿重建的患者和插管困难患者，比容易插管患者发生牙齿损伤的风险高 20 倍。图 138.1 显示了从右上颌磨牙开始的牙齿编号。在研究中，每个牙齿损伤都通过图片中数字记录。侧面文字提示插管导致损伤的相对风险。最常受伤的牙齿是上颌切牙。口腔和牙齿检查应在气管插管完成后进行，也应在气管拔管后再次进行。

- 任何牙齿损伤都应记录在病历中；
- 任何脱落或断裂的牙齿或器具都应收回并查找原因；
- 任何从牙槽脱出的恒牙都应保存在生理盐水或冷却鲜牛奶中，直至可被固定或重新种植；

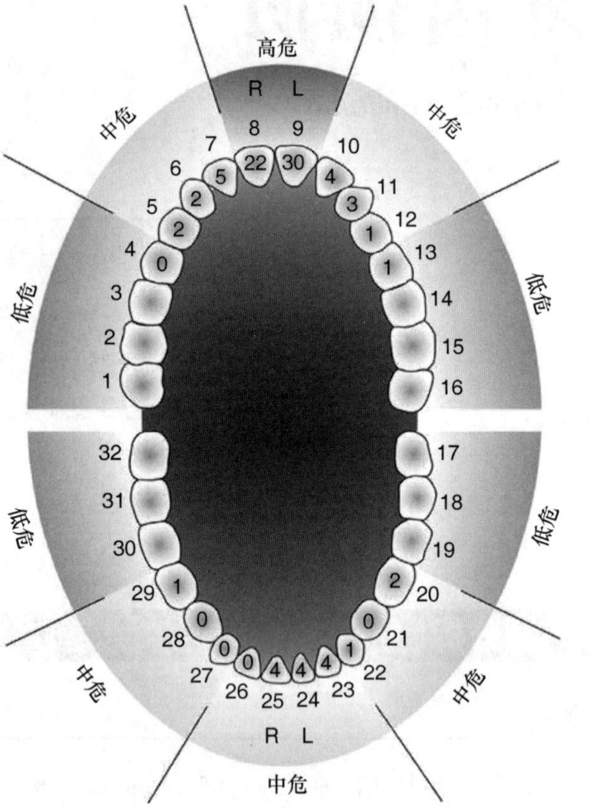

图 138.1 图中牙齿外的数字表示从右上颌磨牙开始的牙齿编号方法。图中个别牙齿内的数字标记了 Newland 等研究中发现损伤的牙齿数量。左上颌中切牙（9 号牙）损伤人数最多（30 人）。8 号牙齿次之（22 人）。这两枚上颌切牙均处于气管插管牙齿损伤的高风险区域（From Newland MC，Ellis SJ，Peters KR，et al.：Dental injury associated with anesthesia：a report of 161，687 anesthetics given over 14 years. *J Clin Anesth* 19[5]：339-345，2007.）

- 如果考虑牙齿再植，应尽早咨询牙科医师；
- 必要时行颈部、胸部或腹部 X 片确定脱落牙齿或植入物位置；
- 误吸入牙齿或牙齿碎片属于麻醉严重并发症，如未及时发现可能导致肺部并发症如肺炎等；
- 应在患者完全清醒后与患者或家属进行讨论；
- 对于不太严重的损伤，如牙釉质骨折，应在患者出院前考虑进行牙科会诊。

预防

Yasny 的一篇关于麻醉科医师围术期保护患者牙齿的综述强烈建议术前应评估患者气道和牙齿。部分患者存在牙齿松动或缺失、多发性龋齿和牙周病等慢性病。在某些情况下，有必要请牙科医师术前会诊。上颌切牙是气管插管时最常损伤的牙齿。

如果用黏结、贴面或牙冠修复，则不如天然牙坚固，更容易发生损伤。松动牙齿容易脱落。病历文书应包括术前牙科评估结果和特定牙齿的风险标记。术前应与患者讨论可能的牙齿损伤，并将讨论内容记录入病例。医师应在术前评估表中的牙科图表上，识别易损牙齿、贴面、种植体或其他矫治器。麻醉从业人员应熟悉美国成人（永久性）牙列的通用编号方法。成人牙列包括上下颌共 32 颗牙齿。从上颌右象限第三磨牙（1 号）开始，牙齿编号从 1 到 32（见图 138.1）。上颌正中切牙右侧标为 8 号，左侧标为 9 号。9 号牙齿是气管插管时最常受伤的牙齿，可能是插管时直接接触喉镜片。儿童最多有 20 颗乳牙。

应考虑处理可能的困难插管的预案。除术前检查患者牙列并在病历中记录外，应识别出所有可能出现插管困难的患者。Aziz 等发现一种可视喉镜相当有效，并有效应用于 71 570 次插管中的 2004 例困难插管中。困难气管插管的常见预测因素有：麦氏评分Ⅲ / Ⅳ级，甲颏距 <6 cm，张口度 <3 cm，颈部病理性包块、手术瘢痕增生或颈部放疗后，颈部肥胖，颈椎活动受限。97% 的病例使用可视喉镜气管插管成功。2004 例患者中有 21 例发生并发症，大多数是轻微的软组织损伤，但仍有 6 种主要并发症，包括声带损伤、气管损伤、下咽外伤、扁桃体贯通伤和两类牙齿损伤（牙齿脱落和既往牙齿脱落史）。

临床上无法预防所有与麻醉相关的牙齿损伤，但可提前干预以将其发生率降至最低。术前对每例患者的牙列进行彻底评估与明确危险因素很有必要。正确的文书记录，与患者的沟通以及与牙科医师的会诊，将在很大程度上减少牙齿损伤的发生率，并减轻由此造成的后果。

（王丽珍　译　吴　倩　校）

延伸阅读

Aziz MF, Healy D, Kheterpal S, et al.: Routine clinical practice effectiveness of the Glidescope in difficult airway management: an analysis of 2,004 Glidescope intubations, complications, and failures from two institutions, *Anesthesiology* 114:34–41, 2011.

Hua M, Brady J, Li G: The epidemiology of upper airway injury in patients undergoing major surgical procedures, *Anesth Analg* 114:148–151, 2012.

Lockhart PB, Feldbau EV, Gabel RA, et al.: Dental complications during and after tracheal intubation, *J Am Dent Assoc* 112:480–483, 1986.

Martin LD, Mhyre JM, Shanks AM, et al.: 3,423 emergency tracheal intubations at a university hospital: airway outcomes and complications, *Anesthesiology* 114:42–48, 2011.

Newland MC, Ellis SJ, Peters KR, et al.: Dental injury associated with anesthesia: a report of 161,687 anesthetics given over 14 years, *J Clin Anesth* 19:339–345, 2007.

Ranum D, Ma H, Shapiro FE, et al.: Analysis of patient injury based on anesthesiology closed claims data from a major malpractice insurer, *J Healthc Risk Manag* 34:31–42, 2014.

Tan TYS, Lim SL, Teo PF, et al.: Peri-anaesthetic dental injury in children: a retrospective audit in a tertiary paediatric centre, *Proc Singapore Healthc* 24:80–85, 2015.

Vallejo MC, Best MW, Phelps AL, et al.: Perioperative dental injury at a tertiary care health system: an eight-year audit of 816,690 anesthetics, *J Healthc Risk Manag* 31:25–32, 2012.

Warner ME, Benenfeld SM, Warner MA, et al.: Perianesthetic dental injuries: frequency, outcomes, and risk factors, *Anesthesiology* 90: 1302–1305, 1999.

Yasny JS: Perioperative dental considerations for the anesthesiologist, *Anesth Analg* 108:1564–1573, 2009.

第 139 章 困难气道和拔管失败

Mohammad El-Orbany

病例概要

患者，男性，肥胖，体重指数 40，从树上坠落造成头部闭合性损伤、肺挫裂伤和颈椎损伤。院前急救人员在现场对患者行气管插管，随后送往医院治疗。3 天后，患者神经功能和呼吸恢复良好（但是带有颈托），达到拔管标准后拔除气管导管。患者立即出现严重呼吸困难，氧饱和度（SpO_2）开始下降，面罩通气失败。患者意识消失时，医师取下颈托并固定头部，随后进行使用喉镜查看，无法看到喉部任何结构。

问题分析

定义

拔管失败

拔管失败是因气道阻塞或通气不足导致患者气管导管拔除后无法维持呼吸。如果缺乏正确及时的处理，会最终导致患者 SpO_2 下降，低氧血症和呼吸衰竭，常常需要立即重新插管，直至病因得到治疗，患者可耐受拔管。重新插管困难或插管失败可能会造成危急情况。美国麻醉科医师协会（American Society of Anesthesiologists，ASA）困难气道管理工作组建议，对可能有拔管失败风险且已知有困难气道的患者应预先制订拔管策略。该指南建议采用“分阶段拔管”策略，建议使用气道装置作为完全拔管的“桥梁”，在需要重新插管时可确保气道连续。

困难气道

困难气道是指接受常规培训的麻醉科医师在面罩通气（facemask ventilation，FMV）或气管插管时遇到困难的临床情况。部分面罩通气困难的患者可能会插管相对容易，反之亦然。框 139.1 列举了气道管理失败的常见原因。

面罩通气困难

独立操作的麻醉科医师在正压通气时不能维持患者 SpO_2 氧饱和度大于 90%（吸入氧浓度为 100%）或通气努力不能阻止或逆转气体交换不足的迹象，则认为发生 FMV 困难。面罩密封不严、气体泄漏过多或气道出入的阻力太大均可造成 FMV 困难。框 139.2 列举了面罩通气困难的征象。

喉镜暴露困难和插管困难

喉镜暴露困难是指使用传统硬质喉镜多次尝试

框 139.1　气道管理失败的潜在原因

- 术前气道评估不准确或不完整
- 预测失败：
  - 面罩通气容易 / 困难
  - 直接喉镜检查和气管插管容易 / 困难
  - 拔管高风险
- 不愿放弃失败的气道管理计划
- 困难气道初次出现时未能尽早寻求帮助
- 备份计划准备不全
- 压力下的操作失败
- 判断错误

框 139.2　面罩通气不足的迹象

- 胸廓运动不足或无运动
- 呼吸音消失或减轻
- 听见气道梗阻的声音，胃内气体吸入或胃扩张
- 氧饱和度下降（晚期）
- 发绀（晚期）
- 呼气末二氧化碳消失、不足或升高
- 呼出气体消失或减少（肺量计测定）
- 高碳酸血症或低氧血症对血流动力学的影响（如心动过速、高血压、心律失常）——发生于后期，不应等到出现这些症状才诊断为面罩通气不足

仍无法看到声门任何部分，需要多次尝试才成功插管称为困难插管，而插管失败是多次尝试也无法置入气管导管。喉镜暴露困难（尝试 2 次以上）的发生率为 0.5% ～ 2%。首次尝试时就应该维持足够的麻醉深度、肌肉松弛、头颈位置合适，必要时进行喉外部按压。更换喉镜片有时可以改善视野，直喉镜片有时有助于暴露喉“前部”，视频喉镜可提供更佳的声门视野。直接喉镜检查不应超过 2 或 3 次，反复尝试可能对患者结局不利（如能够通气转为无法通气，或诱发喉头水肿而导致拔管后声门梗阻）。在多次尝试插管间期进行 FMV，如果 SpO_2 降至 90% ～ 92% 以下，则必须中止喉镜检查（优先保持氧合）。应该让最有经验的麻醉科医师最后一次使用直接喉镜暴露操作。

识别和风险评估

在制订气道管理计划时，回顾患者的麻醉史和气道管理史记录（如果存在）十分重要。对所有患者（包括紧急情况和监护麻醉）均应进行麻醉前气道评估，找出潜在困难气道的预测因素。框 139.3 列举了 FMV 困难的预测因素以及处理建议。喉罩可使大多数 FMV 困难患者维持足够的通气量，因此遇到此类情况时应尽早使用喉罩。框 139.4 列出了喉镜暴露困难相关的预测因素。虽然气道评估的敏感性低且变化幅度大，特异性也不强，但是气道评估的阳性发现，尤其是综合多方面评估的结果，对喉镜暴露 / 插管困难有提示作用。例如，Mallampati 分级高于Ⅱ级，结合其他气道评估结果，提示使用传统硬质喉镜可能会出现喉镜暴露困难。

麻醉科医师须准确记录 FMV 的难易程度、喉镜暴露次数和镜片型号、获得的喉镜下视野情况，最终如何成功插管以及使用的任何特殊操作方法或装置。

FMV 和插管困难，以及其他术前一般情况和术中特殊事件，均提示可能出现拔管困难 / 失败。困难气道患者应符合常规的拔管标准并完全清醒。此类患者在气管导管套囊放气时还应该能够咳嗽和发声。框 139.5 列举了拔管困难 / 失败的预测因素。

对于拔管失败风险高的患者，应在麻醉诱导前制订拔管策略。框 139.6 列出制订拔管策略时需考虑的因素。

框 139.3 面罩通气困难相关的预测因素和患者因素及建议的解决方案

胡须

将塑料膜（嘴和鼻孔开口）粘在面部毛发上，从而获得更好的密封性

尽早放置口（鼻）咽通气道腔或喉罩气道

缺齿

在喉镜操作前，可考虑保留假牙在原位以改善面罩密封性

早期放置喉罩

体重指数 >30

给患者持续气道正压预充氧，反 Trendelenburg 体位 20° ～ 30°，从而增加患者呼吸暂停后或面罩通气困难的耐受时间，反 Trendelenburg 体位可减轻膈肌压力，增加肺顺应性

尽早使用喉罩进行正压通气

打鼾和阻塞性睡眠呼吸暂停

尽早放置口（鼻）咽通气道或喉罩气道

年龄 >55 岁

吸烟史

声门上、声门和声门下病变或喘鸣

强烈建议清醒下气道管理

如果存在喘鸣，避免镇静

支气管痉挛（痉挛活动期或有痉挛风险）

诱导前使用支气管扩张剂雾化吸入

管理

一旦确认“无法通气，不能插管”（cannot ventilate，cannot intubate，CVCI）的情况，必须迅速而果断地进行处理。紧急气道管理包括以下内容。

紧急无创气道通气

根据 ASA 困难气道管理指南，如果初次尝试插管失败且面罩通气不足，如果有条件则应考虑使用声门上气道装置（supraglottic airway device，SAD）。除非气道阻塞部位在声门、声门下或 SAD 位置不当，大多数情况下 SAD 均可充分通气。以下重点介绍 CVCI 情况下最常用的声门上气道急救装置。

喉罩（LMA Classic 或 Unique）可作为通气装置和（或）插管时的引导管。随着喉罩的广泛应用，由 CVCI 引起的病残率和死亡率明显下降，目前已将喉罩纳入 ASA 困难气道管理流程。

喉罩的使用有如下限制：

框 139.4 直接喉镜暴露困难和气管插管困难的预测因素

门齿间距

如果上下门齿间距小于 3 ～ 4 cm，直接喉镜暴露可能发生困难，原因如下：

在不损伤牙齿的前提下，喉镜片置入和“牵引”的空间不足

气管导管置入的空间不足，方向不当

到声门开口的视线受阻

上门齿长度

直接喉镜暴露检查时，切牙过长可阻碍经口轴线和经咽轴线对齐

相对长且突出的上门齿增加插管难度

Mallampati 口咽分级

Mallampati Ⅰ级或Ⅱ级，直接喉镜检查时，舌头应较容易从轴线回缩

Mallampati 分级 > Ⅱ级，插管难度增加

下颌空间

由于舌颏间距以及甲颏间距（可评估下颌空间）分别大于 6 cm 和 7 cm，因此喉镜检查时应将喉头尽量后移，保持良好视线

间距 <3 指（5 cm）时插管难度增加

颈部长度和厚度

直接喉镜检查时，短而粗的颈部不利于上气道各轴线对齐

对于肥胖患者，长颈围和 Mallampati 分级 > Ⅱ级，插管难度增加

头颈部活动范围

寰枕关节伸展或颈部屈曲 <35° 提示喉镜暴露困难；寰枕关节伸展和颈部屈曲对口、咽和喉轴线对齐十分重要

肥胖可能影响口、咽和喉轴线对齐

头、颈和肩部抬高（“堆叠”），使下巴与胸骨齐平有利于肥胖患者进行直接喉镜检查；在正确的定位下，还需纤维支气管镜辅助插管

Mallampati 分级高和颈围大是肥胖患者插管困难的可靠预测指标

下巴不能触碰到胸部时插管难度增加

上颌-下颌咬合困难（龅牙）

直接喉镜检查时，龅牙不利于口腔和咽轴线对齐

下颌移动

下颌能前伸 1 cm 通常提示喉镜直视良好

下门齿可接触到上唇皮肤提示喉镜检查容易

下颌空间顺应性

不利因素包括僵硬、硬结和出现肿块

上颚形态

狭窄或高拱的上腭减少口咽容量，不利于喉镜片和气管导管在口腔的可视化

框 139.5 气管拔管高风险预测因素

1. 气道危险因素

a. 预先存在的困难气道：
 - 面罩通气或插管困难发生史
 - 阻塞性睡眠呼吸暂停
 - 颈部瘢痕、肿块、挛缩或烧伤
 - 颈部手术和放射治疗史
 - 颌面部损伤
 - 颈深部或咽部感染

b. 围术期气道病情恶化：
 - 甲状腺手术后血肿或声带功能障碍
 - 颈前路或颈后路手术（颈椎或颈动脉内膜切除手术）后出现水肿或出血
 - 气管插管或手术造成的气道水肿或损伤
 - 声带和咽喉部手术
 - 悬雍垂腭咽成形术

C. 气道入路受限：
 - Halo 架固定
 - 上-下颌固定
 - 颈椎融合

2. 一般危险因素

a. 呼吸功能受损：阻塞性睡眠呼吸暂停，喉功能不全或声带功能障碍，膈肌固定，喉返神经麻痹

b. 心血管不稳定或失血过多时大量液体复苏

c. 神经系统疾病：可能影响咽部肌肉或声带功能（如帕金森、脑卒中和脱髓鞘）

d. 神经肌肉疾病：先前存在的神经肌肉疾病，残余的神经肌肉阻滞

e. 低体温：可能影响神经肌肉功能，延长药物作用时间，引起的寒战可增加氧耗

f. 电解质酸碱平衡紊乱：影响神经肌肉功能并延长神经肌肉阻滞药物的作用时间

g. 类风湿性关节炎：可影响颈椎、颞下颌关节和环杓关节，限制张口度和颈部活动度

- 喉罩是一种声门上装置，声门或声门下病变时可能无效（如同任何其他 SAD）；
- 不能防止胃内容物反流误吸；
- 正压通气时可能发生胃扩张；
- 对需正压通气的肺顺应性差的患者，可能无法有效密封气道；
- 张口受限或下颌钢丝结扎牵引（除非紧急时剪断钢丝）的患者应用受限。

插管型喉罩（intubating LMA，ILMA）能维持通气并有助于气管内盲探插管（以及光纤辅助）。

当胃扩张或反流是主要问题而又需保持通气时（如产科患者出现 CVCI），LMA Supreme（或 LMA

框 139.6　制定拔管策略时需考虑的因素

清醒拔管对比意识恢复前拔管的优势
- 是否插管困难？
- 是否面罩通气困难？
- 是否误吸风险高？

上呼吸道水肿或出血可能对拔管后的有效通气产生不利影响
- 颈部手术后出血、组织水肿或神经损伤可导致气道阻塞
- 近期颈部感染或放疗导致的水肿风险升高

对气管周围、喉部和声门上结构直接或间接损伤
- 手术期间的操作增加气道阻塞的可能性
- 喉镜暴露困难或多次喉镜检查后可发生水肿，但在拔管后才表现明显

喉返神经损伤

患者拔管后无法维持足量的通气，则按预先制订的气道管理计划实施干预

拔管时使用气道交换导管
- 气道交换导管可用于快速重新插管
- 若交换导管有内腔可用于通气

使用纤维支气管镜穿过气管导管辅助拔管
- 必要时重新推进气管内导管
- 缓慢退出支气管镜时可以检查气管、声门和声门上结构是否异常
- 如果发现气道明显异常，可以停止退出支气管镜查
- 再次推进支气管镜进入气管，随后经支气管镜置入套在其上的气管导管
- 可以在纤维支气管镜逐步退出前通过抽吸通道插入导丝，通过导丝引导再次插管或作为气体交换导管置入气道。

ProSeal）喉罩的作用尤其明显。此类喉罩在作为引导管辅助纤维支气管镜检查（因为管腔较小）方面不如传统喉罩或 ILMA，但对有反流误吸风险的患者，在危急情况下可以用作紧急通气装置。

Air-Q 喉罩除可通气外，还能辅助气管插管（无论是盲探还是光纤辅助）。

喉管（laryngeal tube，LT）是由通气导管和两个低压球囊组成的一种 SAD。采用盲法从口腔插入，远处盲端置于食管上段。远端（食管）球囊密封气道防止反流，近端（咽）球囊密封上咽部防止气体泄漏。两个套囊通过同一个端口充气，通气端口位于两个套囊之间。也可以采用“交换技术”通过 LT 进行光纤引导气管插管。最近有产品增加第二个管腔，用于抽吸“饱胃”患者胃内容物。

LMA CTrach 类似于插管型喉罩，但其尖端配有摄像头，手柄上有一个小型显示屏，用于显示喉部图像，可通过间接可视化辅助通气和气管插管。

建立紧急有创气道

如果不能通过 SAD 建立人工气道（例如，无法放置 SAD，SAD 位置不当伴有漏气，声门或声门下阻塞）则可能迅速发生严重低氧血症，需立即使用侵入性手段进行干预（尤其是伴有心动过缓时）。根据 ASA 困难气道管理流程，可通过手术或经皮环甲膜切开、喷射通气或逆行插管来建立紧急有创气道。环甲膜是声门下最容易进入气道的部位，当其他所有措施都失败时，环甲膜切开可在 CVCI 情况下挽救生命。将装有 3 ml 生理盐水的 5 ml 注射器连接到 14 G 静脉导管上即可进行环甲膜穿刺。将静脉导管刺入环甲膜直到能抽出空气，取下此注射器，将一个不带活塞的 3 ml 注射器连接到静脉导管尾端，并将 7.0 气管导管的接头连接到注射器，然后连接自充气呼吸皮囊或麻醉呼吸回路（图 139.1）。也可以通过静脉导管施行经气管喷射通气，此时必

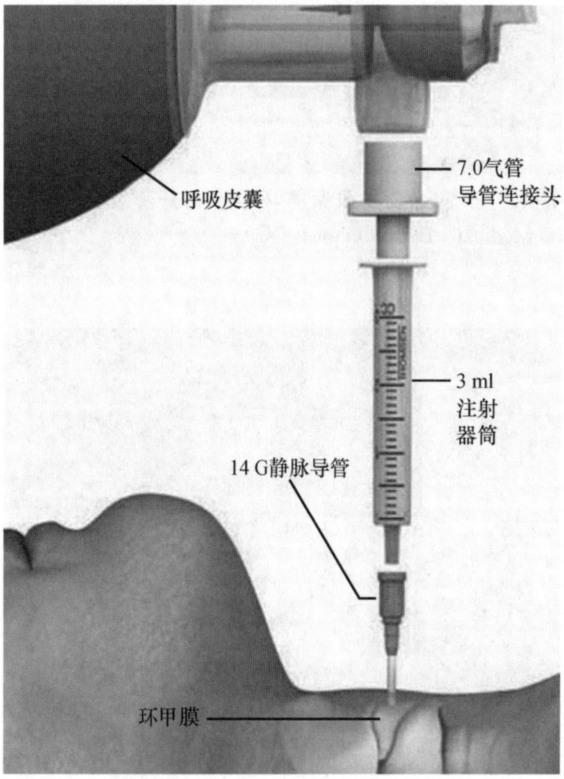

图 139.1　环甲膜穿刺术。在环甲膜上刺入 14 G 静脉导管直到吸出空气并将导管穿入气管腔。然后将导管连接到 3 ml 注射器筒（预先与 7.0 气管导管接头组装在一起）。可以通过使用呼吸皮囊（如图所示）或麻醉机的呼吸回路实现紧急通气

须正确固定静脉导管。如果导管移位可能造成肺气肿，将使病情更复杂。还应允许患者有呼气时间以避免气压伤。一旦氧合改善并且危急情况结束，应该寻求更明确的气道建立方法。也可使用任何市售的经皮扩张环甲膜切开包（percutaneous dilational cricothyrotomy，PDC）进行紧急环甲膜切开术（图 139.2）。经皮扩张环甲膜切开是一种快速、相对简单的手术，与环甲膜切开手术相比，其操作时间短，并发症发生率低。经验丰富的医师可在约 30 s 内使用切开包开展简化的环甲膜切开术（包括触诊、切开和置管）。在尝试对拔管风险高的患者进行气管拔管之前，确保能实施环甲膜切开术的有经验的帮手非常重要。紧急环甲膜切开术是一种临时措施，可以恢复氧合并使患者度过危机。一旦患者病情稳定，应该建立明确气道，例如手术气管切开或尝试其他的气管插管方法。

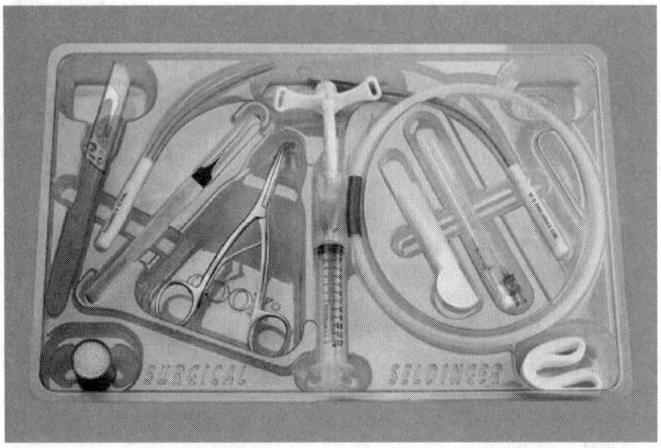

图 139.2 市售经皮扩张紧急环甲膜切开套装包（Courtesy Cook Medical，Bloomington，IN.）

预防

气管拔管是麻醉管理的高风险阶段。根据 ASA 的结案索赔分析：诱导期间气道管理困难导致的死亡和永久性神经损伤的发生率显著下降，而这些严重并发症的发生率在其他麻醉阶段几乎不变，包括拔管和麻醉恢复阶段。在麻醉诱导前应该采取明确的策略（尤其是对困难气道患者）降低拔管相关的发病率和死亡率。第一步是鉴别拔管失败高风险且可能难以重新插管的患者。根据 ASA 困难气道管理工作组和英国困难气道指南的建议，应提前制订分步拔管策略，气管拔管后应在气道中留置气道装置以保证在需要重新插管时保证气道通畅并辅助气管插管。气道交换导管（图 139.3）、纤维支气管镜下拔管或拔管前在气管导管后面插入一个喉罩（图 139.4）（Bailey 技术）可达此目的。框 139.7 和 139.8 简述了英国困难气道学会推荐的高风险拔管情况下，使用气道交换导管和喉罩作为桥接装置的步骤。

“桥接”装置需保留到拔管失败和需要重新插管的风险消失，觉得安全后方可移除桥接装置。通过气道交换导管、支气管镜或喉罩管腔进行抢救性再次插管的成功率高，这是一种可避免患者在气管拔

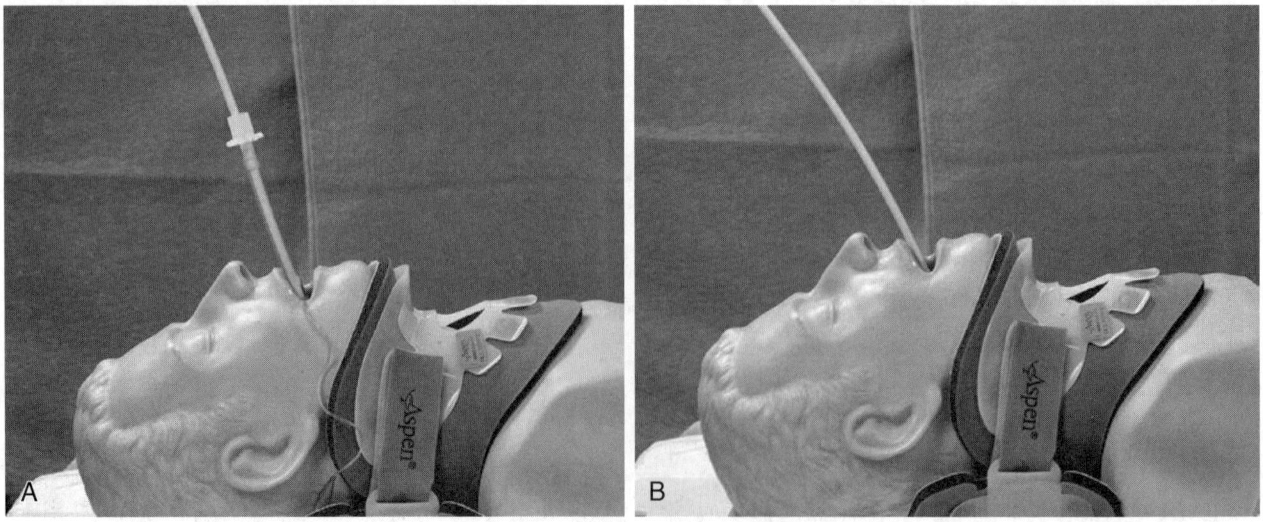

图 139.3 有拔管失败风险的困难气道患者使用气道交换导管作为桥接进行气管拔管。图 A，通过已有的气管导管置入气道交换导管。**图 B，**移除气管导管，并且将气道交换导管固定在原位不动，作为连续气道进入装置，以防需要重新插管

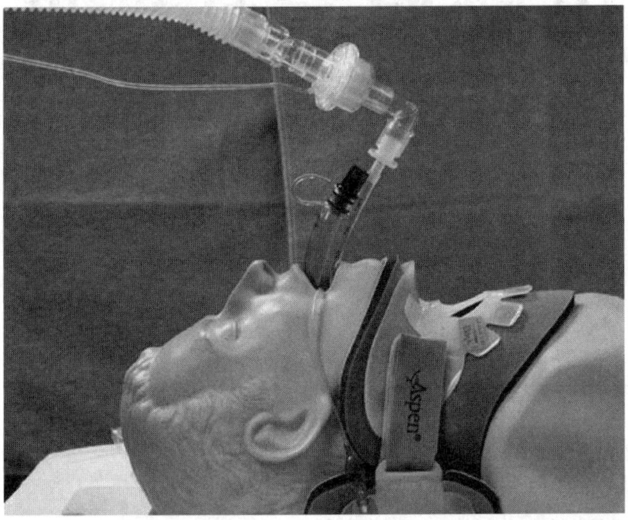

图 139.4 在有拔管失败风险的困难气道患者中使用喉罩作为气管拔管的桥接。在已有的气管导管后面插入喉罩（Bailey 技术），然后拔除气管导管，通过喉罩维持气道通气

框 139.7 使用气道交换导管进行“高风险”拔管的操作顺序

1. 确定气道交换导管（airway exchange catheter，AEC）的置入深度，将导管远端保持在隆突上方至关重要。如果对尖端位置有任何不确定，应在 AEC 插入前用纤维支气管镜检查隆突的相对位置。成年患者 AEC 置入不超过 25 cm
2. 当准备给患者拔管时，将润滑的 AEC 通过气管导管置入预定深度。AEC 置入时遇到阻力时则停止深入
3. 拔出气管导管前将咽部分泌物吸尽
4. 保持 AEC 位置不动的同时，移除 AEC 上的气管导管（不要推进 AEC）
5. 用胶带将 AEC 固定于脸颊或前额
6. 记录 AEC 相对牙齿、嘴唇、鼻的深度
7. 用麻醉回路检查 AEC 周围是否有气体漏出
8. 清楚标记 AEC，防止与鼻胃管混淆
9. 患者应在高度依赖或重症治疗病房接受治疗
10. 可以通过面罩、鼻导管或持续气道正压面罩补充氧气
11. 在移除 AEC 之前，患者应禁食
12. 如果 AEC 导致咳嗽，则检查尖端是否在隆突上方并通过 AEC 注射利多卡因
13. 大多数患者仍可咳嗽和发声
14. 当困难气道风险解除时可拔除 AEC，AEC 留置时间可长达 72 h

管后出现 CVCI 而发生事故的严谨做法。最后但同样重要的一点是，在对已知困难气道的患者进行高风险拔管前，应确保可以随时寻求到紧急建立有创气道经验丰富的医师的帮助。

（王昌理 译 薄禄龙 校）

框 139.8 “高风险”拔管时使用喉罩进行气道交换的操作顺序

1. 吸入纯氧
2. 避免气道刺激：深麻醉或神经肌肉阻滞十分重要
3. 直视下进行喉镜检查和吸引
4. 在气管导管后面置入未充气的喉罩
5. 确保喉罩尖端位置正确
6. 给喉罩气囊充气
7. 保持正压通气，将气管导管套囊放气并移除导管
8. 通过喉罩输送氧气
9. 放置牙垫
10. 让患者坐直
11. 让患者从麻醉中不受干扰地苏醒

延伸阅读

Apfelbaum JL, Hagberg CA, Caplan RA, et al.: Practice guidelines for management of the difficult airway: an updated report by the American Society of Anesthesiologists Task Force on Management of the Difficult Airway, *Anesthesiology* 118:251–270, 2013.

Avitsian R, Doyle DJ, Helfand R, et al.: Successful reintubation after cervical spine exposure using an Aintree intubation catheter and a laryngeal mask airway, *J Clin Anesth* 18:224–225, 2006.

Cavallone LF, Vannucci A: Extubation of the difficult airway and extubation failure, *Anesth Analg* 116:368–383, 2013.

Cooper RM: Extubation and changing endotracheal tubes. In Hagberg CA, editor: *Benumof's airway management*, Philadelphia, 2007, Elsevier, pp 1146–1180.

Difficult Airway Society Guidelines Group, Popat M, Michell V, et al.: Difficult Airway Society Guidelines for the management of tracheal extubation, *Anaesthesia* 67:318–340, 2012.

Ellard L, Brown DH, Wong DT: Extubation of a difficult airway after thyroidectomy: use of a flexible bronchoscope via the LMA-classic, *Can J Anesth* 59:53–57, 2012.

El-Orbany M: The use of supraglottic airway device as an extubation bridge for the difficult airway, *Can J Anesth* 61:387–388, 2014.

El-Orbany M, Woehlck HJ: Difficult mask ventilation, *Anesth Analg* 109:1870–1880, 2009.

Heidegger T: Extubation of the difficult airway—an important but neglected topic, *Anaesthesia* 67:213–215, 2012.

Helm M, Gries A, Mutzbauer T: Surgical approach in difficult airway management, *Best Pract Res Clin Anaesthesiol* 19:623–640, 2005.

Kheterpal S, Martin L, Shanks AM, Tremper KK: Prediction and outcomes of impossible mask ventilation: a review of 50,000 anesthetics, *Anesthesiology* 110:891–897, 2009.

Mace SE, Khan N: Needle cricothyrotomy, *Emerg Med Clin North Am* 26:1085–1101, 2008.

Mort TC: Continuous airway access for the difficult extubation: the efficacy of the airway exchange catheter, *Anesth Analg* 105:1357–1362, 2007.

Nair I, Bailey PM: Use of the laryngeal mask for airway maintenance following tracheal extubation, *Anaesthesia* 50:174–175, 1995.

Peterson GN, Domino KB, Caplan RA, et al.: Management of the difficult airway: a closed claims analysis, *Anesthesiology* 103:33–39, 2005.

Tachibana N, Niiyama Y, Yamakage M: Incidence of cannot intubate–cannot ventilate (CICV): results of a 3-year retrospective multicenter clinical study in a network of university hospitals, *J Anesth* 29:326–330, 2015.

Timmermann A: Supraglottic airways in difficult airway management: successes, failures, use and misuse, *Anaesthesia* 66(Suppl 2):45–56, 2011.

Winterhalter M, Kirchhoff K, Gröschel W, et al.: The laryngeal tube for difficult airway management: a prospective investigation in patients with pharyngeal and laryngeal tumours, *Eur J Anaesthesiol* 22: 678–682, 2005.

Wong DT, Mehta A, Tam AD, et al.: A survey of Canadian anesthesiologists' preferences in difficult intubation and "cannot intubate, cannot ventilate" situations, *Can J Anaesth* 61:717–726, 2014.

第 140 章 水电解质紊乱：低钠血症和高钠血症

Brenda G. Fahy，Arturo G. Torres

低钠血症

病例概要 1

患者，男性，68 岁，拟行右侧全膝关节置换术，既往有高血压病、慢性阻塞性肺疾病、慢性肾功能不全、胰岛素依赖型糖尿病等病史。实验室检查如下：血清钠 130 mEq/L；血浆渗透压 260 mOsm/kg；尿钠 35 mEq/L；血糖、血清尿素氮（blood urea nitrogen，BUN）、甲状腺功能及肾上腺功能均正常。患者否认恶心、嗜睡及乏力等。

问题分析

定义

血清钠浓度及重量渗透摩尔浓度与体内水平衡密切相关，水平衡主要通过渴感、抗利尿激素与肾进行调节。水平衡失调表现为血清钠浓度的异常——低钠血症或高钠血症。低钠血症的定义为血清钠浓度低于 135 mEq/L，当血清钠浓度低于 120 mEq/L 时为严重低钠血症。引起低渗性低钠血症的原因见框 140.1，引起非低渗性低钠血症（曾称为假性低钠血症）的原因见框 140.2。

识别

低钠血症的临床表现与严重程度取决于血清钠的浓度和血清钠下降的速度。钠离子理论上无法通过血脑屏障。因此，血清钠浓度的迅速降低会使水进入脑细胞及其他组织细胞，导致脑组织水肿，进而引起颅内压增高。

进入脑细胞的水的量和速度可以解释与低钠血症相关的中枢神经系统（central nervous system，CNS）的症状以及其严重程度。低钠血症相关的中枢神经系统水潴留的早期症状表现为昏睡、乏力和嗜睡。若低钠血症持续或进一步恶化，症状进展可能导致癫痫发作、昏迷、甚至死亡。因此，任何精神症状疾病的鉴别诊断时都应该考虑低钠血症。

框 140.1　引起真性低渗性低钠血症的原因

细胞外液（ECF）减少
- 肾外钠丢失
  - 消化道疾病：呕吐、腹泻
  - 创伤：失血
  - 皮肤：烧伤、出汗
- 肾性失钠
  - 脑耗盐综合征
  - 利尿剂
  - 肾上腺功能不全
  - 肾病

细胞外液体积正常
- 抗利尿激素分泌不适当综合征
- 利尿剂（如噻嗪类）
- 内分泌疾病（肾上腺功能不全和甲状腺功能减退）
- 原发性烦渴症

细胞外液增加
- 充血性心力衰竭
- 肾病综合征
- 肝硬化

低钠血症的诊断根据实验室检查、发病时间和症状。围术期初步评估低钠血症的主要步骤如图 140.1 所示。必须测量血浆渗透压来排除高血糖和其他原因引起的非低渗性低钠血症。血浆渗透压的正

框 140.2 引起非低渗性低钠血症的原因

血浆渗透压正常
高脂血症
高蛋白血症
经尿道前列腺或膀胱肿瘤切除术；宫腔镜检查术
血浆渗透压升高
高血糖
高尿酸血症
甘露醇利尿

From Rose BD：Hypoosmolal states：hyponatremia. In Jeffers JD，Navrozov M，editors：*Clinical physiology of acid-base and electrolyte disorders*. New York，McGraw-Hill，1994，pp 651-694.

常范围是 274 ～ 290 mOsm/kg。血浆渗透压（P_{osm}）的计算公式为：

$$P_{osm}=（2.0\times[Na^{+}]）+ 葡萄糖（mg/dl）/18 +BUN（mg/dl）/2.8$$

下一步是评估症状的严重程度，以确定是否需要进行干预。如果不需要治疗，则应当进行尿液检查。尿渗透压和钠离子浓度可确定肾是否起作用。肾功能对水平衡和抗利尿激素的作用至关重要。

以往的推荐侧重关注早期容量评估。然而，临床上用于评估容量状态的工具并不准确。因此，一

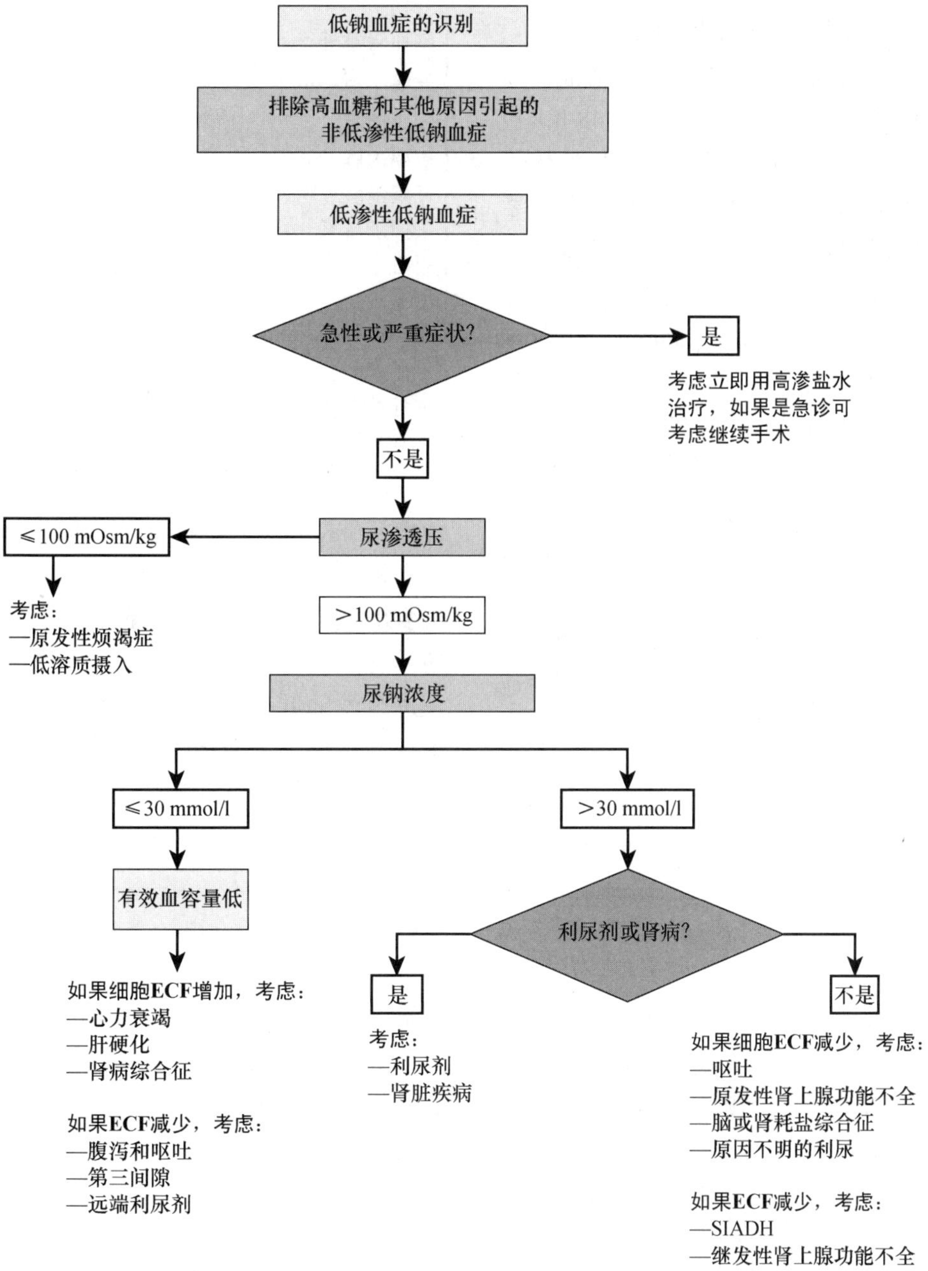

图 140.1 围术期低钠血症初步评估的主要步骤（Adapted from Spasovski G，Vanholder R，Allolio B，et al.：Clinical practice guideline on diagnosis and treatment of hyponatraemia. *Nephrol Dial Transplant* 29[Suppl 2]：i1-i39，2014.）

且测定了尿钠含量，评估有效动脉血容量和细胞外液量，可进一步揭示低渗性低钠血症的原因。最后，其他电解质异常（如：低钾血症、低镁血症）常与低钠血症一样需要被纠正。

风险评估

低钠血症是临床常见的电解质紊乱。15% ～ 22% 的住院患者血清钠离子浓度低于 135 mEq/L，1% ～ 4% 的患者甚至低于 130 mEq/L。近期研究表明，围术期低钠血症患者的术后死亡率较高。死亡原因与血栓栓塞事件、伤口感染及肺炎相关。为此，需要进一步的研究来阐明这一警示性的发现。

围术期低钠血症常表现为低渗性低钠血症。与围术期事件相关的急性低钠血症的原因（<48 h）包括术后管理、前列腺与子宫的内窥镜手术、液体管理、结肠镜检查时肠道准备、催产素和抗利尿激素的使用等。全身麻醉以及所有手术的后遗症（疼痛、呕吐等）都可能导致抗利尿激素分泌不适当综合征（syndrome of inappropriate antidiuretic hormone secretion，SIADH；框 140.3）。术中非低渗性低钠血症可发生在经尿道前列腺或膀胱肿瘤切除术和宫腔镜手术，主要是由于灌洗液（如甘氨酸和山梨醇）向血管内转移所致。临床表现可能是由于溶液代谢产物的积累（如氨和丝氨酸），而不一定是由低钠血症所引起。

术后低钠血症主要是由于抗利尿激素（antidiuretic hormone，ADH）效应的增加，常与术中无限制性地输注等渗液体相关，ADH 使肾通过排出钠离子和重吸收水分子使血液渗透压降低。在 SIADH 状态下，等渗液体（如生理盐水）输入可增加机体对水的重吸收和钠的排泄。另外需要考虑的因素是液体正平衡与住院患者病情恶化之间的关系。围术期以目标为导向的液体管理可能有助于避免其中一些并发症的发生。

另一方面，抗利尿激素基于渗透调节和压力调节进行生理性释放。低血容量或低血压时，压力调节优先于渗透压调节，通常可预防低钠血症，且不管钠离子水平如何，引起抗利尿激素进一步释放。术中推注液体以纠正低血压的常用做法，可能会加重已有的低钠血症。最近的研究亦表明，长期低血压可加重患者围术期的患病率和死亡率。因此，根据生理学原理，术中发生低血压时，给予升压药物治疗及维持容量充足状态优于单纯补液治疗。

框 140.3 引起抗利尿激素分泌不适当综合征的原因

恶性肿瘤
肺（特别是小细胞肺癌）
中枢神经系统
胰腺

肺源性
肺炎
肺结核
真菌感染
肺脓肿
神经源性
感染
外伤
脑血管意外

药物（最常见）
阿米替林
氯磺丙脲
环磷酰胺
去氨加压素
吗啡
尼古丁
非甾体抗炎药
催产素
选择性 5- 羟色胺再摄取抑制剂
长春新碱

神经外科患者经常存在低钠血症的风险。SIADH 是临床最常见的原因。无论病因是 SIADH 还是脑耗盐综合征，神经外科患者的治疗主要是纠正进行性的低钠血症。术中的液体管理、脑灌注压维持与钠离子失衡相互作用。精确的液体管理至关重要，等渗液体可能转化为自由水，可能导致血钠水平进一步降低，加重脑水肿。

启示

低钠血症的危害与血清钠离子绝对浓度相关。因而液体交换所致的血清钠离子浓度降低的速度更为关键。在排除低钠血症的非低渗性原因时，必须确定低钠血症的类型，因为不同类型的治疗方法不一。

低钠血症是否需要纠正及其纠正的速度应根据其症状严重程度而定。当出现急性中枢神经系统症状时，脑水肿的危害比快速纠正的危害更大，因此应及时纠正；然而，同时应该考虑到纠正过快可能导致发病率及死亡率的增加，包括中央脑桥脱髓鞘（稍后讨论）。

治疗

低钠血症的治疗有两个基本原则：一是病因的鉴别和治疗；二是在症状出现时安全地提高血清钠水平。伴有严重的中枢神经系统症状或血清钠低于 110 mEq/L 时，使用高渗盐水（3%）迅速补钠可能有助于避免其死亡。在这种情况下，高渗盐水每小时提高血清钠浓度 1 ～ 2 mEq/L，且不得超过 3 h。整个过程都需要严密监测。24 h 内钠的补充不应超过 8 ～ 10 mEq/L。尽管急性、重症低钠血症存在与之相关的风险，但是血钠纠正过快可引起中央脑桥脱髓鞘改变而使病情在数日内恶化。这被称为**脑桥中央髓鞘溶解**，可导致四肢瘫痪、昏迷、甚至死亡。可以通过计算机断层扫描或磁共振成像进行确诊。**脑桥中央髓鞘溶解**的危险因素见框 140.4。

对于容量状态可以确定的无症状低渗性低钠血症的病例，治疗应集中于确定和治疗其潜在病因。钠离子浓度一定要升高的情况是少见的。更重要的是，应该避免引起低钠血症进一步加重。对于有效动脉血液循环欠佳的患者，目标导向等渗液体输注法比较合理。然而，住院手术患者易出现液体正平衡，应引起注意。如果是因为利尿剂的使用，则应停止使用，并予合适的液体及电解质。如有需要可予盐皮质激素代替治疗。

框 140.4 脑桥中央髓鞘溶解的危险因素

钠离子纠正速率 24 h 大于 12 mEq/L 或 48 h 大于 25 mEq/L
2 天内血清钠离子浓度超过 140 mEq/L 的过度校正
治疗前出现低氧血症或缺氧症状
高凝状态（如烧伤）或营养不良（如慢性酗酒）
慢性而非急性低钠血症

正常血容量的低钠血症患者需要限制自由水。也可能需要类固醇或甲状腺激素的替代治疗。等渗液体不用于治疗因 SIADH（这些可增加自由水的重吸收）引起的低钠血症。应寻找并处理引起 SIADH 的可逆原因（如药物）（见框 140.3）。

由于抗利尿激素（ADH）分泌过多，导致低钠血症患者的细胞外液（extracellular fluid，ECF）增加。这发生于某些疾病的进展过程中（如：肝硬化、肾病综合征或充血性心力衰竭），可使体液总量增加，而与之相关的有效循环容量及肾小球滤过率降低。治疗主要是控制原发疾病的进展及限制自由水。

病例 1 中的患者因使用利尿剂而出现低渗性低钠血症，且伴有潜在的肾功能不全。因不伴有中枢神经系统症状，该患者可能为慢性低钠血症。其麻醉方案应包括目标导向液体疗法、血容量充足时早期应用升压药物治疗低血压，以防进一步加重低钠血症。术后应继续警惕 ADH 对低钠血症的潜在影响。

预防

明确高危患者并高度怀疑低钠血症可有助于预防低钠并发症的发生。治疗主要在于处理其潜在的病因，而非治疗低钠血症本身。更重要的是，对于围术期患者来说，治疗目标在于避免已存在的低钠血症进一步恶化，这需要排除引起非低渗性低钠血症的原因。一旦患者的相关实验室数值（血清和尿渗透压、尿钠）得到评估，则可以判断其容量状态，以寻找低渗性低钠血症的可治疗性的病因。

高钠血症

病例概要 2

患者，男性，50 岁，5 天前因车祸致脑外伤，在重症监护病房（intensive care unit，ICU）初始复苏后因髋关节骨折拟行髋部手术。患者气管插管，护理记录显示“病情平稳”。实验室检查显示血浆钠离子浓度为 155 mEq/L。到达手术室时，患者的尿袋已满。

问题分析

定义

高钠血症的定义是血清钠离子浓度高于 145 mEq/L。这种电解质紊乱在重症患者和神经系统患者中更为常见。高钠血症在住院患者中的发病率为 1%，低于低钠血症。在儿童和成人中，高钠血症主要发生于水摄入受限的患者（极端年龄）。高钠血症可能是医源性的，这是由于摄入过量高钠液体所致。

机体有两种防御机制预防高钠血症：生成浓缩尿液的能力和强大的口渴机制。当血浆渗透压升高至 275 ～ 280 mOsm/kg 时，释放 ADH；当血浆渗透压升高至 290 ～ 295 mOsm/kg 时，尿液达到最大浓度。如果口渴机制正常，自由水摄入不受限制，则很少会发展为持续性高钠血症。

识别

高钠血症的症状和体征主要表现为中枢神经系统功能紊乱。当血清钠离子浓度增加较大或速度较快（即数小时内）时，表现更为显著。

年轻患者的症状主要表现为呼吸过强、躁动、易怒、失眠和典型的高声叫喊。如果未被发现，这些症状会进一步发展为肌无力、精神错乱、萎靡、嗜睡、甚至昏迷。与婴幼儿不同的是，老年患者在血清钠浓度超过 169 mEq/L 前通常很少出现症状。老年人由于口渴反应减弱、尿浓缩能力受损及虚弱（不能摄水）而处于高危状态。意识水平与高钠血症的严重程度相关。肌无力、精神错乱、昏迷可能是其并发疾病的表现，而非高钠血症本身。另外，与门诊高钠血症患者不同，院内获得性类型则包括各个年龄段的患者。此外，由于这些患者通常先前就存在神经功能障碍，因此临床症状更加难以捉摸。

风险评估

高钠血症是指相对于全身钠储备的水缺乏。这可能是由于净失水或高渗钠的增加（见框 140.5）。净失水占多数情况。高钠血症只发生于口渴感觉受损或摄水受限时。婴幼儿出现高钠血症通常的病因是胃肠炎（呕吐和腹泻）；而老年人通常是由于渴觉受损、发热的疾病和虚弱所致。另外一类患者是由于利尿剂（尤其是袢利尿剂）的使用，通常是为了使容量超负荷的 ICU 患者达到液体负平衡。

框 140.5 高钠血症的常见原因

细胞外液（ECF）减少
- 减少水的摄入量
- 肾内失水
  - 尿崩症
    - 中枢性
    - 肾源性
- 肾外失水
  - 通过呼吸道
  - 通过胃肠道
  - 发热

ECF 增加
- 医源性：使用含钠液体
- 盐皮质激素过量
  - 原发性醛固酮增多症
  - 库欣综合征
  - 外源性

大多数低 ECF 的神经性高钠血症、中枢性尿崩症（central diabetes insipidus，CDI）须与脱水相鉴别。神经外科的 CDI 发病率约为 4%。创伤性脑损伤是发生 CDI 的高危因素，如病例 2 所示。

启示

高钠血症使液体从细胞内流出至细胞外间隙，以维持细胞内外渗透压平衡。这导致短暂的脑脱水和脑萎缩。脑细胞体积可急剧减少达 10% ～ 15%，但大脑适应得很快。在 1 h 内，大脑显著增加细胞内钠、钾、氨基酸及未测量的有机物质或特异性渗透分子的含量（即快速适应）。脑体积恢复正常需要 1 周左右，大脑可以恢复大约 98% 的含水量。当发生急性的严重高钠血症时，大脑可能无法通过增加其细胞内溶质维持体积。如果是这样，细胞收缩会导致结构变化。静脉窦血栓形成亦会进展至大脑梗死。动物模型中，急性高钠血症可引起大脑脱髓鞘损伤；人类也有此类报告。肝性脑病患者出现脱髓鞘变的可能性更高。

管理与预防

高钠血症的治疗必须纠正病因，使血清钠离子恢复正常以及恢复正常循环血容量。治疗的根本是提供和保留自由水，以纠正血清钠浓度。当伴有

CDI 时，推荐静脉输注 5% 葡萄糖或水，或经胃管同时给予 1- 去氨基 -8- 精氨酸。

计算出的液体缺失量不包括隐性或持续的尿量和胃肠道丢失量。液体维持量，包括使用低渗液体替代排出的尿量，以补充缺失量。如果存在严重的低血容量或循环衰竭，在纠正自由水缺乏之前，可使用生理盐水、乳酸钠林格液或者胶体液先进行液体复苏。治疗类型主要取决于引起高钠血症的原因，应根据每个患者相关的病理生理事件进行针对性的治疗（表 140.1）。只要患者能够安全耐受，就应尽快进行口服水化治疗。血浆电解质应每 2 ～ 3 h 测量一次，直至患者神经系统稳定。

在数小时内即出现高钠血症的患者中（如意外钠超负荷），快速纠正可改善预后，而不增加脑水肿的风险。这可能是由于累积的电解质迅速从脑细胞中释放的原因。在这些患者中，妥善的做法是，血清钠浓度每小时降低 1 mEq/L。而慢性高钠血症患者和持续时间未知的患者则建议缓慢纠正，因为大脑中累积的电解质会在数天内完全消散。对于这些患者，血清钠浓度降低的速度应低于每小时 0.5 mEq/L 从而预防脑水肿和惊厥。因此，一些专家（如 Adrogué 和 Madias）建议除了那些在数小时内出现紊乱的，其他所有高钠血症患者每天应使血清钠浓度降低 10 mEq/L。治疗的目标是血清钠浓度降低至 145 mEq/L。

表 140.1 高钠血症的治疗

原因	治疗
水钠丢失 [a]；肠胃炎	0.45% 的 NaCl 溶于 5% 的葡萄糖液中
原发性失水 [a]；哺乳不佳；饮水过少	0.2% 的 NaCl 溶于 5% 的葡萄糖液中
肾性尿崩症 [a]	0.1% 的 NaCl 溶于 2.5% 的葡萄糖液中 [b]
中枢性尿崩症 [a]	醋酸加压素
钠超载 [a]	5% 的葡萄糖液 [c]

[a] 另见框 140.5

[b] 紧急处理

[c] 可能需要利尿剂

Adapted from Moritz ML，Ayus JC：Disorders of water metabolism in children. *Pediatr Rev* 23：371-380，2002 and Adrogué HJ，Madias NE：Hypernatremia. *N Engl J Med* 342：1493-1499，2000.

给药方式首选口服或胃管注入。如果均不行，则选择静脉给药。液体的低渗程度越低，输注速度应当越缓慢，以减少脑水肿的风险。最后，除存在明显的循环衰竭外，0.9% 生理盐水和乳酸钠林格液不适合用于治疗高钠血症。

致谢

感谢 J.Tomas Murphy 博士和 John L. Atlee 对本章上一版的贡献。

（孙 莉 译 季 锋 校）

延伸阅读

Adrogué HJ, Madias NE: Hypernatremia, *N Engl J Med* 342:1493–1499, 2000.

Adrogué HJ, Madias NE: Hyponatremia, *N Engl J Med* 342:1581–1589, 2000.

Arieff AI, Llach F, Massry SG: Neurological manifestations and morbidity of hyponatremia: correlation with brain water and electrolytes, *Medicine* 55:121–129, 1976.

Berl T: Treating hyponatremia: damned if we do and damned if we don't, *Kidney Int* 37:1006–1018, 1990.

Brunner JE, Redmond JM, Haggar AM, et al.: Central pontine myelinolysis and pontine lesions after rapid correction of hyponatremia: a prospective magnetic resonance imaging study, *Ann Neurol* 27:61–66, 1990.

Issa MM, Young MR, Bullock AR, et al.: Dilutional hyponatremia of TURP syndrome: a historical event in the 21st century, *Urology* 64:298–301, 2004.

Moritz ML, Ayus JC: Disorders of water metabolism in children, *Pediatr Rev* 23:371–380, 2002.

Nguyen MK, Kurtz I: New insights into the pathophysiology of the dysnatremias: a quantitative analysis, *Am J Physiol Renal Physiol* 287:F172–F180, 2004.

Norenberg MD, Papendick RE: Chronicity of hyponatremia as a factor in experimental myelinolysis, *Ann Neurol* 15:544–547, 1984.

Oster JR, Singer I: Hyponatremia, hypoosmolality and hypotonicity: tables and fables, *Arch Intern Med* 159:333–336, 1999.

Rose BD: Hypoosmolal states: hyponatremia. In Jeffers JD, Navrozov M, editors: *Clinical physiology of acid-base and electrolyte disorders*, New York, 1994, McGraw-Hill, pp 651–694.

Spasovsk G, Vanholder R, Nagler E, et al.: Clinical practice guideline on diagnosis and treatment of hyponatremia, *Eur J Endocrinol* 170:G1–G47, 2014.

Steele A, Gowrishankar M, Abrahamson S, et al.: Postoperative hyponatremia despite near-isotonic saline infusion: a phenomenon of desalination, *Ann Intern Med* 126:20–25, 1997.

Sterns R, Hix J, Silver S: Management of hyponatremia in the ICU, *Chest* 144:672–679, 2013.

Tisdall M, Crocker M, Smith M, et al.: Disturbances of sodium in critically ill adult neurologic patients: a clinical review, *J Neurosurg Anesthesiol* 18:57–63, 2006.

第 141 章 妊娠栓塞事件

Nolan McDonnell

病例概要

患者，孕妇，34 岁，G3P2，孕 29 周时因胎儿出现早产，需行紧急剖宫产手术。脊柱麻醉下新生儿及胎盘娩出后，产妇主诉恶心，继而出现意识消失和呼吸暂停。气管插管后，患者迅速出现血流动力学和凝血障碍。经支持性治疗后，患者顺利拔管，并完全康复。

问题分析

定义

妊娠期栓塞事件是发达国家孕妇发病和致死的主要原因之一。在妊娠期和产后早期，栓塞事件可以表现为急性心血管和呼吸系统衰竭。有多种物质可以导致栓塞性表现，其中绝大多数都继发于血栓形成、空气栓塞和所谓的“羊水栓塞”。其临床表现可以很轻微、无临床症状和体征，直至出现突发性心血管衰竭，需要迅速采取多学科支持治疗。

识别

肺栓塞

肺栓塞的症状见框 141.1。在大面积肺栓塞的情况下，低血压、晕厥或突发循环衰竭等是可能出现的特征性表现。

孕妇肺栓塞的诊断可能较困难。胸部放射检查、心电图和动脉血气对诊断可能有益，但通常不能确诊。由于孕妇血浆 D- 二聚体浓度多已升高，因而其测值的解读可能较困难。最主要的两种影像学诊断技术是通气灌注闪烁扫描术和 CT 肺血管造影术。尽管通气灌注闪烁扫描术的阳性和阴性预测价值取决于患者肺栓塞的预发风险，但其仍可能是有用的初始检查。CT 肺血管造影术尽管能鉴别诊断除肺栓塞以外的其他病理改变（如主动脉疾病），但其代价是患者大剂量的放射线暴露，尤其是孕妇的乳腺组织。

框 141.1 肺栓塞的症状和体征

- 突发心动过速
- 呼吸困难
- 胸膜型胸痛
- 焦虑
- 干咳
- 咯血
- 发绀
- 第二心音亢进

羊水栓塞

羊水栓塞一词多少有点用词不当。传统观念认为本病是由于羊水及其中的碎片进入了肺循环而造成栓塞，但目前的观念提示本病更可能是一种免疫介导的疾病，而羊水进入母体的血液循环是一种相当常见的现象。有建议对此一系列症状和体征采用**妊娠类过敏样综合征**（anaphylactoid syndrome of pregnancy）一词来取代羊水栓塞，但尚未被广泛接受。

羊水栓塞的症状和体征可以从症状隐匿到突发性循环呼吸衰竭等多种多样（框 141.2）。病情恶化前，孕妇可能先出现焦虑和烦躁，胎儿电子心率监测可能出现心脏减速反应、变异性消失和长时间的心动过缓。患者的凝血功能改变表现明显，在罕见

框 141.2 羊水栓塞的症状和体征

- 呼吸困难
- 发绀
- 低血压
- 惊厥
- 心血管衰竭
- 凝血病和大量出血

的情况下，可能是特征性的表现。绝大多数病例的发病都与分娩有关。

羊水栓塞的诊断本质上都是在排除其他可能导致相关临床表现的病因后，依据临床症状和体征做出的临床诊断。此病缺乏特异性的诊断性检查，肥大细胞胰蛋白酶检查可能有助于排除过敏性因素所致。尸检发现母体肺循环中存在羊水碎片有诊断意义，但只有在患者存在相应的临床表现时才能做出诊断。无论经胸或经食管超声心动图均有助于明确诊断和指导治疗。报道的病例中的相关表现包括急性右心室衰竭、严重肺动脉高压和左心室衰竭。

静脉空气栓塞

静脉空气栓塞的症状和体征见框 141.3。其临床表现多变，取决于气栓的容量和栓塞速度、空气栓塞的最终部位以及产妇的基础状况等。若空气滞留在右室流出道，可引起“气阻（air lock）”现象，导致迅速出现低血压和心脏停搏。若空气栓塞在冠状动脉循环中，则出现与急性心肌梗死相似的症状和体征，包括胸痛和心律失常。持续存在右向左分流（如卵圆孔未闭）的患者可能出现脑内空气栓塞，导致视觉障碍、意识改变和惊厥等。后期的病理改变可能与栓塞的空气与内皮细胞和血小板表面的相互作用有关，导致凝血瀑布的激活、血管痉挛和微血栓。

严重的静脉空气栓塞的检测可能很困难。产妇在全身麻醉下，呼气末二氧化碳监测可能是最便捷而敏感的监测方法。出现突发性呼气末二氧化碳浓度急剧下降并伴有氧饱和度的下降对临床医师往往具有警示作用。经食管超声心动图的敏感性可能更高，但出现病情变化时该设备往往并未在床旁备用。某些临床症状可能有助于诊断，例如出现“磨轮样（wheel-mill）”杂音，据信这是由于心脏内的空气喷溅而产生的听诊杂音。亦可见甲床微动脉段和黏膜部位变苍白。

框 141.3 静脉空气栓塞的症状和体征

- 气促
- 呼吸困难
- 胸痛
- 低血压
- 磨轮样杂音
- 发绀
- 中心静脉压升高
- 呼吸末二氧化碳下降
- 心电图改变
- 心脏停搏

风险评估

肺栓塞

大多数妊娠相关的肺栓塞患者都伴有静脉血栓栓塞。妊娠是血栓栓塞的重要危险因素，因为 Virchow 三联征的三大危险因素在孕妇身上都存在，这一风险一直持续到产后 6 周之内。每一例肺栓塞的患者都大约会有 3 ～ 4 处的静脉血栓栓塞。在产前阶段，孕妇发生血栓栓塞的风险是非妊娠妇女的 7 ～ 10 倍，而产后 6 周内的风险更高达 15 ～ 35 倍；这说明大多数的肺栓塞都发生在产后 6 周内。

除了妊娠因素外，还可能存在其他一些预先或并存的与孕妇和分娩相关的危险因素，可导致静脉血栓栓塞及后续的肺栓塞的风险增加。另外，这些危险因素可能会随着妊娠的进展而发生改变，因而一个在刚开始怀孕时的低风险孕妇也可能因为出现了特殊的并发症，而最终演变成了高风险产妇。一些主要的危险因素包括孕产妇的血栓形成倾向、有静脉血栓栓塞的病史、母体体重指数增加、高龄产妇、非择期性剖宫产及出现出血性或感染性并发症等。

羊水栓塞

羊水栓塞是一较少见的并发症，其报道的发病率差异显著。近期的资料提示，发达国家分娩产妇的发病率约为 1∶50 000 ～ 1∶16 000。羊水栓塞绝大多数都发生在分娩期，但在妊娠的各个阶段及产后早期均有报道。据报道，在诸如羊膜穿刺、终止妊娠及创伤等情况下导致子宫胎盘屏障破坏时，也可能发病。已确认的危险因素有很多，包括男性胎儿、多胎妊娠、胎盘早剥、宫颈撕裂及羊水过多；与引产术之间的相关性在报道中尚存争议。重要的是，上述危险因素均非可调控因素。

静脉空气栓塞

静脉空气栓塞的发病率可能要高于临床认知。心前区多普勒检查发现约半数的剖宫产产妇都存在静脉空气栓塞的证据，而更敏感的检查显示产妇几乎普遍存在空气栓子。暴露的子宫血管与心脏之间只需存在很小的压力梯度即可导致空气进入循环，大部分空气入血都发生在剖宫产术中子宫切开至子宫被缝合的时间段内。子宫外置及 Trendelenburg 体位会增大心脏与子宫之间的压力梯度，更易导致空气被吸入。另外，妊娠期的性生活，尤其是口交时吹气，也是一个明确的危险因素。

启示

肺栓塞

尽管针对产妇静脉血栓栓塞的预防已进行了诸多努力，但肺栓塞仍是许多国家导致孕产妇死亡的主要原因。在非致命的病例中，产妇可能残留明显的肺动脉高压，并需要接受长期的抗凝治疗。

羊水栓塞

羊水栓塞尽管较罕见，但仍是许多发达国家孕产妇致死的主要病因。既往该病的病死率很高（超过 80%），近期报道的病死率较低（通常在 20% ～ 40%），若产妇能在最初的心血管打击下存活，则预后一般较好。患者凝血病的发病率很高，因而能否及时获得血液和血制品对患者的生存常常至关重要。新生儿的预后取决于在事件发生时胎儿是否仍在子宫内；若是，则新生儿死亡的风险超过 50%。存活的孕产妇可能出现一系列的并发症，包括多器官衰竭而需要进行积极的危重症治疗。

静脉空气栓塞

分娩过程中空气被吸入虽然相当常见，但仅在少数的产妇中会引起明显的血流动力学障碍。少量的空气可能会导致通气-灌注失调、低氧、右心衰竭、心律失常和低血压。大量的气体（>3 ml/kg）可能致命，患者通常都是死于右室流出道梗阻。

管理

肺栓塞

肺栓塞的治疗应主要集中在早期心血管和呼吸功能的支持上，若无禁忌，则立即开始抗凝治疗。接受抗凝治疗的孕产妇在分娩过程中应制订详细的多学科的诊疗计划。对于血流动力学不稳的患者，尽管存在明显的出血风险，可能仍需进行溶栓治疗（全身性或直接置管溶栓）。其他可以考虑的治疗措施包括放置下腔静脉过滤器或手术取栓。

羊水栓塞

可疑羊水栓塞患者的首要措施是支持治疗，目的在于恢复心排出量、氧合功能，并预防 / 处理任何凝血病。若出现心搏呼吸骤停，则应立即进行复苏，包括气管内插管、100% 氧气行机械通气并开始胸外按压。若胎儿尚未娩出，应将子宫移位，以防造成主动脉腔静脉受压。若产妇经 4 min 心肺复苏后仍无反应，则应考虑行濒死期剖宫产（perimortem cesarean delivery）手术。这样可以缓解子宫对主动脉腔静脉的压迫，有可能改善产妇和胎儿的预后。在医疗机构内出现的心搏骤停患者，该手术应在发生心搏骤停的位置就地进行。

一旦条件允许，则应进行有创监测，并考虑立即进行诸如超声心动图等其他的检查。应预见到患者可能迅速出现凝血功能障碍，因而须立即做好大量输血和血制品的相关准备。出现凝血病的临床证据时，即应开始凝血因子的替代治疗，因为传统的凝血功能检查可能会延误治疗的时机。初始阶段能存活的孕妇一般均需进行危重症支持治疗。

静脉空气栓塞

静脉空气栓塞的成功治疗有赖于尽早诊断和迅速处理，以防空气被进一步吸入。保持产科医师与麻醉科医师团队的良好沟通是治疗的基础。患者应重新放置体位，以使心脏的位置高于手术野（反 Trendelenburg 位），并适当左倾，以促使心脏内任何可能滞留的气泡移行至肺循环的远端。使用氧化亚氮麻醉的患者应立即停用，因其可使气泡的体积增大。使用纯氧通气有助于进一步降低气泡体积，而增加容量负荷可能有助于增加右心前负荷，并进一步促进气泡向肺血管床的远端移行。可能需要使用心脏变力性药物，重症患者在右心房放置中心静脉导管可能抽吸出心脏内的部分空气。高压氧是严重空气栓塞患者的关键性治疗措施之一，为优化患者的预后，应在症状出现的 5 h 之内进行。

预防

肺栓塞

静脉血栓栓塞的预防要求对产妇早期进行妊娠特异性的风险评估（有些女性需要进行孕前咨询），并在妊娠期和产后早期进行反复的再评估。预防措施应包括建立在风险评估基础上，并结合了物理治疗和药物治疗考量的，有关孕产妇活动和适当水化方面的一般性建议。一些女性需要采取产前和产后措施，而另一些则仅需采取产后预防性措施即可。持续存在高危因素的产妇的产后预防措施应持续 6 周或更长时间。应对孕产妇进行有关静脉血栓栓塞的症状和体征方面的宣教，以便其能及时就诊和评估。

羊水栓塞

尽管已经了解了几种羊水栓塞的可能危险因素，但仍未能发现真正有预防作用的可调控的危险因素。目前认为，有妊娠期羊水栓塞病史似乎并非后续妊娠期发生羊水栓塞的危险因素。

静脉空气栓塞

避免头低位和使子宫外置以避免子宫与心脏间出现压力梯度，可以预防静脉空气的吸入。另外，在子宫切开至术毕子宫缝合期间采取适当的反 Trendelenburg 位可以升高静脉压，有助于预防空气吸入。尽早发现、防止空气被进一步吸入，加上适当的处理措施可以有效降低静脉空气栓塞的发病率和病死率。

致谢

感谢 Cheryl DeSimone 博士对本章上一版的贡献。

（陆梁梁　译　倪　文　校）

延伸阅读

Bourjeily G, Paidas M, Khalil H, et al.: Pulmonary embolism in pregnancy, *Lancet* 375:500–512, 2010.

Clark SL: Amniotic fluid embolism, *Obstet Gynecol* 123:337–348, 2014.

Gei AF, Vadhera RB, Hankins GD: Embolism during pregnancy: thrombus, air, and amniotic fluid, *Anesthesiol Clin North Am* 21:165–182, 2003.

McDonnell NJ, Percival V, Paech MJ: Amniotic fluid embolism: a leading cause of maternal death yet still a medical conundrum, *Int J Obstet Anaesth* 22:329–336, 2013.

Royal College of Obstetricians and Gynaecologists: *Greentop guideline no. 37a. Reducing the risk of venous thromboembolism during pregnancy and the puerperium*, April 2015.

Society for Maternal-Fetal Medicine: SMFM clinical guidelines no. 9. Amniotic fluid embolism: diagnosis and management, *Am J Obstet Gynecol* 215:B16–24, August 2016.

第 142 章 脂肪栓塞综合征

Jiabin Liu，Ignacio Badiola

病例概要

患者，男性，29 岁，因摩托车事故致股骨和胫骨骨折，入手术室行两个骨折部位的髓内钉治疗。尽管手术不大，且进行了充分的液体复苏和疼痛管理，但患者在恢复室出现持续性心动过速。次日晨，患者呼吸急促，主诉明显气短。经检查，其在吸空气下脉搏氧饱和度为 88%，胸部和颈部有瘀斑皮疹。胸部 X 线片显示双侧弥漫性浸润影。

问题分析

定义

脂肪栓塞综合征（fat embolism syndrome，FES）的特征是，脂肪栓塞后出现一系列临床症状和体征。目前尚无 FES 定义的金标准。Gurd 系统于 1970 年提出，可能是最为广泛接受的临床诊断系统。FES 包括主要症状和次要症状两类（表 142.1）。除出现脂肪微球蛋白血症外，还出现至少 1 个主要和 4 个次要症状或体征，即可做出诊断。主要症状和体征包括淤斑皮疹、呼吸系统症状伴双侧肺部影像学改变，以及与头部损伤无关的脑部体征。次要症状和体征包括心动过速、发热、视网膜脂肪或淤点、尿脂肪球或少尿、血红蛋白水平骤降、血小板突然减少、红细胞沉降率高和痰中脂肪球。还有基于 Gurd 系统的其他改进，例如 2 个主要特征、2 个主要和 2 个次要特征等。尽管临床常采用 Gurd 诊断系统，但并无科学依据。

表 142.1　Gurd 诊断系统

主要特征	次要特征
淤斑皮疹	心动过速
呼吸系统症状和双侧影像学阳性改变	发热
与头部损伤无关的脑部体征	视网膜脂肪或淤点
	尿脂肪球或少尿症
	血红蛋白水平骤降
	血小板减少
	红细胞沉降率高
	痰中脂肪球

Schonfeld 等开发了 1 个包括 7 项标准的指数系统，每项标准有不同权重。这些标准包括弥漫性淤点、肺浸润、低氧血症（氧分压 <70 mmHg）、意识错乱、体温 >38℃、心率 >120 次 / 分、呼吸频率 >30 次 / 分。≥ 5 分时可诊断 FES。然而，Schonfeld 指数的局限性在于，其不适用于脑部、胸部或腹部损伤患者。Vedrinne 等修订了创伤患者的评分系统，包括肺浸润、神经系统改变、淤点、血小板计数、视网膜改变、总血脂和存在长骨骨折。Weisz 和 Barzilai 进一步修改了适用于儿科患者的标准。

随着影像学和实验室技术的进步，有关 FES 的诊断有可能取得新进展。磁共振成像、高分辨率计算机断层扫描、支气管肺泡灌洗液的细胞研究和其他技术，可能提供更好的诊断工具。然而，这些诊断方式没有特异性，广泛应用于临床时可能导致结果前后不一致。

FES 目前公认的两种主要理论为，机械性脂肪栓塞理论和生化游离脂肪酸理论。尚无法用一种理论解释所有现象。

机械性脂肪栓塞理论

超声检查可见脂肪微栓子的存在。操作和高压扩髓均与微栓事件增多相关，而外固定则较少发生此类事件。脂肪栓子首先进入静脉系统，然后进入肺血管系统。这就解释了一些肺部和心脏症状。然而，部分患者可能出现全身体征，但无明显肺部症状时，机械性脂肪栓塞理论无法很好地解释这种情况。一种理论认为，小脂肪栓子的大小和变形性可能会通过肺部，从而导致全身表现，同时没有明显的临床肺部症状。

生化游离脂肪酸理论

长骨手术与游离脂肪酸水平升高和氧分压下降有关。这可能由于损伤后中性脂肪水解为游离脂肪酸所致。动物模型表明，游离脂肪酸可导致严重血管炎，破坏肺组织结构，从而导致出血和水肿等临床症状。

识别

长骨骨折导致的创伤是最常见原因，约 90% 患者出现脂肪栓塞。然而，只有 2% ～ 5% 患者会有症状，并因此诊断为 FES。其典型表现是在受伤后 12 ～ 36 h 逐渐出现肺部和神经症状。早期持续性心动过速可能是即将出现问题的第一个征兆。患者可能逐渐出现呼吸急促、呼吸困难和低氧血症，甚至进展为急性呼吸窘迫综合征（acute respiratory distress syndrome，ARDS）。血液系统和皮肤系统也常被累及。

术中麻醉状态下可能出现 FES。在长骨手术过程中，任何生命体征的突然改变，在鉴别诊断时都应考虑 FES，特别是出现不明原因的缺氧和（或）低血压时。短时间内可发生相当严重的脂肪栓塞。在心脏储备有限的患者中，急性肺动脉高压可导致右心室衰竭，并伴有低血压、心动过速、低氧血症和心血管衰竭。

风险评估

脂肪栓塞在创伤患者中很常见。其发病率与创伤性质有关，据报道其发生率为 60% ～ 90%。然而，出现临床体征和症状的患者则少得多。20 世纪 70 年代的早期报告表明，约 20% 患者发生了有症状的 FES。在外科技术改进后的 20 年里，这一比例下降近一半。Bulger 等在 3026 例患者中发现 27 例 FES（0.9%）。Fabian 等报道在股骨、胫骨和骨盆骨折患者中，至少 11% 存在 FES。Pinney 等报道股骨骨折的 FES 发生率为 4%。其他研究也报道了 FES 约 2% ～ 5% 的发病率。

许多危险因素已经确定，包括一般因素、损伤相关因素和手术相关因素。一般因素包括男性、年龄在 10 ～ 39 岁、低血容量状态、创伤后事件和心肺储备减少。与损伤相关的因素包括下肢骨折，特别是股骨干或双侧股骨骨折、多发性骨折以及伴有肺损伤的骨折。手术因素包括扩髓、螺钉植入、股骨骨折后的关节成形术、双侧股骨手术和大体积假体的关节成形术。

启示

在现代 ICU 治疗下，FES 死亡率有所下降。FES 主要发病率和死亡率与肺功能障碍、急性肺损伤（acute lung injury，ALI）或 ARDS 有关。由于大多数 FES 患者同时存在其他损伤，因此很难确定与 FES 相关的死亡率。所有出现症状的 FES 患者，死亡率估计为 5% ～ 15%。FES 在骨髓移植、胰腺炎和脂肪肝患者中也有报道。给予支持治疗时，多数患者并存的 FES 肺部后遗症得到缓解。急性神经系统的改变通常在肺部问题解决后几天内出现。长期或永久神经系统后遗症偶见于视力障碍或局灶性神经功能缺损患者。

管理

FES 治疗方案包括预防、早期诊断和支持治疗。早期诊断十分重要，因其可能导致干预提前并改善预后。一旦出现 FES 症状，主要治疗手段为支持治疗。重点是确保氧合、通气和血流动力学稳定。肝素、皮质类固醇和右旋糖酐作为 FES 的治疗手段，在降低死亡率和发病率方面并未显示显著疗效。然而，预防性使用皮质类固醇可能具有保护作用。

FES 导致的呼吸衰竭与 ALI 和 ARDS 相同。其治疗原则是使用呼气末正压，维持有效的气体交换和氧合，同时避免呼吸机相关肺损伤。术中麻醉状态下可能会出现 FES。在这种情况下，治疗策略是与外科团队坦诚沟通，通过容量复苏和正性肌力药物，维持氧合、通气和血流动力学稳定。应实施持续的 ICU 监护以改善预后。

预防

骨折早期固定可有效减少脂肪栓塞，通过减少反复性的脂肪栓子进入循环以减少 FES 发生。24 h

内早期固定可降低单一骨折和多发伤患者 FES 发生率，此外，在已知的其他益处中，早期活动和限制镇静可能通过减少 FES 的发生使患者受益。外科技术的改进，如扩髓后的冲洗，可能有助于减少脂肪栓塞的发生，并降低脂肪栓塞的严重程度。

致谢

感谢 Jennifer T. Fortney 博士对本章上一版的贡献。

（鲁　璐　译　刘　佳　校）

延伸阅读

Akhtar S: Fat embolism, *Anesthesiol Clin* 27(3):533–550, 2009. table of contents.

Aoki N, Soma K, Shindo M, et al.: Evaluation of potential fat emboli during placement of intramedullary nails after orthopedic fractures, *Chest* 113:178–181, 1998.

Bone LB, Johnson KD, Weigelt J, et al.: Early versus delayed stabilization of femoral fractures. A prospective randomized study, *J Bone Joint Surg Am* 71(3):336–340, 1989.

Brundage SI, McGhan R, Jurkovich GJ, et al.: Timing of femur fracture fixation: effect on outcome in patients with thoracic and head injuries, *J Trauma* 52:299–307, 2002.

Bulger EM, Smith DG, Maier RV, et al.: Fat embolism syndrome. A 10-year review, *Arch Surg* 132:435–439, 1997.

Chastre J, Fagon JY, Soler P, et al.: Bronchoalveolar lavage for rapid diagnosis of the fat embolism syndrome in trauma patients, *Ann Intern Med* 113:583–588, 1990.

Christie J, Robinson CM, Pell AC, et al.: Transcardiac echocardiography during invasive intramedullary procedures, *J Bone Joint Surg Br* 77:450–455, 1995.

Dudney TM, Elliott CG: Pulmonary embolism from amniotic fluid, fat, and air, *Prog Cardiovasc Dis* 36:447–474, 1994.

Fabian TC, Hoots AV, Stanford DS, et al.: Fat embolism syndrome: prospective evaluation in 92 fracture patients, *Crit Care Med* 18:42–46, 1990.

Gauss H: The pathology of fat embolism, *Arch Surg* 9:592–605, 1924.

Glover P, Worthley LI: Fat embolism, *Crit Care Resusc* 1:276–284, 1999.

Gurd AR: Fat embolism: an aid to diagnosis, *J Bone Joint Surg Br* 52:732–737, 1970.

Habashi NM, Andrews PL, Scalea TM: Therapeutic aspects of fat embolism syndrome, *Injury* 4)(37(Suppl):S68–S73, 2006.

Jones JG, Minty BD, Beeley JM, et al.: Pulmonary epithelial permeability is immediately increased after embolisation with oleic acid but not with neutral fat, *Thorax* 37:169–174, 1982.

Lehman E, Moore RM: Fat embolism, including experimental production without trauma, *Arch Surg* 14:621–662, 1927.

Levy D: The fat embolism syndrome. A review, *Clin Orthop Relat Res* 261: 281–286, 1990.

Lindeque BG, Schoeman HS, Dommisse GF, et al.: Fat embolism and the fat embolism syndrome. A double-blind therapeutic study, *J Bone Joint Surg Br* 69:128–131, 1987.

Malagari K, Economopoulos N, Stoupis C, et al.: High-resolution CT findings in mild pulmonary fat embolism, *Chest* 123:1196–1201, 2003.

Nixon JR, Brock-Utne JG: Free fatty acid and arterial oxygen changes following major injury: a correlation between hypoxemia and increased free fatty acid levels, *J Trauma* 18:23–26, 1978.

Pell AC, Christie J, Keating JF, Sutherland GR: The detection of fat embolism by transoesophageal echocardiography during reamed intramedullary nailing. A study of 24 patients with femoral and tibial fractures, *J Bone Joint Surg Br* 75:921–925, 1993.

Pinney SJ, Keating JF, Meek RN: Fat embolism syndrome in isolated femoral fractures: does timing of nailing influence incidence? *Injury* 29:131–133, 1998.

Riska EB, Myllynen P: Fat embolism in patients with multiple injuries, *J Trauma* 22:891–894, 1982.

Roger N, Xaubet A, Agusti C, et al.: Role of bronchoalveolar lavage in the diagnosis of fat embolism syndrome, *Eur Respir J* 8:1275–1280, 1995.

Schnaid E, Lamprey JM, Viljoen MJ, et al.: The early biochemical and hormonal profile of patients with long bone fractures at risk of fat embolism syndrome, *J Trauma* 27:309–311, 1987.

Schonfeld SA, Ploysongsang Y, DiLisio R, et al.: Fat embolism prophylaxis with corticosteroids. A prospective study in high-risk patients, *Ann Intern Med* 99:438–443, 1983.

Stanley JD, Hanson RR, Hicklin GA, et al.: Specificity of bronchoalveolar lavage for the diagnosis of fat embolism syndrome, *Am Surg* 60:537–541, 1994.

Stoltenberg JJ, Gustilo RB: The use of methylprednisolone and hypertonic glucose in the prophylaxis of fat embolism syndrome, *Clin Orthop Relat Res*211–221, 1979.

Takahashi M, Suzuki R, Osakabe Y, et al.: Magnetic resonance imaging findings in cerebral fat embolism: correlation with clinical manifestations, *J Trauma* 46:324–327, 1999.

Tanton J: L'embolie graisseuse traumatique, *J de Chir* 12:287–296, 1914.

Taviloglu K, Yanar H: Fat embolism syndrome, *Surg Today* 37:5–8, 2007.

Turillazzi E, Riezzo I, Neri M, et al.: The diagnosis of fatal pulmonary fat embolism using quantitative morphometry and confocal laser scanning microscopy, *Pathol Res Pract* 204:259–266, 2008.

Vedrinne JM, Guillaume C, Gagnieu MC, et al.: Bronchoalveolar lavage in trauma patients for diagnosis of fat embolism syndrome, *Chest* 102: 1323–1327, 1992.

Von Bergmann E: Ein fall todlicher fettembolie, *Berl Klin Wchenschr* 10:385, 1873. Cited in Sevitt S: *Fat embolism*. London, Butterworth, 1962.

Weisz GM, Barzilai A: Nonfulminant fat embolism: review of concepts on its genesis and physiopathology, *Anesth Analg* 52:303–309, 1973.

Wong PS, Aye WM, Lee CN: Pulmonary tumor embolism secondary to osteosarcoma, *Ann Thorac Surg* 77:341, 2004.

Worthley LI, Fisher MM: The fat embolism syndrome treated with oxygen, diuretics, sodium restriction and spontaneous ventilation, *Anaesth Intensive Care* 7:136–142, 1979.

高凝状态：血栓形成和栓塞 第143章

Andrew Disque，*Komal Patel*，*Mark A. Chaney*

病例概要

患者，女性，53岁，肥胖，既往充血性心力衰竭和卵巢癌病史。在全身麻醉下剖腹探查以行肿瘤切除术。术后首日，患者突然出现呼吸急促。

问题分析

定义和识别

150余年前，Virchow提出了导致血管内凝血的三个因素：血管损伤、静脉淤滞和高凝状态。血管损伤如直接外伤、严重烧伤、手术操作或中心静脉穿刺，可引起血管内皮损伤，导致局部血凝块（血栓）形成和随后的蔓延（血栓栓塞）。在麻醉后手术患者或制动患者中可能发生静脉淤滞，导致静脉血流缓慢和血栓形成倾向。要理解高凝状态，需对凝血过程有基本了解。

血栓形成由内皮损伤触发，内皮下胶原被暴露于循环中的血小板。其相互黏附形成血小板栓子。在形成过程中，凝血级联反应通过两种途径被激活。在**内源性途径**中，通过激活Ⅻ因子（需要Ⅷ、Ⅸ、Ⅺ因子）来激活内皮下胶原；在**外源性途径**中，损伤组织释放组织凝血活酶（组织因子）激活Ⅶ因子。最后（共同）途径始于激活Ⅹ（Ⅹa）因子。一旦Ⅹ因子被激活，它就与其辅助因子Ⅴ因子和血小板磷脂结合，形成复合物并激活Ⅱ因子（凝血酶原）形成Ⅱa因子（凝血酶）。凝血酶与血小板磷脂结合，将纤维蛋白原裂解成纤维蛋白单体。聚合形成的纤维蛋白聚合物，通过氢键（可溶性纤维蛋白或纤维蛋白S）松散地保持聚合。随后，由凝血酶和钙离子活化的因子XIII（血纤蛋白稳定因子）介导纤维蛋白单体之间共价肽键的形成，以产生一个稳定的纤维蛋白凝块（不溶性纤维蛋白或纤维蛋白Ⅰ）。

通常，凝血过程由内源性抗凝和溶栓系统相互平衡，限制血栓形成并最终溶解血栓。溶栓过程由纤维蛋白凝块附近受损细胞的组织型纤溶酶原激活剂（tissue-type plasminogen activator，t-PA）启动。当t-PA将循环中的纤溶酶原裂解成纤溶酶时，可溶解凝块基质中的纤维蛋白。

多种生理机制调节凝血过程，从而限制受伤区域的凝块形成，防止过度凝血[即弥散性血管内凝血（disseminated intravascular coagulation，DIC）]：

- 凝血因子以非活性形式存在于循环中。
- 正常的血液流动稀释活化因子的浓度，将其从损伤部位清除。这些细胞随后被肝和网状内皮系统从血液循环中清除。
- 一些凝血因子（如Ⅹa因子）需要磷脂表面（组织因子、血小板磷脂）进行适当的相互作用。
- 抗凝血酶（Antithrombin，AT，以前称为抗凝血酶Ⅲ）能够与凝血酶以及其他循环凝血因子（因子Ⅶ除外）复合并使其失活。抗凝血酶有两个关键的结构域：一个与凝血酶和其他激活的凝血因子结合，另一个与肝素结合。在肝素存在的情况下，AT与凝血酶和其他激活凝血因子的结合速度明显加快。
- 凝血酶与血栓调节蛋白（一种位于血管内皮表面的蛋白）结合，激活蛋白质C，从而使Ⅴa和Ⅷa因子失活。
- 在Ⅴa和Ⅷa因子失活过程中，蛋白质S是一个辅因子（与蛋白质C一起）。
- 组织因子通路抑制剂由血管内皮细胞合成，通过两种方式抑制Ⅹ因子：直接抑制Ⅹa因子，或与

Ⅹa因子形成复合物抑制组织因子Ⅷa，从而抑制外源性途径。

高凝状态是一系列凝血增强、内源性抗凝减弱或溶栓系统活性降低的过程。此类疾病可能是定性的，也可能是定量的，临床表现取决于疾病严重程度。高凝性疾病可分为遗传性疾病（内源性抗凝系统特异性缺陷的疾病见表143.1）或获得性疾病（与一般人群相比，与血栓并发症风险增加有关的疾病或状态；框143.1）

遗传性高凝状态

- **Ⅴ因子莱顿（*Leiden*）突变和对活化蛋白质C产生抵抗**。激活的Ⅴ因子是凝血酶原转化为凝血酶的辅助因子。Ⅴa因子可被活化蛋白质C灭活。Ⅴ因子基因[R506Q（Ⅴ因子莱顿位点）]的单点突变使其对活化蛋白质C的降解产生抵抗，从而增加凝血酶生成，导致机体进入高凝状态。人群中约有3%为这一突变的杂合子。在复发性深静脉血栓形成（deep venous thrombosis，DVT）患者中，这种突变占21%～25%。
- **凝血酶原基因突变**。凝血酶原基因（G20210A）的一个特定位点突变，导致血浆凝血酶原水平增加30%。在复发性DVT患者中，杂合子约占6%～18%。
- **抗凝血酶缺乏症**。AT是在肝中合成的α_2-球蛋白，能够灭活凝血酶、Ⅻa、Ⅺa、Ⅹa、Ⅸa因子及激肽释放酶。AT缺陷是遗传性高凝状态首个被确定的原因。其以常染色体显性方式遗传，约占复发性DVT患者的0.5%～1%。
- **蛋白质C和蛋白质S缺乏**。蛋白质C和S是维生素K依赖的血浆蛋白，可以灭活Ⅴa和Ⅷa因子。常染色体显性遗传，约占复发性DVT患者的5%～10%。

表143.1 导致高凝状态的遗传性疾病

受影响因素	表现
Ⅴ因子基因突变	Ⅴ因子对活化蛋白C产生抵抗
凝血酶原基因突变	凝血酶原生成增加
抗凝血酶	缺陷和功能障碍
人蛋白质C	缺陷和功能障碍
人蛋白质S	缺陷
纤维蛋白原血症	蛋白质功能失调
肝素辅因子Ⅱ	缺陷
促凝血因子	缺陷
纤溶酶原	缺陷或蛋白质功能失调
纤溶酶原激活剂	缺陷
纤溶酶原激活物抑制剂-1	增加

框143.1 获得性疾病易导致血栓形成

静脉淤滞
制动
妊娠
充血性心力衰竭
静脉曲张
肥胖

凝血激活
创伤
外科手术
恶性肿瘤
使用浓缩因子
狼疮抑制剂
心肌梗死
骨髓增生性疾病
肾病综合征
口服避孕药

血管表面异常
动脉粥样硬化，高脂血症
糖尿病
高同型半胱氨酸血症
吸烟
雌激素疗法
人工心血管装置
血管内留置导管

血管闭塞性疾病
高黏血症，红细胞增多症
镰状细胞病
浆细胞失调

血小板反应性增加
血小板增多症
外科手术

获得性高凝状态

- **获得性蛋白质C缺乏**。获得性蛋白质C缺乏可见于DIC、急性白血病、肝病和肾病综合征患者、肾移植患者以及服用华法林或口服避孕药的患者。
- **恶性肿瘤**。据估计，恶性肿瘤患者临床血栓栓塞性疾病的发生率高达11%。血栓发作可先于恶性肿瘤诊断前数月至数年。其可能表现为迁移性浅表血栓性静脉炎（特鲁索综合征）、DVT、DIC、非细菌性血栓性心内膜炎，或极少数表现为动脉血栓形成。肿瘤可分泌促凝剂（半胱氨酸蛋白酶、组织因子样促凝物质等）。肿瘤还可通过压迫、血管侵犯（肾肿瘤）或肝受累和功能障碍，导致静脉血栓形成。

- **妊娠**。妊娠和产后与 Virchow 三联征的 3 个组成部分均有关：下肢静脉内血液淤滞（妊娠子宫阻碍静脉回流），分娩过程中产生的盆腔静脉内皮损伤以及高凝状态。妊娠还与Ⅰ、Ⅱ、Ⅶ、Ⅷ、Ⅸ和Ⅹ因子的增加及蛋白质 S 和 AT 活性的降低有关。此外，妊娠期间，纤溶抑制剂 PAI-1 和 PAI-2 活性增加。
- **手术**。术后可能发生 DVT 和肺栓塞。手术患者血栓形成似乎与手术组织损伤和组织因子的释放导致凝血酶的形成有关。此外，炎症（白细胞反应性）和手术引起的凝血改变，可能导致血栓栓塞（框 143.2）。该改变可能与手术类型和手术干预程度有关，在术后首个 48 h 内最为显著。
- **制动**。静脉淤滞可能通过造成局部缺氧（导致内皮损伤）和激活的促凝蛋白清除不足，导致血栓形成。
- **骨髓增生性疾病**。骨髓增生性疾病患者，如真性红细胞增多症、特发性血小板增多症、骨髓增生性骨髓纤维化、腺样髓样化生、巨核细胞性骨髓增生、慢性粒细胞性白血病，其血栓事件发生率增加。动静脉血栓形成可能发生在非常规解剖部位，包括肠系膜、肾、脾、门静脉和肝（Budd-Chiari 综合征）。
- **高黏滞综合征**。当血液黏度增加（红细胞增多症）、未成熟黏附白细胞增多（再生障碍性贫血）、红细胞膜变形（镰状细胞贫血）和球蛋白浓度升高（浆细胞异常）时，血液黏度增加。与这些病症相关的血液缓慢流动，可导致任何血管床上的血管闭塞。目前认为，未成熟白细胞引起白细胞淤滞，导致蛋白酶释放，促进血栓形成。
- **狼疮抗凝物**。狼疮抗凝物是抗磷脂抗体（通常是免疫球蛋白 Ig G 和少量 IgM）直接抗血浆蛋白（例如，β_2- 糖蛋白Ⅰ、凝血酶原、膜联蛋白Ⅴ）与阴离子磷脂结合。大约 5% ～ 10% 的系统性红斑狼疮患者含有狼疮抗凝物。这些抗凝物阻断了凝血酶原酶复合物的体外组装，导致相关蛋白质检测结果延长，例如活化部分凝血活酶时间、稀释罗素蝰蛇毒液时间、白陶土血浆凝固时间以及凝血酶原时间（较少见）。上述变化提示凝血功能异常，但含有狼疮抗凝物的患者其动脉和静脉血栓形成事件的频率反而增加。其血栓形成机制尚不完全清楚，但可能与 IgG 与磷脂结合相关，这对于蛋白质 C 和蛋白质 S 的正常活化和降解作用至关重要，凝血平衡被打破，转向利于血栓形成。
- **高同型半胱氨酸血症**。高水平的同型半胱氨酸与动静脉血栓形成有关，但高同型半胱氨酸如何促发血栓形成的机制尚不清楚；可能的机制包括内皮活化、平滑肌细胞增殖、内皮一氧化氮生成的变化或内皮甾醇代谢变化。该疾病可以是先天性或获得性的。获得性形式的高同型半胱氨酸血症见于饮食中缺乏叶酸、维生素 B_{12} 或维生素 B_6 的患者。先天性高同型半胱氨酸血症最常见原因是，胱硫醚 β 合酶（cystathion β-synthase，CBS）基因或亚甲基四氢叶酸还原（methylenetetrahydrofolate reductase，MTHFR）基因突变。
- **浓缩因子输注**。几十年来，凝血病的治疗包括维生素 K、血浆、血小板和冷沉淀。考虑到逆转华法林可能需要超过 30 h，并需要大量输注，使

框 143.2 手术引起的止血变化

血小板反应性增强
↑聚集性
↑致密颗粒释放

白细胞反应性增强
↑自由基释放
↑表面黏附分子

增加凝血级联激活
↑纤维蛋白原
↑因子Ⅷ
↑血管性血友病因子
↑凝血酶生成

内源性抗凝剂减少
↓抗凝血酶Ⅲ
↓肝素辅因子Ⅱ
↓组织因子通路抑制剂
↓蛋白质 C、蛋白质 S

纤维蛋白溶解减少
↑纤溶酶原激活物抑制剂 -1

得更新更有效的选择正成为可能，如凝血酶原复合物浓缩物（prothrombin complex concentrates，PCC）、重组活化Ⅶa因子、浓缩Ⅸ因子、浓缩Ⅷ因子、浓缩纤维蛋白原。PCC有3或4种因子组合，含有Ⅱ、Ⅶ、Ⅸ和Ⅹ因子。上述新疗法，尤其是活化Ⅶa因子和PCC，与动静脉血栓形成事件有关。随着上述血制品的使用和研究愈发广泛，血栓形成的风险可能会降低；一些研究表明，当浓缩因子剂量减少时，疗效相似，但血栓形成风险下降。

- **其他因素**。其他可能与高凝状态相关的因素有肾病综合征、口服避孕药、激素替代疗法、长时间旅行、大量吸烟、高血压、阵发性睡眠性血红蛋白尿症、肝素诱导的血小板减少、血小板增多和炎症性肠病。

血栓栓塞

动脉血栓栓塞可导致脑梗死或其他重要脏器梗死。下肢静脉血栓形成的可能性是上肢的10倍，可表现为急性发作的肢体局部血栓或血栓栓塞。静脉血栓栓塞可形成肺栓塞，其病理生理效应如下：

- 血管阻塞、神经体液介质、细胞因子和反射性血管收缩引起的肺血管阻力增加；
- 肺泡死腔增大，通气-血流比失调，肺内右向左分流增加导致气体交换受损；
- 代偿性肺泡过度换气；
- 肺动脉压力、室壁张力、耗氧和缺血增加导致右心功能不全和扩张；
- 支气管收缩和呼吸道阻力增加；
- 水肿、出血引起的肺顺应性降低，以及表面活性物丢失。

风险评估

遗传性高凝状态

DVT患者中，Ⅴ因子Leiden突变和凝血酶原基因突变的发生率分别为21%～25%和6%～18%。然而，这些基因突变的患者，血栓形成的风险相对较低。到65岁时，这些突变的携带者中仅6%出现过静脉血栓形成，大多数血栓形成事件发生在外科手术等高风险时期。Ⅴ因子Leiden突变的频率因种族而异；其在欧洲裔中很常见，但在非洲或亚洲裔中很少见。

AT缺乏仅占DVT患者的0.5%～1%，但超过50%的患者在60岁前发生静脉血栓事件。蛋白质C和蛋白质S缺乏分别占DVT患者的0.5%～4%和1%～7%。

获得性高凝状态

- **恶性肿瘤**。任何恶性肿瘤都可能发生血管内血栓形成，以分泌黏蛋白的器官肿瘤（胃肠道和肺）更常见。高达10%的胰腺癌患者发生移行性浅表血栓性静脉炎。恶性肿瘤患者还存在其他诱发静脉血栓形成的因素，如手术、制动。
- **妊娠**。与未妊娠患者相比，妊娠患者静脉血栓栓塞风险增加约6倍（参见第141章）。栓塞风险在妊娠晚期和产后第一个月最高。据估计，DVT和肺栓塞的发生率高达0.05%～0.1%。妊娠期致死性事件中约12%是由肺栓塞所致。妊娠期血栓形成的危险因素包括，年龄增加、剖宫产、长期制动、肥胖、既往血栓栓塞和并发血栓形成倾向。
- **外科手术**。髋关节、下肢骨科手术是最容易引起血栓的外科手术之一。若无预防措施，全膝关节置换术后深静脉血栓的发生风险约45%～70%，1%～3%的髋关节手术患者可发生致命的肺栓塞。冠状动脉旁路移植手术与约20%的DVT风险和4%的肺栓塞风险相关。血栓栓塞风险以术后2天时最高，但栓塞事件可能发生在膝或髋关节手术后数周至数月。
- **制动**。心力衰竭、卒中、脊髓损伤、老年、肥胖、重大创伤、手术等导致长期制动的病情，会增加高凝状态的风险。据报道，严重创伤后DVT发生率为58%，需要内科重症监护的制动患者DVT发生率为33%。
- **骨髓增生性疾病**。升高的血细胞比容、血液黏度和闭塞性血管事件之间存在相关性。
- **血管内留置导管**。血栓形成并发症常见于中心静脉导管，常伴有导管相关性脓毒症。血栓形成可由纤维蛋白沉积或血管闭塞引起。

启示

肝素的抗凝作用依赖于足够的AT水平，缺乏AT的患者可能对肝素没有适当的反应。使用华法林可能导致蛋白质C和蛋白质S缺乏，在产生抗凝作用前出现华法林诱导的皮肤坏死。对高凝状态患者，肝素治疗可用于存在明显静脉血栓和肺栓塞风险时，如手术、重大创伤和制动。

管理

除 AT 缺乏（参见下述预防）外，对于高凝状态，除抗凝以防止肺栓塞或防止当前血栓扩展、溶栓（链激酶、尿激酶、重组 t-PA）以溶解和治疗形成的血栓外，尚无其他特殊治疗方法。抗凝药物包括肝素（未分级普通肝素或低分子肝素）、磺达肝素或华法林。磺达肝素（一种合成的肝素五糖）通过抗凝血酶发挥作用，其益处是大幅降低肝素诱导的血小板减少症（heparin-induced thrombocytopenia，HIT）的风险。对 HIT 并发血栓的患者，美国胸科医师学会（American College of Chest Physicians，ACCP）推荐使用非肝素类抗凝剂，包括直接凝血酶抑制剂（重组水蛭素、阿加曲班、比伐卢定、达比加群）或直接 X a 抑制剂（达那肝素、阿哌沙班、利伐沙班）。

肺栓塞的治疗包括主要和次要疗法。主要疗法旨在清除血栓，包括溶栓、经导管取栓、碎栓或手术取栓。次要疗法旨在预防复发，包括全身抗凝（肝素、华法林、直接凝血酶抑制剂、Xa 抑制剂）和下腔静脉滤器（如鸟巢或格林菲尔德滤器）。

预防

静脉血栓形成和肺栓塞高危患者的预防措施包括：皮下注射低分子肝素或未分级普通肝素、序贯加压袜和气动加压装置。磺达肝素已被美国食品和药物管理局批准用于预防髋关节骨折、髋关节或膝关节置换术和腹部手术患者 DVT。ACCP 推荐使用阿哌沙班、利伏沙班和达比加群作为髋关节骨折、髋关节置换或膝关节置换手术患者预防 DVT 的其他替代方案。重组水蛭素制剂（如比伐卢定）在欧洲国家已被用作 DVT 的预防药物。在美国，它们目前被批准用于治疗肝素诱导的血小板减少症和经皮冠状动脉介入治疗的抗凝。对获得性或遗传性高凝状态的患者，应考虑以下预防措施：

- **抗凝血酶缺乏**。AT 浓度在手术后常规下降，但在输注血浆 AT 可增加。也可使用重组人 AT，应考虑在围术期用于 AT 缺乏患者，但应注意肝素会降低 AT 浓度。
- **蛋白质 C 和蛋白质 S 缺乏**。输注血浆可提高蛋白质 C 和蛋白质 S 浓度。也可使用特定的蛋白质 C 浓缩物。
- **骨髓增生性疾病**。由于闭塞性血管事件与升高的红细胞比容、血液黏度和白细胞增多相关，这三个指标应通过静脉放血、化学治疗或晶体液的合理应用，以恢复到较为正常的范围。

（王月影　译　李　黛　校）

延伸阅读

Bucur SZ, Levy JH, Despotis GJ, et al.: Uses of antithrombin III concentrate in congenital and acquired deficiency states, *Transfusion* 38:481–498, 1998.

Chou SH-Y, Cai X, Konigsberg RG, et al.: Thromboembolic risks of recombinant factor VIIa use in warfarin-associated intracranial hemorrhage: a case-control study, *BMC Neurol* 12:158, 2012.

Gonsalves WI: The new oral anticoagulants in clinical practice, *Mayo Clin Proc* 88(5):495–511, 2013.

Guyatt GH, Akl EA, Crowther M, et al.: Executive summary: Antithrombotic therapy and prevention of thrombosis, 9th ed: American College of Chest Physicians evidence-based clinical practice guidelines, *Chest* 141(Suppl 2): 7S–47S, 2012.

Loscalzo J, Schafer A: *Thrombosis and hemorrhage*, ed 3, Philadelphia, 2003, JB Lippincott–Williams & Wilkins.

Martinelli I, Mannucci PM, De Stefano VD, et al.: Different risk of thrombosis in four coagulation defects associated with inherited thrombophilia: a study of 150 families, *Blood* 92:2353–2358, 1998.

Mateo J, Oliver A, Borrell M, et al.: Laboratory evaluation and clinical characteristics of 2132 consecutive unselected patients with venous thromboembolism: results of the Spanish Multicentric Study on Thrombophilia (EMET-Study), *Thromb Haemost* 77:444–451, 1997.

Omar HR: Recombinant activated factor VII significantly reduces transfusion requirements in cardiothoracic surgery, *Drugs R D* 15(2):187–194, 2015.

Sanafi M: Low-dose recombinant activated factor VII (rF-VIIa) for excess hemorrhage after cardiac operation, *Ann Thorac Surg* 99(5):2015, 1870.

Santoro SA: Antiphospholipid antibodies and thrombotic predisposition: underlying pathologic mechanisms, *Blood* 83:2389–2391, 1994.

Van Guldener C, Stehouwer CD: Hyperhomocysteinemia, vascular pathology and endothelial dysfunction, *Semin Thromb Hemost* 26:281–289, 2000.

Voils SA, Holder MC, Premraj S, et al.: Comparative effectiveness of 3- versus 4-factor prothrombin complex concentrate for emergent warfarin reversal, *Thromb Res* 136(3):595–598, 2015.

第144章 高血糖与糖尿病酮症酸中毒

Martin L. De Ruyter，*Barry A. Harrison*，*John Bracken*

病例概要

患者，女性，75 岁，合并 2 型糖尿病，每日服用两次 5 mg 格列本脲控制血糖，拟行择期冠状动脉旁路移植术。她患有糖尿病肾病，血清肌酐为 1.8 mg/dl。患者术前未服用降糖药，测空腹血糖为 130 mg/dl。心肺转流开始后，血糖升至 236 mg/dl。术中尿量较多。血钾为 5.8 mEq/L，碱剩余为 -4.0 mEq/dl。在心肺转流期给予呋塞米和甘露醇治疗，并多次给予心脏停搏液。心肺转流术历时 130 min。

问题分析

定义

成人随机血糖大于 200 mg/dl 称为高血糖。尽管最佳血糖范围仍存争议，但普遍认为对未控制的高血糖采取预防措施仍是合理的做法。围术期血糖水平受许多因素影响，包括术前血糖、营养状况、胰岛素水平，以及皮质醇、儿茶酚胺、胰高血糖素、生长激素增多，糖异生和糖原分解增加等。

在疾病或严重的急性应激情况下出现的高血糖，被称为**应激性高血糖**或**应激性糖尿病**。对某些患者来说可能反映其存在糖耐量异常，应采取治疗措施降低发病和死亡风险。手术或急性病恢复后，应对这类患者进行重新评估和分类。类似的方法也适用于妊娠期糖尿病的治疗。

作为最常见的内分泌疾病，糖尿病（diabetes mellitus，DM）是一种慢性多系统疾病，表现为持续存在的与高血糖相关的体征和症状，诊断标准为：随机血糖大于 200 mg/dl，空腹血糖大于 100 mg/dl，餐后 2 h 或口服葡萄糖耐量试验后 2 h 血糖大于或等于 140 mg/dl，随机血糖大于 200 mg/dl。血糖正常值见表 144.1。若无急性代谢性失代偿或严重高血糖，应至少间隔 24 h 再以上述标准明确诊断。糖尿病的患者群体具有异质性，现已有多种糖尿病综合征的分类。糖尿病患者血糖升高是由于胰岛素的相对或绝对缺乏，或者胰高血糖素的相对或绝对过量所致。1 型糖尿病患者胰岛素分泌绝对不足，通常在青春期发病，是因胰腺中胰岛细胞的自身免疫性破坏所致。这类患者通过补充外源性胰岛素防止脂解，最终会发生酮症酸中毒。2 型糖尿病是因胰岛素相对缺乏所致，以胰岛素抵抗为主要表现。2 型糖尿病的典型发病年龄是成年，但有数据显示平均发病年龄呈下降趋势。第三类是妊娠期糖尿病，是首次发病于妊娠期的任何程度的葡萄糖不耐受，在美国约占所有妊娠患者的 4%。

表 144.1　糖尿病前期和非妊娠成人糖尿病的诊断标准

正常值	糖尿病高风险值	糖尿病
空腹血糖（FPG）<100 mg/dl	FPG ≥ 100 ～ 125 mg/dl	FPG ≥ 126 mg/dl
餐后 2 h 血糖（PG）<140 mg/dl	2 h PG ≥ 140 ～ 199 mg/dl	2 h PG ≥ 200 mg/dl 随机血糖≥ 200 mg/dl+ 相应症状
HgbA1C<5.5%	5.5% ～ 6.4%	≥ 6.5%

糖尿病酮症酸中毒（diabetic ketoacidosis，DKA）是一种急症，通常与 1 型糖尿病有关。一般发生在胰岛素缺乏、葡萄糖利用率低和某些病理性应激因素（如疾病、感染、创伤）存在的情况下。机体试图通过糖异生来保证能量储备，动员脂肪和氨基酸向葡萄糖生成途径转变，导致高血糖和酮症（图 144.1）。

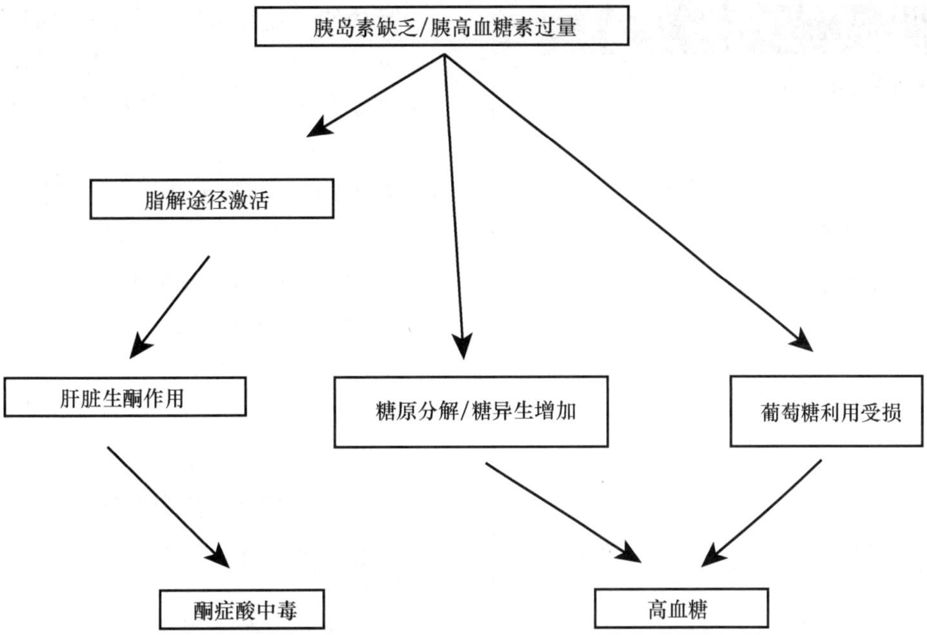

图 144.1 糖尿病酮症酸中毒和高血糖的发病机制

非酮症高渗综合征发生在 2 型糖尿病患者中，通常由生理性应激（如疾病、急性感染、肺炎、脑卒中、心肌梗死）触发。内源性胰岛素的分泌量足以防止酮症酸中毒发生，但可表现为继发于乳酸酸中毒的阴离子隙性代谢性酸中毒。这种酸碱失衡是细胞缺氧的结果，很可能与低血容量、器官灌注不足或休克状态有关。非酮症高渗综合征以严重高渗状态（>320 mOsm/L）、严重高血糖（>600 mg/dl）和严重脱水为特征。

识别

术前，高血糖的症状和体征可能难以发现，也可能变异很大。三分之一的糖尿病患者无自觉症状。糖尿病的症状和体征包括：

- 多食；
- 多饮；
- 多尿；
- 精神错乱；
- 昏迷。

术中体征如下：

- 不明原因的多尿；
- 心动过速和低血压；
- 阴离子隙性代谢性酸中毒；
- 低钠血症和高钾血症。

高血糖首次被发现通常是由于血浆葡萄糖升高。

风险评估

围术期高血糖的原因列于框 144.1 中。急诊手术可增加 1 型糖尿病患者 DKA 的发病风险，增加 2 型糖尿病患者非酮症高渗综合征的发病风险。在创伤等紧急情况下，患者可能会错过每日定时的胰岛素注射，中断正常的热量摄入或面临过度的病理应激，从而改变正常的激素负反馈调节平衡。患者不能增加胰岛素的分泌从而导致高血糖。

糖尿病影响多个器官系统，可导致严重的并发症，包括视网膜病变、神经病变、胃病和肾病等。此外，糖尿病相关并发症对麻醉管理有着至关重要的影响，包括妊娠期糖尿病患者氧输送问题所致的氧饱和度下降，自主神经功能障碍增加术中低体温和直立性低血压的风险。糖尿病还加速动脉粥样硬化，增加冠状动脉疾病、脑血管疾病和外周血管疾病的发病风险。

启示

针对多种患者人群的大样本量的观察性研究表明，高血糖与危重患者的不良预后相关。然而，目前尚未明确高血糖是这些不良后果的原因还是仅仅为严重疾病的标志。

- **创伤**。创伤后血糖过高（≥ 200 mg/dl）的患者死亡率、住院时间、ICU 留滞时间以及医院内感染的发生率均会增加。

框 144.1 围术期高血糖的病因

- 糖尿病（1 型和 2 型）
- 含葡萄糖的静脉输液
  - 维持液或肠外营养
  - 药物治疗
- 儿茶酚胺介导的应激反应
  - 烧伤
  - 创伤
  - 外科手术
  - 脓毒症
  - 脑卒中
  - 疼痛
  - 心肺转流术
- 过度的负反馈激素调节
  - 库欣病与库欣综合征
  - 嗜铬细胞瘤
  - 肢端肥大症
  - 胰高血糖素瘤
- 药物
  - 噻嗪类利尿药
  - 糖皮质激素
  - 苯妥英
  - 喷他脒
  - β- 肾上腺素受体阻滞药
  - 口服避孕药
- 胰腺疾病
  - 胰腺炎或胰腺创伤
  - 血色素沉着症
- 妊娠

- **内科 / 外科**。血糖升高的内外科危重症患者的死亡率高于血糖正常的患者。一项纳入了 1826 例内外科 ICU 患者的回顾性队列研究发现，血糖升高与死亡率之间有成比例的直接相关关系，平均血糖在 80 ～ 99 mg/dl 之间的患者，死亡率为 10%，而平均血糖高于 300 mg/dl 的患者，死亡率增至 43%。
- **细胞功能**。高血糖可导致免疫球蛋白非酶促糖基化、粒细胞功能障碍、CD4 和 CD8 淋巴细胞群减少。高血糖也可加重细胞的缺血再灌注损伤，介导心肌细胞死亡，减少冠状动脉侧支循环等。高血糖还可介导血小板高反应性，促进血栓形成，增加 IL-6、IL-8 和 TNF-α 的水平，有明显的促炎作用。高血糖和胰岛素抵抗可导致内皮细胞功能障碍、一氧化氮失活、前列腺素合成减少、内皮素 -1 合成增加，以上所有均可导致局部血流减少。
- **肾功能**。血糖大于 250 mg/dl 时将超出肾小管重吸收能力，导致继发于渗透性利尿的低血容量。过度利尿可导致肾前性氮质血症、脏器灌注改变、细胞缺氧和乳酸酸中毒。
- **大脑功能**。糖尿病患者或近期发生高血糖的患者罹患严重脑卒中的风险和死亡率都会增加。重型颅脑损伤（traumatic brain injury，TBI）患者被收入 ICU 时，血糖 ≥ 170 mg/dl 是 5 日后低 Glasgow 评分、神经系统不良预后以及颅内压升高的独立预测因子。而且无论入院时血糖是否升高以及 ICU 停留期间血糖是否出现升高或剧烈变化，高血糖与 TBI 不良预后之间的关系在整个住院期间始终存在。不良预后包括死亡率增加、机械通气时间延长、ICU 停留时间和总住院时间延长。此外，血清渗透压大于 330 mOsm/L 与中枢神经功能障碍和昏迷有关。
- **心血管系统功能**。一项对急性心肌梗死入院患者（无论是否诊断糖尿病）的 meta 分析发现，高血糖与住院死亡率增加和充血性心力衰竭的增加相关。
- **住院患者**。新近发现血糖升高的内外科患者住院死亡率可增加 18 倍，且住院时间延长。糖尿病是第七大死亡原因，也是美国出院患者中位列第二的并发症。住院患者高血糖与并发症及死亡率风险增加之间的关系现已明确。高血糖与住院时间延长、感染发生率增加、出院后伤残加重和死亡有关。
- **大手术**。30% ～ 40% 的心脏外科患者合并糖尿病。高血糖可增加心脏外科患者的死亡风险和深部感染的风险。

管理

给予胰岛素纠正高血糖可降低危重症患者以及普通内外科患者的住院并发症和死亡率。但是包括 NICE-SUGAR（normoglycemia in intensive care evaluation and survival using glucose algorithm regulation study）在内的多项随机对照研究和 meta 分析指出：与相对宽松的血糖指标相比，强化胰岛素治疗（血糖目标为 80 ～ 110 mg/dl）可增加严重低血糖的发生率和患者死亡率。2009 年美国临床内分泌医师协会 / 美国糖尿病协会（American Association of Clinical Endocrinologists/American

Diabetes Association，AACE/ADA）就住院患者血糖调控发表共识，支持在 ICU 治疗中应采用更宽松的血糖目标，可达到 140 ～ 180 mg/dl。更重要的是提出，不建议将血糖目标设定到低于 110 mg/dl。此外，不管血糖多高，尽量减少血糖波动可降低危重症患者的并发症发生率和心血管事件死亡率，并可缩短住院时间和降低非 ICU 条件下的死亡率。

术中高血糖

充足的证据表明无论是否有糖尿病病史，住院患者发生高血糖均可增加死亡率和发病率，而目标导向胰岛素治疗可改善预后。在院期间及手术过程中高血糖的治疗面临诸多挑战，包括营养状况的变化和意识水平的改变。鉴于对患者安全的考虑，血糖目标的设定应适当高于门诊糖尿病患者的水平。对于大多数 ICU 危重症患者，建议血糖范围为 140 ～ 180 mg/dl。对于非危重症患者，共识建议餐前血糖低于 140 mg/dl，随机血糖低于 180 mg/dl（表 144.2）。

胰岛素治疗是大多数住院患者控制血糖的首选方法。在 ICU 和围术期，首选途径是静脉输注。有多种胰岛素持续输注方案可有效控制血糖，且低血糖事件发生率低，可改善患者预后。不同的胰岛素静脉输注算法之间无显著的临床差异，只要以规定的频率监测血糖即可。因此，大多数胰岛素给药方案都是合理的，至于如何选择取决于医生的偏好和对成本的考虑。在非重症监护条件下，建议按预定方案皮下注射胰岛素，再结合其他基本的、营养支持和纠正异常等治疗。应当摒弃长期使用梯度胰岛素给药法作为控制血糖的唯一方法。随机对照研究表明，对普通内外科患者使用胰岛素类似物结合基础膳食治疗比单用梯度常规胰岛素注射更有利于血糖控制，且能降低并发症发生率。

表 144.2　非妊娠成人住院期间血糖目标

科室	治疗目标
重症加强治疗病房	
血糖范围（mg/dl）	140 ～ 180
普通内外科（非 ICU）	
餐前血糖（mg/dl）	<140
随机血糖（mg/dl）	<180

糖尿病酮症酸中毒

DKA 是一种内科急症。初步评估包括以下内容：

- 识别诱发事件——感染、缺血，胰岛素给药中断；
- 容量状态：
  - 心动过速、低血压；
  - 尿素和肌酐增加；
- 精神状态——脑水肿；
- 高血糖——血糖和尿糖升高；
- 酮症——血清酮体和 β-羟基丁酸升高；
- 高阴离子隙性酸中毒，表现为：
  - 呼吸频率增加（Kussmaul 呼吸）；
  - 血清碳酸氢根低于 15 mEq/dL；pH 低于 7.3；
- 钾——最初升高是继发于代谢性酸中毒，但总钾储量减少；
- 钠——高血糖后的实验室检查；

液体复苏、静脉注射胰岛素和电解质校正至关重要

- **液体复苏**。通常液体缺失量在 4 ～ 8 L 之间。早期复苏包括输注生理盐水（0.9% NaCl），目标是在最初 2 h 内患者应补充足够的液体以稳定其血流动力学参数（通常为 2 ～ 3 L 非葡萄糖晶体溶液）。血容量恢复后，如果血钠校正值正常或升高，则应开始给予 0.45% 盐水；如果血钠校正值降低，则继续给予等渗盐水。一旦血糖下降到 200 mg/dl 以下，即可在盐水中加入葡萄糖，以保持适宜的血糖水平并降低脑水肿的风险。输注低渗溶液可因反向渗透导致脑水肿。因高渗溶液可能加重酸中毒、脱水和高渗状态，通常并无治疗作用。
- **电解质**。不管最初测得的血钾是多少，DKA 患者总是存在体内钾的大量缺失。高血糖渗透性利尿导致系统性钾丢失（高达 10 mEq/kg），发生代谢性酸中毒后，钾向细胞外转移使血钾浓度升高。如果患者尿量充足，无急性肾衰竭，且血钾正常，应及时补充钾。通常以 20 ～ 30 mEq/h 的速度补充氯化钾应已足够。建议补钾期间监测心电图。实验室检查发现的低钠血症是因高血糖稀释效应所致。一般来说，血糖在正常值基础上每升高 100 mg/dl，血钠就会降低 1.6 ～ 2.0 mEq/L。除了高渗状态需要纠正外，其他情况无需特殊治疗。由于阴离子通过渗透性利尿被排出体外，故

磷酸盐可能会被耗竭。常规补充磷酸盐存在争议，因为快速补充会引起低钙血症。通过定期监测镁、钙和磷酸盐水平以指导磷酸盐的补充。

- **胰岛素治疗**。DKA 患者延迟胰岛素治疗的唯一指征是血钾低于 3.3 mEq/L，防止胰岛素促进钾向细胞内转移，使血钾更低。对中重度 DKA 患者，先行常规胰岛素静脉快速注射（0.1 U/kg），然后静脉维持输注 [0.1 U/（kg·h）]，每小时监测一次血糖。注意避免发生低血糖，有时可能需要额外补充葡萄糖。
- **代谢性酸中毒**。因补碱缺乏有利证据支持且具有潜在危害性，是否输注碳酸氢钠尚存争议。对于动脉血 pH ≤ 6.9 的患者，鉴于其心肌收缩力下降和血管扩张会进一步减少组织灌注，以及潜在的致命性高钾血症，谨慎补碱治疗可能会有益处。

预防

截至 2012 年，约 2910 万美国人（占总人口的 9.3%）患有糖尿病，其中 810 万人未确诊。糖尿病患者需要通过全面的医学评估去发现相关并发症和并存疾病。术前需要停止口服药物。长效磺酰脲类药物或氯磺丙脲类药物至少需术前 72 h 停药，而短效磺酰脲类药物和二甲双胍在术前当晚停药即可。

1 型糖尿病患者和未控制的 2 型糖尿病患者需使用胰岛素治疗。任何治疗方案的目的都是在不发生低血糖的情况下尽量控制好血糖。由于患者要经历从病房到手术室，再到恢复室，最后返回病房的多次转运过程，故治疗方法还须简便实用，频繁地复测血糖也非常重要。故满足上述要求的治疗方案只有连续静脉输注胰岛素。采用胰岛素持续皮下维持的 1 型糖尿病患者的人数在不断增加，建议围术期使用持续静脉输注。对于行中小手术的稳定的 2 型糖尿病患者，口服药物可在术后恢复。

（袁宁平 译 潘 科 校）

延伸阅读

American Diabetes Association: Standards of medical care in diabetes—2014, *Diabetes Care* 37(Suppl 1):S14–S80, 2014.

Griesdale DE, de Souza RJ, van Dam RM, et al.: Intensive insulin therapy and mortality among critically ill patients: a meta-analysis including NICE-SUGAR study data, *CMAJ* 180:821–827, 2009.

Handelsman Y, Bloomgarden ZT, Grunberger G, et al.: American Association of Clinical Endocrinologists and American College of Endocrinology—clinical practice guidelines for developing a diabetes mellitus comprehensive care plan—2015, *Endocr Pract* 21(Suppl 1):1–87, 2015.

Inzucchi SE: Clinical practice. Management of hyperglycemia in the hospital setting, *N Engl J Med* 355:1903–1911, 2006.

Kwon S, Thompson R, Dellinger P, et al.: Importance of perioperative glycemic control in general surgery: a report from the Surgical Care and Outcomes Assessment Program, *Ann Surg* 257:8–14, 2013.

Moghissi ES, Korytkowski MT, DiNardo M, et al.: American Association of Clinical Endocrinologists and American Diabetes Association consensus statement on inpatient glycemic control, *Diabetes Care* 32(6):1119–1131, 2009.

Umpierrez GE, Hellman R, Korytkowski MT, et al.: Management of hyperglycemia in hospitalized patients in non-critical care setting: an Endocrine Society clinical practice guideline, *J Clin Endocrinol Metab* 97:16–38, 2012.

Wiener RS, Weiner DC, Larson RJ: Benefits and risks of tight glucose control in critical adults: a meta-analysis, *JAMA* 300:933–944, 2008.

围术期高热

第 145 章

Vijal N. Patel，David B. Glick

病例概要

患者，女性，23 岁，既往有双相情感障碍病史，服用情绪稳定剂，拟急诊行破裂阑尾切除术。患者既往无手术史，相关家族史不详。术前生命体征为：血压 130/90 mmHg、心率 105 次 / 分、体温 38.5℃、呼吸频率 15 次 / 分。使用琥珀胆碱和丙泊酚快速序列诱导，气管插管顺利，七氟烷吸入及静脉使用阿片类药物维持，30 min 后患者体温升至 40℃。

问题分析

定义

高热是指体温高于正常核心温度（通常为 36.7 ～ 37.0℃ ±0.2 ～ 0.4℃），体温升高会增加代谢需求、耗氧量和一些隐匿性损失，并且可导致高钠血症、癫痫发作、凝血功能障碍（框 145.1）。虽然低体温在围术期更为常见，但术中高热也应值得关注，且有其自身鉴别诊断，比单纯的感染发热和恶性高热更为广泛。

体温调节由下丘脑控制的反馈回路控制来调控热量产生和丢失以维持接近调节调定点的正常体温。体温调定点、阈值范围和下丘脑调节反射，均会受全身和局部麻醉药的影响。高热不同于发热，发热是由于下丘脑调定点升高引起核心体温升高。发热时，调定点升高是由循环中的致热原（如革兰氏阴性菌的内毒素）和细胞因子（白细胞介素 IL-1、IL-6、肿瘤坏死因子、干扰素 -α）所致；因此，发热对退热药（如对乙酰氨基酚）有反应，而高热对这些药物无反应。

框 145.1　高热的影响

- 基础代谢率增加
- 增加耗氧量
- 增加水分的蒸发流失
- 电解质异常（特别是高钠血症）
- 癫痫发作 [和（或）精神状态改变]
- 凝血功能障碍（和 DIC）

DIC，弥散性血管内凝血

识别

识别高热状态需要精确的体温监测。术中可采用多种不同技术监测体温。皮肤表面温度较核心温度更易受环境影响，但监测技术的创伤性最小，通常比核心温度低 2℃。尽管在调整 2℃温差后，额头皮肤温度通常能反映核心温度，若条件许可应优先选择过渡区（直肠、膀胱）监测核心温度。使用带有内置热敏电阻的 Foley 导尿管，便于获得膀胱温度，但低尿流量时所得温度偏低且不准确。其他情况下，可能需要使用肺动脉内（如使用 Swan-Ganz 导管）或食管远端温度探头，以实现更可靠的核心温度监测。

风险评估

高热本身具有多种生理意义。高热可能是医源性的，或继发于低温预防技术，高热也可能是潜在病理过程的一个指标（框 145.2）。通常需要重新评估所有生命体征和监护数据，可能时应进行动脉血气分析。

医源性 / 被动性高热

术中高热最常见的原因是医源性的，继发于为预防低体温而采取的过度隔热和主动加温。由于限制了蒸发和对流热损失，体表面积暴露有限时更易发生术中高热（如全身覆盖的眼科手术）。由于基础代谢率较高、排汗系统不成熟，与复温装置接触的

框 145.2 术中高热的鉴别诊断

医源性 / 被动性高热（尤其是小儿）
神经损伤
脓毒症
疟疾
恶性高热
重度甲状腺毒症
硬膜外镇痛时高热
嗜铬细胞瘤
抗精神病药恶性综合征
肾上腺危象
血清素综合征
输血反应
手术
药物高敏

体表面积比例较大，儿科与新生儿患者更易受到热量积聚医源性高热的影响。

发热 / 脓毒症

如前所述，感染会导致下丘脑体温调定点升高并导致发热。事实上，大多数重症监护室内感染患者均伴有发热。手术指征可明确术中发热的感染病因（如病例概要中的阑尾破裂患者），但无法排除同时导致核心体温升高的其他原因。

恶性高热

与传统教学内容不同的是，恶性高热（malignant hyperthermia，MH）的早期征象是温度升高，而非呼气末二氧化碳（end-tidal carbon dioxide，$ETCO_2$）升高。此外，MH 初始征象在麻醉开始 30 min 后出现（而非普遍认为的在麻醉诱导后很快出现）。MH 详细介绍参见第 195 章。

神经损伤

在颅内手术，甚至是明确合并颅内病变的非颅内手术中，高热可能是神经并发症的临床表现。神经源性高热可能十分隐匿，体温缓慢从 36℃上升至 40℃，且由于体表暴露面积受限，最初易与被动性高热混淆。也可能突发高热，不到 30 min 内体温迅速上升到 40℃以上。无论何种情况，神经源性高热不会同时伴有 $ETCO_2$ 升高（排除恶性高热）。神经源性高热与以下神经损伤相关：急性脑积水、颅内出血和脑室出血（尤其是进入第三或第四脑室）以及下丘脑损伤。

硬膜外镇痛

分娩和非分娩患者硬膜外镇痛时间延长与高热有关，体温可高达 39.5℃。此类患者体温缓慢上升，在硬膜外镇痛约 5 h 后发生，且为孤立体征，无其他生命体征变化。分娩患者高热被认为是代谢率增加和交感神经被阻滞，导致热丢失无法调节，其与发热和炎症不同（使用退热药无效）。然而，非分娩患者也可能出现这些问题，但持续硬膜外镇痛引发高热的潜在机制尚不明确。

抗精神病药恶性综合征

抗精神病药恶性综合征（neuroleptic malignant syndrome，NMS）是抗精神病药物治疗的一种并发症，由于存在肌肉僵硬、高热、横纹肌溶解、自主神经系统不稳定和精神状态改变，NMS 可与 MH 混淆。NMS 的潜在病理生理机制与下丘脑中枢多巴胺能阻滞有关，可由多种抗精神病药 / 抗多巴胺药物触发。通常，高热在开始药物治疗后 2 周内发生。即使经过多年相同剂量的药物治疗，也能首次出现高热。高热也可由多巴胺能药物（如帕金森病治疗药物）的突然停药触发。对接受抗精神病药物治疗且作为唯一药物的患者，氯丙嗪、甲氧氯普胺、氟哌利多和异丙嗪均可触发围术期 NMS。

血清素综合征

血清素综合征与中枢神经系统过量的血清素有关，常被描述为有精神状态改变、自主神经系统兴奋性增加（包括出汗、心动过速、高热和高血压）和神经肌肉异常（从震颤、反射亢进到肌肉僵硬）等症状。近年来，由于使用促血清素分泌药物的门诊患者比例越来越高，特别是选择性 5- 羟色胺再摄取抑制剂类的抗抑郁药，以及单胺氧化酶抑制剂、三环类抗抑郁药、安非他命和可卡因等，血清素综合征的发病率升高。值得注意的是，美国食品和药物监督管理局和世界卫生组织已发布报告指出，5-HT_3 拮抗剂（如昂丹司琼）与其他 5- 羟色胺能药物可能存在相互作用，导致 5- 羟色胺可能过量；然而，使用 5- 羟色胺能药物治疗的患者出现术后恶心时，尚无切实证据支持不使用 5-HT_3 拮抗剂。

内分泌紊乱

严重甲状腺毒症（甲状腺危象）、嗜铬细胞瘤和肾上腺危象等特定的内分泌紊乱或异常，通常与高热有关，这是由潜在的病理原因导致的代谢率增加所致。

输血反应

输血反应也会导致高热，通常发生在刚开始输血时。若仅出现高热，最可能原因是非溶血性输血反应引起的发热。若出现其他症状，如寒战、呼吸频率增加和（或）血流动力学不稳定，则更有可能发生了其他输血反应（如急性溶血性输血反应、输血相关性脓毒症）。更多讨论参见第 101 章。

疟疾

许多病例报告指出，术中发生疟疾的临床表现与恶性高热相似。全身麻醉后，疟疾通常表现为发热、心动过速和寒战；但与 MH 不同的是，疟疾通常对肌松药有反应，且不会引起 $ETCO_2$ 快速上升。

手术因素

某些手术发生的术中高热，与使用的设备和（或）治疗技术相关。腹腔热灌注化疗是将注入腹腔的化疗药液加热至 42 ～ 43℃，术中需主动冷却以缓解手术引起的高热。手术夹闭大血管时，由于夹闭远端的血液淤滞，也可能存在特定的高热风险：灌注不足区域使用加热装置可导致热损伤。

药物高敏

“药物热”唯一症状是体温上升，其在药物高敏患者中的发生率约为 3% ～ 5%。HIV 感染与药物反应的高风险有关。药物热通常与给药呈时间相关性，但亦可能发生于数月后，其平均发作时间为 8 天。在不到 20% 的病例中，药物热也与皮疹（荨麻疹少见）有关，可伴有非特异性的实验室检查结果。

管理

术中高热的处理取决于高热的潜在原因，还应包括缓解高热的干预措施。如前所述，高热可能会导致凝血障碍和弥散性血管内凝血，故应予以正确治疗。

医源性 / 被动性高热

过度隔绝和主动加温是此类高热的主要原因，这些应予以处理。应移除多余的毯子等覆盖物，并停用主动加温装置。

发热 / 脓毒症

若引起高热的可能原因是感染，解热药有一定的效果。此外，还应选择合理的覆盖抗生素并控制感染源。

恶性高热

治疗 MH 可以缓解由此产生的高热。去除 MH 触发剂，给予丹曲林，可中断失控的肌肉收缩。MH 管理详见第 195 章。

神经损伤

神经源性高热的治疗着重于对对神经病损的手术治疗。随着病理过程的结束（或脑室出血时血红素被吸收和分解），高热可持续至术后阶段。

硬膜外镇痛

体温升高常见，无需特别干预。然而，这并不意味着评估过程中无需考虑其他诊断，如硬膜外分娩患者因绒毛膜羊膜炎导致的体温升高。

抗精神病药恶性综合征

若考虑 NMS 是引起术中高热的潜在原因，应避免使用抗精神病药物（以及其他潜在触发剂），支持治疗应注重血流动力学支持和降温。丹曲林、溴隐亭或金刚烷胺等二线治疗药物的使用尚有争议，因其使用证据有限，尤其是术中作为一线药物治疗时时。

血清素综合征

血清素综合征的治疗包括停止 / 避免使用触发剂，并予以适当的血流动力学支持。避免使用间接的拟交感神经药物，如多巴胺和麻黄碱，因其可能会加重血清素综合征。神经肌肉阻滞剂对于限制体温升高有一定的益处和帮助。此外，还需积极降温处理。解热药没有作用，应避免使用。若增加麻醉深度和静脉输液均不能改善自主神经系统紊乱，则有必要使用 5- 羟色胺拮抗剂（经胃管或鼻饲管给予碾碎的赛庚啶 12 mg，之后每 2 h 给予 2 mg，直至血流动力学稳定性得到改善）。

内分泌紊乱

内分泌紊乱的治疗着重于减弱激素失衡的影响，同时予以常规的血流动力学支持。具体来说，治疗甲状腺危象时需立即使用 β - 受体阻滞剂（普萘洛尔或易于滴定的艾司洛尔），以减弱交感神经兴奋性。此外，糖皮质激素已被证明可改善甲状腺危象的预后。硫酰胺（如丙硫脲嘧啶或甲巯咪唑）和碘化钠可限制甲状腺激素的进一步释放并减少外周转化。详见第 11 章。

输血反应

若认为高热是血制品输注后的继发反应，反应严重程度决定了随后治疗步骤。大多数情况下，首先应停止血制品输注。如果表现为发热性非溶血性输血反应，可恢复输血。对于更严重的输血反应，可能需要额外的血流动力学支持及后续针对凝血障碍的处理。详见第 101 章。

药物过敏

停用怀疑有问题的药物至关重要，但取决于反应严重程度和术中所用药物的适应证。

降温技术

各种降温技术，无论是被动还是主动降温，都可用来缓解高热。如果患者体温上升至 39℃以上，应采用主动降温。最简单的第一步是，关闭任何主动加热装置（如压缩空气加热器），甚至将其调到环境温度，启动较冷的空气循环。其他措施包括暴露更多的表面积以增加对流和蒸发损失（尽管在手术环境中，由于无菌原则，实施可能会困难）。主动降温还包括在腹股沟、腋窝及头颈部周围使用冰袋。更具侵入性的主动降温包括使用冷冻过的静脉液体和（或）冰冷的腹腔灌洗（胃和膀胱灌洗效果较差，且并发症发生率较高）。

预防

预防术中高热需要了解促成高热发生的因素，包括识别术中高热风险的患者并予以充分的温度监测，以便及早发现和干预。

（夏博洋　译　查燕萍　校）

延伸阅读

Boyer EW, Shannon M: The serotonin syndrome, *N Engl J Med* 352: 1112–1120, 2005.

Carroll R, Matfin G: Review: Endocrine and metabolic emergencies: thyroid storm, *Ther Adv Endocrinol Metab* 1:139–145, 2010.

Herlich A: Perioperative temperature elevation: not all hyperthermia is malignant hyperthermia, *Paediatr Anaesth* 23:842–850, 2013.

Hrishi AP, Lionel KR: Intraoperative hyperthermia: a harbinger of hypothalamic injury, *J Neurosurg Anesthesiol* 29(3):379–380, 2016.

Kushimoto S, Yamanouchi S, Endo T, et al.: Body temperature abnormalities in non-neurological critically ill patients: a review of the literature, *J Intensive Care* 2:14, 2014.

Larach MG, Brandom BW, Allen GC, et al.: Malignant hyperthermia deaths related to inadequate temperature monitoring, 2007–2012: a report from the North American malignant hyperthermia registry of the malignant hyperthermia association of the United States, *Anesth Analg* 119: 1359–1366, 2014.

Mackowiak PA: Drug fever: mechanisms, maxims and misconceptions, *Am J Med Sci* 294:275–286, 1987.

Reulbach U, Dütsch C, Biermann T, et al.: Managing an effective treatment for neuroleptic malignant syndrome, *Crit Care* 11:R4, 2007.

Stitt JT: Fever versus hyperthermia, *Fed Proc* 38:39–43, 1979.

低体温

第 146 章

Natalie F. Holt

病例概要

患者，女性，74 岁，既往有痴呆和骨质疏松病史，在家中无人目击摔倒后入院。在硬膜外麻醉复合气管插管全身麻醉下行髋部骨折修复术。术中输注 4 单位浓缩红细胞。患者术后在 PACU 内出现精神错乱和定向力障碍。心率 110 次 / 分，血压 160/90 mmHg，体温 33.8℃（口温），动脉血气（鼻导管吸氧，氧流量 6 L/min）：动脉血氧分压（PaO_2）63 mmHg，动脉血二氧化碳分压（$PaCO_2$）54 mmHg。

问题分析

定义

人体正常体温在 36 ～ 38℃，主要由位于下丘脑的体温调节中枢调控。低体温可分为轻度至中度（33 ～ 36℃）、重度（23 ～ 33℃）和深度（<23℃）。意外低体温是一种可预防的围术期并发症，其在麻醉中发生率为 50% ～ 90%。几项重要研究结果显示，即使适度的低体温也会使心源性死亡、手术伤口感染、失血和需要异体血制品的概率增加 2 倍。意外（框 146.1）或医源性（框 146.2）原因可能导致低体温，包括患者、麻醉、手术和环境原因。

框 146.1　低体温的意外原因

环境
风寒
冷水浸泡

温度调节受损
极端年龄（新生儿、老年人）
长期制动
药物
　酒精
　中枢神经系统抑制剂
　药物过量

疾病状态
甲状腺功能减退
大面积烧伤
感染或脓毒症
营养不良
低血糖
下丘脑卒中或肿瘤
意识丧失

框 146.2　低体温的医源性原因

长时间麻醉和手术
长时间心肺复苏术
血液或血制品输注
大量液体复苏[a]

[a] 未充分保温

识别

在全身麻醉中，低体温以特征性模式发生。在第 1 h，中心温度快速下降 0.5 ～ 1.5℃。第 2 ～ 4 h，中心温度呈缓慢线性下降。体温最初快速下降是由麻醉引起血管扩张，导致热量从中心向外周重新分布。体温缓慢线性下降是由热量丢失超过代谢产热。在 3 ～ 4 h 后，中心温度趋于平稳，外周温度继续下降。

阈值区间是不引起生理反应的中心温度变化的范围，该范围非常小（约 0.5℃）。然而，从图 146.1 可明显看出，麻醉将阈值区间扩大到 4℃。例如，中心温度在 34 ～ 38℃时，机体对热量的储存或丢失无任何生理反应。在该范围内，患者呈变温性（即，中心温度直接随环境温度变化）。

热传递有 4 种不同机制：传导、对流、蒸发和辐射。其中，辐射、对流是发生围术期低体温的重要因素。所有物体表面都辐射热量，存在温差的两个不接触表面之间通过辐射传热。热对流损失受温差和风速影响。手术室配备层流和高换气率的专用通风系统，可能导致明显的对流性热量损失。蒸发性热量损失通过出汗、呼吸道和大面积手术伤口发生。这种热量损失方法明显存在于早产儿和大面积手术切口患者。传导是两种相邻物质之间的热传递方法。由于隔热层（如泡沫垫）将患者与手术床隔开，热传导在手术室内可忽略不计。

全身和区域麻醉会干扰生理性体温调节（见图146.1）。全身麻醉药均能轻微增加出汗阈值，同时显著降低血管收缩和寒战阈值，这种反应在老年人中更为明显。血管收缩阈值由正常的37℃下降约2～4℃。全身麻醉药通过直接的外周作用引起血管扩张。非寒战性产热作为婴儿重要的体温调节机制，也被挥发性麻醉药物抑制。麻醉药物还能降低代谢率20%～30%，一定程度上抵消由周围血管收缩调节受损导致的皮肤热损失。

区域麻醉或神经轴索麻醉开始后，中心温度通常降低0.5～1.0℃。类似全身麻醉，早期体温降低是由热量从中心向外周重分布所致。随后，与全身麻醉下体温进入平台期不同，由于外周血管收缩受损，中心温度继续下降。区域麻醉和神经轴索麻醉引起交感神经阻滞，降低所影响皮节的血管收缩和寒战阈值；同时，肌肉活动产生的热量与节段性运动阻滞的程度成比例减少。此外，受影响节段的温度觉传入被阻断，可以解释相关的腿部温度增高。这进一步导致机体对寒冷的血管收缩反应和寒战反应迟钝。矛盾的是，区域麻醉或神经轴索麻醉患者可能感觉不到寒冷。这是由于对寒冷的感知主要取决于皮肤温度，而非中心温度。所以，同全身麻醉一样，在区域麻醉和神经轴索麻醉中监测患者体温非常重要。

风险评估及启示

即使轻度低体温也会引起血小板功能障碍，损害凝血级联反应中酶的功能，增加术中出血风险。这已在几项随机试验中得到证实，即使轻度低体温也会增加术中失血量和异体血输注需求。因为实验室血液样本加温至37℃，所以凝血功能的定量评估有误。目前有证据表明，即使轻度术中低体温也可能增加术后伤口感染风险。这可能是由血管收缩降低组织氧分压并损害趋化作用，从而有助于细菌生长。低体温也会显著影响药物代谢和麻醉药需求。中心温度下降2℃，维库溴铵神经肌肉阻滞时间约增加一倍。中心温度每下降1℃，挥发性麻醉药的最低肺泡有效浓度（minimum alveolar concentration，MAC）下降约5%。在持续输注期间，随着体温降低，丙泊酚血浆浓度也高于正常值。

一些诱发寒冷的因素可能导致麻醉后苏醒延迟，包括中枢神经系统功能损害（如淡漠、精神错乱、

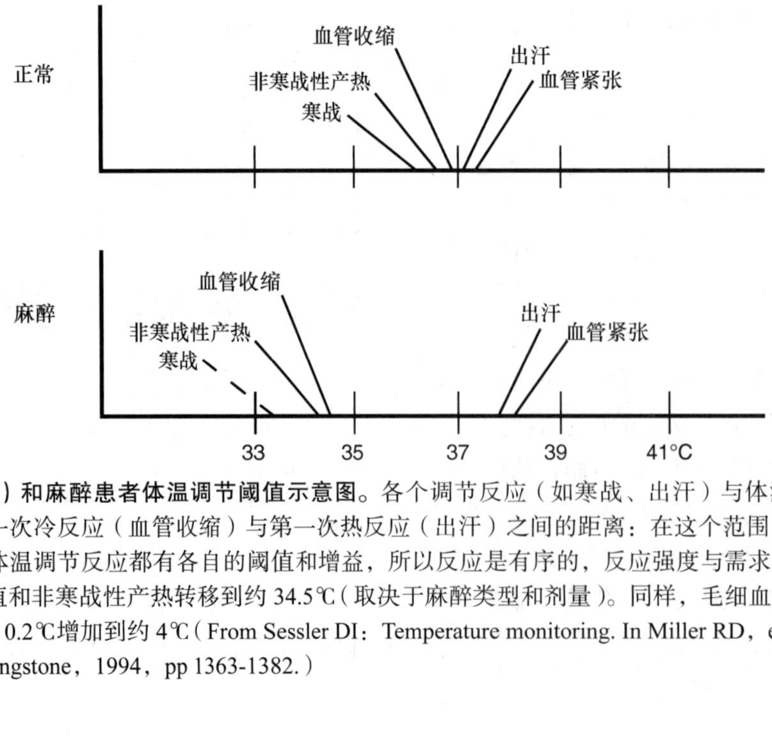

图146.1 未麻醉（正常）和麻醉患者体温调节阈值示意图。各个调节反应（如寒战、出汗）与体温（中心体温）的交点就是阈值。阈值区间是第一次冷反应（血管收缩）与第一次热反应（出汗）之间的距离：在这个范围内的温度不会引起自主体温调节代偿。因为每个体温调节反应都有各自的阈值和增益，所以反应是有序的，反应强度与需求成正比。在全身麻醉（下图）时，血管收缩的阈值和非寒战性产热转移到约34.5℃（取决于麻醉类型和剂量）。同样，毛细血管前血管舒张和出汗阈值增加约1℃，阈值范围从0.2℃增加到约4℃（From Sessler DI：Temperature monitoring. In Miller RD，editor：*Anesthesia*，4th ed. New York，Churchill Livingstone，1994，pp 1363-1382.）

嗜睡）、麻醉药物和神经肌肉阻滞剂的肝或肾清除减慢、对低氧血症和高碳酸血症的通气反应受损。随着低体温严重程度增加（<33℃），几乎所有器官系统都有不良影响（框 146.3、图 146.2）。

寒冷导致血管收缩、全身血管阻力增加，可能加重术后高血压（病例概要中患者血压为 160/90 mmHg）。同时去甲肾上腺素浓度高，这两者都可能导致易感患者心肌缺血。此外，一项前瞻性随机试验显示，心脏病患者行非心脏手术，围术期维持正常体温，其不良心脏事件减少 55%。中度低体温增加心律失常的风险。随着体温降低，心脏电传导受损，致命性室性心律失常风险增加。术后寒战会大大增加需氧量和二氧化碳的产生，从而增加分钟通气量、呼吸功和耗氧量。如果分钟通气量固定（机械通气）或被抑制（麻醉药物或阿片类药物），可能导致高碳酸血症和急性呼吸性酸中毒。当耗氧量增加但心排血量无法代偿时，氧摄取增加，为低氧血症及其后遗症的发生奠定了基础。寒战还会引起患者不适和其他不良后遗症，如伤口裂开、出血增加、颅内压和眼压升高。总的来说，与正常体温患者相比，低体温和温度不适感增加患者术后在麻醉后恢复室的停留时间。

然而，低体温可能避免某些患者器官缺血而使其受益。正常体温每降低 10℃，氧气利用率就减半。轻度低体温（33 ~ 36℃）提供了重要的中枢神经系统保护。越来越多的证据表明，在心室颤动引起的心搏骤停后，低温治疗可能起到保护作用。基于低体温具有降低脑代谢率、颅内压的潜在作用，提出控制性低温治疗作为创伤性脑损伤（traumatic brain injury，TBI）治疗中的一种脑保护方法。TBI 后轻度至中度（33 ~ 35℃）的低温治疗，多项临床试验得出不同的结果。低体温在新生儿窒息的治疗中也可能具有益处，其改善神经系统预后和降低死亡率已经得到证实。最后，在轻度低体温的动物中，

框 146.3 低体温对器官系统功能的不良影响

心血管

早期：心动过速，高血压，心排血量增加，血管收缩（儿茶酚胺释放）

晚期：心动过缓，心排血量减少，低血压

心电图：非特异性传导减慢，窦性心动过缓，T 波倒置，QT 延长，心室异位（32℃，Osborne 波：30℃，心室颤动；见图 146.2）

呼吸

早期：呼吸频率增加

晚期：呼吸频率和潮气量降低，缺氧性肺血管收缩减弱，对低氧血症和高碳酸血症的反应降低，黏液纤毛活动降低。

肾

早期：早期“冷”利尿作用（中心血容量增加，肾血管阻力增加）；由于肾小管钠重吸收受损，利尿持续

晚期：少尿和氮质血症

血液

早期：血液浓缩，黏度增加（淤积、组织灌注不良、缺血），氧利用率降低（血红蛋白氧解离曲线左移）

晚期：弥散性血管内凝血、血小板减少

代谢

早期：低钠血症、高钾血症、高血糖症（抑制胰岛素释放和阻止细胞摄取）

晚期：代谢性酸中毒

神经系统

体温每降低 1℃，脑血流减少 6% ~ 7%：

34℃：遗忘

30℃：反应迟钝

26℃：瞳孔和深腱反射消失

18℃：脑活动消失（脑电图）

胃肠

早期：肠动力下降（饱胃），肝清除减少

晚期：胃、回肠、结肠溃疡；出血性胰腺炎

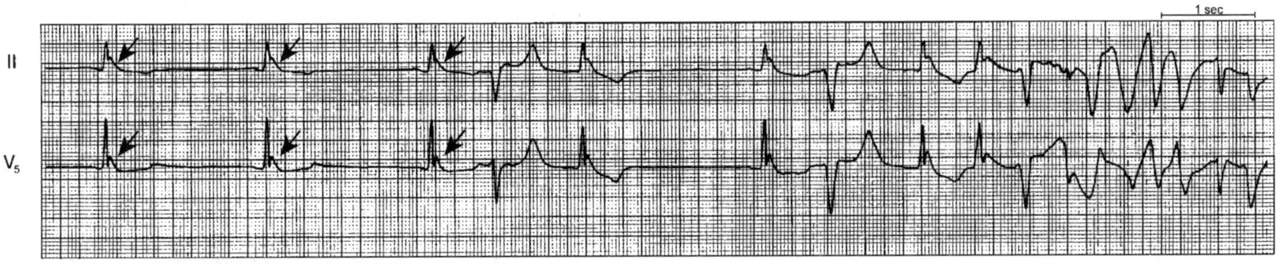

图 146.2 心肺转流低温过程中的两个心电图导联。窦性心动过缓（约 30 bpm）和明显 J 波（Osborne 波，箭头所示）区分了前三个波群。随着患者体温迅速降低，心室异位节律增加并发展为纤维性颤动。膀胱和鼻咽温度分别为 35.8℃和 31.4℃（From Mark JB：*Atlas of cardiovascular monitoring*. New York，Churchill Livingstone，1997，p 331.）

恶性高热更难发生；因此，建议对有恶性高热风险的患者避免主动加温。

管理与预防

术前加温可通过减小患者外周和中心温度差异，有助于防止再分布性低体温。其常可通过在术前等待区或诱导室使用充气温毯实现。手术室内温度是决定皮肤辐射和对流散热速率的最重要因素。为维持正常体温，在麻醉诱导前手术室环境温度应该增加至 23 ～ 26℃。一旦患者被完全覆盖和保护起来后，可以降低室温，以便不影响外科医师或助手的工作。手术结束时应再次提高室温。术前氨基酸输注可增加产热，并可减少术中低体温的发生。

对超过 30 min 的手术都必须进行温度监测。然而，"正常"温度（类似血压）取决于测量位置。中心体温的监测部位包括鼓膜（容易受伤）、鼻咽部（受麻醉气体温度影响）、食管（取决于插入深度；注意，如果热敏电阻位于气管后方，中心温度将比其真实值低 0.2℃）和肺动脉（如果使用的肺动脉导管配备热敏电阻）。当患者体温较高且血管扩张，直肠和膀胱可反映中心体温；当患者体温较低且血管收缩，则反映外周体温。前额皮肤温度比中心温度约低 2℃，变化大，不足以反映中心温度。

约 90% 的热量损失通过皮肤表面流失，因此最有效的加温方法是调节皮肤热量损失。在围术期，充气加温是维持正常体温最经济有效的方法，体温通常平均增加 1℃ /h。全身或半身充气毯可供选择。需要注意的是，在主动脉阻断中不应该在下半身使用，因为这将加剧组织氧供需失衡。放置在患者身下的循环水床垫覆盖相对较小的表面积，对补偿腹侧大量的热损失作用不大。此外，还可能导致压力性热损伤。被动隔离（毯子、洞巾）和电热垫效果有限，主要是通过在患者和绝缘体之间封闭一层空气产生作用。单层毛毯可以减少大约 30% 的热量损失，添加毛毯数量带来的益处有限。虽然辐射加温器经常用于婴幼儿，但患者的皮肤必须暴露在外才能发生热传导。热传导被身处其中的外科或护理人员阻断。此外，位于头部的加温器限制医护人员对患者的接触。

在成人患者中，除为减少已经低体温患者进一步的热量损失，或时间较长的重要手术操作，不常规使用加温和加湿器麻醉回路。这种麻醉回路对提高中心温度作用不大。麻醉诱导后，将新鲜气体流量减少到 2 L/min 以下有助于减少气道热量和水分损失，"人工鼻"（即，热湿交换过滤器或吸湿式冷凝加湿器）也有同样作用。

当输注大量晶体、胶体或血液制品时，应使用液体加温装置。在输入 1 个单位 4℃的冷藏血液或 1 L 室温下的晶体溶液时，成人体温平均减少约 0.25℃。在大量输血中，使用快速输液装置（可提供 1L/min 输注速度）对预防可能危及生命的低体温和不可逆的低温性凝血障碍至关重要。然而，应认识到液体加温并不能有效地使患者变暖，它只能防止液体引起体温降低。发生外伤时，在与酸中毒和危及生命的凝血障碍有关的严重低体温的病例中，可以考虑采用主动体外血液复温，如心肺转流术、动-静脉复温、静-静脉复温或血液透析。这些技术可以使中心温度每 3 ～ 5 min 升高 1 ～ 2℃。

防止术后寒战最有效的方法是给皮肤加温（即使用充气加温毯）。皮肤温度感受器的传入信号控制下丘脑对寒冷的反应；皮肤温度越高，寒战的中心温度阈值就越低。术前给予 α_2- 肾上腺素能受体激动剂（可乐定、右美托咪定）也可能抑制术后寒战。术后寒战除使用皮肤加温治疗，也可以用药物治疗，包括哌替啶（12.5 ～ 25 mg），可乐定（75 μg）和曲马多（0.5 ～ 3.0 mg/kg）。

在麻醉恢复室，根据低体温严重程度，出现不同的复温性血管舒张变化。在周围血管持续收缩时，肌肉张力首先增高（即亚临床寒战）产生热量。因此，中心温度升高，甚至可能"骤升"至 38 ～ 40℃，特别是在低温体外循环后。当发生外周血管扩张，热产生与热损失平衡，在恢复正常前中心温度处于平台期。如果患者血容量过低，复温性血管扩张可引起急性低血压、反射性心动过速和心肌缺血。因此，在术后早期，低体温、血管收缩和高血压患者可能受益于积极的液体治疗联合血管舒张剂合理治疗（如硝普钠、硝酸甘油）。一旦发生复温性血管扩张，就需要补充液体，必要时使用血管升压药。

致谢

感谢 Christopher C. Young 和 Robert N. Sladen 博

士对本章上一版的贡献。

（饶苗苗 译 席 鹏 校）

延伸阅读

Crowley LJ, Buggy DJ: Shivering and neuraxial anesthesia, *Reg Anesth Pain Med* 33:241–252, 2008.

Frank SM, Fleisher LA, Breslow MJ, et al.: Perioperative maintenance of normothermia reduces the incidence of morbid cardiac events. A randomized clinical trial, *JAMA* 277:1127–1134, 1997.

Kurz A, Sessler DI, Lenhardt R: Perioperative normothermia to reduce the incidence of surgical-wound infection and shorten hospitalization, *N Engl J Med* 334:1209–1215, 1996.

Madrid E, Urrútia G, Roqué i Figuls M, et al.: Active body surface warming systems for preventing complications caused by inadvertent perioperative hypothermia in adults, *Cochrane Database Syst Rev* 4:CD009016, 2016.

Melling AC, Ali B, Scott EM, et al.: Effects of preoperative warming on the incidence of wound infection after clean surgery: a randomised controlled trial, *Lancet* 358:876–880, 2001.

Nielsen N, Wetterslev J, Cronberg T, et al.: Targeted temperature management at 33°C versus 36°C after cardiac arrest, *N Eng J Med* 369:2197–2206, 2013.

Sessler DI: Temperature regulation and monitoring. In Miller RD, Cohen NH, Eriksson LI, et al.: *Miller's anesthesia*, ed 8th, Philadelphia, 2015, Elsevier, pp 1622–1646.

Wong PF, Kumar S, Bohra A, et al.: Randomized clinical trial of perioperative systemic warming in major elective abdominal surgery, *Br J Surg* 94:421–426, 2007.

第 147 章 镇痛不足

Charles J. Lin，*Michael L. Kentor*，*Brian A. Williams*

病例概要

患者，男性，30 岁，既往体健，于门诊在气管插管全身麻醉下行踝关节融合术，手术顺利。患者苏醒后，在麻醉后恢复室（postanesthesia care unit，PACU）出现剧烈、顽固性疼痛，使用阿片类药物进行镇痛，出现术后恶心呕吐（postoperative nausea and vomiting，PONV）。患者最终因顽固性疼痛、PONV 和嗜睡而计划外入院，2 日后恢复进食，而后出院。5 日后患者由于便秘、偶发性恶心、伤口开裂伴伤口耐甲氧西林金黄色葡萄球菌和耐万古霉素粪肠球菌阳性而再次于急诊室就诊。1 年后，患者因术后慢性疼痛而就诊于疼痛科医师。

问题分析

定义

一项全国性调查显示，80% 的术后患者从出院至术后 2 周都经历过疼痛，其中有 86% 的患者疼痛无法控制。术后镇痛不足对患者有显著的生理和心理影响，大大增加了整个体系的医疗费用负担。术后镇痛不足有短期和长期的后果（表 147.1）。疼痛控制不佳，导致交感神经兴奋性增加，心脏氧耗和负荷增加，从而增加术后心脏事件的风险。体位固定和通气 / 灌注不足增加了低氧血症和呼吸困难的风险。阿片类药物过量使用会导致 PONV 和术后意识混乱。这些风险的直接后果是延长 PACU 停留时间、延长住院时间、降低患者满意度和增加住院率。

持续性术后疼痛，又称慢性术后疼痛综合征（chronic postsurgical pain syndrome，CPSP），是术后镇痛不足的重要后果。定义是疼痛持续至少术后 2 个月，并且排除其他引起疼痛的诊断。最容易发生 CPSP 的手术包括截肢、开胸、乳房手术、胆囊切除术和腹股沟疝修补术。术后镇痛不足导致的缺勤和工作效率下降所造成的经济成本均较显著。一项横断面研究显示，慢性疼痛患者复工后导致的损伤为每年 612 亿美元，其中主要是因为工作效率下降所造成的。

表 147.1　镇痛不足的全身影响

神经系统	持续性术后疼痛
	术后谵妄和认知障碍
心理	焦虑与抑郁
	患者满意度下降
心血管系统	心动过速
	全身血管阻力增加导致高血压
	心肌收缩力增强
	增加心脏做功
肺	体位固定和膈肌损伤导致通气不足以及肺活量下降
	肺不张和通气 / 灌注不足
	咳嗽和咳痰清除能力下降
	低氧血症
	高碳酸血症
肾	交感神经张力增加引起的尿潴留
胃肠道系统	交感神经张力增加引起的肠梗阻
	术后恶心，呕吐
免疫体统	免疫系统受损和免疫抑制
总体	延长 PACU 停留时间
	延迟恢复
	降低患者满意度
	增加医疗资源的消耗和医疗成本

Adapted from Joshi GP，Ogunnaike BO：Consequences of inadequate postoperative pain relief and chronic persistent postoperative pain. *Anesthesiol Clin North Am* 23（1）：21-36，2005.

风险评估

为每位患者制订充分的镇痛方案时，需要了解患者发生严重术后疼痛的风险、阿片类药物的不良反应以及评估施行周围神经阻滞（peripheral nerve block，PNB）的风险。除了之前列出的最容易发生 CPSP 的手术以外，某些人群有较高的阿片类药物并发症的风险。对于这些人群，优化镇痛的最佳方案是减少麻醉性镇静药技术的多模式镇痛。这一群体包括老年患者、阻塞性睡眠呼吸暂停综合征的患者，以及已存在肺功能不全的患者。

PNB 的风险需要加以考虑，以选择合适的患者接受这种治疗。PNB 绝对禁忌证如下：

- 患者拒绝。应当注意的是，患者拒绝是指在麻醉科医师对患者进行适当的宣教后（某些患者可能需要 10 ～ 15 min），患者仍然拒绝接受 PNB 的情况；常常有些患者一开始拒绝，经过麻醉科医师的宣教后，最终接受 PNB，并且理解体会到 PNB 与他们先前经历的全身麻醉相比的益处。
- 凝血障碍。如需接受 PNB，术前应将全身性抗凝药（如华法林）改为静脉使用的肝素。
- 置针部位感染。
- 全身性菌血症或脓毒症。

实际上，所有上述的情况在当天接受骨科手术的门诊患者几乎不太可能存在。但是，原先已有神经系统问题的患者有时可能是 PNB 的相对禁忌证；所以这类患者要实施 PNB 时，必须仔细记录神经系统状况。

管理

周围神经阻滞

实施 PNB 进行手术麻醉有明显益处，包括出院较早、对疼痛或 PONV 的护理干预较少，而且接受门诊骨科手术的患者实施 PNB 与接受气管插管全身麻醉相比，计划外住院人数更少（框 147.1）。Williams 及其同事在对 1200 例接受门诊膝关节手术的患者进行了连续性案例回顾研究的报告中提到，与实施股神经和坐骨神经阻滞的 PNB 技术相比，发现使用吸入麻醉药物行全身麻醉的患者，当天康复病房对疼痛护理干预增加了 2 倍，非计划入院增加了 3 倍。Williams 及其同事还报告了骨科手术的多模式神经周围麻醉 / 镇痛（Multimodal Perineural Anesthesia/Analgesia，MMPNA）项目的进展，强调了可乐定、丁丙诺啡和地塞米松与局部麻醉剂布比卡因在神经阻滞中的联合使用。这种组合为术后镇痛提供了中位数超过 30 h 的有效阻滞时间。这一结果得到了 Cochrane 回顾性研究的支持，研究显示与全身镇痛相比，辅以周围神经阻滞可减轻疼痛。此外，使用留置导管和便携式输注泵的连续 PNB 技术为门诊手术提供了良好的术后镇痛。在一项关于门诊行择期关节镜下肩袖修复术患者的前瞻性研究中，接受肌间神经阻滞（连续或单次注射）的患者与未接受神经阻滞的患者相比，前者更容易实施快通道，并且在 PACU 停留时间也明显缩短。此外，接受肌间沟神经连续阻滞的患者术后疼痛评分最低，且睡眠时间最长。另一项回顾性研究对 20 000 多名接受肩袖修复术的患者进行了统计，结果显示接受 PNB 的患者比接受全身麻醉的患者住院的风险降低了 18%。研究还指出在住院的费用上，未接受神经阻滞的患者与神经阻滞的患者相比几乎翻了一番。

框 147.1　门诊骨科手术中区域麻醉相对于全身麻醉的优势

- 镇痛效果优于阿片类药物
- PACU 疼痛评分较低
- 术后恶心和呕吐较少
- PACU 镇痛药的消耗更少
- PACU 1 期转出更快
- 快通道 PACU 1 期旁路率更高
- 住院时间更短
- 手术室效率增高
- 患者满意度更高

PACU，麻醉后恢复室

PNB 有两种方法：①单次注射 PNB 技术；②留置导管的连续 PNB 技术。尽管单次注射技术已被证明是有效的，但只能提供从数小时至 24 h 不等的术后镇痛，取决于使用的局部麻醉药和佐剂。由于这些阻滞剂的持续时间太短，可能无法提供持续的或有效的术后镇痛，因此，患者无法积极地开始早期活动。早期理疗对于改善骨科手术后的功能恢复至关重要。留置导管的连续 PNB 与单次注射神经阻滞和（或）椎管内麻醉技术相比具有以下优点：

- 更长的术后镇痛时间；
- 药物剂量可以滴定；
- 术后需要积极理疗动时，可选择性感觉神经阻滞；

- 避免椎管内麻醉及其相关并发症（尤其是在全身抗凝的情况下）。

其他需要考虑的因素包括：用于 PNB 的技术（超声引导，神经刺激器）、阻滞的目标神经及神经阻滞的位置。由于超声在神经阻滞中的可用性和易学性，超声引导的 PNB 技术应用得越来越广泛。神经阻滞的定位取决于相关肢体的皮肤、肌肉和骨骼所处的神经节段。神经阻滞的定位还需要考虑止血带放置的部位和准备手术的区域。在这个案例中，超声引导下放置导管的坐骨神经阻滞是合适的方法（图 147.1）。术后患者携带留置 PNB 导管和便携式输注泵可以出院回家。在出院时向患者及其家属提供并解释导管管理的书面说明，在导管留置期间麻醉护理团队应每天给患者打电话随访。患者也可以及时通过电话咨询麻醉护理团队。神经阻滞导管通常保留 2 ～ 3 天，之后由患者或家属取出。

PNB 技术可以安全地应用于术后需要抗凝以预防深静脉血栓形成的患者。然而，当患者留置 PNB 导管出院回家并可能需要术后抗凝时仍需慎重考虑。术前就已经接受了抗凝治疗的患者需注意这种情况的发生，例如有心房颤动、人工心脏瓣膜或冠状动脉支架的患者。

当术中需要镇静或全凭静脉麻醉时，使用丙泊酚连续输注有利于门诊手术患者减少 PONV 的风险。通常使用 PNB 技术也可以代替全身麻醉，利于术中进行镇静。

多模式镇痛方案

多模式镇痛可以通过不同的机制、不同部位治疗疼痛，可以减少阿片类药物的消耗量。这些镇痛药物包括非甾体抗炎药（nonsteroidal antiinflammatory drugs，NSAIDs，尤其是环氧化酶 -2 特异性抑制剂）；N- 甲基 -D- 天冬氨酸（*N*-methyl-d-aspartate，NMDA）拮抗剂，如氯胺酮；钙通道拮抗剂，如加巴喷丁；对乙酰氨基酚。这些药物的联合使用可以起协同作用，并使每种药物的不良反应降至最低。

预防

周围神经阻滞作为首选

在麻醉科医师熟练掌握这些技术的前提下，重要的是要避免 PNB 技术在门诊骨科手术患者中的**利用不足**。麻醉科医师应积极主动向患者和外科医师宣教，优先把 PNB 技术作为“计划 A”。PNB 无论作为主要麻醉方式，或在有指征时作为丙泊酚全静脉麻醉的辅助麻醉，都有助于快速苏醒和围术期镇痛。

术后恶心呕吐的预防措施

术前制订策略对于术后恶心呕吐的预防很重要，包括多种药物的使用，如血清素受体阻滞剂（如昂丹司琼），多巴胺受体拮抗药（如奋乃静 8 mg 口服，术前和术后），糖皮质激素（如地塞米松 5 mg 静注）。同时丙泊酚输注联合 PNB 亦有益处。在实施 PNB

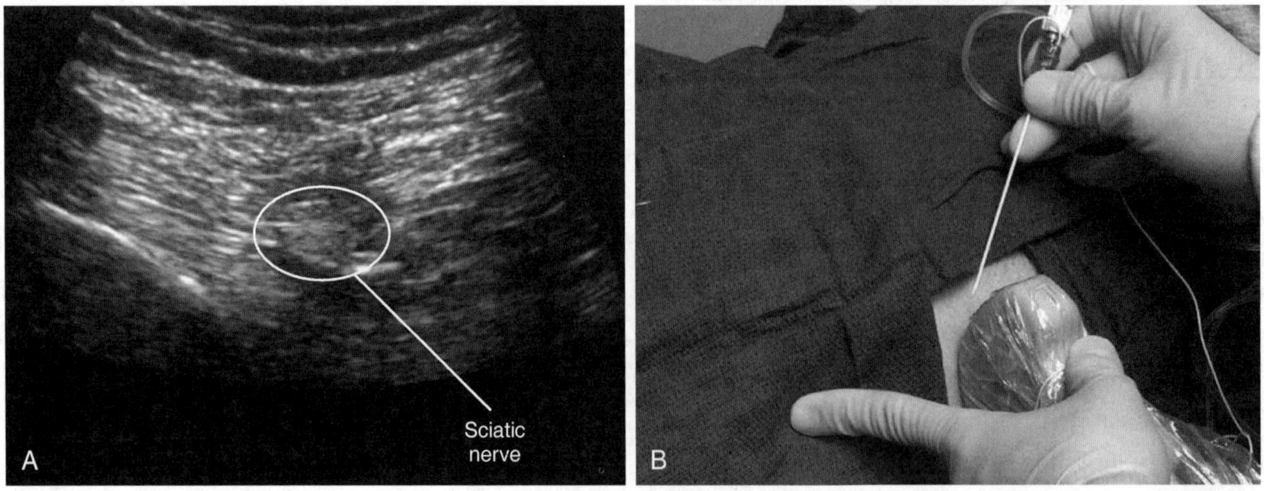

图 147.1　坐骨神经周围神经阻滞。图 A，周围神经阻滞下的坐骨神经超声图像；**图 B，**周围神经阻滞时的针和超声探头

时，尽量减少阿片类药物、除丙泊酚外的诱导药物（如依托咪酯）、挥发性药物、静脉注射或外周注射新斯的明的使用，也有助于降低 PONV 的风险。

便秘

这种不良反应可能是大剂量使用肠外和口服类阿片类药物的一个潜在问题。之前列出的使用节省阿片类药物的技术可有助于预防这种并发症。

医院伤口感染

手术部位感染延长住院时间，增加医疗费用。为了预防与住院相关的院内伤口感染，在手术当天成功出院是很重要的。这需要一个安排有序、全面的症状管理计划，来作为总的麻醉和镇痛治疗方案的一部分。

持续性术后疼痛

早期、有效的镇痛对于降低持续性术后疼痛的风险非常重要。多模式镇痛方案包括非甾体抗炎药、对乙酰氨基酚、PNB、NMDA 拮抗剂，以及尽量少的阿片类药物的使用，有助于避免这种潜在的衰竭性并发症。

（封莉莉　译　季　锋　校）

延伸阅读

Apfelbaum JL, Chen C, Mehta SS, et al.: Postoperative pain experience: results from a national survey suggest postoperative pain continues to be undermanaged, *Anesth Analg* 97:534–540, 2003.

Buvanendran A, Kroin JS: Multimodal analgesia for controlling acute postoperative pain, *Curr Opin Anaesthesiol* 22:588–593, 2009.

Chelly JE, Ben-David B, Williams BA, Kentor ML: Anesthesia and postoperative analgesia: Outcomes following orthopedic surgery, *Orthopedics* 26(Suppl 8):S865–S871, 2003.

Corey JM, Bulka CM, Ehrenfeld JM: Is regional anesthesia associated with reduced PACU length of stay? *Clin Orthop Related Res* 472:1427–1433, 2014.

Danninger T, Stundner O, Rasul R, et al.: Factors associated with hospital admission after rotator cuff repair: the role of peripheral nerve blockade, *J Clin Anesth* 27:566–573, 2015.

Gupta A, Wu CL, Elkassabany N, et al.: Does the routine prophylactic use of antiemetics affect the incidence of postdischarge nausea and vomiting following ambulatory surgery? A systematic review of randomized controlled trials, *Anesthesiology* 99:488–495, 2003.

Ilfeld BM, Morey TE, Enneking FK: Continuous infraclavicular brachial plexus block for postoperative pain control at home: a randomized, double-blinded, placebo-controlled study, *Anesthesiology* 96:1297–1304, 2002.

Ilfeld BM, Morey TE, Wright TW, et al.: Continuous interscalene brachial plexus block for postoperative pain control at home: a randomized, double-blinded, placebo-controlled study, *Anesth Analg* 96:1089–1095, 2003.

Joshi GP, Ogunnaike BO: Consequences of inadequate postoperative pain relief and chronic persistent postoperative pain, *Anesthesiol Clin North Am* 23:21–36, 2005.

Klein SM, Nielsen KC, Greengrass RA, et al.: Ambulatory discharge after long-acting peripheral nerve blockade: 2382 blocks with ropivacaine, *Anesth Analg* 94:65–70, 2001.

Ludwin DB: Setting up an ambulatory regional anesthesia program for orthopedic surgery, *Anesthesiology Clin* 32:911–921, 2014.

Macrae WA: Chronic pain after surgery, *Br J Anaesth* 87:88–98, 2001.

Perkins FM, Kehlet H: Chronic pain as an outcome of surgery. A review of predictive factors, *Anesthesiology* 93:1123–1133, 2000.

Phillips DA, Knizner TL, Williams BA: Economics and practice management issues associated with acute pain management, *Anesthesiology Clin* 29: 213–232, 2011.

Salviz EA, Xu D, Frulla A, et al.: Continuous interscalene block in patients having outpatient rotator cuff repair surgery: a prospective randomized trial, *Anesth Analg* 117:1485–1492, 2013.

Stewart WF, Ricci JA, Chee E, et al.: Lost productive time and cost due to common pain conditions in the US workforce, *JAMA* 290:2443–2454, 2003.

Williams BA, Ibinson JW, Mangione MP, et al.: Research priorities regarding multimodal peripheral nerve blocks for postoperative analgesia and anesthesia based on hospital quality data extracted from over 1,300 cases (2011–2014), *Pain Med* 16:7–12, 2015.

Williams BA, Kentor ML, Vogt ML, et al.: Femoral-sciatic nerve blocks for complex outpatient knee surgery are associated with less postoperative pain before same day discharge: a review of 1200 consecutive cases from the period 1996–1999, *Anesthesiology* 98:1206–1213, 2003.

Williams BA, Kentor ML, Vogt MT, et al.: The economics of nerve block pain management after anterior cruciate ligament reconstruction: significant hospital cost savings via associated PACU bypass and same-day discharge, *Anesthesiology* 100:697–706, 2004.

Williams BA, Vogt MT, Kentor ML, et al.: Nausea and vomiting after outpatient ACL reconstruction with regional anesthesia: are lumbar plexus blocks a risk factor? *J Clin Anesth* 16:276–281, 2004.

Xu J, Chen XM, Ma CK, et al.: Peripheral nerve blocks for postoperative pain after major knee surgery, *Cochrane Database Syst Rev* 12:CD010937,

第 148 章 椎管内阻滞感染性并发症

Stephanie Huang，*Lu Fan Cai*

病例概要

患者，男，58 岁，行膀胱癌根治和分流术，既往有 1 型糖尿病、类风湿性关节炎病史，膀胱癌新辅助化疗后状态。腰段硬膜外置管用于围术期镇痛，泵注罗哌卡因和芬太尼维持术后 3 天镇痛。在拔除硬膜外导管时，发现穿刺点周围皮肤有小块红斑，有少量血清样清亮液体流出。其后患者于急性疼痛服务中心随访 2 天，在此期间胸腰背部疼痛逐渐加重，伴有发热、自觉下肢无力。术后第 5 天背部检查，发现之前硬膜外穿刺置管部位有一硬币大小红斑伴有少量脓性渗出物。神经学检查未见异常，实验室检查显示白细胞升高，胸腰骶椎增强磁共振成像检查显示下段椎体从 T12 到 L4 广泛脊髓硬膜外腔脓肿。行开放式椎板切除术用于脓肿排出，根据细胞培养结果（金黄色葡萄球菌）采取抗生素治疗，患者恢复顺利，于术后第 8 天出院，无神经系统并发症。

问题分析

定义

椎管内麻醉及镇痛出现感染性并发症很少见，但是一旦发生，会造成显著病残，包括硬膜外或椎旁脓肿形成、脑膜炎，甚至导致脓毒症及截瘫发生。高度怀疑、早期诊断和及时治疗干预对良好预后至关重要。

椎管内神经阻滞技术引起的感染性并发症较为多样，从皮下穿刺部位的浅表蜂窝织炎到深部组织感染，如硬膜外脓肿或脑膜炎，都有可能发生。大多数感染并发症与经皮导管穿刺技术相关，但也有报道单次注射麻醉或糖皮质激素注射后引起硬膜外脓肿和脑膜炎。椎管内阻滞相关感染性并发症的潜在机制包括：①在针或导管置入过程中感染源直接接种；②置管部位皮肤感染后沿管道扩散；③注射液污染；④来自远处感染源血源性播散（菌血症种植）。

由于对脊髓或神经根造成压迫，硬膜外或椎旁脓肿可导致肠道、膀胱功能、下肢感觉和运动缺陷的进行性神经功能损害。硬膜外脓肿引起脊髓功能障碍的发病机制被认为与直接机械压迫或血管损伤有关，最终导致脊髓缺血。

识别

浅表感染通常在针和导管穿刺部位出现局部红斑和渗出，深部组织感染除了局部症状外可能同时伴随以下症状：

- 背痛；
- 发热；
- 局部压痛；
- 白细胞升高。

深部组织脓肿伴脊髓或神经根压迫引起神经功能损伤可能出现以下症状：

- 神经根刺激症状；
- 进行性感觉及运动功能缺失；
- 大小便失禁。

脑膜炎的临床特征如下：

- 颈项强直；

- 头痛；
- 白细胞升高和发热；
- 畏光。

对有浅表感染证据的患者进行评估，并监测与深部组织感染相关症状的发展，感染部位引流脓液行细菌学培养有助于指导有效抗生素治疗，在出院前，必须指导患者在发生以下任何情况时通知医护人员或寻求紧急医疗评估：

- 新发背痛；
- 持续发热；
- 穿刺或置管部位红肿酸痛；
- 神经功能损伤的所有症状及体征。

有体征或症状提示脊柱或硬膜外脓肿的患者需行神经系统全面检查和适当的影像学检查，对任何神经功能缺损进行紧急评估。钆增强 MRI 是硬膜外脓肿最佳影像学诊断方法（见图 148.1 和 148.2），需及时诊断及治疗硬膜外脓肿，避免神经功能缺损等症状加重。

风险评估

2016 年一项全国范围的数据库研究显示，1998—2010 年全美 370 多万例硬膜外镇痛手术中非产科患者的硬膜外脓肿发生率为 7.2/100 000。

同样，皇家麻醉科医师学会第三次国家审计项目对椎管内麻醉并发症的前瞻性研究结论是非产科硬膜外置管的硬膜外脓肿发生率为 5.24/100 000。

此外，一项回顾性研究分析了 1993—2010 年期间儿科 10 653 次硬膜外置管，确诊 13 例感染——其中 9 例蜂窝织炎，2 例椎旁肌肉组织感染，1 例硬膜外炎症和 1 例硬膜外脓肿。

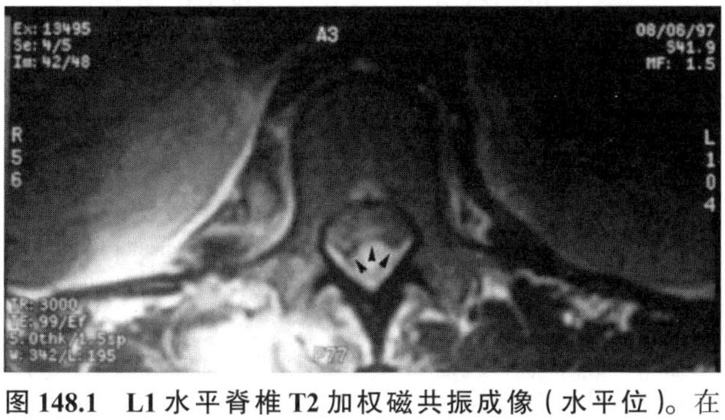

图 148.1　L1 水平脊椎 T2 加权磁共振成像（水平位）。在硬膜外腔后方有一较大高信号液体聚集，脓肿引起硬膜囊前移（箭头），使椎管前后径减小约 30%（From Rathmell JP，Garahan MB，Alsofrom GF：Epidural abscess following epidural analgesia. *Reg Anesth Pain Med* 25[1]：79-82，2000.）

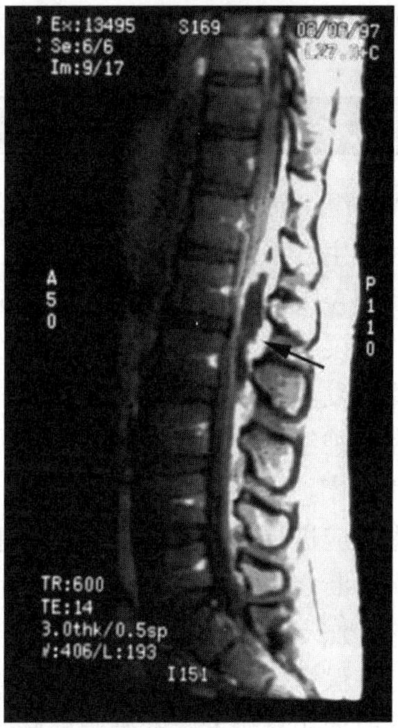

图 148.2　静脉注射钆造影剂后脊椎 T1 加权磁共振成像（矢状位）。后硬膜外腔中有一大钆造影剂增强肿块（箭头），从 T9 延伸到 L3。脓肿内的低信号密度区域代表液化区域灌注不良（From Rathmell JP，Garahan MB，Alsofrom GF：Epidural abscess following epidural analgesia. *Reg Anesth Pain Med* 25[1]：79-82，2000.）

一些其他近来发表的研究，包括回顾性分析和前瞻性临床评价，已报道硬膜外脓肿发生率在 5/10 000 ～ 74/10 000 之间，虽然具体发病率尚未阐明，但任何以下因素的存在表明椎管内阻滞麻醉感染风险较高：

- 免疫功能低下［例如获得性免疫缺陷综合征（acquired immunodefciency syndrome，AIDS）］、癌症、化疗、器官移植、长期透析、静脉毒品滥用、营养不良、长期酗酒）；
- 糖尿病；
- 全身性激素治疗；
- 穿刺点局部感染；
- 全身感染、菌血症或败血症；
- 长期留置导管。

启示

如果不及时治疗，脑膜炎和硬膜外脓肿都可能危及生命或导致永久性神经系统后遗症。再次强调，在发生不可逆神经功能缺损之前，高度怀疑、早期发现、早期诊断和及时内外科治疗是改善预后的关键。

管理

患有浅表组织感染并发症如蜂窝织炎的患者行局部引流和抗生素治疗；密切监测已存在感染风险因素的患者是否出现硬膜外脓肿或脑膜炎的任何体征或症状；建议患者出院后如果出现新发背痛或神经根性疼痛、发热、头痛、畏光、颈项强直或其他先前不存在的神经缺陷，及时就诊，有助于及时发现、诊断和治疗。具有椎管内麻醉病史且出现背痛和发热的患者应进行全面评估，将严重感染性并发症作为鉴别诊断之一。硬膜外脓肿并发症常发生在椎管内麻醉后数天、数周甚至数月。

尽管已有保守治疗的方法报道，但早期手术减压和引流同时使用抗生素治疗硬膜外脓肿仍然是最佳治疗方法。具有神经系统体征或症状的硬膜外脓肿需要紧急手术干预以防止进行性和可能永久性的神经损伤。

需及时启用静脉抗生素治疗。初始药物应对葡萄球菌属包括耐甲氧西林金黄色葡萄球菌（methicillin-resistant *Staphylococcus aureus*，MRSA）有效。最终的抗生素治疗应该依据细菌培养和药敏实验结果，以及临床或不同的单位进行考虑。根据感染的性质和严重程度，可能需要抗生素治疗 4 ～ 6 周或更长时间。

预防

与所有有创性操作一样，必须权衡椎管内阻滞利弊。尽管感染性并发症少见，但行这种麻醉获益最大的患者往往是那些具有并存疾病的患者，因为并存疾病会增加严重感染性并发症的风险。在评估这些患者是否存在潜在的感染并发症时，需要保持高度的怀疑。当术后或外伤后镇痛需长期留置导管时，并发症的风险也会增加，需谨慎对待。

加强无菌操作观念对于减少与椎管内麻醉穿刺或置管相关的感染性并发症至关重要。标准洗手法、无菌手套、手术帽或头罩和口罩，以及无菌麻醉技术都是重要的考虑因素。应该用碘伏、异丁醇碘或氯己定等消毒液行穿刺点周围大面积皮肤消毒，在进行操作之前，必须给足时间保证消毒区域干燥。另外，使用“无接触”技术（即必要时在皮肤消毒前标识穿刺点）有助于降低椎管内麻醉感染性并发症的风险。据报道，与碘伏相比，氯己定和异丁醇碘可提供更好的抗菌皮肤消毒和防止细菌再生。透明塑料铺单的使用具有可在阻滞操作期间直视体表标记的优点，此外，使用透明无菌敷料覆盖硬膜外导管，方便每日评估穿刺点皮肤变化，从而避免揭开敷料所引起的微生物污染。

对于通过导管给药或连续硬膜外泵注更换输液连接，应保持无菌技术。在整个治疗过程中保持紧密关闭的输液系统有助于减少管路或输液更换期间的导管污染，输注液体应由药房人员采用无菌技术和层流罩制备。

菌血症患者椎管内阻滞仍然存在争议。如果认为椎管内麻醉对于菌血症患者是必需的或可行的，则仅在使用适当的抗生素覆盖治疗后才能考虑进行麻醉。对于留置硬膜外导管后引起菌血症的患者，可以考虑拔除导管，提供有适应证的抗生素治疗，如果仍需要连续硬膜外镇痛则需改变置管节段。硬膜外导管尖端的常规细菌培养在诊断感染方面预测价值较低，因此不建议常规检测。然而，如果硬膜外导管置入部位被局部炎症或引流液包围，硬膜外导管尖端的细菌学检查可以指导抗生素治疗。

虽然预防措施很重要，但不能完全消除椎管内阻滞感染性并发症的风险。对感染性并发症的发生予以高度怀疑、及时诊断和治疗是降低患者发病率和永久性神经损伤的重要因素。

致谢

感谢 James C.Crews 博士对本章上一版的贡献。

（黄 婷 译 李斌本 校）

延伸阅读

Aota Y, Onari K, Suga Y: Iliopsoas abscess and persistent radiculopathy: a rare complication of continuous infusion techniques of epidural anesthesia, *Anesthesiology* 96:1023–1025, 2002.

Birnbach DJ, Meadows W, Stein DJ, et al.: Comparison of povidone iodine and DuraPrep, an iodophor-in-isopropyl alcohol solution, for skin disinfection prior to epidural catheter insertion in parturients, *Anesthesiology* 98:164–169, 2003.

Cameron CM, Scott DA, McDonald WM, et al.: A review of neuraxial epidural morbidity: experience of more than 8,000 cases at a single teaching hospital, *Anesthesiology* 106:997–1002, 2007.

Christie IW, McCabe S: Major complications of epidural analgesia after sur-

National Audit Project: Major complications of central neuraxial block: report on the Third National Audit Project of the Royal College of Anaesthetists, *Br J Anaesth* 102:179–190, 2009.

Darouiche R: Spinal epidural abscess, *N Engl J Med* 355:2012–2020, 2006.

Dawson S: Epidural catheter infections, *J Hosp Infect* 47:3–8, 2001.

Du Pen SL, Peterson DG, Williams A, et al.: Infection during chronic epidural catheterization: diagnosis and treatment, *Anesthesiology* 73:905–909, 1990.

Hooten WM, Kinney MO, Huntoon MA: Epidural abscess and meningitis after epidural corticosteroid injection, *Mayo Clin Proc* 79:682–686, 2004.

Huang RC, Shapiro GS, Lim M, et al.: Cervical epidural abscess after epidural steroid injection, *Spine* 29:E7–E9, 2004.

Kindler CH, Seeberger MD, Staender SE: Epidural abscess complicating epidural anesthesia and analgesia: an analysis of the literature, *Acta Anaesthesiol Scand* 42:614–620, 1998.

Kinirons B, Mimoz O, Lafendi L, et al.: Chlorhexidine versus povidone iodine in preventing colonization of continuous epidural catheters in children: a randomized, controlled trial, *Anesthesiology* 94:239–244, 2001.

Koka VK, Potti A: Spinal epidural abscess after corticosteroid injections, *South Med J* 95:772–774, 2002.

Moen V, Dahlgren N, Irestedt L: Severe neurological complications after central neuraxial blockades in Sweden 1990–1999, *Anesthesiology* 101:950–959, 2004.

Popping DM, Zahn PK, Van Aken HK, et al.: Effectiveness and safety of postoperative pain management: a survey of 18 925 consecutive patients between 1998 and 2006 (2nd revision): a database analysis of prospectively raised data, *Br J Anaesth* 101:832–840, 2008.

Rathmell JP, Garahan MB, Alsofrom GF: Epidural abscess following epidural analgesia, *Reg Anesth Pain Med* 25:79–82, 2000.

Reihsaus E, Waldbaur H, Seeling W: Spinal epidural abscess: a meta-analysis of 915 patients, *Neurosurg Rev* 23:175–204, 2000.

Rosero EB, Joshi GP: Nationwide incidence of serious complications of epidural analgesia in the United States, *Acta Anaesthesiol Scand* 60:810–820, 2016.

Sethna NF, Clendenin D, Athiraman U, et al.: Incidence of epidural catheter-associated infections after continuous epidural analgesia in children, *Anesthesiology* 113:224–232, 2010.

Sorensen P: Spinal epidural abscesses: conservative treatment for selected subgroups of patients, *Br J Neurosurg* 17:513–518, 2003.

Steffen P, Seeling W, Essig A, et al.: Bacterial contamination of epidural catheters: microbiological examination of 502 epidural catheters used for postoperative analgesia, *J Clin Anesth* 16:92–97, 2004.

Trautmann M, Lepper PM, Schmitz FJ: Three cases of bacterial meningitis after spinal and epidural anesthesia, *Eur J Clin Microbiol Infect Dis* 21:43–45, 2002.

Von Hosslin T, Imboden P, Luthi A, et al.: Adverse events of postoperative thoracic epidural analgesia: a retrospective analysis of 7273 cases in a tertiary care teaching hospital, *Eur J Anaesthesiol* 33:708–714, 2016.

Wang LP, Hauerberg J, Schmidt JF: Incidence of spinal epidural abscess after epidural analgesia: a national 1-year survey, *Anesthesiology* 91:1928–1936, 1999.

Wittum S, Hofer CK, Rolli U, et al.: Sacral osteomyelitis after single-shot epidural anesthesia via the caudal approach in a child, *Anesthesiology* 99:503–505, 2003.

第 149 章 肌间沟臂丛神经阻滞：潜在严重并发症

Alain Borgeat，Gina Votta-Velis

病例概要

患者，男性，25 岁，拟行肩袖修复手术，遂接受肌间沟神经阻滞和导管置入。借助神经刺激器和 Winnie 入路行肌间沟神经阻滞。在 2.5 cm 深度处获得三头肌反射。导管穿过刺激针尖端 6 cm。除导管置入过程中遇到暂时性阻力外，过程顺利。抽吸血液和脑脊液阴性后，通过导管缓慢注射 0.5% 布比卡因。注射 10 ml 后，患者昏昏欲睡，反应迟钝，呼吸暂停，四肢肌张力消失，瞳孔散大。对患者进行手控辅助通气，随后行气管插管。

问题分析

定义

全脊椎麻醉是进行肌间沟神经阻滞时最严重的并发症之一。其他严重并发症包括意外的血管内（动脉内 / 静脉内）局部麻醉药（局麻药）注射、高位硬膜外麻醉、硬膜下注射、气胸和神经病变。

识别

全脊椎麻醉的体征和症状是由颈胸段椎管内神经阻滞所致。中枢神经系统受累的症状几乎总是存在，其范围从无法发声到意识丧失，以及双侧弛缓性麻痹的迅速发展。常可观察到双侧瞳孔扩张且无反应，与来自 Edinger-Westphal 核的副交感神经传出活动的阻滞相一致。后一迹象表明一定量的局麻药进入了颅内。呼吸暂停通常（但不总是）存在，因为膈神经根（$C_{3\sim5}$）靠近斜角肌注射部位（$C_{6\sim7}$）。心动过缓和低血压发生的原因是颈胸段脊髓心脏加速纤维（$T_{1\sim4}$）被阻滞或局麻药渗入中枢神经系统的髓质区。局麻药进入这种结构会导致低血压、心动过缓和室性心律失常（表 149.1）。

鉴别诊断包括局麻药注射进入椎动脉。当发生这种情况时，癫痫发作和意识丧失几乎立即发生。低血压和心动过缓也可能由局麻药的心脏毒性作用所致。硬膜外注射后，这些体征和阻滞的部位不再向颅内扩散。不太可能出现与颅内局麻药扩散有关的体征和症状。硬膜下注射也是鉴别诊断的一部分。

表 149.1 肌间沟阻滞后意外注射局麻药的体征

动脉内	静脉内	蛛网膜下腔	硬膜下
中枢神经系统毒性→立即 • 癫痫发作 • 意识丧失	全身毒性→延迟（5 ～ 15 min）	双侧麻醉→意识快速丧失 • 呼吸暂停 • 瞳孔散大 • 弛缓性麻痹	与蛛网膜下腔比较→延迟 • 呼吸暂停 • 麻醉不对称 • 瞳孔不对称
血流动力学不稳定 • 低血压 • 心动过缓	血流动力学不稳定 • 低血压 • 心动过缓	血流动力学不稳定 • 低血压 • 心动过缓 • 室性心律失常	血流动力学不稳定 • 低血压 • 心动过缓 • 室性心律失常

在这种情况下，临床阻滞的发展更慢，而且通常不对称和不完全。血管内注射或局部症状的快速再吸收进展较慢。此外，硬膜外麻醉应始终考虑中枢神经系统毒性和血流动力学的不稳定性。然而，双侧弛缓性麻痹的出现使这种诊断非常困难。

肌间沟神经阻滞后出现全脊椎麻醉可能涉及不同的机制（框 149.1）。直接注射到硬膜下或硬膜外间隙可能是将针误入椎间孔的结果。神经周围或神经内注射可能导致药物继发迁移至硬膜下间隙。最后，尸检研究显示，硬脑膜导管延伸至椎间孔外 3 ～ 5 cm 处。将针放置在异常长的硬脑膜根部可能解释了局麻药在鞘内间隙扩散的原因。

风险评估

无论是否在神经周围放置导管，肌间沟神经阻滞后的全脊椎麻醉，都是一种罕见且严重的并发症。这类事件通常以病例报告的形式报道。因此，无法估计这种并发症的具体风险。唯一增加风险的可识别因素是阻滞方法。使用的技术有 Winnie 入路、后入路、改良侧入路和超声引导入路。每种技术的相对优缺点见表 149.2。

启示

全脊椎麻醉是肌间沟阻滞后的一种罕见并发症。

框 149.1　局麻药鞘内迁移的可能机制

椎间孔注射
直接神经内注射
硬膜根部注射

表 149.2　肌间沟神经阻滞技术：相对优势 / 劣势

优势 / 劣势	Winnie 入路	后入路	改良侧入路	超声引导入路
脊髓注射	++	++	–	–
硬膜外注射	++	++	–	–
椎动脉注射	+	+/–	–	–
静脉注射	+	+	+	+
气胸	+	+	+	+
不适	+/–	++	+/–	+
置管便捷性	–	+	++	+

++，最可能 / 最容易；+，可能 / 较容易；+/–，可能；–，不可能 / 困难

然而，由于表 149.1 中提到的机制，即使针在合适位置，若患者存在长的硬脑膜，也可能发生这种情况。及时诊断最为重要。椎动脉或静脉注射的鉴别诊断应该迅速被排除，以便制定妥善的治疗措施。自主呼吸往往会迅速减慢，因此需要手动或机械辅助通气。心动过缓和低血压可能是由血管扩张和心脏交感神经纤维被阻滞引起，如果不予以紧急治疗，可能导致心搏骤停。

管理

需要立即干预：

1. 立即停止局部麻醉注射。
2. 提供纯氧手动或机械辅助通气。通常有必要进行气管插管，但并不强制。
3. 考虑患者的精神状态、用药和手术操作。
4. 可能需要扩容来治疗或预防血流动力学不稳定。
5. 为治疗心动过缓或低血压，可能需要血管升压药、正性变时药或临时起搏。转至重症监护室或恢复室，密切观察患者直至阻滞消失。

预防

最重要的预防措施是缓慢给药，反复抽吸；然而，静脉、动脉或鞘内给药仍可能发生。选择行肌间沟入路的阻滞对并发症的发生是有影响的。自从使用侧向改良入路和超声技术进行神经阻滞以来，肌间沟神经阻滞期间发生全脊椎麻醉的频次一直在下降。

Winnie 入路（图 149.1）使针更多地指向脊柱，因此增加了通过椎间孔注射的风险，尤其当针的水平方向过大时。后路为椎旁阻滞。所有椎旁阻滞至少都有刺穿硬脑膜（无论硬膜是否异常的长）的风险。改良的侧方入路（图 149.2）将针远离脊柱结构，可能是避免椎间或意外硬脑膜穿刺的最安全方法，将导管推进超过刺激针尖端 2～3 cm 并无优势。事实上，因为穿刺更远，麻醉科医师失去对其位置的控制（例如，肌间沟置管被放置在胸膜内）。最后，一个重要的预防措施是只对清醒或轻度镇静的患者实施肌间沟神经阻滞。

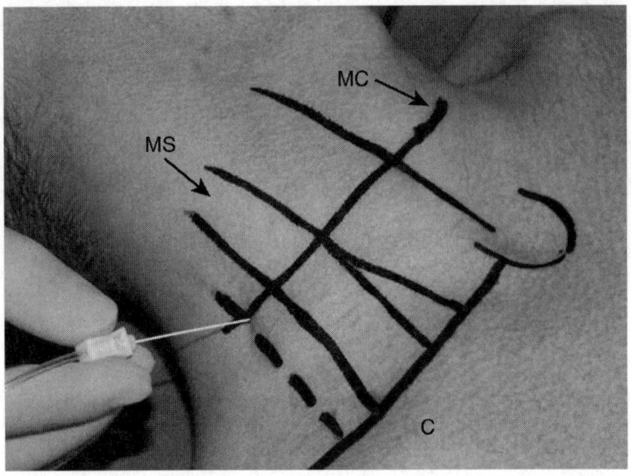

图 149.1 Winnie 技术。针向中央、尾端和稍向后端朝向 C6 横突。针靠近脊柱结构。C，锁骨；MC，环甲膜；MS，胸锁乳突肌锁骨头；虚线，肌间沟

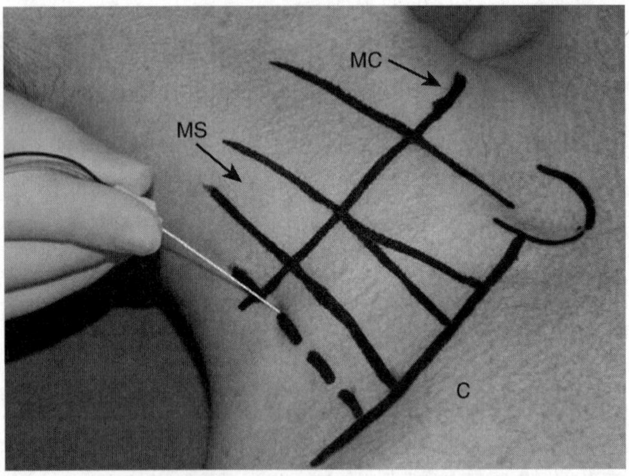

图 149.2 改良侧入路。针头以 45°～ 60°的角度插入到肌间沟间隙平面上。针头避开脊柱结构。C，锁骨；MC，环甲膜；MS，胸锁乳突肌锁骨头；虚线，肌角沟

（顾姣姣 译 王恒跃 校）

延伸阅读

Borgeat A: All roads do not lead to Rome [editorial], *Anesthesiology* 105:1–2, 2006.

Borgeat A, Dullenkopf A, Ekatodramis G, et al.: Evaluation of the lateral modified approach for continuous interscalene block after shoulder surgery, *Anesthesiology* 99:436–442, 2003.

Borgeat A, Ekatodramis G, Kalberer F, et al.: Acute and nonacute complications associated with interscalene block and shoulder surgery: a prospective study, *Anesthesiology* 95:875–880, 2001.

Brown AR: Regional anesthesia for shoulder surgery, *Tech Reg Anesth Pain Manage* 3:64–78, 1999.

Dhir S, Ganapathy S, Lindsay P, Athwal G: Case report: ropivacaine neurotoxicity at clinical doses in interscalene brachial plexus block, *Can J Anaesth* 54:912–916, 2007.

Jocolano CF: Total spinal anesthesia after an interscalene block, *J Perianesth Nurs* 12:163–170, 1997.

Li R, Lasll A, Lai E, et al.: Tension pneumothorax after ultrasound-guided interscalene block and shoulder arthroscopy, *Am J Orthop (Belle Mead NJ)* 44(10):E407–E410, 2015.

Liu SS, Gordon MA, Shaw PM, et al.: A prospective clinical registry of ultrasound-guided regional anesthesia for ambulatory shoulder surgery, *Anesth Analg* 111:617–623, 2010.

Long TR, Wass CT, Burkle CM: Perioperative interscalene blockade: an overview of its history and current clinical use, *J Clin Anesth* 14:546–556, 2002.

Norris D, Klahsen A, Milne B: Delayed bilateral spinal anaesthesia following interscalene brachial plexus block, *Can J Anaesth* 43:303–305, 1996.

Sardesai AM, Patel R, Denny NM, et al.: Interscalene brachial plexus block: can the risk of entering the spinal canal be reduced? A study of needle angles in volunteers undergoing magnetic resonance imaging, *Anesthesiology* 105:9–13, 2006.

颅内高压

第 150 章

Rosemary Hickey

病例概要

患者，男性，64 岁，拟开颅行脑部肿瘤切除术。患者在急诊科临床表现如下：进行性性格改变、记忆紊乱、小便失禁。体格检查表现为意识模糊明显、视神经乳头水肿及左侧轻瘫。CT 扫描显示一巨大肿块，周围水肿，符合胶质母细胞瘤的特点。神经外科团队让其开始每 6 h 口服地塞米松 4 mg。术中脑组织从硬脑膜中膨出，外科医师要求协助脑松弛。

问题分析

定义

当颅内压（intracranial pressure，ICP）持续升高超过 15 ～ 20 mmHg 时则会出现颅内高压。当三种颅内成分——血液、脑组织、脑脊液（cerebrospinal fluid，CSF）——不能再代偿颅内容积变化时则形成颅内高压。CSF 从头部转移至脊髓蛛网膜下腔及其通过蛛网膜绒毛的重吸收，是调节颅内容积增加的主要代偿手段。颅内空间代偿也可通过压缩静脉系统来实现，最终引起毛细血管塌陷，导致脑缺血。

ICP 随颅内容积的变化可用颅内弹性曲线来描述（图 150.1）。曲线第一部分较平坦，因为尽管颅内容积增加，但代偿储备充足。当代偿机制耗竭，由于顺应性急剧降低，即使颅内容积小幅度增加也会导致 ICP 显著升高，曲线迅速升高。ICP 波形有三个明显的峰（图 150.2）。第二峰（P2）被认为与脑组织顺应性密切相关，当其升高或超过 P1 波形水平时，顺应性显著下降。

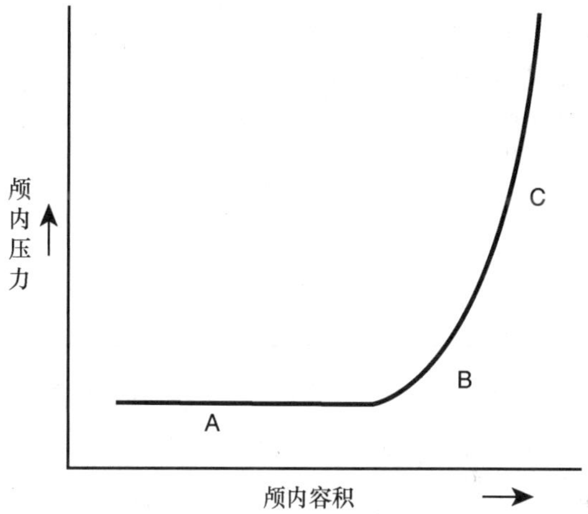

图 150.1　颅内弹性曲线。A，正常弹性；**B**，弹性降低［颅内容积增加，颅内压（ICP）稍有升高］；**C**，弹性耗竭（颅内容积少量增加即可导致 ICP 急剧升高）（From Mahla ME：Neurologic surgery. In Kirby RR，Gravenstein N，editors：*Clinical anesthesia practice*. Philadelphia，WB Saunders，1994，pp 1283-1311.）

识别

颅内高压最常见症状和体征包括头痛、恶心、呕吐、视神经乳头水肿、单侧瞳孔扩大、动眼神经或展神经麻痹。意识改变和不规则呼吸提示颅内高压已较严重。

头痛通常出现在觉醒时，或使患者从睡眠中苏醒。头痛与痛觉敏感性脑血管及硬脑膜牵拉和变形有关。呕吐可能是由局部压迫直接刺激呕吐中枢所致。尽管颅内高压可能不伴有视神经乳头水肿，但视神经乳头水肿却是 ICP 增加最可靠的体征。动眼神经麻痹继发于脑疝或神经压迫，而外展神经麻痹是由于 ICP 增加引起脑干向下移位导致神经牵拉所致。随着 ICP 持续升高，脑血流弥漫性减少，患者精神状态逐渐发生变化。意识水平的进一步恶化，表明患者发生进行性小脑幕切迹疝。随着 ICP 升高及脑干受压，患者生命体征也发生变化（心动过缓、血压升高、呼吸改变）。CT、MRI、血管造影术可提供 ICP 升高的间接证据。ICP 升高指征包括：肿块病变伴中线移位至少 0.5 cm、脑组织扩张侵犯脑

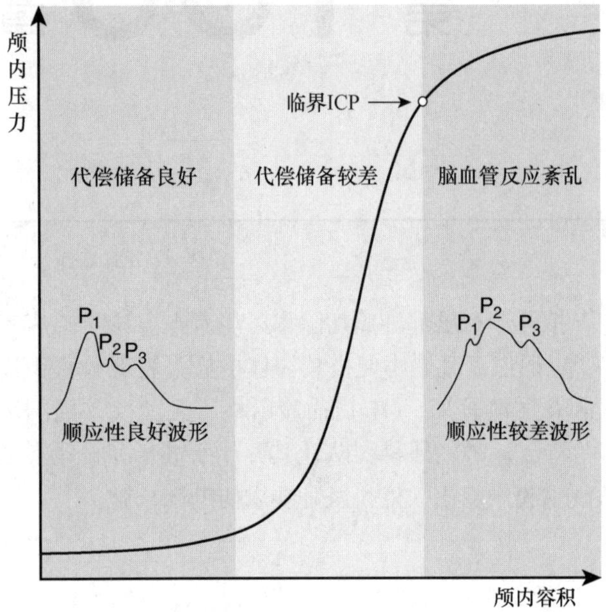

图 150.2 颅内压力-容积曲线（From PerezBarcena J, Llompart-Pou JA, O'Phelan KH：Intracranial pressure monitoring and management of intracranial hypertension. *Crit Care Clin* 30[4]：735-750，2014.）

脊液池，或两者兼有。

风险评估

ICP 升高的三个主要机制：①颅内肿块病变至颅内容积增加（如肿瘤、大面积梗死、创伤、出血、脓肿）、颅外肿块病变（如肿瘤、血肿、脓肿）或急性脑水肿（如缺氧状态、急性肝衰竭、高血压脑病、Reye 综合征）；②心力衰竭、上纵隔梗阻、脑或颈静脉受阻致静脉压升高，使软脑膜静脉和硬脑膜窦血容量增加，并影响脑脊液吸收；③脑脊液流动（脑积水）或吸收（假性脑瘤）障碍。

启示

颅内高压的风险在于脑缺血和脑疝形成的潜在风险。如果 ICP（局部或整体）超过平均动脉压（mean arterial pressure，MAP）水平，即发生脑缺血。有效的脑氧合需要足够的脑灌注压（cerebral perfusion pressure，CPP），而 CPP 取决于 ICP 或脑静脉压（cerebral venous pressure，CVP）提供的阻力，由两者中较高者决定。三者之间的关系为 CPP=MAP-（ICP 或 CVP）。脑缺血是否造成脑组织永久性损伤取决于脑缺血的严重程度和持续时间。当 ICP 升高至阻碍脑静脉回流时，脑动脉流入也可能受到影响。

颅骨内任何固定结构周围都可能发生脑疝。在开放性颅脑损伤中，损伤脑组织可通过颅骨骨折部位膨出。在颅脑闭合性损伤中，脑疝的形成包括三种方式：

1. 大脑镰下疝（又称扣带回疝）：半球可能通过镰状突起向内侧移位，导致镰状疝。
2. 小脑幕切迹疝：颞叶内侧边缘经小脑幕孔膨出，形成小脑幕疝，压迫第三脑神经，导致单侧瞳孔扩大，对光反射消失，当压迫脑干时，患者意识受损。
3. 枕骨大孔疝（又称小脑扁桃体疝）：典型的小脑疝经枕骨大孔膨出，压迫髓质，导致心血管和呼吸衰竭，双侧瞳孔异常。

管理

目前，降低 ICP 升高的治疗干预手段已发展为标准化治疗策略，即采用治疗强度不断提高的方法，即所谓的“阶梯”治疗（表 150.1）。

1. 首先应采用气管插管并通气维持正常二氧化碳水平。由插管经验丰富的麻醉科医师执行，插管前给予镇静及麻醉药，尽量减小 ICP 对气管插管的反应。插管困难或需保持颈椎固定位的患者插管

表 150.1 颅内高压“阶梯”治疗及相关风险

治疗等级	治疗方法	风险
1 级	气管插管 维持正常二氧化碳的通气	呼吸机相关并发症
2 级	增强镇静	低血压 影响神经系统检查
3 级	脑室 CSF 引流	感染
4 级	高渗性治疗（甘露醇或高渗盐水）	低血容量 电解质紊乱
5 级	低碳酸血症	脑缺血
6 级	低温疗法	感染 凝血功能异常
7 级	代谢抑制（巴比妥类）	低血压 苏醒延迟
8 级	去骨瓣减压术	感染 血肿 其他手术并发症

CSF，脑脊液

时，视频喉镜可提供有效帮助。

2. 气管插管后增加镇静以预防动脉血压增高、避免患者-呼吸机非同步化，使癫痫发作风险最低。维持血容量正常以避免镇静引起动脉血压过低。ICU 患者镇静通常选择持续泵注丙泊酚，伴或不伴其他麻醉药物。手术室患者镇静通常采用静脉输注丙泊酚及瑞芬太尼，伴或不伴低浓度吸入麻醉药物。保持头部抬高 15° ～ 30°，避免颈椎过度旋转或弯曲，最大化静脉回流。
3. 脑室 CSF 引流是通过脑室外引流完成的。当 ICP 超过 20 mmHg 时可间断引流。此治疗方法有感染风险。
4. 甘露醇或高渗盐水脱水治疗可降低脑容量和 ICP。此类药物通过在血脑屏障形成渗透梯度从而摄取脑组织水分，甘露醇还能改善脑血流动力学和微循环血流量，但作为一种渗透性利尿剂，甘露醇有引起机体脱水和低血容量的风险，治疗后应监测血清渗透压变化。高渗盐水可能导致血清钠浓度突然升高，治疗中应注意监测血清钠浓度。袢利尿剂（呋塞米）通过利尿-脑脱水作用、减少 CSF 形成和通过改善细胞内水转运缓解脑水肿达到减压目的。
5. 过度通气减少脑血流量、脑血容量降低 ICP。脑缺血患者对脑血流量减少的耐受性较差，需额外监测颈静脉血氧饱和度或脑组织氧合（brain-tissue oxygenation，$pbtO_2$）。颈静脉血氧饱和度监测值大于 75%，提示脑供血充足，过度通气引起的血管收缩有治疗价值；颈静脉血氧饱和度小于 50%，提示脑缺血，进一步诱导脑血管收缩可能对患者有害。临床上通常将微型 Clark 电极置入脑实质来监测 $pbtO_2$。脑严重缺血阈值约为 15 mmHg。
6. 亚低温在降低 ICP 方面有一定效果，对其临床疗效的研究不尽相同，且与其大量不良反应有关。最新临床证据不支持亚低温应用于脑创伤后颅内高压患者。
7. 巴比妥类药物抑制代谢已被应用于降低脑血容量和 ICP。通常用其来治疗其他治疗方法无效的难治性颅内高压，通常在脑电图（electroencephalography，EEG）监测或麻醉深度监测如脑电双频指数监测下治疗。
8. 颅内高压的外科治疗包括清除肿块病变、CSF 引流以及去骨瓣减压术。肿块病变通常包括脑肿瘤或血肿（硬膜外、硬膜下、颅内）。手术切除可减少脑实质所占颅内空间，从而改善颅内顺应性。CSF 引流是降低 ICP 的一种简单有效方法，通过颅室内导管完成（如前所述），不推荐使用腰椎穿刺置入导管，因为 ICP 升高的患者有形成脑疝的风险。外科分流术也能减少 CSF 容量，如脑室-腹腔分流术。去骨瓣减压术为代偿颅内容积增加提供更大的储备，可在清除肿块病变同时进行去骨瓣减压术进行预防，也可在最大限度的内科治疗失败后作为一种抢救手段。外科手术治疗虽能明显降低 ICP，但因缺乏改善临床预后的证据，其在颅内高压治疗中一直存在争议。

脑肿瘤患者降低 ICP 的另一方法是使用皮质类固醇药物，其对减轻肿瘤周围水肿有效，但对头部外伤所致颅内高压无效。

预防

预防颅内高压的关键在于避免升高 ICP 的危险因素。静脉液体治疗旨在维持正常血容量。避免应用降低血浆渗透压的液体（5% 葡萄糖、0.45% 氯化钠、乳酸林格液）。液体治疗对脑水肿最大的影响因素是渗透压。血浆渗透压的急剧下降对脑含水量和 ICP 的影响远大于胶体渗透压的急剧下降。避免使用含糖溶液，高血糖会加重缺血性脑损伤。

其他增加 ICP 且应避免的因素包括：头部位置不当压迫颈静脉，气管内导管刺激引起的咳嗽及牵拉，癫痫发作，高碳酸血症和缺氧。应避免体温升高，因其会增加脑代谢耗氧量。挥发性麻醉药可能会导致脑血流量、脑血容量和 ICP 增加。当发生颅内高压时，适当应用药物治疗配合轻度过度通气及静脉麻醉药（如依托咪酯、丙泊酚等）能有效降低 ICP。氧化亚氮对大脑有刺激作用，能增加脑血流量和脑代谢耗氧量，尤其与挥发性麻醉药联合应用时。颅腔积气（例如近期行开颅手术）时应避免应用氧化亚氮，因其可能进入颅内并扩张其他含气空间。

（谢 韬 译 查燕萍 校）

延伸阅读

Andrews PJD, Sinclair HL, Rodriguez A, et al.: Hypothermia for intracranial hypertension after traumatic brain injury, *N Engl J Med* 373:2403–2412, 2015.

Dostal P, Dostalova V, Schreiberova J, et al.: A comparison of equivolume, equiosmolar solutions of hypertonic saline and mannitol for brain relaxation in patients undergoing elective intracranial tumor surgery: a randomized clinical trial, *J Neurosurg Anesthesiol* 27(1):51–56, 2015.

El Ahmadieh TY, Adel JG, El Tecle NE, et al.: Surgical treatment of elevated intracranial pressure: decompressive craniectomy and intracranial pressure monitoring, *Neurosurg Clin North Am* 24:375–391, 2013.

Imberti R, Bellinzona G, Langer M: Cerebral tissue Po_2 and $Sjvo_2$ changes during moderate hyperventilation in patients with severe traumatic brain injury, *J Neurosurg* 96:97–102, 2002.

Perez-Barcena J, Llompart-Pou JA, O'Phelan KH: Intracranial pressure monitoring and management of intracranial hypertension, *Crit Care Clin* 30:735–750, 2014.

Quentin C, Charbonneau S, Moumdjian R, et al.: A comparison of two doses of mannitol on brain relaxation during supratentorial brain tumor craniotomy: a randomized trial, *Anesth Analg* 116:862–868, 2013.

Stocchetti N, Maas AIR: Traumatic intracranial hypertension, *N Engl J Med* 370:2121–2130, 2014.

Wijayatilake DS, Shepherd SJ: What's new in the management of traumatic brain injury on neuro ICU, *Curr Opin Anesthesiol* 27:459–464, 2014.

Wijayatilake DS, Shepherd SJ, Sherren PB: Updates in the management of intracranial pressure in traumatic brain injury, *Curr Opin Anesthesiol* 25(5):540–547, 2012.

顽固性恶心呕吐

第 151 章

Jennifer L.Stewart，David A.Nakata

病例概要

患者，女性，28 岁，体重 110 kg，在全身麻醉下行腹腔镜胆囊切除术，术后在麻醉恢复室出现了顽固性恶心和呕吐。麻醉除了出现术前焦虑和术后中度上呼吸道阻塞外（通过插入口咽通气道很容易纠正），其他均顺利。既往史中有意义的是既往腹股沟疝修补术后因恶心呕吐而意外入院。

问题分析

定义

术后恶心呕吐（postoperative nausea and vomiting，PONV）是所有类型的麻醉后所患疾病的一个重要原因，通常在麻醉后不久出现，大多数持续不超过 24 h。恶心是通过未知的神经通路介导，是最好由患者自我评估的主观感觉。恶心常常（但不总是）出现在干呕或呕吐之前。呕吐则定义为胃内容物经口腔的强力逆行排出。与呕吐不同的是，干呕缺乏胃内容物的排出。导致 PONV 的原因很多，可分为患者、手术和麻醉相关因素。

识别

恶心的感觉对每个人来说都很熟悉，但由于其主观性，通常很难理解，尤其是在没有判断力的术后患者中。恶心通常伴有胃肠道活动减少或不适，并且可能包括肌肉括约肌张力减退，蠕动迟缓或反向蠕动，以及分泌不足。自主神经系统，尤其是副交感神经系统也可能受到影响，导致皮肤苍白、发汗、唾液分泌增加、血管迷走神经反应和厌食等表现。如果这些症状持续存在，通常就要加重出现干呕和呕吐。

与恶心不同，呕吐根据其表现即可几乎无错误地明确诊断。产生呕吐的神经解剖学途径和介质比恶心已了解得更为透彻。大脑中两个不同区域负责呕吐的发起和协作：第四脑室中的化学感受器触发区和侧网状结构中的呕吐中枢。化学感受器触发区含有高密度的多巴胺能受体，并通过神经通路连接到呕吐中枢。图 151.1 是与负责呕吐的区域相互作用的已知因素的示意图。此外，还会发生许多生理变化，包括胃底和食管下段括约肌松弛以及腹部肌肉组织的强力收缩，导致胃内容物的喷射而出。

风险评估

据报道，术后呕吐的发生率通常在 20% ~ 40%。框 151.1 列出了与 PONV 发生的相关因素。许多因素在普外科患者中广泛存在，每个患者具有多种风险因素较为普遍。这些因素，结合特殊患者的特征，可用于预测那些 PONV 风险最高的患者。不幸的是，没有正式的方案可以让临床医生预测哪种预防性手段成功率最高。

影响恶心呕吐发病率的一些不太明显的因素包括焦虑、性别、肥胖、麻醉科医师的经验和麻醉药物焦虑可能通过释放儿茶酚胺而加剧 PONV。实验模型中存在通过将儿茶酚胺灌注到脑室中可以诱导呕吐的情况。这也可能解释了使用麻醉剂增加循环中儿茶酚胺而导致恶心呕吐发生率增加的原因。女性 PONV 发病率的增加传统上归因于激素。与年龄相近的男性相比，极端年龄（如高龄或低龄）的女性 PONV 发病率下降这种说法也得到了支持。然而，最近的一项研究假设女性 PONV 发病率的增加实际上可能是由于对多巴胺的敏感性增加。肥胖可能会干扰正压通气，导致胃扩张。

病例概要提供了可以增加患者 PONV 风险的常

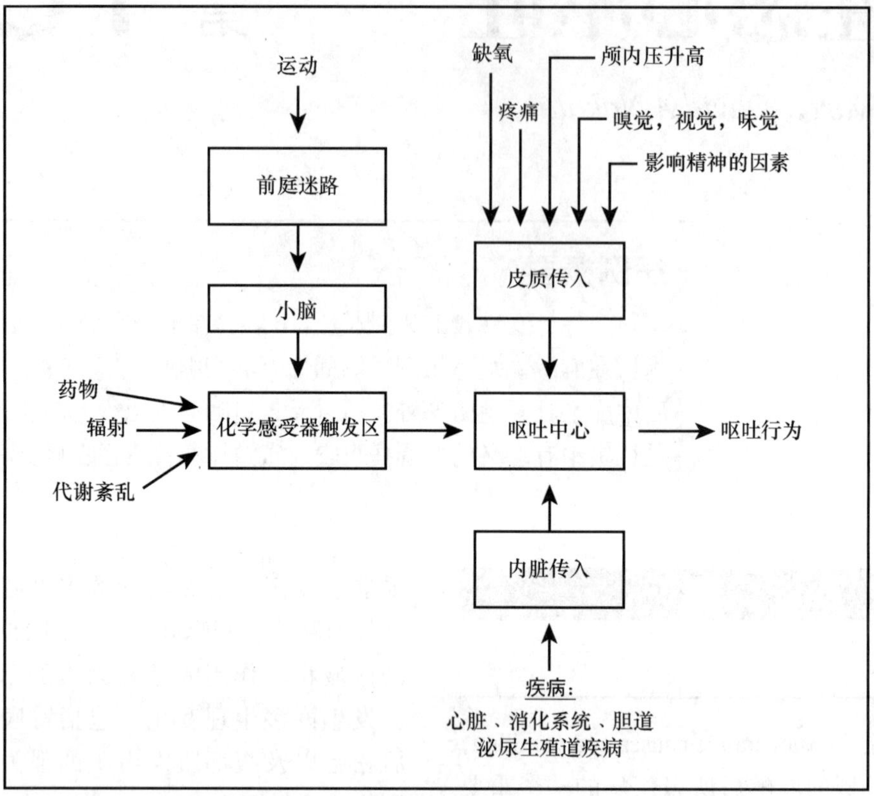

图 151.1 已知与化学受体触发区和呕吐中心相互作用的因素

框 151.1 可能影响术后恶心呕吐风险的因素

年龄：儿童比成人风险更大	药物
麻醉技术	鼻胃管
焦虑	氧化亚氮
并发疾病	肥胖
乙醇中毒	阿片类药物
颅内压增高	疼痛
代谢紊乱	放置人工气道
麻醉科医师的经验	既往有术后恶心呕吐病史
禁食	长时间手术
女性	站立
月经周期	交感神经刺激
胃胀气	患者的转运或运动
高碳酸血症	手术类型
低血压	头颈部手术
吸入麻醉药	腹腔内手术
静脉麻醉药	腹腔镜腹部手术
依托咪酯	斜视手术
美索比妥	
硫喷妥钠	

见诱发因素的例子，包括女性、肥胖、PONV 史、焦虑、腹腔镜腹部手术、放置口咽通气道和全身麻醉。其他因素可能包括由于正压通气困难导致的胃充气增加或低氧血症，以及在腹腔镜操作期间面罩通气不足或腹腔内注入二氧化碳以致增加动脉二氧化碳分压。目前尚且不知道现代挥发性麻醉药物是否会促进恶心和呕吐，但氧化亚氮已被确认会引起恶心呕吐，其机制可能是化学感受器触发区刺激后

导致中耳压力增加或胃肠道扩张。

启示

框 151.2 列出了许多与恶心和呕吐相关的并发症。许多并存疾病和某些外科手术可能使患者容易发生更严重的 PONV 后遗症，包括颅内压增高（导致小脑幕裂孔疝）和食管破裂（Mallory-Weiss 撕裂或 Boerhaave 综合征）。PONV 还可引起伤口裂开，影响复杂手术的修复。由于头颈部的组织比较脆弱，涉及这些部位手术术后发生干呕或呕吐需要特别关注。此外，涉及下颌骨固定于闭合位置的口腔手术特别危险，在这些情况下，如果患者呕吐，可能会误吸大量的胃内容物。

管理

框 151.3 列出了可用于预防和治疗恶心和呕吐的止吐剂。这些药物可分为胃肠动力药、吩噻嗪类、丁酰苯类、抗胆碱能药、抗组胺药、NK_1 拮抗剂，5-羟色胺（serotonin，5-HT3）受体拮抗剂和类固醇。没有一种药物可以普遍有效地预防或治疗 PONV。这些药物中许多都与副作用有关，例如镇静和锥体外系反应。这可能会导致一些临床医师限制使用这些药物，特别是有些人认为 PONV 对整体预后的影响通常可以忽略不计。此外，当考虑到可能影响 PONV 发生的因素较多时，选择最有效的止吐药可能并不容易。

框 151.2　恶心呕吐的相关并发症

- 吸入性肺炎
- 脱水
- 麻醉后恢复室的延迟出室
- 延迟出院
  - 增加成本
  - 不方便
- 电解质不平衡
  - 低钾血症
  - 低氯血症
  - 低钠血症
  - 碱中毒
- 食管破裂（Boerhaave 综合征）
- 术后出血增多
- 颅内压增高
- Mallory-Weiss 撕裂

框 151.3　止吐药

- 抗胆碱能药物
  - 东莨菪碱（静脉注射或透皮贴剂）
  - 阿托品
- 抗组胺药
  - 塞克力嗪（Marezine）
  - 茶苯海明（Dramamine）
  - 苯海拉明（Benadryl）
- 丁酰苯类
  - 氟哌利多（Inapsine，鞘氨醇）
  - 氟哌啶醇（Haldol）
- NK1 拮抗剂
  - 阿瑞吡坦（Emend）
- 吩噻嗪
  - 异丙嗪（Phenergan）
  - 丙氯拉嗪（Compazine）
  - 奋乃静（Trilafon）
- 促动力
  - 甲氧氯普胺（Reglan）
  - 多潘立酮（Motilium）
- 5- 羟色胺（$5\text{-}HT_3$）拮抗剂
  - 昂丹司琼（Zofran）
  - 多拉司琼（Anzemet）
  - 格拉司琼（Kytril）
  - 帕洛诺司琼（Aloxi）
- 类固醇
  - 地塞米松（Decadron）

预防

由于不到 30% 的患者术后会发生呕吐，因此没有必要常规应用止吐药物。呕吐持续的时间通常很短。此外，一些常用的止吐剂引起的镇静和苏醒延迟还可能妨碍它们的有效性。尽管通常不建议进行止吐预防，但必须考虑到 PONV 的治疗通常不如其预防效果的现实，因此可能存在特定情况，对于已知存在风险的患者有必要预防性使用这些药剂。

鉴于 PONV 的发生涉及多种因素，很难提供有关预防的具体建议。PONV 与化放疗相关的恶心和呕吐有所区别，化放疗中的激发剂更容易识别。另外，对于顽固性 PONV 病例，可能需要联合使用药物来增加功效，但联合治疗比单种药物治疗更昂贵，而且即使使用多种药物治疗也不能确保成功。

其他有助于预防 PONV 的因素包括非药物治疗，例如用胃管或鼻胃管进行胃减压。然而，术后胃管的存在可刺激呕吐反射，使胃减压的益处大打折扣。另外，亦有人提倡充分水化可以降低PONV的发生率。该疗法相对成本低和安全性高，考虑使用这种方法似较合理。其他更另类的非药物疗法包括针灸、穴位按摩和特殊的草药。最后，新型药物包括目前正在欧洲上市的5-HT_3拮抗剂托烷司琼（tropisetron）正在美国进行临床试验，NK_1拮抗剂卡索匹坦（casopitant）目前也在临床试验中。

致谢

感谢Robert K. Stoelting博士对本章上一版的贡献。

（凡丽华 译 许 涛 校）

延伸阅读

Apfel CC, Korttila K, Abdulla M, et al.: A factorial trial of six interventions for the prevention of postoperative nausea and vomiting, *N Engl J Med* 350:2441–2451, 2004.

Camu F, Lauwers MH, Verbessem D: Incidence and aetiology of postoperative nausea and vomiting, *Eur J Anaesthesiol* 9(Suppl 6):25–31, 1992.

Diemunsch P, Apfel C, Gan TJ, et al.: Preventing postoperative nausea and vomiting: post hoc analysis of data from two randomized active-controlled trials of aprepitant, *Curr Med Res Opin* 23(10):2559–2565, 2007.

Divatia JV, Vaidya JS, Badwe RA, et al.: Omission of nitrous oxide during anesthesia reduces the incidence of postoperative nausea and vomiting: a meta-analysis, *Anesthesiology* 85:1055–1062, 1996.

Korttila K: The study of postoperative nausea and vomiting, *Br J Anaesth* 69(Suppl 1):20S–23S, 1992.

Moon HY, Baek CW, Choi GJ, et al.: Palonosetron and aprepitant for the prevention of postoperative nausea and vomiting in patients indicated for laparoscopic gynaecologic surgery: a double-blind randomised trial, *BMC Anesthesiol* 14:68, 2014.

Palazzo MGA, Strunin L: Anesthesia and emesis, *Can Anaesth Soc J* 31:178–187, 1984.

Rowbotham DJ: Current management of postoperative nausea and vomiting, *Br J Anaesth* 69(Suppl 1):46S–59S, 1992.

Watcha MF, White PF: Postoperative nausea and vomiting, *Anesthesiology* 77:162–184, 1992.

喉和气管损伤

第 152 章

Michael A. Hall，*Andrew E. Ochroch*

病例概要

患者，女性，58 岁，体重 50 kg，于手术室行经腹全子宫切除术。静脉诱导全身麻醉后，用直接喉镜进行插管，按压环状软骨时仍只能看见杓状软骨。于是使用一次性弯头探条进行盲探直至有顶住迹象（hold-up sign），然后将一根直径 6.5 mm 的气管导管经探头置入气管。通过二氧化碳波形确认气管导管放置的位置。手术中没有发生任何意外。然而在手术结束时掀开手术铺单后发现患者躯干至颈部出现弥漫性皮下气肿。在患者全身麻醉苏醒之前行支气管镜检查，发现气管至右主支气管的气管膜部发生纵向撕裂。

问题分析

定义

喉镜检查和气管插管时，以及气管置管后的不同时期均可发生喉和气管的损伤；表 152.1 列举了一系列临床相关损伤。这些损伤的严重程度差异较大，可从自限性损伤到需要广泛的手术修复。急性损伤很可能与气管插管期间的直接创伤有关。报告的损伤因素包括喉镜（经典直接喉镜和视频喉镜）、单腔和双腔气管导管、气管导管导芯、插管探条和喉罩。

长时间插管造成的伤害更可能是缺血性的，与气管导管（特别是套囊）和气管黏膜之间的接触有关。气管有节段性血液供应，通过滋养血管供养黏膜下血管丛，继续维持软骨环的灌注。黏膜下血管丛的长时间压迫可导致相邻软骨环的缺血。压迫通常由于过度充气的气管导管套囊压在气管黏膜上导致压力大于 25 ～ 30 mmHg 所致。缺血首先会导致水肿，进而进展到溃疡或肉芽肿形成。如果长时间未能察觉，缺血性损伤将导致气管腐蚀，甚至可能发展成气管食管瘘或气管无名血管瘘。拔除气管导管后，严重损伤可能导致气管软化，非严重损伤也可能会因为二期愈合，在 3 ～ 6 周间形成缩窄，导致气管狭窄。

识别

鉴于喉和气管损伤的多样性，最好将气管插管期间或之后损伤的体征和症状按损伤病因分组。

气管插管期间的损伤

大部分气管插管期间造成的损伤相对较轻，包

表 152.1 不同时间阶段喉和气管临床相关损伤的例子

气管插管期间的损伤	插管后的短期损伤（<24 h）	插管后的远期损伤（>24 h）
声带血肿或裂伤	声带和喉头水肿	声带和喉部肉芽肿或溃疡
杓状软骨脱位	声带麻痹	喉气管、声门下或气管狭窄
下咽穿孔	Tapia 综合征（同侧喉返神经和舌下神经的暂时性麻痹）	喉黏膜溃疡和黏膜下出血
气管撕裂、穿孔或破裂	气管水肿或充血	气管溃疡
隆突或支气管裂伤或穿孔		气管软化 气管食管和气管动脉瘘

括声带血肿、咽挫伤和杓状软骨脱位。患者拔管后很快便会主诉喉咙痛并且可能有一定程度的声音变化（声音嘶哑）或刺激性咳嗽。更严重的喉部创伤可能会导致气道阻塞，引起呼吸困难、呼吸急促和喘鸣。清醒患者中其诊断常需通过鼻咽喉镜检查来实现，但通常仅气道存在问题的患者或 1 ～ 2 周内气道损伤症状不能自行缓解的患者才会预约这种检查。气道或上呼吸消化道的任何部分的穿孔、裂伤或破裂最常表现为纵隔和皮下气肿，也可能发生气胸或血胸。极少数情况下，气管或支气管的严重创伤可能导致气管内出血，可在气管导管内发现或从气道中吸出血液。通常用胸部 X 线和纤维支气管镜检查来评估损伤程度。

气管插管后的短期（<24 h）损伤

即使留置气管插管的时间较短，临床上也可能出现一定数量的喉和声带水肿病例，表现为拔管后不久出现的呼吸困难、呼吸急促和喘鸣，并可能发展为部分或完全气道阻塞。在气道受损的情况下，需要用直接间接喉镜进行检查以评估阻塞程度并确定是否需要经喉方式保护气道或进行气管切开以维持通气。也有气管导管导致颅神经损伤的报道，包括喉返神经。这很可能是由于气管导管套囊过度充气导致走行于气管和甲状软骨之间的神经受压所引起。这将导致同侧声带麻痹，这种现象通常是自限性的，需要使用某种形式的喉镜检查进行评估。

气管插管后的远期损伤（>24 h）

长期气管插管时，某些严重的损伤，例如气管动脉瘘和气管软化，可能在拔管前或拔管后不久即可表现出来，但更常见的并发症，如气道缩窄和狭窄，往往需要数周至数月才能完全形成并表现出症状。一方面是因为气管内瘢痕的发生过程缓慢，另一方面是只有当气管的横截面积减少 70% 以上才会在安静状态下产生症状。患者会出现声音嘶哑和咳嗽，进而形成呼吸困难和呼吸急促，最后发生喘鸣并需要使用呼吸机辅助呼吸。虽然肺活量测定可以显示出与气道阻塞相一致的气流受限，但流量-容量环的异常仅在严重狭窄时才会出现。如果临床上怀疑气道狭窄，影像学检查方面可选择 CT 三维重建来评估狭窄部位和程度，还可协助制订手术计划。

风险评估

正如气管插管的并发症有多种形式，增加并发症风险的患者因素也是多种多样的。轻度喉部创伤，包括血肿和水肿增厚，是喉部插管期间最常见的损伤，据报道其在全身麻醉下进行短时间外科手术时的发生率高达 69%。危险因素如下：

- 喉部或上呼吸道的解剖异常；
- 困难插管或喉镜暴露时需要多次尝试；
- 使用双腔或型号过大的气管导管。

对于罕见的，危及生命的插管并发症而言，其真正的发生率很难估计；然而，使用诸如探条的插管辅助装置，以及气管导管的过度移动或操作将增加气管支气管损伤的风险。

对于需要长时间插管的患者，气管缺血性损伤的危险因素包括以下内容：

- 气管导管套囊过度充气；
- 影响气管血流的慢性疾病，包括高血压和糖尿病；
- 影响气管血流的急性病变，包括贫血和低血压。

启示

经口气管插管并发症的范畴包含从普通和自限性损伤到罕见和危及生命的损伤。最常见的并发症，术后声音嘶哑，已经被证明对手术后患者的满意度和患者出院后的活动水平有明显的不良影响。气道任何部位的穿孔均可导致严重感染，并需要进行修复手术。气管狭窄需要患者接受多次支气管镜操作，为行确定性修复还需进行重大手术。任何威胁气道通畅的并发症都可能需要进行气管造口术，有时可能会在紧急情况下实施。

管理

到目前为止，在气管插管期间引起的最常见损伤是喉咙痛和声音嘶哑，它们通常是自限性的损伤并且会在几天内消退。然而对于更严重的损伤，尤其是导致气道阻塞的损伤，一般需要进行紧急干预。对于引起眩晕或呼吸困难的急性喉部或声带水肿，雾化吸入外消旋肾上腺素可能减轻水肿并改善症状。虽然随机性研究并不支持，但是静脉注射地塞米松也经常用于减轻水肿。静脉注射地塞米松也可在拔管前用于减轻水肿，以提高拔管成功率；这已经在儿科重症监护室得到了很好的应用。有症状的杓状软骨脱位可请耳鼻喉科医师进行闭合复位来治疗，用于解决 2 ～ 3 月内的声音改变和声带活动异常。

罕见但可能危及生命的损伤通常需要进行外科手术干预。气管或支气管穿孔或裂伤通常需要右侧开胸术进行修复，如果损伤发生在胸部以外则需要经颈部进行手术。根据损伤或相关症状的严重程度，对于特定患者可进行非手术治疗，并使用广谱抗生素来预防纵隔炎的发生。而气管到邻近结构的瘘管则需要进行手术修复，如果瘘至血管则需行急诊手术治疗。

气道狭窄的治疗取决于损伤的严重程度和位置。急性气道受损的患者，可通过硬性支气管镜检查行一系列扩张治疗。然而，鉴于缺血性损伤的透壁性质，这通常只能作为手术行确定性修复之前的一种临时措施。对于必须延迟手术修复或技术上不可行的患者，可使用 T 管或腔内支架来缓解气道阻塞的症状。但最终还是要切除狭窄段和主要的狭窄部分来重建气管并做好修复，修复时需要仔细关注气管血供和吻合口的张力。

预防

预防喉和气管损伤的重点是在气管插管期间和管理插管患者时减少对气道的损伤。表 152.2 列举了可降低这些损伤风险的具体措施。

（朱 洁 译 王嘉锋 校）

表 152.2 降低气管插管致喉和气管损伤风险的具体措施

气管插管时	管理插管患者
在进行喉镜检查和气管插管通过声门时，尽可能努力减少对声带的直接损伤	保持适当的套囊位置（深度）和充气压力
努力优化插管条件，提高喉镜操作的成功率，减少操作时间，以及使用喉镜的次数	套囊充气时避免导管前进或后退
使用插管探条时应谨慎，应感受气管环而不是使用顶住迹象（hold-up sign）	在 ICU 中，适当使用药物治疗胃食管反流，并使患者处于半卧位（床头抬高 30℃）
确保气管导管套囊充气的压力为保证足够通气的最小值（理想情况下 <20 mmHg）	
将气管导管固定在适当的深度，避免将气囊置于喉内或主支气管内	对于气道或上呼吸消化道穿孔的患者合理使用抗生素治疗
避免使用型号过大的气管导管	
润滑气管导管尖端，特别是双腔或大型号导管	

延伸阅读

Lee DH, Yoon TM, Lee JK, et al.: Clinical characteristics of arytenoid dislocation after endotracheal intubation, *J Craniofac Surg* 26:1358–1360, 2015.

Lui N, Wright C: Intraoperative tracheal injury, *Thorac Surg Clin* 25:249–254, 2015.

Mendels EJ, Brunings JW, Hamaekers AW, et al.: Adverse laryngeal effects following short-term general anesthesia, *Arch Otolaryngol Head Neck Surg* 138:257–264, 2012.

Prasad M, Lim K, Kumar C: Tracheal injury using a gum elastic bougie within a RAE endotracheal tube, *Anaesth Intensive Care* 44:428, 2016.

Stauffer JL: Complications of translaryngeal intubation. In Tobin MJ, editor: *Principles and practice of mechanical ventilation*, 3rd ed, New York, 2013, McGraw-Hill, pp 895–940.

Tesei F, Poveda LM, Strali W, et al.: Unilateral laryngeal and hypoglossal paralysis (Tapia's syndrome) following rhinoplasty in general anaesthesia: case report and review of the literature, *Acta Otorhinolaryngol Ital* 26:219–221, 2006.

Wain JC: Postintubation tracheal stenosis, *Semin Thorac Cardiovasc Surg* 21:284–289, 2009.

第 153 章 医护人员的乳胶反应

Kevin J. Kelly，Robert E. Kettler

病例概要

某麻醉科医师，男性，44 岁，发现右手中指出现皮疹，最近进展为荨麻疹。他平素体健，但对鱼类和花粉过敏，并在小时候因湿疹接受过治疗。近几年，他时常出现皮疹，尤其在佩戴手套进行医疗操作后加重。过去 2 周，他在手术室工作时会发作胸闷和鼻炎。其唯一服用的药物是秋季用于治疗花粉热的抗组胺药。

问题分析

定义

在对患者进行诊疗和护理过程中，天然乳胶过敏（另见第 194 章）对医护人员具有重要的临床意义。橡胶手套的使用可追溯到 19 世纪末，当时 Halsted 发明了橡胶手套保护洗手护士的双手，使其避免经常使用洗手液而造成损害。20 世纪 30 年代医学文献，首次描述了橡胶手套造成的手部皮肤损害。20 世纪 80 年代末，乳胶反应的发生率上升是一系列因素综合作用的结果：肝炎和获得性免疫缺陷综合征（acquired immunodeficiency syndrome，AIDS）的发病率不断上升，需要采取综合预防措施，使得对包括天然乳胶手套在内的防护性装备的需求和使用增加。

橡胶工业满足了这一需求，但最终的产品质量可能受以下因素影响：新加入该领域的制造商、新的橡胶生产地、橡胶生产国的政治动荡以及在满足环境和职业健康要求的前提下，改变生产工艺以增加产量。需求的增加使进口到美国的医疗手套数量增加。

随着乳胶手套使用的增多，不断有患者和医护人员发生过敏反应的报道，引发对该问题的重视，促使人们积极认识和报告该问题。如表 153.1 所示，在 MEDLINE 数据库中以乳胶（latex）为关键词的期刊文章，被引用次数的增加反映了人们医学意识的增强，这些引文的绝对数和占比在都有所增加。

表 153.1 MEDLINE 数据库中有关乳胶的引文

年份	有关乳胶的文献数量（%）	数据库文献总数（百万）[a]
1966—1974	445（0.02）	2.0
1975—1979	241（0.02）	1.3
1980—1984	286（0.02）	1.4
1985—1989	348（0.02）	1.7
1990—1993	472（0.03）	1.5
1994—1997	679（0.07）	1.0
1966—1997	2471（0.03）	8.8

[a] 所有条目按四舍五入计。2004 年 8 月，MEDLINE 数据库包含 1400 万篇文献，其中 14 372 篇（0.1%）与乳胶有关

至 2004 年年中，关于 latex 的文献被引用数量增加到 MEDLINE 数据库的 0.1%。

天然乳胶含数种多肽，可与免疫球蛋白 E（immunoglobulin E，IgE）结合。在生产过程中，这些多肽可能通过变性、聚合或分解过程发生改变。为便于穿戴，大多数乳胶手套都涂有玉米淀粉。这种粉末会与各种乳胶抗原结合，散布到大气中，通过呼吸系统被人体吸收。

识别

乳胶不良反应分为三种（表 153.2）：刺激性皮肤炎、Ⅰ型 IgE 介导的反应、Ⅳ型迟发性接触性超敏反应。

刺激性皮炎

刺激性皮炎是由手套形成的局部环境对皮肤的

表 153.2 乳胶刺激物、即时反应和延迟反应的表现

反应类型	起病时间	临床症状	免疫机制
刺激性皮炎	通常是渐进的（数天）	红斑；热痛；皮肤龟裂、破裂或蜕皮；可能有水泡或小泡	无
IgE 介导反应（Ⅰ型）	数分钟内；很少超过 2 h	肿胀、瘙痒、荨麻疹、鼻结膜炎、哮喘、低血压、过敏反应	IgE 介导释放肥大细胞介质；抗原是天然乳胶蛋白
迟发性接触性超敏反应（Ⅳ型）	接触后 6 ～ 48 h	急性：红斑、瘙痒、水泡，开裂、结痂、脱屑 慢性：皮肤干燥、蜕皮、开裂、增厚或变黑	延迟免疫或细胞介导免疫；T 细胞对充当半抗原的微小橡胶化学物质的反应

From Ownby DR：Manifestations of latex allergy. *Immunol Allergy Clin North Am* 15：34，1995.

物理或化学刺激所致。刺激反应的危险因素包括年龄增加、天气寒冷、出汗过多。数天后皮肤出现破损，受影响区域出现红斑和破裂。这些反应不是免疫介导的，但其可能通过破坏皮肤对过敏原的屏障作用从而成为发生免疫介导反应的危险因素。

Ⅰ型 IgE 介导反应

Ⅰ型反应由 IgE 介导，通常与乳胶蛋白接触后数分钟内发生。过敏原与 IgE 结合，导致肥大细胞释放血管活性物质（组胺、缓激肽、白三烯、前列腺素等）。IgE 介导的反应有多种潜在表现，包括荨麻疹、瘙痒、支气管痉挛、鼻结膜炎、脸红、低血压、血管水肿和过敏反应。

Ⅳ型迟发性超敏反应

乳胶手套引起的Ⅳ型反应由细胞介导的对手套残留的化学物质的反应。症状在几天内出现，包括红斑、瘙痒、小泡、开裂、蜕皮和增厚。皮疹通常会延伸到接触部位外。Ⅳ型反应通常不由天然胶乳引起，而是制造过程中的添加剂所致，如硫脲和巯基苯并咪唑等。

风险评估

关于天然胶乳反应的自然史和临床过程的研究较少。此外，由于其研究方法的不同，报道的发生率也不同。即便如此，普通人群中乳胶过敏的发生率一直不到 1%。一项针对献血者的研究显示，6.5% 受试者可检测到抗体，但并不表明临床上就会发生过敏现象。据估计，儿童脊柱裂患者中乳胶过敏发生率为 28% ～ 67%。医护人员乳胶过敏发生率为 5% ～ 17%，而过敏性体质医护人员中其发生率为 24% ～ 36%。

乳胶反应的危险因素包括环境过敏史、食品过敏史（尤指香蕉、猕猴桃或鳄梨）、花粉热、湿疹、哮喘和长期乳胶暴露史（无论是职业性还是治疗性，暴露频率和强度均为影响因素）。皮肤相对不易受乳胶蛋白影响，但刺激或接触反应对皮肤的破坏可能使患者易于发展成 IgE 介导的免疫反应和随后的全身反应。玉米淀粉润滑剂结合乳胶蛋白，分散在大气中增加了呼吸暴露量。如患者既往史存在乳胶过敏的风险因素，应进行血清 IgE 对乳胶过敏原的反应水平检测或专业的皮肤测试。如表 153.3 所示，可以进行进一步的检查。

表 153.3 乳胶刺激性反应、即时反应和延迟反应的表现

阴性	阳性
有乳胶过敏风险的患者 [a]	
无症状，无乳胶过敏，无需检测	有症状；可能的乳胶过敏；进行诊断试验
血清试验	
阴性；做进一步测试	阳性；不需要进一步检测（确认乳胶过敏）
乳胶使用试验	
阴性；做进一步的测试	阳性；不需要进一步检测（确认乳胶过敏）
皮肤反应测验	
阴性；无乳胶过敏	阳性；不需要进一步检测（确认乳胶过敏）

[a] 一些研究者主张，对所有脊柱裂患者进行乳胶试验。这一方法可识别无症状但血清测试结果阳性者。进一步检测前，此类患者应被视为对乳胶过敏。

From Kelly KJ，Kurup VP，Reijula KE，et al：The diagnosis of natural rubber latex allergy. *J Allergy Clin Immunol* 93：814，1994.

启示

乳胶反应的严重程度可从小烦恼到危及生命的过敏反应甚至可致残（例如哮喘）。除医学并发症外，还会产生社会影响例如需要改换岗位或职业以及支付残疾津贴的费用。机构和个人可能必须改变其医疗实践的各个方面，以降低乳胶反应的发生风险。

治疗

治疗方法如下：

- 避免过敏原；
- 局部治疗；
- 全身性治疗（见第 129 章）。

天然橡胶制品普遍存在，医疗卫生领域避免过敏原可能较为困难。然而，仍可采取一些措施，如佩戴非乳胶手套或在乳胶手套和皮肤之间使用某种屏障（例如乙烯基手套）。仅在必要时使用乳胶手套也可减少暴露。个人发生严重反应而又无法避免过敏原时，可能不得不改换岗位或职业。只使用无粉、低过敏原乳胶手套或合成手套，可使空气中的过敏原完全消除或降低到无临床意义的水平。局部使用类固醇和保湿剂治疗可缓解刺激症状和Ⅳ型反应。针对 IgE 介导反应的全身治疗包括气道管理、必要时的通气和循环支持（包括使用肾上腺素）、抗组胺药和支气管扩张剂。

预防

建议易感个体避免接触乳胶制品，但通常较难实行。此类个体应佩戴过敏警示识别标志，并携带可自动注射装置，以便紧急情况时使用肾上腺素。各机构应考虑设立多学科委员会进行管理和预防，为患者、医护人员及其他雇员制定指导方案。该委员会应在鉴别含乳胶的医疗产品、识别和购买不含乳胶的替代品、为易感个体建立无乳胶处理区和使用无粉手套等方面提供指导意见。

（张莹莹 译 盛 颖 校）

延伸阅读

Garabrant DH, Schweitzer S: Epidemiology of latex sensitization and allergies in health care workers, *J Allergy Clin Immunol* 110:S82–S95, 2002.

Kelly KJ: Management of the latex-allergic patient, *Immunol Allergy Clin North Am* 15:139–157, 1995.

Kelly KJ, Kurup VP, Reijula KE, et al.: The diagnosis of natural rubber latex allergy, *J Allergy Clin Immunol* 93:813–816, 1994.

Landwehr LP, Boguniewicz M: Current perspectives on latex allergy, *J Pediatr* 128:305–312, 1996.

Ownby DR: Manifestations of latex allergy, *Immunol Allergy Clin North Am* 15:31–43, 1995.

Ranta PM, Owenby DR: A review of natural-rubber latex allergy in health care workers, *Clin Infect Dis* 38:252–256, 2004.

Sussman GL, Beezhold DH: Allergy to latex rubber, *Ann Intern Med* 122:43–46, 1995.

Truscott W: The industry perspective on latex, *Immunol Allergy Clin North Am* 15:89–121, 1995.

局部麻醉药神经毒性：马尾综合征 第 154 章

Christina M. Spofford

病例概要

患者，男性，48 岁，脊椎麻醉（腰麻）下行右腹股沟疝修补术。患者取坐位，在 L4 ～ L5 间隙用 24 号无损伤（笔尖）腰麻针进行穿刺。脊椎麻醉药物包括 75 mg 5% 盐酸利多卡因和 7.5% 葡萄糖、0.1 mg 肾上腺素和 25 μg 芬太尼，5 min 后阻滞平面达 L3 水平。然后将患者置于右侧卧位，鞘内追加 50 mg 5% 利多卡因和葡萄糖。阻滞平面达 T10 水平，手术顺利进行。术后 12 h，患者会阴部麻木感持续存在，排空障碍。肛门括约肌张力减弱，肛门反射消失。腰骶部磁共振成像结果正常，没有脓肿或血肿证据。术后 6 个月，患者小便失禁，无法自发排便，且 S3 ～ S5 区域持续存在双侧感觉减弱。

问题分析

定义

正如该术语所提示，马尾综合征（cauda equina syndrome，CES）临床表现为脊髓圆锥以下神经根损伤有关的症状。因此，CES 可导致不同程度的肠道和膀胱功能障碍，会阴感觉丧失和下肢运动无力。尽管存在多种潜在原因，麻醉科医师仍应关注以下两个问题：①压迫性损伤（例如硬膜外或脊髓血肿 / 脓肿）；②鞘内药物的直接毒性。临床经验和实验数据表明，在某些情况下，目前临床上使用的局部麻醉药有可能诱发神经毒性损伤和 CES。我们将在本章中回顾该问题。

识别

医学文献中偶有与脊椎麻醉和硬膜外麻醉相关的明显神经损伤的报道，并进一步探究局部麻醉的神经毒性。早期报道认为，CES 与持续脊椎麻醉（continuous spinal anesthesia，CSA）的微导管有关。这些与 CSA 相关的病例有两个共同因素：局限于骶部阻滞，其需要重复剂量的局部麻醉药以实现充分的外科手术麻醉；累积剂量远超过单次脊椎麻醉的常用剂量。有人提出，分布不均和高剂量麻醉药二者导致蛛网膜下腔狭窄区域局部麻醉药达到神经毒性浓度，该机制被随后的体内、外试验数据所支持。尽管大部分损伤涉及通过小口径微导管给予 5% 利多卡因，但并非都与利多卡因有关，有些则涉及通过硬膜外导管鞘内给予局部麻醉药。因此，临床中不再使用导管并未消除 CES 风险，从业者仍可使用硬膜外导管进行 CSA。此外，如果在尝试硬膜外导管放置期间发生硬脊膜意外穿破，部分临床医师通常会改为 CSA。

并非只有 CSA 技术会导致神经毒性损伤；它们也存在于单次注药脊椎麻醉。具体而言，单次注药脊椎麻醉时，阻滞不全通常由药物分布不均所致。这种情况下，重复给药可能以相同模式分布，导致蛛网膜下腔局限范围内局部麻醉药达到神经毒性浓度。病例报告和已结案索赔数据库审查结果似乎支持这一考虑。

第三种机制是高剂量局部麻醉药被注入蛛网膜下腔。如果操作者未能意识到硬膜外针或导管穿破硬脊膜或蛛网膜而常规使用硬膜外局部麻醉药，则施用药量可使蛛网膜下腔药物达到神经毒性浓度。正如病例概要所述，即使在没有分布不均的情况下，上述剂量也足以诱发损伤。

CSA、脊椎麻醉失败后重复注药以及无意中鞘内注射硬膜外麻醉药量引起神经损伤的报道表明，超过脊椎麻醉常规临床剂量范围的局部麻醉药具有潜在毒性。更令人惊讶的是，有两份报告指出在单次脊椎麻醉中给予推荐剂量的利多卡因也可能导致神经功能损伤。其中一份为鞘内注射混有肾上腺素的利多卡因 100 mg 后发生 CES，另一份来自法国区域麻醉前瞻性研究。两份报告中存在其他因素无法解释的单次推注利多卡因后持续神经损伤。所有病例均使用相对较高的剂量（≥ 75 mg），但永久性损伤仅发生在注射最大临床推荐剂量（100 mg）之后。

风险评估

前瞻性研究、回顾性研究和流行病学研究所报道的局部麻醉药神经毒性反应所致 CES 发生率各不相同。鉴于临床模式等原因，这些信息可能具有误导性。前述法国的研究指出，单次注射利多卡因脊椎麻醉后永久性损伤发生率约为 1/5000，这可能高估了其风险，因当前已更改临床模式以降低损伤风险（见“预防”部分）。尽管如此，在评估术后 CES 可能是药物神经毒性反应时，应考虑与已知临床毒性相关的因素（例如，意外鞘内注射预估的硬膜外麻醉药剂量）。

除脊椎或硬膜外麻醉后发生罕见 CES 外，利多卡因脊椎麻醉后多达 1/3 患者可能出现短暂的神经系统症状（transient neurologic symptoms，TNS），即臀部和下肢疼痛或感觉迟钝。TNS 已知风险因素包括门诊患者和手术体位（例如，接受膝关节镜检查或处于截石位的患者）。然而，TNS 较易与 CES 区分开，因为前者与感觉、运动缺陷或膀胱、肠道功能紊乱无关。

启示

CES 是一种罕见但具有灾难性的并发症，可能与脊髓圆锥以下神经根毒性损伤有关。因其严重性和缺乏有效的治疗，必须注意采用最小化风险的临床策略（见“预防”部分）。

管理

虽然有观点主张使用大剂量类固醇药物，但没有任何证据证明这些药物对局部麻醉药引起的神经根损伤有益处。如前所述，CES 有许多潜在原因，包括压迫性病变（例如血肿、脓肿）。与神经毒性损伤不同，压迫导致的损伤容易逆转，恢复程度与功能丧失程度以及从损伤出现到手术减压的时间有关。临床情况（凝血功能、阻滞困难等）可用于指导区分其他病因的可能性。此外，神经毒性表现为无持续使用局部麻醉药时神经阻滞并未消退，而压迫性病变表现为术后神经功能恢复一段时间后又逐渐丧失。因为时间至关重要，任何疑似病例都应通过急诊磁共振成像来判断。

预防

分析脊椎麻醉和硬膜外麻醉发生 CES 的临床报告以及神经毒性实验研究的数据，可识别出可能加剧 CES 风险的因素。这些因素构成了改进临床实践的基础。

连续脊椎麻醉

CSA 时因阻滞不全而鞘内注射大剂量局部麻醉药会导致损伤。当单次给予正常剂量范围却未达到足够阻滞平面的局部麻醉药时，指南强调应采用给予测试剂量、调整技术或放弃该技术（框 154.1）。

脊椎麻醉失败后重复给药

与 CSA 类似，已经提出针对脊椎麻醉阻滞失败的指南。包括评估技术错误的可能性（例如，鞘内注药失败）和适当减少重复注射的剂量。然而，更有效（并且可能更安全）的策略是，简单地将使用的麻醉药总量限定为临床医师认为合理的单次鞘内注射的最大量。

硬膜外麻醉

因意外鞘内注射硬膜外麻醉剂量导致的神经毒性，业已强调测试剂量和分次给药的重要性。此外，如果通过位置错误的鞘内导管给予大剂量麻醉药，无论何种麻醉药，均应考虑反复回抽少量脑脊液并用盐水填充。

利多卡因脊椎麻醉

最近，大多数与脊椎麻醉和硬膜外麻醉相关的损伤，与使用利多卡因有关。实验研究结果更增加了对这种麻醉药的担忧，表明其固有毒性超过布比卡因。在动物实验中，鞘内注射利多卡因可引起脊髓背根神经节细胞凋亡。框 154.2 概述了使用该药的改进指南，并在以下段落中详述（尽管利多卡因是重点，但大多数建议适用于任何鞘内麻醉药）。

剂量

大多数研究表明，利多卡因与布比卡因的效能比约为 1∶4。然而，最大推荐剂量分别为 100 mg 和 20 mg，或给予这些药剂的整支安瓿（100 mg 和 15 mg），所得到比例为 5∶1 或 6.7∶1。除相对毒性的问题，100 mg 利多卡因已超过可靠的脊椎麻醉所需剂量。这与剂量范围上限可能的神经毒性病例报告相符，因此没有理由继续使用 100 mg 极量。尽管这些数据不足以对最大安全剂量提出强有力的质疑，但许多人使用 3 ml 2% 利多卡因（60 mg）即可获得可靠的脊椎麻醉。

框 154.1 连续脊椎麻醉：给药指南

将导管置入足够深度以确认位置并固定
使用最低有效麻醉浓度
给予测试剂量，并评估阻滞范围
如果怀疑分布不均，使用下述操作增加局部麻醉药扩散（例如，改变患者体位，改变腰骶曲率，换成不同比重的溶液）
若在达到限制剂量前未达到满意的感觉阻滞平面，则放弃该技术

Adapted from Rigler ML，Drasner K，Krejcie TC，et al：Cauda equina syndrome after continuous spinal anesthesia. *Anesth Analg* 72（3）：275-281，1991.

框 154.2 利多卡因脊椎麻醉：常规指南

剂量应限制在 60 mg
浓度不应超过 2%
使用布比卡因或甲哌卡因延长阻滞时间

Data from Drasner K：Lidocaine spinal anesthesia：a vanishing therapeutic index? *Anesthesiology* 87（3）：469-472，1997.

浓度

大量数据表明，麻醉药的神经毒性某种程度上取决于药物浓度。因此很难证明持续使用远超达到充分阻滞所需要的药物浓度是合理的。利多卡因的注射浓度不应超过 2%，因其临床上产生相当于 5% 溶液的感觉麻醉。

葡萄糖

新近临床损伤病例的共同特征是，使用混有高浓度葡萄糖的麻醉药溶液，其张力远超过正常生理范围。尽管存在这种相关性，但 7.5% 葡萄糖不会影响体外复合动作电位或增强麻醉导致的传导阻滞。此外，7.5% 葡萄糖也不会影响在体鞘内利多卡因产生的剂量依赖性感觉功能消失，10% 葡萄糖也不会引起功能障碍或形态学损伤。这些研究表明，葡萄糖可安全用于增加药液比重。

血管收缩药

血管收缩药可能通过促进组织缺血，减少麻醉药摄取或直接影响神经元而产生毒性。肾上腺素可增强鞘内注射利多卡因导致的感觉神经阻滞。最近的在体动物实验表明，5% 或 7.5% 利多卡因中加入肾上腺素，未显示组织病理学变化，与之前报道结果相反。在该问题得到最终解决之前，如果麻醉目的是提供更长的手术麻醉持续时间，可使用布比卡因或甲哌卡因。

（王 委 译 许 涛 校）

延伸阅读

Auroy Y, Narchi P, Messiah A, et al.: Serious complications related to regional anesthesia: results of a prospective survey in France, *Anesthesiology* 87:479–486, 1997.

Drasner K: Lidocaine spinal anesthesia: a vanishing therapeutic index? *Anesthesiology* 87:469–472, 1997.

Drasner K, Rigler M: Repeat injection after a "failed spinal"—at times, a potentially unsafe practice, *Anesthesiology* 75:713–714, 1991.

Drasner K, Rigler M, Sessler D, et al.: Cauda equina syndrome following intended epidural anesthesia, *Anesthesiology* 77:582–585, 1992.

Freedman J, Li D, Drasner K, et al.: Transient neurologic symptoms after spinal anesthesia: an epidemiologic study of 1863 patients, *Anesthesiology* 89:633–694, 1998.

Hampl KF, Schneider MC, Ummenhofer W, et al.: Transient neurologic symptoms after spinal anesthesia, *Anesth Analg* 81:1148–1153, 1995.

Hashimoto K, Bollen A, Ciriales R, et al.: Comparative toxicity of glucose and lidocaine administered intrathecally in the rat, *Reg Anesth Pain Med* 23:444–450, 1998.

Hashimoto K, Hampl K, Nakamura Y, et al.: Epinephrine increases the neurotoxic potential of intrathecally administered local anesthetic in the rat, *Anesthesiology* 94:876–883, 2001.

Komatsu T, Takenami T, Nara Y, et al.: Epinephrine administered with lidocaine solution does not worsen intrathecal lidocaine neurotoxicity in rats, *Reg Anesth Pain Med* 38(2):140–144, 2013.

Lambert L, Lambert D, Strichartz G: Irreversible conduction block in isolated nerve by high concentrations of local anesthetics, *Anesthesiology* 80:1082–1093, 1994.

Li Y, Jia Z, Zhang L, et al.: Caspase-2 and microRNA34a/c regulate lidocaine-induced dorsal root ganglia apoptosis in vitro, *Eur J Pharmacol* 767:61–66, 2015.

Pollock JE, Neal JM, Stephenson CA, et al.: Prospective study of the incidence of transient radicular irritation in patients undergoing spinal anesthesia, *Anesthesiology* 84:1361–1367, 1996.

Rigler M, Drasner K: Distribution of catheter-injected local anesthetic in a model of the subarachnoid space, *Anesthesiology* 75:684–692, 1991.

Rigler M, Drasner K, Krejcie T, et al.: Cauda equina syndrome after continuous spinal anesthesia, *Anesth Analg* 72:275–281, 1991.

长 QT 综合征与尖端扭转性室速 第 155 章

Mohammed E. Haque，*Rajamani Sethuraman*

病例概要

患者，女性，65 岁，在全身麻醉下行腹腔镜子宫切除术。患者有阵发性心房颤动（简称房颤）史，服用索他洛尔治疗，近期因足部水肿开始使用利尿剂。手术平稳完成后，给予昂丹司琼，不久即出现突发性多形性室性心动过速（ventricular tachycardia，VT，简称室速）。因血流动力学不稳，采用了心脏非同步直流电复律治疗，并开始输注镁剂。心脏复律成功后，12 导联心电图（electrocardiogram，ECG）显示 QTc 为 490 ms，动脉血气分析示血钾为 3.0 mmol/L。

问题分析

定义和病因

长 QT 综合征（long QT syndrome，LQTS）是一种以 QT 间期延长并伴有特征性的、被称为**尖端扭转**（Torsades de Pointes，TdP）的多形性室速为特征的心脏传导疾病。这种异质性疾病的统一机制是心脏复极化延长，合并早期后去极化（early after depolarization，EAD），在达到一定的阈值时，触发诸如室性心律失常等事件。此类心律失常可自行终止或进展为心室颤动（ventricular fibrillation，VF，简称室颤）和心源性猝死（sudden cardiac death，SCD）。

LQTS 可分为先天性（congenital-LQTS，c-LQTS）和获得性（acquired-LQTS，a-LQTS）两类。部分 a-LQTS 患者存在潜在的遗传突变，导致“复极化储备（repolarization reserve）”降低，而未达到 c-LQTS 的诊断标准。Jervell Lange-Nielsen 综合征（一种与感觉神经性听力障碍有关的常染色体隐性遗传性疾病）是第一种被认知的 c-LQTS，随后发现的是常染色体显性遗传性疾病 Romano-Ward 综合征。此后又鉴定出了多种相关的基因突变，目前已知 c-LQTS 存在 13 种亚型。LQT 1、LQT2 和 LQT3 占了遗传学确诊病例的 92% 以上。

药物诱发的 LQTS 的假定机制是相关药物抑制由 *KCNH2*/*HERG* 基因编码的钾通道。流经该通道的离子产生快速作用的外向整流钾电流（IKr），负责心脏动作电位的 3 相电位变化。其功能障碍导致复极化延长，表现为 QTc 延长。*KCNH2* 基因突变导致 LQT2，并可能存在类似的发病机制。值得注意的是，许多药物可阻断 IKr 但不引起 TdP。

LQT1 由 *KVLQT1* 基因突变引起，该基因编码的是一种能影响慢性延迟性整流钾电流（IKs）的蛋白质组分。此类患者占 c-LQTS 的 30% ～ 35%，对交感神经刺激敏感，在刺激时出现 QTc 延长。此特点可用于诊断。采用 β - 受体阻滞剂和交感神经切除术对此型患者有显效。

复极化的延长也可能由不当的内向钠电流引起，如 LQT3，此类患者因 *SCN5A* 基因突变导致钠通道失活障碍。

LQT1 的 TdP 触发是由儿茶酚胺介导的；而在 LQT3 和 a-LQTS 中，心率慢、缓慢性心律失常和期前收缩后的心搏停顿可触发 TdP（“暂停依赖，pause dependent”）。实际上，LQT3 患者的 TdP 和 SCD 主要发生于睡眠期间。在这种情况下，增加心率可降低 QTc（逆使用依赖性，reverse use-dependence），并可用于治疗（见“管理”部分）。

识别

ECG 上 QT 间期延长代表的是心肌细胞复极化时间的延长（图 155.1）。虽然它是 LQTS 的特征，但在静息时可能并不出现。心室复极化的异质性被认为可能为 EAD 和折返回路提供了必要的条件，从而引发 TdP，并使其持续存在。这种异质性的 ECG 特征包括 QT 离散度（QT_{max}-QT_{min}）的增加、T 波形态的异常和 T 波交替（图 155.2）。

通过 Bazett 公式（QTc=QT 间期 / $\sqrt{RR\text{ 间期}}$）进行心率校正后的正常 QT 间期范围为男性 <430 ms、女性 <450 ms（性激素效应）；QT 延长分别是指男性 >450 ms，女性 >470 ms。QTc 随自主状态、药物和昼夜节律的变化而变化。

TdP 的 ECG 特征如下（图 155.3）：

- QRS 波的在波幅变化的同时，围绕等电位基线扭住；
- 心率在 200 ～ 250 bpm；
- 伴有心动过缓和心脏阻滞（特别是 a-LQTS）。

TdP 可能发作短暂且耐受良好，或持续发作并伴有血流动力学障碍，甚至进展为室颤。

风险评估

c–LQTS

病史采集可能发现患者存在晕厥、晕厥先兆、心悸和心搏骤停等病史，或存在心源性猝死家族史。实际上，大多数患者（60%）是在家庭成员出现相关事件后经 ECG 筛查确诊的。有症状的心律失常预示着心脏事件的风险高。患者可使用 β- 受体阻滞剂治疗，高风险患者可植入心脏复律除颤器（implantable cardioverter defibrillator，ICD）和（或）行左心交感神经切除术。

心脏事件最有效的单个预测因素是 QT>500 ms。出现明显的 T 波交替（见图 155.2）是心电不稳定的另一迹象，需要进行干预。

Jervell Lange-Nielsen 综合征的病程凶险。QTc>500 ms 的 LQT1 和 LQT2 患者以及男性 LQT3 患者的相关风险最高。女性患者产后期的风险增高。

a–LQTS

药物

尽管抗心律失常药物是主要病因之一，但许多药物都与 QTc 延长有关（表 155.1）。QTc 延长与 TdP 风险有关，但并非完全相关。已知有两个药物例外，如胺碘酮能延长 QTc，但很少引起 TdP；特非那定与 TdP 强烈相关，但对 QTc 影响不大。

与 QTc 延长药物相关的风险因素包括：同时使用两种或两种以上的药物、药物浓度高、快速静脉内给药，以及联合使用相关药物的代谢抑制剂。

患者因素

许多患者因素能增加对药物诱发 LQTS 的易感性。女性患者居多，占 TdP 报道病例的 70%，表

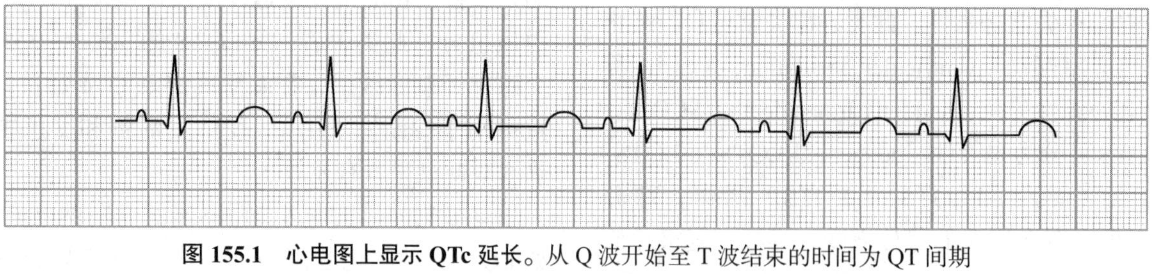

图 155.1　心电图上显示 QTc 延长。从 Q 波开始至 T 波结束的时间为 QT 间期

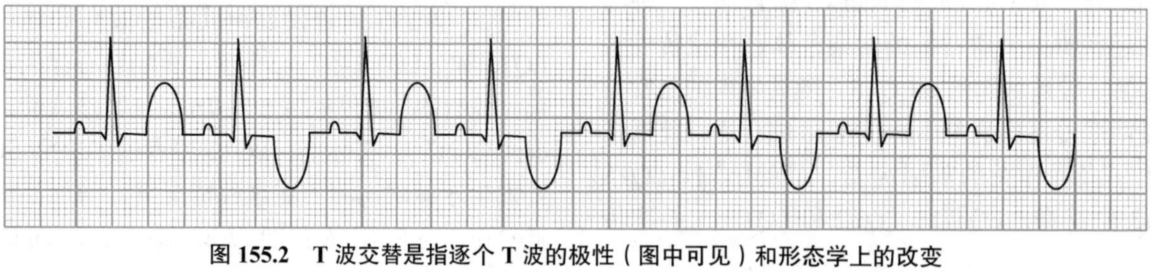

图 155.2　T 波交替是指逐个 T 波的极性（图中可见）和形态学上的改变

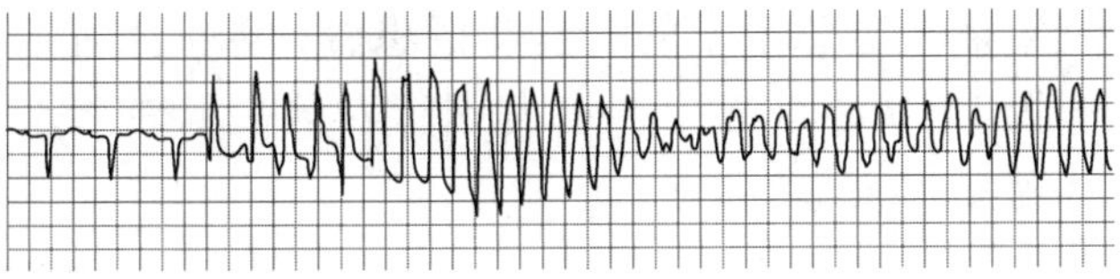

图 155.3 TdP 之前为窦性心律，伴 QTc 延长。注意室速发生时"尖端的扭转"是 TdP 的特征（From Compton SJ: Ventricular tachycardia workup. 2015. Available at http://emedicine.medscape.com/article/159075-workup#c8. Accessed September 6, 2016.）

观因素是女性的基础 QTc 较长，因而降低了其复极化储备。其他一些心脏疾病也可增加患者的易感性（框 155.1）。

电解质

电解质紊乱可延长 QTc，使 TdP 更易发生。重要的是：

- 低镁血症；
- 低钾血症；
- 低钙血症；

利尿治疗、腹泻和呕吐、代谢紊乱、非均衡性饮食（神经性厌食症、绝食、液态蛋白质饮食）都可能是病因或促进因素。

启示

有关 c-LQTS 的预后方面的信息主要来自前瞻性的国际 LQTS 登记数据库。统计结果表明，c-LQTS 的各亚型都有其独特的病史特点。

LQT1 和 LQT2 出现心脏事件（晕厥、心搏骤停或猝死）的年龄较小，且容易反复发作。到 15 岁时，相应有 53% 和 29% 的患者发生过心脏事件；而在 LQT3 中这一比例仅为 6%。LQT1 和 LQT2 患者分别有 37% 和 36% 有过反复发作，而 LQT3 仅有 5%。

尽管存在这些差异，所有亚型病死率都在 3% ～ 4%，40 年的累积病死率为 6% ～ 8%。部分原因是因为 LQT3 患者发生心脏事件后的相关病死率较高（20% vs. 4%）。

该病案登记数据库是将发病者（先证者）及其家属（受影响者）都登记在了同一个组，因此受影响者的病死率可能会显著提高。实际上，当把 479 名发病者（先证者）和 1041 名受影响家庭成员分别进行单独的统计分析，则表明，两组心脏事件的发病率分别为 76% 和 22%。

虽然 a-LQTS 更常见，但其意义却不太清楚。

表 155.1 已知具有诱发 TdP 风险的药物分类

抗心律失常药物	胺碘酮
	丙吡胺
	多非利特
	屈奈达隆
	氟卡尼
	伊布利特
	普鲁卡因胺
	奎尼丁
	索他洛尔
抗生素	阿奇霉素
	环丙沙星
	克拉霉素
	红霉素
	加替沙星[a]
	左氧氟沙星
	莫西沙星
	司帕沙星[a]
抗真菌药物	氟康唑
	喷他脒
抗疟药	氯奎
	卤泛群
止吐药	氯丙嗪
	多潘立酮
	氟哌利多
	昂丹司琼
抗精神病药物	氟哌啶醇
	左美丙嗪
	美索达嗪[a]
	匹莫齐特
	舒必利
	硫利达嗪
抗抑郁药，选择性 5- 羟色胺再摄取抑制剂	西酞普兰
	艾司西酞普兰
抗组胺药	阿司咪唑[a]
	特非那定[a]
阿片受体激动剂	左旋乙酰美沙酮[a]
	美沙酮
磷酸二酯酶 3 抑制剂	阿那格雷
	西洛他唑
抗肿瘤药	三氧化二砷
	奥沙利铂
	凡他尼布（凡德他尼）
其他药物	苄普地尔[a]
	西沙比利[a]
	多奈哌齐
	盐酸罂粟碱
	普罗布考[a]

其他药物有"可能的"和"有条件的"风险——参见 www.crediblemeds.org：Arizona Center for Education and Research on Therapeutics。

[a] 已从美国市场撤除。

框 155.1 增加药物诱发 TdP 风险的因素

女性
高龄
膳食失调
心动过缓
房颤近期转复
充血性心力衰竭
地高辛治疗
基线 QT 延长
室性心律失常
左心室肥大

抗心律失常药物引起的 TdP 发病率估计在 1% 到 10% 之间，而非心血管药物的相关发病率则要更低得多。

在两组回顾性队列研究中，c-LQTS 儿童患者围术期 TdP 的发病率分别为 2.6%（3/114）和 3.2%（5/158）。对所有年龄段的病案报道进行系统性回顾发现，发生围术期 TdP 的有 46 例，病案总体病死率为 4%（2/46）。

管理

c-LQTS

c-LQTS 的一般处理包括适当改变生活方式和避免触发因素。随着认识的提高，基因特异性治疗逐渐可行。抗肾上腺素能治疗策略对 LQT1 和 LQT2（儿茶酚胺敏感）患者特别有效；钠通道阻滞剂对 LQT3 特别有效；而对 LQT3 和 a-LQTS（暂停依赖的 TdP 易感性）患者，变时性治疗策略特别有效。

- 建议所有患者使用 β- 受体阻滞剂（虽然对 LQT3 效果较差），能降低心脏事件风险，特别是在产后期（风险从 1/50 降低到 1/2500）；
- ICD 适用于心搏骤停幸存者和使用 β 受体阻滞剂后症状仍持续存在的患者；
- 心脏起搏联合 β 受体阻滞剂对 LQT3 特别适用（该类患者的 QTc 随心率增加而缩短）。
- 对 β 受体阻滞剂和 / 或 ICD 不耐受或无效的高风险患者，禁忌行左心交感神经切除术。
- LQT3 用美沙利汀（慢心律）、氟卡尼或雷诺嗪等钠通道阻滞剂治疗。
- 对需要紧急手术的有症状的患者，如无条件放置 ICD/ 心脏起搏，可考虑行左侧星状神经节阻滞。

a-LQTS

首要原则是撤除致病药物和纠正电解质紊乱。

- 停止使用致病药物，并酌情使用适当的药物替换；
- 纠正电解质，特别是钾、镁和钙离子紊乱；可能伴有腹泻、呕吐或利尿剂的使用；
- 纠正膳食不均衡。

TdP

a-LQTS 和 c-LQTS 患者中 TdP 的处理大体相似。血流动力学不稳定患者应使用非同步直流电复律。虽然 TdP 通常是暂时性的，但依然可以进行医疗干预。

- 镁 2 g 静脉滴注：
  - 首选治疗；
  - 给药时间超过 15 min，或心搏骤停患者 1 ～ 2 min 内给药；
  - 考虑以 3 ～ 20 mg/min 的速率持续给药。
- 经静脉起搏，使心率达到 100 bpm：
  - **仅限 a-LQTS 患者**：异丙肾上腺素开始以 2 μg/min 的速率逐步滴定（c-LQTS 患者禁忌）。
- 使用 1B 类抗心律失常药物（尽管其作用有限）：
  - 利多卡因、苯妥英或美西律。
- 将钾纠正至 4.5 ～ 5.0 mmol/L。
  - 证据尚不肯定，但很容易实现。

多形性室性心动过速

TdP 的主要鉴别诊断是多形性室性心动过速（polymorphic ventricular tachycardia，PMVT）。虽然在室性心律失常期间两者很难区分，但 PMVT 在发作间期的 QTc 是正常的。PMVT 最常见的原因是心肌缺血，其也可能会有明显的临床表现。PMVT 的治疗包括 β- 受体阻滞剂、利多卡因和胺碘酮（TdP 禁忌）。随后应急诊行冠状动脉造影。

与 TdP 一样，应纠正镁和钾，如果血液动力不稳定，则应行非同步直流电复律。

预防

关于 LQTS 围术期处理的证据很少，且多是以病案报道和病例系列为基础的。目前尚不清楚 c-LQTS 患者术中 TdP 的真实发病率，尽管回顾性研究认为儿童 TdP 发病率为 2.6% ～ 3.2%。麻醉苏醒期似乎是一个关键时期，一项研究中 3 个病例（共 114 例全身麻醉）的 TdP 均发生在这段时间。有关相关药物和挥发性麻醉药的研究结论存在分歧，即使使用相同的药物，不同报道的结论也不尽相同。在应激反应最大时，麻醉技术和麻醉药物选择的重要性可能要低于提供适当而均衡的麻醉。方法如下。

术前

- 提供安静的环境，术前用药使用镇静药 / 抗焦虑药（如咪达唑仑或芬太尼）；
- 继续使用 β - 受体阻滞剂和抗心律失常治疗。若尚未开始使用 β 受体阻滞剂，围术期可考虑使用（c-LQTS）；
- 检查和纠正电解质紊乱（Mg^{2+}、K^{+}、Ca^{2+}）。治疗前考虑使用镁剂；
- 复查 ECG 以确定 QTc 是否延长；
- 处理获得性因素（如药物诱发、营养不均衡），在适当情况下可推迟手术，尤其是有晕厥和晕厥先兆病史的患者；
- ICD：停用，并准备好体外除颤器；
- 起搏器：常规术前检查。如未放置，应做好迅速放置临时经静脉起搏器的准备。

术中

- 监测 QTc，大手术患者（可能导致液体和电解质转移）考虑采用有创监测；
- 全身麻醉和区域麻醉技术都是合适的；后者具有

表 155.2　麻醉药物与作者建议

	安全[a]	谨慎使用[b]	避免使用 / 不安全[c]
诱导药物	硫喷妥钠 咪达唑仑	丙泊酚	氯胺酮
肌松药	维库溴铵 罗库溴铵 阿曲库铵 米库氯铵	泮库溴铵	琥珀胆碱
挥发性麻醉药	异氟烷	七氟烷	恩氟烷 氟烷 二氧化氮
局部麻醉药	利多卡因 布比卡因		可卡因 避免添加肾上腺素
阿片类药物	吗啡 芬太尼	舒芬太尼	美沙酮
止吐药	地塞米松 甲氧氯普胺	赛克力嗪	5-HT_3 拮抗剂（如，昂丹司琼） 达哌啶醇 左美丙嗪
拟交感神经药	间羟胺	麻黄碱 去氧肾上腺素	异丙肾上腺素 肾上腺素 多巴酚丁胺
抗胆碱能药		阿托品 格隆溴铵	
其他	可乐定 右美托咪定	新斯的明 / 格隆溴铵	

[a] 由于存在文献冲突，此处仅是指导意见而非专家共识。避免心动过速和心动过缓是安全使用的关键。
[b] 存在病例报道和（或）警告，但已被安全使用。应尽可能避免使用。
[c] 大量病例报道或致病的药效学影响。也许可安全使用。建议避免使用。

镇痛完善和避免应激反应的优点。可以采用全凭静脉麻醉技术；

- 维持体温正常：低体温将延迟失活的钠通道的恢复并延长 QTc；
- 避免交感神经反应：
  - 减轻喉镜的刺激，考虑加用表面麻醉；
  - 维持血二氧化碳、血糖、和氧分压正常；
  - 完善地镇痛；
- 避免浅麻醉。
- 刺激迷走神经可引起心动过缓，易引发暂停依赖性 TdP，并延长 QTc。因此应：
  - 避免心动过缓；
  - 避免胸腔内通气压力过高；
  - 在已知的手术操作刺激期间（例如腹腔镜操作）保持高度警惕。
- 避免使用已知可致 LQTS 的药物（见表 155.1）和相关的麻醉药物（表 155.2），应具备选择适当的替代性药物的经验。

术后

- 术后仍应避免出现应激，并监测电解质和 QTc，继续使用 β- 受体阻滞剂。

致谢

感谢 John L. Atlee 博士对本章上一版的贡献。

（王　芷　译　倪　文　校）

延伸阅读

Berul CI, Seslar SP, Zimetbaum PJ, et al.: Acquired long QT syndrome. In: Triedman JK, Lévy S, Asirvatham S, et al., editors: *UpToDate*, Waltham, MA. (Accessed August 26, 2016).

Booker PD, Whyte SD, Ladusans EJ: Long QT syndrome and anaesthesia, *Br J Anaesth* 90(3):349–366, 2003.

Drew BJ, Ackerman MJ, Funk M, et al.: Prevention of torsade de pointes in hospital settings: a scientific statement from the American Heart Association and the American College of Cardiology Foundation, *J Am Coll Cardiol* 55(9):934–947, 2010.

Fazio G, Vernuccio F, Grutta G, Re GL: Drugs to be avoided in patients with long QT syndrome: focus on the anaesthesiological management, *World J Cardiol* 5(4):87, 2013.

Johnston J, Pal S, Nagele P: Perioperative torsade de pointes: a systematic review of published case reports, *Anesth Analg* 117(3):559–564, 2013.

Kies SJ, Pabelick CM, Hurley HA, et al.: Anesthesia for patients with congenital long QT syndrome, *Anesthesiology* 102(1):204–210, 2005.

Nathan AT, Berkowitz DH, Montenegro LM, et al.: Implications of anesthesia in children with long QT syndrome, *Anesth Analg* 112(5):1163–1168, 2011.

Priori SG, Wilde AA, Horie M, et al.: Executive summary: HRS/EHRA/APHRS expert consensus statement on the diagnosis and management of patients with inherited primary arrhythmia syndromes, *Europace* 15(10):1389–1406, 2013.

Roden DM: Drug-induced prolongation of the QT interval, *N Engl J Med* 350(10):1013–1022, 2004.

Staikou C, Chondrogiannis K, Mani A: Perioperative management of hereditary arrhythmogenic syndromes, *Br J Anaesth* 108(5):730–744, 2012.

Woosley RL, Romero KA: QTDrugs list. Available at www.Crediblemeds.org. Accessed February 1, 2016.

Zareba W, Moss AJ, Schwartz PJ, et al.: Influence of the genotype on the clinical course of the long-QT syndrome, *N Engl J Med* 339(14):960–965, 1998.

Zipes DP, Camm AJ, Borggrefe M, et al.: Guidelines for management of patients with ventricular arrhythmias and the prevention of sudden cardiac death. Executive summary, *Rev Esp Cardiol* 59(12):1328, 2006.

代谢性酸中毒和碱中毒 第156章

Patrick J. Neligan

病例概要

患者，男性，56岁，出租车司机，因腹痛和顽固性呕吐2天去急诊室（emergency department，ED）就诊，诊断为急性小肠梗阻。到达急诊室时，其血气和生化检查显示pH 7.38，$PaCO_2$ 28 mmHg，PaO_2 100 mmHg，Na^+ 145 mEq/L，K^+ 3.8 mEq/L，Cl^- 90 mEq/L，HCO^-_3 21 mEq/L，碱剩余（BD）−3 mmol/L，乳酸12 mEq/L，白蛋白4.2 g/dl，肌酐1.5 mg/dl，酮体+++。

患者入手术室前，在急诊室输注3 L等渗盐水溶液[生理盐水（normal saline，NS），0.9%NaCl]，并进行胃肠减压，引流出1000 ml胃液。在手术过程中，从患者肠中吸出3 L液体，补充3 L生理盐水和3 L乳酸林格液（lactated Ringer's，LR）。

患者术后被送去重症加强医疗病房，进行全套实验室检查（FiO_2 0.4），结果显示pH 7.38，$PaCO_2$ 40 mmHg，PO_2 100 mmHg，HCO^-_3 14 mEq/L，BD −10 mmol/L，Na^+ 145 mEq/L，K^+ 4.9 mEq/L，Cl^- 117 mEq/L，乳酸1.2 mEq/L，白蛋白18 g/dl，肌酐2.5 mg/dl，尿素25 mg/dl，葡萄糖145 mg/dl，酮体呈阴性，少尿。

问题分析

动脉血气分析是麻醉科医师的有用工具，可提供人体重要系统的功能和储备情况及其对治疗的动态反应。例如，氧分压（pressure of oxygen，PaO_2）可用来计算肺泡气体方程和调整吸入人体中的氧浓度分数（FiO_2）和呼气末正压。二氧化碳分压（pressure of carbon dioxide，$PaCO_2$）可用于调整肺泡通气，并寻找动脉血和呼气末CO_2的关系，以此反映死腔比例。对患有慢性阻塞性肺病的患者，对血气的预先了解可明确是否存在慢性低氧血症和高碳酸血症。后者可以通过查看$PaCO^-_2[HCO^-_3]$关系（框156.1）来实现。

在临床医学中，酸碱平衡作为一种可靠、可重复的急性疾病生物标志物已有100余年历史。急性代谢性酸中毒的存在，表明患者存在体液和电解质异常、系统性应激和器官功能障碍的症状、严重性和持续时间。对需要急诊手术的患者，酸碱状态可提醒麻醉科医师患者是否存在器官衰竭，是否需要复苏以及生理储备状态等。麻醉科医师必须充分了解患者体内酸碱生理状况，掌握数据解读的方法，从而制订术前优化患者的决策方案。

框156.1 $[HCO^-_3]$和$PaCO_2$与各种酸碱紊乱相关变化的公式：六条规则

$PaCO_2$值以mmHg，$[HCO^-_3]$以mEq/L或mmol/L计。

1. 急性呼吸性酸中毒：预期$[HCO^-_3]=24+(PaCO_2-40)/10$
2. 慢性呼吸性酸中毒：预期$[HCO^-_3]=24+4\times(PaCO_2-40)/10$
3. 急性呼吸性碱中毒：预期$[HCO^-_3]=24-2\times(40-PaCO_2)/10$
4. 慢性呼吸性碱中毒：预期$[HCO^-_3]=2-5\times(40-PaCO_2)/10$
5. 代谢性酸中毒：预期$PaCO_2=1.5[HCO^-_3]+8$
6. 代谢性碱中毒：预期$PaCO_2=0.9[HCO^-_3]+9$

酸碱化学主要指动脉或静脉氢离子浓度，简

单表示为 pH。pH 改变表明存在潜在的急性或慢性异常生理和疾病。如果动脉 pH 小于 7.35，则存在酸中毒状态。如果 pH 大于 7.45，则为碱中毒状态。动脉 pH 变化由 $PaCO_2$ 变化、呼吸异常或细胞外液完全或部分解离的离子化合物的相对浓度变化造成。其中，不能在体内自由结合成盐的离子最为重要，被称为“强离子”。强离子在全身传递电化学电荷，其相对浓度显著影响酸碱平衡。强离子分为阳离子—钠（Na^+）、钾（K^+）、镁（Mg^{2+}）和钙（Ca^{2+}）和阴离子—主要是氯（Cl^-）。它们总是存在于细胞外液，但也可能被代谢过程中产生的各种通常无法测量的阴离子所补充，使强阴离子与强阳离子的相对比例失衡，即所谓的**强离子差异**（strong ion difference，SID）。这些代谢产物的阴离子包括乳酸、酮体和由肾排泄的各种代谢副产物，通常称为“肾酸”。就功能而言，细胞外液中新的阴离子出现与相应的相关氢离子有关（必须保持电中性），这会导致 SID 变窄（通常为 44 mEq/L），并与代谢性酸中毒有关（框 156.2）。三个部分解离的“弱”酸也可能影响酸碱化学—血清磷酸盐水平（$PO^{2-}{}_4$）、血清白蛋白和细胞外碳酸氢盐（HCO^-_3）。后者主要反映体内二氧化碳总储量并提供大部分细胞外缓冲代谢酸。体内二氧化碳在功能上是碳酸：$PaCO_2$ 升高导致酸中毒，CO_2 将氢离子输送到细胞外液（呼吸性酸中毒），$PaCO_2$ 降低导致碱中毒。

从这个范例中的三个观察，可以构建对酸碱化学的理解：所有的酸碱异常都可能由于① $PaCO_2$ 的变化，可能发生酸碱异常；② SID；③弱酸的总浓度，主要是白蛋白和磷酸盐。

通过观察动脉血气三个相互关联的数据，来检测是否存在酸中毒或碱中毒：pH、$PaCO_2$ 和 HCO_3^-。一般而言，pH 范围是 7.35 ～ 7.45。若 pH 小于 7.35，则存在酸中毒；若 pH 大于 7.45，则为碱中毒。然而，如果酸中毒或碱中毒在生理上得到纠正（代偿）或多个过程同时引起酸中毒和碱中毒，则 pH 可以在正常范围内。因此，临床医师必须查看与二氧化碳相关的变量，$PaCO_2$ 大于 40 mmHg 是异常的，如果 $PaCO_2$ 高且 HCO_3^- 也升高，则患者存在呼吸性酸中毒。如果 $PaCO_2$ 低于 40 mmHg 且 HCO_3^- 也低，则患者过度通气。如果 pH 大于 7.5，则是原发性呼吸性碱中毒，通常由疼痛或焦虑（以及某些中毒，如水杨酸盐）所致。如果 pH 小于 7.35，则表示对急性代谢性酸中毒的补偿。如果 pH 大于 7.5 且 $PaCO_2$ 和（或）HCO_3^- 升高，则患者出现急性代谢性碱中毒

框 156.1 代谢性酸中毒的原因

降低强离子差异（SID）

稀释性酸中毒（↓ Na^+：Cl^-）

1. 输注低渗液体
2. 渗透间隙增加
   a. 乙醇
   b. 乙二醇中毒
3. 钠损失增加
   a. 腹泻
4. 水超载（急性）
   a. 充血性心力衰竭
   b. 肝硬化
   c. 急性肾损伤

高氯血症（↑ Cl^-：Na^+）

1. 输注增加
   a. 0.9%NaCl
2. 排泄减少
   a. 肾小管酸中毒
   b. 输尿管植入术

未测定的阴离子

1. 乳酸酸中毒
   a. A 型无氧糖酵解
   b. B 型有氧糖酵解
2. 酮症酸中毒
   a. 糖尿病酮症酸中毒
   b. 饥饿 / 酒精性酮症酸中毒
3. “肾酸中毒”
   a. 高氯血症
   b. 高磷血症
   c. “肾酸”
   d. 低钠血症

弱酸增加

高蛋白血症

1. 白蛋白给药
2. 霍乱

高磷血症

1. 清除率降低—急性肾损伤
2. 产生增加：
   a. 再喂养综合征
   b. 肿瘤溶解综合征
   c. 横纹肌溶解症
   d. 肠缺血
   e. 恶性精神抑制药综合征
3. 摄入量增加
   a. 静脉注入
   b. 磷酸盐灌肠

（框 156.3）。

在血气中发现的最终变量称为碱缺失（base deficit，BD）（负数）或碱剩余（base excess，BE）（正数）——BD/BE。BD/BE 通过计算来标准化 pH、呼吸成分和温度，以构建代谢性酸中毒或碱中毒程度的数值。例如，若 BD 为 -5 mmol/L，意味着细胞外液中存在 5 mEq/L 阴离子过剩，需要 5 mmol/L 阳离子（如 Na^+）才能将 pH 恢复到 7.4。如果 BE 为 +5 mmol/L，这意味着阳离子剩余量为 5 mEq/L，细胞外液中需要 5 mmol/L 阴离子（如作为 Cl^-）将 pH 恢复至 7.4。当然，在同时进行多次酸化和碱化过程时，BD/BE 没有差异，而主要表现为整体酸碱异常。

阴离子间隙（anion gap，AG）于 20 世纪 70 年代引入，作为区分高氯血症引起的代谢性酸中毒与未测量阴离子引起的代谢性酸中毒的方法。它是基于电中性的概念，在代谢性碱中毒的研究中没有作用。AG 的计算公式如下：

$$AG（简单）=[Na^+]-（[Cl^-]+[HCO_3^-]）=12 \sim 14\ mEq/L$$

临床实践中钾离子测量比较普遍，因此应将其添加到 AG 计算中：

$$AG（常规）=[Na^+]+[K^+]-（[Cl^-]+[HCO_3^-]）=14 \sim 18\ mEq/L$$

“间隙”是指白蛋白和磷酸盐携带的电荷，通常约 8 ～ 18 mEq/L。无论酸中毒原因如何，随着 $[HCO_3^-]$ 下降，$[Cl^-]$ 的增加都与 $[HCO_3^-]$ 的下降相关：间隙保持不变（“无间隙”酸中毒）。如果系统中存在未测定的阴离子，则 AG 似乎变宽（“阴离子间隙增加”的酸中毒）。由于大多数医院现在直接测量乳酸，因此将乳酸盐测量值添加到 AG 是合适的：

$$AG（现代）=[Na^+]+[K^+]-（[Cl^-]+[HCO_3^-]+[lac^-]）=14 \sim 18\ mEq/L$$

尽管 AG 非常受欢迎，但当应用于重症患者或液体复苏时，AG 有缺陷且经常误导计算。通常这些患者血清白蛋白较低，掩盖了未测定阴离子的存在。因此应该校正白蛋白和乳酸来计算 AG：

$$AG(校正)=[(Na^++K^+)-(Cl^-+HCO_3^-+lac^-)]-[2.5\times（40-白蛋白，单位为\ g/L）]$$

如上所述，BD/BE 是存在酸碱显著异常时的有用筛选工具，但它缺乏特定原因和识别多种原因的能力。幸运的是，有许多“数据背后”的信息可以看出酸中毒或碱中毒的原因，并检测出未测量阴离子的存在。计算被称为碱缺失间隙（base deficit gap，BDG），BDG 的计算参见框 156.4。

计算酸碱明显异常更复杂但更准确的方法是使用强离子间隙（strong ion gap，SIG），实际上是 AG 的“豪华”版本。**明显的**强离子差异（strong ion difference *apparent*，SIDa）反映了所有强阳离子之间的电荷差异减去强阴离子：$[(Na^++Mg^{2+}+Ca^{2+}=K^+)-(Cl^-+A^-)]$。SIDa 始终为正，其强度为 40 ～ 44 mEq/L。这种电荷由等量的阴离子平衡——白蛋白、磷酸盐和碳酸氢盐携带的电荷反映——**有效的**强离子差异（strong ion difference effective，SIDe）。SIDa 和 SIDe（SIG）之间存在微小的差异，它可以量化存在的未测量阴离子的量。

框 156.3 代谢性碱中毒的原因

增加强离子差异（SID）

浓缩性碱中毒（↑ Na^+：Cl^-）

1. 输注高渗液体
2. 因出汗、肠梗阻等引起的水分流失
3. 袢利尿剂

高钠性碱中毒

用弱酸缓冲液给予 Na^+：

1. 碳酸氢钠
2. 柠檬酸钠
3. 醋酸钠

次氯酸血症（↓ Cl^-：Na^+）

1. 呕吐
2. 幽门梗阻

弱酸增加

低蛋白血症

1. 晶体液复苏
2. 营养不良
3. 脓毒症

低磷血症

1. 营养不良
2. 利尿
3. 过度清除（透析）

框 156.4 自由水和白蛋白的碱缺乏 / 剩余计算

$BDE_{NaCl}=（[Na^+]-[Cl^-]）-38$

$BDE_{Alb}=0.25（42-白蛋白\ g/L）$

$BDE_{NaCl}-BDE_{Alb}=BDE_{calc}$

$BDE-BDE_{calc}$=BDE 间隙 = 未测量的阴离子或阳离子的影响

$$SIDa=([Na^+]+[K^+]+[Mg^{2+}]+[Ca^{2+}])-[Cl^-]$$

$$SIDe=[HCO_3^-]+[白蛋白上的电荷]+[磷酸盐上的电荷]（以 mmol/L 计）$$

弱酸的离子化程度取决于 pH，因此必须这样做。为此计算：

$$[alb^-]=[alb\ g/L]\times(0.123\times pH-0.631)$$

$$[Pi](mg/dL)=[Pi]/10\times pH-0.47$$

$$SIG=SIDa-SIDe$$

临床情景

该患者既有手术问题（肠梗阻）又有内科问题（脱水和明显的电解质紊乱）。表面上，pH 为 7.38（正常范围）。然而，使用前面描述的各种方法将发现许多酸碱异常问题。最简单和最高效的技术是使用框 156.4 中描述的 BDG 方法。术前患者的碱缺失为 −10，代偿性代谢性酸中毒（$PaCO_2$ 为 28 mmHg，pH“正常”范围），存在高钠血症、低氯血症以及乳酸增加。钠、氯和游离水的 BD/BE 为 +17，这意味着该患者患有严重的代谢性碱中毒（低氯血症）和游离水流失（浓缩性碱中毒）——NaCl 的 SID 为 55 mEq/L（表 156.1）。白蛋白水平正常——无低蛋白性碱中毒。计算出的碱缺乏为 −3，但碱剩余为 +17：碱剩余间隙为 20。乳酸是 12，这意味着细胞外液中有 8 mEq/L 的未测量阴离子——可能是酮体和肾酸的组合。因此，该患者术前有乳酸酸中毒、饥饿酮症酸中毒、肾性酸中毒（可能）、浓缩性碱中毒和低氯性碱中毒。其主要问题是体液不足和低氯血症，术中使用了大量 0.9% 氯化钠治疗。

这导致了一个不同但同样复杂的术后问题。使用相同的方法，人们注意到酮症酸中毒和乳酸酸中毒已基本解决（表 156.2）。然而，由于所使用静脉输注的液体的特点，患者已经出现明显的高氯血症性酸中毒。使用 BD/BE 间隙方法显示存在危险的继发性酸中毒，由白蛋白稀释的碱化作用引起。存在 15.2 mEq/L 的未测量阴离子；在无酮体的情况下，这可能是肾性酸中毒。在术后少尿和严重肾性酸中毒的情况下，患者可能需要肾脏替代疗法。

管理

乳酸酸中毒

为制定复杂酸碱异常患者的管理方案，了解潜

表 156.1 使用碱缺失-剩余间隙术前评估患者酸碱状态

酸化过程	幅度	BDC	碱化过程	幅度	BEC
乳酸	12mEq/L	−12	高钠血症	145 mEq/L	+5
酮体	++++	?	低氯血症	90 mEq/L	+12
肾损伤	肌酐	?	低蛋白血症	4.2g/L	0
总体		−12+ 未测定的未知阴离子	总体		+17

BDC，校正的碱缺失；BEC，校正的碱剩余

BDC-BEC= 测定的 BDE=（−12+17）=+5.

计算的 BD/BE- 测定的 BDE=BD/BE 间隙 =−3+5=−8 mmol/L=BDE 间隙 − 未测定阴离子（酮体和肾酸）所致 BDE 间隙 .

表 156.2 使用碱缺失-剩余间隙术后评估患者酸碱状态

酸化过程	幅度	BDC	碱化过程	幅度	BEC
乳酸	1.2	−12	高钠血症	145mEq/L	+5
高氯血症	117	−15	低蛋白血症	1.8	+6
肾损伤	肌酐 2.5 mg/dl	?			
总体		−16.2+ 未测定的未知阴离子	总体		+11

BDC，校正的碱缺失；BEC，校正的碱剩余

BDC-BEC= 测定的 BDE=（−16.2+11）=−5.2.

计算的 BD/BE- 测定的 BDE=BD/BE 间隙 =−10+（−5.2）=−15.2 mmol/L=BDE 间隙 − 未测定阴离子（肾酸）

在的疾病过程非常重要。

乳酸是糖酵解代谢的生理产物，由丙酮酸在乳酸脱氢酶的作用下持续产生。在厌氧条件下，如剧烈运动，[LA^-] 可能会大幅提升。LA^- 也在有氧条件下产生。应激（循环儿茶酚胺增加）或儿茶酚胺输注时，β- 肾上腺素能受体激活增加 [LA^-]。LA^- 在肝中被代谢为二氧化碳和水，或通过 Cori 循环再生为葡萄糖。这通常称为乳酸清除过程。乳酸酸中毒发生在 LA^- 产生大于肝对其清除能力时，因此 [LA^-] 可能反映过度生成或清除不足。2 mmol/L[LA^-] 具有临床意义，5 mmol/L 或以上被认为是严重的乳酸酸中毒。该例患者乳酸酸中毒可能源于两种不同机制。首先是血容量缺失，末梢循环差，并且由于肝血流灌注不足而降低了乳酸的肝清除率。第二种是由肾上腺素能受体激活引起的“有氧糖酵解”增加——血清乳酸水平反映了循环中的肾上腺素水平。该乳酸酸中毒的初始治疗是液体补充至正常循环量（很难评估术前晶体液的缺乏），本例是几升液体。在手术室中，现代化的循环容量动态监测（如脉压或每搏量变异度监测装置、脉冲轮廓分析）有助于恢复血容量。乳酸是复苏不佳的指标—肝分解相对缓慢，高乳酸血症可能需数天才能消失。通常，预期血清乳酸浓度每小时降低 10%。乳酸增高是一种预后不良的信号。

酮症酸中毒

酮体在肝细胞的线粒体中产生，是脂肪代谢的最终产物。脂肪酸被 β 氧化成乙酰辅酶 A。乙酰辅酶 A 通常进入柠檬酸（Krebs）循环并代谢为二氧化碳和水。但是，这个过程需要胰岛素，而胰岛素由葡萄糖刺激产生。在没有胰岛素时，产生酮体——乙酰乙酸酮、β- 羟基丁酸酮和丙酮。酮症常见于饥饿、食物供应有限（营养不良）、肠道疾病或酗酒。当产生的酮体量超过肝清除率时，酮症酸中毒就会发生，通常是当血清酮体水平超过 2 mmol/L 时。尽管大多数临床医师熟悉糖尿病酮症酸中毒，但由于胰岛素绝对缺乏，酮症酸中毒可能发生在危重的外科患者（如本例），缘于饮食中缺乏碳水化合物，肝低灌注减少酮体清除率，以及潜在的肝脂肪变性（如肥胖和酗酒）。治疗该患者酮症酸中毒的方法是液体复苏，包括抑制酮类产生的葡萄糖和促进酮类代谢的胰岛素疗法。

肾酸中毒

急性肾损伤的特征在于肾单位不能排泄代谢副产物，主要是蛋白质代谢物和过量的电解质。通常，患者发生尿毒症、高钾血症、高氯血症、高磷血症和水超负荷，导致低钠血症。因此与代谢性酸中毒有关的肾损伤由多因素所致，与测量和未测量的阴离子和血液稀释相关。当肾小球滤过率 <25 mL/（min · 1.73m^2），通常会出现酸中毒。虽然血清肌酐广泛用于急性肾损伤的诊断，但在大容量液体复苏背景下，血清肌酐可能会被稀释，导致测量值偏低。因此，少尿且存在代谢性酸中毒应警示临床医师尿毒症、体液超负荷和腹腔间隔室综合征的可能性。在这种情况下，特别是术后，可以采用保守的治疗方法，包括限制液体和利尿剂治疗。然而，如果患者出现显著的高钾血症、循环不稳定、明显的液体超负荷（如明显的肺水肿或气体交换障碍）或无尿，则有指征进行肾脏替代治疗。碳酸氢钠治疗有助于稳定心血管状态，可用作血液透析滤过的桥接治疗

低氯性碱中毒 / 高氯性酸中毒

细胞外液中钠与氯的相对比例约为 1.4 : 1。该比例的增加通常伴随着游离水的缺乏，增加 SID，导致代谢性碱中毒（在本例中为“浓缩性”碱中毒）。在本病例简介中，血清钠在正常范围，但血清氯已被耗尽，这可能是患者有继发于胃液丢失、呕吐后低氯血症性碱中毒。治疗方法是给予富含氯离子的液体直至血清氯浓度在正常范围。等渗盐水（“正常”0.9%）含有 154 mmol/L 钠和 154 mmol/L 氯化物，SID 为 0。因此，每升生理盐水有效地将 50 mmol/L 的 HCl 输送到细胞外液，并迅速逆转低氯碱中毒。然而，当过量使用 0.9% 氯化钠时，会导致高钠血症和进行性高氯血症性酸中毒，如本病例所述。高氯血症是不良征兆，高氯血症性酸中毒与肾损伤有关。在围术期和重症监护中，患有高氯性酸中毒的患者预后更差，包括死亡率升高。

预防

这位患者可以处理得更好吗？在这例患者中，小肠梗阻导致明显的液体和电解质缺乏，发生了低

氯性碱中毒。鼻胃管引流对降低吸入性肺炎的风险至关重要。采用等渗盐溶液进行初始液体复苏可以迅速纠正低氯血症。然而，肠梗阻时大多数电解质和游离水严重不足。乳酸林格液（Lactated Ringer's solution，LR）虽然略微低渗（取代游离水），但可补充钠、钾和钙并补充细胞外缓冲液（乳酸转化为碳酸氢盐）。LR 的 Na：Cl SID 为 20，该液体可用于纠正低氯性碱中毒，但患者不太可能出现明显的高氯性酸中毒。持续使用 0.9%NaCl 肯定会导致高氯性酸中毒，并且可能诱发急性肾损伤的发展。

也有观点强烈建议，应推迟手术直至患者代谢状态得到解决。液体复苏和镇痛可改善患者整体血流动力学，降低肾上腺素能活性，限制乳酸生成，加快乳酸代谢。除补液和补充电解质外，静脉输注葡萄糖和胰岛素可在术前迅速消除酮症酸中毒。

术中采用目标导向的液体复苏方法，动态监测容量变化，例如经食管多普勒、每搏量变异度、脉压变异度、液体冲击治疗后的脉冲轮廓分析、直腿抬高或呼气末阻塞试验等，可以精细滴定术中液体治疗，有助于预防术后腹腔间隔室综合征和急性肾损伤。

（朱 洁 译 汪 惠 校）

延伸阅读

Davies SJ, Minhas S, Wilson RJ, et al.: Comparison of stroke volume and fluid responsiveness measurements in commonly used technologies for goal-directed therapy, *J Clin Anesth* 25(6):466–474, 2013.

Fencl V, Jabor A, Kazda A, et al.: Diagnosis of metabolic acid-base disturbances in critically ill patients, *Am J Respir Crit Care Med* 162(6):2246–2251, 2000.

Kellum JA: Reunification of acid-base physiology, *Crit Care* 9(5):500–507, 2005.

Malbrain ML, De Laet IE: Intra-abdominal hypertension: evolving concepts, *Crit Care Nurs Clin North Am* 24:275–309, 2012.

Malbrain ML, Marik PE, Witters I, et al.: Fluid overload, de-resuscitation, and outcomes in critically ill or injured patients: a systematic review with suggestions for clinical practice, *Anaesthesiol Intensive Ther* 46(5):361–380, 2014.

McCluskey SA, Karkouti K, Wijeysundera D, et al.: Hyperchloremia after noncardiac surgery is independently associated with increased morbidity and mortality: a propensity-matched cohort study, *Anesth Analg* 117(2):412–421, 2013.

McDermid RC, Raghunathan K, Romanovsky A, et al.: Controversies in fluid therapy: type, dose and toxicity, *World J Crit Care Med* 3(1):24–33, 2014.

Moviat M, van den Boogaard M, Intven F, et al.: Stewart analysis of apparently normal acid-base state in the critically ill, *J Crit Care* 28(6):1048–1054, 2013.

Shaw AD, Bagshaw SM, Goldstein SL, et al.: Major complications, mortality, and resource utilization after open abdominal surgery: 0.9% saline compared to Plasma-Lyte, *Ann Surg* 255(5):821–829, 2012.

Story DA, Morimatsu H, Bellomo R: Strong ions, weak acids and base excess: a simplified Fencl-Stewart approach to clinical acid-base disorders, *Br J Anaesth* 92(1):54–60, 2004.

Yunos N: Association between a chloride-liberal vs chloride-restrictive intravenous fluid administration strategy and kidney injury in critically ill adults, *JAMA* 308(15):1566–1572, 2012.

Yunos NM, Bellomo R, Story D, Kellum J: Bench-to-bedside review: chloride in critical illness, *Crit Care* 14(4):226, 2010.

患者的错误识别

第 157 章

Kenneth Kuchta

病例概要

患者，男性，12 岁，于周日夜间入手术室行肝移植手术。整个手术过程行多次抽血，并在手术室床旁检测仪器上进行检测。该仪器可手动或是以扫描条形码的方式输入患者的病历号。然而，由于工作人员发现触摸屏小键盘使用不便，出现了几起实验室检查输入至错误患者的情况，几年前该手术室全面禁用了手动输入病历号的方式。由于术中需包裹患者手臂以至于无法读取手腕识别带，所以麻醉科医师需从患者手腕部取下条形码以便扫描。虽然已经多次用于实验室检查，但是这个条形码依然难以扫描，因此请巡回护士提供患者资料，其中也包含条形码。经过几组检测后发现个人资料有误，进一步调查发现这是 2 天前上一位肝移植患者手术时落在巡回护士工作台的条形码。麻醉团队追踪该患者至儿童重症监护室（pediatric intensive care unit，PICU），并将该错误通知了整个团队。这时候一名细心的护士注意到，她在近期的几个小时内并未送检过实验室检测血样，PICU 的研究小组也注意到病历中的实验室检测结果，并对血红蛋白降低和其他几个临界值进行调查。经过数次与医院技术支持进行长时间电话沟通后，错误的检查结果最终到达了正确的患者病历中。

问题分析

定义

在患者接触医疗保健系统的整个过程中都必须确认其身份，以匹配对应的干预措施和检查结果。尽管患者进入手术室的主要原因是手术，但其与当地医疗保健系统的交互要复杂得多。

因此，患者在围术期的错误识别可导致以下结果：

- 患者接受了非预期的内科或外科干预；
- 患者接受了不匹配或错误的血液制品；
- 患者接受了错误的药物或未使用预期的药物；
- 患者被检测出错误的实验室检查或检验结果；
- 在错误的肢体上实施了计划性手术或未获患者知情同意而实施了手术。

如病例概要所示，这些错误会影响到后一个患者，而他往往是医生当时未曾注意的患者。任何与医疗保健系统的交互都有可能影响我们患者的治疗，即使是远离手术室的患者亦可能会影响我们的患者的治疗（如院外某医疗单位提供的其他患者的病史和体检信息被错误地输入我们患者的电子病历）。

识别

在麻醉下接受手术的患者通常被认为是最脆弱的，并且非常依赖于那些临时照看他们的人。镇静和全身麻醉使他们无法注意和拒绝这些错误识别的事件。在这些错误识别产生影响前及时发现的任务通常落在医务人员身上（在发生重大影响前及时发现这些未遂错误）。尽管如此，患者和患者家属仍起着重要作用，让患者参与到他们自身医疗保健系统中来，不仅要参与确定患者的身份，而且要对正在进行的手术、实验室检查以及治疗进行核对。其中大部分工作通常在手术前完成，由医疗团队的各成员多次询问患者身份、病史和过敏史等信息。开放式问题能更好地让患者积极参与其中（如“你做什么手术”与“你做腔内动脉瘤修复手术，对吗？”）。最后，当所有的障碍都消除后，患者、家庭成员或医务人员就可能在尚未产生影响前发现未被发现的错误识别。

风险评估

患者的错误识别是一组异质性事件；因此，报告的发生率因定义不同导致差异很大。灾难性部位错误的手术非常罕见，发生率介于 1/100 000～1/25 000 之间。一般来说，患者错误识别的可能性要大得多。一家儿童医院发现腕部识别带的错误率达 20.4%，错误定义相当广泛：腕带丢失、放置不当、难以辨认和数据不准确。然而，不当和难以辨认的含义和临床意义却没有进一步阐明。尽管事件报告不够全面，但美国退伍军人事务部对患者安全和事件报告的强调促成了 2000 年 1 月至 2003 年 1 月间 100 余项根本原因分析，其中也包括了患者的错误识别。英国 2006 年 2 月至 2007 年 1 月期间就有 24 382 例患者接受了错误的治疗，其中 2900 例（>10%）与腕带及其使用有关。而在 2003 年 11 月至 2005 年 7 月，同一机构只有 236 份关于腕带丢失或腕带信息错误的报告，这可能表明报告数量在增加或该问题的定义存在差异。尽管手术部位错误可能会被当作错误识别出来，但与患者身份识别相关的几近发生的错误事件往往被医务人员纠正或补救，并仅被当作现代医疗行为中另一个烦心事件而已。

启示

很多患者的错误识别的情况即使被发现，也只是造成轻微的烦恼和尴尬（例如，一个医疗工作者在拥挤的术前区域走错了床，但当患者注意到其被称呼为错误姓名时才会发现错误）。即使是这样的事件，也可能会导致患者对医疗保健行为的安全性产生长久的不信任感（尽管患者会因为礼貌而克制这种情绪）。而另一个极端影响就是当错误识别出现不良结局时，后果可能会非常严重。识别错误对患者和家庭的潜在影响是显而易见的，进一步仔细检查能预料到会产生进一步后果。我们只需关注大众媒体就可以看到其影响，如巨额医疗事故赔付、执照或认证丢失，以及个人或机构名誉受损等。不管医疗保健系统多复杂，显然公众希望所有的手术、药品和血液制品输注都能被准确地实施。

管理

尽管重点在于减少识别错误以防止不良后果的发生，但也应制订管理计划。这种错误，特别是导致了严重后果的错误，会对患者、家属和医疗工作者造成毁灭性的影响。有必要进行适当的支持和指导，尤其是对造成严重影响的事件。

一般情况下，如果出现患者识别错误，应做好以下工作：

- 直面此事件（原因不确定时不揣测）；
- 及时通知各方和相应的风险管理 / 质量改进委员会；
- 在病历中清晰记录患者发生的情况（以避免妄加揣测原因）；
- 继续随访患者，并记录就诊事件；
- 立即进行调查，防止再次发生。

当发生识别错误时，我们在道德和伦理上有义务对患者坦诚，尤其是这些错误可能与重大不良后果有关时。这一方案已被编入医疗政策中［自 2001 起，医疗保健认证联合委员会（Joint Commission on Accreditation of Health Care Organizations，JCAHO）已要求将意外结果告知患者］，而且被告知患者的接受程度往往比我们预期的更好。事实上，对患者坦白可减少诉讼的可能性。对患者的健康表现出同情心和持续的关注肯定比完全逃避这种情况更好。如果案件被提出诉讼，事后访视记录不仅仅是一种医疗行为，而且也表明了医生的持续关注。毫无疑问，犯识别错误的从业者在一段时间内会牢记此事。

本案例所涉及的所有人员都应当立即被告知识别错误的发生。这包括医院风险管理和质量保证委员会以及任何可能被涉及的保险公司。患者病历中必须清楚记录所发生的事情。对于识别错误应立即进行调查，以确认错误是如何发生的，以及必须立即采取预防措施以避免此类错误再次发生。有趣的是，随着对“公平文化”的重视，此类调查对犯错者的关注越来越少，而更多地关注导致错误发生的原因。

预防

考虑到现代医疗服务的复杂性，患者错误识别的可能性一直存在。传统来说，当此类错误发生时，通常的解决办法是忠告与发生事件最相关的医务人员在未来需更小心，并教育他人提高警惕。这种方法往往忽略了该事件中包含潜在错误的系统缺陷，这种缺陷可使主动错误的发生成为可能。最近，卫生保健机构对导致这一事件的整个过程进行了较为结构化的审查，通常手段是根本原因分析。审查的目的是发现系统中可导致未来其他从业人员发生失误事件的潜在错误和缺陷。然后该机构会制定相应的政策并改变程序来减少再发生的可能。

回顾事件时，随着对系统问题的强调不断变化，JCAHO 继续强调了患者识别错误。2016 年美国患者安全目标要求在手术、治疗、用药或输血制品，或者标本采样时（包括血液样本），至少使用两个患者识别号（既不是房间号也不是患者位置）。血液和标本的容器不能预先标记。输血时须经两个人验证（或一个人加自动鉴定标记，如条形码）。联合委员会关于“预防手术部位错误、手术错误和手术患者错误的通用流程”将继续出现在新的安全目标中。该协议包含三大类要素。第一类要素为术前核查以确认患者正确、手术正确、部位正确，以及其他必要的信息和设备已准备到位。这可以在术前多个时间或场合实施，强调采用标准化的方法，并且在可能的情况下让患者一起加入进来。第二类要素为部位标记，要求机构确定何时需要进行部位标记（定义为在另一部位实施手术可能会对质量或安全产生不利影响）。当然，如果可能的话术前手术部位标记也需患者参与。理想情况下，标记要求有执照的从业人员完成，且该从业人员手术时应在场且最终对该手术负责，但也列出了允许委托他人完成的例外情况。标记必须清楚并与制度规定的相一致。例外情况需要提供文字材料（患者拒绝、不可能或不切实际的部位）。最后一个要素是术前核查（time-out），要求手术团队所有成员在手术前即刻进行标准化主动交流。JCAHO 的最基本要素是确认患者正确、部位正确和手术正确，在核查结束后必须记录在案。如果另一个外科医师在同一个患者中实施第二次手术，也需进行第二次核查。

2016 年 JCAHO 患者安全目标中，包括具体实施要素在内的许多细节都留给了医疗保健机构自行制订。这些目标的成功可能依赖于实施的具体细节。例如，美国退伍军人管理局作为一家大型机构把这些推荐扩展到具体实施细则。其手术准确性政策将范围延伸至包含外科手术的所有有创操作。知情同意和术前核查的内容非常广泛，操作部位和项目的核查分为两部分过程：第一步是部位标识时，第二步为手术室外即刻，与一同进入手术室的工作人员一起进行核查。

幸运的是，人们越来越重视患者识别错误的预防，尽管对患者造成重大伤害的事件很少见。预防或杜绝此类错误的方法已广泛推广于整个医疗系统，但这些方法的有效性一直难以被证明。2015 年一篇关于减少手术部位错误干预措施的 Cochrane 综述更新只筛选了两篇相关的高质量出版物。第一篇是前文提到的牙科文献。另一项最近的研究显示一所大学附属医院神经外科的错误发生率有所下降，但可能存在混杂因素，因为在干预前不久，这一错误发生率已经下降至接近于零。最近一篇关于外科核查表有效性的文章也没有显示出对患者结局存在影响（尽管该核查表不单纯是为了患者识别错误而设立）。

尽管研究结果令人失望，但临床医师还是在寻找干预措施以解决患者识别错误的问题。2009 年一项在急诊室进行的模拟研究可能可说明这种困境。面对三名患者，当其中一名患者的识别带不正确时，只有 61% 的医务人员发现了错误。尽管提出的解决方案尚未广泛实施，但人们认为技术可以为解决这一问题提供帮助。使用射频识别标签追踪测试患者在手术室的位置被认为具有一定前景。标签中的信息与手术室电子日程表相关联，当错误的患者被带到手术室时可通过传呼机生成警报。该方案需要对系统进行更新，将射频识别标签添加至手术室人员的传呼机号码中，以便最接近患者的工作人员能够收到寻呼机警报。不幸的是，尽管这种技术支持方案被提出，但在实施方面进展缓慢。最后，我们仍需提高认识，继续保持警惕，增加事件或几近错误的报告，开展全面的质量评估，开展结局研究以最终解决患者识别错误的问题。

（郭　玉　译　王嘉锋　校）

延伸阅读

Department of Veterans Affairs: Ensuring correct surgery and invasive procedures: VHA directive 1039: Ensuring correct surgery and invasive procedures. July 26, 2013. Available at http://www.va.gov/vhapublications/ViewPublication.asp?pub_ID=2922. Accessed August 26, 2016.

Hain PD, Joers B, Rush M, et al.: An intervention to decrease patient identification band errors in a children's hospital, *Qual Saf Health Care* 19:244–247, 2010.

Henneman PL, Fisher DL, Henneman EA, et al.: Patient identification errors are common in a simulated setting, *Ann Emerg Med* 55:503–509, 2010.

The Joint Commission: 2016 National Patient Safety Goals. January 1, 2016. Hospital Accreditation Program. Available at http://www.jointcommission.org/standards_information/npsgs.aspx. Accessed August 26, 2016.

Michaels RK, Makary MA, Dahab Y, et al.: Achieving the National Quality Forum's "Never Events": prevention of wrong site, wrong procedure, and wrong patient operations, *Ann Surg* 245:526–532, 2007.

Sandberg WS, Häkkinen M, Egan M, et al.: Automatic detection and notification of "wrong patient–wrong location" errors in the operating room, *Surg Innov* 12:253–260, 2005.

World Health Organization; WHO Collaborating Centre for Patient Safety Solutions: Patient identification. Vol. 1, sol. 2, May 2007. Available at http://www.who.int/patientsafety/solutions/patientsafety/PS-Solution2.pdf. Accessed August 26, 2016.

围术期高血压

第 158 章

Jerrold H. Levy

病例概要

患者，男性，58 岁，在行开腹腹主动脉瘤修复术后立即出现高血压，血压达 160/110 mmHg，窦性心律 72 次 / 分，肺动脉压 45/25 mmHg，肺动脉闭塞压 6 mmHg，中心静脉压 5 mmHg。心前区心电图导联出现 ST 段压低。术前评估患者既往无高血压病史，但有外周血管疾病史。

问题分析

定义

围术期高血压的定义与慢性高血压病的定义不同。围术期静脉容量快速更换、手术刺激诱发的交感神经张力改变、应激反应或疼痛刺激都可能造成患者血压剧烈变化。基于这些因素，血压正常的患者在围术期也可发生高血压。此外，该患者有外周血管疾病病史，还有弥漫性动脉粥样硬化，这与血管内皮和血管功能障碍相关。由于此时患者不能口服抗高血压药物，因此采用非口服药物治疗。高血压是心脏和非心脏手术后的一个主要问题。非心脏手术患者术后高血压发生率为 6% ～ 20%，术前高血压患者的发生率更高，但是与麻醉方案无关。

识别

血压监测是围术期管理的重要组成部分，有创或无创方法均可用于高血压的诊断和治疗。心脏手术患者通常保持较低的血压以避免移植物或缝合处破裂和出血。依据国际研究结果，心脏手术后高血压的定义为血压持续高于 140/90 mmHg。当血压超过此值时，大多数麻醉科医师会对高血压进行治疗。最近美国高血压预防、检测、评估与治疗联合委会员第 8 次报告发布后系统阐述了内科患者新的血压指南。

风险评估

有研究报道患者在麻醉后恢复室发生高血压的危险因素包括年龄、吸烟和肾脏疾病。患者术前有心绞痛病史或术后通气不足均增加术后高血压风险。高血压和心动过速与远期病死率增加相关。患者高血压病史也是围术期高血压的一个危险因素。

据报道，30% ～ 80% 的冠状动脉旁路移植患者术后发生高血压。心肺转流诱发的放大的应激反应被认为是患者血管阻力增加的病理生理学基础。其他相关因素包括心脏手术后快速撤除机械通气和冠状动脉移植物痉挛。术前心脏功能正常的患者术后也常发生心室功能障碍。

启示

何时治疗围术期高血压以及如何迅速降低血压，这两个问题仍未得到很好的解决。维持血流动力学稳定的治疗目标取决于许多因素，尤其是术前血压——即患者的“正常”血压。目前可以指导围术期血压管理的数据较少，对某些患者（如神经外科和心脏外科手术患者）而言，术后血压常维持较低水平，以避免出血、缝合处破裂、脑血管意外、心肌缺血和心律失常等并发症。

治疗

围术期高血压治疗方法包括以下：

- 静脉扩张剂、二氢吡啶类钙通道阻滞剂（如氯维地平和尼卡地平）、多巴胺受体激动剂（非诺多泮）、肼屈嗪或具潜力的血管紧张素转换酶（angiotensinconverting enzyme，ACE）抑制剂（如依那普利）；

- 静脉注射 β-肾上腺素受体阻滞剂；
- 术中加深麻醉。

血管扩张剂

硝普钠和硝酸甘油释放的一氧化氮可舒张动脉和静脉，对血流动力学不稳定的患者，尤其是血容量相对不足有显著作用，如本病例概要所描述。对于血容量不足的高血压患者，常先补充静脉血容量，随后输注硝普钠*。虽然硝普钠常用于控制术后高血压，但是它可非特异性诱发冠状动脉扩张和冠状动脉窃血而导致心肌缺血。肼屈嗪是一种动脉选择性血管扩张剂，也可用于产科和围术期患者，常与 β-肾上腺素受体阻滞剂同时使用。

钙通道阻滞剂

钙通道阻滞剂有三种类型：维拉帕米、地尔硫卓和二氢吡啶类（如尼卡地平）。这些药物可以减少钙离子进入血管平滑肌而舒张血管。二氢吡啶类钙通道阻滞剂与 L- 型钙通道亲和力高，二者结合后能调节电压依赖的钙离子流动。二氢吡啶主要扩张外周阻力动脉。在降低血压的有效剂量范围内，二氢吡啶对心肌收缩力或传导很少有或没有直接的负性影响。二氢吡啶类药物缺乏负性变时效应，在用药早期可反射性增加心率，而长期使用会降低心率。与硝酸甘油类不同的是钙离子通道阻滞剂不影响静脉平滑肌，不扩张静脉，对充盈压和前负荷几乎没有影响。因此，钙通道阻滞剂在降低动脉压时可维持或增加心排出量。尼卡地平还是一种冠状动脉和脑血管的强效扩张剂，在神经外科和心脏外科患者中具有重要应用。

其他药物

虽然 ACE 抑制剂广泛用于心力衰竭治疗，但唯一可静脉注射的是依那普利，其为一种间接发挥作用的药物，偶可用于治疗围术期高血压。ACE 抑制剂是一类复杂的干扰血管紧张素Ⅱ合成的药物，可通过增加缓激肽水平而促进血管内一氧化氮释放。特异性多巴胺受体激动剂是处于临床研究阶段的一类新药。非诺多泮是外周 1 型多巴胺受体的选择性激动剂，可舒张血管，增加肾灌注，促进尿钠排出，但对血压和心率的影响可能差异较大。

β-肾上腺素能受体阻滞剂

β-肾上腺素能受体阻滞剂可降低心率和心肌收缩力，减少心排出量，从而同时降低收缩压和舒张压。因此，对于心动过速的围术期高血压患者，应考虑使用 β-肾上腺素能受体阻滞剂。心率是心肌血供的主要决定性因素之一，因此对缺血性心脏病患者必须积极治疗心动过速，应将 β-肾上腺素能受体阻滞剂用作一线用药。下列几种 β-肾上腺素能受体阻滞剂可静脉注射，在围术期可用作抗高血压药：普萘洛尔、美托洛尔、阿替洛尔、艾司洛尔和拉贝洛尔。拉贝洛尔的优点是能同时阻断 α-和 β-受体，艾司洛尔的消除半衰期短（<10 min）以及具有 β_1-受体选择性。

加深麻醉

加深麻醉是治疗术中高血压的潜在方法，但需要考虑可行性和有效性。区域麻醉也可有效预防围术期高血压。正压通气或持续气道正压对静脉回流的阻碍作用亦不可忽视，这能显著降低前负荷和全身血压。

预防

围术期高血压的发生常常是对麻醉诱导、手术、麻醉苏醒和疼痛刺激的正常反应。持续治疗慢性高血压对于围术期血流动力学稳定至关重要。通过区域麻醉技术更好地控制围术期疼痛得到越来越广泛的运用，这也可能对围术期高血压有重要的预防作用。虽然加深麻醉能有效控制血流动力学稳定，但是此技术有时并非总是可行；因此，可能需要使用本文列举的抗高血压药物治疗围术期高血压。

（王昌理 译 卞金俊 校）

* 除了其动脉扩张效应外，硝普钠主要以扩张静脉容量床为主，是一种强效静脉扩张剂。静脉舒张可减少静脉回流和心脏前负荷。慢性高血压患者通常前负荷受限——对全身血管阻力和心室壁压力（后负荷）慢性增加的适应性反应；当给予以扩张静脉为主的抗高血压药物时，患者可能会出现相对低血容量状态。从 2015 年起，硝普钠十分昂贵，每瓶价格暴涨至近 1000 美元（这是临床医生可能意识不到的一个重要因素），此外，使用硝普钠时还需要动脉置管监测血压。

延伸阅读

Aronson S, Boisvert D, Lapp W: Isolated systolic hypertension is associated with adverse outcomes from coronary artery bypass grafting surgery, *Anesth Analg* 94:1079–1084, 2002.

Fleisher LA, Fleischmann KE, Auerbach AD, et al.: 2014 ACC/AHA guideline on perioperative cardiovascular evaluation and management of patients undergoing noncardiac surgery: a report of the American College of Cardiology/American Heart Association Task Force on practice guidelines, *J Am Coll Cardiol* 64(22):e77–e137, 2014.

James PA, Oparil S, Carter BL, et al.: 2014 evidence-based guideline for the management of high blood pressure in adults. Report from the panel members appointed to the Eighth Joint National Committee (JNC 8), *JAMA* 311(5):507–520, 2014.

Levy JH, Tanaka K, Ramsay JG: Cardiac surgical pharmacology. In Cohn LH, editor: *Adult cardiac surgery*, ed 4, New York, 2012, McGraw-Hill, pp 85–118.

Tanaka KA, Tsuda A, Yamaguchi K, et al.: In vitro effects of antihypertensive drugs on thromboxane agonist (U46619)-induced vasoconstriction in human internal mammary artery, *Br J Anaesth* 93:257–262, 2004.

Vuylsteke A, Feneck RO, Jolin-Mellgard A, et al.: Perioperative blood pressure control: a prospective survey of patient management in cardiac surgery, *J Cardiothorac Vasc Anesth* 14:269–273, 2000.

第159章 围术期缺氧

Taras Grosh，Diana Ayubcha

病例概要

患者，男，42岁，178 cm（70英寸），95 kg，既往有慢性阻塞性肺疾病和高血压病史，拟行腹腔镜下阑尾切除术。予丙泊酚和琥珀胆碱行快速序贯诱导，并合理应用抗生素，建立气腹。手术开始15 min后，麻醉机氧气压力低报警，FiO_2为16%，脉搏血氧饱和度（saturation by pulse oximetry，SpO_2）显示为99%，但逐渐下降。气道峰压、潮气量和分钟通气量无明显变化。

问题分析

定义

缺氧是指组织或器官中氧含量异常降低，不能满足机体的需要。氧梯度是指从大气到线粒体的局部氧气压力逐级降低（图159.1），其任何一个环节的中断均可导致终末器官氧供不足。缺氧可分为低氧血症（低氧性缺氧）、贫血性缺氧、循环性缺氧和组织细胞性缺氧。

低氧血症/低氧性缺氧

低氧血症是氧气（oxygen，O_2）与血红蛋白结合失败或者不能溶于血浆中导致血液中的O_2含量降低。图159.2列出了低氧血症的原因。肺泡气体方程式主要用于预测肺泡中的氧分压，可用于计算A-a梯度以确定低氧血症的原因。

$$PaO_2=FiO_2\%（PB-PiH_2O）-PaCO_2/RQ$$

PaO_2和$PaCO_2$分别是肺泡内O_2和CO_2的分压；FiO_2是吸入氧浓度；PB是大气压；PiH_2O为饱和H_2O蒸汽压力；RQ是呼吸熵（0.8）。

当氧气从肺泡向血液扩散时存在一个正常的梯度。

$$A\text{-}a梯度=PAO_2-PaO_2$$

PAO_2是肺泡氧分压；PaO_2是血氧分压。A-a梯度随着年龄的增长而增加，年龄每增加10岁A-a梯度增加1 mmHg。

$$标准预计A\text{-}a梯度=年龄/4+4$$

低氧血症可分为A-a梯度正常（<15 mmHg）或A-a梯度升高（>15 mmHg）（表159.1）。

导致正常A-a梯度（<15 mmHg）低氧血症的原因如下：

1. 吸入氧浓度低，例如由于吸入过量的氧化亚氮或氮气导致的低氧混合气体（FiO_2<21%），流量计设置不正确，供氧管连接错误，中心气体供应错误或吸入气体压力低于760 mmHg。
2. 中枢性（药物使用过量导致的中枢神经系统毒性）或外周性（肥胖、脊柱后凸、肌无力）通气不足导致动脉血和肺泡中CO_2蓄积，在吸入O_2浓度恒定的情况下所导致的缺氧。

导致高A-a梯度（>15 mmHg）低氧血症的原因：

1. 肺泡通气量（Ventilation/perfusion，V/Q）失调是最常见的原因（图159.3）。血液通过灌注良好、灌注不足以及完全无灌注的肺泡，因此动脉氧含量是所有这些部分混合后的平均值。V/Q失调极端表现为**死腔通气和分流**。
   - 死腔通气（V>Q），即仅有通气而无血流灌注，常见于肺尖、COPD或肺栓塞。在肺尖，PA>Pa>Pv。膨胀的肺泡会导致毛细血管塌陷、通气浪费以及与血液进行气体交换的有效通气极少。通过补充O_2可纠正这一情况但会进一步扩大A-a梯度（图159.4）。这些区域具有高

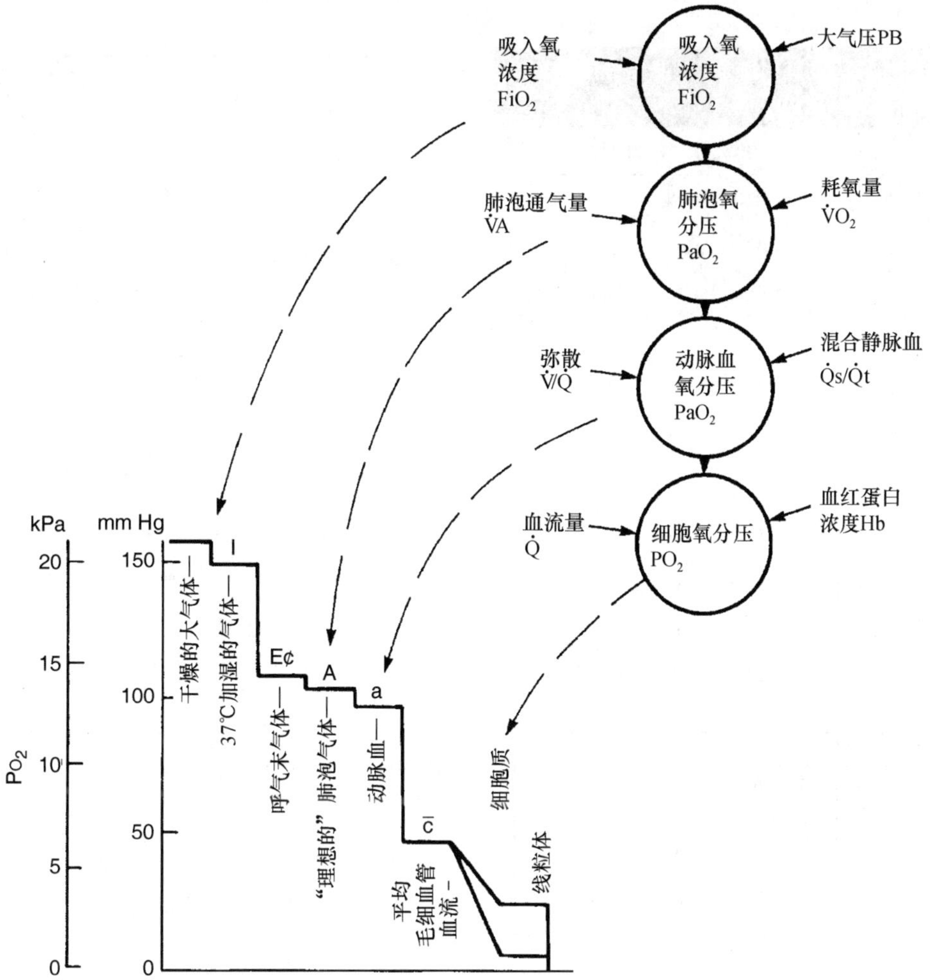

图 159.1 从一个大气压的干燥气体（160 mmHg）到线粒体（3 ~ 20 mmHg）的氧分压梯度（From Lumb AB：Nunn's applied respiratory physiology，5th ed. London，Butterworth-Heinemann，2000，p 250.）

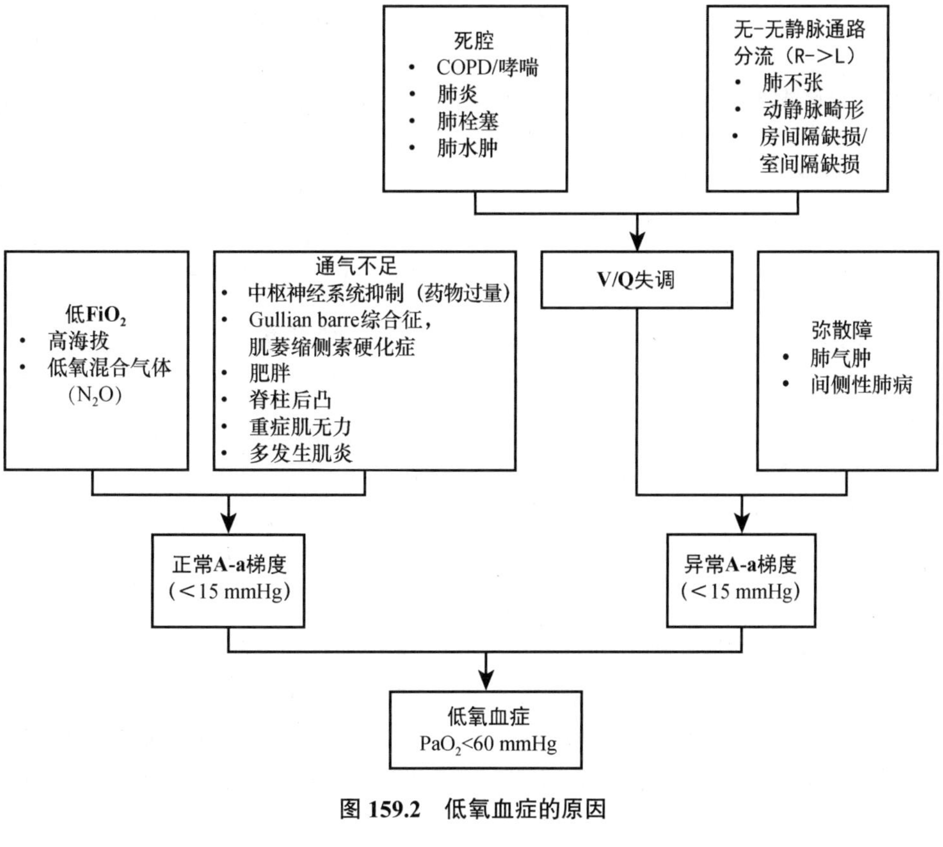

图 159.2 低氧血症的原因

表 159.1 低氧血症的原因及其对肺泡-动脉氧分压差、对 100% 氧和动脉二氧化碳分压的反应

原因	P(A-a)O_2	100%O_2	$PaCO_2$
低 FiO_2	正常	增加 PaO_2	正常
低通气	正常	增加 PaO_2	增加
V/Q 失调	增加	增加 PaO_2	正常
分流(Vs/Qt)	增加	不变	正常
弥散障碍	增加	增加 PaO_2	正常

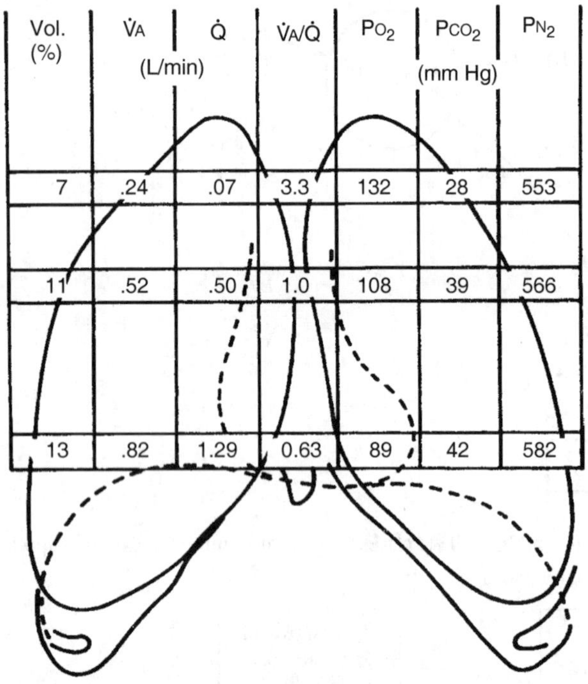

图 159.3 直立体位时三个肺区域肺泡通气血流(V/Q)比值及气体组成(From West JB: *Pulmonary pathophysiology*: the essentials. Baltimore, Williams & Wilkins, 1980.)

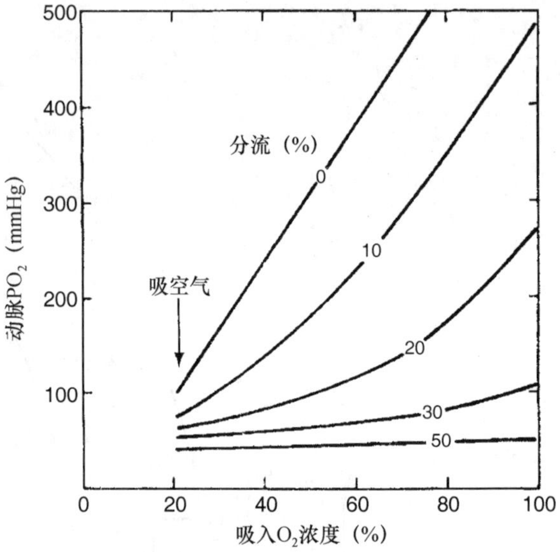

图 159.4 等分流图显示了在不同程度的单纯分流量下,改变吸入氧浓度(FiO_2)对动脉血氧合(PaO_2)的影响。等分流线适用于血红蛋白 100 ~ 140 g/L 和动脉血二氧化碳分压($PaCO_2$)为 25 ~ 40 mmHg(Modified from Nunn JF: *Applied respiratory physiology*, 4th ed. London, Butterworth-Heinemann, 1993, p 184.)

PO_2 和低 PCO_2 的特点。

- 分流 Q>V,灌注良好但通气不足,最常发生在肺底部。此区域 Pa>Pv>PA,最常见于术后肺不张,肺炎或肺水肿。静脉和肺毛细血管氧含量几乎相同(低 PO_2 和 O_2 含量)。在肺底部,混合静脉血通过肺毛细血管床时不能得到氧合,进一步加重 V/Q 比例失调。这些区域表现为低 PO_2 和高 PCO_2。提高 FiO_2 无法改善氧合。

2. 如果 Hb 分子已饱和或功能不佳,可用于气体交换的表面积减少或扩散屏障增厚,则会导致肺泡到毛细血管的 PO_2 梯度丧失,出现弥散功能障碍。常见于间质性肺病、肺气肿、纤维化或急性呼吸窘迫综合征。肺泡-毛细血管气体交换受限于特定气体穿过肺泡毛细管膜的能力(D)。O_2 的扩散能力(Diffusing capacity for O_2, Do_2)从静止状态下 21 ml/min 至运动时 65 ml/min 不等。PaO_2/FiO_2 比值是机械通气患者常用的氧合指标。其正常值为 300 ~ 500 mmHg。小于 300 mmHg 提示气体交换异常;低于 200 mmHg 表示严重的低氧血症。在机械通气的过程中,a-A 氧比值对于撤机是一个有用的参数。正常的 a/A 比(PaO_2/PAO_2)大于 0.75,大于 0.25 提示可成功脱机。有中心静脉置管的患者,混合静脉饱和度(mixed venous saturation, SVO_2)可有效排除贫血或低心排血量导致的 A-a 梯度升高。

贫血性缺氧

贫血性缺氧是由低血红蛋白或血红蛋白功能异常从而显著影响其携氧能力所致。以下几点与贫血性缺氧有关:

- 血红蛋白结构-功能关系;
- 氧-血红蛋白(O_2-Hb)解离曲线;
- 氧含量;
- 其他血红蛋白种类;
- 血红蛋白最低浓度。

血红蛋白(hemoglobin, Hb)结构。Hb 由 4 个蛋白亚基形成四聚体分子。有几种不同的亚基

（用 α 至 ε 来表示），但一个 Hb 分子只包含两种亚基。正常成人 Hb 有两个 α 和两个 β 亚基。含铁的血红素嵌入 Hb 的每一个亚基，允许它结合一个 O_2 分子（氧化作用）。Hb 亚基之间的相互作用（亚基协同性）导致随着每个 O_2 分子与 Hb 结合而产生 O_2 亲和力增加。这一特征解释了为何 O_2-Hb 氧离曲线呈 S 形。

氧离曲线。O_2-Hb 离解曲线呈 S 形，描述了血红蛋白对 O_2 的亲和力。每个 O_2 分子依次与血红蛋白中的铁分子结合后促进后续的氧分子以更大的亲和力与血红蛋白结合。P50 为 50% 的血红蛋白分子达到饱和的氧分压；正常成人 P50 为 26.6 mmHg。曲线向右移动意味着更容易将 O_2 释放到组织中，向左移动意味着更难释放 O_2。四个因素调节 Hb 对 O_2 的亲和力：氢离子（玻尔效应）、2,3- 二磷酸甘油酸、CO_2（霍尔登效应）和温度。任何一个这些因素的增加都会降低 Hb 对 O_2 的亲和力，使 O_2-Hb 的离解曲线向右移动（即增加 P50），即在给定的 PO_2 下会有更多的 O_2 释放到组织中。反之，这些因素的降低会使 O_2-Hb 解离曲线向左移动，即在任何给定的 PO_2 下向组织中释放的 O_2 均减少。

血氧含量。根据标准命名法，正常血红蛋白浓度约为 150 g/L 或 15 g/dL。1 g 血红蛋白结合 1.39 ml O_2；然而，由于通常存在少量的高铁血红蛋白和碳氧血红蛋白，这一数字通常略低（约为 1.34 ml/g）。此外，血浆中存在物理溶解的氧气 [0.03 ml/（L·mmHg）的 PO_2]，约占血液中总氧气浓度的 2%。CaO_2 代表血液种氧气完全饱和时的动脉氧含量，大约为 200 ml/L。

$$CaO_2 =（SaO_2 \times Hb \times 1.34）+0.003（PaO_2）$$

随着血红蛋白浓度的变化，氧含量也随之变化，但每克血红蛋白的氧含量不变。

其他血红蛋白种类。肌红蛋白既可以作为氧气缓冲液，也可以在肌肉中储存氧气。所有已知的脊椎动物的肌红蛋白和 β- 血红蛋白亚基的结构很相似，但在低 PO_2 时肌红蛋白结合 O_2 的能力更强，因为它是一种单体（即，它不会随着氧合发生明显的构象变化）。因此，肌红蛋白在 15 ～ 30 mmHg 的氧分压下保持完全饱和，仅在极低的氧分压下将 O_2 卸载至肌肉线粒体。注意，胎儿血红蛋白在低 PO_2 水平时功能也强于成人血红蛋白，P50 为 19 mmHg。

最低血红蛋白浓度。2015 年美国麻醉科医师协会（American Society of Anesthesiologists，ASA）和 2016 年美国血库协会在其血液成分治疗实践指南中提出了最佳血红蛋白浓度。建议采用两级标准：对于血流动力学稳定的成人，血红蛋白浓度低于 70 g/L 需要输血；对于合并心血管疾病或接受心脏或骨科手术的患者，低于 80 g/L 需要输血。对于无明显出

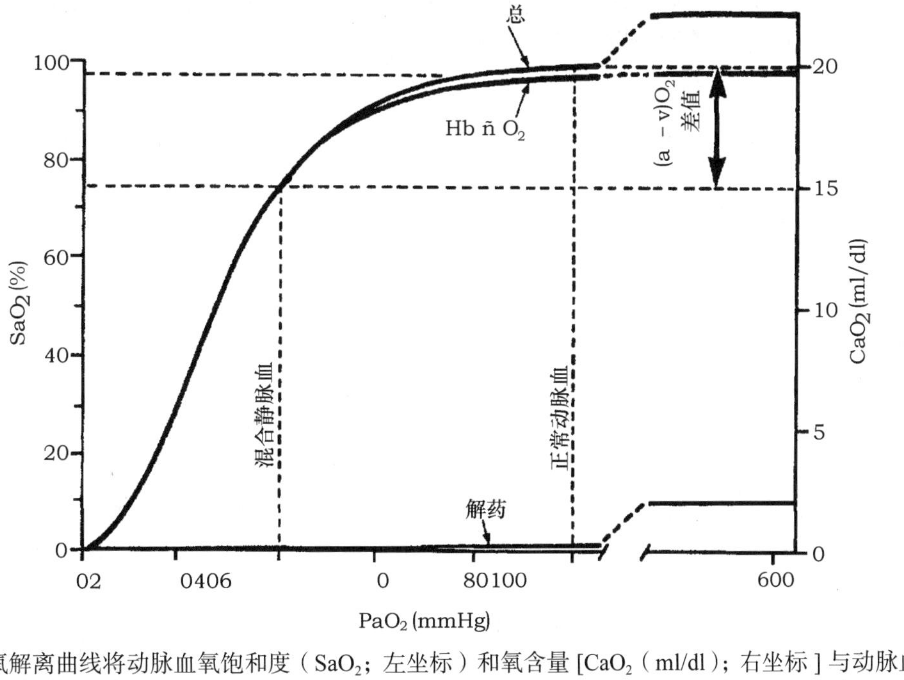

图 159.5 血红蛋白氧解离曲线将动脉血氧饱和度（SaO_2；左坐标）和氧含量 [CaO_2（ml/dl）；右坐标] 与动脉血氧分压（PaO_2；横坐标）联系起来。假定血红蛋白 =150 g/L，CaO_2=20 ml/dl，动静脉 CaO_2 差值 =5 ml/dl（From Luce JM，Pierson DJ，Tyler ML：*Intensive respiratory care*，2nd ed. Philadelphia，WB Saunders，1993，p 27.）

血的患者应从给予 1 单位红细胞开始补充，每次输血后复查血红蛋白水平，目标分别为 70 ～ 90 g/L 和 80 ～ 100 g/L。此外，强调使用药物疗法以尽量减少输血，如贫血患者给予促红细胞生成素；基于血栓弹力图检测的输血流程、血液预订计划表和限制性输血策略来制定。

循环性缺氧

循环性缺氧或淤血性缺氧是由于流经器官毛细血管床的流量不足，导致组织供氧不足；这可能是全身的，也可以局部的。全身循环性缺氧是心率或每搏量降低从而导致心排血量减少或休克时导致的严重全身循环停止的结果。局部淤血性缺氧发生于周围血流受阻的情况：Raynaud 病、Beurger 病或使用止血带。75 kg 男性的耗氧量（oxygen consumption，VO_2）约为 250 ml/min，基础氧供（O_2 delivery，DO_2）约为每分钟每升心排血量 200 ml 氧气（或心排血量为 5 L/min 时 1000 ml 氧）；这足以满足正常有氧代谢过程中的需求。FTE 氧摄取率（oxygen extraction ratio，O_2ER）为 VO_2/DO_2 的比值，其正常值休息时为 25%，最高为 75%。

$$O_2ER=VO_2/DO_2=(SaO_2-SvO_2)/SaO_2$$

图 159.6 描绘了临界 DO_2（critical DO_2，cDO_2）或最大 O_2ER，在此之后，细胞转变为无氧代谢，组织缺氧表现为乳酸产量增加。但什么是生命的临界氧供？一项针对清醒静息志愿者的研究报告认为其

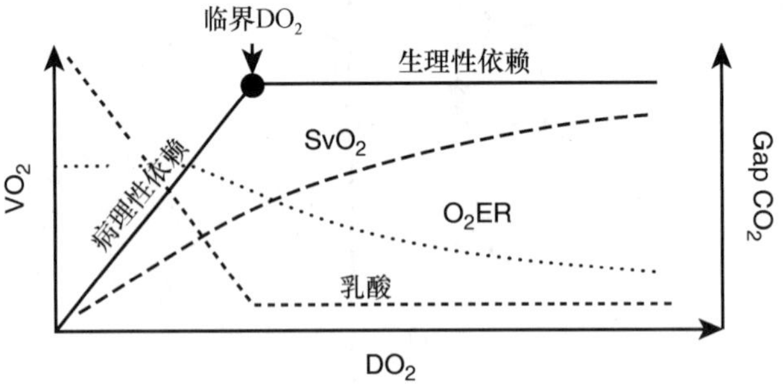

图 159.6 代谢需求（VO_2）和氧供（DO_2）的关系。当 VO_2 增加，或 DO_2 降低时，O_2ER 增加以维持有氧代谢。在临界 DO_2（cDO_2）时 O_2ER 达到最大，为 70%，在此之前 VO_2 与 DO_2 无关；在此之后，VO_2 增加或 DO_2 降低均会导致组织缺氧和无氧代谢（乳酸升高）。DO_2，氧供；VO_2，耗氧量；O_2ER，氧摄取率；SvO_2，混合静脉氧饱和度；Gap CO_2，胃黏膜二氧化碳分压差（From Assuncao MS，Corrêa TD，Bravim Bde A，Silva E：How to choose the therapeutic goals to improve tissue perfusion in septic shock. *Einstein*（*São Paulo*）13[3]：441-447，2015.）

值为每分钟 7.5 ml/kg（70 kg 成人为 525 ml/min）。一例耶和华见证会（Jehovah’s Witness）患者的病例报告发现临界 DO_2 为每平方米 184 ml/min。

组织细胞性缺氧

组织细胞性缺氧是指尽管 DO_2 正常，但在细胞水平无法利用氧从而影响 ATP 生成。氰化物（CN^-）中毒是一个典型的例子，可发生于使用大量硝普钠时。CN^- 与线粒体细胞色素氧化酶结合，破坏有氧代谢，从而导致无氧代谢。CN^- 毒性的早期症状是心动过速、O_2ER 降低但混合静脉血氧饱和度升高（SVO_2 正常值为 70%）、静脉血颜色鲜红以及乳酸酸中毒；所有这些都是由于组织无法利用氧。杀虫剂鱼藤酮和抗霉素 A 也会中断电子传递链，从而导致类似的缺氧。

一氧化碳（carbon monoxide，CO）与细胞色素 C 结合并干扰线粒体水平的氧化代谢。一旦结合 CO 将 Hb 分子转化为碳氧血红蛋白，由于 CO 结合导致 COHb 构象变化从而使与其结合的氧具有极强的亲和力，氧离曲线左移，尽管 PaO_2 和双通道脉搏血氧测定为正常值，仍可导致组织缺氧。CO 对血红蛋白的亲和力极高（是氧气的 200 倍），因此需要高浓度的氧（在 1 ～ 3 个大气压下为 100%）才能有效地治疗 CO 中毒。CO 与 O_2 置换后功能性细胞色素 C 的再生可能是防止神经元死亡的机制。高铁血红蛋白是血红蛋白的另一种异常形式，由于血红蛋白中的铁部分处于铁（Fe^{3+} 氧化）状态，而不是亚铁（2+ 还原）状态；因此，预计曲线会左移。高铁血红蛋白可遗传或见于 G6PD 缺乏症、接触丙胺卡因、苯甲卡因、硝酸盐和亚硝酸盐。另外，它也被应用氰化物中毒的治疗。

识别

发绀

在脉搏血氧仪普及之前，低氧血症是导致麻醉相关死亡的主要原因。在此之后，与麻醉相关的死亡率降低了 20 倍。麻醉患者的低氧血症（PaO_2<60 mmHg）的临床识别较困难，因为麻醉药会削弱由缺氧引起的生理状态（心动过速、高血压、呼吸急促）和精神状态（躁动、嗜睡）的改变。对于麻醉患者，术野中黏膜发绀或血液呈现暗红色往往是最早的预警。然而，只有当 15% 或 2 ～ 3 g 血

红蛋白去饱和时才会出现发绀，而合并贫血使发绀的识别更加困难。诊断低氧血症的金标准是用 Clark 电极直接测定 PaO_2；但这一操作为有创性，且不是一个连续的参数。

脉搏血氧测量

脉搏血氧仪发出 660 nm（红色）和 940 nm（红外）的光，另一侧有一个光电探测器。利用 Beer-Lambert 定律，分析脉动血液与非脉动血液吸收光的变化，并以此作为饱和度的估计值。在血红蛋白只有还原或含氧血红蛋白存在的情况下，脉搏血氧仪可提供低氧血症的早期预警（SpO_2 从 70% 到 100%），耳和前额探头对血氧饱和度变化的反应比手指探头快。碳氧血红蛋白和高铁血红蛋白的吸收光谱与氧血红蛋白相似，可能提供错误信息；事实上，碳氧血红蛋白和氧合血红蛋白是无法区分的。在存在碳氧血红蛋白时，脉搏血氧仪读数偏高。随着高铁血红蛋白浓度的增加，脉搏血氧测定读数趋于接近 85%。荧光也可能导致 SpO_2 的假性升高。蓝色指甲油、胶带、亚甲蓝、靛蓝胭脂红和异磺胺蓝可能会导致血氧饱和度测量值假性降低。协测仪可测量血液样本中异常血红蛋白的量：脱氧血红蛋白、氧合血红蛋白、碳氧血红蛋白和高铁血红蛋白。如果血氧饱和度读数可疑（如静脉注射或浸润染料进行手术标测），或怀疑一氧化碳中毒时，则应进行此类测试。一家大会制造商开发了一种使用八个波长的脉搏分析仪，能够测量脱氧血红蛋白、氧合血红蛋白、碳氧血红蛋白和高铁血红蛋白。

特定的器官

评估器官和组织氧供是否充分的方法总结见表 159.2。

表 159.2 评估器官和组织氧供是否充分的方法

器官 / 组织	方法
大脑	脑灌注压（CPP=MAP-ICP），经颅多普勒监测，脑电图，颈静脉血氧饱和度，近红外光谱检查，SSEP/MEP
心脏	心电图，经食管超声心动图，冠状窦血氧饱和度，肺动脉导管
肺	PaO_2/FiO_2 比值，肺损伤评分，肺动脉压，气道压（肺顺应性和阻力），支气管肺泡灌洗
肝、肾、肠	乳酸生成，肝酶，尿量和比重，血尿素氮和肌酐，胃张力测定

CPP，脑灌注压；FiO_2，吸入氧浓度；ICP，颅内压；MAP，平均动脉压；MEP，运动诱发电位；PaO_2，动脉血氧分压；SSEP，躯体感觉诱发电位

风险评估

吸入和静脉麻醉剂（氯胺酮除外）可使二氧化碳-通气反应曲线的斜率减缓，且与剂量成正比。吸入麻醉药、丙泊酚和右美托咪定，即使在低剂量下依然被证明可抑制机体对低氧的通气的反应。麻醉诱导后功能残气量下降，直到麻醉结束后数小时后才恢复正常，可导致肺不张。吸入麻醉药的最低肺泡有效浓度（minimum alveolar concentration，MAC）大于等于 1.0 时缺氧性肺血管收缩反应消失，从而增加因通气血流不匹配而导致缺氧的风险，但静脉麻醉药无此反应。在麻醉恢复过程中，氧化亚氮消除可使 PAO_2 降低数分钟，这是由于弥散性缺氧所致。麻醉剂还可降低参与维持咽部通畅的肌肉张力，增加部分或完全气道梗阻的风险。基于这些原因，任何使用麻醉剂的患者都存在缺氧风险。

缺氧风险增加的患者包括患有严重心肺疾病、功能残气量严重降低（妊娠和病态肥胖）、严重创伤、血栓形成、脓毒症、头部创伤、肺误吸和药物过量。当患者在静脉注射镇静剂的情况下进行诊断或治疗（如放射介入治疗或心脏及磁共振成像）时，如若负责监测的人员不专心、未经培训或过于繁忙，发生缺氧的风险也会增加。使用长效麻醉药或神经肌肉阻滞剂也会增加术后缺氧的风险，而低温则会导致不受控制的寒战及药物代谢和消除障碍。

启示

严重缺氧会导致缺血或死亡。中枢神经系统最不耐受缺氧（正常体温下耐受时间≤ 5 min）。缺氧时，无氧代谢会取代有氧代谢，从而导致细胞内高能量化合物不足和酸中毒。高能量化合物不足会导致细胞内泵失能和细胞内储存的钙释放，破坏细胞内结构。酸中毒和随后的葡萄糖无氧代谢（导致乳酸酸中毒）会进一步损害细胞。如前所述，大脑最易受损，其次是心脏、肝和肾。

管理

- 确定并纠正根本原因；
- 提供给氧；提高 FiO_2；

- 增加氧供（输血、强心或两者兼有）。
- 治疗通气血流失调（呼气末正压、叹息、吸入一氧化氮、体位）；
- 保护重要器官（低体温、药物、脊髓引流、类固醇）；
- 使用硝酸戊酯、亚硝酸钠或硫代硫酸盐进行 CN-毒性试验。

预防

表 159.3 列出了本文讨论的降低围术期缺氧风险的措施。

表 159.3 针对原因降低围术期缺氧风险的措施

原因	措施
低氧血症	确认氧气供应（检查麻醉机），确认故障保护功能；使用主路氧分析仪；预给氧；增加 FiO_2
通气不足	确认呼吸音和呼气末二氧化碳；增加 FiO_2；评估肺顺应性；使用支气管扩张剂；保持支气管通畅
V/Q 失调	增加 FiO_2；限制挥发性麻醉药的使用（抑制低氧性肺血管收缩）
分流	使用大潮气量（10～15 ml/kg），间歇叹息通气，频繁吸痰；高危患者增加 PEEP（低 FRC、肥胖、低蛋白血症）
弥散障碍[a]	增加 FiO_2
贫血	持续评估红细胞比容；输血；增加 FiO_2
循环衰竭	增加心排血量（容量、正心肌力药，心脏循环辅助装置）；减轻手术压迫或牵拉；增加 FiO_2
氧利用	限制 1～3 h 内 SNP ≤ 1 mg/kg 和 24 h 内 0.5 mg/kg，使用其他血管舒张剂[b]，或合并使用另一种血管扩张剂或 SNP 和 β 受体阻滞剂减少 SNP 的用量；增加 FiO_2（特别对于 CO 中毒）

CO，一氧化碳；CO_2，二氧化碳；FiO_2，吸入氧浓度；FRC，功能残气量；PEEP，呼气末正压通气；SNP，硝普钠；V/Q，肺泡通气量。

[a] 正常患者的非常见原因：肺泡毛细血管床减少（肺气肿）和高心排血量患者行肺切除术后可能导致缺氧。

[b] 静脉使用氯维地平 / 尼卡地平可能优于 SNP，由于后者大剂量使用时可能导致氰化物中毒。

致谢

感谢 John C. Boncyk 博士对本章上一版的贡献。

（李海莲　译　孟　岩　校）

延伸阅读

Carson JL, Guyatt G, Heddle NM, et al.: Clinical practice guidelines from the AABB: red blood cell transfusion thresholds and storage, *JAMA* 316(19):2025–2035, 2016.

Chan ED, Chan MM, Chan MM: Pulse oximetry: understanding its basic principles facilitates appreciation of its limitations, *Respir Med* 107(6):789–799, 2013.

Comroe JH, Botehlo S: The unreliability of cyanosis in the recognition of arterial hypoxemia, *Am J Med Sci* 124(1):1–6, 1947.

Comroe JH, Forster RE, Dubois AB, et al.: Diffusion. In *The lung: clinical physiology and pulmonary function tests*, ed 2, Chicago, 1962, Year Book Medical Publishers, pp 111–139.

Hall AH: Systemic asphyxiants. In Irwin RS, Rippe JM, editors: *Intensive care medicine*, ed 5, Philadelphia, 2003, JB Lippincott–Williams & Wilkins, pp 1608–1616.

Hébert PC, Wells G, Blajchman MA, et al.: A multicenter, randomized, controlled clinical trial of transfusion requirements in critical care, *N Engl J Med* 340(6):409–417, 1999.

Jubran A: Pulse oximetry, *Intensive Care Med* 30(11):2017–2020, 2004.

Kelly SD, Lieberman J, Feiner JR, et al.: Critical oxygen delivery in resting conscious humans is less than 7.5 mL O_2/kg/min [abstract], *Anesthesiology* 87:58, 1997.

Lumb AB: Anaesthesia. In *Nunn's applied respiratory physiology*, ed 5, London, 2000, Butterworth Heinemann, pp 420–459.

Lundsgaard C, Van Slyke DD: Cyanosis, *Medicine* 2:1, 1923.

Martin RL, Lloyd HGE, Cowan AI: The early events of oxygen and glucose deprivation: setting the scene for neuronal death? *Trends Neurosci* 17(6):251–256, 1994.

Moon RE, Camporesi EM: Clinical care at altered environmental pressure. In Miller RD, editor: *Anesthesia*, ed 5, Philadelphia, 2000, Churchill Livingstone, pp 2271–2301.

Moon RE, Camporesi EM: Respiratory monitoring. In Miller RD, editor: *Anesthesia*, ed 5, Philadelphia, 2000, Churchill Livingstone, pp 1255–1295.

Stehling LC, Doherty DO, Faust RJ, et al.: Practice guidelines for blood component therapy, *Anesthesiology* 84:732–747, 1996.

van Woerkens EC, Trouwborst A, van Lanshot JJ: Profound hemodilution: what is the critical hemodilution at which oxygen delivery-dependent oxygen consumption starts in an anesthetized human? *Anesth Analg* 75(5):818–821, 1992.

Wilson WC, Shapiro B: Perioperative hypoxia: the clinical spectrum and current oxygen monitoring methodology, *Anesthesiol Clin North Am* 19(4):769–812, 2001.

围术期心肌缺血和梗死

第 160 章

Jennifer M. Banayan，BobbieJean Sweitzer，Mark A. Chaney

病例概要

患者，男性，62 岁，拟行胆囊切除术。因冠状动脉疾病（coronary artery disease，CAD）于 8 年前行冠状动脉搭桥术，有糖尿病、高血压、高脂血症病史。目前服用阿司匹林、阿替洛尔、普伐他汀和氯沙坦。患者可爬一层楼且无任何不适。术中平稳，在麻醉后恢复室拔管时出现心动过速，心率达 110 次 / 分，但未引发胸痛，予以测定肌钙蛋白水平，并发现其结果升高。

问题分析

定义

心肌缺血是由心肌氧供需不平衡所致。心肌需氧量取决于前负荷、后负荷、心肌收缩力和心率。心肌供氧量取决于冠状动脉血管床的容量。冠状动脉粥样硬化限制冠状动脉血流，从而限制心肌供氧量。心肌氧供需不平衡可导致心肌缺血（框 160.1），持续长时间的缺血可导致心肌梗死（myocardial infarction，MI）。

框 160.1　导致心肌缺血的因素

心肌需氧量增加
- 心率增快
- 心肌收缩力增加
- 左心室舒张末期容积增加
- 室壁张力（后负荷）增加

心肌供氧量降低
- 冠状动脉血流减少
  - 血管收缩
  - 血栓形成
  - 舒张期缩短
  - 主动脉舒张压降低
  - 心室舒张末期压力增加
- 血氧含量下降
  - 血细胞比容降低
  - 血氧饱和度降低

围术期心肌梗死（Perioperative myocardial infarction，PMI）分为两个亚型：1 型和 2 型。1 型是典型的原发性冠状动脉事件，例如冠状动脉血栓形成。2 型是氧供需不平衡造成的缺血，95% 以上的 PMI 由 2 型引发。动脉粥样硬化和冠心病患者发病的主要因素是围术期氧需求量增加和血流量受限。围术期心肌氧供需不平衡的常见原因包括低血压、心动过速、低氧血症、出血和发热。在临床中，2 型 MI 通常类似于非 ST 段抬高型 MI，心肌标志物的增加幅度比 1 型 MI 小。急性冠状动脉血栓形成导致 MI 的发生率较低，但心源性死亡风险显著增加。血栓形成的原因包括炎症等手术应激、心动过速、围术期高凝状态、后负荷增加、斑块破裂和停用抗血小板治疗。

识别

围术期心肌缺血或 PMI 的最佳诊断方法，目前尚无共识。围术期患者被麻醉并给予阿片类药物，可掩盖胸痛症状，故很难识别心肌缺血。心电图（electrocardiogram，ECG）的变化可能细微难以发现。PMI 的确诊通常需下列三个标准中的两个：临床症状如胸痛、心电图改变和心肌标志物升高。

心电图是诊断心肌缺血和急性 MI 的最常依赖

的方法。心肌缺血（表 160.1）和既往 MI 的患者（表 160.2），其心电图变化可能不如想象中那么有用，因这些改变短暂、细微，甚至没有改变。其他筛查工具，如经食管超声心动图（transesophageal echocardiography，TEE）和心肌标志物，提高了 PMI 诊断的特异性。

TEE 检测节段性室壁运动异常，被认为是一种比心电图更敏感的检测心肌缺血的方法。多普勒检查可发现，二尖瓣口左心室流入道收缩期室壁增厚程度减少或舒张期充盈异常。然而，不伴有血流动力学或心电图改变的一过性收缩期室壁运动异常并不总与心肌缺血相关。因此，术中发生 ST 段改变时，使用 TEE 辅助确诊更有效。与室壁运动正常的患者相比，围术期新发持续性室壁运动异常者更易出现术后心脏不良事件。

肌钙蛋白I、肌钙蛋白T、肌酸激酶-MB（CK-MB）等心肌标志物的升高对 MI 的诊断有重要价值。血 CK 在急性 MI 后 4 h ～ 8 h 内升高，2 ～ 3 天恢复正常。CK 有三种同工酶（BB、MM、MB）。脑和肾主要含有 BB，骨骼肌主要为 MM（含 1% ～ 3%MB），心肌有 MM 和 MB（MB1 和 MB2 异构体）。一项研究发现，当 CKMB2>1U/L 或 CKMB2/CKMB1>1.5 时，发病 2 ～ 4 h 和 4 ～ 6 h 诊断急性 MI 敏感性分别为 59% 和 92%。

心肌钙蛋白是心肌坏死高度敏感和特异的化学标志物，预示急性冠状动脉综合征的患者死亡和再梗死的风险增加。肌钙蛋白（troponin，Tn）复合物由三个亚基（TnC、TnI、TnT）组成，调节钙介导的横纹肌收缩。TnC 与钙结合，TnI 与肌动蛋白结合，TnT 与原肌球蛋白结合。骨骼肌和心肌中均存在 TnI 和 TnT，但它们的编码基因和氨基酸序列不同，产生心肌钙蛋白（cardiac Tn，cTn）特异性抗体，并可定量检测 cTnI 和 cTnT。在急性 MI 患者中，cTnT 和 cTnI 在胸痛或其他缺血相关症状出现后 3 h 开始高于正常值，cTnI 持续 7 ～ 10 天，cTnT 持续 10 ～ 14 天。急性 MI 后，Q 波型和非 Q 波型急性 MI 患者生物学指标的释放动力学相似。cTnI 是目前最敏感、最特异的心肌损伤标志物。cTnT 可能检测出低于 CKMB 检测限度的心肌坏死。因此，“微小心肌损伤”和“微梗死”被用来描述胸痛、TnT 升高但 CKMB 正常的心肌变化。这类患者的不良临床结果（如复发 MI、需要血运重建或死亡）风险增加。30 天死亡率增加与术后 3 天 TnT 的升高直接相关。

无心肌标志物升高的围术期心肌损伤难以识别。在 2014 年非心脏手术患者血管事件队列评估（Vascular Events in Noncardiac Surgery Patients Cohort Evaluation，VISION）的研究中，19% 的患者无心脏症状，但肌钙蛋白升高并死于 PMI，70% 以上出现缺血相关的心电图改变。因此，尽管常规评估肌钙蛋白存在争议，但建议在高危手术后应用心肌标志物筛查高危患者，发现缺血并早期干预。

表 160.1　可提示心肌缺血的心电图变化

心电图改变	心电图描述
ST 段抬高	≥ 2 个相邻导联 J 点 ST 段抬高。V2、V3 导联，男性应≥ 0.2 mV，女性应≥ 0.15 mV；其他导联应≥ 0.1 mV
ST 段压低	新发两个相邻导联 T 波水平或下斜性压低≥ 0.05 mV
T 波异常	两个相邻导联 T 波倒置≥ 0.1 mV 且 R 波显著或 R/S 大于 1
左束支传导阻滞	新发左束支传导阻滞

表 160.2　心肌梗死的心电图变化

心电图变化	心电图描述
Q 波	V1 ～ V3 导联的任意 Q 波，或 Ⅰ、Ⅱ、aVL、aVF、V4、V5 或 V6 导联出现 Q 波或 5 ～ 30 ms（0.03 s）。Q 波变化必须存在于任意两个相邻导联，深度为 0.5 ～ 1 mm

风险评估

改良心脏风险指数（revised cardiac risk index，RCRI），也称为 Lee 指数，是评估围术期重大心脏并发症风险有效且常用的工具（框 160.2）。患者有≥ 2 个 RCRI 危险因素，其发生重大心脏不良事件（major adverse cardiac event，MACE）的风险增加，在接受大手术时应常规行心脏标记物监测，以明确围术期心肌损伤。目前已有的另外两种预测 MACE 的工具：美国外科医师学会全国科质量改进计划（National Surgical Quality Improvement Program，NSQIP）心肌梗死和心搏骤停（Myocardial Infarction and Cardiac Arrest，MICA）（http://www.surgicalriskcalculator.com/miorcardiacarrest）和美国外

框 160.2 改良心脏风险指数

腹股沟以上的血管、腹腔内和胸腔内手术
缺血性心脏病
心力衰竭
脑血管疾病
需胰岛素治疗的糖尿病
术前血肌酐 >2.0 mg/dl

科医师学会 NSQIP 手术风险计算器（http://www.riskcalculator.facs.org/）。使用这些计算方式，当 MACE 风险超过 1% 则认为风险增加，需要进一步干预降低风险。功能贮备是心脏病患者行非心脏手术术前评估的重要组成部分。对接受重大非心脏手术的患者，不能爬两层楼对术后 30 天死亡有 82% 的阳性预测值。此外，不能爬两层楼是围术期并发症增多的独立预测因素。相反，能爬两层楼是预测低风险患者简单且有效的筛选测试。

对接受低风险非心脏手术的患者，不建议采用无创应激试验进行常规筛查，但无诱发性缺血症状的患者发生围术期心脏并发症概率低。不推荐为减少围术期心脏事件而常规进行术前冠状动脉造影。

冠状动脉粥样硬化性疾病是 PMI 的重要危险因素，但狭窄最严重的部位不一定是梗死部位。通常，心肌缺血或梗死的部位是狭窄程度小于临界值的冠状动脉供应的范围。

启示

美国每年进行 2 亿例非心脏手术，其中 800 万例在 30 天内发生心肌缺血。在 POISE 试验的安慰剂组中，5.7% 的患者在非心脏手术后 30 天内发生 MI。PMI 是非心脏手术相关病残率和死亡率最可靠的预测指标之一，死亡率近 25%。围术期发生心肌缺血的患者常合并 CAD。美国心脏病学会（The American College of Cardiology，ACC）和美国心脏协会（American Heart Association，AHA）推荐近期 MI 患者行非心脏手术时应推迟至少 60 天以降低 PMI 的风险。

由于心肌缺血发生于 PMI 前，早期发现围术期心肌缺血应及时采取治疗措施来解除缺血，从而降低随后 MI 的发生率或程度。

管理

围术期心肌缺血的处理可分为术前、术中和术后干预。

术前，麻醉科医师使用 RCRI 或 NSQIP 手术风险计算器识别高危患者。此外，确定手术是否为紧急、急诊或择期，是否允许推迟手术，给予 β- 受体阻滞剂、补铁避免贫血、阿司匹林和他汀类药物进行围术期优化治疗。

术中，临床医师必须防止哪怕是轻度的心率增加，并避免术中低血压。平均动脉压下降超过 20%，术后并发症（包括 PMI、脑卒中和死亡）风险显著增加。所有引起心动过速、低血压、贫血、低氧血症和疼痛的因素均为 2 型 MI 的常见原因，并可能导致 1 型 MI，故均应积极治疗。减少心肌耗氧量或增加供氧量是控制 PMI 的干预措施（框 160.3）。

麻醉期间，术中应维持稳定的血流动力学参数。对于哪种类型的麻醉（全身麻醉、区域麻醉或椎管内麻醉，吸入麻醉与静脉麻醉）降低高危患者围术期缺血或 PMI 发生率，目前尚无明确共识。大量研究表明，椎管内麻醉时深静脉血栓、肺炎、致命性肺栓塞或术后低氧血症的发生率较低。一项接受关节置换患者的研究显示，非全身麻醉者死亡率较低。最近更多研究发现，与椎管内麻醉相比，接受全身麻醉的患者持续低血压时间更长。因此，需要积极治疗低血压，预防 PMI 的发生。

在接受心脏和非心脏手术的患者中，采用区域

框 160.3 心肌缺血处理

减少心肌需氧量
降低心率
降低心肌收缩力
减少左心室舒张末期容积
减少后负荷
增加心肌供氧量
增加冠脉血流量
　减少血管收缩
　减少血栓形成
　延长舒张期
　增加主动脉舒张压
　降低心室舒张末期压力
提高血氧含量
　提高血细胞比容
　增加血氧饱和度

麻醉或多模式镇痛积极控制术后疼痛，减轻相关应激，可降低心脏事件病残率和死亡率。应始终考虑凝血功能异常、影响凝血的药物和患者的偏好。

高危患者术后需要监测 24 ～ 48 h。因为大多数 PMI 无症状，或有不典型的症状和微小的心电图变化。对至少有一个 RCRI 因素且接受高风险手术的患者，推荐常规检测肌钙蛋白。

预防

预防策略仍存在争议。预防性冠状动脉血管重建（Coronary Artery Revascularization Prophylaxis，CARP）试验比较了近 6000 例缺血性心脏病患者在大血管手术前药物治疗和血管重建。研究结果显示，在死亡率和 PMI 发生率上，二者没有差别，预防性血管重建不能改善患者预后。阿司匹林、β-受体阻滞剂和他汀类药物的使用是最佳干预方案。大量研究表明，阿司匹林和他汀类药物可以降低患者 30 天死亡率。

血管紧张素转换酶抑制剂（angiotensin-converting enzyme inhibitor，ACEI）和血管紧张素受体阻滞剂（angiotensin receptor blocker，ARB）是治疗慢性高血压和心力衰竭的常用药物。它们改善低射血分数患者的症状，提高患者的存活率，并降低有 MI 史患者的死亡风险。术中 ACEI 和 ARB 可引起低血压，特别是接受全身麻醉的患者。因此，一些医师建议在术前 24 h 停用 ACEI 和 ARB，避免低血压。然而，有证据表明，围术期继续使用这些药物是有益的。原因可能在于，在及时干预下，与 ACEI、ARB 和麻醉相关的低血压并未带来严重后果，如 MI、脑卒中或肾衰竭。事实上，如果在术前停用且术后未立即重新使用 ACEI 或 ARB，患者 30 天死亡率增加。

多年来，阿司匹林一直被用于 CAD、脑血管病患者 MI 或脑卒中的预防，其疗效已被普遍认可。尽管有证据表明阿司匹林治疗有益，但为防止出血，围术期常停用阿司匹林。临床医师应综合考虑出血风险与持续服用阿司匹林预防 CAD、脑血管病或外周动脉疾病的益处。当在手术前停用阿司匹林时，突然停药可能增加重大血栓栓塞事件的发生风险。当出血风险低于围术期心脏事件风险时，患者应继续服用阿司匹林。另一方面，对服用阿司匹林作为一级预防措施的患者，术前 5 ～ 7 天应停止服药。

β-受体阻滞剂通过降低心率和心肌收缩力来降低心肌耗氧量，通过增加舒张期时间和降低心室壁张力来增加氧供应，是预防 MI 的金标准。围术期缺血评估（Perioperative Ischemic Evaluation，POISE）试验是一项大型随机对照研究，共有 8000 多例患者参加。该试验显示，在大手术当天服用 β-受体阻滞剂的患者，围术期非致死性 MI 减少，但脑卒中增加。脑卒中和死亡率的增加可能由持续的、未经治疗的低血压所致。Wallace 等的研究显示，术前开始使用 β-受体阻滞剂的患者，30 天和 1 年死亡率降低。他们制定降低的围术期心脏风险治疗方案，对患有 CAD、周围血管疾病或有两种 CAD 危险因素（年龄 >60 岁、吸烟、糖尿病、高血压、胆固醇 >240 mg/dl）的患者，应开始使用 β-受体阻滞剂。总之，长期服用 β 受体阻滞剂者不应停用，低血压应在围术期积极治疗。如需要，β-受体阻滞剂应在手术前开始使用，并滴定给药，以防止低血压。

围术期继续使用钙通道阻滞剂和 α_2-受体激动剂治疗高血压。目前尚无证据支持其应用可以减少围术期缺血。

3-羟基-3-甲基戊二酰辅酶 A 还原酶抑制剂（他汀类药物）可以稳定冠状动脉斑块，降低围术期斑块破裂、MI 和死亡风险。他汀类药物也可以降低急性肾衰竭的风险。突然停用他汀类药物可导致斑块不稳定，增加 PMI 风险。对接受血管手术或其他增加心肌梗死风险手术的患者，围术期应用他汀类药物是合理的。

贫血状态下心肌供氧量减少，而心排血量增加使需氧量增加，导致心肌缺血。输血与各种并发症有关，关于输血的血红蛋白水平存在争议。无 CAD 且无症状患者，血红蛋白 <6 g/dl 时采用限制性输血策略。缺血性心脏病患者可以考虑更宽松的输血策略：将血红蛋白保持在 9 g/dl 以上。对于贫血患者，术前应考虑铁剂治疗。推迟手术来评估和治疗贫血可以改善预后。

曾经接受过经皮冠状动脉介入治疗的患者，有发生心脏事件的风险。关于冠状动脉支架的详细内容见第 22 章。

在过去 20 年里，预防围术期心肌缺血和心肌梗死的建议已发生变化。管理重点更多在于管理，而非干预。阿司匹林、他汀类药物和 β-受体阻滞剂治疗心动过速和低血压，术前纠正贫血，可降低预后不良的可能性。

（胡琍琍 译 席 鹏 校）

延伸阅读

Archan S, Fleisher LA: From creatine kinase-MB to troponin: the adoption of a new standard, *Anesthesiology* 112:1005–1012, 2010.

Biccard BM, Rodseth RN: The pathophysiology of peri-operative myocardial infarction, *Anaesthesia* 65:733–741, 2010.

Biccard BM: Relationship between the inability to climb two flights of stairs and outcome after major non-cardiac surgery: implications for the preoperative assessment of functional capacity, *Anaesthesia* 60:588–593, 2005.

Botto F, Alonso-Coello P, Chan MTV, et al.: Myocardial injury after noncardiac surgery: a large, international, prospective cohort study establishing diagnostic criteria, characteristics, predictors, and 30-day outcomes, *Anesthesiology* 120:564–578, 2014.

Cohen ME, Ko CY, Bilimoria KY, et al.: Optimizing ACS NSQIP modeling for evaluation of surgical quality and risk: patient risk adjustment, procedure mix adjustment, shrinkage adjustment, and surgical focus, *J Am Coll Surg* 217:336–346.e1, 2013.

Devereaux PJ, Mrkobrada M, Sessler DI, et al.: Aspirin in patients undergoing noncardiac surgery, *N Engl J Med* 370:1494–1503, 2014.

Devereaux PJ, Chan MT, Alonso-Coello P, et al.: Association between postoperative troponin levels and 30-day mortality among patients undergoing noncardiac surgery, *JAMA* 307:2295–2304, 2012.

Devereaux PJ, Xavier D, Pogue J, et al.: Characteristics and short-term prognosis of perioperative myocardial infarction in patients undergoing noncardiac surgery: a cohort study, *Ann Intern Med* 154:523–528, 2011.

Devereaux PJ, Yang H, Guyatt GH, et al.: Rationale, design, and organization of the PeriOperative ISchemic Evaluation (POISE) trial: a randomised controlled trial of metoprolol versus placebo in patients undergoing noncardiac surgery, *Am Heart J* 152:223–230, 2006.

Fleisher LA, Fleischmann KE, Auerbach AD, et al.: 2014 ACC/AHA guideline on perioperative cardiovascular evaluation and management of patients undergoing noncardiac surgery: a report of the American College of Cardiology/American Heart Association Task Force on Practice Guidelines, *J Am Coll Cardiol* 64(22):e77–e137, 2014.

Ford MK, Beattie WS, Wijeysundera DN: Systematic review: prediction of perioperative cardiac complications and mortality by the revised cardiac risk index, *Ann Intern Med* 152:26–35, 2010.

Gerstein NS, Carey MC, Cigarroa JE, et al.: Perioperative aspirin management after POISE-2: some answers, but questions remain, *Anesth Analg* 120:570–575, 2015.

Gupta PK, Gupta H, Sundaram A, et al.: Development and validation of a risk calculator for prediction of cardiac risk after surgery, *Circulation* 124:381–387, 2011.

Keller T, Zeller T, Ojeda F, et al.: Serial changes in highly sensitive troponin I assay and early diagnosis of myocardial infarction, *JAMA* 306:2684–2693, 2011.

Kristensen SD, Knuuti JSO: New ESC/ESA guidelines on non-cardiac surgery: cardiovascular assessment and management, *Eur Heart J* 35(35):234–235, 2014.

McFalls EO, Ward HB, Moritz TE, et al.: Coronary-artery revascularization before elective major vascular surgery, *N Engl J Med* 351:2795–2804, 2004.

Raju MG, Pachika A, Punnam SR, et al.: Statin therapy in the reduction of cardiovascular events in patients undergoing intermediate-risk noncardiac, nonvascular surgery, *Clin Cardiol* 36:456–461, 2013.

Van Kuijk J-P, Flu W-J, Schouten O, et al.: Timing of noncardiac surgery after coronary artery stenting with bare metal or drug-eluting stents, *Am J Cardiol* 104:1229–1234, 2009.

Wallace AW, Au S, Cason BA: Association of the pattern of use of perioperative β-blockade and postoperative mortality, *Anesthesiology* 113:794–805, 2010.

第 161 章 围术期快速性心律失常

Alexander Michael Stewart，James Bromilow

病例概要

患者，男性，68 岁，因小肠缺血性坏死在全身麻醉下急诊行剖腹探查术时突发快速心房颤动。患者血压下降，伴有不规则的窄 QRS 波心动过速，心室率为 140 次 / 分。快速静脉补液、给予升压药、补充电解质以及输注胺碘酮后循环恢复稳定。患者术后被转送至 ICU 后突发室性心动过速，立即行电复律，进一步给予负荷剂量的胺碘酮和调整电解质。

问题分析

定义

心率在 100 次 / 分以上的异常心律被归为快速性心律失常。围术期心律失常发作时，应根据心律失常的性质、程度以及患者病史去寻找并明确其可逆性发病因素。

心房颤动（atrial fibrillation，AF）和心房扑动（atrial flutter，AFl）是围术期最常见的心律失常，发病高峰在术后 1 ～ 3 天，可能与炎症和组织创伤相关的交感兴奋有关。其发病率与患者年龄和术前心率正相关，且男性患者高发。

识别

在术前评估过程中，系统问诊可使临床医师了解心律失常的病史。突发性心悸是一种指示性症状，相关症状（如气短、胸痛、头昏和晕厥）可能对分析心律失常的严重程度有指导作用。伴有上述症状的择期手术患者应推迟手术并请心脏科医师会诊。

术中心律失常一般通过心电图（electrocardiogram，ECG）诊断，快速性心律失常的诊断特征见表 161.1。根据心肌内的兴奋位点，可大致分为室上性（窄 QRS 波）和室性（宽 QRS 波）心律失常。规则的宽 QRS 波心动过速应被视为心室来源性的，除非已明确诊断为室上性心动过速（supraventricular tachycardia，SVT）伴室内差异传导或逆向性房室折返性心动过速（antidromic atrioventricular reentrant tachycardia，AVRT）（表 161.1）。给予腺苷等阻滞房室结传导的药物治疗室性心动过速（antidromic atrioventricular，VT）不仅无效而且具有潜在危险性。同样，在静态心电图上识别预激和 Wolf-Parkinson-White 综合征也至关重要。患者心脏传导通路存在不应期比房室结更短的旁路，当出现房性快速性心律失常时可危及生命。禁用阻滞房室结传导的药物（腺苷、地尔硫卓、维拉帕米、β-受体阻滞药和地高辛），因其阻断房室结传导后会加重旁路传导，有导致心室颤动的可能。

风险评估

快速性心律失常的危险因素见表 161.2。有助于明确心律失常危险因素的围术期检查见表 161.3。

启示

因手术和麻醉可加重心律失常，故需在术前对心律失常进行控制和调整。由于心室充盈有赖于心房收缩，SVT 患者突然失去有效的心房收缩将影响其心排血量。随着心室率增加，舒张期心室充盈进一步减少，该情况在舒张功能障碍和瓣膜性心脏病的患者中尤其有害。

单发的室性异位心律或非持续性 VT 通常不需要抗心律失常治疗，但可提示存在需要治疗的可逆性触发因素。而持续性 VT 是潜在的致命性心律失常，需要紧急诊断和治疗。

表 161.1 快速性心律失常的分类及诊断特征 [a]

心律失常	原因	ECG 特征	心室率（次 / 分）	起病	治疗注意事项	ECG
窦性心动过速	应激反应、拟交感神经药、抗胆碱能药、甲状腺功能亢进、恶性高热、特发性	R-R 间期规则，P-R 间期正常，类似于静息 ECG	220 减去患者年龄（最大值）	逐渐发作	对因治疗	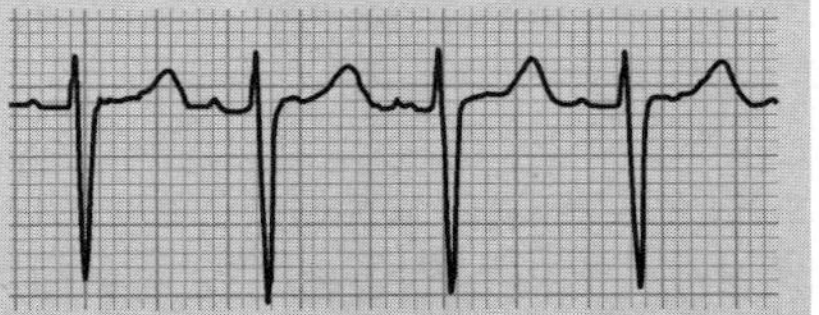
心房颤动	心血管疾病、心脏手术、COPD、炎症、甲状腺功能亢进、电解质紊乱	R-R 间期不规则，心房活动不协调伴 P 波缺失	100 ～ 220	突然发作（新发）或逐渐发作（慢性）	对因治疗，在围术期难以行早期复率，故需开始心率控制治疗	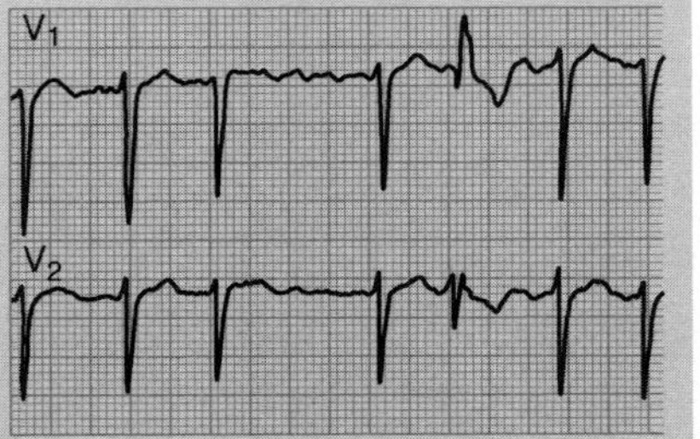
心房扑动	见心房颤动	R-R 间期规则（若有变异性 AV 传导，可不规则），规则的扑动样波形，典型频率为 300 次 / 分伴 2：1 下传	150	突然发作	与心室颤动相比，心房扑动更易于复律，腺苷有助于诊断，但不能用于复律	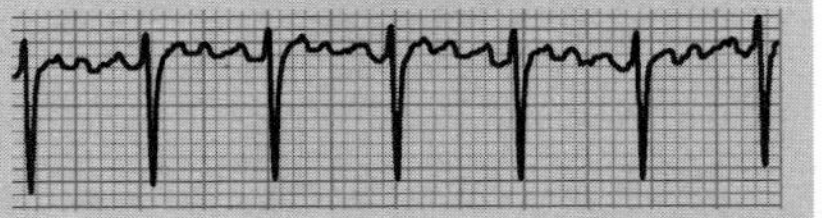
局灶性房性心动过速	心肺疾病、洋地黄中毒	R-R 间期规则，P 波形态单一且不同于窦性心律	150 ～ 250	突然发作超过 3 ～ 4 次	对因治疗，启动心率控制治疗	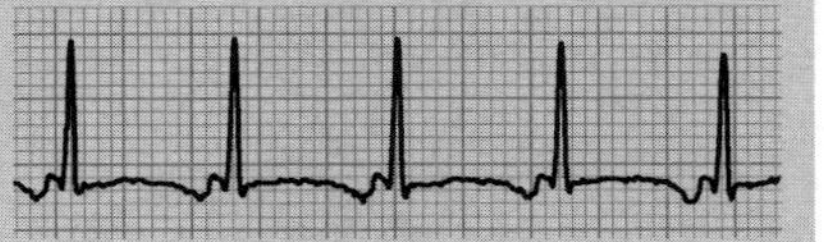
多源性房性心动过速	肺病、茶碱中毒	R-R 间期不规则，P 波形态多样	100 ～ 150	逐渐发作	对因治疗，启动心率控制治疗，很难复律	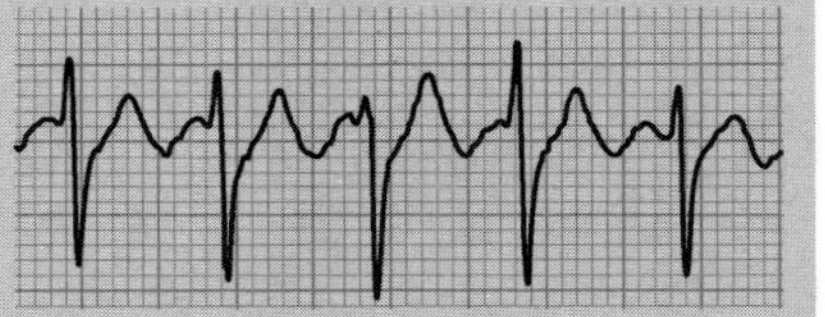
AV 结折返性心动过速	通常发生于年轻患者，AV 结内有折返回路，但无旁路	R-R 间期规则，心房和心室同时激动时 P 波隐藏在 QRS 波中	150 ～ 250	突然发作	清醒状态下可刺激迷走神经或予腺苷治疗	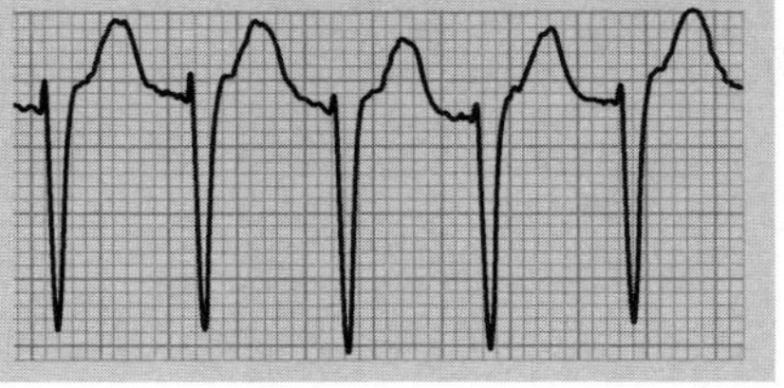

续表

心律失常	原因	ECG 特征	心室率（次/分）	起病	治疗注意事项	ECG
AV 结性心动过速	先天性旁路	R-R 间期规则，经 AV 结下传时为窄 QRS 波，经旁路下传时为宽 QRS 波	150 ～ 250	突然发作	窄 QRS 波时，清醒状态下可刺激迷走神经或予腺苷治疗；宽 QRS 波时，予胺碘酮或普鲁卡因胺治疗	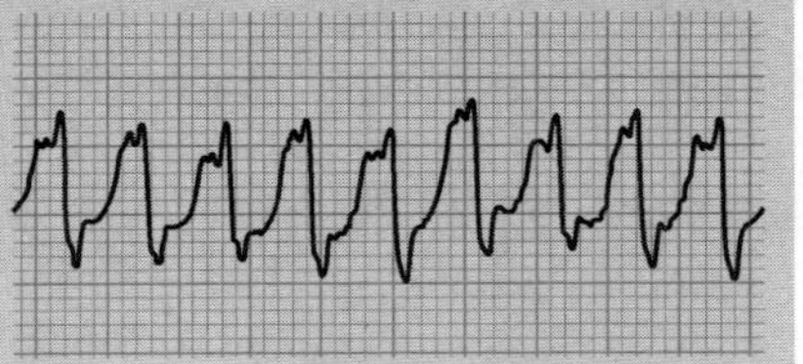
AF 合并预激	上述引起 AF 的原因，并同时伴有先天性旁路	R-R 间期不规则，经旁路下传时为宽 QRS 波，静息 ECG 有 Wolff-Parkinson-White 综合征的表现	150 ～ 250	突然发作	对因治疗，应考虑早期电复律，可予胺碘酮或普鲁卡因胺	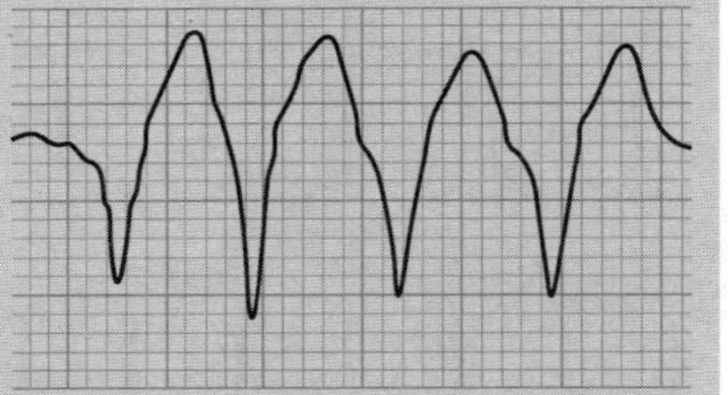
单形室性心动过速	心血管疾病、心肌缺血、直接刺激心肌、再灌注、严重电解质紊乱	R-R 间期规则，宽 QRS 波，静态 ECG 上 QT 间期正常	110 ～ 250	突然发作	对因治疗，若电复律效果不稳定，可考虑胺碘酮或利多卡因	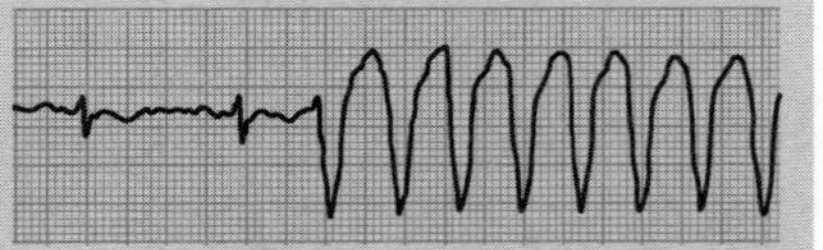
多形室性心动过速	心肌缺血，尖端扭转型室速的起因是 QT 间期延长	QT 间期正常或延长，QRS 波的振幅、轴向和持续时间呈多样	110 ～ 250	突然发作	有关长 QT 综合征和室性心律失常的更多详情参见第 155 章	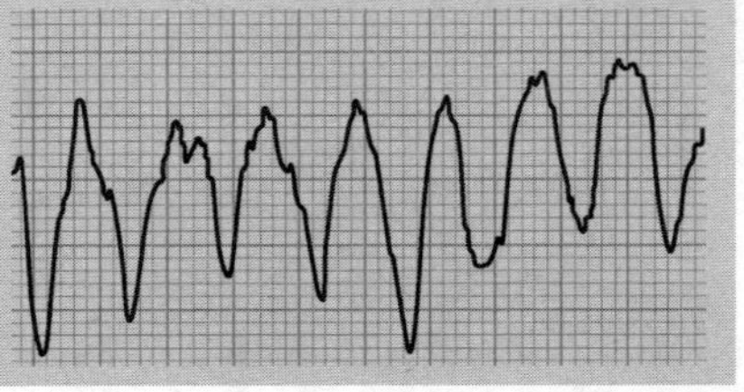

[a] 这是围术期快速性心律失常的经典 ECG 特征及治疗方案。注意会存在变异的情况，如患者可能既往有束支传导阻滞，在这种情况下窦性心动过速实际上可表现为宽 QRS 波。应注意养成查看术前心电图的习惯。

AF，心房颤动；AV，房室的；COPD，慢性阻塞性肺疾病；ECG，心电图

表 161.2　围术期快速性心律失常的危险因素[a]	
麻醉相关的急性因素	**急性外科因素**
高血容量和急性心房牵张	休克
麻醉引起的心脏抑制	疼痛
内源性 PEEP	创伤
正性肌力药	贫血
局部麻醉药中毒	局部和全身性炎症
放置肺动脉导管 / 中心静脉导管位置异常	纵隔或心脏操作
急性内科因素	**慢性内科因素**
缺氧	衰老（纤维化和炎症）
低血容量	心房扩张（心力衰竭、瓣膜病）
电解质紊乱	缺血性心脏病
心肌缺血	充血性心力衰竭
代谢性 / 呼吸性酸中毒	慢性缺氧（如 COPD、OSA）
脓毒症	心肌病
肺栓塞	持续性心动过速引起的心房重构
低血糖 / 高血糖	旁路
低体温 / 体温过高	先天性心脏病
心肌炎 / 心包炎	心脏术后瘢痕形成
气胸	肺动脉高压
过量摄入酒精或咖啡因	甲状腺功能亢进 / 甲状腺功能减退
致幻剂	恶性肿瘤

[a] 这些因素可触发围术期快速性心律失常，并加重心血管的不稳定性，应尽可能识别并干预。

COPD，慢性阻塞性肺疾病；OSA，阻塞性睡眠呼吸暂停；PEEP，呼气末正压

表 161.3　快速性心律失常相关的围术期检查[a]	
检查项目	**需关注的结果**
心电图	节律是否规整、有无缺血和传导旁路
超声心动图	容量状态、瓣膜性心脏病、心房大小、心室大小和功能、心肌病、既往心脏手术、先天性心脏病、心包积液、肺动脉高压
胸片	肺炎、气胸、肺水肿
全血计数	贫血
动脉血气	缺氧、酸血症
血电解质	电解质紊乱（特别是低钾血症、低镁血症）
甲状腺功能检查	甲状腺功能亢进
药物筛查	致幻性拟交感神经药物的使用

[a] 有指征的情况下应在术前完善这些检查。术中新发的心律失常需彻底检查以降低其发病率并据此指导围术期治疗。

管理

对突发的快速性心律失常，应分析病因并立即纠正诱发因素。在血流动力学极度不稳定的情况下，可能需要电复律，但如果根本原因没有得到解决，可能会复律失败。给予氧疗、保持良好的通气、纠正低血容量、维持电解质平衡及适当镇痛，可能会改善血流动力学，而无需再使用抗心律失常药物。图 161.1 是术中突发快速性心律失常的治疗流程。

预防

对于病情稳定的 AF 或 AFl 患者，除调整抗凝外，一般不需在围术期更改治疗方案或进行特殊评估。对高血栓栓塞风险的患者，可能需要低分子肝素桥接治疗。

术前有 VT 病史和心脏植入式电子设备的患者，需参考心脏科医师的评估和建议。

患者正在服用的控制心率的药物应在围术期继续使用，可以降低心律失常的发生率，但可能需要根据临床情况（如术后低血压）调整剂量。接受利尿剂治疗的患者或有慢性肾病病史的患者，应在术前检查血电解质并维持平衡。

（张程程　译　潘　科　校）

延伸阅读

Amar D: Perioperative atrial tachyarrhythmias, *Anesthesiology* 97(6):1618–1623, 2002.

Atlee JL: Perioperative cardiac dysrhythmias: diagnosis and management, *Anesthesiology* 86(6):1397–1424, 1997.

Fleisher LA, Fleischmann KE, Auerbach AD, et al.: 2014 ACC/AHA guideline on perioperative cardiovascular evaluation and management of patients undergoing noncardiac surgery: executive summary: a report of the American College of Cardiology/American Heart Association Task Force on practice guidelines. Developed in collaboration with the American College of Surgeons, American Society of Anesthesiologists, American Society of Echocardiography, American Society of Nuclear Cardiology, Heart Rhythm Society, Society for Cardiovascular Angiography and Interventions, Society of Cardiovascular Anesthesiologists, and Society of Vascular Medicine Endorsed by the Society of Hospital Medicine, *J Nucl Cardiol* 22(1):162–215, 2015.

Link MS, Berkow LC, Kudenchuk PJ, et al.: Part 7: Adult Advanced Cardiovascular Life Support: 2015 American Heart Association Guidelines Update for Cardiopulmonary Resuscitation and Emergency Cardiovascular Care, *Circulation* 132(18 Suppl 2):S444–S464, 2015.

Page RL, Joglar JA, Caldwell MA, et al.: 2015 ACC/AHA/HRS guideline for the management of adult patients with supraventricular tachycardia: a report of the American College of Cardiology/American Heart Association Task Force on Clinical Practice Guidelines and the Heart Rhythm Society, *J Am Coll Cardiol* 67(13):e27–e115, 2016.

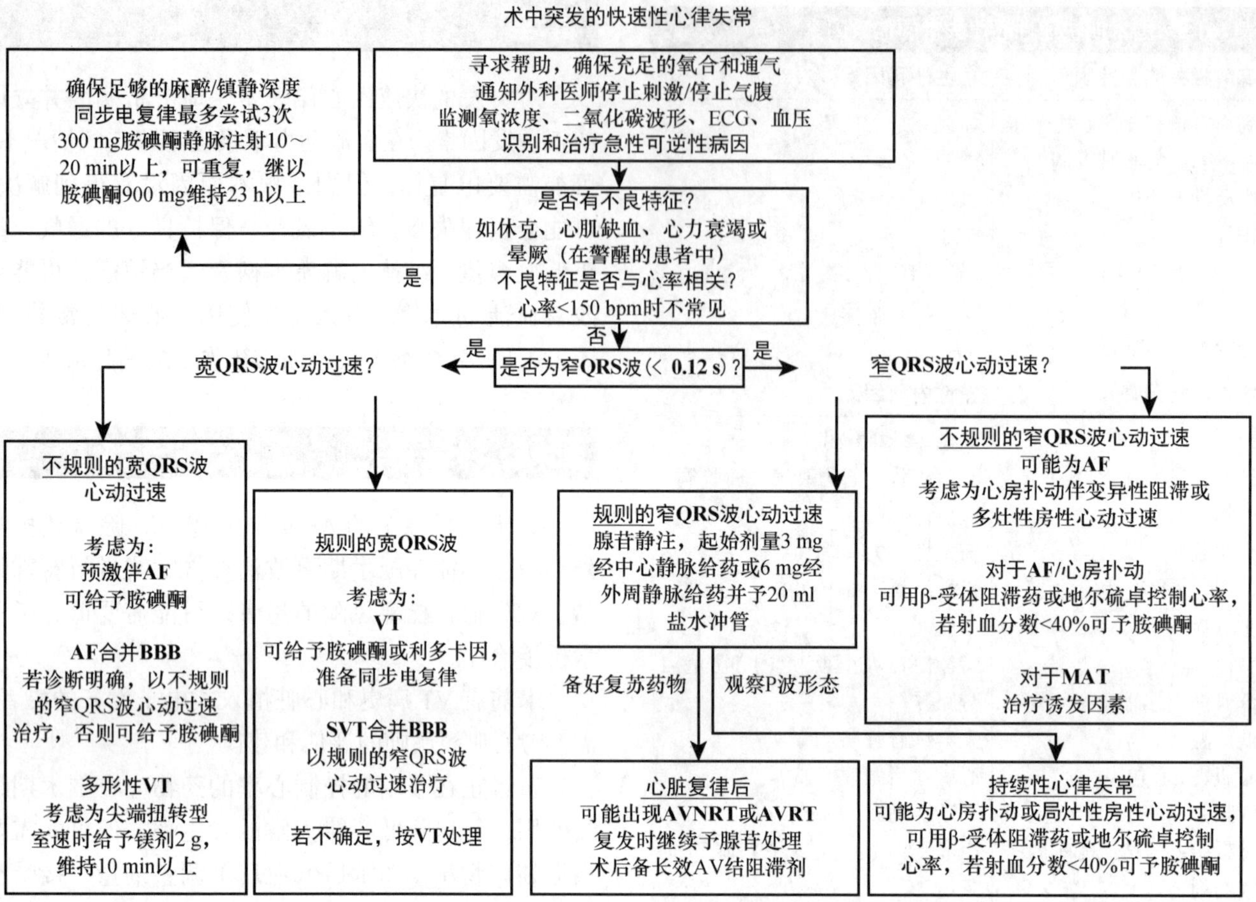

图 161.1　心动过速治疗流程。围术期使用药物纠正心律通常无效，抗心律失常药物如氟卡尼或普鲁卡因胺的不良反应在病情严重或全身麻醉时可能会更加明显。应将重点放在逆转触发因素和控制心率上

Stewart AM, Greaves K, Bromilow J: Supraventricular tachyarrhythmias and their management in the perioperative period, *Contin Educ Anaesth Crit Care Pain* 15(2):90–97, 2015.

Tracy C, Boushahri A: Managing arrhythmias in the intensive care unit, *Crit Care Clin* 30(3):365–390, 2014.

Zipes DP, Camm AJ, Borggrefe M, et al.: ACC/AHA/ESC 2006 guidelines for management of patients with ventricular arrhythmias and the prevention of sudden cardiac death: a report of the American College of Cardiology/American Heart Association Task Force and the European Society of Cardiology Committee for Practice Guidelines (Writing Committee to Develop guidelines for management of patients with ventricular arrhythmias and the prevention of sudden cardiac death) developed in collaboration with the European Heart Rhythm Association and the Heart Rhythm Society, *Europace* 8(9):746–837, 2006.

围产期神经系统并发症

第 162 章

Nathaniel Hsu

病例概要

患者，女性，32 岁，初次怀孕，予 0.125% 的布比卡因和 2 μg/ml 的芬太尼进行硬膜外无痛分娩镇痛。先予 10 ml 硬膜外推注，随后同样的混合药物以 10 ml/h 的速度输注。接着，需手法翻转胎位以纠正枕后位，并行中位产钳分娩。在新生儿转位和娩出之前，给予 2% 利多卡因混合 1∶200 000 的肾上腺素共 20 ml。产后第 2 天，患者主诉双下肢感觉丧失，无法移动，大便失禁。两天后，患者下肢部分运动和感觉功能恢复，但仍有大便失禁，随后出现尿潴留伴尿失禁。产后第 4 天神经科会诊，诊断马尾综合征可能。产后 6 个月，患者仍需靠轮椅生活，但肠道和膀胱功能已有所改善。

问题分析

定义

尽管许多研究试图确定围产期神经并发症的发生率，但实际发病率可能由于从业医师的熟练度以及当时麻醉技术的不同而有很大差异。2006 年的最新数据显示，产科患者短暂神经并发症的发生率为 1/6700，而持续性神经损伤的发生率为 1/240 000。持续性并发症通常并非麻醉药本身所致，更常与分娩时的产科创伤有关。在一项已完结的索赔项目中，Lee 及其同事对 1005 例区域麻醉进行分析，对其中 368 例产科患者，以及 637 例非产科患者中的 453 例患者均实施椎管内阻滞，产科组中 51% 和非产科组中 41% 的损伤均与椎管内阻滞有关。与非产科组（38%）相比，产科组发生短暂性和低度损伤的索赔率（71%）明显较高，但其发生严重不良结局（包括死亡或永久性脑损伤）的索赔率明显较低。这些不良结局的原因包括心血管衰竭、呼吸停止和凝血障碍患者发生椎管内血肿。2009 年，英国国家审计显示，在产科患者中，脊椎–硬膜外联合（combined spinal-epidural，CSE）麻醉风险最高，硬膜外麻醉风险最低。

Wong 及其同事研究调查了 60 057 名平安生下婴儿的产妇，随后对其中 6048 人进行随访，发现 56 例产妇（0.92%）出现新诊断的下肢周围神经损伤。通过逻辑回归分析，多胎和第二产程延长与神经损伤显著相关。神经损伤的患者在半斜坡截石位“用力”的时间更长。症状的持续时间平均为 2 个月，而损伤常涉及下肢单侧周围神经或腰骶神经丛。因此，这些发现表明，与分娩有关的神经损伤可能更多地与分娩本身有关，而不是麻醉药物。

识别

在评估疑似神经系统并发症的患者时，常涉及以下几个问题：

- 分娩的持续时间是多少？
- 患者“用力”的时间？
- 用力时患者是否处于极度的截石体位？
- 产科医师是否使用产钳协助分娩？
- 新生儿的体重是多少？
- 先露部位（例如枕后位）是什么？
- 患者是否有背部疾患或神经功能缺损的既往史

[例如多发性硬化症，人类免疫缺陷病毒（human immunodefciency virus，HIV）]？

- 使用局部麻醉药的类型和剂量？
- 患者出现新症状前是否恢复了感觉或运动功能？

如果发生围产期神经并发症，通常涉及硬膜外镇痛或麻醉。一定要咨询麻醉科医师。产后神经损伤的潜在原因很多，硬膜外损伤只是其中之一。这种神经损伤通常是由于胎头或产钳直接损伤了支配下肢的主要神经根或神经干。下脊髓的直接缺血损伤也是可能的原因之一。如果胎头压迫髂内动脉脊髓升支，也可能会发生这种情况。还应考虑椎管内血肿的可能性（见第 179 章）。一旦发现广泛的神经功能缺损时，必须请神经学专家会诊。此外，应立即获取脊髓的磁共振成像或计算机断层扫描。

风险评估

在计算围产期神经损伤的风险时，考虑相关的解剖结构是很重要的。分娩引起的神经损伤可累及腰骶神经丛的分支（即髂腹下神经、髂腹股沟神经、生殖股神经、股外侧皮神经、胫前神经、股神经、闭孔神经和坐骨神经）。也可能涉及来自骶（S3 和 S4）神经根的阴部神经，以及来自 S4、S5 和尾神经根的尾丛。广泛的神经损伤偶尔可能导致马尾综合征。损伤若涉及大神经丛（腰椎和骶椎），就可能会造成这种范围较广泛的损伤，需要数周或数月才能恢复。

腰丛或骶丛的分支（图 162.1）包括坐骨神经（包含腓总神经和胫骨神经），这些分支在胎儿出生时可能会被胎头挤压，因为胎头在出生时穿过骨盆后缘。75% 的病例为单侧损伤，其余病例为双侧损伤。压迫性损伤在骨盆扁平、巨大儿、头盆不称、顶先露及产钳分娩的初产妇中更常见。这些损伤可能涉及多个神经根水平，或表现为股神经或闭孔神经损伤，L4 ～ L5 皮肤节段感觉受损。表 162.1 列举出了分娩过程中常见的一些周围神经损伤，图 162.2 为腰骶神经丛分支支配的皮肤节段。

关于特定神经损伤的机制（见表 162.1），多发性硬化症复发往往导致股外侧皮神经损伤。股外侧皮神经损伤引起的大腿前部麻木称为“**感觉异常性股痛**”。在剖宫产时，这种神经也可能因过度伸展的截石位，胎头压力或剖宫产术中不当的手术牵引而受伤。当股骨神经损伤时，髋关节屈曲和膝关节伸展变得困难。损伤是由于第二产程中髋部主动屈曲，导致腹股沟韧带压迫神经所致。因此在“用力”时应避免髋关节过度弯曲。双腿应在宫缩和用力之间休息。此外，在第二产程中使用“蹲杆”体位髋关节过度弯曲，可能会导致股神经损伤。胎头压迫腰骶丛也会使股神经损伤。

大内收肌接受闭孔神经和坐骨神经的双重神经支配。如果闭孔神经受累，大腿外展减弱，大腿内侧感觉丧失。坐骨神经是人体最大的周围神经。腓总神经是其重要的分支之一，支配小腿运动和感觉。这条神经缠绕在腓骨颈部，是下肢唯一手可触及的神经（图 162.3），故易受损伤，尤其易受产床脚蹬的伤害。这种损伤会导致踝关节和足部瘫痪，导致足下垂、内翻以及足背部感觉受损。

梨状肌的炎症或痉挛（妊娠期长时间坐姿或大量负重引起）偶尔可引起坐骨神经刺激。当大腿伸展并向内侧旋转时，就会产生臀部放射至膝部的疼痛。

脊髓的血液供应通常不稳定，且存在一些重要的变异（图 162.4）。如果血液供应中断，就会对脊髓造成损伤。脊髓由一条脊髓前动脉和两条脊髓后动脉供血。在脊髓的某些部位，有许多来自其他动脉的补充供血，其中之一是 Adamkiewicz 动脉（根大动脉）；这通常起源于 T9 的主动脉，但也可以出现在 T9 和 T12 之间的任何节段。供应下脊髓的动脉通常起源于胸腰椎节段动脉（T9 至 L2）的左侧。因此，这些动脉的损伤可能导致脊髓下段损伤。在大约 15% 的病例中，根大动脉起源于 T5 水平。在这种情况下，下脊髓的主要血液供应是由髂内动脉的腰椎分支提供的，髂内动脉位于骶髂前，通过 L5 ～ S1 椎间孔进入脊髓。胎头压迫此支，可导致脊髓圆锥缺血。此外，由于同一椎间孔较硬的硬膜外导管压迫根大动脉，可能损害脊髓的血液供应，导致脊髓前动脉综合征。常规 MRI 往往无法检测到急性脊髓缺血。超声平面扩散加权 MRI 可用于诊断急性脊髓缺血，硬膜外血肿或脓肿。

启示

局部麻醉药毒性（化学损伤）、直接创伤、硬膜外血肿的缺血性压迫，以及硬膜外脓肿和脑膜炎等

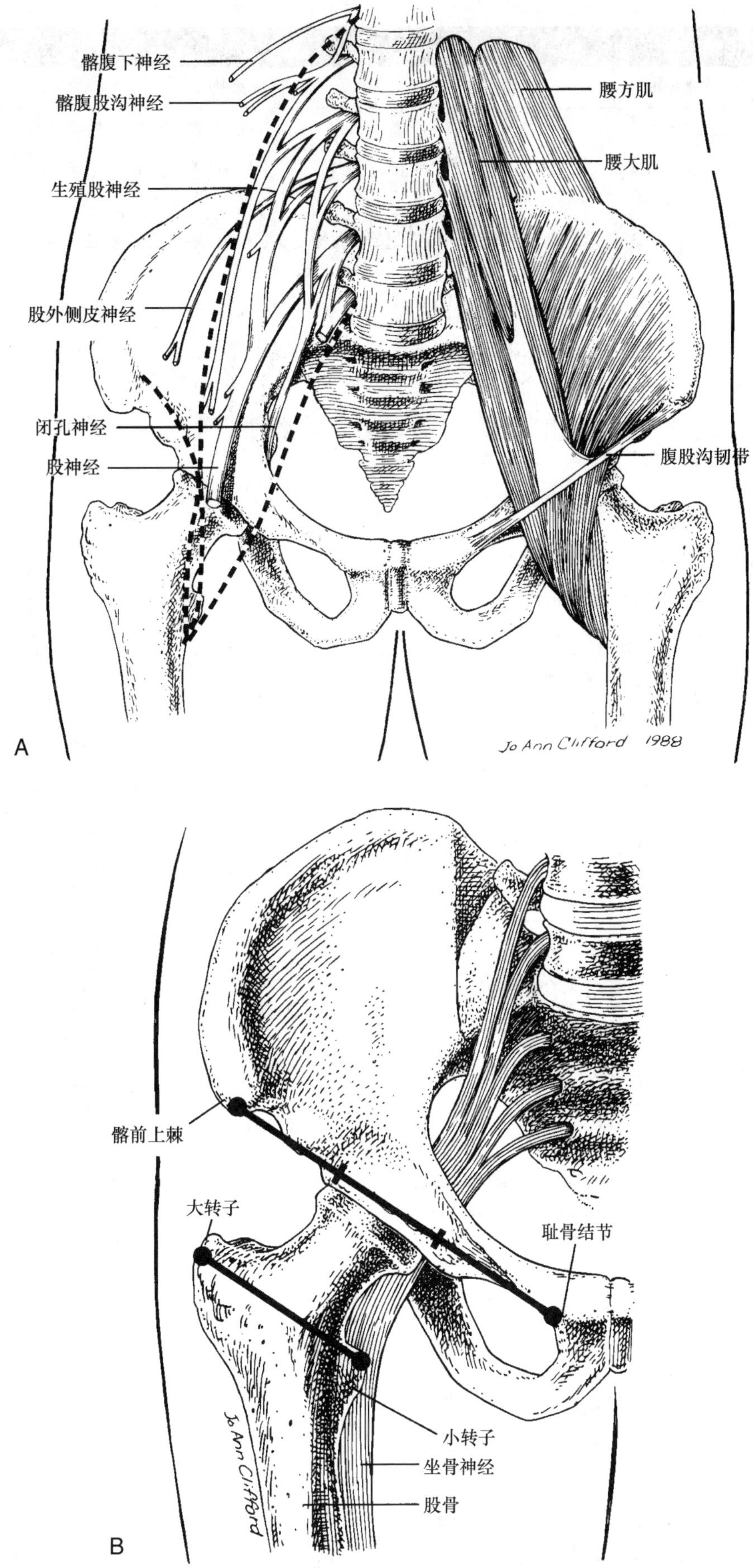

图 162.1　图 A，腰丛来源于 L1 ～ L5 神经根，位于腰大肌和腰方肌之间的腰大肌间隙。**图 B**，骶丛由 L4,L5 和 S1 ～ S3 形成。未显示出的阴部神经和尾神经丛则分别来源于第 3、4 骶神经根的分支以及第 4、5 骶神经和尾神经

表 162.1 产科患者周围神经损伤

神经	神经根	可能的机制	临床表现
腰骶干	L4 ~ L5，S1	产钳伤	足下垂；股四头肌和内收肌受到影响
股神经	L2 ~ L4	胎头；剖宫产时的牵开拉钩	股四头肌无力；髋关节无力；髌骨反射缺失；大腿和小腿感觉受损
股外侧皮神经	L2 ~ L3	产床脚蹬；用力时长时间极度的截石位	大腿前外侧的感觉减退
腓总神经（坐骨神经）[a]	L4 ~ S2	产床脚蹬或床栏	足下垂；小腿外侧和足背部感觉减退
胫骨神经（坐骨神经）	L4 ~ S2	产床脚蹬或床栏	足下垂（腓肠肌和比目鱼肌）；内侧（腓肠肌）分支导致小腿感觉丧失
闭孔神经	L2 ~ L4	胎头	大腿内收肌无力；大腿内侧感觉减退

[a] 由于其位置表浅，容易受到损伤的神经

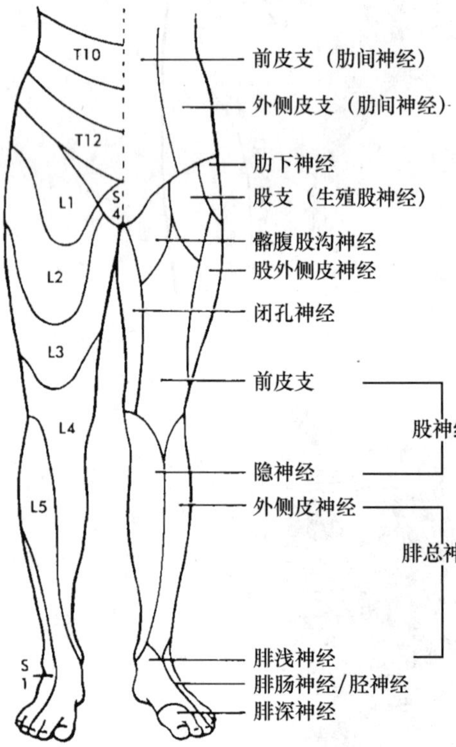

图 162.2 节段性和周围神经分布有助于区分中枢神经损伤和周围神经损伤（From Redick LF：Maternal perinatal nerve palsies. *Postgrad Obstet Gynecol* 12：1-6，1992.）

椎管内感染可能损伤神经组织。

化学损伤

化学损伤通常是由于意外将刺激物注入硬膜外或蛛网膜下腔造成的。防腐剂和亚硫酸氢钠等抗氧化剂与粘连性蛛网膜炎或马尾综合征的发生有关。直接的局部麻醉药毒性会导致任何一种疾病，两者都可以使蛛网膜下腔闭塞。这种毒性被认为是由于局部麻醉药在脑脊液中分布不佳，随后毒性药物浓度在神经根处聚集沉积所致。因此，鞘内注射利多卡因，尤其是 5% 重比重，已经有大量导致马尾综合征的报道。建议鞘内注射利多卡因的上限为 60 mg。对于微导管持续脊椎麻醉也有相关马尾综合征的报道。尽管美国食品药物管理局建议不要常规

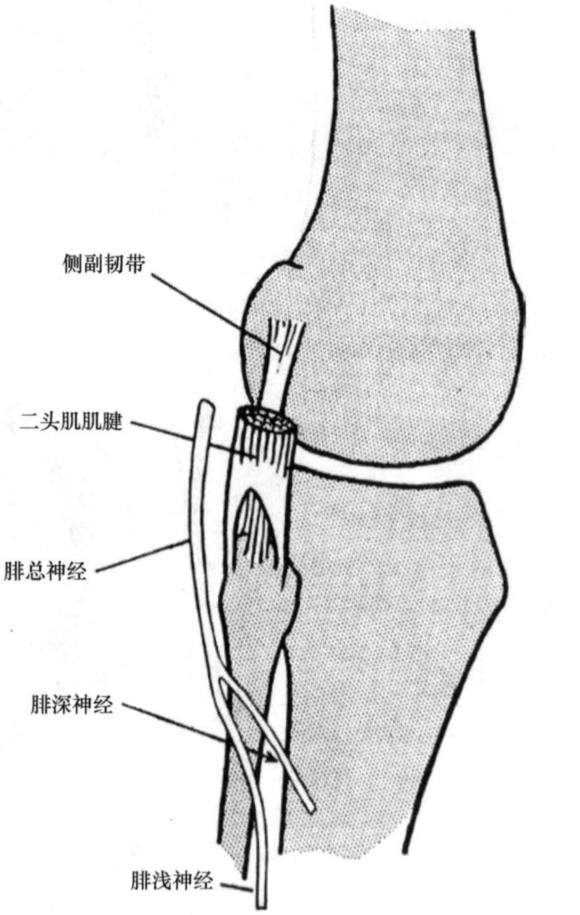

图 162.3 腓总神经的解剖位置使其易受直接压力（例如产床脚蹬）的损伤。这是产妇中最常受损的神经

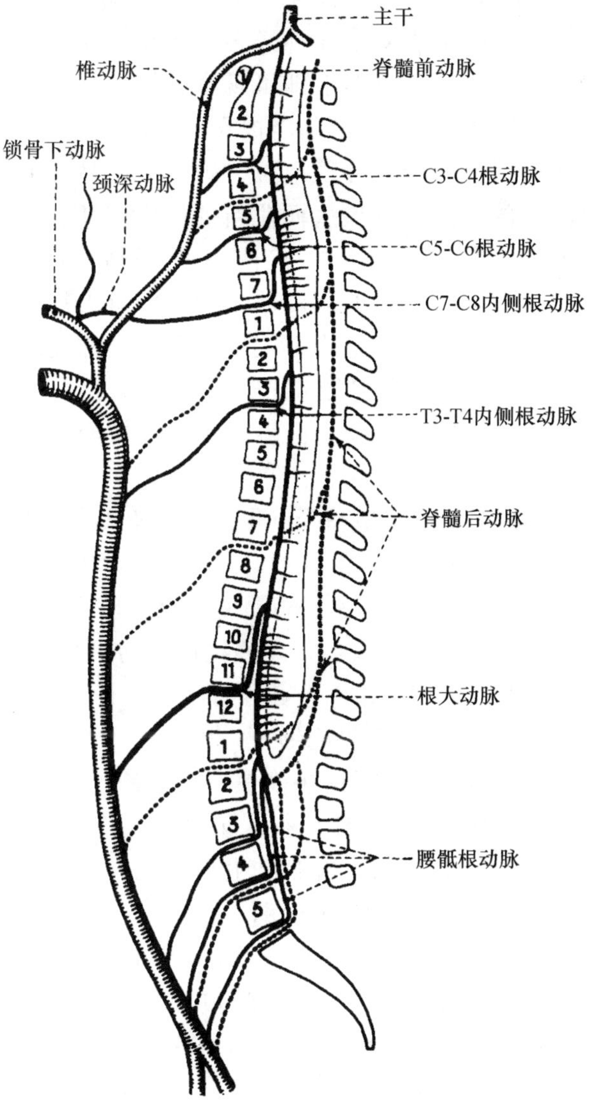

图 162.4　脊髓供血侧视图，展示前、后脊髓神经根的分支。 胸腰椎脊髓段的主要供血是 Adamkiewicz 动脉，如图所示，它起源于 T9，但也可以出现在 T9 和 T12 之间的任何节段。当根大动脉起源较高时，脊髓圆锥主要的血供通常源自腰动脉（From Djindjian R：Arteriography of the spinal cord. *Am J Roentgenol Radium Ther Nucl Med* 107：461-478，1969.）

使用微导管进行蛛网膜下腔连续输注，但大家因评估其在产科麻醉中的效用重新对其产生了兴趣。急性椎间盘突出也可能导致马尾综合征，需要立即手术治疗。

由于有害的鞘内注射引起的另一种类似形式的神经损伤是短暂性神经系统综合征（transient neurologic syndrome，TNS），表现为背部、臀部疼痛，可能还有下肢放射痛。这种并发症的危险因素与马尾综合征类似，但 TNS 在外科手术中比在产科患者中更为常见。

直接神经损伤

局部麻醉时直接神经损伤较少引起神经功能缺损。使用针或导管注射时的疼痛或感觉异常应引起注意。重新定位至关重要。持续硬膜外麻醉的刚性尼龙导管比软尖端导管更容易导致感觉异常。此外，与硬膜外麻醉相比，脊椎麻醉更容易导致神经损伤。如果在椎管内神经阻滞期间出现感觉异常，麻醉科医师应记录感觉异常的严重程度和位置。若症状持续时间较长，且分布有多个脊髓节段，则可能是脊髓直接损伤的征兆。由于在椎管内神经阻滞期间发生直接神经损伤，从神经病变中完全恢复可能需要 48 h 至 3 个月。

对神经组织的直接损伤可能发生在脊髓、神经根或周围神经的水平。硬膜外针或导管更容易损伤神经根。蛛网膜下腔穿刺针可损伤蛛网膜下腔内的神经根或脊髓本身以及蛛网膜下腔外的神经根。2/3 的神经后遗症发生在感觉异常（直接神经损伤）或注射过程中的疼痛（神经内注射）之前。神经内注射局部麻醉药更容易导致长期的神经功能缺损。在一系列超过 10.3 万的区域麻醉案例中，34 例患者出现神经系统后遗症，其中 29 例为短暂性神经功能缺陷，神经功能在 48 h 至 3 个月间完全恢复。有趣的是，脊椎麻醉明显比硬膜外麻醉更容易引起神经损伤（5.9/10 000 vs. 2/10 000）或神经根病变（4.7/10 000 vs.1.7/10 000）。脊椎麻醉过程中脊髓圆锥的损伤可能与对腰椎间隙的定位不准确或脊髓异常长有关。对于病态肥胖的人来说，以 Tuffier 线水平作为体表标志线可能难以触及，会导致定位不确切。因此，利用超声椎管内定位可以提高椎间隙识别的准确性。

轻度神经损伤时，传导阻滞仅发生在受损的神经段（即神经麻痹）。如果情况得到纠正，神经功能便得以恢复。但是，必须告知患者，根据最初症状的严重程度，恢复可能需要数周。严重损伤会导致轴突变性（轴突断伤），永远不会完全恢复，受损区域功能完全或部分丧失。神经断伤意味着神经外膜的破坏。手术修复是必要的，但神经功能不可能完全恢复。

感染

感染相关并发症包括硬膜外脓肿和脑膜炎。Green 和 Paech 在一项回顾性研究中发现，与硬膜外导管相关的深部组织感染发生率为1/2371，而产科患者在CSE和腰麻后发生脑膜炎的概率为1/39 000。硬膜外脓肿的症状通常开始于硬膜外导管拔除后4～10天，如果不及时治疗，可能最终导致马尾综合征。较轻的症状可以用抗生素保守治疗，但完全引流脓肿可能需要手术干预。脑膜炎症状可能在产后12 h至数天就会出现，在微生物培养结果出来之前应开始抗生素治疗。合理的治疗通常能促进患者完全康复。

脊髓血肿

脊髓血肿（硬膜外血肿、硬膜下血肿、蛛网膜下血肿）作为占位性病变，可压迫附近的神经和血管结构，导致缺血。尽管在产科人群中椎管内血肿的发生率非常罕见，但如果神经系统检查考虑椎管内血肿，则应立即寻求进一步的影像学检查。在症状出现后，手术减压延迟超过6～12 h可能导致永久性残疾（更多详见第179章）。

管理

当患者出现产后神经系统问题时，必须警惕其他原因，包括糖尿病、获得性免疫缺陷综合征（艾滋病）和多发性硬化症。尽管糖尿病性神经病变众所周知，但艾滋病相关的神经病变知之甚少，尽管其是1型艾滋病毒感染和晚期艾滋病最常见的神经并发症，表现为远端对称性多发性神经病变，主要发生于免疫抑制晚期。患有晚期艾滋病的产妇人数正在增加，一些抗逆转录病毒的药物也可能导致神经毒性。进行性多发性神经根病变发生于免疫抑制晚期，通常由巨细胞病毒感染引起。

在初步评估中，麻醉科医师应记录所有的感觉和运动缺陷，并请熟悉产科神经损伤的神经学专家会诊。其他影像学检查行包括计算机断层扫描或MRI扫描等，这些必须立即实施，不可延误。如果需要紧急行椎板切除术以避免永久性神经损伤，则应立即请外科会诊。

进一步的神经肌肉电生理检查包括肌电图（electromyography，EMG）和神经传导检查。肌电图对周围神经损伤程度的诊断非常有用；然而，时机非常关键。在静息肌肉中出现异常自发活动（纤颤电位）或在记录针插入肌肉时活动增加（插入活动）通常表明存在神经系统疾病。在神经受损后数天内，肌电图上即可观察到插入活动，而纤颤电位则需2～4周才能被测出。如果在所谓的损伤后很快记录到纤颤电位，则更可能是先前未诊断出的神经系统疾病而非新的损伤。神经损伤的另一个肌电图征象是，当肌肉受到刺激时，肌电图无法募集更多的运动单位。在完全去神经支配的肌肉中，不发生再募集。然而，当神经受到损伤时，由于传导速度减慢，就会发生部分的再募集。肌电图也有助于区分是否存在神经丛或神经根病变。

根据损伤的类型和严重程度，神经系统损伤完全恢复可能需要长达8周的时间。为了评估损伤的进展或消退，需要经常进行重复的电生理检查。此外，需要请理疗师会诊，以确定最佳的康复方案，以防止肌肉萎缩。如果患者有明显的足下垂，可能需要夹板来防止永久性畸形。

病例概要中描述的患者具有广泛的神经损伤，表明腰骶神经丛或脊髓受损。肠道或膀胱功能障碍通常提示脊髓损伤。虽然电生理学检查表明存在脊髓根部或更高水平的病变，但分娩2 d后脊髓的MRI扫描显示正常。然而，1周后进行的增强MRI与脊髓缺血情况保持一致。这很可能是由于骶骨水平的腰椎动脉受压所致。框162.1列出了产妇长期神经功能缺失的其他潜在原因。

预防

对于患有系统性疾病的产妇，麻醉科医师应全面记录任何既往的神经功能病变，以避免潜在的医学法律问题。多发性硬化症尤其容易在产后复发。对于有凝血障碍危险因素的患者，应在置入和拔除硬膜外导管时检查凝血状态。在预防感染性并发症方面，椎管内技术相关的感染性并发症ASA工作组的2010年的实务公告为预防和管理提供了循证建议。此外，分娩室的麻醉从业人员必须确保患者在被送至产后病房前已经完全从区域阻滞麻醉中恢复。如果患者在麻醉后感觉和运动完全恢复后出现神经功能缺损，则与椎管阻滞或与阻滞药物的相关性不大。

框 162.1 神经阻滞延长的鉴别诊断

药物作用
局部麻醉药作用时间长
　阻滞作用减退缓慢
　多次给药后更常见
　在局部麻醉注射期间，针或导管尖端靠近神经根
直接神经毒性
　常用药物的罕见效果（如 5% 重比重利多卡因）
　用药不当（如氯化钾）

外伤
周围神经
　体位不当造成的神经压迫
　已知的周围神经模式
椎管内神经
　由针或导管引起的神经组织的直接创伤
神经根或脊髓的外部压迫
　椎间盘突出
　硬膜外血肿（早期）
　硬膜外脓肿（晚期）
　椎管狭窄

血管
出血——脊髓动静脉畸形
血液供应减少——没有恢复的证据；永久性伤害
脊髓前动脉综合征
　胎头压迫动脉血供
　严重的低血压
心脏骤停后
　栓子（例如空气、血栓、羊水）

神经系统疾病（原有或新发）
多发性硬化症
HIV，免疫抑制治疗
巨细胞病毒
Landry-Guillain-Barré 综合征

其他原因
占位性病变
　硬膜外血肿
　硬膜外脓肿

致谢

感谢 Zakowski、Vallejo 和 Ra-manathan 博士对本章上一版的贡献。

（叶偲敏　译　卜　岚　校）

延伸阅读

American Society of Anesthesiologists Task Force on Infectious Complications Associated with Neuraxial Techniques: Practice advisory for the prevention, diagnosis, and management of infectious complications associated with neuraxial techniques, *Anesthesiology* 112:530–545, 2010.

Aminoff MJ: Electrophysiologic testing for the diagnosis of peripheral nerve injuries, *Anesthesiology* 100:1298–1303, 2004.

Auroy Y, Benhamou D, Bargues L, et al.: Major complications of regional anesthesia in France: the SOS regional anesthesia hotline service, *Anesthesiology* 97:1274–1280, 2002.

Biglioli P, Roberto M, Cannata A, et al.: Upper and lower spinal cord blood supply: the continuity of the anterior spinal artery and the relevance of the lumber arteries, *J Thorac Cardiovasc Surg* 127:1188–1192, 2004.

Bromage PR: Neurologic complications of regional anesthesia in obstetrics. In Hughes SC, Levinson G, Rosen MA, editors: *Obstetric anesthesia*, ed 2, Philadelphia, 1999, JB Lippincott–Williams & Wilkins, pp 723–748.

Confavreux C, Hutchinson M, Hours MM, et al.: Rate of pregnancy-related relapse in multiple sclerosis: pregnancy in Multiple Sclerosis Group, *N Engl J Med* 339:285–291, 1998.

Cook TM, Counsell D, Wildsmith JA: Royal College of Anaesthetists Third National Audit Project: Major complications of central neuraxial block: report on the Third National Audit Project of the Royal College of Anaesthetists, *Br J Anaesth* 102:179–190, 2009.

Faccenda KA, Finucane BT: Complications of regional anaesthesia: incidence and prevention, *Drug Saf* 24:413–442, 2001.

Gray H: *Gray's anatomy*, ed 27, Philadelphia, 1959, Lea & Febiger, pp 1036–1057.

Green LK, Paech MJ: Obstetric epidural catheter-related infections at a major teaching hospital: a retrospective case series, *Int J Obstet Anesth* 19:38–43, 2010.

Jaime F, Mandell GL, Vallejo MC, et al.: Uniport soft-tip, open-ended catheters versus multiport firm-tipped close-ended catheters for epidural labor analgesia: a quality assurance study, *J Clin Anesth* 12:89–93, 2000.

Kuczkowski KM: Neurologic complications of labor analgesia: facts and fiction, *Obstet Gynecol Surv* 59:47–51, 2004.

Lee LA, Posner KL, Domino KB, et al.: Injuries associated with regional anesthesia in the 1980s and 1990s: a closed claim analysis, *Anesthesiology* 101:143–152, 2004.

Loher TJ, Bassetti CL, Lovblad KO, et al.: Diffusion-weighted MRI in acute spinal cord ischemia, *Neuroradiology* 45:557–561, 2003.

Reynolds F: Neurologic complications of pregnancy and neuraxial anesthesia. In Chestnut DH, Wong CA, Tsen LC, et al.: *Chestnut's obstetric anesthesia: principles and practice*, ed 5, Philadelphia, 2014, Elsevier, pp 739–784.

Ruppen W, Derry S, McQuay H, et al.: Incidence of epidural hematoma, infection, and neurologic injury in obstetric patients with epidural analgesia/anesthesia, *Anesthesiology* 105:394–399, 2006.

Vallejo M, Mariano D, Kaul B, et al.: Piriformis syndrome in a patient after cesarean section under spinal anesthesia, *Reg Anesth Pain Med* 29:364–367, 2004.

Wedel DJ, Horlocker TT: Nerve blocks. In Miller RD, editor: *Miller's anesthesia*, ed 6, Philadelphia, 2005, Churchill Livingstone, pp 1685–1717.

Wlody D: Complications of regional anesthesia in obstetrics, *Clin Obstet Gynecol* 46:667–678, 2003.

Wong CA, Scavone BM, Dugan S, et al.: Incidence of postpartum lumbosacral spine and lower extremity nerve injuries, *Obstet Gynecol* 101:279–288, 2003.

Wulff EA, Wang AK, Simpson DM: HIV-associated peripheral neuropathy: epidemiology, pathophysiology and treatment, *Drugs* 59:1251–1260, 2000.

Zakowski MI: Complications associated with regional anesthesia in the obstetric patient, *Semin Perinatol* 26:154–168, 2002.

第163章 持续性感觉异常

Miguel A. Yaport，Ignacio Badiola

病例概要

患者，女性，63岁，乳腺癌化疗后，拟行左侧腕掌关节成形术。麻醉方式为锁骨下臂丛神经阻滞，给予0.5%罗哌卡因30 ml。术后随访发现，患者主诉手外侧出现麻木症状。术后12周行肌电图和神经传导功能检查提示，左上肢感觉运动混合性神经元病变。随着时间推移，患者症状有所改善，直至5个月后症状完全消失。

问题分析

定义

区域阻滞麻醉存在神经损伤的潜在风险。虽然总体认为区域麻醉比较安全，但也有出现严重或灾难性并发症的报道。Cheney等利用美国麻醉科医师协会终审索赔数据库，回顾分析并评估围术期麻醉操作不当致神经损伤的相关索赔事件。在4183例索赔案例中，有670例与麻醉导致的神经损伤有关。常见损伤包括尺神经、臂丛、腰骶神经根和脊髓。

现有数据愈发强烈地显示，围术期神经系统损伤继发于其他原因，而非区域麻醉所致。Horlocker等报道了1614例腋路臂丛神经阻滞的上肢手术中发生61例神经损伤，其中7例由麻醉所致，54例由手术所致。Brull等回顾过去10年区域麻醉致神经系统并发症的32项调查研究，估算得出外周神经阻滞相关神经损伤风险约为3%。与椎管内麻醉有关的神经损伤，虽然在并发症方面比较严重，但风险较低，据估计发生率不到万分之四。

识别

持续性感觉异常是指神经阻滞后区域麻醉不完全消退，或术后出现无力和（或）感觉异常等新的神经病理症状。这些症状平均持续时间通常为2～4个月。其他更严重并发症包括永久性神经损伤，罕见的如完全性肢体功能丧失或严重脊髓损伤。围术期神经系统并发症可能与手术创伤造成的神经损伤、患者体位、长时间使用止血带造成的缺血以及石膏/敷料造成的压迫有关。虽然持续性感觉异常发生于区域麻醉阻滞后，但上述原因显然与区域麻醉无关。直接由区域麻醉导致的损伤，可能由阻滞针或神经周围导管所引起的神经损伤、局部麻醉药/辅助药物的神经毒性和（或）神经缺血。

风险评估

持续性感觉异常的危险因素包括手术本身、患者并存疾病、药物和麻醉相关因素。

暴露、体位和手术入路等手术相关因素与损伤风险相关。肩关节镜检查为改善术野暴露会采用外科牵引，损伤风险为0.1%～10%。使用“candy-cane stirrups”（译者注：一种牵引器械）的膝关节镜手术常与腓神经损伤有关。经前路全髋关节置换术造成股外侧皮神经损伤的风险明显高于后路。

数项患者因素与实施区域麻醉后发生围术期并发症的风险有关。椎管内病变，如椎管狭窄、神经根管异常和肿块占位等病变，与椎管内麻醉后神经损伤的高风险相关。伴有Guillain-Barré综合征、重症肌无力等原有神经功能障碍疾病的患者，在实施椎管内麻醉或外周神经阻滞麻醉后更容易出现神经损伤。已有神经系统疾病的患者，由于局部麻醉药的神经毒性效应或直接针刺损伤，也更容易发生神经损伤。这种“双重打击”伤，是指先前已异常的神经系统遭受第二次“打击”而导致的更严重结果。患者服用的药物也可能与外周神经损伤有关。抗凝治疗所带来的损伤风险为 1/15 000 ～ 1/4000。同样，可产生神经毒性的化疗药物（顺铂、长春新碱、紫杉醇等）、神经血管性疾病、高血压和糖尿病也会增加患者神经损伤风险。糖尿病患者神经损伤风险可能至少是普通人群的 10 倍。糖尿病等罹患微血管病变的患者，神经血流供应减少，进而对区域麻醉药的摄取减少、清除能力降低。因此，对存在周围神经病变的患者，应减少神经阻滞和毒性局部麻醉药的用量。综上所述，这些患者对局部麻醉药更为敏感。

大量数据表明，由神经阻滞本身导致的围术期神经损伤并不常见，但麻醉科医师在实施可能增加神经损伤风险的阻滞时，仍须作出一些选择。局部麻醉药、血管收缩剂及注射剂量可能与直接的神经毒性或缺血风险增加有关。然而，目前还没有令人信服的证据来支持某一具体做法。局部麻醉药可能直接有神经毒性作用。有证据表明，利多卡因和丁卡因等药物可能比布比卡因更具有神经毒性。肾上腺素和碳酸氢盐等辅助药物也可能增强局部麻醉药的毒性。

神经内即使注射了小量的局部麻醉药也会明显增加压力，进而超过血流灌注压力而导致神经缺血。最后，对患有微血管疾病或神经组织已受损的患者，当使用含有肾上腺素的药液时，理论上会导致血流进一步减少，可能造成局部神经缺血。

技术的选择也会影响风险。Moayeri 等提出，神经近端比远端包含更多的神经组织（远端包含更多的结缔组织），在考虑外周神经阻滞时，近端神经阻滞可能比远端更具风险。对椎管内麻醉而言，硬膜外比蛛网膜下腔穿刺有更高的血肿风险。

实施神经阻滞麻醉时诱发的异感，可能表示出现直接的针刺损伤，增加持续性感觉异常的风险。Selander 等报道了一组差异无统计学意义的研究数据：腋路臂丛神经阻滞穿刺中出现异感的患者，术后神经损伤的发生率为 2.8%，而采用血管旁穿刺技术的患者，其发生率为 0.8%。

Liguori 等比较了针刺异感引导和神经刺激仪引导技术在肌间沟臂丛神经阻滞中的作用，发现两者在导致神经损伤症状上没有差异。同样，超声引导目前也并不比周围神经刺激引导更能降低神经损伤风险。Orebaugh 等评估了两种不同技术导致的不良事件，结果表明超声技术可降低局部麻醉药中毒的发生率，但在神经损伤发生率方面没有差异。超声引导理论上具有优势，但也可能与麻醉科医师试图将神经阻滞针更为靠近神经，意外注射至神经外膜下的风险增加有关，而这种操作趋势可能引起不必要的危险。因有研究表明，在臂丛附近而非筋膜鞘内注射局部麻醉药，可产生等效的神经阻滞效果。

最后，留置导管也可能与损伤并发症有关。损伤通常来自于直接的神经损伤、感染、意外的血管穿刺和血肿形成，或需要手术切开取出的残留导管碎片。幸运的是，后遗症比较罕见。虽然细菌定植率高达 57%，但感染率不到 3.2%。在导管留置过程中刺破血管的发生率为 6%。

启示

最初 24 h 内出现的神经系统受损，与 24 h 后再出现的情况，在病因上可能存在不同。即刻出现症状的原因包括神经内水肿或血肿，或真正的神经损伤。而后期出现的症状可能是神经周围瘢痕形成等其他原因所致。

围术期炎症性神经损伤受到越来越多的关注，其特点是发病延迟，可在 30 天内出现，早期可存在一段无症状期。患者会在术后经历一段时间的剧烈疼痛，通常与手术创伤不成比例。疼痛可能自行消失，随后会出现无力。

患者出院后也需要关注。据报道，在接受下肢关节置换术的患者中，直至出院时还没有进行日间手术后随访以及识别延迟的比例高达 90%。识别延迟常与神经损伤的非手术原因相关，如制动、敷料压迫、感染或炎症。

管理

虽然区域麻醉后发生神经损伤并不常见，但一旦发生对患者来说可能具有毁灭性影响，甚至从此改变生活。在神经阻滞实施前就应该开始进行管理。必须全面了解病史，进行体格检查，重点是神经功能。应该告知，患有神经系统疾病者并发症风险可能更高，或加重其潜在疾病，导致神经功能障碍。在这些患者中，与记录术前功能相比，完整的术前评估显得更为重要。然而，稳定的基础病情不是使用区域麻醉的绝对禁忌证。和医学上的其他情形一样，我们需要权衡利与弊。

预防

预防神经损伤和持续性感觉异常的要点包括选择合适的患者，避免直接针刺伤及神经和神经内注射，使用适当浓度的局部麻醉药，以及对术后新发或恶化的神经病变进行快速评估。

术后出现神经功能障碍的患者应尽快进行评估，并采取多学科联合的管理方法。

越来越多的证据表明，患者预后受不同医院系统的独立影响。如果医院采取保持警惕和循证的管理方法，则患者可获得快速诊断和早期治疗。这意味着，医院开发评估和危险因素分层系统并实施诊断和治疗途径，可以降低损伤发生率并改善患者预后。

致谢

感谢 Horlocker 博士对本章上一版的贡献。

（钱晓春　译　陈　辉　校）

延伸阅读

Auroy Y, Benhamou D, Bargues L, et al.: Major complications of regional anesthesia in France: the SOS Regional Anesthesia Hotline Service, *Anesthesiology* 97(5):1274–1280, 2002.

Auroy Y, Narchi P, Messiah A, et al.: Serious complications related to regional anesthesia: results of a prospective survey in France, *Anesthesiology* 87:479–486, 1997.

Barrington MJ, Watts SA, Gledhill SR, et al.: Preliminary results of the Australasian Regional Anaesthesia Collaboration: a prospective audit of more than 7000 peripheral nerve and plexus blocks for neurologic and other complications, *Reg Anesth Pain Med* 34(6):534–541, 2009.

Bergman BD, Hebl JR, Kent J, et al.: Neurologic complications of 405 consecutive continuous axillary catheters, *Anesth Analg* 96:247–252, 2003.

Brull R, McCartney CJ, Chan VW, et al.: Neurological complications after regional anesthesia: contemporary estimates of risk, *Anesth Analg* 104(4):965–974, 2007.

Capdevila X, Bringuier S, Borgeat A: Infectious risk of continuous peripheral nerve blocks, *Anesthesiology* 110:182–188, 2009.

Capdevila X, Pirat P, Bringuier S, et al.: Continuous peripheral nerve blocks in hospital wards after orthopedic surgery: a multicenter prospective analysis of the quality of postoperative analgesia and complications in 1,416 patients, *Anesthesiology* 103(5):1035–1045, 2005.

Cheney FW, Domino KB, Caplan RA, et al.: Nerve injury associated with anesthesia: a closed claims analysis, *Anesthesiology* 90:1062–1069, 1999.

Fanelli G, Casati A, Garancini P, et al.: Nerve stimulator and multiple injection technique for upper and lower limb blockade: failure rate, patient acceptance, and neurologic complications, *Anesth Analg* 88:847–852, 1999.

Goldberg ME, Gregg C, Larijani GE, et al.: A comparison of three methods of axillary approach to brachial plexus blockade for upper extremity surgery, *Anesthesiology* 66(6):814–816, 1987.

Hadzic A, Vloka J, Hadzic N, et al.: Nerve stimulators used for peripheral nerve blocks vary in their electrical characteristics, *Anesthesiology* 98:969–974, 2003.

Hogan QH: Pathophysiology of peripheral nerve injury during regional anesthesia, *Reg Anesth Pain Med* 33(5):435–441, 2008.

Horlocker TT, Kufner RP, Bishop AT, et al.: The risk of persistent paresthesia is not increased with repeated axillary block, *Anesth Analg* 88:382–387, 1999.

Jacob AK, Mantilla CB, Sviggum HP, et al.: Perioperative nerve injury after total knee arthroplasty: regional anesthesia risk during a 20-year cohort study, *Anesthesiology* 114(2):311–317, 2011.

Jacob AK, Mantilla CB, Sviggum HP, et al.: Perioperative nerve injury after total hip arthroplasty: regional anesthesia risk during a 20-year cohort study, *Anesthesiology* 115(6):1172–1178, 2011.

Kalichman MW, Calcutt NA: Local anesthetic-induced conduction block and nerve fiber injury in streptozotocin-diabetic rats, *Anesthesiology* 77:941–947, 1992.

Kopp SL, Jacob AK, Hebl JR: Regional anesthesia in patients with preexisting neurologic disease, *Reg Anesth Pain Med* 40(5):467–478, 2015.

Liguori GA, Zayas VM, YaDeau JT, et al.: Nerve localization techniques for interscalene brachial plexus blockade: a prospective, randomized comparison of mechanical paresthesia versus electrical stimulation, *Anesth Analg* 103(3):761–767, 2006.

Moayeri N, Bigeleisen PE, Groen GJ: Quantitative architecture of the brachial plexus and surrounding compartments, and their possible significance for plexus blocks, *Anesthesiology* 108(2):299–304, 2008.

Neal JM: Effects of epinephrine in local anesthetics on the central and peripheral nervous systems: neurotoxicity and neural blood flow, *Reg Anesth Pain Med* 28:124–134, 2003.

Neal JM, Barrington MJ, Brull R, et al.: The second ASRA practice advisory on neurologic complications associated with regional anesthesia and pain medicine: executive summary 2015, *Reg Anesth Pain Med* 40(5):401–430, 2015.

Neal JM, Hebl JR, Gerancher JC, et al.: Brachial plexus anesthesia: Essentials of our current understanding, *Reg Anesth Pain Med* 27:402–428, 2002.

Orebaugh SL, Kentor ML, Williams BA: Adverse outcomes associated with nerve stimulator-guided and ultrasound-guided peripheral nerve blocks by supervised trainees: update of a single-site database, *Reg Anesth Pain Med* 37(6):577–582, 2012.

Rice ASC, McMahon SB: Peripheral nerve injury caused by injection needles used in regional anaesthesia: influence of bevel configuration, studied in a rat model, *Br J Anaesth* 69:433–438, 1992.

Selander D, Dhuner KG, Lundborg G: Peripheral nerve injury due to injection needles used for regional anesthesia, *Acta Anaesthesiol Scand* 21:182–188, 1977.

Selander D, Edshage S, Wolff T: Paresthesiae or no paresthesiae? *Acta Anaesthesiol Scand* 23:27–33, 1979.

Selander D, Sjostrang J: Longitudinal spread of intraneurally injected local anesthetics, *Acta Anaesthesiol Scand* 22:622–634, 1978.

Spence BC, Beach ML, Gallagher JD, Sites BD: Ultrasound-guided interscalene blocks: understanding where to inject the local anaesthetic, *Anaesthesia* 66(6):509–514, 2011.

Stan TC, Krantz MA, Solomon DL, et al.: The incidence of neurovascular complications following axillary brachial plexus block using a transarterial approach: a prospective study of 1000 consecutive patients, *Reg Anesth* 20:486–492, 1995.

Verlinde M, Hollmann MW, Stevens MF, et al.: Local anesthetic-induced neurotoxicity, *Int J Mol Sci* 17(3):339, 2016.

Weeks L, Barry A, Wolff T, et al.: Regional anaesthesia and subsequent long-term pain, *J Hand Surg Br* 19(3):342–346, 1994.

Welch MB, Brummett CM, Welch TD, et al.: Perioperative peripheral nerve injuries: a retrospective study of 380,680 cases during a 10-year period at a single institution, *Anesthesiology* 111(3):490–497, 2009.

Wiegel M, Gottschaldt U, Hennebach R, et al.: Complications and adverse effects associated with continuous peripheral nerve blocks in orthopedic patients, *Anesth Analg* 104:1578–1582, 2007.

Winfree CJ, Kline DG: Intraoperative positioning nerve injuries, *Surg Neurol* 63(1):5–18, 2005.

梗阻后肺水肿

第 164 章

Katarzyna Luba

病例概要

患者，男性，37 岁，体重 77 kg，既往体健，在全身麻醉下行眶底骨折修复术。患者术中平稳，气管拔管后即刻发生喉痉挛。在尝试球囊面罩正压通气失败后，静脉注射琥珀胆碱控制喉痉挛。15 min 后，患者自主呼吸，潮气量充足，但患者咳嗽，鼻导管吸氧条件下氧饱和度为 92%，心率 110 次 / 分。肺部听诊显示弥漫性粗啰音。胸部 X 线片提示急性双侧肺水肿，心脏轮廓正常。

问题分析

定义

梗阻后肺水肿（postobstruction pulmonary edema，POPE），又称负压性肺水肿，是一种非心源性肺水肿，在急性上呼吸道梗阻（1 型 POPE）后或慢性部分气道梗阻（2 型 POPE）缓解后立即发生。

1 型 POPE 是因尝试用力吸气对抗闭合的声门（Mueller 检查法）或其他方式阻塞上呼吸道而产生。年轻、健康患者可产生吸气负压（negative inspiratory pressure，NIP），其最大水平为 −140 cmH_2O。NIP 持续极度升高可增加静脉回流、肺血流量和毛细血管压力，并降低肺间质压力。与此同时，气道梗阻相关的高肾上腺素能状态，引起外周血管收缩，进一步增加静脉回流和肺血流量。右心室扩张及体循环阻力增加共同抑制左心室射血，并使左心室舒张压、左心房压力和肺静脉压升高，进而使肺毛细血管静水压升高。跨毛细血管静水压梯度的增加有利于流体从肺毛细血管渗透到间质中。肺淋巴系统的清除能力最终不堪重负，导致间质性和肺泡内肺水肿。

2 型 POPE 可能与慢性气道梗阻的突然缓解有关。部分气道慢性梗阻时伴有内源性呼气末正压（positive end-expiratory pressure，PEEP）和胸腔内压的慢性升高。梗阻的缓解导致胸膜腔内压急剧下降，静脉回流和肺血流量增加。由此产生的肺毛细血管和间质之间的流体力学失衡，将使急性肺水肿形成，其机制类似于 1 型 POPE 所假设的机制。

识别

当慢性或急性气道梗阻缓解后迅速出现呼吸窘迫为主的急性肺水肿的临床特征时，便可能诊断 POPE。其临床表现包括躁动、心动过速、呼吸急促、咳嗽、弥漫性湿啰音和干啰音，以及缺氧。气管插管后才能观察到典型肺水肿的表现，即粉红色泡沫样分泌物。胸片显示双侧肺门周围斑片状浸润影（图 164.1）。POPE 通常即刻发病，也有报道称其延迟至 24 h，故在发生气道梗阻后需要延长观察时间。

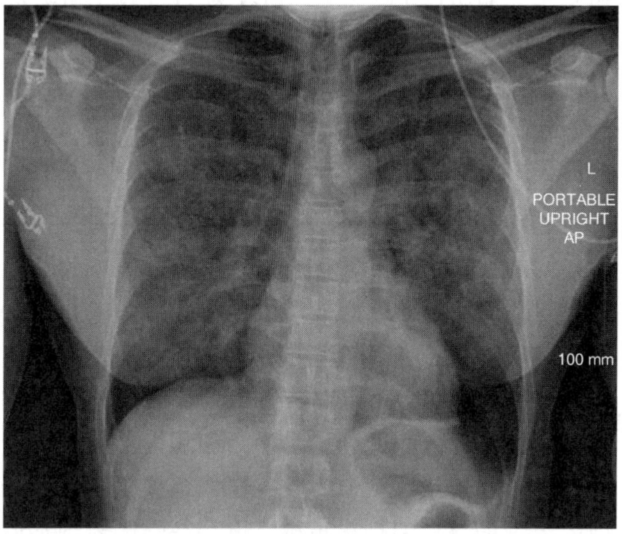

图 164.1　阻塞后肺水肿的胸片表现

可能导致2型POPE发生的外科手术包括，腺样体切除术/扁桃体切除术、巨大甲状腺肿物切除术或上呼吸道肿瘤切除术。1型POPE见于多种临床情况，如气道异物窒息、压迫、悬吊、会厌炎、喉炎、气管导管阻塞、术后声带麻痹、困难插管或在肌松残余下过早拔管。但成人围术期POPE最常见原因是喉痉挛。喉痉挛可能发生在麻醉诱导期间、拔管后即刻或在未采取气道保护的麻醉期间。

围术期急性呼吸窘迫原因的鉴别诊断，应包括误吸、过敏反应、容量超负荷、肺栓塞，以及心源性或神经源性肺水肿。回顾患者的既往史和导致呼吸窘迫发作的一系列事件，可能有助于明确诊断。由喉痉挛或其他原因导致的气道阻塞，伴随着剧烈的用力吸气，故POPE成为最可能的诊断。可能需要超声心动图、有创血流动力学监测或两者同时，以排除其他原因，尤其是心源性肺水肿、液体超负荷或肺栓塞。POPE患者在缓解上呼吸道阻塞后通常显示正常的血流动力学参数。POPE还可能伴有引起呼吸窘迫或衰竭的其他原因（如误吸或残余肌松）。

风险评估

任何急性气道阻塞或严重慢性气道损害缓解后都可能发展为POPE。然而，该并发症更可能发生于年轻、健康的成年人或儿童。这类患者更容易发生喉痉挛，并能产生足以对抗上呼吸道梗阻的极大胸腔内负压。因上呼吸道梗阻而需紧急插管的成人和儿童患者，POPE发生率估计为11%～12%。成人患者中，麻醉后出现喉痉挛是POPE最常见原因，占报道病例的50%。在10岁以下儿童中，50%以上的POPE病例与喉炎和会厌炎有关。

启示

POPE是一种常发生于健康儿童或青年的常见并发症。应在短时间内及早识别和恰当处理POPE，患者症状常在24 h内缓解而不产生进一步后果。但在POPE急性期，患者存在显著的病残风险，严重时可危及生命。因此，尽早诊断和积极治疗至关重要。呼吸窘迫或衰竭通常在急性气道梗阻发作数分钟内表现明显。但据报道称，也存在临床表现延迟达24 h的病例。因此，有必要对发生急性气道梗阻的任何患者进行长期观察，门诊发生气道阻塞时应收治入院。

管理

POPE以支持治疗为主，POPE 1型和2型的临床处理类似。保持呼吸道通畅、吸氧和气道正压通气是主要措施。维持气道的方法和气道正压通气的方式取决于肺水肿严重程度、缺氧和呼吸窘迫程度、患者精神状态以及是否有麻醉残余。大多数患者（近85%）需要气管插管或再插管，其中一半患者需要机械通气，其余患者可采用无创正压通气治疗。通常，机械通气或持续气道正压通气患者使用PEEP可迅速缓解肺水肿。利尿剂常被使用，但其使用存在争议；利尿剂在POPE中的应用缺乏证据，且可能导致低血容量和终末器官灌注不足。轻度POPE患者可能仅需吸氧。轻度且治疗及时的POPE可在12～48 h内缓解，严重者尤其是需转入ICU治疗的患者，可能需要数天才能完全康复。

预防

大多数POPE由意外的急性上呼吸道阻塞引起。某些临床情况下POPE发生风险更高。对POPE保持警惕，并预测发生气道阻塞和POPE的可能性，可提前做好准备并采取预防措施。

任何气道操作，例如球囊面罩通气、放置口咽或鼻咽通气道、口咽吸痰、置入声门上通气装置（supraglottic airway，SGA）以及喉镜检查和插管等，如果在浅麻醉下进行操作，可能导致喉痉挛。因此，上述操作均应在足够麻醉深度下进行。SGA管理的气道或气道未受保护的患者，浅麻醉下的气道或手术操作可能导致喉痉挛，前述预防措施也适用。拔除气管导管或SGA应在深麻醉或患者完全清醒时进行。患者麻醉苏醒前放置牙垫可防止咬合引起气管导管阻塞。儿童、青少年和年轻健康的成年人发生喉痉挛和POPE的风险更高。肌松残余可能会影响气管拔管后的气道通畅，但患者仍可用力呼吸对抗梗阻气道。对已知或怀疑存在困难气道的患者，应考虑清醒气管插管，以避免在麻醉诱导期间发生插管失败和灾难性气道梗阻。清醒气管插管本身可能会诱发喉痉挛和 POPE。使用局部麻醉和谨慎的静脉镇静可预防该并发症，同时最大限度地减少患者不适并有用力于手术实施。

（金培培 译 许 涛 校）

延伸阅读

Dolinski SY, MacGregor DA, Scuderi PE: Pulmonary hemorrhage associated with negative-pressure pulmonary edema, *Anesthesiology* 93:888–890, 2000.

Guffin TN, Har-El G, Sanders A, et al.: Acute postobstructive pulmonary edema, *Otolaryngol Head Neck Surg* 112:235–237, 1995.

Krodel DJ, Bittner EA, Abdulnour R: Case scenario: acute postoperative negative pressure pulmonary edema, *Anesthesiology* 113:200–207, 2010.

Lemyze M, Mallat J: Understanding negative pressure pulmonary edema, *Intensive Care Med* 40:1140–1143, 2014.

Maxwell BG, Mihm FG: Questioning diuretic use in acute negative-pressure pulmonary edema, *Anesthesiology* 114(2):461, 2011.

Udeshi A, Cantie SM, Pierre E: Postobstructive pulmonary edema, *J Crit Care* 25:508.e1–508.e5, 2010.

第 165 章 术后急性肾衰竭

David Roberts，*Andrew Shaw*

病例概要

患者，男性，75 岁，既往高血压多年，2 型糖尿病，拟行肾下型腹主动脉瘤开放修补术。术前肌酐 1.6 mg/dl，术后第二天肌酐 2.0 mg/dl，术后第 5 天出现低氧血症、发热、低血压。肺血管增强造影显示并非肺栓塞，于是开始按肺炎治疗，应用 β - 内酰胺类及氨基糖苷类抗生素。在接下来的 12 h 内，患者出现低血压、无尿，予以肾替代治疗，抗生素改为喹诺酮类。患者肾功能在几周后恢复并出院。

问题分析

定义

术后急性肾损伤（postoperative acute kidney injury，AKI）是描述术后发生肾功能减退的术语，目前公认的指南是由改善全球肾脏疾病预后组织（Kidney Disease Improving Global Outcomes，KDIGO）提出的，其根据血肌酐值与尿量对 AKI 进行了定义。这个定义综合了 RIFLE 与 AKIN 标准，应用于临床实践与研究中。

符合下列任一标准即可诊断 AKI，分级见表 165.1：

- 48 h 内 S_{Cr} 升高≥ 0.3 mg/dl（26.5 μmol/l）；
- 7 天内 S_{Cr} 增长≤ 1.5 倍基础值；
- 尿量 <0.5 ml/（kg · h）且持续 6 h 以上。

引起 AKI 的原因习惯上分为肾前性（灌注降低）、肾性（实质损伤）、肾后性（泌尿道阻塞）。尽管这些区别在概念理解上有一定帮助，但他们不能描述相关的复杂的病理生理学特征，所以现在 AKI 定义不依赖于这些。在许多情况下，术后 AKI 是持续肾前性损伤的一种极端形式的后果：缺血性急性肾小管坏死（ischemic acute tubular necrosis，ATN）。

表 165.1 KDIGO 急性肾损伤分级

分级	血肌酐值	尿量
1	基线值 1.5 ～ 1.9 倍或 48 h 内 S_{Cr} 升高≥ 0.3 mg/dl	<0.5 mL/（kg · h），6 ～ 12 h
2	基础值 2.0 ～ 2.9 倍	<0.5 mL/（kg · h），≥ 12 h
3	基础值 3 倍或 S_{Cr} ≥ 4 mg/dl，或开始肾替代治疗（RRT），或年龄 <18 岁者肾小球滤过率降至 <35 ml/（min · 1.73 m^2）	<0.3 mL/（kg · h），≥ 24 h 或无尿≥ 12 h

在动物模型中，短时间低灌注产生了表现为少尿、低尿钠、水钠潴留的肾前状态。这是肾对血容量减少的正常反应，由肾素-血管紧张素-醛固酮系统（renin-angiotensin-aldosterone system，RAAS）、其他神经体液因子和内在的管球反馈所介导。增加灌注，尿量恢复正常，因此这是一种保护肾小管功能的血流动力学保护性措施，当血流动力学恢复正常，肾小管功能可被逆转，长期灌注不足导致少尿（高尿钠）时，则灌注增加时仍不能逆转其作用。这种情况下发生内在损害，特点是超滤液经中断的肾小管基底膜回漏，细胞碎片阻塞管腔更促进了其回漏，后者是持续血流动力学状态且伴有肾小管功能丧失，血流恢复后不可逆转。

AKI 的发病机制反映了肾对损伤的独特敏感性。图 165.1 列出了几个肾单位的高危区域。髓质和内层皮质有轻微氧合作用，因此肾内氧供减少会导致缺血性 ATN，其可能是由于血容量降低、低血压、心排血量减少或贫血所致。对于肾毒性 ATN，炎症信号、自由基损伤、干扰细胞内代谢、抑制前列腺素和一氧化氮释放而使得肾血管持续收缩都会引起肾小管损伤。肾小管细胞坏死和细胞凋亡导致功能

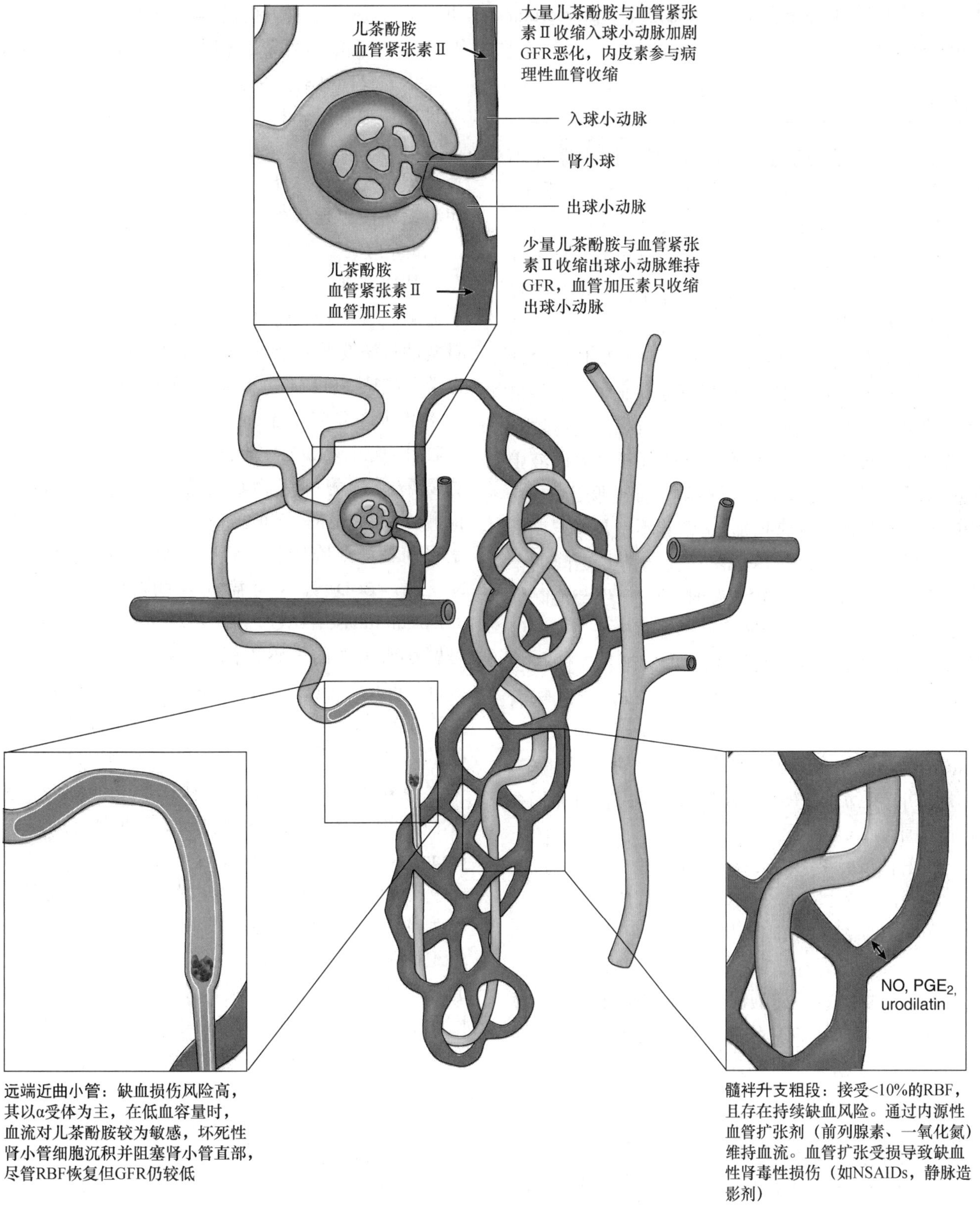

图 165.1 近曲小管和髓袢升支粗段是存在潜在缺血风险和毒性肾小管损伤的部位。这两段肾小管都是耗氧高并存在供需不平衡的风险。GFR，肾小球滤过率；NO，一氧化氮；NSAIDs，非甾体抗炎药；PGE_2，前列腺素 E_2；RBF，肾血流量

丧失、细胞结构破坏、肾小管阻塞，一旦发生，恢复肾血流量将不能恢复肾小球滤过率（glomerular filtration rate，GFR）。

识别

尽管术中常规监测尿量，但围术期少尿并不是体液平衡的可靠指标。应激时交感肾腺素系统、RAAS 系统、抗利尿激素系统被激活，继而导致血管收缩、钠潴留，这些因素影响医师使用尿量判断容量状态的能力。此外，术中少尿与术后 AKI 并没有必然联系。当 AKI 发生时，肾溶质清除下降开始导致血中电解质浓度的增加，水、尿素及其他渗透性分子蓄积（氮质血症）。血尿素氮和血肌酐值是最常见的肾功能检查实验室指标。尿素在肾小管排出，但其水平可能误导对肾小管功能的判断，因血液中尿素水平可受非肾性病理学影响，如胃肠道出血、蛋白质分解代谢（异常增加）、营养不良及终末期肝病（异常下降）。S_{Cr} 反映肌酐产生与清除之间的平衡，当肾功能在一个稳定状态时，S_{Cr} 产生与清除保持平衡。但是，S_{Cr} 和 GFR 之间并非直接关系亦非线性关系，而是呈指数倒数关系，即 S_{Cr} 增长 2 倍 GFR 降低一半，S_{Cr} 从 0.6 mg/dl 增长到 1.2 mg/dl 意味着 GFR 下降了 50%。此外，在 GFR 下降至 <50 ml/min 之前，S_{Cr} 增长不会超过正常范围。在恶病质患者中，由于肌酐产生量低，GFR<30 ml/min 时 S_{Cr} 可能仍在正常范围。

肌酐清除率提供了一个实时评估 GFR 的方法，因为它的计算公式（$U \times V/S_{Cr}$，U 是尿肌酐，V 是尿流速）包含肌酐的排泄率（$U \times V$），其直接与 GFR 成正比。如果患者有导尿管，并且仔细测量尿流速，可收集 2 h 或更短时间的尿液准确的估计 GFR。常用于围术期肾功能研究的简便方法是通过公式代替尿液收集计算 GFR，如 Cockroft-Gault 公式：

$$\text{肌酐清除率} = \frac{[140 - \text{年龄（岁）}] \times \text{体重（kg）} \times 1.73\ m^2 \times 0.85^*}{72 \times S_{Cr}\text{（mg/dl）} \times \text{体表面积（}m^2\text{）}}$$

（* 注释：0.85 仅适用于女性）

存在少尿时，评估肾小管功能有助于区分肾前综合征与 AKI。肾前性的特点是过度的肾小管内水钠潴留，导致少量尿浓缩及低尿钠（<10 mEq/L），钠排泄分数（FE_{Na}）低于 1%。肾前状态导致钠排泄增多，肾小管功能正常（如代谢性碱中毒，利尿剂使用）可将 FE_{Na} 虚假提高至大于 3%。在这种情况下，高 FE_{Na} 并不可靠，但持续性 FE_{Na} 低于 1% 高度提示为肾前状态。尿素氮排泄分数是区分肾前性 ATN 氮质血症的一种更敏感和特异的指标，尤其是在使用利尿剂时。

AKI 发生后，肾小管功能丧失，肾不能潴留钠和浓缩尿液，导致少量稀释尿及高尿钠（>80 mEq/L）和高 FE_{Na}（>3%）。

其他客观数据可能来自电解质紊乱和血流动力学监测。肾血管、肾及泌尿系统超声可以帮助排除阻塞性肾病变及确定 ATN 的诊断（正常的肾血流动力学）或缺血性损伤（局部或整体缺血）。

目前许多应用于研究的生物标记物尚未应用于临床实践，最终可能证明其临床诊断价值。半胱氨酸蛋白酶抑制物 C 与 GFR 相关，尤其在 S_{Cr} 检测不到变化的区间时（GFR 在 60 ～ 90），可能是目前检测亚临床急性肾损伤最好的敏感标志物。N- 乙酰 -β-D- 氨基葡萄糖苷酶（N-acetyl-beta-D-glucosaminidase，NAG）源于近端小管细胞的溶酶体，是肾小管损伤的敏感指标。肾损伤因子 -1（kidney injury molecule-1，KIM-1）是一种膜糖蛋白，参与受伤的管状上皮细胞免疫反应，出现在缺血性损伤的最初 12 h 尿中，S_{Cr} 在肾损伤后 48 h 内明显上升，与其相比，KIM-1 为肾损伤的早期预警指标。中性粒细胞明胶酶相关脂质运载蛋白（neutrophil gelatinase associated lipocalin，NGAL）水平增高，是一个很好的生物标志物，尿液和血中都可检测，作为预测 AKI 的一个独立的研究指标。金属蛋白酶组织抑制剂 2（tissue inhibitor of metalloproteinase 2，TIMP-2）和胰岛素样生长因子结合蛋白 7（insulin-like growth factor–binding protein，IGFBP7）联合检测是目前灵敏度和特异性最高的预测 AKI 风险的方法，并已投入市场。这些只是许多生物标志物中的一小部分，可能有一天进入临床实践并提供早期 AKI 预警及肾单位–肾节段–特异定位。

风险评估

鉴别高危患者可以更准确的预测术后 AKI，术后 AKI 发生风险取决于患者个体差异和手术相关风险因素。对于非心脏手术，术后 AKI 的整体风险为

1% 左右。存在 3 个或 3 个以上危险因素（框 165.1）会增加围术期 AKI 发生的风险。在接受心脏手术的患者中，围术期发生 AKI 的风险接近 30%。接受心脏手术的患者存在额外的肾损伤风险和一组扩展的风险因素（框 165.2）。由于危险因素叠加，潜在的急性肾损伤发生风险呈指数倍数增加。例如，暴露于单一肾毒性因素（例如，酮咯酸）很少会引起问题，但在高风险手术时，如果联合其他肾毒性因素（如庆大霉素）且灌注下降（低血容量），AKI 发生的可能性将会变得非常高。

术前危险因素中最具有预测性的是既往肾功能障碍，其他重要的风险因素包括高龄、血管疾病及终末器官损伤的标志，如糖尿病、胆固醇代谢异常、高血压等。严重的阻塞性黄疸和肝肾综合征与门静脉异常吸收内毒素相关，导致肾血管收缩及难治性低尿钠特征的肾前状态。脓毒症诱发类似的状态，且伴有低血压、系统性炎症、交感性肾血管收缩。

框 165.1　非心脏手术患者 AKI 危险因素

危险因素

年龄≥ 56 岁
男性
充血性心力衰竭活跃期
腹水
高血压
急诊手术
腹腔内手术
肾功能不全——轻、中度[a]
糖尿病——口服药物或胰岛素治疗

危险指数取决于危险因素存在的数量：1 级（0 ～ 2 个危险因素），2 级（3 个危险因素），3 级（4 个危险因素），4 级（5 个危险因素），5 级（6 个或更多的风险因素）

[a] 术前血肌酐值 >1.2 mg/dl

From Kheterpal S，Tremper KK，Heung M，et al：Development and validation of an acute kidney injury risk index for patients undergoing general surgery：results from a national data set. *Anesthesiology* 110(3)：505-515，2009.

框 165.2　心脏手术后发生 AKI 危险因素

危险因素

慢性肾病
复杂的手术（冠状动脉旁路移植术 + 瓣膜手术）
心肺转流持续时间
主动阻断时间
输血（剂量依赖）
静脉淤血
栓子
升压药及正心肌力药
术后心源性休克
高龄

术中危险因素与手术类型（潜在的并发症，如出血、低血压或低心排血量状态）和特殊的干预措施（例如主动脉阻断、心肺转流术）相关。肾上主动脉阻断导致 GFR 完全停止，恢复可能需要 24 ～ 48 h，肾下主动脉钳闭通过反射性血管收缩也会导致 GFR 下降，无论什么情况，阻断时间都与 AKI 发生风险相关。

心肺转流术也会增加 AKI 的风险，但肾功能正常、病程不复杂的患者对此具有良好的耐受性。尽管早期较为乐观，但非体外循环冠状动脉旁路移植术并不能持续降低围术期肾功能损伤的发病率。心脏手术最重要的风险因素仍然是术前持续肾功能不全、手术复杂及术后心功能障碍。

对于所有类型的手术，最重要的可改变的围术期风险因素是循环不稳定。脓毒症本身可通过局部血管收缩和肾毒性诱发肾损伤，而无明显的血流动力学波动。伴随其他肾毒素明显加剧肾损伤风险，包括横纹肌溶解引起的色素肾病、血管内溶血、严重阻塞性黄疸、造影剂肾病、毒品。在病例概述中，患者存在术前肾功能障碍（即高 S_{Cr}），接受高风险手术（主动脉动脉瘤修复，虽然是肾下主动脉阻断），之后暴露于其他几个肾损伤风险（脓毒症、造影剂、氨基糖苷类抗生素）。

启示

数据表明血肌酐水平增加符合 AKI 的标准是与死亡率增加和慢性肾病进展相关的独立因素。AKI 恶化期显著增加死亡风险，肾替代治疗（renal replacement therapy，RRT）包括持续血液透析（continuous venovenous hemodiafiltration，CVVH）并没有改善死亡率。尽管 RRT 可以持续调节电解质水平、酸碱失衡、循环超负荷、急性尿毒症，但却不能改善已存在的肾损伤，也不能消除脓毒症、多器官系统功能障碍发生风险或改善受损的伤口愈合，这些都是影响术后病死率的因素。此外有证据表明，符合 AKI 标准的患者中有很大一部分不会恢复正常肾功能，且其发展为慢性肾病的风险更高。

管理

目前急性肾损伤尚无明确的治疗策略。因此，消除或治疗引起 AKI 的原因，维持机体稳态，同时在恢复期预防未来可能发生的肾损伤是治疗的关键。一旦判断患者存在 AKI 发生风险或根据 KDIGO 标准诊断为 AKI，临床医师可采取预防和支持性疗法（表 165.2），及时启动肾脏替代治疗预防酸中毒、电解质失衡、容量超负荷、尿毒症（所谓的 AEIOU 指征）引起的肾损伤。尽管有证据表明早期启动 RRT 是获益的，但目前并没有明确的启动阈值。

预防

预防的第一步是明确如前所述的 AKI 高危患者，然后尽量减少围术期的肾功能损伤。虽然目前仍无法准确的监测血容量状态，但避免围术期低血压和肾毒性药物也许是最容易改变的危险因素。存在血流动力学风险的患者可采取有创动脉监测实时血压，数据表明短暂低血压与围术期急性肾功能障碍有关。

避免应用肾毒素药物如氨基糖苷类、两性霉素、造影剂，是一个获益高的干预措施。

虽然临床试验还没有证实各种高氯晶体液如生理盐水、平衡液（Plasma-Lyte 或乳酸林格液）的差别，但应用高氯晶体液可降低动物模型和人类肾灌注压。围术期频繁应用高氯溶液也会引起高氯性代谢性酸中毒。鉴于潜在的电解质和酸碱平衡的干扰有加剧肾血流量恶化的风险，目前合理的建议是平衡晶体液应选择不含氯溶液以减少肾损伤的风险。

目前还没有明确的药物治疗可改善急性肾衰竭的预后。袢利尿剂理论上可通过阻断氯通道降低外部肾髓质缺氧环境中的代谢活动，对急性肾损伤有效，但临床试验未能证明此可改善结局。渗透性利尿剂和甘露醇同样没有证实在尿量或死亡率方面有明显差别。利尿剂可能用于容量超负荷的少尿性肾损伤，但使少尿 AKI 转变为非少尿 AKI 事实上并不能改善肾损伤，过度减少循环血量反而可能会加重急性肾损伤。

随机对照研究发现小剂量多巴胺对改善肾功能无益。潜在不利因素是多巴胺可引起快速性心律失常和心肌缺血，所以应该放弃其在预防和治疗急性肾损伤中的应用。此外，一些证据表明在急性肾损伤时，应用多巴胺可加剧肾血管舒缩失调而导致灌注减少。非诺多泮是一种选择性 DA-1 受体激动剂，但它既没有减少需要肾替代治疗的患者数量，也不能降低心脏手术后死亡率。非诺多泮的血管舒张特性可能导致患者低血压的风险，因此它也不是急性肾损伤治疗的推荐用药。

利钠肽在临床应用于充血性心力衰竭，理论上对急性肾损伤有益。有一小部分研究证明利钠肽对 AKI 有潜在作用，但目前尚未有充足证据推荐其在临床实践中常规使用。

没有明确的随机对照试验证据支持 N- 乙酰半胱氨酸、碳酸氢钠、前列腺素类似物、人类生长因子等药物应用于术后急性肾损伤患者。

小结

术后急性肾损伤是一种严重的围术期并发症，具有高发病率、高死亡率和发展为慢性肾病的风险。急性肾损伤药物应用缺乏循证药理学证据，主要强

表 165.2 急性肾损伤的治疗

危险因素	1 级	2 级	3 级
停止使用肾毒性药物	无创诊断检查	密切关注出血和感染	尽可能避免锁骨下置管
功能性血流动力学监测	有创诊断检查	肾替代治疗	准备好供血液透析或 CVVH 的血管通路
定期监测 S_{Cr} 和尿量	容量超负荷时应用利尿剂	ICU 治疗	
避免高血糖	定期监测电解质和 pH		
考虑避免造影剂操作的其他方式	依据 GFR 调整药物剂量		
	营养支持		

Data from Kidney Disease：Improving Global Outcomes（KDIGO），Acute Kidney Injury Work Group：KDIGO clinical practice guideline for acute kidney injury. *Kidney Int Suppl* 2（1）：1-138，2012.

调术前风险分层的重要性，调整可更改的危险因素，术后加强监测和支持治疗。在未来，新型生物标志物可能提高我们对于 AKI 的诊断和早期预警。

致谢

感谢 Mark Nunnally 和 Robert Sladen 博士对本章上一版的贡献。

（李荣岩　译　赵珍珍　校）

延伸阅读

Bellomo R, Kellum JA, Ronco C: Acute kidney injury, *Lancet* 380:756–766, 2012.

Bove T, Zangrillo A, Guarracino F, et al.: Effect of fenoldopam on use of renal replacement therapy among patients with acute kidney injury after cardiac surgery: a randomized clinical trial, *JAMA* 312:2244–2253, 2014.

Brezis M, Rosen S: Hypoxia of the renal medulla—its implications for disease, *N Engl J Med* 332:647–655, 1995.

Bucaloiu ID, Kirchner HL, Norfolk ER, et al.: Increased risk of death and de novo chronic kidney disease following reversible acute kidney injury, *Kidney Int* 81:477–485, 2012.

Carvounis CP, Nisar S, Guro-Razuman S: Significance of the fractional excretion of urea in the differential diagnosis of acute renal failure, *Kidney Int* 62:2223–2229, 2002.

Charlton JR, Portilla D, Okusa MD: A basic science view of acute kidney injury biomarkers, *Nephrol Dial Transplant* 29:1301–1311, 2014.

Chowdhury AH, Cox EF, Francis ST, et al.: A randomized, controlled, double-blind crossover study on the effects of 2-L infusions of 0.9% saline and Plasma-Lyte(R) 148 on renal blood flow velocity and renal cortical tissue perfusion in healthy volunteers, *Ann Surg* 256:18–24, 2012.

Cockcroft DW, Gault MH: Prediction of creatinine clearance from serum creatinine, *Nephron* 16:31–41, 1976.

Goren O, Matot I: Update on perioperative acute kidney injury, *Curr Opin Crit Care* 22:370–378, 2016.

Jha V, Kumar V: Acute kidney injury: validating the KDIGO definition and staging—one step at a time, *Nat Rev Nephrol* 10:550–551, 2014.

Kheterpal S, Tremper KK, Heung M, et al.: Development and validation of an acute kidney injury risk index for patients undergoing general surgery: results from a national data set, *Anesthesiology* 110:505–515, 2009.

Kidney Disease: Improving Global Outcomes (KDIGO), Acute Kidney Injury Work Group: KDIGO clinical practice guideline for acute kidney injury, *Kidney Int Suppl* 2(1):1–138, 2012.

Lassnigg A, Schmidlin D, Mouhieddine M, et al.: Minimal changes of serum creatinine predict prognosis in patients after cardiothoracic surgery: a prospective cohort study, *J Am Soc Nephrol* 15:1597–1605, 2004.

Luo X, Jiang L, Du B, et al.: A comparison of different diagnostic criteria of acute kidney injury in critically ill patients, *Crit Care* 18:R144, 2014.

O'Neal JB, Shaw AD, Billings FT: 4th: acute kidney injury following cardiac surgery: current understanding and future directions, *Crit Care* 20:187, 2016.

Raghunathan K, Murray PT, Beattie WS, et al.: Choice of fluid in acute illness: what should be given? An international consensus, *Br J Anaesth* 113:772–783, 2014.

Zacharias M, Mugawar M, Herbison GP, et al.: Interventions for protecting renal function in the perioperative period, *Cochrane Database Syst Rev* 9:CD003590, 2013.

第 166 章 术后谵妄

Philip R. Levin

病例概要

患者，男性，90 岁，有稳定性心绞痛、肾功能不全、慢性阻塞性肺疾病、高血压、抑郁和听力障碍病史，在全身麻醉下行股骨骨折固定术。手术和麻醉都很顺利。在麻醉后恢复室（postanesthesia care unit，PACU），患者失去定向力并出现攻击行为。

病例分析

定义

术后谵妄是一种急性发作的注意力和认知功能障碍，通常在 PACU 中出现典型症状，可持续到术后 3 天。患者通常会出现意识改变以及定向障碍。

识别

引起术后谵妄的原因很多，PACU 的麻醉科医师应及时评估患者是否存在术后谵妄。评估患者呼吸和循环情况对于排除缺氧、高碳酸血症及气道梗阻等危及生命的问题极其重要。应详细询问患者病史，围术期用药列表，回顾麻醉和手术过程（包括麻醉的类型），进行详细的体格检查以及相关实验室检查。

严重的疼痛（手术、尿道刺激或胃扩张等）可引起精神状态改变，应及时处理。某些代谢、内分泌和传染性疾病也会导致精神状态的改变，必须排除。存在局灶性神经系统异常和步态障碍的患者应排除颅内病变。此外，麻醉药的残留作用也可产生与术后谵妄类似的表现。难以区分由镇静药、止吐剂或导致去抑制的麻醉药产生的残留镇静作用与需要镇静治疗的病因。

术后谵妄患者存在伤害自身以及 PACU 工作人员的危险。患者可能会撕开绷带、伤口或拉出静脉输液导管。术后谵妄的患者同样也存在摔倒和骨折的风险。

风险评估

已有研究确认了以下引起术后谵妄的主要术前危险因素：年龄大于 65 岁，已有痴呆或慢性认知功能减退、听力或视力损害、酒精滥用史、有多种内科并存疾病以及感染。

术中危险因素包括手术类型。术后谵妄最常见于心胸外科手术、髋部骨折以及其他大手术。与择期手术相比，急诊手术也是一个危险因素。某些麻醉药物，包括抗胆碱能药物、苯二氮䓬类药物和抗组胺药物均与术后谵妄相关。有趣的是，数项研究均表明不同的麻醉方法如全身麻醉、硬膜外麻醉或脊椎麻醉对术后谵妄的发生率无影响。

启示

术后谵妄延长患者的恢复时间及住院时间，增加医疗费用及患者与患者家属的心理负担。

管理

确定并纠正潜在的病因

首先，确定和纠正潜在的原因很重要。详细询问患者病史，包括任何一个的家庭成员或看护人员提供的资料（例如平时的行为和精神状态）。仔细进行体格检查，包括详细的神经和精神病学检查。密切监护患者的生命体征和身体状况，直至发现并纠正潜在的致病因素（例如呼吸状态异常、感染、体液或电解质失衡）。回顾相关的实验室和影像学检查结果。充分镇痛同样很重要。

药物治疗

确认和纠正潜在致病因素可能足以逆转谵妄。可能需要特异性的药物干预以减少谵妄的强度和持续时间。许多研究已经证实了抗精神病药物的安全性和有效性。在这类药物中，氟哌啶醇是首选药物，因为与其他抗精神病药物相比，其心血管和呼吸系统不良反应小，且其抗胆碱能作用几乎可以忽略。氟哌啶醇可口服、肌注或静脉注射，剂量从 0.25 mg 到 2 mg 不等。每 30 ~ 60 min 重复使用或剂量加倍，直到患者镇静并安静下来。氯丙嗪对术后谵妄也有效，但会导致严重的低血压。抗精神病药物可延长 QT 间期，从而增加尖端扭转性室性心动过速的风险。接受这种治疗的患者应在治疗前做基线心电图。如果患者的 QT 间期超过服药前的 25% 或超过 450 ms，可能需要减少剂量或停止治疗。关于该问题尚需进一步的研究。

苯二氮䓬类药物并非术后谵妄的有效药物，但对酒精或镇静催眠药物停用引起的戒断症状有效。劳拉西泮是最常用的苯二氮䓬类药物；可口服、肌内注射或静脉注射，剂量从 0.5 mg 到 2 mg 不等。可根据患者的镇静水平，每 30 ~ 60 min 重复使用或剂量加倍。

毒扁豆碱用于治疗术后谵妄目前仍有争议，但一些特定情况可用。该药物过去常用于治疗术后谵妄，尤其是中枢胆碱能危象所致的谵妄。与第四代抗胆碱能药物（如阿托品、甘氯苯酯）相比，毒扁豆碱（一种叔胺）更容易透过血脑屏障。

环境干预

支持治疗对缓解谵妄症状有效。包括调整患者对时间、地点和人物的重新定向，并尽量减少过多噪音。家属床旁陪护可有助于患者安静。由于感觉障碍会加重谵妄，恢复患者原有的视力（近视的患者戴眼镜或隐形眼镜）或听力（更换助听器）可能会有效。尽量减少患者的身体约束，因为它给人一种被束缚住的感觉，可能会加重患者的精神错乱。

精神和神经学治疗

如果以上治疗均失败，或需要更积极的治疗，则需要精神科医师会诊。如果怀疑术后谵妄是神经系统问题引起，应请神经内科或神经外科会诊。

预防

目前，对于如何预防术后谵妄知之甚少。有证据表明，积极减少相关风险因素对预防谵妄有效。术中一些可能有效的措施包括维持良好的氧合和正常的血压，使用正确的药物剂量，维持正常的电解质水平。限制药物数量，因为使用 5 种或 5 种以上的药物（多药）会增加谵妄的风险。引起精神异常的药物应谨慎使用。如果使用抗胆碱能药物，则应使用季胺类药物（如胃长宁）。一般来说，消除半衰期短的药物比长效药物有利。最近的一些研究表明，使用术中脑电图监测有助于临床医师控制麻醉深度。研究证明深度镇静增加术后谵妄的风险。术后充分的镇痛对预防术后谵妄也很重要。

（姜 静 译 赵珍珍 校）

延伸阅读

American Geriatrics Society Expert Panel on Postoperative Delirium in Older Adults: American Geriatrics Society abstracted clinical practice guideline for postoperative delirium in older adults, *J Am Coll Surg* 220(2):136–149, 2015.

American Psychiatric Association: *Diagnostic and statistical manual of mental disorders (DSM-5)*, ed 5, Washington, DC, 2013, American Psychiatric Association.

Fritz BA, Kalarickal PL, Maybrier HR, et al.: Intraoperative electroencephalogram suppression predicts postoperative delirium, *Anesth Analg* 121(1):234–242, 2016.

Krenk L, Rasmussen LS, Kehlet H: Delirium in the fast-track surgery setting, *Best Pract Res Clin Anaesthesiol* 26:345–353, 2012.

Lee HB, Mears SC, Rosenberg PB, et al.: Predisposing factors for postoperative delirium after hip fracture repair in individuals with and without dementia, *J Am Geriatr Soc* 59:2306–2313, 2011.

Litaker D, Locala J, Franco K, et al.: Preoperative risk factors for postoperative delirium, *Gen Hosp Psychiatry* 23:84–89, 2001.

National Institute for Health and Care Excellence (NICE): Delirium: prevention, diagnosis and management, Clinical guideline [CG103], July 2010. Available at https://www.nice.org.uk/guidance/cg103. Accessed September 26, 2016.

Whitlock EL, Torres BA, Lin N, et al.: Postoperative delirium in a substudy of cardiothoracic surgical patients in the BAG-RECALL clinical trial, *Anesth Analg* 118:809–817, 2014.

第167章 术后血流动力学不稳定

Elizabeth Mahanna Gabrielli，Andrea Gabriell

病例概要

患者，男性，75岁，90 kg（体重指数35），既往有吸烟史，高血压控制良好，早年接受过肺癌化疗，患者接受了6 h的复杂手部手术后带气管插管转运至麻醉后恢复室（postanesthesia care unit，PACU）。术前用药包括美托洛尔和氢氯噻嗪。术中尿量300 ml。留置动脉导管。在PACU期间，静脉注射2 mg吗啡和1 g对乙酰氨基酚。随后测量无创血压为70/40 mmHg，心率80次/分且律齐。吸入氧浓度（fraction of inspiration，FiO_2）为0.6时氧饱和度为92%，呼气末正压（positive end expiratory pressure，PEEP）为5 cmH_2O，呼气末二氧化碳为50 mmHg。

问题分析

定义

随着全球手术量持续增长超过3.12亿，术后并发症也不断增多。在近200万的医疗保险受益人中，包括我们提供的案例在内，有24%～50%的病例发生了严重并发症，“救援失败”事件——国家质量论坛将其定义为未能识别出而导致预后恶化的不良事件——发生率从4%到41%不等。

识别

避免危重患者“救援失败”需要医护人员判断出患者处于危急状态并采取有效措施。心率、心律和血压，作为后负荷、前负荷以及左、右心室功能的一般指标，都需要结合临床表现和近期手术进行快速评估。

心率

心动过速是交感传出增加后对休克最常见的代偿性反应。当前负荷或收缩力较低时，心率增加可补偿双心室每搏输出量的减少。然而，残留的麻醉药物影响迷走神经张力、区域麻醉作用残余和术前使用β-受体阻滞剂往往会干扰这一代偿反应。

心率超过40次/分时，窦性心动过缓很少引起血流动力学不稳定。迷走张力突然增高可导致严重的心动过缓和低血压，需要应用正性变时性药物或起搏。如果存在充血性心力衰竭或正性变时性药物效果不佳，需要迅速升级为正性肌力药物。术后合并全身性高血压的心动过速通常因切口疼痛引起，很少由急性高碳酸血症引起，而后者与肺动脉高压有关。

心律

阵发性不稳定心律失常通常是严重潜在病程、心脏并存疾病和（或）严重并发症的一个标志。不稳定、低血压、非窦性心动过速且对液体复苏无反应是进行心脏复律的指征，因为任何药物干预都可能使心律更加恶化。心脏复律有时可能使患者转变为需要紧急起搏的心动过缓。应快速识别无脉性恶性心律失常，排除导联断开或功能障碍后，随即正确实施高级生命支持方案。

后负荷

体循环血压虽然测量的是中心血压，但血压在每个器官和不同休克状态下的自动调节是不同的。重症患者的目标是将平均动脉压控制在 65 ～ 70 mmHg，证据来源为特殊种类休克、分布性或脓毒性休克低血压时，通常仍具有正常的心室功能和高输出量。最近有证据表明，对分布性休克应采取更加个体化的血压控制方法。对长期高血压而脑自动调节功能右移的患者，或在较高压力下自动调节功能的肾而言，这可能意味着需要维持稍高的血压。术后低血压应得到合理且系统的治疗。血管麻痹、第三间隙转移和急性失血通常是低血压的最初原因，或伴发其他低血压因素。在这些患者中，充分的静脉回流往往是器官灌注的背压（back pressure）。在某些非分布性休克（如心源性休克）中，通过使用血管升压药增加全身血管阻力不仅不会增加器官灌注，而可能适得其反。因此，对术后低血压患者的治疗必须始终遵循对前负荷的功能评价。

25% 高血压患者会出现术后高血压，这是术后不良事件的另一个独立预测因素。应排除假性高血压的原因，如动脉校准漂移和袖带过紧。术后血压升高通常由手术应激或切口疼痛引起的内源性儿茶酚胺增加所致。血压急剧升高（收缩压 >180 mmHg，舒张压 >110 mmHg）时左心室舒张末期压力和心肌耗氧量增加，引起心肌缺血。高血压危象可加剧其他并存疾病，如收缩性心力衰竭、颅内高压、主动脉夹层或术后出血。当需要时，理想的术后抗高血压药物应起效快速、易于静滴且作用短暂。

前负荷

在循环休克的早期阶段，容量不足通常表现为尿量减少、心率加快和血压下降。大手术常常通过第三间隙、隐形液体丢失或出血导致血管内容量的持续减少。根据 Frank-Starling 定律，液体复苏后积极的血压反应和尿量增加是由于心脏前负荷增加而导致的每搏量的增加。然而这种反应也依赖于心室收缩力，而在无心排血量监测仪或超声心动图时心室收缩力并不容易评估。一些简单的操作，如 15 s 呼气末阻断、少量补液试验，以及被动抬腿引发的前负荷重力性转移，都是建议在患者大量液体冲击治疗（臭名昭著的“一升液体冲击”）之前使用的，可限制不必要的液体负荷。当心室收缩力受损时，大量液体冲击会导致肺水肿（左心室）或肝充血（右心室）。

正压通气插管患者周期性呼吸脉压变异性（pulse pressure variability，PPV）是近年来研究的热点。尽管体积描记仪大幅波动可能提示容量不足，但 PPV 只有在具备动脉监测时才能被检测到。在某些特定条件下，PPV 在 10% 到 15% 之间，能够可靠地预测容量复苏的反应和血流动力学参数的改善情况。然而应用 PPV 的局限性仍有很多：低心率 / 呼吸频率比值、心律失常、低潮气量通气（<8 ml/kg，理想体重）、自主呼吸、腹内压升高和开胸均会影响其准确性。尽管有这些限制，旨在增加氧供的干预过程中，该前负荷反应性“动态”预测因子仍能提供生理性反馈。除严重分布性休克外，若术后低血压患者对前负荷增加没有反应，麻醉科医师应将心室功能作为低血流动力学状态的主要考虑因素。如果怀疑“泵衰竭”，及时加强有创监测能够更有效地指导麻醉科医师进行复苏，并可以显著改善结局。对心源性休克监测的详细回顾在本书的其他章节进行了介绍，不在本章讨论范围之内。血浆乳酸水平、静脉-动脉二氧化碳分压差和直接床旁超声已越来越多被用作组织灌注不足的替代检测指标。

左心室衰竭

左心室衰竭（left ventricular failure，LVF）是由收缩力丧失、严重心律失常引起的，少数患者由于张力性气胸或心脏压塞所致的梗阻引起。大多数病例中，术后 LVF 是由心肌缺血引起的，可通过心电图和检测心肌酶谱标志物诊断。大量的专家共识可用于指导麻醉科医师进行心室功能支持治疗和准备冠状动脉血运重建。

右心室衰竭

右心室（right ventricle，RV）的主要作用是通过调节进入右心室的流量变异极大的血流来维持右心房（right atrial，RA）的低压。正常情况下，肺血管可以通过血管迅速收缩和扩张，适应不断变化的血流和容量，从而使肺动脉压力保持最小限度地增加。右心室后负荷由肺泡压、血管舒缩张力增加和肺血流分布决定。与 LVF 相反，右心室衰竭（right ventricular failure，RVF）多发生在右室流出道急性梗阻时。可能伴随有肺动脉压升高或肺动脉系统顺应性降低，常见原因有急性左侧心力衰竭、肺栓塞（血栓、空气、脂肪、羊水）、严重缺氧性肺血管收缩和胸腔内压力升高（胸腔内容积增加、过度 PEEP 或内源性 PEEP、张力性气胸）。在急性肺心病患者，右心室扩张和舒张末期容积增加时，导致左心室舒张末期容积因心室相互依赖作用而减少。随后出现全身性低血压，导致右冠状动脉灌注压下降、RVF进一步加重。此外，在急性RVF和心室扩张时，右心房压力升高，如果不与系统充盈压力相匹配，静脉回流将随之减少。如果任由这种恶性循环继续，将导致双心室衰竭和心脏停搏。

只有临床高度怀疑时，才能认识到RVF是系统性低血压的原因之一。除非能直接测量心排血量和肺动脉压，否则有创血压监测也无法鉴别低血压的原因。床边经胸超声心动图（transthoracic echocardiogram，TTE）或经食管超声心动图（transesophageal echocardiogram，TEE）显示右心室扩张、室间隔反常移位、三尖瓣反流、右心房压力增高，偶尔发现血栓可快速做出诊断。RVF治疗侧重于减轻流出阻力和强心支持。

风险评估

术后血流动力学不稳定与预后不良相关。低血压、平均动脉压（mean arterial pressure，MAP）降低40%或小于50 mmHg造成的心血管和肾发病率比高血压更高。原已存在的血压自动调节和低血压持续时间是影响围术期发病率和死亡率的其他因素。

启示

当组织耗氧量与氧供不匹配时，术后血流动力学不稳定将演变为休克状态，最初表现为最敏感器官的灌注不足。如不及时改善，休克将不可逆转、发生心脏停搏。

管理

该病例简要描述了由肺栓子引起RVF导致的心源性休克。危险因素包括手术和恶性肿瘤。在PaO_2/FiO_2降低、乳酸持续升高、对前负荷冲击无反应后，经TTE可进行确诊。在PACU时留置了中心静脉测压导管，中心静脉压（central venous pressure，CVP）为20 cmH_2O，动-静脉CO_2间隙增大。肺动脉导管替换CVP后，显示心脏指数为1.2，肺动脉平均压力为40 mmHg，TTE证实了RVF。患者在接受小剂量肾上腺素、米力农、血管加压素并吸入依普列烯醇后，血压有所改善。患者术前使用了β受体阻滞剂，所以未发生心动过速。在与手术小组讨论后，患者被转到介入放射科，经血管造影证实了肺栓塞的诊断。采用选择性肺溶栓治疗，缓解了血流动力学危象。

预防

判断术后血流动力学不稳定的系统方法必须包括对休克状态决定因素的快速鉴别诊断。通过应用选择性干预和评估功能性血流动力学监测来评估患者的生理储备，可预测休克状态是否可逆转。最近引入的TTE和TEE，虽应用还未普及，但提供了明确的鉴别诊断，能够直接显示自然或病理状态下的心脏结构，以及前负荷、左心室和右心室功能。

（王 芷 译 赵珍珍 校）

延伸阅读

Asfar P, Meziani F, Hamel J-F, et al.: High versus low blood-pressure target in patients with septic shock, *N Engl J Med* 370(17):1583–1593, 2014.

Bose EL, Hravnak M, Pinsky MR: The interface between monitoring and physiology at the bedside, *Crit Care Clin* 31(1):1–24, 2015.

Breitkreutz R, Walcher F, Seeger FH: Focused echocardiographic evaluation in resuscitation management: concept of an advanced life support–conformed algorithm, *Crit Care Med* 35(5):S150–S161, 2007.

Di Giantomasso D, May CN, Bellomo R: Vital organ blood flow during hyperdynamic sepsis, *Chest* 124(3):1053–1059, 2003.

Jabot J, Teboul J-L, Richard C, et al.: Passive leg raising for predicting fluid responsiveness: importance of the postural change, *Intensive Care Med* 35(1):85–90, 2009.

Kheterpal S, O'Reilly M, Englesbe MJ, et al.: Preoperative and intraoperative predictors of cardiac adverse events after general, vascular, and urological surgery, *Anesthesiology* 110(1):58–66, 2009.

Kiely DG, Cargill RI, Lipworth BJ: Effects of hypercapnia on hemodynamic, inotropic, lusitropic, and electrophysiologic indices in humans, *Chest* 109(5):1215–1221, 1996.

Levy B, Bastien O, Bendjelid K, et al.: Experts' recommendations for the management of adult patients with cardiogenic shock, *Ann Intensive Care* 5(1):52, 2015.

Michard F, Chemla D, Teboul JL: Applicability of pulse pressure variation: how many shades of grey? *Crit Care* 19:144, 2015.

Monnet X, Osman D, Ridel C, et al.: Predicting volume responsiveness by using the end-expiratory occlusion in mechanically ventilated intensive care unit patients, *Crit Care Med* 37(3):951–956, 2009.

Monnet X, Teboul JL: Invasive measures of left ventricular preload, *Curr Opin Crit Care* 12(3):235–240, 2006.

Muller L, Toumi M, Bousquet PJ, et al.: An increase in aortic blood flow after an infusion of 100 ml colloid over 1 minute can predict fluid responsiveness: the mini-fluid challenge study, *Anesthesiology* 115(3):541–547, 2001.

Pinsky MR: The right ventricle: interaction with the pulmonary circulation, *Crit Care* 20(1):266, 2016.

Pizov R, Eden A, Bystritski D, et al.: Arterial and plethysmographic waveform analysis in anesthetized patients with hypovolemia, *Anesthesiology* 113(1):83–91, 2010.

Silber JH, Williams SV, Krakauer H, et al.: Hospital and patient characteristics associated with death after surgery: a study of adverse occurrence and failure to rescue, *Med Care* 30(7):615–629, 1992.

Varon J, Marik PE: Perioperative hypertension management, *Vasc Health Risk Manag* 4(3):615–627, 2008.

Varpula M, Tallgren M, Saukkonen K, et al.: Hemodynamic variables related to outcome in septic shock, *Intensive Care Med* 31(8):1066–1071, 2005.

Vincent JL, Rhodes A, Perel A, et al.: Clinical review: update on hemodynamic monitoring—a consensus of 16, *Crit Care* 15(4):229, 2011.

Walsh M, Devereaux PJ, Garg AX, et al.: Relationship between intraoperative mean arterial pressure and clinical outcomes after noncardiac surgery: toward an empirical definition of hypotension, *Anesthesiology* 119(3):507–515, 2013.

Weiser TG, Haynes AB, Molina G, et al.: Size and distribution of the global volume of surgery in 2012, *Bull World Health Organ* 94(3):201–209F, 2016.

第168章 术后肝功能障碍

Kerri M. Wahl

病例概要

患者，男性，60 岁，有丙型肝炎和肝细胞肝癌病史，拟择期行部分肝切除术。术前血红蛋白为 10 g/dl。白蛋白、肌酐、转氨酶和凝血酶原时间（prothrombin time，PT）均在正常范围内。术中出血 2000 ml，输浓缩红细胞 5 U，手术过程顺利。术后患者因少尿及高钾血症（6.1 mmol/L）转至外科 ICU 接受治疗，患者恢复顺利，但在术后第 5 天出现黄疸。

问题分析

定义

临床上严重的急性肝功能障碍在麻醉和手术后较为常见。主要危险因素包括先前既往肝病（肝硬化、肝纤维化或脂肪性肝炎）、大量输血、肝大部切除术后残肝体积小和围术期肝损伤（缺氧、脓毒症、药物毒性、营养不良）。技术难度大伴胆道引流或胆漏也可能是原因之一。大多数术后黄疸是多因素起源，并且难以诊断，往往需要支持治疗。择期腹部手术后肝功能异常的发生率为 25% ～ 75%，而术后肝功能障碍的发生率低于 1%。

术后黄疸通常在术后第一周内明显，与急性肝衰竭无关。正常血清胆红素水平为 0.3 ～ 1.1 mg/dl。当血清胆红素超过 3 ～ 5 mg/dl 时或患者出现巩膜和皮肤黄染时，可在临床上检测到黄疸。结合胆红素的增加反映了肝细胞功能障碍、肝内胆汁淤积或胆道梗阻导致胆红素分泌的问题。如果总胆红素的增加主要是由非结合胆红素引起，那么最有可能的原因是红细胞溶血，导致大量胆红素生成或肝脏对胆红素的摄取、转运或结合方面出现缺陷。

研究表明，术后功能性肝体积大小与发生临床明显肝衰竭的可能性之间存在明确的关系。一个健康的肝，切除 75% 的肝体积几乎不影响肝功能。据报道，术后肝衰竭（postresectional liver failure，PLF）的发生率在 0.7% ～ 9.1%。近十年来，肝部分切除术后死亡率为 0% ～ 5%，PLF 是主要的死亡原因。不幸的是，对于 PLF 的定义还没有达成共识。一般来说，PLF 的特征是一种或多种肝脏合成和排泄功能障碍，导致高胆红素血症、低白蛋白血症、PT 延长、血清乳酸增加以及不同级别的肝性脑病。术后第 5 天，凝血酶原指数 <50%[国际标准化比值（international normalized ratio，INR）>1.7] 和血清胆红素大于 2.9 mg/dl 对于预测既往无肝病的患者肝大部切除术后死亡风险为 59%（敏感性 69.6% 和特异性 98.5%）。此外，峰值胆红素 7.0 mg/dl 已被认为是 PLF 相关死亡的预测指标。

识别

由于肝具有巨大的储备功能，尽管有严重的基础疾病，但常规实验室检查仍可能为正常。几种常见实验室检查的异常结果可大致反映肝功能障碍情况（框 168.1）。在急性肝损伤中，PT 及总胆红素水平是判断病情严重程度的最佳指标。

传统上，PT 一直在 Child Pugh 评分中用来评估肝损伤的严重程度，或在 MELD 评分中代替 INR（在本章后面讨论）。PT 测定外源性凝血途径的活性，需要在肝中合成的纤维蛋白原、凝血酶原和因子Ⅴ、Ⅶ和Ⅹ参与。如果 PT 延长超过 3 s，这可能反映严重的肝功能障碍，因为凝血只需要 20% ～ 30% 的正常因子活性。实际上凝血是一个复杂的过程，涉及促凝和抗凝因子的相互作用与纤溶系统。由于抗凝血因子和促凝因子均减少，急性和慢性肝病患者的凝血功能检测可能是正常的。对于梗阻性胆道疾病，

框 168.1　评估肝功能的检查

合成功能障碍引起的肝实质损伤

凝血功能：PT 或 INR 升高，血小板计数及纤维蛋白原减少

肝功能检查：转氨酶升高（天冬氨酸转氨酶、丙氨酸转氨酶）、碱性磷酸酶、胆红素和血氨

血乳酸升高

低磷血症

病毒性肝炎和自身免疫性疾病标志物的筛选

疑似感染患者的血液培养

腹部超声或 CT

肝组织活检

胆汁淤积或胆道疾病

胆红素（总胆红素、结合和非结合胆红素）：尿液和血清水平

碱性磷酸酶

腹部超声或 CT

内镜逆行胰胆管造影或经皮肝胆管造影

INR，国际标准化比值；PT，凝血酶原时间

胆汁盐分泌障碍可能导致维生素 K 的吸收不良，这是转录后 γ- 羧化和激活因子Ⅱ、Ⅶ、Ⅸ和Ⅹ所必需的辅助因子。24 h 内未经维生素 K 纠正的 INR 大于 1.5 提示存在严重的肝病。多种更特异的凝血试验可用于检测肝功能异常（如活化部分凝血活酶时间、凝血时间、出血时间、凝血酶时间、全血凝块溶解时间、血浆纤维蛋白原、血清纤维蛋白原降解产物、血浆 D- 二聚体、球蛋白溶解时间、F XIII、蛋白质 C、蛋白质 S、抗凝血酶Ⅲ等）。以及整体止血试验 [血栓弹力图，旋转式血栓弹力计（rotational thrombeolastometry，ROTEM），INR 肝]。

PT/INR、部分凝血活酶时间、血小板计数等常规凝血指标异常与肝切除程度有关。手术后 12 h 内 PT/INR 明显增加。血小板计数和纤维蛋白原也相应减少。残存肝合成功能下降，血液稀释和凝血因子消耗很可能是造成这种术后凝血障碍的主要原因，这种情况在手术后 2 ~ 5 天达到高峰。

虽然测定血清肝酶水平的试验通常称为肝功能试验，但它们通常反映肝细胞完整性或胆汁淤积，而不是肝功能。肝大部切除后，大多数患者肝功能测试异常的模式大多是可预测的（图 168.1）。肝中的丙氨酸转氨酶（alanine aminotransferase，ALT）和天冬氨酸转氨酶（aspartate aminotransferase，AST）因缺血性肝损伤即刻升高并逐渐下降，胆红素升高

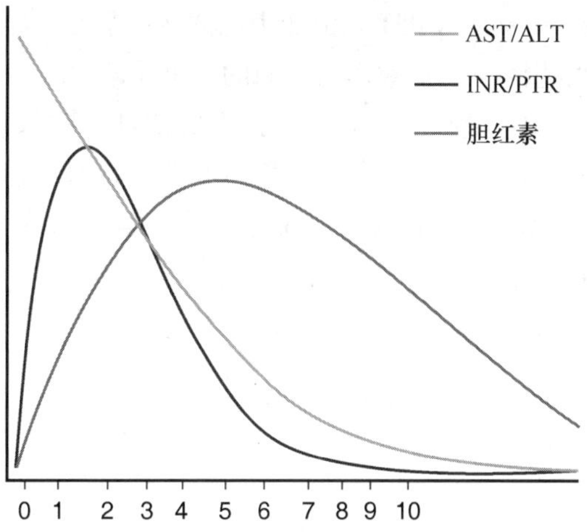

图 168.1　部分肝切除后肝功能检查异常的类型（From Wigmore S：Why do people develop jaundice after liver resection? Prof Steve Wigmore [blog] 2012. Available at https://profstevewigmore.wordpress.com/2012/12/19/why-do-people-develop-jaundice-after-liver-resection/. Accessed September 26，2016.）

常在第 4 ～ 6 天达到峰值。在肝转氨酶中，ALT 是肝细胞损伤的金标准，因为它仅局限于胞质内。对酶异常的全面评估包括①酶改变的主要模式（肝细胞与胆汁淤积）；②血药浓度变化幅度（轻度，< 上限 5 倍；中度 5 ～ 10 倍，上限 5 ～ 10 倍；重度，> 上限 10 倍）；③变化的速率（随时间增加或减少）；④变化过程的性质（轻度波动或递增）。

血清氨浓度代表氨的产生（主要在肠道和肾）与肝尿素合成之间的平衡。由于正常肝对尿素合成的储备能力大，血氨浓度升高通常表明肝功能明显下降。高乳酸血症和低磷血症是肝切除术后常见的疾病。肝中糖异生通常消耗 40% ～ 60% 的乳酸。在切除或应激期间，乳酸通常是产生多于代谢。因此，动脉血乳酸浓度是一个独立的预测病残率和死亡率的指标，这在死亡患者中尤为突出。肝切除术后几乎所有患者都会出现低磷血症。人们对这一疾病的发病机制知之甚少，普遍认为这是由于肝细胞再生或过多的尿丢失而导致的磷酸盐增加所致。

黄疸是最常见且最容易识别的肝功能障碍症状。胆红素是血红蛋白代谢的主要最终产物。非结合胆红素摄取和转运进入肝细胞后与葡萄糖醛酸盐结合，然后排泄到胆管，总胆红素浓度 >1.5 mg/dl 者为异常。诊断高胆红素血症包括病史、体格检查、生化检查和肝胆管造影。碱性磷酸酶（alkaline phosphatase，ALP）和胆红素水平是评估肝功能的常规指标，而 γ- 谷氨酰转移酶（gamma-glutamyl transferase，γ-GT）由于其敏感性高但特异性低，在某些情况下常被作为诊断的辅助手段。

术后黄疸可分为三类：①肝前性（胆红素产生大于排泄）；②肝内性（急性或亚急性肝细胞损伤，有或无既往肝病史）；③肝后性（胆管阻塞引起胆汁淤积）。

肝前原因

术后黄疸肝前原因的分类

1. 淤血的再吸收。
2. 溶血：
   a. 药物、感染或禁食后血管内溶血；
   b. 溶血性贫血：先天性（酶缺乏症或血红蛋白病）或获得性（输血相关，ABO 或 Rh 血型不合，机械性红细胞破裂）。
3. 特发性高胆红素血症。
   a. 肝细胞摄取减少：吉尔伯特综合征（Gilbert），克里格勒–纳贾尔综合征（Crigler-Najjar）；
   b. 结合胆汁排泄障碍：杜宾–约翰逊综合征（Dubin-Johnson syndrome）。

术后患者非结合（间接）胆红素水平的单独升高很可能是由于肝前机制引起的。肝前原因是胆红素分泌过多所致，通常是内出血患者溶血（红细胞破裂）或吸收外渗血所致。通常情况下，胆红素浓度在术后前几天达到峰值，并在几天到几周内逐渐降低。除了减少红细胞持续崩解的治疗外，没有任何特定的治疗方法。

严重的术后黄疸在外科创伤患者中普遍存在。这些患者中的多数存在肌肉和软组织多重损伤，需要行大手术干预和液体复苏，通常需要输入大量红细胞和其他血液制品。在输注红细胞时，每单位血液中多达 10% 的红细胞在最初 24 h 内发生溶血，产生 250 mg/100 ml 血液的胆红素负荷。当胆红素水平超过正常胆红素的 3 倍（成人为 250 ～ 400 mg）时，肝分泌和（或）结合胆红素的能力可能暂时不堪重负，黄疸可能会出现。

溶血性贫血的诊断需要与网织红细胞增多症、非结合高胆红素血症、乳酸脱氢酶升高以及结合珠蛋白浓度低或缺乏等相鉴别。患者可表现为苍白、疲劳、发热和虚弱无力，尿色变深，皮肤和巩膜变黄。如果患者有潜在的慢性肝病、肝急性缺血性损伤或肾功能受损，则溶血引起的临床表现可能更加突出。

外科手术可加重因应激、感染和禁食而产生的溶血病或遗传性溶血倾向（如镰状细胞病、遗传性球形细胞增多症或葡萄糖 -6- 磷酸脱氢酶缺乏症）患者的溶血症状。最有可能发生机械性红细胞破裂的患者是心脏手术加体外循环、长时间手术或左室辅助装置、主动脉球囊反搏或体外膜氧合的血流动力学支持。由链球菌、大肠杆菌、类杆菌和梭菌引起的脓毒症也可引起溶血。其机制虽尚不清楚，但很可能是由于细菌溶血素和肝吸收胆红素与低血压有关。药物性溶血性贫血最常见的原因是头孢菌素，其他药物包括左旋多巴、左氧氟沙星、甲基多巴、呋喃妥因、非甾体抗炎药、青霉素、吡啶和奎尼丁等。

肝内原因

肝内黄疸是由炎症、缺血再灌注、坏死或肝切除等过程所介导的肝细胞损伤或胆管上皮细胞损伤所致，其功能储备不足。临床过程取决于先前存在的肝病、其严重程度、手术方法和麻醉类型，围术期肝损伤的主要原因包括缺血、药物毒性（包括吸入麻醉药和抗生素）、脓毒症、新发病毒性肝炎和全肠外营养（total parenteral nutrition，TPN）。

术后黄疸肝内原因的分类

1. 急性：
   a. 缺血性损伤（缺氧，肝血流量减少，贫血）；
   b. 药物毒性；
   c. 感染；
   d. 新获得的病毒性肝炎；
   e. 全肠外营养；
   f. 残余肝体积。
2. 慢性
   a. 肝炎、肝纤维化、肝硬化；
   b. 原发性胆汁性肝硬化、原发性硬化性胆管炎。
3. 良性术后胆汁淤积症。

缺血性肝损伤是围术期急性低灌注和缺氧所致。肝血供复杂，代谢活性高，易受血流动力学影响所致的弥漫性缺血损伤。肝总血流量为 1.5 L/min，占正常成人心排血量的 25% ～ 30%。肝动脉供应肝总血流量的 25%，门静脉供应 75%。然而，两者对肝的氧合贡献相同。实质上，门静脉系统是一个被动的血管床，其流量取决于灌注压、心排血量和内脏血管阻力。门静脉血流的减少通常与肝动脉的舒张相互影响，从而维持肝的总血流量和供氧。

缺血性损伤

全身麻醉和手术期间降低心排血量和血压会减少肝血流量并危及肝氧合。影响因素包括麻醉药物和其他治疗药物、低血容量、低氧血症、贫血、酸中毒和通气模式（高二氧化碳 / 持续气道正压）。由于交感神经刺激或直接压迫腔静脉和内脏血管，右上腹的手术操作可使肝血流量减少 60%。挥发性麻醉药以剂量依赖性方式对抗代偿性肝动脉血管扩张和门静脉流入减少。因此，门静脉灌注依赖于压力。

肝硬化患者由于先前存在的灌注受损，以及细胞炎症介质释放导致的多器官系统衰竭，故使缺血性肝损伤的风险增加。缺血性肝炎导致肝小叶中央坏死，而非炎性坏死。通常情况下，在肝损伤被确诊之前，血流动力学受损的临床表现已经出现。黄疸发生于术后 1 ～ 5 天，9 ～ 18 天达高峰。肝功能检测显示胆红素升高，乳酸脱氢酶水平大幅升高，转氨酶浓度通常是正常上限的 25 ～ 250 倍。临床研究表明，仅低灌注压不足以导致既往无肝病或心脏病的患者产生上述临床表现，而中心静脉压升高和门静脉充血可能导致肝血流进一步减少。

药物毒性

药物性肝损伤可能很难诊断，因为药物与肝毒性之间的关系并不十分明确。丙泊酚、咪达唑仑和芬太尼这三种麻醉药尚未被证明能显著改变肝功能，而大剂量硫喷妥钠（>750 mg）可引起肝功能障碍。吸入麻醉剂的肝代谢程度与发生毒性反应的可能性有关。异氟烷、地氟烷和七氟烷的肝代谢低于氟烷或安氟烷，且肝炎风险最低。有证据表明这些药物之间存在“交叉致敏”现象。

氟烷肝炎是众所周知的，这仍然是成人患者术后黄疸的常见外科诊断，尽管氟烷在大多数医院已经过时。在挥发性药物中，氟烷导致肝血流量减少变化最大，这与心排血量的减少一致，并且可能在 10 000 次暴露中导致 1 次轻度的、自限性肝炎。临床特征包括暴露后第 3 ～ 14 天高热，并在 1 ～ 2 天后出现黄疸。白细胞增多伴嗜酸性粒细胞增多的病例占 20%。暴发性肝坏死很少见（大约 35 000 例中有 1 例），但死亡率为 40%。不良结局与年龄大于 60 岁、肥胖、短时间反复暴露、血清胆红素 >10 mg/dl 和 PT>20 s 有关。最有可能的损伤机制是直接肝毒性、肝血流量减少和免疫反应。

常见的肝毒性药物包括口服避孕药、类固醇类激素、氯丙嗪、苯妥英钠、酒精、胺碘酮、他汀类、肼屈嗪、对乙酰氨基酚、阿司匹林、异烟肼、甲基多巴和抗生素。四环素与脂肪浸润、青霉素和头孢菌素合并肝炎、磺胺类药物引起过敏性和局灶性肝细胞坏死有关。

危重患者的 TPN 与肝坏死和胆汁淤积有关，可引起黄疸。摄入过多热量可能是肝功能不全的一个危险因素。

严重的细菌感染或腹腔内脓毒症通常与胆汁淤积有关。致病因素包括低血压、溶血、药物治疗和内毒素介导的细胞因子释放的影响，导致胆红素和胆盐运输受损。与此相似，创伤患者的小肠梗阻可能会中断肠道和肝之间正常的内源性胆汁酸循环，这将使肝细胞对胆红素超载的胆汁淤积作用更加敏感。在早期脓毒症中，内脏血流量增加是由于肝氧摄取增加用以支持细菌内毒素的吞噬作用。在脓毒性休克中，尽管内脏血管收缩，但全身容量血管扩张可导致低血压，并且肝动脉缓冲反应失调导致乳酸酸中毒。

病毒性肝炎

急性病毒性肝炎是术后黄疸的罕见原因，但可发生在术前暴露于甲型、乙型或丙型病毒的患者，较少见的原因是丁型或 EB 病毒或巨细胞病毒。确诊需要检测抗原和抗体，因为许多种类的药物都会引起与病毒性肝炎相同的临床和组织学表现。其一般症状包括尿色变深、疲劳、食欲缺乏、呕吐、脱水、低热、肌萎缩和右上腹疼痛，且肝炎早期肝酶的升高先于黄疸出现。

严重急性炎症性肝炎患者腹部手术死亡率为 15%（病毒性肝炎）～ 55%（酒精相关性肝炎）。因此，所有的择期手术应该推迟到感染得到控制，以正常的肝功能检查结果为指标。恢复到接近正常值可能需要 4 个月左右的时间。任何病因所致输血后肝炎的发病率均可忽略不计，根据临床报告显示，自 2004 年以来，85% 的输血后感染是由丙型肝炎病毒引起的，但其发生率每 100 万单位输血或血液制品中不足一例。

慢性肝炎

慢性肝炎有两种类型：慢性持续性肝炎和慢性

活动性肝炎，后者更严重，也更容易进展为肝硬化和肝衰竭。肝硬化患者，无论其病因如何，预期寿命都会缩短。虽然肝功能失代偿的可能性相对较低，但在出现第一次主要并发症（即腹水、静脉曲张出血、黄疸、肝性脑病）之后，死亡风险很高。麻醉和手术与肝脏失代偿有关，影响肝硬化患者围术期肝并发症和死亡率的重要因素（多因素分析）包括性别、较高的Child-Pugh评分（或MELD评分）、原发性胆汁性肝硬化以外的肝硬化（尤其是隐匿性肝硬化）、肾功能不全、慢性阻塞性肺疾病、糖尿病、充血性心力衰竭、术前脓毒症、消化道出血或腹水，手术严重程度评分高的急诊手术，以及明确的术中低血压。

良性术后胆汁淤积症

良性术后肝内胆汁淤积是一种排除性诊断。病程通常自限，在3～4周内消退，在长时间手术和危重手术后发生，这可能是导致术后黄疸的多种可能原因。重度黄疸，结合胆红素高达40 mg/dl，血清碱性磷酸酶升高，转氨酶正常至轻度升高是典型表现。病理活检典型表现为中央小叶充血和胆汁淤积。

肝后原因

肝外梗阻很少引起术后黄疸，但应排除此病因，因为黄疸是可以纠正的。原因包括胆管损伤、肿瘤、结石或狭窄；急性胆囊炎、胆管炎或胰腺炎。

风险评估

大多数外科手术，无论是在全身麻醉、脊椎麻醉或硬膜外麻醉下进行，都会伴随着血清肝生化检测水平的轻微升高。无基础肝病患者术后血清转氨酶、碱性磷酸酶或胆红素水平轻微升高，临床上无太大意义。然而，在基础肝病患者，尤其是肝脏合成功能受损的患者中，外科手术可导致肝功能失代偿。

手术风险与基础肝病的严重程度、内科并存疾病和手术操作的性质有关。在肝硬化患者中，Child-Pugh分级 [Child-Turcott-Pugh（CTP）评分] 和终末期肝病（Model for End-stage Liver Disease，MELD）评分可合理预估围术期死亡率。CTP评分系统是根据患者的血清胆红素和白蛋白水平、PT以及肝性脑病和腹水的严重程度来评估。病例回顾统计，接受手术的Child分级A级患者死亡率为10%，B级为30%，C级为76%～82%。除预测围术期死亡率外，Child分级还与术后并发症的发生率相关，包括肝衰竭、恶化的脑病、出血、感染、肾衰竭、缺氧和顽固性腹水。一般共识是Child A级肝硬化患者可耐受择期手术，无门脉高压的B级肝硬化患者（除大范围肝切除或心脏手术外）术前准备充分也可允许手术，C级肝硬化患者则禁忌手术。

MELD评分的建立是用于预测经颈静脉肝内门体分流术后的死亡率，后来该评分用来对等待肝移植的患者进行风险分层，近来也可用于预测围术期死亡率。MELD评分是基于患者血清胆红素、肌酐和INR的线性回归模型。MELD评分作为围术期死亡率预测指标的最大回顾性研究评估了772例接受开腹、矫形和心血管手术的代偿性肝硬化患者。患者术前MELD评分中位数为8分，少数患者MELD评分>15分（相当于Child C级）。MELD评分≥7分者死亡率为5.7%；MELD评分为8～11的患者死亡率为10.3%，MELD评分为12～15的患者死亡率为25.4%。MELD评分>8分时，相对死亡风险的增加几乎呈线性。基于这项研究，Mayo开发了一个死亡风险预测模型（http://www.mayoclinic.org/meld/mayomodel9.html），根据患者的年龄、ASA分级和MELD评分，计算术后7天、30天、90天、1年和5年患者的外科手术死亡风险。MELD评分和Child分级的使用并不是相互排斥，而是可以相互补充，但MELD评分可能是最精确的围术期死亡率预测指标。

肝切除术

肝硬化患者肝部分切除术后死亡率高达25%。根据Child分级和MELD评分进行风险分级，可以更合理地筛查患者，从而降低病死率。对82例肝硬化肝切除术患者进行分析，MELD评分≥9分者围术期死亡率为29%，MELD评分≤8分者为0%。MELD评分除了能预测死亡率外，还能预测肝切除术后的病残率。在一项研究中，MELD评分小于9、9～10和大于10分的患者肝切除术后肝衰竭的发生率分别为0%、3.6%和37.5%。肝切除的程度也是死亡率的预测因素，低血钠也是如此。肝切除术后INR大>1.7，血清胆红素>2.9 mg/dl可诊断肝功能衰竭，这就是所谓的“50-50”标准。当符合这些标准时，术后死亡率为60%，而不符合这些标准的患者为1.2%。

术后肝功能障碍和单纯高胆红素血症的外科危

险因素包括急诊手术和严重程度评分高的外科手术，包括：

- 心脏直视手术（体外循环效应，充血性心力衰竭，血管升压药）；
- 开腹胆囊切除术与腹腔镜胆囊切除术；
- 创伤手术，尤指涉及肝脏或胆道损伤的手术；
- 腹部大手术（特别是胆道手术、肝切除术）；
- 需要大量输注血液或血制品。

肝硬化患者胆石症的发生率是非肝硬化患者的 2 倍。尽管腹腔镜手术和开放手术技术都取得了进展，但肝硬化和门静脉高压患者的围术期死亡率（7% ～ 20%）和病残率（出血、肾衰竭和脓毒症）仍然很高。腹腔镜胆囊切除术可以最大限度地减少炎症介质的释放和肝脏缺血。然而术中头高位，重力依赖性静脉池和 CO_2 气腹压升高仍然会导致肝灌注下降。此外，上腹部手术中肝的外科操作、高碳酸血症和神经体液应激反应等增加了多器官系统衰竭的风险。

急性炎症性肝衰竭与慢性肝病急性加重期的鉴别与患者的预后相关。肝病患者择期手术的禁忌证包括急性病毒性肝炎、药物性肝炎、酒精性肝炎、急性肝衰竭、急性肾衰竭、心肌病、低氧血症和严重的凝血功能障碍。

无症状的慢性肝炎患者几乎不增加麻醉风险。然而，有症状的肝硬化或慢性肝炎患者术后并发症的风险显著增加，其风险程度与其疾病的严重程度相关。

重度梗阻性黄疸患者外周阻力降低，内脏储血减少。此外，肾盐消耗，左心室功能下降，以及窦房结功能不全引起心律失常的风险，导致低血压风险增加，但失血量减少到最小。围术期死亡率的危险因素包括血细胞比容 <30%、胆红素 >11 mg/dl、恶性胆道梗阻、胆管炎、肾功能不全、血清白蛋白水平降低。严重梗阻性黄疸患者术后并发症包括感染、肾衰竭、弥散性血管内凝血及肝功能进一步恶化等。

启示

大多数术后黄疸通常为自限性，一般支持治疗即可消散。诊断最可能病因的重要性在于判断能否通过内镜或外科干预纠正黄疸。急性炎症性肝炎、肝细胞坏死或代偿性肝硬化伴门脉高压和 MELD 评分 >15 分（Child C）的患者，外科手术并非最佳治疗方式。慢性肝病患者和仍有储备功能的患者几乎不增加手术风险。临床上胆汁淤积患者与代偿性肝硬化患者相比，前者的病残率和死亡率更低。

术前重点评估对于识别高危患者很有必要。在选择手术方法和麻醉方式时，应认识到慢性肝细胞损伤的急性损害可能导致肝衰竭。肝功能不佳的临床指标可能包括持续低体温、凝血功能障碍性疾病、酸中毒或高血糖（晚期为低血糖）、少尿、肾功能不全、血流动力学不稳定、肺泡-动脉氧分压差降低和术后苏醒延迟。

管理

对于有术后黄疸的成年患者，其评估是基于对患者的病史、药物治疗、围术期、实验室检查和影像学结果的全面回顾。最重要的问题如下：

1. 胆红素升高的方式、肝功能改变或影像学检查是否反映肝细胞损伤、胆汁淤积或胆道梗阻？黄疸发作的病史是什么？
2. 患者是否有肝病或肝病危险因素？
3. 药物、酒精或脓毒症引起急性肝炎的可能性有多大？
4. 有溶血的迹象吗？
5. 手术方式是什么？是否有明显软组织出血的证据？
6. 患者接受何种麻醉方式？是否应用吸入性麻醉气体？确定低血压、低氧血症和需要输血的时期，并回顾围术期使用的药物清单，包括升压药物。

如果尿检胆红素阴性，且血清非结合胆红素升高，则提示为胆红素负荷过大所致的肝前原因。然而，如果尿液中胆红素呈阳性，总胆红素和结合胆红素升高，这可能是肝内或肝后原因之一。如果碱性磷酸酶和肝转氨酶均升高，则提示应行肝胆管造影。若阴性，则提示应查肝炎血清学、甲胎蛋白、抗线粒体抗体和内镜逆行胰胆管造影。胆管扩张需要行胆道造影检查。局灶性病变需要进一步行腹部超声、CT、MRCP、MRI、超声内镜等检查，必要时肝活检。根据 Child 分级或 MELD 评分对患者进行分级。

治疗方案包括以下建议：

1. 一般支持治疗；

2. 确保稳态环境（如正常的电解质、酸碱状态和血细胞比容）；
3. 循环系统的稳定性（维持容量稳定，平均动脉压 >60 ～ 75 mmHg）；
4. 治疗细菌性感染和与肝病相关的并发症（如肝性脑病、腹水、低钠血症、静脉曲张出血、凝血相关性疾病）；
5. 避免使用肝毒性和肾毒性药物。若有溶血的迹象，应立即终止输血；
6. 优化肾灌注：鉴别肾实质疾病，血管内扩容，采用内脏血管收缩剂或肾血管扩张剂；通过碱化尿液和利尿的应用治疗血红蛋白尿。

患者的治疗和预后取决于对高危患者的识别，并明确可能采取特定干预措施的病因。经过一般治疗和支持治疗后，黄疸将在几周到数月内消退。对于大多数暴发性肝衰竭患者，其生存完全取决于药物能否控制其稳定和紧急肝移植术。

（朱立鹏 译 赵珍珍 校）

延伸阅读

Amarapurkar PD, Amarapurkar DN: Management of coagulopathy in patients with decompensated liver cirrhosis, *Int J Hepatol* 2011:695470, 2011.

Dufour DR, Lott JA, Nolte FS, et al.: Diagnosis and monitoring of hepatic injury. I. Performance characteristics of laboratory tests, *Clin Chem* 46:2027–2049, 2000.

Fink SA: Approach to the patient with postoperative jaundice. In: Brown RS, Travis AC, editors. *UpToDate*. Waltham, MA. Available at www.uptodate.com/contents/approach-to-the-patient-with-postoperative-jaundice. Accessed September 26, 2016.

Teh SH, Nagorney DM, Stevens SR, et al.: Postoperative mortality of patients with cirrhosis, *Gastroenterology* 132(4):1261–1269, 2007.

van den Broek MA, Olde Damink SW, Dejong CH, et al.: Liver failure after partial hepatic resection: definition, pathophysiology, risk factors and treatment, *Liver Int* 26:767–780, 2009.

Wrighton LJ, O'Bosky KR, Namm JP, Senthil M: Postoperative management after hepatic resection, *J Gastrointest Oncol* 3(1):41–47, 2012.

术后周围神经病变 第 169 章

David A. Nakata，*Adam J. Lemmon*

病例概要

患者，男性，28 岁，患有胰岛素依赖型糖尿病 15 年，被诊断为睾丸癌。其化疗方案包括博来霉素和顺铂。患者化疗后在全身麻醉下行腹膜后淋巴结清扫术。手术历时 2 h，术中及术后麻醉恢复均无异常。术后第 3 天，患者发现左手第四和第五手指感觉减退。既往无周围神经病变史。随后患者被诊断为左侧尺神经病变。

问题分析

定义

神经病变分为三种组织学类型，其严重程度逐渐增加：神经失用、轴突断裂和神经断裂。临床上，任何或所有这些损伤模式都可以出现在受累神经中。对于神经失用，神经元解剖结构没有发生实质性断裂。然而，在缺血或一定程度脱髓鞘时可能导致暂时性传导阻滞，对大纤维功能（即运动、关节位置感知、柔软的触感）的影响更大。神经失用通常会在几周内消退，可完全恢复。轴突断裂，轴突被破坏，但神经鞘保持完好无损，Wallerian 变性随之而来，但是轴突再生使得功能恢复需数周至数月。即便如此，某种程度的感觉或运动缺失可能会持续存在。神经断裂是最严重的损伤，整个神经受到破坏，包括轴突和髓鞘的横断。这通常会阻碍再生和恢复，导致功能恢复不良。神经常被纤维瘢痕组织取代。

术后神经病变多为神经缺血所致。最常见的原因是牵拉或压迫。直接机械压迫显然会导致血流减少，而牵拉会使神经结构的横截面积减小，导致血管受压（图 169.1）。

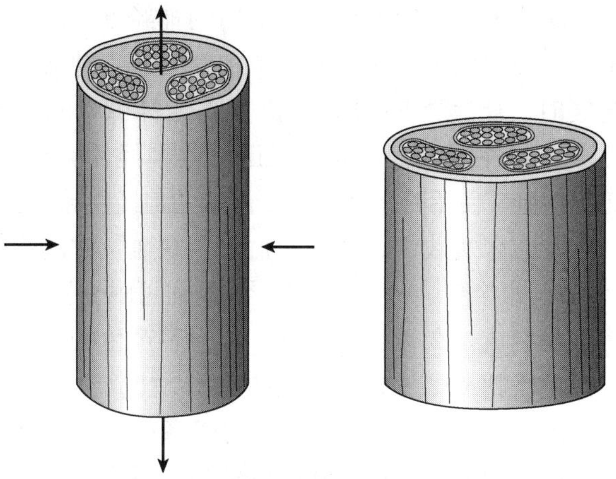

图 169.1 神经牵拉和横截面积减少与神经内压力增加有关（From Butler DS：*Mobilization of the nervous system*. New York，Churchill Livingstone，1991.）

识别

术后神经病变通常归咎于术中发生的事件。然而，在许多病例中，尽管进行了密切的随访，但直到术后数天症状才被报告。显然，如果术中事件是这些神经病变发生的原因，那么症状应于麻醉苏醒后不久出现。鉴于症状报告的延迟性，必须要考虑到许多神经病变可能由术后发生的事件引起。这与许多人仍然持有的传统观点形成鲜明的对比，既往多数认为神经病变发生表示术中医疗治疗偏离了标准。

风险评估

许多已知的因素与术后神经病变存在相关性（框 169.1）。本病例概要介绍的患者，其性别（男性）、术前化疗和糖尿病是与神经病变相关的已知风险因素。

由于不同性别之间的解剖学差异，男性尺神经损伤的风险似乎更高。男性冠状突结节约是女性的 1.5 倍，这可能导致对神经的骨性压迫增加。另外，女性通常在肘内侧有较大脂肪垫，有助于保护尺神

框 169.1 增加围术期神经病变的风险因素

酗酒	直接神经创伤
淀粉样变	性别（男性）
关节炎	肝衰竭
动脉粥样硬化	甲状腺功能减退
自身免疫紊乱	感染性疾病
Bell 麻痹	营养不良
恶性肿瘤	神经卡压综合征
化疗	肾衰竭
结缔组织病变	邻近组织创伤
糖尿病	维生素缺乏

经（图 169.2）。此外，有研究表明男性的肘管支持带更加强健，拉伸时可能尺神经会受到更大的压力（图 169.3）。

周围神经比中枢神经系统内的神经更能耐受缺血。使用止血带止血时，周围神经常发生缺血。当充气时，所施加的力通常比收缩压高 100 mmHg。已证实此种压力直接使受压区域的神经传导减慢，随着止血带使用时间增加，更远端的神经传导减慢。

在临床实践中，使用止血带“缺血”时间小于 2 h 被普遍接受。动物研究表明，缺血可耐受长达 4 h 而不会造成永久性神经损伤。止血带产生的压力通常比把胳膊或腿放在带衬垫的手术台上产生的压力大。因此，手术时间小于 2 h 的患者应该几乎不会因为止血带的应用或可接受的体位而发生术后神经病变。

本文病例概要中所描述的患者具有多种神经病变发生的危险因素，包括长期糖尿病病史和近期化

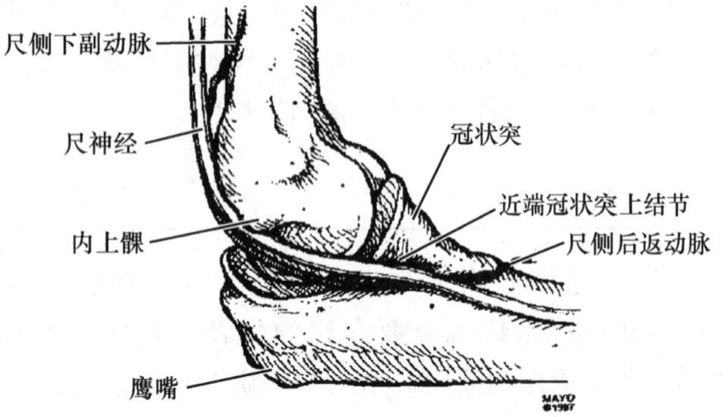

图 169.2 肘部尺神经和尺侧副动脉相对浅表，易受压迫，男性冠状突大于女性，脂肪层不明显，这些因素增加了男性尺神经受压的风险（From Warner M：Perioperative neuropathies，blindness，and positioning problems. American Society of Anesthesiologists 53rd Annual Refresher Course Lectures，2002，Orlando，FL.）

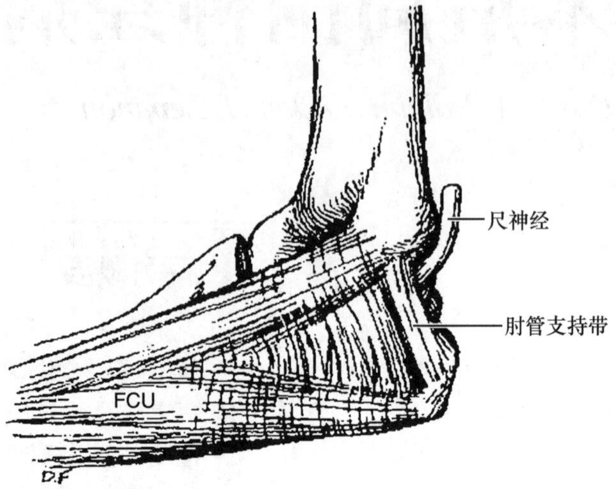

图 169.3 肘管支持带是一种坚韧的纤维带，靠近尺神经，尺神经受压可能发生于肘管支持带和内侧上髁之间。FCU，尺侧腕屈肌（尺骨头）（From Warner M：Perioperative neuropathies，blindness，and positioning problems. American Society of Anesthesiologists 53rd Annual Refresher Course Lectures，2002，Orlando，FL.）

疗史。在许多患者中，既往存在的情况可能在神经病变的发生中起重要作用。本例患者既往无周围神经受累症状，但与代谢（例如糖尿病、化疗）相关的神经病变通常起病隐匿。这种渐进性发病为亚临床神经病在症状出现前能够确诊提供了机会，而且它还增加了有症状性神经病变出现的敏感性。造成这种危险因素增加的研究比较透彻的潜在原因是双重挤压综合征。

双重挤压综合征是一种周围神经系统疾病，在这一疾病中，同一神经受到双重病变的协同作用从而增加各自的严重程度。Nemoto 等研究发现，在狗的周围神经上放置低压钳可能会产生不完全传导阻滞。这只是造成轻度的轴索变性，没有明显的临床后遗症。如果在同一外周神经的更远端放置第二个同样的低压钳，则表现为完全传导阻滞伴有明显的轴索变性。这种双重挤压损伤模型为并存疾病如何增加围术期神经病变的风险提供了一个很好的解释。该模型也可解释尽管使用相同体位预防措施，为什么某些患者会出现神经病变，而某些患者却不会。

双重挤压综合征可能在既往存在神经卡压综合征的患者发生神经病变的过程中发挥重要作用。例如，肘管综合征是一种常见的神经卡压综合征，发病率仅次于腕管综合征。肘管是一个封闭空间，周围是坚韧的纤维组织和骨骼。由于存在这些解剖学

边界，肘管在流体积聚时其扩张能力有限。术后，患者第三间隙（即间质）液体潴留，其中一些积聚在肘管内，可能增加肘管内压力，导致尺神经受到双侧挤压。众所周知，妊娠会引起腕管综合征，液体潴留可导致临床上显著的周围神经病变。

启示

美国麻醉科医师学会已结案的索赔分析认为，术后尺神经病变是术后最常见的周围神经病变之一。1999 年，所有此类神经损伤的索赔中，有 28% 涉及尺神经。最近一项对涉及麻醉护理索赔的分析表明，一些神经损伤直到麻醉护理结束后才发生。

在一项前瞻性研究中，Warner 及其同事发现报告尺神经病变症状的时间的中位时间是术后第 4 天（范围在 2 至 7 天）。该团队的另一项前瞻性研究显示，尺神经病变也发生在未行手术的内科患者中。根据以上研究，假设所有围术期神经病变发生在术中和围麻醉治疗期间是不合理的。因此，需要探寻周围神经病变的其他机制。

术后患者常规接受阿片类药物来控制疼痛。这些药物不仅可以缓解疼痛，还可能钝化其他异常感觉。镇痛药也会产生镇静作用，因此患者的活动能力较差。这种制动状态使患者在可能导致神经牵拉或压迫受损的体位上保持太长的时间。

最后，在术后查房中，通常会发现患者双臂交叉放在胸部或腹部休息。肘部弯曲已知也会增加肘管内压力，牵拉尺神经，这两种情况都会增加神经缺血的可能性（图 169.4）。通常这种手臂交叉的姿势使肘管直接与床接触，进一步压迫尺神经。当患者坐在扶手椅上，双臂弯曲，这样肘管与扶手直接接触，可能造成尺神经损伤。

管理

对于周围神经病变的主诉，何时应咨询神经科医师，尚无明确的指南。需要考虑症状持续时间和严重程度。如果疑似的周围神经病变在短时间内消退，那么最可能的诊断是神经失用症，并且有望完全恢复。然而，如果症状持续而没有改善，应考虑神经内科会诊，以协助诊断和治疗。在某些情况下，可能需要进行神经传导检查。

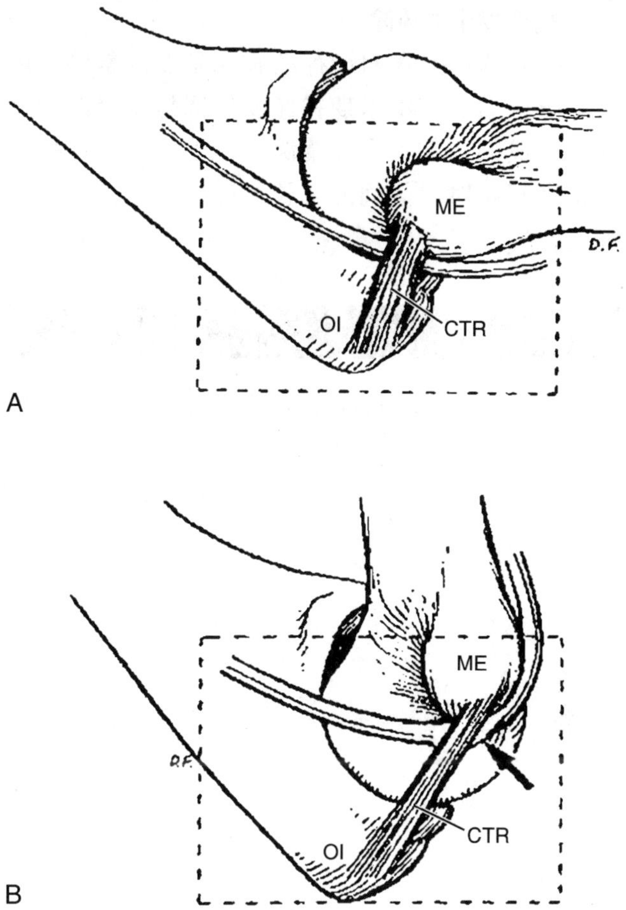

图 169.4　图 A，肘部伸展解剖；**图 B，**肘部屈曲时，肘管支持带（CTR）在内侧外髁（ME）和鹰嘴（OL）之间伸展，导致尺神经受压（箭头所指）。此外，尺神经在肘关节屈曲期间被物理拉伸，导致横截面积和血流减少（From Warner M：Perioperative neuropathies，blindness，and positioning problems. American Society of Anesthesiologists 53rd Annual Refresher Course Lectures，2002，Orlando，FL.）

预防

2000 年，美国麻醉科医师协会发布了一项关于预防围术期周围神经病变的实践建议。该建议提出了几项可能降低尺神经病变发生率的推荐意见：

- 仰卧位患者手臂外展应限制在 90° 内；俯卧位患者可承受手臂外展大于 90°；
- 应将手臂放置在正确的位置以减小肱骨后髁沟（尺神经沟）的压力。当双臂向两侧收拢时，建议前臂保持中立位。当手臂放在搁手板上外展时，可以采用仰卧位或前臂中立位；
- 带衬垫的搁手板可以降低上肢神经病变发生的风险；
- 肘部和腓骨头处的衬垫可分别降低上肢和下肢神

经病变发生的风险。

鉴于导致围术期尺神经病变是多因素的，因此不能认为所有围术期神经损伤都是违反医护标准而造成的。在大多数情况下，手术与最初症状报告之间相对时间间隔较长，进一步支持了这一观点。

致谢

感谢 Robert K.Stoelting 博士对本章上一版的贡献。

（黄 婷 译 韩 烨 校）

延伸阅读

Bentley FH, Schlapp W: Experiments on the blood supply of nerves, *J Physiol* 102:62, 1943.

Cheney FW, Domino KB, Caplan RA, et al.: Nerve injury associated with anesthesia: a closed claims analysis, *Anesthesiology* 90:1062–1069, 1999.

Gelberman RH, Yamaguchi K, Hollstien SB, et al.: Changes in interstitial pressure and cross-sectional area of the cubital tunnel and of the ulnar nerve with flexion of the elbow: an experimental study in human cadavera, *J Bone Joint Surg Am* 80:492–501, 1998.

Nemoto K, Matsumoto N, Tazaki K, et al.: An experimental study on the "double crush" hypothesis, *J Hand Surg [Am]* 12:552–559, 1987.

Practice advisory for the prevention of perioperative peripheral neuropathies: a report by the American Society of Anesthesiologists Task Force on Prevention of Perioperative Peripheral Neuropathies, *Anesthesiology* 92:1168–1182, 2000.

Warner MA, Warner DO, Harper C, et al.: Ulnar neuropathy in medical patients, *Anesthesiology* 92:613–617, 2000.

Warner MA, Warner DO, Matsumoto JY, et al.: Ulnar neuropathy in surgical patients, *Anesthesiology* 90:54–59, 1999.

术后肺动脉高压

第 170 章

Regina E. Linganna，Jiri Horak

病例概要

患者，女性，50 岁，伴有慢性栓塞性肺动脉高压，因结肠腺癌拟行开腹结肠部分切除术和一期再吻合术。患者接受华法林治疗，术前被要求停药 7 天，未服用其他治疗肺动脉高压的药物。由于呼吸困难，患者行走不到一个街区就需要停下休息。患者术前超声心动图显示中重度肺动脉高压。最近一次右心导管检查是 6 年前，当时的平均肺动脉压为 40 mmHg。由于患者的既往病史，麻醉诱导后放置了肺动脉导管。该病例术中平稳，在麻醉后恢复室（postanesthesia care unit，PACU）苏醒。患者进入麻醉后恢复室观察 20 min 后，心率从 85 次 / 分升至 120 次 / 分，目前血压为 70/35 mmHg。吸入 10L/min 纯氧时的脉搏氧饱和度为 92%，体温 36.5℃。肺动脉导管显示肺动脉压从基线值 45/28 mmHg 升至 75/45 mmHg。在麻醉后恢复室重新插管，行经食管超声心动图（transesophogeal echocardiogram，TEE）检查示右心室严重扩张，室间隔凸向左心室，左心室容量不足。

问题分析

定义

肺血管系统为一高流量、高顺应性、低压系统。因此，肺动脉压（pulmonary artery pressure，PAP）通常远低于全身动脉血压。肺动脉高压是一种可能在临床上被怀疑的疾病，最初经超声心动图诊断，再经右心导管检查（right-sided cardiac catheterization，RHC）确诊。症状通常是非特异性的，最常见的症状为呼吸困难，但也可能有胸痛、心悸或晕厥。一旦怀疑肺动脉高压，需行 RHC 确诊。平均 PAP 大于 25 mmHg，或峰值压力大于 40 mmHg，就可诊断为肺动脉高压。肺动脉高压程度不一，可分为轻度（肺动脉收缩压 40 ～ 49 mmHg）、中度（肺动脉收缩压 50 ～ 59 mmHg）或重度（肺动脉收缩压 60 mmHg 或以上）。

肺动脉高压分为五类（表 170.1）。第 1 类是肺动脉高压，是原发于肺动脉本身的疾病。第 2 类至第 5 类是继发于其他病因的肺动脉高压。

表 170.1　肺动脉高压的分类

		举例
第 1 类	肺动脉高压（PAH）	遗传性肺动脉高压 结缔组织病 中毒
第 2 类	继发于左心疾病	二尖瓣疾病 体循环高血压
第 3 类	继发于肺疾病	慢性阻塞性肺疾患 间质性肺疾患 阻塞性睡眠呼吸暂停
第 4 类	继发于慢性血栓栓塞性疾病	凝血因子 V Leiden 基因突变 蛋白质 C 缺乏 蛋白质 S 缺乏 抗磷脂综合征
第 5 类	混杂因素	真性红细胞增多症 结节病 组织细胞增多症 X

识别和风险评估

在术前阶段，辨别患者可能有未诊断的肺动脉高压非常重要。任何患有与肺高压第 2 类至第 5 类相关疾病之一的患者应怀疑有 PAP 升高。例如，已知患有结节病并伴有活动后进行性呼吸困难的患者应怀疑存在肺动脉高压。同样，二尖瓣狭窄患者症状恶化也应怀疑除了瓣膜病变进展外有新发的肺动脉高压。此外，吸烟者总是有肺动脉高压的风险，除了经常被诊断为慢性阻塞性肺疾患外，一种已知的肺血管收缩剂内皮素 -1 水平会升高，内皮素 -1 作为肺血管收缩剂发挥作用，从而增加肺血管阻力（pulmonary vascular resistance，PVR）。

如果已知或怀疑患者有肺动脉高压，行择期手术前有客观数据非常重要。如上所述，肺动脉高压最准确的诊断手段的金标准是 RHL，直接测量 PAP。然而，术前超声心动图通常是唯一术前可参考的客观数据，能提供关于 PVR 和右心室功能的有价值信息。长期患有肺动脉高压患者的右心室扩张伴肥厚，可能有轻度收缩力降低。另外，由于右心室压力升高，右心房将会扩张。随着肺血管系统压力的升高，右心室需适应并克服这种压力向肺提供前向血流。因此，患者的超声心动图也将提示有右心室收缩压升高。如果存在三尖瓣反流，也可在超声心动图上估测肺动脉收缩压。

常规胸部 X 线片可能显示右侧心影扩大，结合之前提到的其他风险因素，应引起临床医师怀疑肺动脉高压。心电图伴电轴右偏应提出相似的疑问。也应获取动脉血气确定患者的基本氧合情况和通气状态。

患者之前存在肺动脉高压的严重程度可基于前面描述的客观数据、患者的症状、药物治疗方案和对氧气的需求做出评估。每天步行 20 min 并采用前列环素患者的治疗方案与持续依前列醇滴注和 6 L/min 氧患者的治疗方案大不相同。

急性或慢性右心室收缩功能失代偿急性发作表现为右心室收缩力降低、急剧扩张和三尖瓣反流程度加重。右心室压力增加将导致室间隔移向左心室，进一步加重右心室衰竭。接着将引起左心功能障碍，每搏量显著降低，心排血量取决于心率。

启示

肺动脉高压最可怕的并发症是继发于不能适应肺循环后负荷增加的右心室衰竭造成的心血管衰竭。当右心室衰竭时，室间隔移向左侧，随后左心室功能因舒张期充盈不足和收缩期收缩力下降而受损。由于室壁扩张和腔内高压，右心室冠状动脉灌注减少，导致右心室缺血，进一步加重右心室衰竭。随着右心衰竭不断恶化，心排血量将持续降低。每搏量降低，心排血量取决于心率。

因心排血量降低发生低血压时，右心室冠状动脉灌注压进一步降低，进行性右心室缺血最终导致心血管性衰竭。

管理

除了之前提到的术前评估，行择期手术前应使用药物优化患者病情。术前也应讨论完善的疼痛治疗方案，降低术中患者对交感神经刺激的反应非常重要，以免加重肺动脉高压，可以通过全身和区域或椎管内技术相结合来实现良好的镇痛。对于本例患者，硬膜外麻醉可降低其术中和术后的交感神经反应。

由于血流动力学参数必须保持在很窄的范围内，这些患者的术中管理极具挑战。必须全程仔细调节呼吸机参数进行治疗，与所有患者一样，避免低氧血症很重要，对这类患者尤为重要，因为其对缺氧性血管收缩非常敏感，缺氧性血管收缩会增加 PAP，增加右心室后负荷，这是这类患者无法耐受的。避免高碳酸血症也很重要，因为产生的酸中毒会增加肺血管阻力。由于肺泡压增加，过度呼气末正压也会使 PVR 升高。另外，有必要避免肺不张，这会增加缺氧性血管收缩的可能性。呼吸机可通过多种途径对右心室产生不利影响，因此全程仔细调节呼吸参数设置以优化右心室做功非常重要。

非药物治疗包括避免脓毒症和导致 PVR 增加的酸中毒的其他病因。维持正常体温也很重要，因为体温过高会导致 PVR 增加，体温过低会导致心肌收缩力降低。另外需避免任何继发于喉镜或手术刺激的交感神经反应增高。

药物治疗可分为两大类：降低 PVR 的药物和提供右心室正性肌力支持的药物。降低 PVR 的药物通常是那些门诊患者服用的药物，包括前列环素、内皮素受体拮抗剂、磷酸二酯酶抑制剂、鸟苷酸环化酶激活剂和重组脑利钠肽（表 170.2）。此外，吸入用一氧化氮（inhaled nitric oxide，iNO）和吸入用依前列醇也可降低 PVR。一氧化氮是直接肺血管扩张剂，可被肺血管系统迅速降解，几乎没有体循环血

表 170.2 降低肺血管阻力的药物

药物分类	示例
前列环素	依前列醇（持续静注）
内皮素受体拮抗剂	波生坦 安立生坦
磷酸二酯酶抑制剂	西地那非 他达拉非
鸟苷酸环化酶激活剂	Rocociguat Cinaciguat
重组脑钠肽	奈西立肽

流动力学效应，iNO 的使用很昂贵且有多种不良反应，包括由代谢产物 N_2O 引起的高铁血红蛋白生成和支气管痉挛。米力农也是一种肺血管扩张剂，与 iNO 不同，米力农不具有肺血管特异性，有体循环低血压的不良反应，因此米力农通常与血管加压素同时给药。由于肺没有血管加压素受体，血管加压素能在不增加 PVR 的情况下抵消米力农在体循环中的扩血管作用。

提供右心室正性肌力支持的药物包括肾上腺素和多巴酚丁胺。肾上腺素直接作用于右心室增加心肌收缩力。多巴酚丁胺也能直接作用于右心，但伴有体循环低血压的不良反应。与肾上腺素不同，多巴酚丁胺主要刺激 β 受体，使其成为强心扩血管药。因此，体循环血管收缩药如血管升压素或去氧肾上腺素需与多巴酚丁胺同时给药以避免体循环低血压。为此，多巴酚丁胺作为治疗肺动脉高压一线药物的吸引力较小。

液体治疗对于这类患者也很重要。尽管患者在 PVR 急剧增加的情况下依赖于前负荷，但右心室容量负荷进一步增加也可能导致不利的室间隔移位。TEE 是指导液体治疗的重要方法。扩张、肥厚和收缩力增高的右心室可能对液体负荷作出心排血量增加的反应，这是因为心室已适应了升高的 PVR 而泵血，该心室的心排血量依赖于前负荷。相反，扩张和收缩力低下的心室对液体负荷反应不佳，因为这是新发病或肺动脉压急剧增高的急性右心室衰竭患者。在这种情况下过多的液体负荷只会加剧右心室衰竭，因为右心室不能处理增加的前负荷。从这两个例子中明显可以看出，根据病程不同，肺动脉高压患者的液体治疗可能存在很大差异。

这些患者的术后治疗应包括尽快重启家庭用药。如果患者有第 4 类肺动脉高压，从手术角度出发尽快重启患者的抗凝治疗非常重要，由于围术期患者血栓栓塞事件风险增加，因此抗凝治疗，包括桥接，应是最重要的。围术期血栓栓塞事件可能引起病例概要中的患者急性右心室衰竭。刺激性肺量仪锻炼设备也应在术后阶段开始，以降低可能导致的缺氧性血管收缩和由此导致肺血管阻力增加的肺不张的发生率。

预防

肺动脉高压是一种没有许多可改变的危险因素的疾病。然而，吸烟就是其中一种危险因素。除外戒烟的许多其他好处，戒烟可降低内皮素 -1 的水平，减少血管收缩的刺激。对于第 4 类肺动脉高压患者，术前桥接抗凝可减少患者未进行治疗性抗凝的时间，因此存在额外血栓栓塞事件的风险。患者还可以在术前放置下腔静脉滤器，以防止亚治疗抗凝期间意外发生肺栓塞。

（耿长振 译 朱文忠 校）

延伸阅读

Fischer LG, Van Aken H, Burkle H: Management of pulmonary hypertension: Physiological and pharmacological considerations for anesthesiologists, *Anesth Analg* 96:1603–1616, 2003.

Galiè N, Humbert M, Vachiery JL, et al.: 2015 Guidelines for the diagnosis and treatment of pulmonary hypertension, *Eur Heart J* 37(1):67–119, 2015.

Meyer KC, Love RB, Zimmerman JJ: The therapeutic potential of nitric oxide in lung transplantation, *Chest* 113:1360–1371, 1998.

第 171 章 术后呼吸衰竭

Michael J. Stentz，*Maurizio Cereda*

病例概要

患者，男性，75 岁，拟行急诊胆囊切除术。尽管已进行充分的液体复苏，但术中仍出现低血压。手术结束时，其动脉氧分压（arterial partial pressure of oxygen，PaO_2）为 80 mmHg，吸入氧浓度（fraction of inspired oxygen，FiO_2）为 100%。术后患者被送至重症监护室，胸部 X 线片显示双肺弥漫性浸润。患者术后留置气管导管 5 天，最终延长住院时间后出院，进入亚急性康复机构。

问题分析

定义

术后呼吸衰竭是指术后需要延长机械通气 48 h 或更长时间，或术后需计划外再插管。术后呼吸衰竭最常见原因是急性呼吸窘迫综合征（acute respiratory distress syndrome，ARDS）、肺不张、肺水肿和肺炎。正确识别和治疗潜在病因，对逆转术后呼吸衰竭至关重要。细致的术中管理在降低术后呼吸衰竭的风险中发挥了重要作用。

识别

术后呼吸衰竭的临床表现，很大程度上取决于潜在病因。除后述将讨论的肺部原因外，上呼吸道阻塞或麻醉引起的呼吸抑制也是术后再次气管插管的指征。术后第 3 天夜间血氧水平达最低点，提示患者在此期间再次插管的风险很大。

几乎所有患者术后均存在肺不张，但 1/5 的患者术后持续存在肺不张。其通常表现为低氧血症和胸部 X 线片上肺基底实变。尽管过去将术后发热归因于肺不张，但多项研究未能证实两者之间存在关联。

术后肺炎的诊断可能具有挑战性。任何术后需氧量增加的患者都应怀疑肺炎。胸部 X 线片提示浸润、发热和白细胞增多的症状组合高度提示肺炎，尽管这些体征是非特异性的。进展性肺炎的其他征象包括，脓性痰或对气道吸引的需求增加，咳嗽或呼吸困难症状恶化，以及胸膜炎性胸痛。体格检查结果可能再次证明诊断，但同样是非特异性的。实验室检查，包括革兰氏染色和呼吸道分泌物培养，例如军团菌等免疫染色，可能有助于诊断并指导抗生素治疗。

术后肺水肿可分为静水压性和渗透性两大类，取决于其表现和诱发危险因素。静水压性肺水肿是肺毛细血管壁上的压力增加，迫使水分脱离毛细血管并进入肺泡和间质。静水压性肺水肿常见于心室衰竭或瓣膜病，称为心源性肺水肿。即使没有心脏病，急性液体超负荷也会导致术后健康的患者出现静水压性肺水肿。间质和肺泡气腔内过量的液体损害气体交换，减少可用于通气的肺泡总量，表现为呼吸困难和低氧血症。胸部 X 线片显示为典型的肺血管头侧化（肺上管血管比下部粗），“蝙蝠翼”状肺阴影，支气管袖套征和胸膜渗出。

ARDS 是一种炎症导致肺毛细血管通透性增加的临床病症。其引起的肺泡与间质弥漫性水肿，降低了肺顺应性并严重影响氧合。ARDS 的发病机制复杂且因素多样，可由肺内或肺外因素触发。ARDS 表现为呼吸困难，呼吸做功增加，氧合功能受损，胸部 X 线片双侧斑片状渗出影（图 171.1）。2012 年的一份共识声明，更新了 ARDS 的临床诊断标准，并在框 171.1 中列出。半数医院获得性 ARDS 发生于外科手术患者，其中绝大多数（近 80%）与严重脓毒症有关；其他原因包括创伤、输血、误吸和胰腺炎，仅占少数病例。

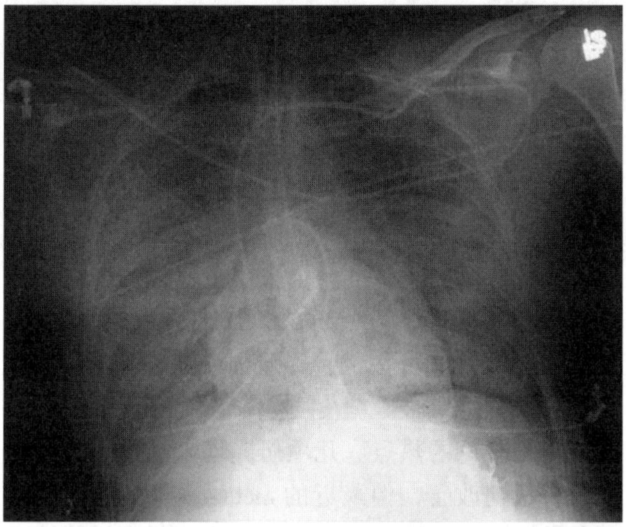

图 171.1 胸片显示弥漫性双侧肺浸润，符合急性呼吸窘迫综合征

框 171.1 急性呼吸窘迫综合征诊断标准
在病因损伤后 7 天内急性起病
胸部影像学呈双侧模糊影，并非由渗出、肺萎陷或结节所致
呼吸衰竭不能完全由心力衰竭或容量超负荷来解释
PaO_2：FiO_2 ≤ 300 且 PEEP ≥ 5 cmH_2O
轻度（PaO_2：FiO_2>200 ～ 300）
中度（PaO_2：FiO_2>100 ～ 200）
重度（PaO_2：FiO_2 ≤ 100）

Data from ARDS Definition Task Force，Ranieri VM，Rubenfeld GD，et al：Acute respiratory distress syndrome：the Berlin definition. *JAMA* 307（23）：2526-2533，2012.

FiO_2，吸入氧浓度；PaO_2，动脉氧分压；PEEP，呼气末正压

风险评估

呼吸模式的术后改变导致呼吸衰竭的风险增加。疼痛导致呼吸变浅而无周期性深“叹息”样呼吸，促进了肺基底不张。膈肌功能障碍亦可观察到，尤其是在上腹部切口的患者中。黏膜纤毛功能受损以及长期卧床休息导致肺部分泌物清除不佳。长效肌松药与术后呼吸衰竭也有一定的联系，提示残余肌无力会导致气道保护和分泌物清除不足。综上所述，这些变化导致大量患者存在术后肺部并发症的风险，并且大大增加了那些氧储备功能已经较差的患者的风险。

最近，学术界内对术后呼吸衰竭的诊断和研究的兴趣促进了多种评分系统的发展，以确定有肺部并发症风险的患者。毫无疑问，并存疾病较多的患者术后呼吸衰竭的风险增加。接受大血管、胸腔或上腹部手术的患者术后呼吸衰竭的风险也增加，因为这类患者术后疼痛、浅呼吸和膈肌功能障碍的风险高于其他患者。其中许多评分系统包含相似的风险因素，见表 171.1。

启示

3% ～ 5% 患者发生术后呼吸衰竭，其所致术后死亡率约 30%。与其他并发症相比，术后肺部并发症导致总住院费用增加，住院时间延长。早期识别有呼吸衰竭风险的患者，可更及时实施治疗并调动资源，因这些患者术后常需要机械通气和重症监护。

管理

肺不张

呼气末正压（positive end-expiratory pressure，PEEP）和连续的复张手法已证明可消除肺不张。但在正压停止后，肺不张会频繁地再次发生。术后早期持续气道正压通气可改善术后肺不张，减少再次插管的需要。目前，已提出多种肺不张治疗方法，包括深呼吸训练、间歇正压呼吸和激励性肺量仪锻炼。目前文献认为，这三种方式在减少术后肺不张中的作用效果相同。

表 171.1 易致术后呼吸衰竭的危险因素[a]

患者危险因素	手术危险因素	麻醉危险因素
年龄（>60 岁）	上腹部、胸部、血管、颈部或神经外科手术	较高的潮气量
术前 SpO_2 低	手术时长 >2 h	高驱动压力，高吸入氧浓度
术前 30 天内呼吸道感染	急诊外科手术	输血
术前贫血		晶体液过量
白蛋白 <30 g/L		
尿素氮 >30 mg/dl		
COPD		
ASA 分级 ≥ 3		

[a] 这些危险因素基于数个预测术后呼吸衰竭、术后 ARDS 和（或）术后早期再插管的评分系统

ASA，美国麻醉科医师协会；COPD，慢性阻塞性肺疾病；SpO_2，血氧饱和度

肺炎

若怀疑肺炎是术后呼吸衰竭的原因，早期开始合理的抗生素覆盖对提高患者生存率至关重要。现已证明，延迟使用抗生素或选择不够强效的抗生素，可使患者死亡率增加数倍。手术前已入住医院或接受长期护理的患者，发生医疗机构相关性肺炎（health care-associated pneumonia，HCAP）和多重耐药菌的风险增加。经验性抗生素的初始应用应选择广泛，应针对已知可引起 HCAP 的病原微生物，如金黄色葡萄球菌（包括耐甲氧西林金黄色葡萄球菌）、铜绿假单胞菌、不动杆菌、肠杆菌和肺炎克雷伯菌。在合理选择抗生素治疗时，也应考虑当地的耐药菌情况。一旦获得培养和敏感性数据，抗生素选择范围应相应缩小。

肺水肿

术后肺水肿的处理在很大程度上取决于潜在病因。正压通气增加胸膜腔内压，减少心脏前负荷和后负荷，从而改善心排血量。液体量超负荷时，使用利尿剂或超滤可能会有益处。心源性肺水肿可能需要正性肌力药物支持，通常需要更加有创性的监测，如中心静脉压与肺动脉压监测。一旦肺水肿的潜在病因得到解决，随着淋巴系统清除多余的水肿，氧合会得到改善。

急性呼吸窘迫综合征

ARDS 的治疗主要以支持为主，重点是避免进一步肺损伤，同时维持足够的氧合。尽管无创通气在轻度 ARDS 患者中的应用日趋广泛，但大多数患者仍需要气管插管和机械通气来维持氧合并减少呼吸做功。吸入氧浓度过高会增加肺泡炎症，加重肺损伤，要尽可能将 FiO_2 降至维持氧合所需的最低水平。考虑到肺泡充血导致可用于通气的肺容量较小，并伴随死腔通气比增加，此类患者必须使用比健康对照组小得多的潮气量进行通气。基于 ARDS 网络试验的结果，应根据理想体重予以小潮气量通气 6 ～ 8ml/kg；男性理想体重（kg）计算：2.3×[身高（in）-60]+50；女性理想体重（kg）计算：2.3×[身高（in）-60]+45.5 已成为标准治疗。ARDS 网络试验显示，与高潮气量通气相比，小潮气量通气的患者死亡率显著降低。PEEP 通常用于改善氧合，但使用高水平 PEEP（≥ 12 cmH_2O）似乎并不能改善预后并且很可能导致血流动力学不稳定。然而，许多医师在管理 ARDS 患者时仍采用适度的高 PEEP 策略。

在严重 ARDS 患者中，正确的呼吸机管理可能不足以确保充足的氧供。由于 ARDS 肺水肿和肺实质病变部位倾向于肺的重力依赖下垂区域，将患者长期置于俯卧位（≥ 16 h/d）可改善氧合并降低死亡风险。最初 48 h 内的神经肌肉松弛也可减少需氧量并降低死亡风险。糖皮质激素在 ARDS 治疗中的地位仍是争论的热点。几项研究均未能显示患者结局上有任何改善，但最近的 meta 分析表明，ARDS 患者早期使用甲泼尼龙后死亡率会降低。尽管糖皮质激素可能在 ARDS 治疗中有一席之地，鉴于缺乏前瞻性研究数据，很难予以强烈推荐。

尽管数据有限，其他高级疗法已建议用于术后呼吸衰竭。吸入型前列环素（依前列醇、伊洛前列素）和吸入型一氧化氮是强效肺血管扩张剂，已显示可略微改善氧合，但进一步研究未能显示两种疗法的益处。此外，这两种疗法非常昂贵，限制了其应用。近年来，呼吸衰竭患者应用体外膜氧合（ECMO）支持的数量也有大幅度增加。尽管接受 ECMO 支持的患者结局有所改善，但其仍是一种侵入性治疗，具有自身的相关风险，通常仅适用于已接受其他所有治疗方案但无效的患者。

预防

术中管理可对术后肺部结局产生显著影响。即便是既往体健的患者，小潮气量和中等 PEEP 的术中肺保护性通气策略，与术后呼吸衰竭发生率的降低和住院时间缩短相关。与长效药物相比，使用短效肌松药可降低术后肺部并发症。神经肌肉阻滞不完全逆转、术后呼吸衰竭和死亡率的关系，已在文献中被证实。然而，相当比例的麻醉科医师在拮抗神经肌肉阻滞时，未依照循证指南来监测 TOF 比值。

麻醉性镇痛药引起的呼吸抑制在术后 24 h 最明显。睡眠呼吸紊乱的患者，对阿片类药物引起的呼吸抑制特别敏感，故应密切监测有无即将发生呼吸衰竭的迹象。椎管内麻醉可能降低术后肺部并发症风险，现有数据尚有矛盾之处。

尽管没有一种方法可消除术后呼吸衰竭，但审慎仔细的麻醉技术可降低风险，尤其是存在易感并存疾病或外科手术的患者。鉴于术后呼吸衰竭的高发病率、高死亡率和高治疗费用，即使适度的风险降低也可能对个体患者和整个医疗系统产生重要影响。

（袁 炜 译 薄禄龙 校）

延伸阅读

Amato MB, Meade MO, Slutsky AS, et al.: Driving pressure and survival in the acute respiratory distress syndrome, *N Engl J Med* 372(8):747–755, 2015.

Arozullah AM, Daley J, Henderson WG, et al.: Multifactorial risk index for predicting postoperative respiratory failure in men after major noncardiac surgery, *Ann Surg* 232(2):242–253, 2000.

Blum JM, Stentz MJ, Dechert R, et al.: Preoperative and intraoperative predictors of postoperative acute respiratory distress syndrome in a general surgical population, *Anesthesiology* 118(1):19–29, 2013.

Brooks-Brunn JA: Postoperative atelectasis and pneumonia, *Heart Lung* 24:94–115, 1995.

Brower RG, Lanken PN, MacIntyre N, et al.: Higher versus lower positive end-expiratory pressures in patients with the acute respiratory distress syndrome, *N Engl J Med* 351(4):327–336, 2004.

Chaiwat O, Vavilala MS, Philip S, et al.: Intraoperative adherence to a low tidal volume ventilation strategy in critically ill patients with preexisting acute lung injury, *J Crit Care* 26(2):144–151, 2011.

Definition Task Force ARDS, Ranieri VM, Rubenfeld GD, et al.: Acute respiratory distress syndrome: the Berlin definition, *JAMA* 307(23):2526–2533, 2012.

Fernández-Pérez ER, Keegan MT, Brown DR, et al.: Intraoperative tidal volume as a risk factor for respiratory failure after pneumonectomy, *Anesthesiology* 105(1):14–18, 2006.

Fernández-Pérez ER, Sprung J, Afessa B, et al.: Intraoperative ventilator settings and acute lung injury after elective surgery: a nested case control study, *Thorax* 64(2):121–127, 2009.

Futier E, Constantin J-M, Paugam-Burtz C, et al.: A trial of intraoperative low-tidal volume ventilation in abdominal surgery, *N Engl J Med* 369:428–437, 2013.

Guerin C, Reignier J, Richard J-C, et al.: Prone positioning in severe acute respiratory distress syndrome, *N Engl J Med* 368(23):2159–2168, 2013.

Lawrence VA, Cornell JE, Smetana GW: Strategies to reduce postoperative pulmonary complications after noncardiothoracic surgery: systematic review for the American College of Physicians, *Ann Intern Med* 144:596–608, 2006.

Licker M, Diaper J, Villiger Y, et al.: Impact of intraoperative lung-protective interventions in patients undergoing lung cancer surgery, *Crit Care* 13(2):R41, 2009.

Naughton MT, Rahman MA, Hara K, et al.: Effect of continuous positive airway pressure on intrathoracic and left ventricular transmural pressures in patients with congestive heart failure, *Circulation* 91(6):1725–1731, 1995.

Overend TJ, Anderson CM, Lucy SD, et al.: The effect of incentive spirometry on postoperative pulmonary complications: a systematic review, *Chest* 120:971–978, 2001.

Papazian L, Forel J-M, Gacouin A, et al.: Neuromuscular blockers in early acute respiratory distress syndrome, *N Engl J Med* 363(12):1107–1116, 2010.

Ramachandran SK, Nafiu OO, Ghaferi A, et al.: Independent predictors and outcomes of unanticipated early postoperative tracheal intubation after nonemergent, noncardiac surgery, *Anesthesiology* 115(1):44–53, 2011.

Rubenfeld GD, Caldwell E, Peabody E, et al.: Incidence and outcomes of acute lung injury, *N Engl J Med* 353:1685–1693, 2005.

Sachdev G, Napolitano LM: Postoperative pulmonary complications: pneumonia and acute respiratory failure, *Surg Clin North Am* 92(2):321–344, ix. 2012.

Shari G, Kojicic M, Li G, et al.: Timing of the onset of acute respiratory distress syndrome: a population-based study, *Respir Care* 56(5):576–582, 2011.

Squadrone V, Coha M, Cerutti E, et al.: Continuous positive airway pressure for treatment of postoperative hypoxemia: a randomized controlled trial, *J Am Med Assoc* 293(5):589–595, 2005.

第172章 术后尿潴留

Eric Pan，D.Janet Pavlin

病例概要

患者，男性，73岁，脊椎麻醉（腰麻）下行全髋关节置换术[麻醉使用了1.5 ml 0.75%布比卡因（11.25 mg）和100 μg吗啡]。手术历时2 h，静脉输液约1500 ml。入苏醒室3 h后，患者主诉膀胱中度饱胀，并用力排出了150 ml尿液。排尿完毕后超声评估提示残余尿量约为700 ml，并同时留置导尿管。24 h后移除导尿管，患者恢复足量的自主排尿。患者出院后，无其他并发症。

问题分析

定义

术后尿潴留（postoperative urinary retention，POUR）的主要原因是膀胱充盈时不能充分排尿。正常成人膀胱容量约为400～600 ml。POUR的危险因素包括手术的性质和部位、使用的麻醉方式、药物以及患者的基础生理和内科病情。如不及时治疗，可引起尿失禁，当延长数小时后，可引起膀胱壁缺血。

对正常膀胱功能的知晓是了解尿潴留发生的方式和原因的先决条件。正常排尿是对膀胱充盈的反射反应，称为排尿反射（框172.1）。它需要膀胱膨胀，然后将感觉输入从膀胱传递到脊髓的骶中部，膀胱不自主地同时收缩，以及尿道内括约肌反射性抑制。尿道外括约肌自主松弛后排尿。来自膀胱的内脏感觉主要在骨盆内脏神经和骶中脊髓突触（S2～S4）中传播，并投射到大脑的排尿中枢。反射支传出包括以下内容：

- 起源于S2～S4的节前副交感神经纤维在盆腔内脏神经中走行至膀胱壁的外周胆碱能受体中，并在排尿活跃期刺激膀胱收缩。
- 起源于T10～L2的交感传出纤维通过上、下腹下神经丛到达尿道内括约肌。其在控尿时保持括约肌张力，排尿时反射性抑制。
- 躯体传出纤维穿行于阴部神经中，支配尿道外括约肌的横纹肌，在排尿时横纹肌必须主动放松。

框172.1　排尿的神经控制

膀胱膨胀

内脏传入纤维经盆腔内脏神经

骶中段束排尿中枢突触（S2～S4）

副交感神经传出胆碱能纤维（于S2～S4发出，与盆腔内脏神经伴行，在膀胱壁胆碱能部位形成突触，并刺激收缩）

交感传出纤维（于T10～L2发出，通过下腹丛走行至尿道内括约肌，排尿时不自主地被抑制）

躯体传出纤维（经阴部神经走行至尿道外括约肌横纹肌，排尿时自主放松）

整个反射弧通过脊髓延髓束受脑桥排尿中枢和大脑高级中枢的控制

排尿反射受高级脑中枢的调节，包括脑桥排尿中枢（背外侧脑桥）、间脑区域和大脑皮层。该通路脊髓部分的受体易受阿片类、乙酰胆碱、多巴胺、5-羟色胺、去甲肾上腺素、γ-氨基丁酸、兴奋性和抑制性氨基酸以及其他神经肽等物质的调控。

识别

诊断POUR的三种主要方法是病史或体检、导尿和超声检查。尽管不同的研究中，定义POUR的特定的标准各不相同（框172.2），但诊断一般是在不能完全排空饱胀膀胱的情况下进行的，和（或）通过导尿或超声检查确认存在大量的膀胱残余量。

病史和体格检查，特别是出现下腹部疼痛不适，伴或不伴有可以触及到的膀胱常用来鉴别是否存在POUR，尽管这两种方法对检测尿潴留都不是非常敏

框 172.2 定义 POUR 的常用标准

患者不适，膀胱膨胀感
可触及的膨胀膀胱
膨胀膀胱无法排空
Foley 导尿管拔除后 6 h 内不能排空膀胱
手术结束后 6 h 内不能排空膀胱
术后首个 24 ～ 48 h 内需要膀胱内插入导尿管
超声评估：
  无法排尿时膀胱内尿量≥ 600 ml
  残余尿量≥ 300 ～ 500 ml
排空膀胱后导尿，膀胱内尿量≥ 200 ml

感。此外，患者先前存在的并存疾病以及麻醉和手术因素可能掩盖 POUR 的常规体征和症状。事实上，一项研究报告提示，超过 60% 全身麻醉患者尽管其膀胱内容量超过 600 ml，在进入麻醉后监护室后并未表现出任何支持诊断的症状。

间歇导尿和留置导尿都可以作为诊断和治疗的工具，尽管这种操作并非没有风险。可能的并发症包括尿道创伤、感染和患者不适，在进行导尿前应予以考虑。

膀胱容量很容易通过超声评估，目前的证据通常支持其使用。在无意识患者中，便携式超声扫描可能是诊断尿潴留的唯一实用、可靠、无创的手段。然而，需要注意的是，当同一个人进行评估时，变异性似乎减小，这表明一致和可靠的测量需要标准化的方法。

尽管手术持续时间和术中给予的补液量与手术结束时的膀胱容量相关，但这些关系的变化足以限制其在预测个别患者膀胱容量方面的价值。在一项研究中，手术时间与手术后膀胱容量的相关性为 0.32（P=0.0002）。术中静脉内补液容量与膀胱容量的相关性为 0.26（P=0.0021）。有趣的是，Pavlin 及其同事研究发现，当超声测量的膀胱容积与膀胱的空虚、中度充盈或过度充盈的特征相比较时，56% 病例中患者的容量估计值不正确，46% 病例中护士出现差错。

风险评估

POUR 的风险因素列于框 172.3。尿潴留常与使用椎管内阻滞有关，使用长效局部麻醉药时发生率可能大于 60%。10 mg 布比卡因腰麻后对膀胱功能的影响可持续约 10 h。硬膜外吗啡作用可持续 16 h。但

框 172.3 尿潴留的危险因素

椎管内局部麻醉药
椎管内或全身性阿片类药物治疗
抗胆碱能类药物
原有梗阻症状（即良性前列腺肥大）
下尿路或周围区域的手术
腰骶神经分布区手术（腹股沟、直肠周围、阴茎）
尿潴留的既往史
脊髓疾病或功能障碍
半卧位
过量补液治疗
年龄≥ 50 岁
男性
手术时间过长
既往盆腔手术史

使用不含血管收缩剂或阿片类药物（即普通利多卡因或 2- 氯普鲁卡因）的低剂量、短效局部麻醉药，发生率相对较低。Mulroy 及其同事发现，201 名患者中有 3 例在使用短效脊椎或硬膜外麻醉后发生了 POUR。Brouwer 及其同事最近比较了椎管内麻醉与全身麻醉的结果，并证实使用短效局部麻醉药进行椎管内麻醉后导尿管置入术的风险增加 2 倍，使用长效局部麻醉药时增加 10 倍。

腰骶神经分布范围内的手术也可导致尿潴留。疝修补术和直肠手术常合并尿潴留（疝修补术为 14% ～ 35%；直肠手术为 1% ～ 52%）。此外，尿潴留可由手术疼痛和腰骶神经分布区交感神经活性增强引起。尿道的机械性创伤或原有的出口梗阻占泌尿外科手术后尿潴留的大多数比例。腰骶部脊髓病变与脊髓损伤患者一样，可出现排尿的干扰或排尿中枢协调的障碍。

强制性卧位与一些患者不能排尿有关，在足部手术后卧床的患者中 POUR 报告的发生率为 18%。其他因素，包括全身性阿片类药物、抗胆碱能药物和静脉大量补液也可导致排尿困难和 POUR。尿潴留病史也增加了 POUR 的可能性。机制包括上述任何原因，可能同时与易发生排尿受损的敏感性固有差异有关。

启示

膀胱过度膨胀可引起疼痛，并可随之发生尿失禁。它还可反射性引起交感神经活性增加，导致全

身性高血压；这在脊髓横断患者中更可能发生（自主神经反射亢进）。动物模型的研究也表明，膀胱过度膨胀可导致膀胱壁缺血。如持续超过 3 ～ 10 h，可发生尿路上皮细胞损伤、出血和水肿，最终可导致副交感神经末梢丧失，副交感神经活性降低，最终逼尿肌不能正常收缩。

副交感神经活动受损的症状包括不能充分排空膀胱，导致尿频、小尿（尿频、夜尿）、尿流无力、犹豫、尿淋漓不尽和膀胱不稳定。长期尿滞留可导致尿脓毒症。大多数情况下，细胞再生将发生在数周后，最终恢复正常的膀胱功能。然而，细胞间连接破裂和间质胶原沉积可导致整个膀胱壁冲动传递的永久性损害。

抛开 POUR 的并发症不谈，留置导尿管本身的并发症包括感染和医源性尿道损伤。一家机构报道的尿道损伤发生率为 3.2‰，其中一些患者出现了显著的病残率，包括需要多次扩张的复发性缩窄。长期留置导尿管也与感染发生率相关，感染发生率与留置导尿时间直接相关。Zaouter 及其同事报告称，在整个使用胸段硬膜外镇痛期间，使用留置导尿管的患者尿路感染率为 14%。在手术当天拔除导尿管可以使这个比例下降到 2%。

管理

当排尿反射因麻醉或手术而受损时，膀胱的过度膨胀通常导致 POUR。因为这通常是暂时的，一些尿潴留的发生可以通过简单地确保患者术前排空膀胱和避免过多的围术期液体治疗来预防。当已知手术或麻醉药物易致尿潴留或有尿潴留病史时，这一点尤其重要。

考虑到成人正常的尿生成速率约为 75 ml/h，因此膀胱充盈的时间（约 600 ml）约为 8 h。基于动物研究，为避免潜在神经损伤，膀胱过度膨胀的临界持续时间为 4 h。由此临床医师可以认为膀胱过度膨胀超过 4 h 是不可取的。

表 172.1 显示了 4 h 膀胱容量超过 600 ml 所需的估计时间，假设尿液形成率为 50 ml/h 或 100 ml/h。假设在开始时排空膀胱，则临界时间为 10 h（速率为 100 ml/h）和 16 h（速率为 50 ml/h）。然而，如果初始容积为 400 ml，则临界时间分别为 6 h 和 8 h。因此，为避免与术后尿潴留相关的并发症，应谨慎采取以下步骤：

- 确保所有患者在术前排尿。
- 确保术后患者在最后一次排尿后约 8 ～ 10 h 内排尿或导尿。
- 使用留置导管进行预期持续 5 ～ 6 h 以上的手术，并且假设患者在术后 1 ～ 2 h 内不能排尿。

表 172.1 达到临界膀胱容量的预计时间

膀胱初始容量	4 h 后达到 >600 ml 尿量所需要的时间（h）	
	尿量生成速度 50 ml/h	尿量生成速度 100 ml/h
0	16	10
100	14	9
200	12	8
400	8	6
600	4	4

虽然大多数麻醉科医师通常不负责 POUR 的药物治疗，值得一提的是已有数种药物正在使用，包括胆碱能药物、α-受体阻滞剂、镇静药物和前列腺素。在 Cochrane 协作网最近发表的一篇综述中提及，使用胆碱能药物、α-受体阻滞剂或镇静药物作为单药治疗时，未观察到显著改善。然而，前列腺素以及胆碱能药物，当与镇静药物联合膀胱内注射时，与成功治疗存在显著相关性。

预防

如果患者在最后一次排尿后 6 ～ 8 h 内未排尿，应在患者离开恢复室之前评估膀胱容量。膀胱容积可通过超声无创测定，若容积超过约 600 ml 则应引流。或者，如果不能使用超声，则可通过触诊评估膀胱容量，并通过插入导尿管引流排空膀胱。这在已知有 POUR 风险因素的患者中尤其重要。

值得注意的是，需要进行导尿的膀胱容量并不明确。在一项量化患者个体膀胱容量的研究中，为了明确患者是否需要导尿，Brouwer 及其同事测量患者手术前几周的最大膀胱容量。以此为触发因素，而不是任意的容量阈值（500 ml），结果发现导尿术的发生率显著降低，在年龄小于 60 岁的患者中效果最明显。

对于门诊手术，必须决定是否应要求患者在出院前进行排尿。至少有两项研究表明，不存在尿潴留潜在危险因素的患者应允许其可以在出院前不排尿就回家。在此类患者中，尿潴留的发生率小于 1%。对于存在尿潴留危险因素的患者，应谨慎要求其在出院前排尿，并检查残余尿量，以证实膀胱确实排空。当患者未能及时就医的情况下。这样做可以防止潜在的膀胱过度膨胀。因此直肠、腹股沟或泌尿道手术的患者和（或）有脊髓疾病或尿潴留病史的患者应要求在出院前排尿或导尿。

在脊椎或硬膜外麻醉后，应要求患者排尿或导尿，但有一些可能的例外。使用短效局部麻醉药（即利多卡因或 2- 氯普鲁卡因）进行过椎管内阻滞的患者，如果出院时膀胱检查显示膀胱容量小于 400 ml，可以安全出院而不排尿。由于这两种药物的作用持续时间较短，几乎可以肯定，任何局部麻醉药的残留效应都会在超过临界容量超过 4 h 之前消退。然而，接受过长效药物（例如布比卡因）或椎管内阿片类药物的患者在排尿或膀胱置管引流之前不应出院。

如上所述，排尿的高危患者应检查排尿后残余量，以确保膀胱确实排空。在许多情况下，用力排尿导致少量尿液排出，残余量仍可能超过 400 ～ 600 ml，因为排尿反射可能尚未完全恢复。如果超声扫描不可用，患者排尿少于 300 ml，则有理由怀疑残余尿量偏高（>400 ml）。应要求患者留观直至再次排尿并完全排空膀胱。或者，膀胱可以通过插入导尿管后再拔出，以确保在出院前排空膀胱。最后，如果所有门诊患者在出院后 8 ～ 10 h 内无法排尿，无论风险高低，均应指导他们返回医疗机构。对于离开恢复室后入住医院病房的患者，也应采用类似的方案。

（顾士杰　译　范晓华　校）

延伸阅读

Azadzoi KM, Pontari M, Vlachiotis J, et al.: Canine bladder blood flow and oxygenation: changes induced by filling, contraction and outlet obstruction, *J Urol* 155:1459–1465, 1996.

Baldini G, Bagry H, Aprikian A, et al.: Postoperative urinary retention: anesthetic and perioperative considerations, *Anesthesiology* 110:1139–1157, 2009.

Brouwer TA, Rosier PF, Moons KG, et al.: Postoperative bladder catheterization based on individual bladder capacity, *Anesthesiology* 122:46–54, 2015.

Buckley BS, Lapitan MC: Drugs for treatment of urinary retention after surgery in adults, *Cochrane Database Syst Rev* 10, 2010. CD008023.

DeGroat WC, Yoshimura N: Pharmacology of the lower urinary tract, *Ann Rev Pharmacol Toxicol* 41:691–721, 2001.

Kamphuis ET, Ionescu TI, Kuipers PW, et al.: Recovery of storage and emptying functions of the urinary bladder after spinal anesthesia with lidocaine and with bupivacaine in men, *Anesthesiology* 88:310–316, 1998.

Lamonerie L, Marret E, Deleuze A, et al.: Prevalence of postoperative bladder distension and urinary retention detected by ultrasound measurement, *Br J Anaesth* 92:544–546, 2004.

Lasanen LT, Tammela TL, Kallioinen M, et al.: Effect of acute distension on cholinergic innervation of the rat urinary bladder, *Urol Res* 20:59–62, 1992.

Lloyd-Davies RW, Clark AE, Prout WG, et al.: The effects of stretching the rabbit bladder, *Invest Urol* 8:145–152, 1980.

Lumen N, Hoebke P, Willemsen P, et al.: Etiology of urethral stricture disease in the 21st century, *J Urol* 182(3):983–987, 2009.

Mulroy MF, Salinas FV, Larkin KL, et al.: Ambulatory surgery patients may be discharged before voiding after short-acting spinal and epidural anesthesia, *Anesthesiology* 97:315–319, 2002.

Pavlin DJ, Pavlin EG, Fitzgibbon DR, et al.: Management of bladder function after outpatient surgery, *Anesthesiology* 91:42–50, 1999.

Pavlin DJ, Pavlin EG, Gunn HC, et al.: Voiding in patients managed with or without ultrasound monitoring of bladder volume after outpatient surgery, *Anesth Analg* 89:90–97, 1999.

Wu AK, Auerbach AD, Aaronson DS: National incidence and outcomes of postoperative urinary retention in the surgical care improvement project, *Am J Surg* 204:167–171, 2012.

Zaouter C, Kaneva P, Carli F: Less urinary infection by earlier removal of bladder catheter in surgical patients receiving thoracic epidural analgesia, *Reg Anesth Pain Med* 34(6):542–548, 2009.

第 173 章 围术期视力丧失

Kerri M. Wahl

病例概要

患者，男性，49 岁，体重 125 kg，拟行腰椎椎板减压切除术及多节段椎间融合术来治疗腰椎管狭窄症。患者全身麻醉期间顺利，术中采用俯卧位，用马蹄形头枕保护患者的面部和眼睛免受直接压力。术中监测体感诱发电位。手术总共持续了 8 h，术中预计出血约 2.5 L，静脉输注血液、晶体液补充血容量并进行抗纤维蛋白溶解治疗，术中最低血细胞比容为 25%。术后第二天，患者主诉双眼视力模糊。

问题分析

定义

据报道，脊柱外科手术每 500 例有 1 例（0.2%）出现围术期视力丧失（perioperative visual loss，POVL）。围术期视力丧失是指在实施全身麻醉的手术过程中出现的永久性视力损伤或完全失明。围术期包括从术前评估到从医疗机构出院的期间。

美国麻醉科医师协会（American Society of Anesthesiologists，ASA）结案索赔项目（www.asaclosed-claims.org）于 1999 年建立了术后视力损失登记处，旨在鉴定非眼科手术后 7 天内患者出现视力缺陷的危险因素。眼外伤最常见的原因是角膜擦伤，这可能与视力下降有关或没有关联。造成永久性 POVL 损伤常见原因是缺血性视神经病变（ischemic optic neuropath，ION）、视网膜中央动脉阻塞和大脑视觉丧失。归纳其各种原因及促成因素，包括以下几点：

- 术前情况如血管危险因素（动脉粥样硬化、糖尿病、高血压、冠心病）；贫血、病态肥胖、男性、年龄大于 50 岁；眼睛、视神经及其血供的解剖异常；
- 长时间的头颈部静脉压力升高（俯卧位手术或头低位）；
- 特定类型的手术架可能会增加头部静脉压力；
- 俯卧或头低位时手术时间过长（超过 6.5 h），大量失血（平均为估计血容量的 44.7%），并给予大量晶体液；
- 低血压；
- 贫血。

自 1996 年美国食品和药物管理局（Food and Drug Administration，FDA）批准使用脊柱椎间融合器以来，使脊柱椎体成形手术时间延长，手术失血量增加。其他的围术期危险因素包括使用氨甲环酸、液体管理（晶体液或胶体液）、面部肿胀、眼球受压、栓子、药物不良反应、使用血管收缩药物（如肾上腺素）和偶见控制性降压。在随机对照试验或动物研究中，这些因素均未发现与视觉丧失存在因果关系。

POVL 不常见的原因包括急性闭角型青光眼、球后血肿、垂体卒中、可逆性脑后部白质病变综合征和甘氨酸诱导的视力丧失。

识别

以眼部疼痛为表现的角膜擦伤是围术期最常见的眼部并发症。据报道，其在全身麻醉中发病率达 0.1‰～1‰。围术期视力损伤的机制是由于角膜上皮直接损伤（角膜擦伤）、角膜干燥或房水流出受阻伴眼压急剧升高（闭角型青光眼）。眼睑闭合不全或眼球突出的患者风险可能会增加。据报道，麻醉从业人员的类型不同导致结果存在显著差异，与有资质的麻醉护士和住院医师相比，见习麻醉护士导致受伤的比例更高。

ION 是非眼部手术后成人永久性 POVL 最常

见的原因，与腹部手术相比，心脏、脊柱和骨科手术后更为常见。也有报道称在双侧根治性颈清术和在极度头低脚高体位的手术后发生，如腹腔镜妇科和泌尿外科手术。大部分的三级医疗中心报告行多节段的脊柱重建手术患者中的 ION 发生率为 0.28‰～ 1.2‰。

ION 可能是动脉性的（如系统性血管炎引起的巨细胞性动脉炎）或非动脉性的（如术后缺血性视神经病变）。术后 ION 有两种类型：前部缺血性视神经病变（anterior ischemic optic neuropathy，AION），缺血从视神经前段，至睫状体后短动脉和瞳孔周围脉络膜血供；以及后部缺血性视神经病变（posterior ischemic optic neuropathy，PION），它是由球后视神经梗死引起的，其血供来自软膜的毛细血管丛。

术后 AION 最常见于心脏手术后，但也好发于大血管手术后、脊柱融合手术后以及头颈部手术后。受累患者表现出广泛的视力和视野缺陷。视盘最初肿胀，随后一个月逐渐发展成视神经萎缩。这是一种多因素疾病，它影响着神经乳头形态较小或拥挤，即所谓的"高危视盘"结构的中年患者。视神经缺血性损伤的其他危险因素包括糖尿病、高胆固醇、吸烟、生理性夜间动脉性低血压、视神经乳头血流不能正常自动调节以及视神经乳头血管供应的个体间变异。

脊柱手术后 PION 较 AION 更为常见。患者表现为视力范围从正常到无光感或视神经相关的视野缺陷。PION 早期眼底检查是正常的，但大约 5 ～ 6 周后视盘因萎缩而变苍白，瞳孔光反射延迟或消失，50% 以上的患者双侧受累，40% ～ 45% 的患者有一定程度的康复。诊断研究包括眼科检查（视力、眼压、颜色测试、视野、瞳孔反射、扩瞳后眼底镜检查），荧光眼底血管造影，以及视神经增强磁共振（magnetic resonance imaging，MRI）。计算机断层扫描（computed tomography，CT）对 ION 的诊断并无帮助。视觉诱发电位在检测到视盘苍白前是有用的，但由于全身麻醉（静脉或吸入麻醉）的影响，视神经诱发电位不能作为视神经功能的术中监测。

在 90% 的患者中，视网膜中央动脉阻塞（central retinal artery occlusion，CRAO）会导致手指计数到光知觉范围内的视力突然、急性、持续性和无痛性丧失。在每 1 万名门诊患者中发现 1 例 CRAO。在这些患者中，有 1% ～ 2% 的患者出现双侧受累。典型的眼底镜检查表现为"樱桃红点"，数小时可能形成视网膜周围苍白。CRAO 的最可能的原因是胆固醇栓塞，但它也有可能有静脉药物滥用导致形成的钙化、细菌或滑石粉栓有关。严重低血压和长时间的眼球压迫亦可导致 CRAO。

脑或皮质视觉丧失通常是由枕叶皮质栓塞性梗死（通常为单侧）或由严重低血压和（或）低血容量导致枕叶上分水岭区（双侧）缺血引起。术后脑视力丧失在小于 18 岁的患者中更为常见（4.3/10 000），而在心脏、脊柱融合、非融合骨科和腹部手术后，10 000 例脑视力丧失病例中的发生率为 0.38。双侧梗死时，患者可能完全失明或只有小部分中心视力得以保留；单侧梗死时，患者表现为对侧对称性偏盲，瞳孔光反射及眼底镜检查正常。脑 CT 或 MRI 显示脑后动脉或枕旁分水岭区梗死。

风险评估

对于"预期手术时间延长、大量失血的患者，或者两者都兼而有之的患者，围术期视力损失有着难以预测的风险"（ASA 工作组，2012）。

ION 的病因尚不清楚，大部分关于脊柱手术围术期 ION 的文献是基于病例报告和回顾性研究得到的。2006 年，ASA 专业责任委员会发表了一份来自 ASA 下面 POVL 登记处的 93 例（占所有登记病例的 72%）与俯卧位脊柱手术相关病例的深入分析报告。其中 83 例（89%）（56 例为 PION，19 例为 AION，8 例为未明确的）失明的原因是缺血性视神经病变，其余 10 例 POVL 为 CRAO。ION 患者的平均年龄是 50 ± 14 岁，大多数患者是相对健康的男性，96% 的患者失血量在 1000 ml 以上或麻醉时间在 6 h 以上。在 83 例病例中，采用梅菲尔德（Mayfield）神经外科头架的有 16 例，这表明 ION 是在眼球未受压的情况下发生的。这一结果与 ION 眼科检查视网膜不存在缺血是一致的。而且，大多数病例（55 例）双眼 ION 的发生更符合系统性病因，而不是通常只影响一只眼的眼球受压。47 例患者患眼视力完全丧失。ASA 专责小组（2012）认为面部水肿在围术期不存在引起 ION 的病理生理机制。此外，没有证据表明眼部压迫会导致围术期孤立的 AION 或 PION。但应避免眼睛直接受压，以免引起 CRAO。

大脑循环中血流自动调节已经在人类身上得到了很好的证实。但目前尚不清楚视神经是否也具有前后区域自动调节的能力。27% 的病例使用控制性降压来降低血压以减少术中失血。很多 ION 病例并没有出现很明显的低血压，这使血压在该过程中的作用不明确。有假设认为俯卧位可能会增加视神经的静脉压力和眼内压力。高静脉压和间质组织水肿可能会影响视神经的血流导致“筋膜室综合征”。这一假说的支持者推荐：在容易发生此类的手术中采用头高位和胶体液体复苏，以减少视神经周围组织水肿的可能性。

启示

2012 年，ASA 围术期视力丧失专题小组发布了一份最新的实践咨询意见，推荐如下：

术前患者评估及准备：

1. 可识别的术前危险因素包括贫血、手术时间过长和 / 或大量失血。
2. 没有易患 POVL 的患者可识别特征。
3. 尚无证据表明眼科或神经眼科检查在鉴别高危患者方面是有用的。

术中管理：

1. 血压管理：高危患者应持续监测全身血压；脊柱外科手术中控制性降压技术的使用尚未被证明与 POVL 有关，应根据患者的具体情况加以确定。
2. 术中液体处理：高危患者应考虑持续中心静脉压力监测；在大量失血的患者中，胶体液应与晶体液一起用于维持血容量。
3. 贫血的处理：应监测血红蛋白或血细胞比容；预防 POVL 的输血阈值目前尚不清楚。
4. 升压药的使用：应视患者的个体情况而定是否长时间使用大剂量的 α - 肾上腺素能受体激动剂。
5. 患者体位：避免直接压迫眼睛，高危患者应将头部置于正中前向位置，与心脏平齐或高于心脏。
6. 分期手术：高危患者应予以考虑。

术后管理：

工作组的共识是：当患者值得我们警惕时，应对高危患者的视力进行评估。如果怀疑有 ION 和潜在的视力丧失，应立即进行眼科会诊以确定其原因。术后其他管理可包括提高血红蛋白或血细胞比容、提升血压、吸氧。为了排除视觉损伤的颅内原因，考虑 MRI。该工作组认为，抗血小板药物、类固醇或降眼压药物对于围术期 ION 治疗没有作用。

控制性降压技术：

高危患者的血压管理取决于患者的多个特性，如术前慢性高血压、心功能障碍、肾脏和血管疾病等。此外，术中有许多影响血压管理的因素，如液体管理、失血速度、低血压和影响血压管理的升压药的使用。病例报告显示，对于无高血压或控制良好的慢性高血压患者，在术中维持低血压的患者在手术后易发生 POVL。在这个患者群体中使用控制性降压技术是有争议的。建议如果患者的血压平均维持在预估基线平均动脉压的 24%（0% ～ 40%）以内，或收缩压最低为 84 mmHg，控制性降压可以用于术前无慢性高血压的患者。

管理

围术期视力丧失是最常见于脊柱俯卧融合术后、体外循环术后、下肢关节置换术后一种严重并发症。缺血性视神经病变是最常见的病因。强烈建议尽早眼科医师会诊。在这一点上，预防策略似乎是减少这一并发症的最佳选择，因为目前尚无确定有效的治疗策略。脊柱融合术后与 ION 相关的独立危险因素包括男性、使用 Wilson 头架、长时间麻醉、估计失血量较大和较低的胶体比例（ASA 专责小组，2012）。

（林安琪　译　沈　镀　校）

延伸阅读

American Society of Anesthesiologists Task Force on Perioperative Visual Loss: Practice advisory for perioperative visual loss associated with spine surgery: an updated report by the American Society of Anesthesiologists Task Force on Perioperative Visual Loss, *Anesthesiology* 116(2):274–285, 2012.

Holy SE, Tsai JH, McAllister RK, et al.: Perioperative ischemic optic neuropathy: a case control analysis of 126,666 surgical procedures at a single institution, *Anesthesiology* 110(2):246–253, 2009.

Lee LA, Newman NJ: Postoperative visual loss after anesthesia for nonocular surgery. In Pasternak JJ, Crowley M, editors: *UpToDate*, Waltham, MA. Accessed September 29, 2016.

Lee LA, Roth S, Posner KL, et al.: The American Society of Anesthesiologists Postoperative Visual Loss Registry: analysis of 93 spine surgery cases with postoperative visual loss, *Anesthesiology* 105(4):652–659, 2006.

Postoperative Visual Loss Study Group: Risk factors associated with ischemic optic neuropathy after spinal fusion surgery, *Anesthesiology* 116(1):15–24, 2012.

非硬脊膜穿刺后导致的产后头痛

第 174 章

David Wlody

病例概要

患者，24 岁，初产妇，因胎儿臀先露使用 27 号 Whitacre 针行简单的蛛网膜下腔麻醉后行剖宫产术。产后第二天，产妇自述有严重的弥漫性头痛。产后第三天，产妇突然癫痫大发作。产科医师认为可能是脊髓性头痛并请麻醉科医师会诊。

问题分析

定义

产后头痛的定义为分娩后 6 周内发生的任何头痛。这种头痛可能是由产前早已存在的情况引起的，也可能是产程中相关事件的表现，或由产后偶发的一种不相关的疾病引起。存在一种自然倾向，特别是患者和产科医师将产后头痛归咎于椎管内麻醉，即使已知使用了大口径针进行硬膜穿刺，但并非所有的产后头痛都是硬脊膜穿破后头痛。本章讨论产后头痛最常见的原因，以及一些不太常见的情况，它的误诊可能会导致灾难性的结局。

识别

虽然特殊类型的头痛的发生率在近期分娩的妇女中可能有所不同，但在普通人群中出现的任何头痛都可能在产后发生。2013 年，国际头痛协会发布了第三版头痛诊断和分类标准的测试版。对这些标准的完整讨论超出了本文的讨论范围，但是为将头痛分为原发性和继发性提供了一个有用的讨论框架（表 174.1）。

原发性头痛（即无其他诱发疾病）

偏头痛

偏头痛分为两大类：有先兆偏头痛和无先兆偏头痛，前者为可逆的神经系统症状逐渐发生超过 5 min 或更长，持续不到 60 min。这些症状通常是视觉上的，包括闪光、边缘闪烁的盲点（“闪烁的暗点”）、曲线形成。面部麻木或手臂或腿无力也可能发生。包括失语症在内的语言障碍也偶有发生。下面这两个亚型的其他方面的特征相似：

- 单侧定位；

框 174.1　产后头痛的分类

原发性头痛
- 偏头痛（有无先兆）
- 紧张型头痛

继发性头痛
- 由脑血管疾病引起的头痛
  - 颅内出血
  - 脑静脉与静脉窦血栓形成
- 非血管性颅内疾病引起的头痛
  - 肿瘤
  - 特发性颅内压增高
  - 颅内积气
- 由某种物质或者其戒断引起的头痛
- 由体内稳态失衡引起的头痛
  - 子痫前期
  - 代谢紊乱
- 感染性头痛
  - 脑膜炎
  - 鼻窦炎

Data from Headache Classiflcation Committee of the International Headache Society（IHS）：The International Classiflcation of Headache Disorders，3rd edition（beta version）. *Cephalalgia* 33（9）：629-808，2013.

- 搏动性；
- 日常活动后加重；
- 与恶心和（或）畏光和恐声有关。

偏头痛通常开始发生于青春期，男性和女性的发病率分别为6%和17%。虽然与孟德尔遗传定律不一致，但有明显的家族性倾向；偏头痛在有偏头痛亲属的人群中的发病率是无偏头痛家族史的人群的3倍。

女性偏头痛的增加表明偏头痛受激素的影响。多达50%的女性描述偏头痛和月经之间有关系，这似乎与雌激素水平的变化有关。大多数妇女在妊娠期间偏头痛的发作频率降低，尤其是在妊娠中期和晚期。这种效应在无先兆偏头痛妇女中最为明显。偏头痛在产后早期复发较为常见。妊娠期或产后新发偏头痛不常见，需要密切调查，确保没有其他不良原因。

紧张型头痛

这是最常见的头痛类型，据报道男性终生患病率高达69%，女性高达88%。它是原发性头痛中研究最少的一种类型，曾经被认为主要是由心理因素引起，现在认为它的发生是有器质性基础的，可能通过肌筋膜痛觉感受器的外周激活，以及对慢性紧张型头痛的患者中枢致敏。紧张型头痛又分为偶发、频发和慢性三种亚型，根据每月发作的次数定义。除此之外，具有以下特征：

- 双侧性；
- 压迫感、非搏动性；
- 不因日常活动加重；
- 轻到中等强度；
- 无恶心、畏光和恐声。

与偏头痛一样，紧张型头痛在女性中更为常见。不像偏头痛，他们很少在青春期开始，但更可能在中年发生。并且还与慢性焦虑或抑郁相关。紧张型头痛与妊娠的关系尚未得到广泛研究，尽管一些研究表明妊娠期间紧张型头痛的发作频率有所降低，但这种降低的程度与偏头痛不同。

继发性头痛（即与已知可引起头痛的疾病密切相关的新发头痛）

由脑血管疾病引起的头痛

颅内出血，包括蛛网膜下腔出血、颅内（脑实质）出血或硬膜下血肿。颅内出血继发头痛的特点如下：

- 突然发病；
- 程度剧烈；
- 可能与局灶性体征或意识水平改变相关。

孕妇自发性蛛网膜下腔出血的发生率似乎并不比其他人群高。大约75%是由于颅内小动脉瘤破裂所致，其余是由于动静脉畸形破裂引起的。常伴有高血压和蛋白尿，因此蛛网膜下腔出血可与子痫前期相混淆。脑出血通常见于重度子痫前期或子痫。硬膜下血肿在硬脊膜穿破后头痛中有报道；颅内压降低可能导致桥静脉破裂。

脑静脉与静脉窦血栓形成。据估计，每2500～10 000例分娩中就有1例发生脑静脉血栓。事实上，孕妇在脑静脉血栓形成的患者中占有非常大的比例。妊娠引起的高凝状态是一个影响因素；还应评价患者是否存在遗传性血栓形成倾向（蛋白质S或C缺乏，Leiden第Ⅴ因子）。近80%的病例发生在产后前两周，但有报道可晚至产后3个月发生。继发于颅内血栓形成的头痛的特征各不相同，取决于血栓形成于大静脉窦还是孤立的皮质静脉。对于前者，头痛、癫痫、颅内压增高（由于脑脊液吸收受阻）和意识水平改变较为常见。当皮质静脉血栓形成时，更容易出现局灶性运动和感觉障碍以及癫痫发作。有趣的是，有几例报告的颅内血栓形成的病例最初是被当作硬脊膜穿破后头痛治疗的；在行硬膜外血补片之前症状和体征提示颅内高压应该进行更积极的检查。磁共振成像和磁共振血管造影被认为是诊断颅内血栓形成的金标准。尽管存在争议，但有一些证据表明D-二聚体水平正常可以排除脑静脉血栓形成。

静脉血栓闭塞导致毛细血管压力增高，常引起出血性梗死。随着血管的再通，毛细血管压力降低，可防止进一步出血。尽管肝素无溶栓特性，但可防止血栓进一步蔓延；因此，即使对于已存在出血的患者，它的应用也是有意义的。抗惊厥药物通常用于有出血或局灶性神经功能损伤的患者

非血管性颅内疾病引起的头痛

颅内肿瘤。与颅内肿瘤相关的头痛特征包括：

- 弥漫性、无搏动性；
- 常伴有恶心、呕吐；
- 因体力活动、Valsalva动作、咳嗽或打喷嚏而加重。

颅脑肿瘤的发病率在妊娠期并不增加，但症状在妊娠期首次出现并不罕见，继发于细胞外液增多。已确认激素对某些肿瘤也有影响，特别是脑膜瘤和垂体腺瘤。症状将受肿瘤位置、大小和颅内压升高程度影响。

特发性颅内压增高（idiopathic intracranial hypertension，IIH）。以前被称为良性颅内压增高或假性脑瘤，这种疾病最常见于青年肥胖女性，提示与激素成分相关。其特点如下：

- 弥漫性、非搏动性疼痛；
- 每天发生；
- 咳嗽加重。

患者警醒，神经系统检查可能正常。最常见的神经病学表现是视神经乳头水肿、第Ⅵ对脑神经麻痹和视野缺损，如果患者不及时治疗，这些症状会逐渐加重。IIH 是一种排除性诊断，必须排除其他颅内的、代谢性、中毒性或内分泌疾病。IIH 在妊娠期首次出现并不罕见，且在既往已确诊疾病的患者中症状通常会恶化。分娩后可有望改善。

颅内积气。通过非正常的蛛网膜下腔注射空气确定硬膜外腔有时较复杂。头痛通常在注射后立即发生，可相当强烈，直立位时加重。普通颅骨平片可轻松识别颅内积气。吸入 100% 的氧气可以加速气体吸收。

药物或其戒断引起的头痛

在硫酸镁治疗期间头痛很常见，特别是在使用负荷剂量时。对于每天摄入超过 200 mg 咖啡因的患者来说，突然停止摄入咖啡因会导致头痛，服用咖啡因 1 h 后头痛就会缓解。慢性阿片类药物治疗停止可在 24 h 内导致头痛。有研究表明，突然停用皮质类固醇、三环抗抑郁药和非甾体抗炎药会导致头痛。

体内稳态异常导致的头痛

子痫前期 / 子痫。头痛当然是重度子痫前期的标志，也可能是子痫发生的先兆。典型特征如下：

- 双侧，搏动性；
- 体力活动后加重；
- 伴有高血压和蛋白尿；
- 视觉障碍（视力模糊或出现盲点）。

与子痫前期相关的头痛一般发生在分娩前，但也可能在产后出现。此类患者有发生子痫的危险，应密切监护。

代谢紊乱。即使没有发生低血糖，禁食也会导致头痛发生。大约 30% 的慢性甲状腺功能减退患者对甲状腺替代疗法有反应，出现广泛的、非搏动性头痛。

感染性头痛

脑膜炎，继发于脑膜炎的头痛的特点如下：

- 弥漫性，逐渐加重的疼痛；
- 意识状态改变；
- 发热；
- 颈项强直；
- 恶心、呕吐、畏光。

脑膜炎是一种极为罕见的区域麻醉并发症，若不及时诊断和治疗，可造成灾难性后果。硬脊膜穿破后头痛与脑膜炎引起的头痛有许多共同的特点。对于推测的硬脊膜穿破后头痛伴发热、白细胞增多和脑膜刺激征的患者，应认真考虑进行诊断性腰椎穿刺；在明确致病菌之前，应考虑开始广谱抗生素治疗。

鼻窦炎。鼻窦炎引起的头痛常伴有脓性鼻涕和发热。受累鼻窦压痛常见。没有急性加重的情况下，慢性鼻窦炎不被认为是头痛的可能原因。

风险评估

头痛可发生在围产期的任何时候，产后极为常见。有头痛或抑郁病史的患者发生风险特别高。子痫前期或已知有颅内病变的患者必须仔细评估，特别是当头痛的严重程度超过通常严重程度时，以及尤其是伴有任何神经功能损伤时。

启示

产后头痛不一定与区域麻醉有关，即使是那些已知使用大口径硬膜穿刺针的患者。在进行硬膜外血补片前一定要考虑头痛的其他原因，特别是当出现不典型特征时，如发热、白细胞增多或局灶性神经功能损伤。当头痛对血补片反应不佳时，必须特别警惕。

管理

产后头痛的处理取决于病因，总结见表 174.1。

表 174.1 产后头痛的治疗

病因	治疗
偏头痛	β-受体阻滞剂、三环类抗抑郁药、5-羟色胺受体激动剂；避免已知的诱发因素；哺乳期母亲避免使用麦角生物碱
紧张型头痛	镇痛药、三环类抗抑郁药
颅内出血	减压手术
脑静脉和静脉窦血栓形成	抗惊厥药、抗凝药
颅内肿瘤	甘露醇、糖皮质激素、手术
特发性颅内压增高	糖皮质激素、碳酸酐酶抑制剂、腰椎穿刺
颅内积气	镇痛药、去氮
药物或其戒断引起的头痛	避免或调整诱发物质的剂量
子痫前期	抗高血压药、硫酸镁
与代谢紊乱有关的头痛	纠正代谢紊乱
感染性头痛	抗生素

预防

- 偏头痛患者应该避免食用如红酒、奶酪和腌肉等已知的诱发食物；
- 应维持慢性镇痛治疗，以避免头痛复发；
- 子痫前期患者应积极控制血压；
- 在实施椎管内麻醉时采用严格的无菌技术，以最大限度地降低感染并发症的风险。

（韩风瑞 译 韩 烨 校）

延伸阅读

Alons IM, Jellema K, Wermer MJ, et al.: D-dimer for the exclusion of cerebral venous thrombosis: a meta-analysis of low risk patients with isolated headache, *BMC Neurol* 15:118–125, 2015.

Aminoff MJ, Douglas VC: Neurologic disorders. In Creasy RK, Iams JD, et al.: *Creasy and Resnik's maternal-fetal medicine: principles and practice*, ed 7th, Philadelphia, 2013, Elsevier, pp 1100–1121.

Benzon HT, Iqbal M, Tallman MS, et al.: Superior saggital sinus thrombosis in a patient with postdural puncture headache, *Reg Anesth Pain Med* 28:64–67, 2003.

Cutrer FM, Bajwa FM: Pathophysiology, clinical manifestations, and diagnosis of migraine in adults. In Swanson JW, Dashe JF, editors: *UpToDate*, Waltham, MA. Accessed September 30, 2016.

Donaldson JO: *Headache. Neurology of pregnancy*, ed 2nd, Philadelphia, 1989, WB Saunders, pp 217–227.

Ferro JM, Canhão P: Etiology, clinical features, and diagnosis of cerebral venous thrombosis. In Kasner SE, Dashe JF, editors: *UpToDate*, Waltham, MA. Accessed September 30, 2016.

Headache Classification Subcommittee of the International Headache Society: The International Classification of Headache Disorders, 3rd edition (beta version), *Cephalalgia* 33:629–808, 2013.

Lim SY, Evangelou N, Jurgens S: Postpartum headache: diagnostic considerations, *Pract Neurol* 14:92–99, 2014.

Macarthur A: Postpartum headache. In Chestnut DH, Wong CA, Tsen LC, et al.: *Chestnut's obstetric anesthesia: principles and practice*, ed 5th, Philadelphia, 2014, Elsevier, pp 713–738.

MacGregor EA: Headache in pregnancy, *Neurol Clin* 30:835–866, 2012.

MacGregor EA, Frith A, Ellis J, et al.: Incidence of migraine relative to menstrual cycle phases of rising and falling estrogen, *Neurology* 67:2154–2158, 2006.

Masuhr F, Mehraein S, Einhäupl K: Cerebral venous and sinus thrombosis, *J Neurol* 251:11–23, 2004.

Ropper AH, Samuels MA, Klein JP: Headache and other craniofacial pains. In Ropper AH, Samuels MA, Klein JP, editors: *Adams and Victor's principles of neurology*, ed 10th, New York, 2014, McGraw-Hill, pp 175–203.

Taylor FR: Tension-type headache in adults: pathophysiology, clinical features, and diagnosis. In Swanson JW, Dashe JF, editors: *UpToDate*, Waltham, MA. Accessed September 30, 2016.

腰肌间隙阻滞的潜在并发症

第 175 章

Daryl S. Henshaw，Robert S. Weller

病例概要

患者，男性，68 岁，既往有心房颤动病史，拟行左侧髋关节置换术。患者每天服用抗凝药物利伐沙班（Xarelto）10 mg，以降低脑卒中和血管栓塞的发生风险，术前 72 h 停用。术前实验室检查结果显示：血红蛋白 13 g/dl，血小板计数为 $175 \times 10^3/\mu l$，肌酐为 0.9 mg/dl，肾小球滤过率大于 60 ml/（min · 1.73m²）。术前行后路腰丛神经阻滞（腰肌间隙阻滞）用于术后镇痛，手术麻醉采取蛛网膜下腔阻滞；两项操作均顺利实施。患者生命体征平稳，术中失血量约为 300 ml，手术顺利，术后安返病房。术后 18 h，即次日（术后第 1 日）早晨，重新开始服用利伐沙班 10 mg。当日，患者血压逐渐从 140/90 mmHg 下降至 95/55 mmHg，并且患者出现意识模糊和少尿的现象。外科医师随即反复给予 500 ml 生理盐水补液，随后血压得以改善，但尿量依旧很少。术后第 2 天上午，患者血红蛋白为 7.3 g/dl，立即给予红细胞悬液 2 个单位。复查血红蛋白为 7.7 g/dl。患者遂被转移到重症监护室，并停止服用利伐沙班，腹部 CT 检查结果提示左侧腹膜后巨大血肿。

问题分析

定义

腹膜后出血（retroperitoneal hemorrhage，RPH）是出血流至壁层腹膜后的潜在腔隙中，常发生在腰肌间隙阻滞（psoas compartment block，PCB）后，可由于动脉损伤合并凝血功能异常所致。腹膜后潜在间隙较大，含有松散的结缔组织并从膈肌延伸至骨盆，在压塞效应发生之前可以容纳大量的血液。

RPH 的发生主要是创伤性和医源性因素导致。此外，也可能发生自发性 RPH，最常见于接受抗凝治疗或血液透析以及有潜在凝血功能异常的患者。事实上，伴有股神经麻痹的自发性髂腰肌出血是引起血友病患者出现神经麻痹症状最常见的自发性出血种类。口服抗凝药物治疗的患者自发性 RPH 发生率显著增加。所有报道的病例显示，PCB 后 RPH 与凝血异常和（或）使用抗凝药物有关。

识别

腹膜后出血部位深且较为隐蔽，直到发生明显的失血才被发现。RPH 的症状和体征取决于出血的速度和程度以及血肿是否压迫邻近结构。

腹膜后出血的最常见体征是由于血管容量减少以及贫血导致的低血压和心动过速（框 175.1）。最初，通过补液可以改善低血压和心动过速。最终，患者可能会出现少尿和精神状态改变等失血性休克的表现。虽然少尿可能是因为输尿管梗阻，但腹膜后血肿通常不会延伸越过中线，且理论上不会同时压迫双侧输尿管，所以前期少尿更常见于血容量不足。

腹膜后血肿的其他症状可能包括腹部、侧腹、腹股沟或腿部疼痛，可触及的腹部肿块，以及腰丛

框 175.1 腹膜后出血的症状和体征

低血压
贫血
休克
腹部、侧腹、腹股沟或腿部疼痛
可触及的肿物
股神经病变
体侧淤斑（Gray Turner 征）
脐周淤斑（Cullen 征）

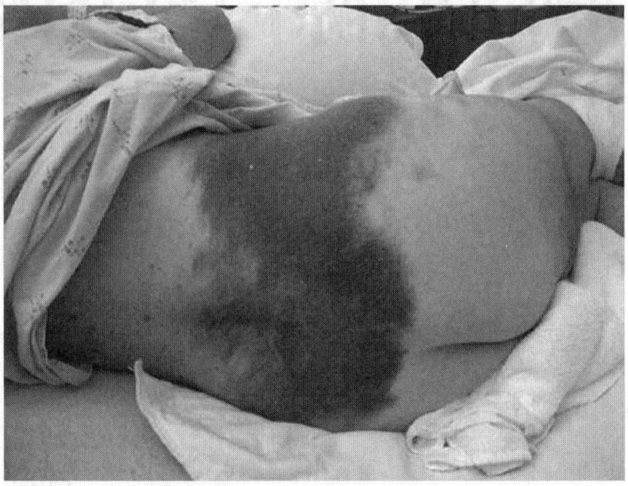

图 175.1 患者处于左侧卧位，由于腰肌间隙阻滞后出现的腹膜后血肿而引起广泛的体侧淤斑（Gray Turner 征）

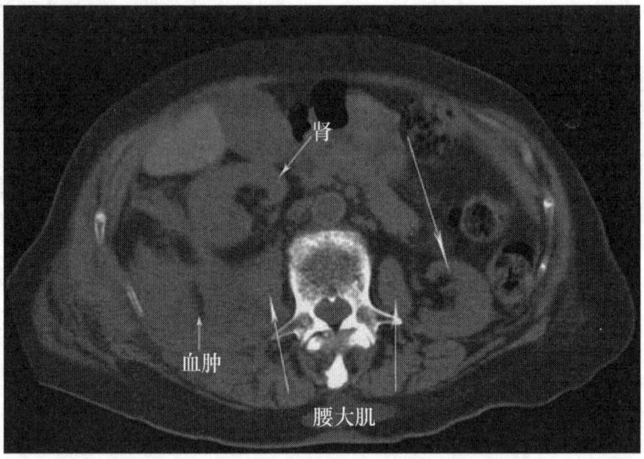

图 175.2 腹部 CT 扫描显示腰肌间隙阻滞后形成的巨大腹膜后血肿

神经刺激或功能障碍。肾起源的自发性 RPH，称为 Wünderlich 综合征，与经典的 Lenk 侧腹痛，可触及的腹部肿物和低血容量性休克有关。随着时间的推移，病症可能发展为脐周（Cullen 征）或体侧淤斑（Gray Turner 征；图 175.1），但这些往往是晚期的后遗症。

在一项涉及抗凝治疗后发生自发性 RPH 的病例系列中，腹痛发生率为 83%，严重低血压或休克发生率为 44%，40% 可触及腹部肿物，神经病变发生率为 29%。在另一项观察心导管术后 RPH 的病例系列中，低血压（收缩压 <90 mmHg）发生率为 64%，进行性贫血发生率为 73%。此外，该组中 45% 的患者主诉下肢疼痛，55% 出现股神经麻痹。

因为 RPH 的症状和体征主要是非特异性且缓慢出现，只有具有丰富临床经验的临床医师才能对 PCB 后 RPH 进行早期发现与诊断。对于髋关节术后 PCB 导致的低血压和贫血，更常见的病因包括手术持续出血以及术中输血不足。围术期低血压和心动过速也可能由脓毒症所致，通常表现为发热但无贫血症状。在患者复苏并去除围术期低血压或血容量不足的因素后，应进行腹部 CT 检查，因为 CT 对于诊断 RPH 敏感性较高（图 175.2）。

风险评估

1974 年首次提出了经腰肌后路腰丛神经阻滞或 PCB。自此，阻滞方法和进针入路经过数次改进。现在最流行的 PCB 方法需要使用神经刺激器通过股四头肌的运动反射来识别腰丛的股神经部分。近年报道了超声引导下腰丛神经阻滞的多种入路与方法，但是对于过度肥胖的患者，由于受限于深度和分辨率等因素，超声引导也并不总是可行。

如果考虑将 PCB 作为手术麻醉或术后镇痛的一部分时，必须考虑到与替代技术相比其成功率以及可能带来的风险。髋关节置换手术后 PCB 的镇痛效果已经获得研究证实。与全身性使用阿片类药物进行镇痛相比，PCB 已被证实可降低术后疼痛评分、减少阿片类药物消耗量，并可减少围术期失血。但在风险方面，一项与区域麻醉相关的主要并发症调查中，Auroy 及其同事提醒 PCB 相比其他外周神经阻滞可能会出现危及生命的并发症，比如发生全脊椎麻醉、全身毒性反应和心脏停搏（8：1000）。然而，这项调查仅包括 394 例 PCB 操作病例，所占外周神经阻滞总数的比例很小。另一个重要的并发症是局部麻醉药的硬膜外间隙扩散，成人和儿童发生率分别为 27% 和 92%。尽管以前认为 PCB 方法会影响硬膜外扩散的发生率，但并非所有研究都支持这种解释。最近，有研究表明高注射压力增加了椎管内扩散的可能性。在尝试连续 PCB 期间也发生过药液扩散到硬膜外甚至蛛网膜下腔的情况。考虑到椎间孔的解剖学结构特征与 PCB 穿刺的入路与部位，发生此类并发症并不意外。PCB 的并发症在框 175.2 中列出。

虽然 PCB 通常情况下安全且有效，但 RPH 存在潜在致病和死亡的风险。腹膜后空间包含丰富的动静脉网。腰椎的动脉起源于主动脉，沿着椎体走行，穿行在腰大肌和腰丛神经后方、腰椎横突之间。髂腰动脉起源于下腹部动脉并上行与腰大肌内侧边缘的第四腰椎动脉汇合。节段性的腰椎静脉通过上行腰静脉相互连接（图 175.3），进入下腔静脉。鉴于腰丛神经附近存在丰富的血管供应，在 PCB 操作期间发生穿刺针进入或损伤血管、并进一步造成出血或全身局部麻醉药中毒也就不足为奇了。

腰段交感神经阻滞和 PCB 后，已有数例 RPH 的报道。每一个病例均涉及同时采用单次注射和留置导管连续阻滞技术，并且在阻滞前、后进行过抗凝治疗。随着抗凝程度的增加，这种并发症的风险也会增加。

框 175.2　腰肌间隙阻滞的并发症

- 腹膜后血肿
- 肾损伤和包膜下血肿
- 蛛网膜下腔、硬膜外、椎间盘内或腹腔内置管
- 股神经病变
- 硬膜外扩散
- 全脊椎麻醉伴心脏停搏
- 全身毒性反应导致心脏停搏
- 死亡

单次注射或连续 PCB 操作后，临床上出现显著腹膜后出血的真实发生率与用于围术期血栓预防或抗凝治疗的药物使用剂量之间的关系尚不清楚。然而，有报道显示在通过股动脉进行心脏导管置入术后此发生率为 0.49%，并且在慢性肾功能不全、动脉穿刺部位更靠近心脏或在接受糖蛋白Ⅱ b/ Ⅲ a 抑制剂治疗的患者中发生率更高。

在考虑每例患者的 PCB 操作的风险效益比数时，必须考虑发生隐匿性大出血的可能性。在分析过程中必须包括备用方案、抗凝血或抗血小板药物的使用情况以及抗凝程度。美国区域麻醉和疼痛医学学会（American Society of Regional Anesthesia and Pain Medicine，ASRAPM）已就正在接受抗凝治疗的患者进行椎管内麻醉的医疗操作规范制定了共识指南，并建议将这些指南同样应用于深部神经丛阻滞，如 PCB。然而，一些临床医师建议在进行 PCB 操作时或在移除 PCB 所留置的导管时不必参照 ASRAPM 指南要求。一项研究结果显示，200 例接受连续性 PCB 操作的患者，术后使用利伐沙班进行抗凝治疗，并且在使用了 1 ～ 2 个剂量的利伐沙班后拔除导管，然而这些患者中并无明显出血并发症

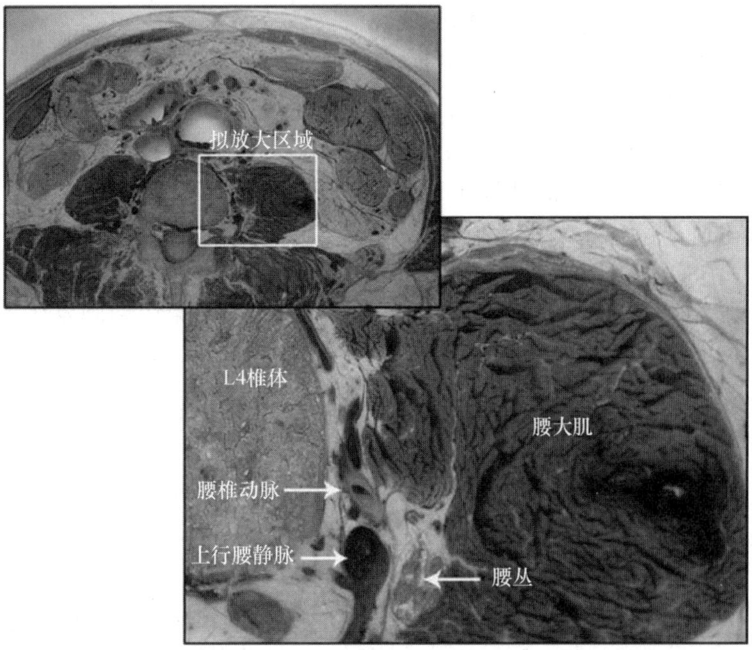

图 175.3　L4 椎体的横截面解剖图示。放大的图像显示了靠近腰丛神经的腰动脉和更大的上行腰静脉

的病例报道。但在这项研究中，导管放置和移除的确切时机并未报道或标准化，同时也没有描述在放置导管时发生出血的处理措施。此外，即便在此200例患者中发生的出血事件为零，但出血的统计学风险也可能大于1%。事实上，即便排除了阻滞操作的因素，这项研究中发生大出血的概率仍为1.9%。

启示

PCB导致的腹膜后出血，如果早期诊断并接受输血或支持治疗，通常可以完全康复并不需要手术治疗。然而，这种并发症的治疗仍然需要昂贵的成本，并且也存在很多风险，比如大量输血、延长住院时间以及抗凝措施的拮抗等。更为严重的是，PCB后腹膜出血可引起持续性股神经病变甚至死亡。

尽管PCB后RPH导致的确切死亡率尚不清楚，但有报道显示心脏导管术后RPH的死亡率为4%～12%。此外，在一项针对接受抗凝治疗患者的系列报道发现，与自发性RPH相关的死亡率高达20%。因此，在使用PCB操作时应权衡利弊。

管理

早期诊断对于快速启动治疗非常重要。框175.3详细介绍了PCB后RPH的处理方案。首要任务是补充血容量，同时进行实验室检查，包括血红蛋白浓度、血小板计数和凝血指标的测定，以指导输血和其他治疗措施的开展。有时可能需要停止抗凝措施，或需将患者转运至ICU直至循环状况稳定。一旦患者恢复生命体征平稳，可进行CT扫描确定诊断并评测出血的程度。如果存在持续活动性出血，锝-99扫描可助于确定出血部位并指导出血血管的栓塞治疗。放置血管内支架或移植物是对于持续性出血的另一种治疗选择。

框175.3 腰肌间隙阻滞后腹膜出血的管理

恢复血容量
检查血细胞计数和凝血功能
根据指征输注血液和凝血因子
药理学上进行抗凝治疗的拮抗措施
转至ICU，直到患者循环功能稳定
进行腹部CT扫描以明确诊断
对持续性出血考虑介入放射会诊
对持续性出血、股骨麻痹或腹腔间隔室综合征考虑手术探查

许多权威人士认为，因腰丛神经受压导致的持续性或进行性神经功能障碍应进行紧急减压手术。也有人认为手术干预应是最后的选择，并建议更加积极地治疗股骨神经病变，尤其对于存在先天性凝血障碍的患者。手术治疗虽可以减轻血肿但会导致再出血。对于保守治疗或血管内介入治疗措施无效仍持续出血，以及出现腹腔间隔室综合征的患者，通常应选择开放式手术治疗。

预防

腰大肌旁的组织血管分布特点使得穿刺针不可能完全避开动脉或静脉。即使在超声引导下也无法完全避免血管损伤，并且没有证据表明超声引导下PCB操作减少血管损伤的发生。因为与单次阻滞所使用的穿刺针相比，连续硬膜外麻醉所使用的穿刺针和留置导管较粗，后者具有更高的硬膜外血肿发生风险，所以对于类似PCB的周围神经阻滞操作也同样遵循这一规律。

当使用神经刺激器和绝缘穿刺针来定位PCB的腰丛神经时，即便操作过程中保持间断负压回抽的操作，血管损伤也可能无法及时发现。即使使用空心针，血管损伤也可能不明显。无论使用何种针头，都有关于PCB后发生RPH的报道。因此应注意以下事项：

- 遵循ASRAPM关于抗凝或溶栓治疗患者进行区域麻醉的循证操作指南；
- 如后续有需要进行溶栓治疗的可能性，应避免使用PCB；
- 对接受过PCB治疗且术后抗凝的患者，对隐性出血保持高度警惕；
- 如在PCB操作期间发生明确的血管损伤，应及时告知手术团队，并考虑推迟术后强效血栓预防性治疗措施。建议对患者保持仔细随访和并持续监测血细胞比容。
- 拔除PCB导管应按照ASRAPM指南要求进行，并在出血风险可能增加的患者（例如接受多种抗凝药物治疗的患者）中保持高度警惕。
- 与基层手术机构的医师沟通隐匿性出血的可能性，使其能够对PCB后出血相关并发症保持警

惕，特别是在术后发生预期外的贫血或血容量不足时。

（郑 敏 译 杨 涛 校）

延伸阅读

Auroy Y, Benhamou D, Bargues L, et al.: Major complications of regional anesthesia in France: the SOS Regional Anesthesia Hotline Service, *Anesthesiology* 97:1274–1280, 2002.

Aveline C, Bonnet F: Delayed retroperitoneal haematoma after failed lumbar plexus block, *Br J Anaesth* 93(4):589–591, 2004.

Capdevila X, Biboulet P, Morau D, et al.: Continuous three-in-one block for postoperative pain after lower limb orthopedic surgery: where do the catheters go? *Anesth Analg* 94:1001–1006, 2002.

Capdevila X, Marcaire P, Dadure C, et al.: Continuous psoas compartment block for postoperative analgesia after total hip arthroplasty: new landmarks, technical guidelines, and clinical evaluation, *Anesth Analg* 94: 1606–1613, 2002.

Chan YC, Morales JP, Reidy JF, et al.: Management of spontaneous and iatrogenic retroperitoneal haemorrhage: conservative management, endovascular intervention or open surgery? *Int J Clin Pract* 62(10):1604–1613, 2008.

Chudinov A, Berkenstadt H, Salai M, et al.: Continuous psoas compartment block for anesthesia and perioperative analgesia in patients with hip fractures, *Reg Anesth Pain Med* 24:563–568, 1999.

Dauri M, Faria S, Celidonio L, et al.: Retroperitoneal haematoma in a patient with continuous psoas compartment block and enoxaparin administration for total knee replacement, *Br J Anaesth* 103(2):309–310, 2009.

Gadsden JC, Lindenmuth DM, Hadzic A, et al.: Lumbar plexus block using high-pressure injection leads to contralateral and epidural spread, *Anesthesiology* 109(4):683–688, 2008.

González C, Penado S, Llata L, et al.: The clinical spectrum of retroperitoneal hematoma in anticoagulated patients, *Medicine (Baltimore)* 82(4): 257–262, 2003.

Horlocker TT, Wedel DJ, Rowlingson JC, et al.: Regional anesthesia in the patient receiving antithrombotic or thrombolytic therapy: American Society of Regional Anesthesia and Pain Medicine Evidence-Based Guidelines (ed 3), *Reg Anesth Pain Med* 35(1):64–101, 2010.

Kaloul I, Guay J, Cote C, et al.: The posterior lumbar plexus (psoas compartment) block and the three-in-one femoral nerve block provide similar postoperative analgesia after total knee replacement, *Can J Anaesth* 51:45–51, 2004.

Karmakar MK, Li JW, Kwok WH, et al.: Ultrasound-guided lumbar plexus block using a transverse scan through the lumbar intertransverse space: a prospective case series, *Reg Anesth Pain Med* 40(1):75–81, 2015.

Klein SM, D'Ercole F, Greengrass RA, et al.: Enoxaparin associated with psoas hematoma and lumbar plexopathy after lumbar plexus block, *Anesthesiology* 87:1576–1579, 1997.

Macalou D, Trueck S, Meuret P, et al.: Postoperative analgesia after total knee replacement: the effect of an obturator nerve block added to the femoral 3-in-1 nerve block, *Anesth Analg* 99(1):251–254, 2004.

Maier C, Gleim M, Weiss T, et al.: Severe bleeding following lumbar sympathetic blockade in two patients under medication with irreversible platelet aggregation inhibitors, *Anesthesiology* 97:740–743, 2002.

Narouze S, Benzon HT, Provenzano DA, et al.: Interventional spine and pain procedures in patients on antiplatelet and anticoagulant medications: guidelines from the American Society of Regional Anesthesia and Pain Medicine, the European Society of Regional Anaesthesia and Pain Therapy, the American Academy of Pain Medicine, the International Neuromodulation Society, the North American Neuromodulation Society, and the World Institute of Pain, *Reg Anesth Pain Med* 40(3):182–212, 2015.

Schulman S, Beyth RJ, Kearon C, et al.: Hemorrhagic complications of anticoagulant and thrombolytic treatment: American College of Chest Physicians Evidence-Based Clinical Practice Guidelines (ed 8), *Chest* 133(Suppl 6):257S–298S, 2008.

Souron V, Delaunay L, Schifrine P: Intrathecal morphine provides better postoperative analgesia than psoas compartment block after primary hip arthroplasty, *Can J Anaesth* 50:574–579, 2003.

Sreeram S, Lumsden AB, Miller JS, et al.: Retroperitoneal hematoma following femoral artery catheterization: a serious and often fatal complication, *Am Surg* 59:94–98, 1993.

Stevens RD, Van Gessel E, Flory N, et al.: Lumbar plexus block reduces pain and blood loss associated with total hip arthroplasty, *Anesthesiology* 93(1):115–121, 2000.

Tiroch KA, Arora N, Matheny ME, et al.: Risk predictors of retroperitoneal hemorrhage following percutaneous coronary intervention, *Am J Cardiol* 102(11):1473–1476, 2008.

Tokarz VA, McGrory JE, Stewart JD, et al.: Femoral neuropathy and iliopsoas hematoma as a result of postpartum factor-VIII inhibitor syndrome, *J Bone Joint Surg Am* 85:1812–1815, 2003.

Turker G, Uckunkaya N, Yavascaoglu B: Comparison of the catheter-technique psoas compartment block and the epidural block for analgesia in partial hip replacement surgery, *Acta Anaesthesiol Scand* 47:30–36, 2003.

Weller R, Gerancher JC, Crews JC, et al.: Extensive retroperitoneal hematoma without neurologic deficit in two patients who underwent lumbar plexus block and were later anticoagulated, *Anesthesiology* 98:581–585, 2003.

Williams P: *Gray's anatomy: the anatomical basis of medicine and surgery*, ed38, New York, 1995, Churchill Livingstone, pp 1562, 1558, 1600.

Wilson MW, Fidelman N, Lull RJ, et al.: Evaluation of active bleeding into hematomas by technetium-99m red blood cell scintigraphy before angiography, *Clin Nucl Med* 27:763–766, 2002.

Winnie A, Ramamurthy S, Durrani Z, et al.: Plexus blocks for lower extremity surgery: new answers to old problems, *Anesthesiol Rev* 1:11–16, 1974.

第176章 肺部误吸

Andrew Davidson, Michael Robinson

病例概要

患者，女性，76岁，既往有高血压病史，因坠落机械性造成股骨颈骨折，拟行全髋关节置换术。在平稳静脉麻醉诱导后，在保留自主呼吸状态下置入声门上气道装置，通过吸入挥发性麻醉剂维持麻醉。在手术台上摆好体位后不久，患者开始呼吸急促。手术开始后几分钟，患者出现低氧血症，呼吸变得不规则，在呼吸回路和患者口腔里发现黄色液体。

问题分析

定义

肺部误吸的定义是吸入口咽或胃食管的内容物通过声门进入支气管树。在麻醉期间由于正常的保护性喉反射减弱，如咳嗽、呼气和喉痉挛导致肺部误吸发生。误吸最常发生于麻醉下未实施气道保护的反流患者，这意味着反流风险越大的患者肺部误吸风险也大。

识别

误吸可引起轻微的呼吸障碍，如呼吸急促或短暂性喉痉挛，严重的低氧血症和心血管虚脱或多器官功能衰竭而死亡。

误吸物的数量、物理性质和酸度决定了可能的临床进程。牙齿、固体食物碎片或可能随后凝结的血液，有可能导致快速的致命性窒息。大量强酸性胃液可诱发严重的化学性肺炎，表现为进行性呼吸困难、低氧血症、支气管喘鸣和胸部X线显示的肺部浸润。

在大量胃内容物呕吐后呼吸突然恶化时，很显然可能发生了误吸，但在更多不明显的情况下，在无气道保护的麻醉患者发生呼吸道并发症时，则需要高度怀疑是否发生了误吸并进行识别。

风险评估

肺部误吸的可能性很大程度上取决于患者的风险因素。这些风险因素决定了在全身麻醉误吸并发症的风险在1/10 000～1/900之间。虽然肺部误吸在急诊麻醉中发生的可能性要高出3～4倍，但由于择期手术的患者比急诊手术的患者多得多，因此在择期手术中会出现更多的吸入性病例。

最近的证据表明，大约50%与气道相关的麻醉死亡是由于误吸导致。由于风险评估或气道管理不当而发生的误吸仍然是诉讼的一个重要原因。

在对风险进行准确和全面的评估之后，必须采取适当的措施，这对于减少肺部误吸的可能性和严重程度至关重要。一致的证据表明，在一些肺部误吸的病例中，尽管进行了恰当的风险评估，但麻醉的实施并没有考虑到患者反流风险的增加而做出改变。

表176.1根据患者、手术和麻醉列出了风险因素。如果发现误吸的风险增加，则应相应地改变麻醉技术。

患者的风险因素可能与饱胃有关，如急诊手术、胃排空延迟、食管下段括约肌功能不全导致的逆流和潜在的反流。手术风险因素包括腹腔镜、反屈氏体位（Trendelenburg体位）和胃肠疾病包括肠梗阻等。麻醉风险因素包括在高危患者中使用不恰当的气道技术，饱胃患者实施镇静，以及麻醉深度过浅。误吸通常发生于不能使用带套囊的气管插管保护气道或在实施快速顺序诱导时插管失败。

虽然患者的风险因素明确且众所周知，并且保持不变，但肥胖的发病率和严重程度的增加，以及腹腔镜手术的开展和长时间的屈氏体位，这些均增加了总的发病率。先前的严格和长时间的禁食固体

表 176.1 误吸的风险因素

患者因素	外科	麻醉
饱胃 • 急诊手术 • 禁食时间不充分 • 胃肠道梗阻	体位 • 头低脚高位 • 截石位	术前评估 • 急诊手术 • 不能进行风险评估 • 不能改变麻醉技术
胃排空延迟 • 糖尿病性胃轻瘫 • 自主神经病变 • 慢性肾病 • 近期创伤 • 颅内压升高 • 阿片类药物 • 妊娠和主动分娩	外科疾病 • 胃肠道梗阻 • 上消化道手术史 • 病态肥胖	气道 • 困难气道 • 声门上气道装置（很大可能使用一代声门上气道装置）
食管下段括约肌功能不全 • 裂孔疝 • 复发性反流 • 消化不良 • 胃食管反流	手术 • 腹腔镜 • 胆囊切除术 • 上消化道手术	麻醉期间 • 过浅的麻醉 • 手术时间超过 2 h • 正压通气

食物或液体的规定最近有所放宽，但这本身并没有增加肺部误吸的风险。关于术前禁食的建议仍然是 6 h，包括手术饮料和非母乳；4 h 的母乳；2 h 的清亮液体。

预防

当确定误吸风险升高时，应更改麻醉方式以降低风险。减少误吸风险的策略见表 176.2，包括通过使用椎管内阻滞、区域或局部麻醉技术而避免全身麻醉。术前准备包括充分的术前禁食或使用术前药物减少胃容量和胃内容物酸度。

如果需要全身麻醉，则应采用减少误吸风险的气道管理策略，所采用的策略应与风险程度相匹配。例如，如果患者存在轻度的误吸风险，可考虑使用第二代声门上气道装置；但如果患者有较高的误吸风险，则应使用带套囊的气管插管。当存在非常高的风险时，例如在紧急情况下，强烈建议使用快速序贯诱导下进行气管插管。

环状软骨加压（Sellick 手法）常被推荐作为快速序贯诱导时防止食管上括约肌上方胃内容物被动反流的一种方法，但应注意的是，它可能会妨碍直接喉镜检查时喉部的显示，并可能会导致

表 176.2 可使用的降低误吸风险的策略汇总

减少胃容量	• 术前充分禁食 • 如留置胃管则通过胃管吸引 • 术前服用促动力药（如甲氧氯普胺）
避免全身麻醉	• 区域麻醉
降低胃内容物的 pH	• 抗酸剂（如柠檬酸钠） • H_2 组胺拮抗剂（如雷尼替丁） • 质子泵抑制剂（如奥美拉唑）
气道保护	• 气管插管 • 第二代声门上气道装置
防止反流	• 环状软骨压迫 • 快速序贯诱导
拔管	• 苏醒后气道反射恢复 • 体位（侧卧位、头低位或近似坐位）

一部分患者呕吐。环状软骨压迫时若发生主动性呕吐，应立即释放，否则可能导致食管破裂伴纵隔炎。

误吸风险不仅存在麻醉诱导中，而且在整个麻醉维持过程中、拔管期间，甚至可能在麻醉苏醒后仍然存在。应该在拔管前吸出口腔和口咽的分泌物，以防止随后发生误吸；例如扁桃体切除或拔牙后可能存在出血时，应该特别小心。如果风险评估要求使用快速序贯诱导，则麻醉苏醒时应在患者意识和气道反射完全恢复，在侧卧位或近似坐位下，才能拔除导管。框 176.1 提供了关于如何防止误吸的最新临床建议。

框 176.1 预防和管理误吸的最新临床建议

1. 确保术前彻底准确评估误吸风险。如果有疑问，就假设风险更高
2. 选择符合已识别风险的气道策略
3. 在任何时候都有设备、技能和经验丰富的援助来发现和管理反流和误吸
4. 在下列情况下气管插管（或强烈考虑插管）
   - 所有紧急情况
   - 胃排空延迟（糖尿病性胃轻瘫、妊娠、阿片类药物、慢性肾病）
   - 腹内压升高（肥胖、腹水、腹部肿块）
5. 对包括紧急情况在内的高风险人群使用快速序贯诱导
6. 轻度反流风险的患者考虑使用第二代声门上气道装置
7. 在可能有出血的情况下，拔管前确保仔细地吸引口腔
8. 记住，如果患者在麻醉前被认为存在风险，那么应该使用一些策略来最大限度地减少苏醒 / 拔管时误吸风险（例如清醒拔管、侧卧位、抬头或近似坐位）

管理

一旦确认误吸，治疗以支持治疗和器官支持为主。使用快速作用的肌肉松弛药如琥珀胆碱行气管插管。在开始正压通气之前，最好应对气管进行吸引以尝试将上呼吸道中误吸物吸除。

维持氧合的方法是确保充足的吸入氧浓度（FiO_2），并通过使用呼气末正压和调整呼吸频率和吸气时间来优化通气。

低血压可能提示循环性休克，应积极静脉输液和（或）使用血管加压药物进行治疗。

只有在患者没有需要持续的器官支持治疗的迹象，且临床医师认为这样做是安全的操作时，才可以考虑苏醒和拔管。然而，对于在麻醉后治疗单元或重症治疗病房的患者，应考虑在苏醒后进行一段较长时间的观察。如果患者需要持续的器官支持治疗，可能需要长时间的机械通气和镇静，并需要转移到合适的危重治疗病房。如果患者出现休克的迹象，应插入导尿管及有创动脉和中心静脉导管。

氧合和通气的充分性应通过连续脉搏血氧、二氧化碳描记图和多次动脉血气测定来监测。胸部X线片在大多数情况下都能发现肺部实变，在仰卧位误吸的患者中，由于右主支气管走行方向较垂直，胸部X线片显示误吸通常是对右侧的影响更大。早期治疗性支气管镜检查有助于预防远端肺不张和肺塌陷，特别是在吸入微粒物质的情况下。硬质支气管镜检查可用于去除气管和上支气管气道中的固体物质比如牙齿。

抗生素仅在出现肺炎后才能使用，因为抗生素的不合理应用可能会导致耐药性或毒性细菌的定植，如铜绿假单胞菌。尽管使用糖皮质激素理论上可以减少炎症，但没有证据表明它们可以改善预后或降低死亡风险。事实上，它们可能是有害的，因为它们的免疫抑制作用增加了继发感染的风险。

（王月影 译 杨宇光 校）

延伸阅读

American Society of Anesthesiologists Committee: Practice guidelines for preoperative fasting and the use of pharmacologic agents to reduce the risk of pulmonary aspiration: application to healthy patients undergoing elective procedures: an updated report by the American Society of Anaesthesiologists Committee on Standards and Practice Parameters, *Anaesthesiology* 114(3):495–511, 2011.

Asai T: Who is at risk of pulmonary aspiration? *Br J Anaesth* 93:497–500, 2004.

Cook T, Frerk C: 4th National Audit Project (NAP 4): Major Complications of Airway Management in the United Kingdom Report and Findings—Chapter 19. Aspiration of gastric contents and of blood, The Royal College of Anaesthetists and The Difficult Airway Society, 2011.

Frerk C, Mitchell VS, McNarry AF, et al.: Difficult Airway Society guidelines for management of unanticipated difficult intubation in adults, *Br J Anaesth* 115(6):827–848, 2015.

Kluger MT, Short TG: Aspiration during anaesthesia: a review of 133 cases from the Australian Anaesthetic Incident Monitoring Study (AIMS), *Anaesthesia* 54:19–26, 1999.

Mendelson CL: The aspiration of stomach contents into the lungs during obstetric anaesthesia, *Am J Obstet Gynecol* 52:191–205, 1946.

Ng A, Smith G: Gastroesophageal reflux and aspiration of gastric contents in anesthetic practice, *Anesth Analg* 93:494–513, 2001.

Robinson M, Davidson A: Aspiration under anaesthesia: risk assessment and decision-making, *Contin Educ Crit Care Pain* 14(4):171–175, 2014.

Sellick BA: Cricoid pressure to control regurgitation of stomach contents during induction of anaesthesia, *Lancet* 2:404–406, 1961.

Smith I, Kranke P, Murat I, et al.: Perioperative fasting in adults and children: guidelines from the European Society of Anaesthesiology, *Eur J Anaesthesiology* 28(8):556–569, 2011.

Warner MA, Warner ME, Weber JG: Clinical significance of pulmonary aspiration during the perioperative period, *Anesthesiology* 78:56–62, 1993.

产妇肺误吸

第 177 章

Laura J. Alexander，*William R. Camann*

病例概要

患者，女性，32 岁，G2P1，足月妊娠，因胎儿持续心动过缓在全身麻醉下行紧急剖宫产。给予丙泊酚和琥珀胆碱行快速序贯诱导后，使用 3.0 Macintosh 喉镜，压迫环状软骨，插入带导丝的型号为 6.5 的气管导管。剖宫产后，拔除患者气管导管并将其转运至麻醉后恢复室。患者在吸氧下自主呼吸。生命体征为血压 110/78 mmHg，心率 96 次 / 分，在面罩给氧，氧流量为 6 L/min 的情况下，动脉血氧饱和度为 88%。体检时发现患者双肺有哮鸣音，胸部 X 线片提示右下肺叶浸润。

问题分析

定义

长期以来，麻醉科医师一直对分娩过程中的镇痛感兴趣。随着对分娩最佳镇痛和麻醉探索的继续，预防和管理最重要的围产期并发症之一：胃内容物的肺误吸也从未停止。Hall 在 1940 年首先注意到产科患者中这种并发症的发生率增加。用于描述这种肺误吸的术语——化学性肺炎很快就流行起来。1946 年，Mendelson 对这种情况进行更完整的定义。

产妇是一类特殊的患者，其插管困难或失败以及误吸的风险增加。据估计，产科患者插管失败的发生率高于一般手术患者，尽管这种增高是一个动态问题并无确切答案。吸入性肺炎最常见于插管困难或失败。然而，有一些妊娠特异性因素导致误吸风险增加，包括以下因素：

- 黄体酮水平升高；
- 胃食管交接处括约肌张力降低；
- 妊娠子宫上移抵住胃；
- 由胃引起的十二指肠机械性梗阻。

由于胃食管之间的角度扭曲，妊娠子宫进一步影响食管括约肌张力。此外，在第二产程“用力”期间，下腹部人为施压和截石体位协同作用增加腹内压力并减少胃排空（表 177.1）。

促胃动素是一种加速胃排空的激素，它的产生在整个妊娠期间受到抑制，在产后 1 周恢复到接近正常水平。然而，在孕期大部分时间胃排空似乎是正常的。虽然硬膜外镇痛效果令人满意，但是分娩晚期胃排空延迟的原因尚不清楚。然而，最近的研究表明，妊娠期胃容量和胃酸浓度与非妊娠期，妊娠早期或产后并无差异。

表 177.1 与分娩有关的误吸危险因素

原因	影响
胃容量和胃液酸度	在妊娠足月妊娠早期没有变化
黄体酮水平升高	胃食管括约肌张力降低
降低促胃动素水平	分娩晚期胃排空延迟
妊娠子宫	食管括约肌的机械性影响
肠外或硬膜外阿片类药物	胃动力降低和镇静
抗胆碱药	食管括约肌张力下降

可能增加胃误吸风险的医源性因素包括胃肠外或硬膜外应用阿片类药物和抗胆碱能药物（例如格隆溴铵）。阿片类药物减缓胃动力，抗胆碱能药降低食管括约肌张力。

识别

化学性肺误吸的体征和症状非常多变，很大程度上取决于吸入物的容量和 pH（框 177.1）；然而，这种误吸也可能是“无症状的”。此外，麻醉科医师可能无法看到口咽后部的吸入物。咳嗽和支气管痉

框 177.1 化学性吸入性肺炎的体征和症状

无
口咽部的胃内容物
咳嗽
支气管痉挛
氧饱和度下降
循环性休克
胸部 X 线片有浸润

挛也可能是不常见的症状。通常，影像学的改变可提供误吸的一手证据；这种变化见于肺的下垂部位，通常在右肺下叶。

化学性肺误吸的患者结局可分为以下几类：约 10% ～ 15% 的患者临床病情迅速恶化，伴有缺氧和早期循环性休克。其余患者中，约有 2/3 在 1 ～ 4 天内迅速改善；他们可能需要通气支持。另外 1/3 的患者出现肺部细菌性感染，需要抗生素治疗。大多数肺损伤最终会痊愈。

风险评估

产妇化学性误吸的实际发生率尚不清楚。程度较轻的误吸可能常常被忽视，只有因误吸使产妇死亡或引起其他严重并发症时才被报道。在一项对 185 000 例麻醉诱导病例的回顾性研究中，Olsson 及其同事发现，非产科患者麻醉诱导中肺误吸的发生率为 1/2131（0.047%），剖宫产患者麻醉诱导中肺误吸的发生率为 1/661（0.15%）(即妊娠期间误吸风险增加 3 倍)。Warner 及其同事发现全身麻醉患者中肺误吸的发生率为 1/3216（0.031%），急诊手术患者中肺误吸的发生率为 1/895（0.11%）。Warner 团队评估了所有类型的紧急情况，剖宫产往往是紧急的。最近，Ezri 及其同事回顾性研究了 1979—1993 年在分娩时（如手动分离胎盘）或在分娩后即刻（如修复撕裂伤）立即进行全身麻醉的患者。他们发现误吸的发生率为 0.05%（1/1870）。所有患者均为自主呼吸，未插管，全身麻醉诱导和维持使用静脉药物。该组误吸发生率低于普通外科手术人群，这可能与腹内压降低有关。此外，许多化学性肺误吸发生在插管困难或者插管失败需要面罩通气时。可用的最新数据来自 SCORE 项目。美国于 2014 年发布的这项多机构调查，研究了超过 250 000 种用于分娩的麻醉药和大约 5000 例全身麻醉。作者报告的误吸发生率为 0%。

并非所有的产科全身麻醉都需要气管插管，喉罩（laryngeal mask airway，LMA）可能是气管插管困难或失败的情况下的一个有用的辅助工具。Han 及其同事报道了 1060 例择期剖宫产患者使用 LMA 的情况。然而没有报道误吸病例，这一成功可能归功于对患者的谨慎选择。在被排除的患者中有胃反流症状，美国麻醉科医师协会（American Society of Anesthesiologists，ASA）分级高于Ⅱ级，已知的困难气道，或妊娠前体重指数大于 30，以及禁食少于 6 h 的患者。此外，术前应用抗酸药物预防，环状软骨加压。然而，在实践中，几乎所有需要全身麻醉的产妇都是产科急症患者，尤其是那些意外需要剖宫产的产妇。我们认为这些非空腹患者需要快速序贯诱导和气管插管。然而，在气管插管失败的情况下，即使是情况紧急的产科患者，LMA 也可以实现挽救生命的氧合，并应予以考虑。

最后，近年来，由于区域麻醉使用的增加，与麻醉有关的产妇死亡率有所下降。即便如此，Hawkins 及其同事报道产科患者中与麻醉有关的死亡中有 23% 直接由误吸造成。虽然关于围术期产妇误吸发生率的数据通常未见报道，但现在的一些研究表明，产科患者中与此情况相关的发病率仍然较显著。尽管所有产妇发生化学性肺误吸的风险增加，但在解读围产期化学性肺误吸发生率的研究时，必须考虑围产期手术的时机和性质，以及实施全身麻醉的情况。

启示

误吸的胃内容物的容量、含量和特性决定了肺误吸后肺炎的严重程度。许多人认为，在判断肺误吸后肺损伤的严重程度方面误吸的胃内容物的 pH 比实际误吸的容量（假如少于 25 ml）更为关键。其他人，尤其是 James 及其同事，认为无论误吸的容量多少，低 pH 与高死亡率相关。

吸入颗粒物会增加误吸后肺损伤的风险，因为大颗粒会嵌顿在主支气管中，在几分钟内导致窒息。然而，非酸性吸入物可能只产生轻微的短暂的缺氧，没有实质损伤的迹象；这种缺氧可能是由支气管痉挛和轻微的肺不张所致。随着吸入物酸度的增加，肺实质损伤和肺出血的可能性增加。这种反应的增强可能导致急性呼吸窘迫综合征，其特点是持续的肺部炎症，并伴有双肺浸润的影像学改变。这些浸润是由于血管通透性增加和动脉氧分压降低（不受吸入氧浓度或呼气末正压的使用的影响），而左心房压力没有增加。通过采取更好的支持治疗和通气策略，生存率有所提高，而由胃吸入物引起的及与其相关的急性呼吸窘迫综合征导致的死亡率仍然非常高，目前估计从 35% 到 40% 不等。

管理

误吸后立即进行气道管理至关重要（框 177.2）。任何在口咽后部发现的吸入物都应迅速排出，并确保气道安全。尽管有几位作者建议采用头低位或左侧卧位来减少吸入物的扩散，但这种体位并没有被证明能够减少这种扩散。建议在不使用生理盐水冲洗的情况下进行气管内吸引，以去除吸入物。生理盐水灌洗可能使吸入物扩散到更远端的气道，使病情恶化。可以通过测量吸入物的 pH 来帮助确定胃内容物的性质。

降低病残率的最重要的因素是快速识别吸入物、迅速气管插管以及补充氧气和呼气末正压通气。静脉注射 β 受体激动剂可以缓解支气管痉挛。虽然酸损伤的肺更容易受到细菌感染，但没有证据表明预防性使用抗生素会改变感染的发生率，也不会影响结局。预防性使用抗生素甚至可能促进耐药微生物感染的发生。同样，全身性糖皮质激素使用是有争议的。一些动物模型表明，受到损伤后立即使用类固醇，可以减少肺损伤。其他数据表明，类固醇引起的巨噬细胞活性降低以及随后对革兰氏阴性肺炎的易感性增加可能会抵消任何益处。尽管使用甲泼尼龙（30 mg/kg）或地塞米松（1 mg/kg）并不少见，但目前的意见并不提倡这种做法。必须限制液体的使用。受损的肺内皮渗出富含蛋白质的水肿液，过于积极的静脉输液可能进一步加重患者肺水肿。

框 177.2 疑似肺误吸后的指导性疗法

确保气道安全；补充氧气和呼气末正压通气
使患者头低位，头转向一侧
或者，将患者置于左侧卧位。
气管内吸引（如果还未插管，行气管插管以保护气道）
一旦气道得到保护，考虑用口胃管或鼻胃管进行胃肠减压。
开始使用 β 受体激动剂治疗支气管痉挛
考虑全身使用类固醇（地塞米松 1 mg/kg 或甲泼尼龙 30 mg/kg）
制定保守的液体管理方案

预防

也许唯一最重要的单一治疗措施就是预防。预防措施包括以下内容：

- 根据 ASA 禁食指南指导分娩患者禁食；
- 区域麻醉；
- 环状软骨压迫；
- 使用非颗粒抗酸药；
- 使用甲氧氯普胺；
- 使用 H_2 受体拮抗剂。

预防方法可分为药物性和非药物性。非药理性方法包括根据 ASA 禁食指南指导分娩患者禁食，通过适当使用区域麻醉技术，尽量减少全身麻醉。然而，可能会出现紧急情况，在插管条件不佳的情况下需要全身麻醉。在这些情况下，预防通常是采取药物性预防措施和经典的饱胃预防措施相结合。

近期的趋势鼓励分娩时口服液体，ASA 产科麻醉工作组支持这一做法。值得注意的是，其他国家级的学会指南，如欧洲麻醉学学会的指南，也支持在整个分娩过程中摄入清亮液体。由于产程中长时间饥饿会带来代谢不良的后果，推荐非复杂分娩的患者少量饮用透明液体，包括等渗“运动饮料”。有数据表明分娩患者胃排空透明液体的能力与非分娩患者的基础排空水平没有区别，支持了这一做法。事实上，对于摄入液体较少的分娩患者来说，排空大量液体的半衰期甚至可能更短。然而，对于有额外误吸风险因素（如病态肥胖、糖尿病、困难气道）或手术分娩风险增加的患者，可能需要更严格地限制经口摄入；这应该根据每名患者的具体情况来决定。值得注意的是，有证据表明，咀嚼口香糖不仅能提高患者的满意度，而且还能促进胃排空。尽管仍有争议，但许多临床医师不会因为不久前嚼口香糖而取消或推迟择期手术，我们同意这一做法。所有进入产程活跃期的患者和接受过含有阿片类镇痛药物的患者应避免进食固体食物。

环状软骨压迫是一种简单的技术，可以帮助预防全身麻醉诱导期间的被动反流。必须持续加压，直到气管插管，气管内导管套囊充气，且确认插管。应该注意的是，环状软骨加压可能不会完全闭塞食管，可能会降低食管下括约肌的张力，并且可能无法防止误吸。

一些产科患者存在气管插管困难。如果预计会出现困难气道，则清醒气管插管可能是合理的选择。正如这些患者在诱导期间有误吸风险一样，拔管期间也必须采取类似的预防措施。只有当患者意识清醒并能正确地执行指令时才能拔管。区分复苏的兴奋阶段和实际的苏醒非常重要。在全身麻醉诱导前，应复习气道评估、插管失败的处理以及气道管理的替代技术。

降低误吸风险的药物方法通常是开始于非微粒抗酸剂的应用。抗酸药是改变胃液 pH 的最有效、最实用的方法之一。然而，非微粒抗酸剂的最大作用时间限制在大约 30 min。同样，静脉注射甲氧氯普胺 10 mg 具有益处。虽然甲氧氯普胺不直接影响胃液的 pH，但它具有止吐作用，能增加食管下括约肌张力，减少胃排空时间。静脉给药约 20 min 后可观察到胃容量减少。H_2 受体拮抗剂如西咪替丁、雷尼替丁和法莫替丁能有效减少胃壁细胞产生盐酸。对于组胺阻断剂，使用时机很重要；静脉给药后 30 min 就可以看到效果，但要想达到最大效果，需要 60 ～ 90 min。这种延迟起效限制了它们在紧急情况下的疗效。除了组胺和胃泌素，乙酰胆碱是另一种内源性促分泌素。抗胆碱能药物可抑制胃液分泌，但效果不尽相同。在抗胆碱能药物中，格隆溴铵对胃液分泌和 pH 的影响最为显著，但其同时具有降低食管下括约肌张力和延迟胃排空的作用，使它的优势相形见绌。因此，这些药物不推荐用于预防误吸。

（方　亚　译　韩　烨　校）

延伸阅读

American Society of Anesthesiologists Committee: Practice guidelines for preoperative fasting and the use of pharmacologic agents to reduce the risk of pulmonary aspiration: application to healthy patients undergoing elective procedures: an updated report by the American Society of Anesthesiologists Committee on Standards and Practice Parameters, *Anesthesiology* 114(3):495–511, 2011.

American Society of Anesthesiologists Task Force on Obstetric Anesthesia: Practice guidelines for obstetric anesthesia: an updated report by the American Society of Anesthesiologists Task Force on Obstetric Anesthesia and the Society for Obstetric Anesthesia and Perinatology. *Anesthesiology* 124:270–300, 2016.

Downs JB, Chapman Jr RL, Modell JH, et al.: An evaluation of steroid therapy in aspiration pneumonitis, *Anesthesiology* 40(2):129–135, 1994.

Ezri T, Szmuk P, Stein A, et al.: Peripartum general anesthesia without tracheal intubation: incidence of pulmonary aspiration, *Anaesthesia* 55(5):421–426, 2000.

Gibbs CP: Gastric aspiration prevention and treatment, *Clin Anesth* 4:47, 1986.

Hall GC: Aspiration pneumonitis as an obstetric hazard, *JAMA* 114:728, 1940.

Han TH, Brimacombe J, Lee EJ, et al.: The laryngeal mask airway is effective (and probably safe) in selected healthy parturients for elective cesarean section: a prospective study of 1067 cases, *Can J Anaesth* 48(11):1117–1121, 2001.

Hawkins JL: Excess in moderation: general anesthesia for cesarean delivery, *Anesth Analg* 120(6):1175–1177, 2015.

Hawkins JL, Koonin L, Palmer SK, Gibbs CP: Anesthesia-related deaths during obstetric delivery in the United States, 1979–1990, *Anesthesiology* 86(2):277–284, 1997.

James CF, Modell JH, Gibbs CP, et al.: Pulmonary aspiration effects of volume and pH in the rat, *Anesth Analg* 63(7):665–668, 1984.

King TA, Adams AP: Failed tracheal intubation, *Br J Anaesth* 65(3):400–414, 1990.

Kubli M, Scrutton MJ, Seed PT, et al.: An evaluation of "isotonic sports drinks" during labor, *Anesth Analg* 94(2):404–408, 2002.

Malinow AM, Ostheimer GW: Anesthesia for the high-risk parturient, *Obstet Gynecol* 69(6):951–964, 1987.

Mendelson CL: Aspiration of stomach contents into lungs during obstetric anesthesia, *Am J Obstet Gynecol* 52:191–205, 1946.

Olsson GL, Hallen B, Hambraeus-Jonzon K: Aspiration during anaesthesia: a computer-aided study of 185,358 anesthetics, *Acta Anaesthesiol Scand* 30(1):84–92, 1986.

O'Sullivan G, Scrutton M: NPO during labor: is there any scientific validation? *Anesthesiol Clin North Am* 21(1):87–98, 2003.

Poulton TJ: Gum chewing during pre-anesthetic fasting, *Paediatr Anaesth* 22(3):288–296, 2012.

Schwartz DJ, Wynne JW, Gibbs CP, et al.: The pulmonary consequences of aspiration of gastric contents at pH values greater than 2.5, *Am Rev Respir Dis* 121(1):119–126, 1980.

Smith I, Kranke P, Murat I: Perioperative fasting in adults and children: guidelines from the European Society of Anaesthesiology, *Eur J Anaesthesiol* 28(8):556–569, 2011.

Warner MA, Warner ME, Webber JG: Clinical significance of pulmonary aspiration during the perioperative period, *Anesthesiology* 78(1):56–62, 1993.

Wong CA, McCarthy RJ, Fitzgerald PC, et al.: Gastric emptying of water in obese pregnant women at term, *Anesth Analg* 105(3):751–755, 2007.

脊椎麻醉：硬脊膜穿刺后的头痛

第 178 章

Christina M. Spofford

病例概要

患者，女性，25 岁，在门诊接受宫腔镜检查时，使用 25 号腰麻 Quincke 针进行脊椎麻醉。次日，患者自述头痛，直立时头痛加重，仰卧时头痛消失。

问题分析

定义

硬膜穿刺后头痛（post-dural puncture headache、PDPH）是脊椎麻醉的常见并发症。通常发生在硬膜穿刺后 24 ～ 48 h（92% 的患者），但表现可延迟长达 5 天。穿刺部位脑脊液（cerebrospinal fluid，CSF）丢失引起的脑脊液量和压力减少是关键的始动因素（图 178.1）。当患者直立时，大脑和支撑结构下垂。脑下垂直接牵拉疼痛敏感结构，也可引起疼痛反射性脑血管舒张。PDPH 的病理特征性表现——即直立位发病或加重以及仰卧位消退也支持了这一理论。一般情况下，70% 的 PDPH 在硬膜穿刺后 1 周自行消退，95% 在 6 周时自行消退。

识别

PDPH 应被视为排除性诊断。易被误诊为 PDPH 的疾病包括下丘脑肿瘤、子痫、脊髓脑膜炎和上矢状窦血栓。

PDPH 的临床特征包括以下几点：

- 硬脊膜穿刺史；
- 体位相关性的头痛（直立 15 min 后加重并且仰卧位 15 min 后缓解）；
- 头痛部位通常位于额部或枕部；
- 头痛通常会伴随以下症状：颈部僵硬、耳鸣、视力减退、畏光；

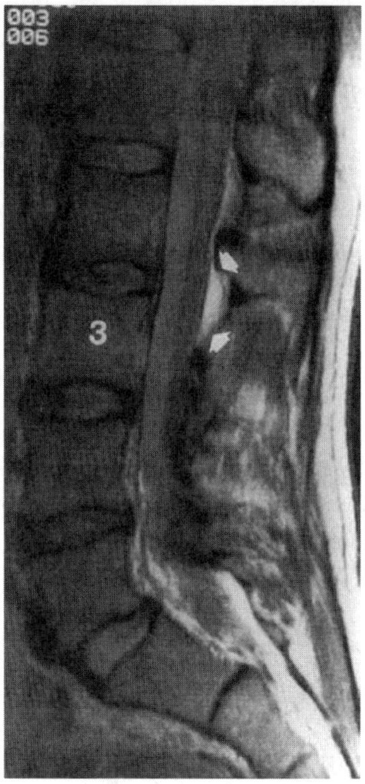

图 178.1　硬脊膜穿刺后头痛患者在使用硬膜外血液填充前的腰椎磁共振图像，L2 L3（箭头）处的液体信号与硬脊膜穿刺部位脑脊液漏有关（From Vakharia SB，Thomas PS，Rosenbaum AE，et al：Magnetic resonance imaging of cerebrospinal fluid leak and tamponade effect of blood patch in postdural puncture headache. *Anesth Analg* 84[3]：585-590，1997.）

- 95% 的病例在硬膜穿刺后 1 周内自然缓解（如果头痛持续，应考虑其他诊断）；
- 48 h 内硬膜外注射血补丁多数可改善。

风险评估

在目前的麻醉实践中，脊椎麻醉后 PDPH 的发生率一般在 1% ～ 7%。患者特征和麻醉技术都被认为是 PDPH 发生的危险因素。

增加风险的患者因素包括：

- 低龄，可能是由于硬脊膜的弹性随着年龄的增长而变化；
- 女性；
- 既往 PDPH 病史。

减少 PDPH 发生的麻醉因素包括：

- 使用直径较小的脊髓穿刺针（图 178.2 和 178.3）；

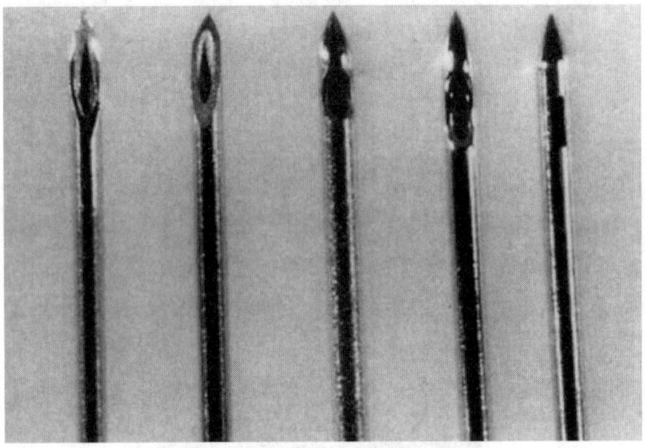

图 178.2 从左起：Atraucan、Quincke、Gertie Marx、Sprotte 和 Whitacre 针。注意 Atraucan 和 Quincke 针上的切割点。同样，笔尖式针的侧孔各不相同。Gertie Marx 针的注药口是最小的且离针尖最近。左起水平标记以 2 mm 递增（From Vallejo MC，Mandell GL，Sabo DP，et al：Postdural puncture headache：a randomized comparison of fve spinal needles in obstetric patients. *Anesth Analg* 91[4]：916-920，2000.）

- 体外研究发现使用笔尖穿刺针较使用斜面穿刺针减少脑脊液外漏（见图 178.2 和 178.3）；
- 与直接横向切割相反，穿刺针的斜面与蛛网膜长轴平行穿刺时，由于纤维的纵向切割，可以在组织中产生较小的裂口。

启示

PDPH 可导致明显的不适和活动受限。对于产后患者，这可能会造成护理和照顾新生儿的困难。大多数患者可以口服镇痛药物或者辅助其他药物治疗，直到症状自然消退。在这些患者中，大约 18% 的人会有轻微的活动受限，31% 的人会因活动受限需要卧床休息，51% 的人则完全卧床不起。

管理

PDPH 的治疗包括全身性治疗和有创性治疗。在实施进一步的有创治疗前应先尝试全身性治疗（图 178.4）。

全身性治疗

咖啡因

静脉注射咖啡因（500 mg）可使 PDPH 患者的脑血流减少 22%。静脉注射咖啡因治疗的成功率在 40% ～ 80%，但有轻微的不良反应（头晕、脸红）。口服咖啡因也是一种有效的治疗方法，口服 300 mg

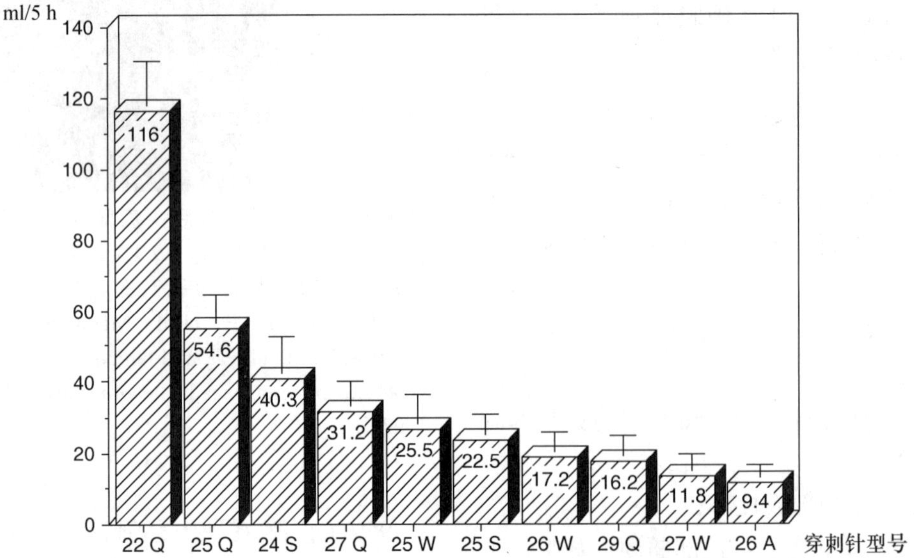

图 178.3 实验室模型硬脊膜穿刺针直径、针尖切面与脑脊液漏的关系（From Holst D，Möllmann M，Ebel C，et al：In vitro investigation of cerebrospinal fluid leakage after dural puncture with various spinal needles. *Anesth Analg* 87[6]：1331-1335，1998.）

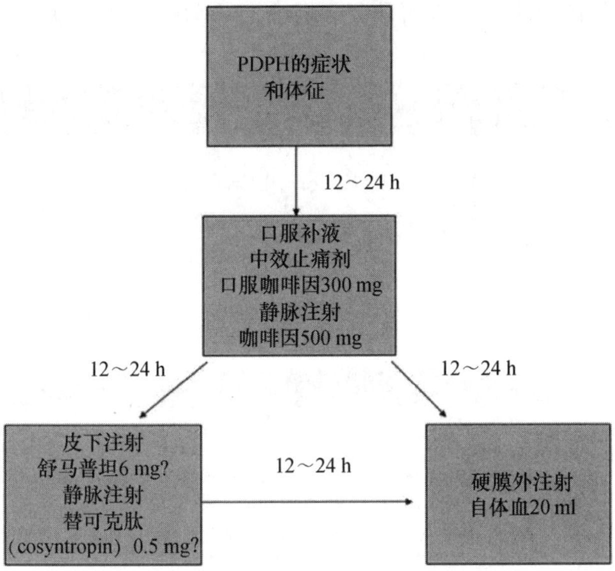

图 178.4　硬膜穿刺后头痛的建议治疗流程

咖啡因的成功率约为 50%。

促肾上腺皮质激素和舒马曲坦

铁事型证据表明使用促肾上腺皮质激素（adreno-cortico-tropic-hormone，ACTH）的成功率约为 70%～95%，但是迄今为止唯一的一项随机对照试验显示其并无任何益处。已有产科患者使用 ACTH 类药后发作癫痫的病例报告。同样的，舒马曲坦虽然对其他类型的头痛有益，但对 PDPH 尚无确切益处。一项 Cochrane 综述对 7 个随机对照试验进行了回顾，并无支持使用 ACTH 或舒马曲坦的结论性证据。然而，与安慰剂相比，加巴喷丁、茶碱和氢化可的松可降低疼痛评分。

体位和液体治疗

一旦发生 PDPH，应长期卧床休息和积极的液体扩容治疗。在一项涵盖 23 项试验的 Cochrane 综述显示，与立即活动相比，术后卧床休息对 PDPH 的发生率没有任何益处。同样，补液对预防 PDPH 的发生没有任何益处。

有创治疗

硬膜外血补丁

硬膜外自体血液注射在 1960 年首次被提出作为治疗 PDPH 的一种方法，在此之前轶事性观察报道称，硬脊膜穿刺若带血 PDPH 的发病率有所降低。当保守治疗失败时，硬膜外血补丁（epidural blood patch，EBP）是目前 PDPH 治疗的金标准。EBP 的成功率大于 90%。其机制被认为是由于团块效应增加了颅内脑脊液压力和硬脊膜穿刺处纤维蛋白凝块封堵了硬脊膜上的穿刺口（图 178.5）。将血液注入硬膜外腔即刻就可产生至少持续 3 h 的团块效应。注射后 7 h 即可形成成熟的血块并封闭硬脊膜上的破口。最初的 EBP 报告使用的是小容量的血液（2～3 ml），但近来推荐使用大容量的血液（15～20 ml）。注射容量越大，凝块扩散范围越广（5～9 个脊柱节段），团块效应越强，治疗的成功率也越高。虽然使用 EBP 安全有效，但也存在一定的风险。EBP 的禁忌证包括全身感染、背部局部感染和活动性神经系统疾病。报道的 EBP 并发症包括短暂性背痛（发病率 35%～100%）、轻度体温升高（5%）、突发心动过缓和神经根性疼痛。EBP 也可能造成长期后遗症。据报道 EBP 治疗后会降低硬膜外麻醉成功率。

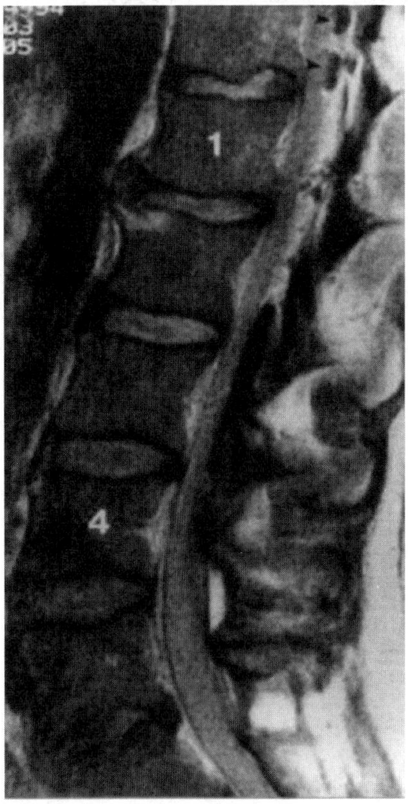

图 178.5　硬膜外注射 20 ml 血补丁的磁共振图像显示硬膜外漏被封堵，血补丁从 L4 扩散至 T12（From Vakharia SB，Thomas PS，Rosenbaum AE，et al：Magnetic resonance imaging of cerebrospinal fluid leak and tamponade effect of blood patch in postdural puncture headache. *Anesth Analg* 84[3]：585-590，1997.）

其他硬膜外液体注射治疗

硬膜外注射生理盐水和右旋糖苷都已被用于治疗 PDPH。报道的成功率差异很大，从完全无效到 90% 成功。由于注射生理盐水和右旋糖苷的成功率不定，通常只是暂时性缓解，再加上硬膜外注射本身的风险，使得其应用仍受到质疑。有个案报道，PDPH 患者进行 3 次 EBP 无效后注射了 3 ml 纤维蛋白，获得成功。

预防

预防 PDPH 的关键是选择纤细、无切割头的硬脊膜穿刺针。全身预防性用药和有创性治疗尚未得到充分研究，并非所有的硬脊膜穿刺患者都会出现 PDPH，所以大多数患者只在出现症状后才推荐使用 EBP。另一种反对预防性使用 EBP 的观点认为，早期（硬脊膜穿刺后 24 h 内）使用 EBP 的有效性值得怀疑。数项研究表明，早期经硬膜外导管给予相对少量血液（7 ～ 10ml）对于因大口径 Tuohy 穿刺针穿破硬脊膜后引起的 PDPH 的后续发展几乎没有影响。但这些研究因为使用少量的血液，效果受到质疑。最近的一项研究显示，经硬膜外导管注射更大容量的血液（15 ml）可显著降低被大口径 Tuohy 针穿破硬脊膜的产科患者 PDPH 的发生率（治疗组为 5%，而未治疗组为 88%）。最近的另一项对照试验显示，意外硬膜穿刺后立即注射 10 ml 生理盐水，治疗组 32% 患者发生 PDPH，未治疗组 62% 患者发生 PDPH。因此，如果认为患者和麻醉的危险因素大到足以需要采取预防性治疗，大剂量的 EBP 或立即注射适量生理盐水可能是一种合理有效的治疗方法。

致谢

感谢 Matthew P. Feuer 和 Spencer S. Liu 博士对本章上一版的贡献。

（韩风瑞 译 盛 颖 校）

延伸阅读

Arevalo-Rodriguez I, Ciapponi A, Munoz L, et al.: Posture and fluids for preventing post–dural puncture headache, *Cochrane Database Syst Rev*(7), 2013. CD009199.

Basurto Ona X, Martínez García L, Solà I, et al.: Drug therapy for treating post–dural puncture headache, *Cochrane Database Syst Rev*(8), 2011. CD007887.

Basurto Ona X, Uriona Tuma SM, Martínez García L, et al.: Drug therapy for preventing post–dural puncture headache, *Cochrane Database Syst Rev*(2), 2013. CD001792.

Baysinger CL: Accidental dural puncture and postdural puncture headache management, *International Anesth Clin* 52:18–39, 2014.

Boonmak P, Boonmak S: Epidural blood patching for preventing and treating post–dural puncture headache, *Cochrane Database Syst Rev*(1), 2010. CD001791.

Canovas L, Barros C, Gómez A, et al.: Use of intravenous tetracosactin in the treatment of postdural puncture headache: our experience in forty cases, *Anesth Analg* 94(5):1369, 2002.

Connelly NR, Parker RK, Rahimi A, et al.: Sumatriptan in patients with postdural puncture headache, *Headache* 40:316–319, 2000.

Halpern S, Preston R: Postdural puncture headache and spinal needle design: metaanalyses, *Anesthesiology* 81:1376–1383, 1994.

Harrington BE: Postdural puncture headache and the development of the epidural blood patch, *Reg Anesth Pain Med* 29:136–163, 2004.

Kroin JS, Nagalla SK, Buvanendran A, et al.: The mechanisms of intracranial pressure modulation by epidural blood and other injectates in a postdural puncture rat model, *Anesth Analg* 95:423–429, 2002.

Lybecker H, Djernes M, Schmidt J: Postdural puncture headache (PDPH): onset, duration, severity, and associated symptoms, *Acta Anaesthesiol Scand* 39:605–612, 1995.

第 179 章 脊髓血肿

Mahmoud I. Wagih

病例概要

患者，男性，69 岁，在全身麻醉下行腹主动脉瘤修补术。诱导前置入硬膜外导管以实施术后镇痛。麻醉科医师在尝试三次后，成功地放置了硬膜外导管。导管置入后回抽产生发现回血，导管拔出 2 cm 后回血消失。尽管使用了相对稀释的局部麻醉药（0.125% 的布比卡因和 1 μg/ml 的芬太尼），但患者术后 2 h 出现了完全的单侧运动阻滞；尽管停止了硬膜外输注，但这种阻滞仍然持续存在。磁共振图像显示 T10 有硬膜外血肿。立即手术减压，最后神经系统完全恢复。

问题分析

定义

1850 年，Tellegen 首次描述了脊髓血肿（spinal cord hematoma，SCH）的临床症状。从解剖学上讲，血肿可发生在脊髓的硬膜外、硬膜下或脊髓髓内区域。由于中枢椎管内阻滞（central neuraxial blockade，CNB）相关的神经并发症很少，因此很难准确估计与其相关的 SCH。不同的作者根据不同的患者数量 / 队列得出他们的研究结果，但是由皇家麻醉科医师学院和其他组织实施的国家审计项目 3（the National Audit Project 3，NAP3）在 700 000 例 CNB 中发现了 8 例 SCH。硬膜外及腰硬联合麻醉的 SCH 发生率（17/100 000，18/100 000）明显高于脊椎麻醉或骶管麻醉（2/100 000）。在纳入统计的 707 425 例患者中有 5 例出现永久性神经功能障碍。当 CNB 用于分娩、小儿镇痛或慢性疼痛管理时，SCH 很少见。70 岁以上患者的发病率显著增加。这一增加是由于相关的并存疾病还是由于技术原因尚不清楚。

大约 50% 的 SCH 与拔除导管有关，多达 13% 的病例出现在无任何术前危险因素的患者中。SCH 有多种病因（框 179.1），偶尔也会自发发生。

框 179.1 脊髓血肿的病因

- 血管畸形
- 凝血性疾病（先天性 / 后天性）
- 脊髓炎 / 血管炎
- 脊髓空洞症
- 机械性创伤
- 腰穿 / 硬膜外穿刺
- 肿瘤
- 手术后
- 特发性

识别

典型的 SCH 表现为不同强度的局限性背痛和神经压迫症状（运动、感觉和自主神经）。较大比例发生于 CNB 导管拔除后。与运动无力相比，背痛不是主要的临床特征。单侧症状是脊髓血肿的危险信号。停止 CNB 输注或单次给药后，感觉或运动阻滞的不完全缓解者均应该被随访和检查。

风险评估

导致 SCH 发生的因素可分为患者相关因素、技术相关因素和药物相关因素。

患者相关因素：

- 老年人群（>70 岁）；
- 女性比男性多见；
- 非产科（1/505 000）、非儿科适应证；
- 凝血功能异常；
- 脊髓畸形。

技术相关因素：

- 腰硬联合麻醉 > 硬膜外麻醉 > 脊椎麻醉（腰麻）> 骶管麻醉；
- 导管技术；
- 操作难度；
- 多次尝试；
- 导管中出现血迹。

药物相关因素：

在接受围术期抗凝 / 抗血小板治疗的患者中，SCH 的发生率显著增加。抗凝剂主要包括：

- 普通（未分级）肝素；
- 低分子肝素（low-molecular-weight heparin，LMWH）；
- 口服抗凝药物，包括新一代药物如达比加群（Pradaxa）、利伐沙班（Xarelto）、阿哌沙班（Eliquis）；
- 抗血小板药物（不同代）。

普通（未分级）肝素

使用普通肝素进行完全抗凝和心肺转流（如在血管和心脏外科手术中）已得到充分的实践。Sanchez 和 Nygard 报告了一项共 558 例无并发症的大型前瞻性系列研究。尽管如此，尚无足够数据来确定并发症的确切发生率。一般建议术前 24 h 置入硬膜外导管。

在 NAP3 中，15 例患者在拔除导管后数小时内发生 SCH，其中 9 例使用了肝素治疗。这与 Vandermeulen 及其同事在 1906—1994 年对他们的患者队列记录中对 SCH 的回顾中所描述的情况相一致。

当技术性置管困难或在置管后 1 h 内即开始完全抗凝时的术中抗凝（如血管手术）可能与 SCH 的发生风险增加有关。目前临床上当硬膜外置管有损伤时，倾向于取消手术，尽管尚无循证依据支持这种做法，与外科团队公开沟通并进行个体风险评估较为明智。如果术后需继续抗凝，停用肝素和硬膜外导管拔除之间应间隔 4 h。如果在使用肝素后进行硬膜外麻醉，应观察同样的 4 h[最好是在部分凝血活酶时间（partial thromboplastin time，PTT）正常的情况下]。皮下肝素与极少数 SCH 病例相关，确切的时间间隔很难确定，但 4 h 间隔可避免血浆峰值。

低分子肝素

LMWH 具有不同于普通肝素的药理作用，除了作用时间较长之外，它们只能被鱼精蛋白部分拮抗，其清除依赖于肾功能，且很难密切监测（即使在测量抗 -Xa 水平时也是如此）。自美国 FDA 首次批准使用每日两次的治疗方案以来，SCH 的发病率一直很高。

美国区域麻醉和疼痛医学协会（the American Society of Regional Anesthesia and Pain Medicine，ASRAPM）提出以下建议：

- 给予预防剂量后 12 h 和治疗剂量后 24 h 允许 CNB；
- 如果同时联合使用抗血小板药物，考虑使用替代 CNB 的其他止痛方法。
- 每日两次使用 LMWH 治疗的患者切勿留置导管；
- 如果导管置入时出血或损伤，则延迟至术后 24 h 使用 LMWH；
- 硬膜外导管拔出后 2 h 可开始术后 LMWH 每日两次的治疗方案（通常为术后 24 h）。

口服抗凝药

华法林在不同程度上作用于维生素 K 依赖因子（Ⅱ，Ⅶ，Ⅸ，Ⅹ）。国际标准化比值（the international normalized ratio，INR）准确反映了华法林对Ⅶ因子的影响，但在评估华法林对Ⅱ因子和Ⅹ因子的影响方面作用有限。ASRAPM 提出以下建议：

- 长期使用华法林治疗的患者在 CNB 之前必须停用华法林 4 ～ 5 天且 INR 正常。
- INR 小于 1.5 才推荐拔除 CNB 导管。
- 如果 INR 为 1.5 ～ 3，则强烈建议谨慎拔除 CNB 导管，同时应严密进行神经功能监测。
- 服用华法林的患者不建议同时使用影响凝血途径的其他药物（阿司匹林、LMWH）。

新型口服抗凝剂达比加群、利伐沙班及阿哌沙班的使用时间不够长，在计划 CNB 时关于其如何使用的临床数据积累尚不够充分。Benzon 及其同事们的建议是立足于它们的药代动力学特性，因为 INR 并不能反映它们的活性水平。对于静脉血栓栓塞或卒中高危患者，在停药和椎管内阻滞之间间隔 2 ～ 3 个半衰期。对于大多数血栓形成低风险患者，应该增加到 4 ～ 6 个半衰期。慢性肾功能损害的患者应根据肌酐清除率来调整剂量。抗凝药可在 CNB 或硬膜外导管拔除后 24 ～ 48 h 内恢复使用。

抗血小板药物

- 氯吡格雷：理想的是在椎管内阻滞前 7 天停用，

但 5 天可能也安全；如果出现隐患，应获取并确认血小板检测正常。

- 新型药物：普拉格雷应在腰麻或硬膜外麻醉前 7 ～ 10 天停用；替格瑞洛应停用 5 天。

预防

考虑到可能造成灾难性后果，应投入最大的努力进行预防。

如果考虑区域阻滞，术前评估应包括凝血异常、药物治疗及其时机（出血倾向史 / 易淤伤、既往手术出血史、抗凝药 / 抗血栓药物）的详细信息。在 CNB 前的手术当天可能需要 INR 或 PTT（偶尔需要血栓弹性图）等检查。CNB 的时机应遵循上述指南（表 179.1）。应制订方案，不仅在术后早期监测这些患者，而且在置入导管及导管拔除后也能监测这些患者。该方案应确定负责患者治疗的团队 / 个人以及所有干预的时机。70% 的 SCH 伴有永久性神经损伤。应建立持续的审查和培训体系。

积极治疗

单侧运动阻滞或持续性感觉丧失

一些“危险信号”应警示麻醉科医师关注潜在的并发症（框 179.2）。及早发现至关重要，即使及时进行椎板切除术（治疗椎管脓肿更有效）并不意味着一定能完全恢复 SCH 后的神经功能，但早期干预总有一定效果。在腰麻后的一段时间内，只要腰椎硬膜外注射持续，就会出现下肢无力，胸段硬膜外阻滞中，阻滞的节段性排除了下肢运动阻滞的可能性，对出现的任何运动障碍应进行彻底积极的检查。用稀释的局部麻醉药和阿片类药物或不加阿片类药物的混合剂可以早期发现神经系统并发症，而深度的运动阻滞则是例外。任何深度的运动阻滞都应向麻醉科主管医师汇报，应停止输注局部麻醉药，运动功能应在 4 h 内恢复。任何部位持续无力都应该被标记为“有意义”，并需要进一步检查。因此，已证实 Bromage 腿无力评分是实用且易于使用和教学。如果不能维持这种监测标准，则认为进行 CNB 是不安全的。如果在患者出现不明原因的或持续的无力后拔除硬膜外导管，则应在拔除导管后

表 179.1 使用抗凝药和抗血小板药的中枢神经阻滞

药物	使用中枢神经阻滞
普通肝素-预防剂量	最后一次肝素剂量至少间隔 4 h 后尝试 CNB CNB 或导管拔除后间隔 4 h（理想情况下为 6 h）给予肝素
普通肝素-完全抗凝	在心脏 / 复杂血管手术中，完全抗凝前 24 h 置入 CNB 导管
普通肝素-术中抗凝	CNB 1 h 后可给予单次任何剂量的肝素 如果阻滞过程中有出血迹象，需评估权衡患者抗凝的风险效益
低分子肝素（LMWH）	预防剂量 LMWH 间隔 12 h 后再行 CNB 治疗剂量 LMWH 间隔 24 h 后再行 CNB 尽可能每日给予一次 LMWH 如果与抗血小板药联合使用，考虑使用 CNB 以外的其他替代方法控制疼痛； 每天两次 LMWH 治疗的患者不可留置导管 如果导管置入出血或有创伤，术后延迟 24 h 给予 LMWH 硬膜外导管拔除 2 h 后开始 LMWH 治疗
华法林	CNB 前必须停用华法林 4 ～ 5 天和 INR 正常 推荐在拔除 CNB 导管前 INR 小于 1.5
达比加群、利伐沙班、阿哌沙班	在停药和 CNB 之间应有 3 个半衰期（利伐沙班和阿哌沙班需 3 天，达比加群需 5 天） 抗凝药可在 CNB 或硬膜外导管拔除后 24 ～ 48 h 内恢复使用
抗血小板药	氯吡格雷：停 7 天 普拉格雷：停 7 ～ 10 天 替格瑞洛：停 5 天

INR，国际标准化比值。

框 179.2 中枢神经阻滞后出现的危险信号

显著的胸段硬膜外运动阻滞
意外的深度运动阻滞，包括单侧阻滞
硬膜外输注时运动阻滞显著增加
硬膜外停止用药后运动阻滞不能恢复
由于运动阻滞而停止硬膜外输注，在重新开始硬膜外输注后，再次出现意外的运动阻滞

进行 24 h 的持续神经监测（见表 179.1）。

（段盼盼　译　查燕萍　校）

延伸阅读

Bateman BT, Mhyre JM, Ehrenfeld J, et al.: The risk and outcomes of epidural hematomas after perioperative and obstetric epidural catheterization: a report from the Multicenter Perioperative Outcomes Group Research Consortium, *Anesth Analg* 116(6):1380–1385, 2013.

Benzon HT, Avram MJ, Green D, et al.: New oral anticoagulants and regional anaesthesia, *Br J Anaesth* 111(Suppl 1):i96–i113, 2013.

Cook TM, Counsell D, Wildsmith JA: Royal College of Anaesthetists Third National Audit Project: Major complications of central neuraxial block: report on the Third National Audit of The Royal College of Anaesthetists, *Br J Anaesth* 102(2):179–190, 2009.

Horlocker TT, Wedel DJ, Rowlingson JC, et al.: Regional anesthesia in the patient receiving antithrombotic or thrombolytic therapy: American Society of Regional Anesthesia and Pain Medicine evidence-based guidelines (ed.3), *Reg Anesth Pain Med* 35(1):64–101, 2010.

Sanchez R, Nygard E: Epidural anesthesia in cardiac surgery: is there an increased risk? *J Cardiothorac Vasc Anesth* 12(2):170–173, 1998.

Vandermeulen EP, Van Aken H, Vermylen J: Anticoagulants and spinal–epidural anesthesia, *Anesth Analg* 79(6):1165–1177, 1994.

Wysokinski WE, McBane 2nd RD: Periprocedural bridging management of anticoagulation, *Circulation* 126(4):486–490, 2012.

锁骨上及锁骨下神经阻滞的并发症：气胸

第 180 章

David A. Olsen，*Sandra L. Kopp*

病例概要

患者，男性，42 岁，行右腕关节融合术后不久，在门诊恢复室内主诉呼吸短促和右侧轻微的胸痛。术前实施了超声引导下锁骨上入路的臂丛神经阻滞。检查发现患者呼吸频率 20 次 / 分，吸室内空气氧饱和度为 94%，血压和心率正常。胸部 X 线片示：右侧少量气胸。

问题分析

定义

气胸是肺和胸壁（胸膜腔）之间的空气或气体的积聚。采用锁骨上入路，臂丛神经阻滞在近端分支水平，此处神经排列紧密（图 180.1）。锁骨上臂丛神经阻滞技术有几个优点：包括手臂的中立位，阻滞起效快，进针浅超声影像清晰和各神经阻滞非常均匀。它的局限性包括潜在的膈神经阻滞和气胸的风险。神经阻滞的一般风险，包括神经损伤、感染、血肿和局部麻醉药中毒等，在此暂不讨论。需要特别注意已患有严重呼吸道疾病的患者，这类患者无法耐受气胸或膈神经阻滞等并发症。

而锁骨下入路臂丛神经阻滞的局部麻醉药注射位置在肌皮神经和腋神经的分支水平以上。锁骨下入路比腋路更靠近臂丛发出处，但其又比锁骨上入路更远离，可以阻滞来自神经丛的所有神经，而气胸或膈神经阻滞的发生率较低（图 180.2）。与锁骨上入路一样，手臂可以保持在中立位。锁骨下入路尤其适合需要行导管置入的连续阻滞的患者，因为该部位比在腋窝更方便覆盖无菌敷料。

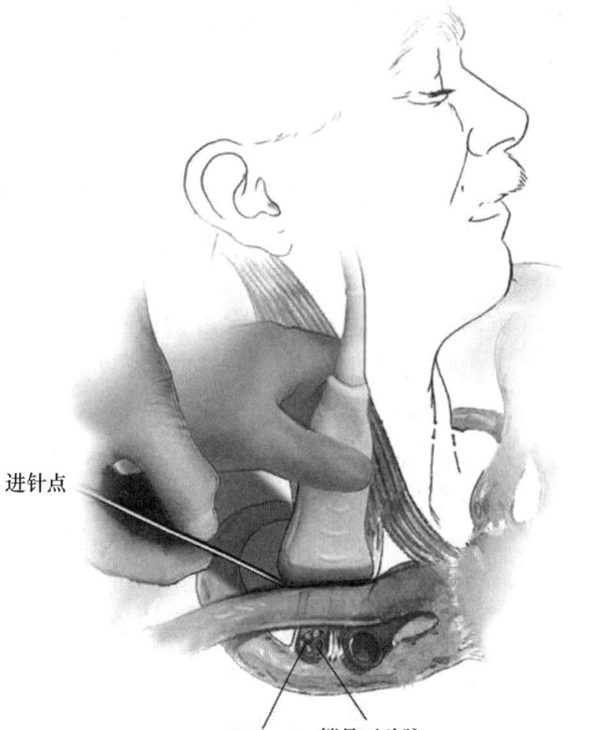

图 180.1 锁骨上阻滞，该针在平面内向前推进，朝向位于第一肋骨水平的排列紧凑的臂丛的后部（From Brown DL，Sites BD，Spence BC：Supraclavicular block. In Brown DL，editor：*Atlas of regional anesthesia*，4th ed. Philadelphia，Saunders，2010，p 57.）

识别

对气胸的识别主要根据临床表现。气胸可能发生在阻滞即时，或者在数小时后。如患者在阻滞过程中通过阻滞针吸入空气、或在进针过程中咳嗽、或阻滞后出现呼吸急促，则应怀疑是否存在气胸。在近端臂丛（如肌间沟入路）神经阻滞时，单侧的膈神经麻痹和一侧膈肌上抬非常常见，必需予以排

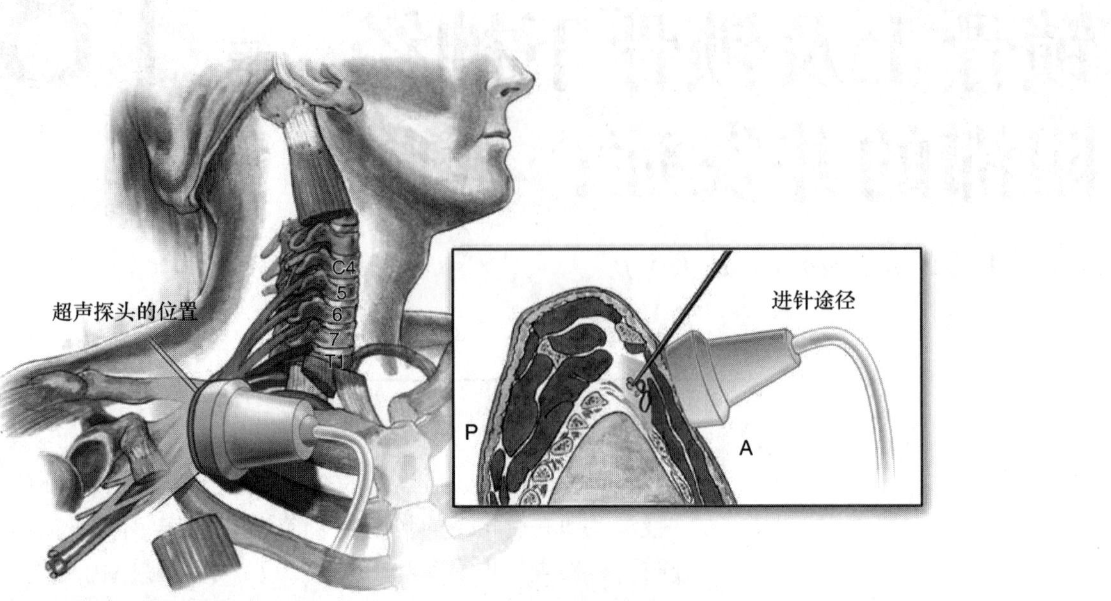

图 180.2 锁骨下阻滞，臂丛位于声带的水平（From Infraclavicular block. In Brown DL，editor：*Atlas of regional anesthesia*，4th ed. Philadelphia，Saunders，2010，p 65.）

除。尽管与肌间沟阻滞相比，锁骨上入路的膈肌麻痹发生率明显降低，但估计仍有高达 50% 的患者可能发生。锁骨下入路臂丛神经阻滞与肺功能的改变关系不大。如在机械通气期间，患者的临床状态突然恶化，则必须考虑是否发生气胸。发生气胸时，行容量控制模式机械通气的患者的气道峰值和平台压力均增加，而使用压力控制模式机械通气的患者的潮气量则减少。

气胸时，患者胸部可能有过清音或叩诊出现鼓音。患侧呼吸声可能消失。当肺容量减少不低于 25% 时，这些体征最为明显。

虽然计算机断层扫描是最敏感的检查，但通常胸片即可诊断。在呼气末时的 X 线片更容易显影，因为气胸在呼吸周期的这一期间占据患侧肺的比例更大。气胸的主要影像学特征是白色脏层胸膜线，通过无血管的积聚气体与壁层胸膜分开。大多数情况下，脏层胸膜边缘以外肺血管是不可见的（图 180.3）。

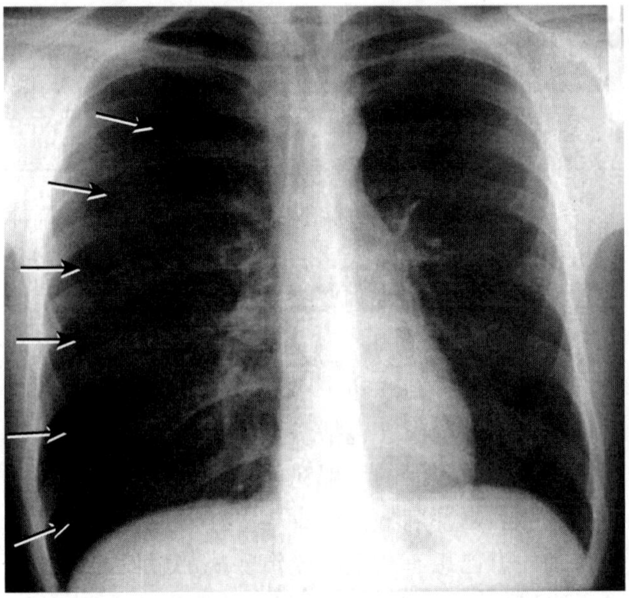

图 180.3 右侧 40% 气胸。箭头标出内脏胸膜线

在气胸的诊断中接受程度越来越高的方式是肺部超声检查。在接受过相关培训的内科医师中，肺部超声检查的敏感性可能超过了胸部 X 线。由于超声设备现在可以在大多数区域阻滞时方便地使用，因此肺部超声可以在临床怀疑气胸时进行快速检查。在患者仰卧位时，气胸患者的前胸壁的超声特征是肺滑行征和彗尾征均消失。

风险评估

随着超声的使用，锁骨上入路臂丛神经阻滞再度流行。在没有超声的情况下，锁骨上入路气胸的风险为 0.5% ～ 6.1%，而在超声引导下气胸发生率降低至 0.04% ～ 0.06%。由于气胸发生率低以及其症状的出现可能长达 24 h，因此行锁骨上入路臂丛神经阻滞后无需进行常规胸部 X 线检查。

启示

在整个呼吸周期期间，胸膜腔中的压力相对于肺泡压通常为负压。如果在穿刺时阻滞针刺穿胸壁，则会在大气和胸膜腔之间形成通路。空气开始进入胸膜腔，直到压力梯度消失或者通路被修复。气胸引起的主要生理变化是动脉氧分压（PO_2）降低和肺活量减少。肺功能差的患者症状更为明显，因为肺活量减少可导致呼吸功能不全，表现为肺通气不足并最终导致呼吸性酸中毒。

虽然在自主呼吸的患者中不太可能出现张力性气胸，但行正压机械通气的患者的风险则显著增加。吸气的正压使更多的空气进入胸膜腔，超过了呼气时排出的气体，导致张力性气胸。如果患者心肺功能突然下降应该怀疑是否存在张力性气胸。心肺状态的恶化可能是由于静脉回流减少引起的心排血量减少和通气-灌注失调导致的极度缺氧共同造成的。

管理

如果患者症状轻微且气胸小于肺容量的 15%，可以继续观察。患者还有必要有吸氧，这可以加快气胸的吸收速率。因为氮气是胸膜腔中的主要气体，所以氮气吸收到血液中的梯度是决定气胸重吸收速率的主要因素。通过吸入 100% 的氧气可以加速气胸的重吸收，因为提高氧浓度降低了血液中氮气的分压，从而增加了从胸膜腔吸收氮气的梯度压力。

如果患者的症状明显或气胸占据单胸腔的 15% 以上，那么用空针抽吸是首选治疗方法。如果抽吸无法防止气胸进一步扩张，应行胸腔置管闭式引流术。

行正压机械通气的患者治疗气胸，应行胸腔引流术以防止发展为张力性气胸。最常见的方法是在腋前线或腋中线水平、第四或第五肋间隙切开置入胸管，并且导管朝向胸腔顶部。

张力性气胸是一种急症。当怀疑患者有张力性气胸时，应立即吸入 100% 的氧气，以缓解缺氧。并沿锁骨中线第二肋间隙置入大口径的导管进入胸膜腔。如果通过导管吸出空气确诊后，患者应立即行胸腔闭式引流术。

预防

为了降低并发症的发生率，锁骨上和锁骨下入路的臂丛神经阻滞已经得到了许多改进。1949 年，Bonica 及其同事首先提出了一种细致轻柔的技巧，首先需要熟悉解剖关系，使用第一根肋骨作为肺部的保护盾；并使用一种短而细的针头来预防并发症，包括气胸的发生。现在是超声引导下神经阻滞的时代，针尖和胸膜的实时可视化能进一步降低气胸的发生率。与所有超声操作程序一样，保持针尖影像，使针与超声束位置良好，优化超声束与针的入射角，并且只在超声直接引导下进针，应该可以减少并发症的发生。间歇性水分离和可回声针可以增强针尖可见度。虽然这些技术自 Bonica 描述以来已经发生了变化，但使用第一根肋骨作为保护结构以及小心轻柔的操作技术，在当下超声引导的时代，仍然是很好的建议。

（李之娥 译 季 锋 校）

延伸阅读

Abell DJ, Barrington MJ: Pneumothorax after ultrasound-guided supraclavicular block: presenting features, risk, and related training, *Reg Anesth Pain Med* 39:164–167, 2014.

Bonica JJ, Moore DC, Orlov M: Brachial plexus block anesthesia, *Am J Surg 65*, 1949.

Brown DL: *Atlas of regional anesthesia*, ed 4th., Philadelphia, 2010, Saunders.

Gauss A, Tugtekin I, Georgieff M, et al.: Incidence of clinically symptomatic pneumothorax in ultrasound-guided infraclavicular and supraclavicular brachial plexus block, *Anaesthesia* 69:327–336, 2014.

Husain LF, Hagopian L, Wayman D, et al.: Sonographic diagnosis of pneumothorax, *J Emerg Trauma Shock* 5(1):76–81, 2012.

Light RW, Gary Lee YC: Pneumothorax, chylothorax, hemothorax, and fibrothorax. In Broaddus VC, editor: *Murray and Nadel's textbook of respiratory medicine*, ed 6th, Philadelphia, 2016, Elsevier, pp 1439–1460.

Neal JM, Moore JM, Kopacz DJ, et al.: Quantitative analysis of respiratory, motor, and sensory function after supraclavicular block, *Anesth Analg* 86:1239–1244, 1998.

Rodriquez J, Barcena M, Rodriguez V, et al.: Infraclavicular brachial plexus block effects on respiratory function and extent of the block, *Reg Anesth Pain Med* 23:564–568, 1998.

第181章 注射器互换

Carsten Nadjat-Haiem，*Michael J. Sopher*

病例概要

患者，女性，32岁，平素体健，拟行“子宫肌瘤摘除术”，全身麻醉诱导后行气管插管，外科医师要求预防性使用抗生素头孢唑啉。麻醉科医师用10 ml注射器进行给药，但立马意识到他给的是去氧肾上腺素，因此他转换注射器给予递增剂量的硝酸甘油，以减少预期性高血压，患者无明显不良后果。

问题分析

定义

注射器互换造成相当一批患者出现给药错误。给药错误发生率为每10万剂麻醉药中有18例，其中注射器互换约占6.4%。当注射器贴错标签或正确标记但误认为是不同的药物时，会发生注射器互换。给药错误的其他常见原因是药物过量或选择错误，无意中发生的脊椎麻醉（腰麻）平面过高和局部麻醉药中毒，这类问题本章节在这里不做过多讨论。

识别

当给药后出现意想不到的结果或当事件发生且没有明显的解释时，通常可以识别为注射器互换。在观察到任何效果之前，也可以对这种交换进行确认。最常见的错误是在需要肌松恢复时再追加一剂肌松药。

风险评估

任何患者都有互换注射器的危险。尽管研究表明，由互换注射器造成的死亡很罕见，但其仍然会导致严重的病死率。有趣的是，大多数注射器互换都发生在美国麻醉科医师协会ASA Ⅰ级和ASA Ⅱ级患者的“简单”麻醉药中，这只能解释为大部分麻醉药通用于ASA Ⅰ级和ASA Ⅱ级患者身上。然而，对于健康程度较差的患者而言，注射器互换将会使其受到更为不利影响。尽管注射器互换仅构成所有药物错用的一小部分，但并非罕见事件。在受访者中85%～94%承认其职业生涯中至少进行过一次注射器互换，而且有相当一部分如实地报告对患者造成了伤害。

常见互换注射器的原因包括以下方面：

- 在抽药时缺乏警惕性；
- 在给药时缺乏警惕性（实际未认真阅读标签）；
- 注射器未贴标签或贴错标签；
- 未用带颜色编码的标签标记注射器；
- 药瓶和注射器外观相似；
- 药品托盘摆放不合理；
- 疲劳（睡眠剥夺、无聊、晚夜班交替、工作超负荷）；
- 应激性环境，进展性压力；陌生环境；
- 班次变化；
- 沟通问题；
- 经验不足；知识不足；
- 分心（电脑、手机、嘈杂的音乐）。

管理

注射器交换的管理包括以下几个方面：

- 识别错误；
- 处理后果；
- 调查事件；
- 制定防止再次发生的措施。

如果给患者使用了不正确的药物，首先应识别错误和治疗任何急性后果。如果失误很快被发现，就像案例概述一样，执行者应该对结果进行预期性的处理。如果错误不易立即发现，且发生了不良事件，应立即在手术室内进行调查。封闭房间，随后的患者应推迟或转移到其他房间，以防止再次发生。通过系统的调查，包括事件中使用的药物。检查当天使用的药瓶，也可能还需要分析注射器的内容物。麻醉科应立即制定预防措施，确保不再出现类似的错误。

如果失误导致并发症，应告知患者以及与患者治疗近期直接相关的所有人员。所有事件也应清楚地记录在图表中。还应通知风险管理 / 质量保证委员会以及可能涉及的其部门，如药房。如果互换注射器是由于药物标签相同造成的，应将问题通知相关的制药公司。麻醉科或责任药房也应采取措施进一步区分药瓶。

从法医的角度来看，互换注射器违反了治疗标准，是一个明显的过失案例。应在早期阶段征求风险管理部门的建议。

预防

预防的方法包括三大类：

- 提高警惕；
- 检查和复查；
- 具体措施。

防止注射器互换的最佳方法是麻醉科医师在准备和使用药物时保持警惕性。用药前应严格按常规进行药物的配制和复查。以下具体建议有助于防止用药错误：

1. 仔细检查所有药瓶后再将其抽吸入注射器。包括检查药瓶上标签的药品名称、有效期和浓度。最近的一份报告指出，0.2% 和 0.75% 的罗哌卡因的外观几乎相同。还应检查溶液中是否有异常的外观或气味。
2. 在配制抽取药物前，所有注射器都应贴上标签。在推车上应配备有条理的、预先打印好彩色编码的标签系统（图 181.1）。空白标签可用于不常使用的药物。注射器应该被环向标记，这样无论注射器的方向如何，都能辨认出药物。
3. 使用不同规格的注射器会有所帮助。例如，诱导药放在较大的 20 ml 注射器中，肌松药放在 10 ml 注射器中，麻醉性镇痛药和其他镇静药放在较小的 3 ml 或 5 ml 注射器中。大多数注射器交换发生在相同尺寸的注射器之间。

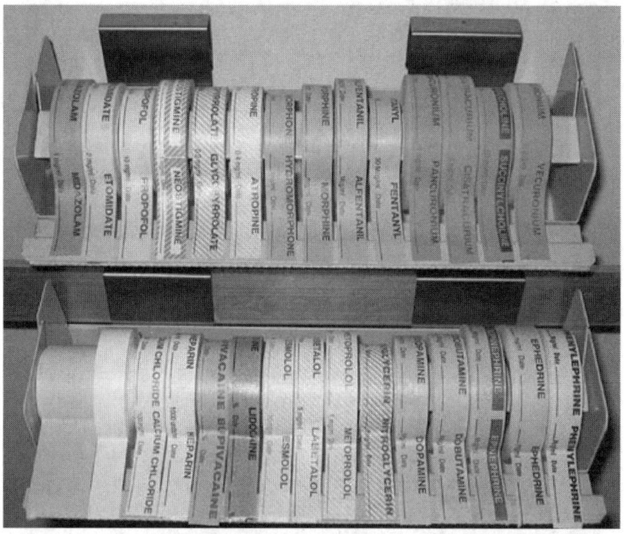

图 181.1 彩色编码标签。应用摆放有序、储备充足的彩色标签托盘有助于快速标记药物注射器。麻醉药物使用标签的标准 D4774 于 1983 年推出，目前仍在使用。这些标签降低了注射器互换的发生率，但肯定没有消除这个问题

4. 避免将药物包装在具有类似外观的预混合注射器中。例如，利多卡因和肾上腺素都装在预先贴上标签的玻璃注射器中，具有非常相似的外观。在光线不好的环境中，这些标签尤其难以读取。如果药物使用这种类型的包装，请在注射器的塑料部分另外贴上一个容易识别的标签，或仅限使用一种预先包装的药物（如肾上腺素）。
5. 避免使用具有外观相似的药物容器。如果将带有类似包装的药物放在推车上，应在药瓶上放置明亮的警告标签。强效的药物应该通过附加标签来识别，或者不要常规地放在药物托盘上。药物应按类别堆放在药物托盘上。
6. 切勿使用未贴标签的注射器注射任何药物。
7. 麻醉车储存方式的一致性尤为重要。药物应始终放置在推车的相同位置，并按类堆放（例如，拮抗剂、降压药、肌松药）（图 181.2）。
8. 住院医师教育应包括技能培训，确保在处理药物时能做到一丝不苟。住院医师在麻醉车顶端标记和摆放注射器时，要鼓励他们制定严格的常规。将注射器分离成诱导药、肌松药、阿片类药物和其他药物可能会有所帮助。
9. 最近的证据表明，系统改进措施可以显著降低注射器互换的发生率。其中一个系统利用条形码扫

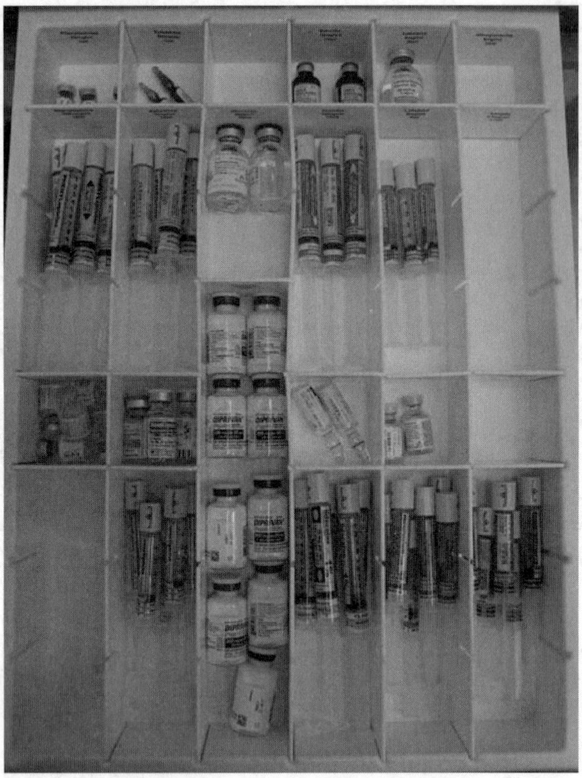

图 181.2 药物托盘摆放。将药物统一分为升压药（左上）、拮抗剂（左下）、诱导药（中）、降压药（右上）和麻醉药（右下）可降低更换注射器的风险。特别重要的是拮抗剂和肌松药物在空间上要隔离开来。相同外观的药瓶上的附加标签可以进一步降低风险（上图的药盘上没有这类附加标签）。还应注意托盘中的商用预抽药注射器，水平和垂直双标记，以降低在一定角度观察时标签“不可见”的风险

描药物，然后通过计算机 / 分配装置对药物进行听觉和视觉确认（图 181.3）。这已被证明可以将注射器交换的发生率降低 35% 或更多，且用户的满意度很高。

（夏博洋 译 王恒跃 校）

延伸阅读

Bastien JL, Bailey PD: Ropivacaine packaging: a potential for drug error, *Anesthesiology* 101(2):551, 2004.

Fastings S, Gisvold SE: Adverse drug errors in anesthesia, and the impact of coloured syringe labels, *Can J Anaesth* 47(11):1006–1007, 2000.

Gordon PC, Llewellyn RL, James MF: Drug administration errors by South African anesthetists—a survey, *S Afr Med J* 96(7):630–632, 2006.

Irita K, Tsuzaki K, Sawa T, et al.: Critical incidents due to drug administration error in the operating room: an analysis of 4,291,925 anesthetics over a four year period, *Masui* 53(5):577–584, 2004.

Liang BA, Bramhall J, Cullen B: Which syringe did I use? Anesthesiologist confusion and potential liability for a medical error, *J Clin Anesth* 14(5):371–374, 2002.

Orser BA, Chen RJ, Yee DA: Medication errors in anesthetic practice: a survey of 687 practitioners, *Can J Anaesth* 48(2):139–146, 2001.

Warltier DC, Howard SK, Rosekind MR, et al.: Fatigue in anesthesia: implications and strategies for patient and provider safety, *Anesthesiology* 97(5):1281–1294, 2002.

Webster CS, Larson L, Frampton CM, et al.: Clinical assessment of a new drug administration system. A prospective, controlled, longitudinal incident monitoring study, *Anesthesia* 65(5):490–499, 2010.

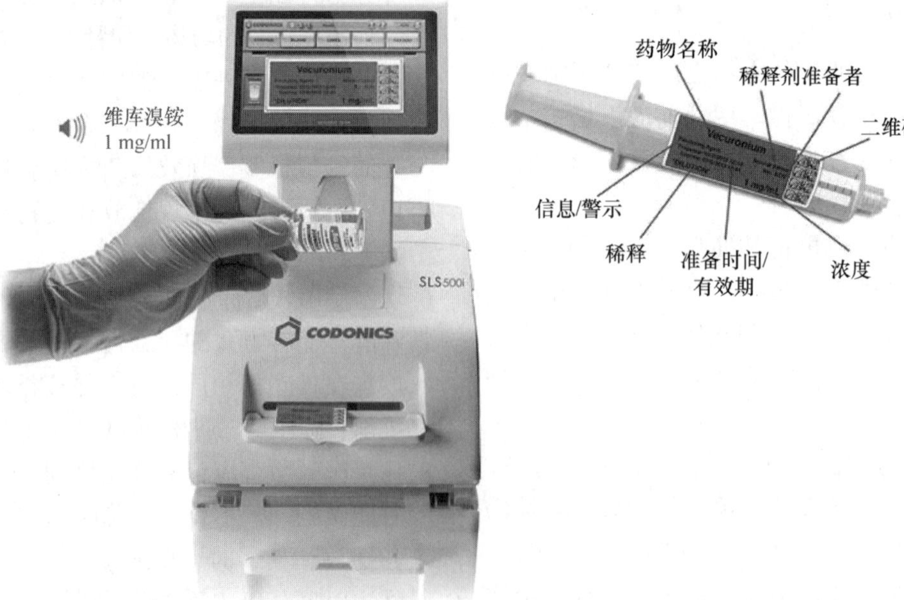

图 181.3 现代彩色编码标签系统。市场上最新推出的系统可以扫描药物，打印适当的标签，并帮助确认（在设备监视器上）和听觉识别（通过装置报出药物名称）正在配置的药物。早期研究表明，这些装置显著降低了注射器交换的发生率

有恶意攻击行为的患者 第 182 章

Krzysztof Laudanski

病例概要

患者，男，14 岁，确诊为自闭症谱系障碍，他在 5 岁时因烧伤致手部挛缩，计划行限期手部挛缩松解术。他曾接受过三次手术，据了解手术期间出现过苏醒困难。目前，他正在等候区内痴迷地玩着平板电脑上的游戏，忽略了需要前往手术室做手术这件事。他的父母对这种情况感到苦恼和担忧，不断怀疑工作人员是否有能力妥善处理这种情况。

问题分析

定义

一般的假设是，患者来手术就医的目的就是配合好让手术得以顺利完成。但这种假设并非普遍适用。有恶意的患者是指与医护人员的建议不合作的个体。不合作行为可能发生在初次访谈期间，诱导时或在麻醉后恢复室（postanesthesia care unit, PACU）中。

一些患者由于理解手术及其后果（如智力残疾）的能力有限、缺乏心理技巧来应对手术压力（如自闭症）或不适应的应对策略而积极抵制治疗。另外还有一些患者由于摄入了精神刺激物质而出现药物中毒从而表现出攻击性行为。有些人可能因为与他们的原发性疾病或并存疾病（疼痛）有关的不适而显得不合作。最后，麻醉科医师可能面临一个敌对和暴力的患者，他们有明确和坚定的意图破坏治疗，造成自我伤害或伤害医务人员（暴力囚犯）。由于陪伴的第三方（父母、警察、朋友、护理人员）的出现，使得临床状况更加复杂，有时甚至使本已复杂的情况更加复杂化。总之，患者可能会拒绝治疗的原因似乎有很多。麻醉科医师必须具有足够的灵活性，以解决几种特殊的临床状况（表 182.1）。

识别

仔细检查以往的记录通常可以发现先前出现过的困难情况。定期与照顾患者的医务人员或者与他的父母交谈也同样有帮助。此外，初次访谈可以评估患者在治疗过程的潜在困难。来自监狱或赡养院的患者应该仔细评估他们接受手术的知情同意和一般意愿的能力。

在初次访谈期间，尊重患者的权利和偏好至关重要，因为对患者行为的错误解读可能会导致不好

表 182.1 有恶意攻击性患者的可能原因

药理学因素	器官学因素	行为学因素	发育学因素	社会学因素
戒断综合征	谵妄	注意力缺失症	智力障碍	监禁
药物滥用	痴呆	自闭症	幼龄	
谵妄	脑病	创伤后应激障碍		
麻醉后苏醒	无法控制的疼痛	焦虑		
	尿潴留（术后）	精神病		

表 182.2 不易相处的患者麻醉计划的关键部分

组织	环境	药理	心理
与父母 / 看护人面谈	术前访视	使用非静脉方法进行预防	广泛的交流沟通
安慰以消除恐惧	避免中断和意外	吸入麻醉	
保证其他工作人员的安全	昏暗的环境		
情景预演			

的第一印象。患有创伤后应激障碍或经历过严重医院相关创伤的患者可能尤其会这样。他们对心理伤害导致的类似情况的高度焦虑或反应可能会被医护人员误解。

风险评估

与不易相处的患者互动的相关风险可分为与患者本人、患者陪护人员和医务人员相关的风险。此外，不配合的行为在任何时候都可能出现，有时会让 PACU 的工作人员感到惊讶，但大部分情况下，这种行为都发生在转运患者的过程中。通常，患者父母可以详细说明引发不配合行为的潜在诱因，其严重程度以及处理这些行为的最佳策略。警方通常可以提供一些有关预期问题的细节。在紧急情况下，此类评估更难以预测。

启示

对有恶意的患者进行麻醉可能具有挑战性，并具有一些严重的影响。获得知情同意可能并不容易。对于未成年人或有指定监护人的患者，如果文件明确，则可以相对容易地获得麻醉许可。但通常情况并非如此。医院管理部门或社会工作者可以帮助确定责任方并获取联系信息。必要时可能需要寻求紧急法院命令，并且所有州都明确规定了如何获得法院命令的程序。如果是谵妄、脑病（例如肝衰竭、创伤后脑损伤）或痴呆患者，责任方的寻找可能颇具挑战。如果有恶意的患者有能力就非急诊手术做出知情决策，并且拒绝同意该手术，则必须取消该手术。

在急诊手术时，应考虑患者的普通诉求。例如，拒绝输血的患者应该尽力避免患者出血过多，预防贫血，但不应该拒绝手术或麻醉。如果是未成年人，可以寻求法律上的紧急同意。有时患者可能坚持一种麻醉方式。如果患者理解决定的影响，并且不会对患者造成任何不合理的伤害，则应满足患者的要求。但是，如果麻醉科医师不能同意患者的要求，则应推迟手术直到问题得到解决。

麻醉方案的选择至关重要，因为它将决定患者的安全和满意度以及医务人员的安全。区域麻醉可能因为需要患者的积极配合，因而不可能考虑应用，但是对于一些对全身麻醉心存焦虑的患者来说，这可能是一种合适的麻醉方法。静脉通路的建立可能会是一大难题。使用复方利多卡因麻醉乳膏（EMLA），转移注意力和肌内注射抗焦虑药物都可以考虑使用。另一种选择是吸入诱导，随后建立静脉通路或使用吸入麻醉剂来减轻焦虑。

敌视的患者可能不配合气道检查。因此，应该预料到患者可能会存在困难气道。有困难气道病史的不合作患者将会面临真正的挑战，以往的医疗记录对于确定建立安全气道的策略至关重要。患者可能无法达到最佳的脱氮条件，特别是在闭合能力增加的有攻击行为的患者（如肥胖、阻塞性睡眠呼吸暂停）。在麻醉科医师使患者失去知觉之前，通常难以对患者进行适当的监测或只能推迟监测。

如果不合作的患者发生跌倒也会有受伤的风险。自我伤害可能不易被发现，患者突然活动可能会使工作人员感到惊讶。通常，在极端年龄如老人和小孩中的具有严重认知障碍的患者往往表现出这种行为。在运送过程中或准备转移患者时，这些行为往往会吓到工作人员。与照顾者的交谈是预料到此类行为的关键。合计的计划包括持续监测患者行为，床铺以柔软衬垫，使用个人防护设备，配备专门的工作人员对病人进行观察，最后，采取身体或药物约束措施。

表现出攻击性行为的药物中毒患者应从手术安排表中删除。经常性的急性中毒可导致血流动力学不稳定和苏醒期谵妄的高发病率。如果计划手术的患者不是急诊手术，这些风险超过了潜在的益处。在紧急情况下，应预料到出现苏醒期谵妄的可能，患者可预先服用辅助药物（如抗精神病药、可乐定）。

有故意攻击行为的患者应有保安或警察的陪同。通常情况下，根据监狱规定，手术室或 PACU 中这些官员必须在场。因此，必须进行充分的计划以满足他们的需要和要求。

管理

建议与护士、手术室工作人员和患者的陪护人员一起讨论处理策略以应对任何可能会发生的情况。有预见性的计划可以减少混乱，特别是在局势失控的情况下。如果局势迅速升级，获得额外资源以提供帮助始终是一种很好的做法。

成功地处理困难的、不合作的患者的关键是耐心、计划和保持警惕。意外和急躁会进一步增加理解的缺乏。因此，避免迅速中断应成为一项规则。说服、推理和公开是成功的关键。这取决于麻醉科医师和困难患者之间交流的情况。

在本病例中，父母是信息和支持的主要来源。考虑到父母的陪伴可减轻患儿应激，且可避免使用以前出现反常反应的药物，他们可能会陪伴孩子到手术室直到诱导。然而，我们必须记住，过度焦虑的父母可能是分散注意力的源头，而明智的麻醉科医师应能同时关注孩子和父母的需求。通常情况下，有既往病史儿童的父母会感到压力大，并且精通医学术语。如果这方面处理得不好，这可能使本已很困难的情况更具有挑战性。由于认知或应对能力受损的儿童对抗焦虑药物更常出现躁动反应，因此术前用药应保留作为最后的手段之一。在某些情况下，通过组织患儿术前对手术室访视可以减轻孩子的应激。这种方法可以让孩子适应手术室的环境。但由于日程繁忙，此解决方案可能无法实现。

玩具可以用来分散注意力，即使患者没有静脉通路也可以有多种药物可以应用。若患者同意接受术前用药，通常首选口服用药。否则可以使用静脉内或（更常见）肌内注射方法。一些人主张使用身体束缚，但这是最后的手段，因为它可能会使情况更加恶化。身体束缚应仅用于患者明显会伤害自己或工作人员的情况。诱导后，麻醉维持期间可为工作人员提供了休息的机会。麻醉苏醒可能比较困难，有时建议使用右美托咪定或丙泊酚，但反应可能会有所差异。治疗过程中对任何药物的反应良好意味着最好的预后。因此，不能过高估计与父母面谈和审查医疗记录的价值。假设患者气道条件良好，深麻醉下拔管可能是避免躁动的一种方法，但无论如何都可能出现苏醒期谵妄。父母的在场和安慰往往是最好的措施。有时可能有指征需要使用抗精神病药物。困难患者出现苏醒期谵妄时者不应该取消对其行为的其他原因的探究（过剧疼痛、代谢紊乱、膀胱充盈、缺血等）。

预防

充分准备是对有恶意攻击行为患者麻醉成功的关键。让父母、孩子和所有医务人员参与是成功的首要条件。在一个安静的环境中提供最喜欢的娱乐消遣方式很有帮助。对于麻醉开始时管理困难患者的最佳方法，目前还缺乏结论性的研究。麻醉科医师的经验是成功解决问题的关键。

（方　亚　译　陆　军　校）

延伸阅读

Bhat R, Santhosh MC, Annigeri VM, et al.: Comparison of intranasal dexmedetomidine and dexmedetomidine-ketamine for premedication in pediatrics patients: a randomized double-blind study, *Anesth Essays Res* 10(2):349–355, 2016.

Done V, Kotha R, Vasa AA, et al.: A comparison of the effectiveness of oral midazolam–N_2O versus oral ketamine—N_2O in pediatric patients—an in-vivo study, *J Clin Diagn Res* 10:ZC45–ZC48, 2016.

McKelvey VA, Morgaine KC, Thomson WM: Adults with intellectual disability: a mixed-methods investigation of their experiences of dental treatment under general anaesthetic, *N Z Dent J* 110(2):58–64, 2014.

Snow SL, Smith IM, Bird SJ, et al.: A call to solve the puzzle together by building an evidence base for perioperative management of children with autism spectrum disorder, *Paediatr Anaesth* 26(7):772–773, 2016.

Vlassakova BG, Emmanouil DE: Perioperative considerations in children with autism spectrum disorder, *Curr Opin Anaesthesiol* 29(3):359–366, 2016.

Vulser H, Airagnes G, Lahlou-Laforêt K, et al.: Psychiatric consequences of intraoperative awareness: short review and case series, *Gen Hosp Psychiatry* 37(1):94–95, 2015.

White SM: Ethical and legal aspects of anaesthesia for the elderly, *Anaesthesia* 69(Suppl 1):45–53, 2014.

第183章 血栓栓塞性并发症

Gerard R. Manecke

病例概要

患者，男性，53岁，接受了L1～L4节段后路椎体内固定融合手术。患者有蛋白质S缺乏症病史并接受华法林治疗。手术前2周停用了华法林，但没有告知医务人员。手术时长8 h，期间患者生命体征基本平稳。但在术后1 h，他开始呼吸急促，血压从130/80 mmHg降至88/50 mmHg，血氧饱和度从99%降至88%。患者被诊断为急性肺栓塞。

问题分析

血栓栓塞事件是围术期最令人畏惧的并发症，是住院患者最常见的死亡原因。它通常危及生命（肺栓塞），威胁肢体安全（外周动脉栓塞），或对中枢神经系统（脑血管栓塞）有更大危险。麻醉科医师作为围术期外科之家的领导者，作用变得日益重要。血栓栓塞等并发症的预防和治疗也越来越依赖麻醉科医师。

定义

血栓栓塞是一系列涉及血管内血液凝固的血管闭塞性疾病。血栓症是指血凝块形成，以及血凝块或其他物质的播散至血管树的某处。除了凝块之外，诸如血管内气体和骨髓等物质都成为栓子（表183.1）。循环中的静脉或动脉均可能受累，包括脑血管、心腔、冠状动脉和肺动脉（表183.2）。本章的重点是静脉血栓栓塞（venous thromboembolism，VTE）的两种表现：深静脉血栓形成（deep venous thrombosis，DVT）和肺栓塞（pulmonary embolism，PE）。

表183.1　栓子的来源

栓塞来源	临床情景
静脉血栓	深静脉血栓形成，制动，高凝状态
空气	坐位手术；背部手术且手术部位高于心脏水平；静脉输液中的意外空气；开腔心脏手术；冠状动脉手术中气体意外夹带
二氧化碳（CO_2）	腹腔镜手术中的气体栓塞
	开腔心脏手术中使用CO_2
氧气	骨科使用过氧化氢作为长骨手术中的冲洗剂
导管，导管碎片，导丝，导丝碎片	开放血管通路的并发症
化脓性栓子	长期感染（导管部位，心内膜炎，脓肿）
肿瘤栓子	肾细胞癌，心腔肿瘤
脂肪栓子	长骨骨折，手术

风险评估与管理

据估计，普通外科患者发生DVT的风险高达30%，不过支持这一点的数据包含了部分旧数据，即该部分并不反映更新、更有效的预防手段。普通外科患者的PE风险可能高达1%。手术患者通常表现为由癌症、化疗、妊娠和遗传性疾病（如蛋白质C缺乏症）等引起的高凝状态。既往患有DVT或PE是高风险因素，此外，吸烟和肥胖也是风险因素之一。重要的是，大手术和创伤本身会导致高凝状态，使这些患者处于围术期血栓栓塞并发症的极高风险之中。

所有接受手术的患者都应考虑VTE的风险，时间越长、创伤越大的手术带来的风险也越高，具有其他危险因素（表183.3）的患者更应该特别注意。对住院患者进行风险分级的方法有很多种，其中Caprini评分系统应用较广（图183.1）。基于该

表 183.2 特定的血栓栓塞现象及其临床表现		
位置	诱发因素	临床结果和后遗症
深静脉血栓形成	静脉淤滞	肺栓塞，下腔静脉血栓形成，上腔静脉综合征
肺栓塞	深静脉血栓形成，高凝状态	休克，死亡，残余肺动脉高压
外周动脉血栓形成或栓子	房间隔或室间隔缺损，胸主动脉或外周动脉手术	器官、肢体缺血或梗死
脑动脉血栓形成或栓子	动脉粥样硬化，房间隔或室间隔缺损，手术涉及颈动脉或主动脉弓	脑卒中
冠状动脉血栓形成	冠状动脉支架，停用抗血小板药物，严重的冠状动脉疾病	突发性心肌梗死
冠状动脉栓塞	动脉粥样硬化，房间隔或室间隔缺损，手术涉及主动脉弓	心肌缺血或梗死
心室血栓形成	心房颤动，心力衰竭	动脉栓塞

表 183.3 围术期血栓栓塞的危险因素	
遗传性高凝状态	蛋白质 C 缺乏症 蛋白质 S 缺乏症 Ⅴ因子 Leiden 病变 抗磷脂综合征 异常纤维蛋白原血症 抗凝血酶缺乏症
获得性高凝状态	大手术，创伤 癌症 化疗 口服避孕药 激素替代疗法 真性红细胞增多症 急性疾病
其他风险	静脉淤滞，深静脉血栓形成或肺栓塞史 吸烟 心房颤动 高龄 制动，骨科石膏，肥胖 中心静脉导管 房间隔缺损：反常栓塞

评分系统，可以使用诸如早期下床活动、低剂量普通肝素、序贯加压袜和弹力袜等预防措施。由于接受手术的患者有罹患风险，比较常见的围术期方案包括气动序贯加压袜、药物预防和早期运动。可使用“三步法”模型预防围术期 VTE，低风险患者需要简单预防，中等风险患者接受气动加压设备或低剂量肝素（分级肝素或未分级普通肝素），高风险患者同时接受气动加压和低剂量普通肝素（表 183.4）。低剂量的血栓预防导致出血风险增加的可能性很低，因此“三步法”模型适用于大多数手术。

静脉血栓栓塞

深静脉血栓形成

DVT 在临床上相对常见，临床表现为小腿腓部疼痛和下肢肿胀。其危险因素包括：高凝状态、静脉淤滞和内皮损伤（“Virchow 三要素”）。脊髓损伤、旅行或手术等因素引起的长时间制动已被确定为重要的危险因素，可能是因为引起静脉淤滞所致。此外，手术的体液应激反应会导致机体高凝状态。

DVT 的诊断是通过在围术期保持高度警惕，检测其常见的体征和症状，并通过超声或放射影像学检查确认。深静脉血栓的常见症状包括通常沿着腿部静脉路径发生的下肢肿胀，以及疼痛、发红和发热。经下肢超声探查、静脉造影或磁共振成像（magnetic resonance imaging，MRI）可证实诊断。静脉血栓一般在四肢近端静脉和骨盆形成，越大、越近心端的血栓具有越大的血管损害和栓塞风险。接受大手术的患者通常会因为手术出血的风险而“持续”应用抗凝剂，但这种“双刃剑”的另一面则是患者因此被置于增加血栓形成和栓子的风险中。

当 DVT 在围术期发生时，必须迅速诊断，并用抗凝和活动进行积极治疗，因为它会导致左右心存在循环交通的患者出现 PE 和动脉（反常）栓子（如房间隔缺损、卵圆孔未闭）。在接受高剂量抗凝剂治疗的外科患者中，出血是一种风险，这使围术期 VTE 的管理非常具有挑战性。肝素输注或溶栓治疗这些积极方法，虽然常适用于非手术患者，但可能会使手术患者面临很大的出血风险。因此，应与外科医师讨论应用抗凝剂的时间和剂量，以及延迟治

深静脉血栓形成（DVT）

预防医嘱
（适用于择期普外科患者）

血栓形成风险因素评估
（选择所有适用项）

出生日期

姓名

住院号

性别 男 女 访问号________________

每个风险因素代表1分

- ☐ 年龄41～60岁
- ☐ 急性心肌梗死
- ☐ 腿部肿胀（当前）
- ☐ 充血性心力衰竭（<1个月）
- ☐ 静脉曲张
- ☐ 长期卧床
- ☐ 肥胖（BMI>25）
- ☐ 炎症性肠病史
- ☐ 计划进行小手术
- ☐ 既往大手术史（<1个月）
- ☐ 脓毒症（<1个月）
- ☐ 肺功能异常（COPD）
- ☐ 严重的肺部疾病，包括肺炎（<1个月）
- ☐ 口服避孕药或激素替代疗法
- ☐ 妊娠或产后（<1个月）
- ☐ 不明原因的死胎史，反复发作的自发性流产（≥3），早产合并毒血症或婴儿生长受限
- ☐ 其他风险因素 ________________

小计：

每个风险因素代表2分

- ☐ 年龄61～74岁
- ☐ 建立中心静脉通路
- ☐ 关节镜手术
- ☐ 大手术（>45分钟）
- ☐ 恶性肿瘤（现在或既往）
- ☐ 腹腔镜手术（>45分钟）
- ☐ 床上制动（>72 h）
- ☐ 固定石膏模型（<1个月）

小计：

每个风险因素代表3分

- ☐ 年龄75岁或以上
- ☐ 血栓形成的家族史*
- ☐ DVT/PE病史
- ☐ 凝血酶原阳性20210A
- ☐ V因子Leiden病变阳性
- ☐ 狼疮抗凝剂阳性
- ☐ 血清同型半胱氨酸升高
- ☐ 肝素诱导的血小板减少症（Heparin-induced thrombocytopenia，HIT）（不要使用肝素或任何低分子量肝素）
- ☐ 抗心磷脂抗体升高
- ☐ 其他先天性或获得性血栓形成倾向

如果有：类型 ________________

* 最常漏掉的风险因素

小计：

每个风险因素代表5分

- ☐ 卒中（<1个月）
- ☐ 多发伤（<1个月）
- ☐ 择期下肢大关节成形术
- ☐ 髋，骨盆或腿部骨折（<1个月）
- ☐ 急性脊髓损伤（瘫痪）（<1个月）

小计：

总计风险得分：

图 183.1 可对静脉血栓栓塞的发生进行风险分层的 Caprini 评分系统

表 183.4 外科患者血栓预防的“三步法”

低风险：小手术，早期下床活动	最简单的预防：抗血栓栓塞袜
中等风险：最常见，胸科、妇科、腹腔镜或开放手术	气动压力袜或低剂量肝素（普通肝素 5000 U 皮下注射 q 8～12 h，或依诺肝素 40 U 皮下注射 qd 或 30 U 皮下注射 q 12 h）
高风险：髋关节或膝关节成形术、创伤、脊髓损伤、腹部和盆腔手术治疗癌症	气动压力袜和低剂量肝素（普通肝素 5000 U 皮下注射 q 8～12 h，或依诺肝素 40 U 皮下注射 q d 或 30 U 皮下注射 q 12 h）

疗的潜在风险。请血液科医师会诊或许有帮助。下腔静脉滤器可以用来降低 PE 的风险，特别是对于抗凝剂禁忌的患者。围术期 DVT 患者需要在事件发生后的几个月内持续进行术后治疗，并且应在出院前进行合理规划。

出血的患者如外伤或肝病患者通常使用新鲜冰冻血浆、血小板浓缩物、冷沉淀和凝血因子Ⅶ或Ⅸ浓缩物等血液制品进行治疗。这些患者在治疗过程中出现高凝状态并不罕见。这种高凝状态加上低心排血量，可使患者容易发生下腔静脉（inferior vena cava，IVC）血栓形成。这种状态由于静脉回心血量减少，导致心排血量急剧下降从而危及生命。在治疗凝血障碍的过程中，最好通过仔细监测凝血系统来预防 IVC 的血栓形成，凝血因子Ⅶ或Ⅸ浓缩物应分次应用。可采用腹部超声、计算机断层扫描或 MRI 实施诊断。

静脉血栓形成也可能在上肢或上腔静脉中形成，导致上腔静脉综合征。其特征在于面部、颈部和上肢肿胀，并且可能导致气道和血管损害。

肺栓塞

PE 是一种潜在的危及生命的疾病，是由于静脉血栓形成并栓塞到肺循环所致。如果栓子较大，肺循环可能大部分甚至完全被阻塞，导致右心衰竭以及肺部气体交换中断。可能发生低血压伴休克或心搏骤停，同时伴有高碳酸血症、低氧血症和酸中毒。如果栓子较小，可能出现肺梗死伴咯血。

清醒的患者，例如本章病例概要中描述的患者，可能会主诉呼吸困难，偶尔会出现胸膜痛。也可伴发气喘、颈静脉怒张、低血压和发绀。

在麻醉患者中，突然发生的低血压伴呼气末二氧化碳（end-tidal carbon dioxide，$ETCO_2$）的骤减可能是大面积 PE 的第一个征象。动脉血气可显示高碳酸血症以及动脉血 PCO_2 与 $ETCO_2$ 梯度大，提示肺栓塞具有显著的死腔通气特征。经食管多普勒或基

于动脉系统的微创心排血量监测，可以显示心排血量减少，有助于区分 PE 与血管扩张（如过敏反应）引起的高心排血量休克状态。中心静脉压升高可以区分 PE 和低血容量。休克状态的鉴别诊断相当广泛（表 183.5），因此高度的怀疑有助于 PE 的诊断。患者易患 DVT 的危险因素与 PE 的危险因素相同，既往或目前有 DVT 的患者风险特别高。

超声心动图是帮助鉴别突发性休克的最快床边检查。可以使用经胸超声心动图（transthoracic echocardiography，TTE）或经食管超声心动图（transesophageal echocardiography，TEE）。由于对肺动脉的优质显像，TEE 可能更胜一筹。在大面积 PE 中，TTE 或 TEE 都会显示右侧心力衰竭的征象，包括右心房扩张、右心室扩张和室间隔向左移位（图 183.2）。右心腔内或近端肺动脉可能会发现栓子，

表 183.5 休克的常见原因

↓左心室前负荷	↓后负荷	↓收缩性
低血容量	血管舒张	心肌梗死
• 出血	• 麻醉药	心肌缺血
	• 降压	心脏创伤，挫伤
右心室衰竭	过敏	
• PE	• 乳胶	
• 支气管痉挛	• 抗生素	
• 脂肪栓塞	• 肌肉松弛药	
• 气胸		
• 鱼精蛋白		
心脏压塞	过敏样反应	缺氧
	• 万古霉素	心肌病
	• 鱼精蛋白	

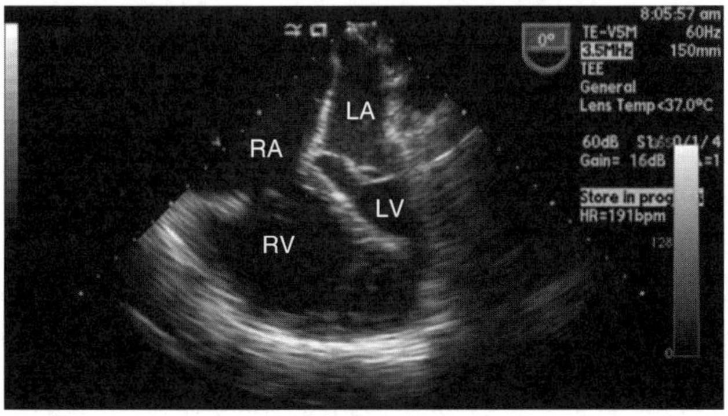

图 183.2 一例急性肺栓塞患者经食管超声心动图。食管中段四腔心切面显示右心室（RV）和右心房（RA）严重扩张，表明 RV 功能衰竭。室间隔和房间隔分别向左心室（LV）和左心房（LA）弯曲。LA 和 LV 严重受压导致其充盈下降且功能严重受损

不过是否发现栓子存在对诊断不是绝对必要的，因其在超声心动图检查时可能会向远端迁移。PE 通常可以通过胸部 MRI 确认，其来源或可通过腹部 MRI 或其他四肢成像方式找到。实验室检查可以包括 D- 二聚体，其是一种敏感但非特异性的 PE 标志物。

PE 的处理可能需要充分地心肺复苏。随后必须针对抗凝和溶栓做出决策。最好与外科医师和其他会诊专家一起讨论并决定，因为这些治疗出血的风险很高，特别是围术期患者。也有医院实施肺栓子切除手术，但这并不常见。

慢性血栓栓塞性肺动脉高压（chronic thromboembolic pulmonary hypertension，CTEPH）是一种常见的、未被重视的 PE 长期后遗症。肺血栓内膜切除术是这种情况最有效的治疗方法，目前在世界各地的应用越来越广泛。CTEPH 患者在接受其他手术时应长期抗凝，抗凝必须在尽可能短的中断时间后继续。这些患者常有残余肺动脉高压，因此必须尽可能充分了解肺循环的功能状态和条件以获得全面的术前评估。对于接受肺血管扩张剂治疗的患者，建议在整个围术期继续这种治疗，因为停药（特别是前列腺素）可能导致严重的反跳性肺动脉高血压。

反常栓子

有静脉血栓栓塞疾病或有静脉血栓栓塞风险的患者，如果其循环的左心与右心系统之间有交通，如房间隔缺损、室间隔缺损或动脉导管未闭，则存在栓塞物质从循环的右心系统进入左心系统的风险。这会导致各种器官的卒中或梗死，如脊髓、肠系膜以及肾脏。存在此类缺损的患者在计划进行大型非心脏手术前应接受心脏学评估，考虑通过介入心脏学或外科手术来闭合缺损。这对已经有反常栓塞病史的患者尤为重要。

动脉血栓形成

患有严重外周血管疾病、低心排血量和高凝状态的患者有动脉血栓或左心室血栓从而导致栓塞的风险。应对这些患者进行预防血栓和能耐受的早期活动等相应的管理。

冠状动脉血栓形成

冠状动脉支架患者，特别是药物洗脱支架，在

围术期存在冠状动脉支架内血栓形成的风险。这是一种由迅速进展的心肌梗死引起的潜在致命性并发症。药物洗脱支架患者通常接受抗血小板治疗。该治疗应在围术期持续进行，并尽可能缩短中断时间。麻醉科医师、外科医师和心脏病专家之间的密切合作至关重要，应提供有关解剖结构，放置日期和支架类型的完整信息。理想情况下，每个机构都应制订一个管理冠状动脉支架患者的方案，由麻醉科医师，心脏病专家和外科医师组成的多学科团队监督过程并就方法达成一致。

（孙媛媛 译 包 睿 校）

延伸阅读

Agnelli G: Prevention of venous thromboembolism in surgical patients, *Circulation* 110:IV4–IV12, 2004.

Bates SM, Ginsberg JS: Clinical practice. Treatment of deep-vein thrombosis, *N Engl J Med* 351:268–277, 2004.

Diaz-Gomez JL, Perez-Protto S, Hargrave J, et al.: Impact of a focused transthoracic echocardiography training course for rescue applications among anesthesiology and critical care medicine practitioners: a prospective study, *J Cardiothorac Vasc Anesth* 29:576–581, 2015.

Dresden S, Mitchell P, Rahimi L, et al.: Right ventricular dilatation on bedside echocardiography performed by emergency physicians aids in the diagnosis of pulmonary embolism, *Ann Emerg Med* 63:16–24, 2014.

Maynard GA: *Preventing hospital-associated venous thromboembolism: a guide for effective quality improvement*, ed 2, Agency for Healthcare Research and Quality, 2016.

Maynard GA, Morris TA, Jenkins IH, et al.: Optimizing prevention of hospital-acquired venous thromboembolism (VTE): prospective validation of a VTE risk assessment model, *J Hosp Med* 5:10–18, 2010.

Pavlidis AN, Kallistratos MS, Karamasis GV, et al.: Diagnosis and risk stratification in acute pulmonary embolism: the role of echocardiography, *Rev Cardiovasc Med* 14:56–65, 2013.

Tapson VF: Acute pulmonary embolism, *N Engl J Med* 358:1037–1052, 2008.

意外入院和再入院 第184章

Zhuang T. Fang

病例概要

患者，女性，45岁，体重指数（body mass index，BMI）24，美国麻醉科医师协会（ASA）评分2级，在独立的门诊手术中心于全身麻醉下行左眼眼眶切开术以矫正甲状腺突眼，患者对手术的耐受性良好，无麻醉并发症。但是，手术异常困难，持续了2 h以上。估计出血量（estimated blood loss，EBL）约为50 ml。术后，患者主诉左眼严重疼痛，经多次静脉注射芬太尼和氢吗啡酮后没有改善。手术小组被叫到麻醉后恢复室（postanesthesia care unit，PACU）检查患者情况。他们发现患者的左眼眶肿胀，眼压升高，怀疑是因为眼眶内出血所致。患者在下午晚些的时候被推到手术房间内进行眼眶内探查。从眼眶内去除一个血块，但仍有渗血，估计手术出血量为300 ml。患者被救护车送往医院进行血管造影，以确定出血的来源和进行进一步治疗。手术没有发现活动性出血，但术侧眼睛失明，住院观察和治疗数日后患者视力最终得到了恢复。

问题分析

定义

意外入院是指患者在预定的门诊手术后，在术前没有计划住院的情况下入院。总的来说，根据手术中心的设置（附属医院与独立诊所）、手术类型和患者群体的不同，意外住院的发生率从0.6%到9.4%不等。意外再入院还包括出院后30天内再次入院的患者，占0.15%～1.3%。

意外入院

在过去的30年里，门诊手术一直在稳步增加，占所有手术的65%，在美国每年门诊手术超过5330万例。门诊手术的优势是能够为医生和患者提供更大的便利，且节约大量的成本。但由于手术或麻醉并发症需要意外入院时，这些优势则不复存在。从管理的角度来看，门诊手术后的意外入院不仅是患者发病率，而且也是门诊手术中心质量和安全的重要衡量指标。

意外再入院

大多数患者在门诊手术后恢复良好。当然，也有约1%～3%的患者在出院回家后30天内会到急诊室就医，这些患者中，46%～85%的患者会被要求入院治疗，再入院的主要原因往往是出血、疼痛、尿潴留、发热和感染。

识别

在过去的10年里，外科手术越来越复杂，越来越多过去被认为不适合门诊手术的患者现在都被认为可以接受手术。这主要是由于无创手术技术的进步，不良反应降低的新型麻醉剂的使用和区域麻醉联合监护麻醉（monitored anesthesia care，MAC）的开展。研究表明，高龄、高ASA评分、长时间的手术、复杂的内科疾病，这些与术中和术后并发症相关，是导致意外入院的原因。在术前评估期间，确定外科手术、麻醉和社会经济风险等因素对于预防这些事件至关重要。在PACU中进行充分干预和治疗仍无效的外科和麻醉并发症需警惕监测和早期发现，并及时将患者转移至更高级一级治疗机构进行治疗以防止更大的伤害。此外，对出院患者进行认真评估，识别风险因素也是预防再入院的重要措施。

风险评估

手术并发症导致约 40% 的门诊手术后的意外住院；20% 为麻醉并发症所致。这些并发症包括术后恶心呕吐（postoperative nausea and vomiting，PONV），嗜睡和误吸，与糖尿病、缺血性心脏病、睡眠呼吸暂停相关的内科并发症以及社会经济原因等。

如病例概要所示，手术大出血、渗出和剧烈的疼痛等是导致大部分由于手术并发症而意外入院的原因。对于该名不吸烟的年轻女性患者来说，由于难以控制的疼痛而引起的恶心和呕吐进一步增加了入院的可能性。暂时性或永久性视力丧失是眼眶手术的严重并发症，可能是神经的直接损伤、血肿压迫神经导致局部缺血或眼压增高所致。

一般而言，以下危险因素已被确定与意外入院有关：

1. 手术时间超过 120 min；
2. 未预料的大范围手术；
3. ASA Ⅲ级或以上；
4. 高龄（>80 岁）；
5. 全身麻醉；
6. BMI 大于 30。

具有复杂内科疾病的老年患者在术中、术后可能面临更高的手术、麻醉并发症发生率。门诊手术入院指数（Outpatient Surgery Admission Index，OSAI）用于评估门诊手术患者由于并存疾病而导致入院的风险（表 184.1）。OSAI 得分为 3 的患者在门诊手术后入院的可能性是得分为 0 或 1 的患者的 21 倍；得分为 4 分、5 分或 6 分的患者意外入院的概率将增加到 32 倍。然而，OSAI 得分高的患者不一定不能进行门诊手术，因为意外入院的总发生率仍然很低。

比值比将每项因素分为 0 和 1，以下每项危险因素各得 1 分：手术时间超过 120 min，以下每项内科并存疾病（心脏病、外周血管疾病、脑血管疾病、恶性肿瘤和血清反应为阳性的人类免疫缺陷病毒），区域阻滞麻醉，年龄 65 岁以上。全身麻醉得 2 分。

表 184.1　基于门诊手术入院指数（OSAI）的短期住院比值比

OSAI	意外入院的比值比
0 和 1	
2	9.5
3	20.6
4、5 和 6	31.96

Adapted from Fleisher LA，Pasternak LR，Lyles A：A novel index of elevated risk of inpatient hospital admission immediately following outpatient surgery. *Arch Surg* 142（3）：263-268，2007.

肥胖和阻塞性睡眠呼吸暂停（obstructive sleep apnea，OSA）不是门诊手术后意入院的独立危险因素，但是，如果 OSA 患者在家中持续使用气道正压通气（continuous positive airway pressure，CPAP），且患者进行的是气道手术或面部手术，术后无法使用 CPAP，则不适合门诊手术。在一项门诊整形外科的研究中，与非肥胖患者相比，肥胖患者在出院后 30 天内至少有过一次医院急诊治疗（7.3% vs. 3.6%）或严重不良事件（3.2% vs. 0.9%）。肥胖患者的平均住院费用也比非肥胖患者高 3700 ～ 7400 美元。此外，由于肥胖患者的内科并存疾病较多，包括高血压、糖尿病、精神健康问题、慢性呼吸道疾病和睡眠呼吸暂停，故肥胖患者手术和麻醉并发症的发生率更高。在全身麻醉、MAC 手术或 PACU 恢复期间，呼吸系统并发症的增加可能需要延长在 PACU 的停留时间，如果患者持续通气不足或缺氧，则可能需要住院治疗。一项研究发现，在有或没有 OSA 的肥胖患者中，意外入院率分别为 7.0% 和 5.6%。

启示

转院 / 住院是门诊手术的意外结局，可能的原因包括对患者或手术选择的准确性不够。医院转诊 / 入院可能导致患者和支付方承担意外的费用和时间。它也反映了门诊手术服务的质量。除此之外，患者及其家属均受意外入院的影响，特别是对于儿科患者和他们的父母来说，工作日程计划不得不改变。

管理

当预期到会发生手术或麻醉并发症时，应积极治疗以防止患者受到伤害。如需意外入院时，应及时、有序启动入院流程以确保转运期间患者的安全。麻醉科医师、外科医师、PACU 护士、患者和家属之间的充分沟通是流程顺利的必要条件。在不具备高水平的外科或内科治疗仅需夜间观察的外科中心，比如治疗 PONV 或疼痛，这通常是最便宜的选择。但由于护理人员和设备的支持不足，小儿呼吸并发症患者通常不适合在独立的外科中心停留 23 h，因此必须住院。详细记录并发症、治疗和入院必要性的文件对于保险和医疗法律依据是必不可少的。

外科医师通常是治疗门诊手术后意外入院患者的主要团队。和病例概要里的患者类似，大多数患者再次入院接受额外的手术。普外科手术意外入院的风险最高，其次是妇产科、泌尿科和耳鼻咽喉科。在住院期间，患者无论是手术并发症还是麻醉并发症，都需要积极的治疗，尤其是疼痛，是再次入院的常见原因。

预防

术前对患者和手术的仔细评估是预防门诊手术后意外入院的关键。患者的选择应侧重于风险因素的识别和手术地点的确定（如门诊手术中心 *vs.* 医院手术室），以及当发生手术和麻醉并发症时，对治疗和医院转院的充分规划。

术前考虑的关键因素

1. 评估意外住院的危险因素；
2. 特别注意手术的创伤性和手术时间；
3. 全面评估老年患者的并存疾病；
4. 将高风险病例转诊至医院住院患者的手术室。

术中管理的关键因素

1. 尽可能使用区域麻醉或 MAC。
2. 避免使用导致过度镇静和改变精神状态的药物。
3. 对有既往史或 PONV 的高危患者进行 PONV 预防：
   a. 使用全静脉麻醉技术，或联合使用丙泊酚与除氧化亚氮以外的挥发性吸入药物。
   b. 多模式止吐治疗（水化、地塞米松、5- 羟色胺抑制剂、甲氧氯普胺、H_2 受体抑制剂）。
   c. 充分水化。
   d. 考虑使用辅助镇痛药物（如静脉注射对乙酰氨基酚、布洛芬、酮咯酸）。
4. 对于术后疼痛风险较高的患者，采用多模式镇痛：
   a. 区域阻滞或伤口局部浸润。
   b. 非甾体抗炎药和阿片类药物。
5. 小儿上呼吸道轻度感染应避免插管。

术后管理的关键因素

1. 对通气不足和缺氧早期进行干预。
2. 积极治疗低血压。
3. 及早有效地治疗疼痛。
4. 尽早和充分治疗 PONV。
5. 保持充分水化，但对于充血性心力衰竭或血液透析患者则要谨慎。

预防意外入院需要一种系统的方法，包括术前筛查期间的风险因素评估，早期识别不适合门诊手术的高危患者，并将其手术推迟至住院病房手术室进行。早期干预术中及术后患者的潜在疾病，在 PACU 早期识别手术并发症，积极治疗疼痛及 PONV。对于肥胖患者，尤其是 OSA 患者，或者 OSAI 评分高的患者，进行大范围手术时，门诊手术可能不是合适的选择。通过这些方法，可能避免或减少意外入院以及门诊手术的发病率和死亡率。

（王靖云 译 卜 岚 校）

延伸阅读

Bryson GL, Gomez CP, Jee RM, et al.: Unplanned admission after day surgery: a historical cohort study in patients with obstructive sleep apnea, *Can J Anesth* 59(9):842–851, 2012.

Fleisher LA, Pasternak LR, Lyles A: A novel index of elevated risk of inpatient hospital admission immediately following outpatient surgery, *Arch Surg* 142(3):263–268, 2007.

Imasogie N, Chung F: Effect of return hospital visits on economics of ambulatory surgery, *Curr Opin Anaesthesiol* 14(5):573–578, 2001.

Katasia T, Cutter TW, Apfelbaum JL: Patient selection in outpatient surgery, *Clin Plastic Surg* 40(3):371–382, 2013.

Mathis MR, Naughton NN, Shanks AM, et al.: Patient selection for day case-eligible surgery, *Anesthesiology* 119(6):1310–1321, 2013.

Morales R, Esteve N, Casas I, et al.: Why are ambulatory surgical patients admitted to hospital? Prospective study, *Ambul Surg* 9(4):197–205, 2002.

Sieffert MR, Fox JP, Abbott LE, et al.: Obesity is associated with increased health care charges in patients undergoing outpatient plastic surgery, *Plast Reconstr Surg* 135(5):1396–1404, 2015.

Whippey A, Kostandoff G, Paul J, et al.: Predictors of unanticipated admission following ambulatory surgery: a retrospective case-control study, *Can J Anaesth* 60(7):675–683, 2013.

第 185 章 失控的急性术后疼痛

Ronnie H. Zeidan，Peter K. Yi

病例概要

患者，女性，35 岁，因溃疡性结肠炎并发症拟行部分结肠切除术。患者既往有偏头痛、子宫内膜异位症、纤维肌痛和非特异性下腰痛病史，目前口服大剂量阿片类药物治疗。患者十分紧张，有大祸临头的感觉，担心术后会出现难以治愈的长期慢性疼痛。

问题分析

定义

国际疼痛研究协会（International Association for the Study of Pain，IASP）将**疼痛**定义为“一种不愉快的主观感觉和情感体验，伴随着现有的或潜在的组织损伤（或描述的类似损伤）。每个人在生命的早期就通过损伤的经历学会了表达疼痛的词汇的用法。”

术后疼痛可分为两大类：术后急性疼痛和术后慢性疼痛。**急性疼痛**定义为“近期发生的与创伤和疾病有明确关系的疼痛，持续时间可能有限，通常预期持续时间为 7 天。”相比之下，**慢性疼痛**“常没有明确具体的原因（IASP，2014），通常在伤口愈合后仍然持续疼痛，并持续超过 3 个月。”

识别

评估患者术后疼痛是正确处理术后急性疼痛的第一步。疼痛是一种主观体验，包含生理和心理构成的不能客观量化的多变量的综合结果。但是，目前全国普遍认可的是 10 分制的疼痛评估量表，总分为 10 分，其中 1 分是没有疼痛，10 分是所能想到的最严重的疼痛。患者的疼痛评分取决于患者本人和评估者。为便于在疼痛转为失控的疼痛之前进行早期干预，需要对疼痛治疗的效果以及患者满意度的随访评估进行记录，这是评估的重要组成部分。

风险评估

失控的急性术后疼痛的风险几乎适用于任何与手术相关的不愉快的主观感觉和情感体验。根据美国疾病控制与预防中心（Centers for Disease Control and Prevention，CDCP）的数据，2010 年美国共实施了 5140 万例住院外科手术，该数据与术后急性疼痛这个问题非常相关。研究表明，术后 24 h 内，60% 的患者活动时疼痛评分为 5 分或 5 分以上（0= 无疼痛；10= 无法忍受或非常严重）；术后 7 天，39% 的患者活动时疼痛评分为 5 分或 5 分以上；8% 的患者的疼痛评分为 8 ～ 10 分。框 185.1 列出了最易转化为失控的术后疼痛的危险因素。

框 185.1 术后疼痛的危险因素

术前因素
- 疼痛，中度至重度，持续 >1 个月
- 重复手术
- 心理脆弱
- 术前焦虑
- 女性
- 年轻（成人）
- 工人的赔偿问题
- 遗传易感性
- 伤害性抑制控制的无效扩散

术中因素
- 手术入路有神经损伤的风险
- 避免使用 N_2O 麻醉

术后因素
- 疼痛（急性、中度至重度）
- 手术部位放射治疗
- 化疗引起的神经毒性
- 抑郁 / 心理脆弱
- 神经质
- 焦虑

启示

围术期疼痛是由组织损伤（即外科手术、解剖分离、烧伤）或直接神经损伤（即神经横断、神经伸展或受压迫）等引起的炎症所致。组织损伤释放局部炎症介质，炎症介质的刺激可使损伤外周区域的敏感性增强（hyperalgesia，痛觉过敏）或对非伤害性刺激的错觉疼痛（allodynia，痛觉超敏）。其他导致痛觉过敏和痛觉超敏的机制包括：对周围疼痛受体的敏化（原发性痛觉过敏）和中枢神经系统神经元的兴奋性增加（继发性痛觉过敏）。这些生理反应可能导致术后失控的疼痛反应，疼痛控制不佳，同时增加术后的病死率（表 185.1）。

交感神经传出活动的激增会增快心率，增强心肌收缩力和升高血压。随着交感神经兴奋，心肌需氧量增加，心肌缺血的风险提高。必须特别关注并采取适当的干预措施，以确保患有心脏疾病患者的术后急性疼痛得到充分控制。交感神经活动增强也会减少胃肠蠕动导致肠梗阻。上腹部和胸科手术后的剧烈疼痛使患者咳嗽能力受限，功能残气量降低，导致肺不张、通气血流比例异常、低氧血症和增加肺部并发症的发病率。术后的损伤反应也导致细胞和体液免疫功能的抑制和高凝状态的发生，这两者都可能导致术后并发症的发生。有证据表明，外科手术可依据手术创伤的程度成比例地抑制免疫系统。

表 185.1 未控制的术后疼痛的不良影响

短期影响	长期影响
• 心血管影响 • 肠道运动受损 • 呼吸功能的影响 • 延迟下床活动 • 深静脉血栓形成的风险增加	• 急性疼痛可导致慢性疼痛 • 行为变化 　• 抑郁、焦虑、阿片类药物成瘾

框 185.2 美国麻醉科医师学会急性疼痛工作组管理指南推荐（2012 年）

麻醉科医师在处理围术期疼痛时，应充分考虑每个患者的风险和疗效，采用以下治疗方案：

- 硬膜外或鞘内应用阿片类药物
- 全身性应用阿片类药物患者自控镇痛
- 区域技术

除非有禁忌，患者应接受 NSAIDs 类药物、COX-2 抑制剂或对乙酰氨基酚的 24 h 治疗

剂量方案应在优化疗效的同时尽量减少不良事件的风险

药物的选择、剂量、治疗途径和疗程应当个体化

管理

疼痛是复杂和多因素的，因此需要一种平衡多模式的方法进行适当的管理。多模式治疗的定义是同时给予两种以上的药物或治疗方法，每一种药物或治疗方法的作用机制不同。美国麻醉科医师协会急性疼痛工作组在制定围术期实践指南的中推荐“条件允许的情况下麻醉科医师应使用多模式镇痛方法进行疼痛管理”（框 185.2）。

全身性应用阿片类药物

阿片类药物是应用最广泛的治疗术后疼痛的药物。其在中枢和外周的阿片类受体中起激动剂的作用。给药途径多种多样，可通过口服给药、直肠栓剂、舌下含服、透皮贴剂、皮下注射、肌内注射、静脉注射或椎管内麻醉。由于各种给药途径的药物浓度水平难以预测，静脉输注使血药浓度更稳定，可更准确地预测药物疗效；但是发生副作用的风险更高。所有阿片类药物都有共同的副作用，包括嗜睡、抑郁脑干控制的呼吸冲动、尿潴留和由于对化学感受器触发区的直接刺激引起的恶心呕吐。阿片类药物给药后常伴随组胺的释放，可引起颜面潮红、心动过速、低血压、瘙痒和支气管痉挛。患者自控镇痛（patient-controlled analgesia，PCA）的使用可能在降低危害风险的同时，提高患者对疼痛控制的满意度。

非阿片类药物辅助治疗

全身性非阿片类药物辅助治疗是多模式镇痛方法的一部分。这类药物类型众多，包括 NSAIDs、NMDA 和对乙酰氨基酚。这些药物是管理急性疼痛的重要组成部分，因为它们针对不同的疼痛通路；与其他各类治疗疼痛的药物（包括阿片类药物）一起应用具有协同作用，可以减少某个单一药物的使用剂量，同时降低不良反应发生的风险。

区域技术

椎管内和其他区域技术可能是术后疼痛的有效

治疗方法，与全身性应用阿片类药物相比，疼痛的控制效果更佳。硬膜外和蛛网膜下腔镇痛已被证明可以通过减少术中出血量、降低术后分解代谢和血栓栓塞事件的发生率来改善手术结局，并可改善血管移植物的血流和术后肺功能。对于阿片类药物的应用，尽管硬膜外和蛛网膜下腔给药的镇痛效果优于全身性给药，但使用中仍存在副作用和内在风险，因此监测方案很有必要。椎管内应用麻醉性镇痛药可存在迟发性呼吸抑制的隐患，大量的患者可出现瘙痒（表 185.2）。

预防

如果可能，术后疼痛的处理应在手术刺激前开始。“超前”镇痛的概念是指在手术切皮前即根据所选择的镇痛策略开始给药。可以改变对外周神经系统和中枢神经系统有害刺激的处理进程，从而减少中枢敏化、痛觉过敏和异位疼痛。研究表明，同样的治疗方法，术前治疗比切皮后或术中同样的治疗措施更加有效。

（吴 巧 译 卞金俊 校）

延伸阅读

American Society of Anesthesiologists Task Force on Acute Pain Management: Practice guidelines for acute pain management in the perioperative setting: an updated report by the American Society of Anesthesiologists Task Force on Acute Pain Management, *Anesthesiology* 116(2):248–273, 2012.

Blackburn GL: Metabolic considerations in management of surgical patients, *Surg Clin North Am* 91(3):467–480, 2011.

表 185.2 治疗技术小结

技术	范例	优点	缺点
外周区域镇痛	局部麻醉药行外周神经阻滞（如布比卡因、罗哌卡因）	与生理盐水相比，可改善疼痛缓解和降低麻醉性镇痛药的消耗量	短暂性的运动功能阻滞
	手术部位浸润	一般来说，与生理盐水相比，可改善疼痛缓解和降低麻醉性镇痛药的消耗量	未提及
椎管内	鞘内或硬膜外应用阿片类药物	改善缓解疼痛	瘙痒频率增加，迟发性呼吸抑制
	硬膜外腔应用阿片类药物 + 局部麻醉药	改善疼痛评分	运动无力的发生增加
全身性应用阿片类药物	医护人员静脉注射阿片类药物	疼痛控制效果类似于 PCA	疼痛缓解仍有漏洞，阿片类药物不良反应
	PCA	与口服相比，疼痛控制的效果和患者满意度更高	与口服相比，增加了阿片类药物的消耗和皮肤瘙痒发生
非阿片类药物的全身性应用	对乙酰氨基酚	与静脉注射和 PCA 使用阿片类药物疗效相似，但药物不良反应少	未提及
	NSAIDs	改善疼痛评分，减少麻醉性镇痛药使用	与 NSAIDs 类药物相关的消化系统、神经系统、泌尿系统、凝血和过敏反应方面的副作用增加
	抗惊厥药（加巴喷丁和普瑞巴林）	当与阿片类药物联合使用时，可改善疼痛评分并减少镇痛药物的使用	镇静和眩晕
	α_2- 受体激动剂	当与阿片类药物联合使用时，可减少由于阿片类药物戒断引起的不良生理和心理的反应	当静脉快速给药时可能发生心动过缓、低血压和窦性停搏
	NMDA 拮抗剂（氯胺酮）	当与阿片类药物联合使用时，可降低痛觉过敏和阿片类药物耐受性，从而降低术后对阿片类药物的需求，并可能降低术后慢性疼痛	可能引起幻觉和精神分裂状态

注：IV，静脉注射；NMDA，N- 甲基 -D- 天冬氨酸；NSAIDs，非甾体抗炎药；PCA，患者自控镇痛；PO，口服

Cardinale F, Chinellato I, Caimmi S, et al.: Perioperative period: immunological modifications, *Int J Immunopathol Pharmacol* 24(Suppl 3):S3–S12, 2011.

Carli F, Schricker T: Modification of metabolic response to surgery by neural blockade. In Cousins MJ, Bridenbaugh PO, Carr D, et al.: *Neural blockade in clinical anesthesia and pain medicine*, ed 4, Philadelphia, 2008, Lippincott Williams & Wilkins.

Centers for Disease Control and Prevention: National Center for Health Statistics. Available at www.cdc.gov/nchs/faststats/inpatient-surgery. Accessed September 1, 2014.

International Association for the Study of Pain: *IASP taxonomy by Task Force on Taxonomy*, Available at http://www.iasp-pain.org/Educa on/Content.aspx?ItemNumber=1698, 2014. Accessed September 17, 2014.

Kelly DJ, Ahmad M, Brull SJ: Preemptive analgesia I: physiological pathways and pharmacological modalities, *Can J Anaesth* 48(10):1000–1010, 2001.

Lennard TW, Shenton BK, Borzotta A, et al.: The influence of surgical operations on components of the human immune system, *Br J Surg* 72:771–776, 1985.

Moore A, Edwards J, Barden J, et al.: *Bandolier's little book of pain*, Oxford, 2003, Oxford University Press.

Moss E, Taverner T, Norton P, et al.: A survey of postoperative pain management in fourteen hospitals in the UK, *Acute Pain* 7:13–20, 2005.

Pollock RE, Lotzova E, Stanford SD: Mechanism of surgical stress impairment of human perioperative natural killer cell cytotoxicity, *Arch Surg* 126:338–342, 1991.

Prabhakar A, Mancuso KF, Owen CP, et al.: Perioperative analgesia outcomes and strategies, *Best Pract Res Clin Anaesthesiol* 28(2):105–115, 2014.

Woolf CJ, Chong MS: Preemptive analgesia—treating postoperative pain by preventing the establishment of central sensitization, *Anesth Analg* 77:362–379, 1993.

Suzuki H: Recent topics in the management of pain: development of the concept of preemptive analgesia, *Cell Transplant* 4(Suppl 1):S3–S6, 1995.

Yeager MP, Glass DD, Neff RK, et al.: Epidural anesthesia and analgesia in high-risk surgical patients, *Anesthesiology* 66:729–736, 1987.

第 186 章 静脉气体栓塞

Maurice S. Albin，Gwendolyn L. Boyd

病例概要

重力压力梯度 10.0 cmH_2O

患者，女性，43 岁，于俯卧位下再次行 L4 ～ L5 椎板切除术，手术开始后 45 min 突然出现心脏骤停，血压（blood pressure，BP）测不出，呼气末 CO_2（end-tidal CO_2，$ETCO_2$）下降至 15 mmHg。紧急给予心肺复苏成功，$ETCO_2$ 升至 36 mmHg，血压升至 82/60 mmHg，心率达到 90 次 / 分，抬高的 ST 段恢复正常。快速关闭切口后，将患者转成仰卧位，BP 又降至 40/30 mmHg，进行心前区多普勒超声检查发现探头位置有气体流经。再次给予患者复苏处理，但宣告失败。尸检发现右心房内有中等大小的气泡。该患者无卵圆孔未闭病史。

重力压力梯度 22.0 cmH_2O

患儿，女性，6 岁，体重 20.0 kg，因右侧小脑肿块接受麻醉，麻醉时身上有用于脑脊液引流的脑室导管。给予其心前区多普勒超声监测，并且准备了 20 号的桡动脉导管和 Bunegin-Albin 中心静脉气体抽吸导管。手术体位为 90° 竖直体位。手术开始后 30 min，多普勒超声的音调发生变化，表明有静脉空气栓塞（venous air embolism，VAE）可能，经中心导管抽出了 1.0 ml 空气。此后的 1.5 h 内，又接连发生了四次多普勒超声报警，从中心导管共吸出了 4.0ml 空气。前三次患者血流动力学始终稳定，但最后一次 VAE 发生时，$PaCO_2$ 从 36 mmHg 下降到 31 mmHg，同时 BP 下降到 60/30 mmHg。前后从中心导管排出空气共计 11.0 ml，救治措施宣告成功。然而，在该手术即将完成的剩余的短时间内，多普勒超声仍间歇性地发出报警。术者在缝合头皮时发现有根开放的静脉，经结扎后多普勒超声报警终于消失。患者进入复苏区时反应正常，自主呼吸正常并且未出现神经功能缺损。

经内镜行逆行胰胆管造影术（Endoscopic Retrograde Cholangiopancreatography，ERCP）中的 VAE

患者，男性，78 岁，气管插管全身麻醉，术中突发心脏骤停并最终心肺复苏失败。死后尸检发现肺动脉（pulmonary artery，PA），右心，上、下腔静脉，肝静脉和右大脑半球内存在气体。本病例中所用气体的充气压力和种类都未注明。

玻璃体视网膜手术中的 VAE

患者，男性，63 岁，因脉络膜黑色素瘤行玻璃体切割术，麻醉方式为全身麻醉，吸入氧浓度为 50%，手术野暴露于空气中。在空气 / 液体交换时，患者 $ETCO_2$ 陡然下降，出现心脏骤停，最终心肺复苏失败而死亡。死后行 X 线检查发现心脏内有大量气体，进一步行尸体解剖发现心脏有浮力，当心包在水下打开时，有气泡产生。该患者的输液管路中未发现气体。

问题分析

定义

当右心房和切口上方或气体入口间存在负压梯度时，气体可能进入静脉循环。压力可由重力引起，Albin 及其同事曾报道：5.0 cmH_2O 的重力梯度足以在神经外科手术中携带空气进入循环。负压梯度也可由环境压力增加所引起，如各种内镜手术（胃肠道，眼科等）中使用气体作为加压介质，或者除升高的周围压力对组织产生压迫作用外，即使是窄束的流体或气体也可能对组织产生破坏性（射流）作用。向静脉中一次性输入 100 ml 气体即可致命，并且经计算该体积的气体可通过 14 号针头以 5.0 cmH_2O 的压力梯度在数秒内输入完成。与气体被携带入静脉相关的因素有：体位、充气深度、气体进入血管的体积、气体进入速率、气体成分以及吸入性麻醉混合气体中的浓度。动物研究和人类病例已经表明，即使没有卵圆孔未闭的情况，气体仍可跨过肺途径造成栓塞。由血容量下降（出血性血容量减少）导致的中心静脉压降低，或者由于使用手术台或支架减少了腹部压迫而导致胸内压力降低，均有助于增加重力压力梯度和促进气体被携带进入循环。

气体进入循环后的转归如图 186.1 所示。在第一个病例中，重力梯度可能低于 10.0 cmH_2O，但由于失血和使用降低腹压的矫形架导致了压力梯度增加，从而使得呼气相胸内负压变大。由于使用了 50% 的氧化亚氮（N_2O），这使气体体积增加了约 2 倍。尸检结果提示右心内有气体。

在第二个病例中，一名 6 岁儿童在进行后颅窝探查时共经受了四次单独发作的 VAE，该手术具有相当大的重力梯度。尽管该病例中麻醉药物的管理近乎完美，但似乎头皮切缘的止血并未做到无可挑剔。Hagen 及其同事研究了 965 例正常人群超声探头检测下心脏卵圆孔未闭（patent foramen ovale，PFO）的发现率，结果为 27.3%，PFO 平均直径为 5.0 mm，因此并不是只有儿科患者才是气体栓塞高风险人群。必须强调的是，由于溶解度的原因，应用氧化亚氮可能增加气泡体积，并且在 50%N_2O-O_2 浓度下，进入循环的气体体积会加倍，该情况有可能发生于第一个病案。在第二个病案中，由于重力梯度较大，我们担心 VAE 如果发生于存在 PFO 的情况，空气可能会进入左心并进入冠状动脉和 / 或脑血管。

这些病例证明 VAE 可以来源于任何体位，只要手术区域和心脏之间的压力梯度允许气体侵入。有证据表明，在俯卧位手术的患者中，VAE 远非罕见，尤其是脊柱手术，据报道至少有 22 例病例发生（13 例死亡），其中 10 例属于儿科年龄组（Albin 及其同事，2006 年报道）。包括神经外科手术，几乎各科手术以及内镜检查中都有发生 VAE 的可能。在心脏

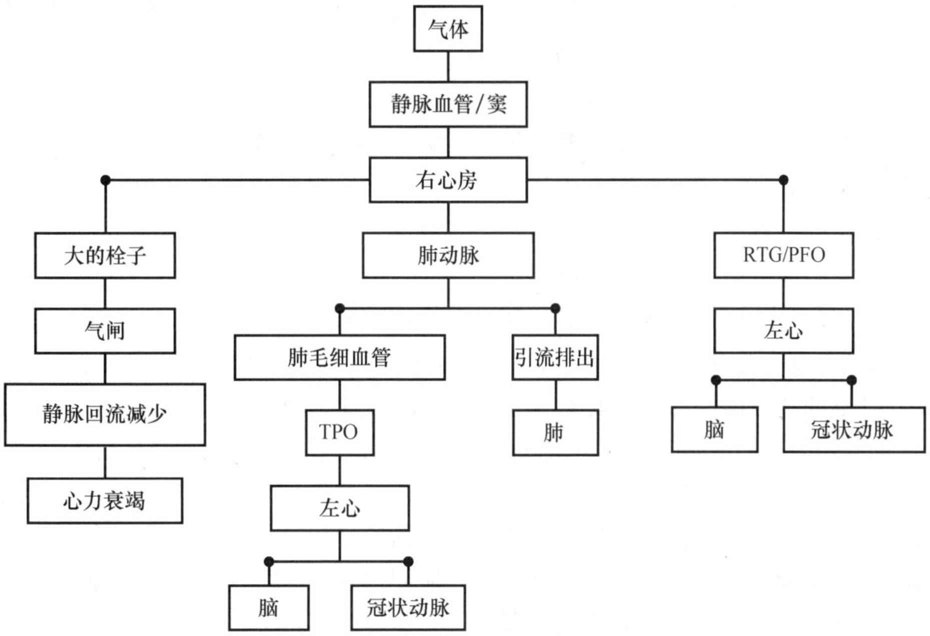

图 186.1 气体侵入静脉后的转归。PFO，卵圆孔未闭；TPO，跨肺流动；RTG，反向心房梯度

或中心血管置管，动静脉分流置管，静脉输液和输血治疗时也可以发生。

识别

症状和体征包括：自主呼吸的患者出现喘息样呼吸，中心静脉压和肺动脉压升高，心律失常，心电图（electrocardiographic，ECG）改变，低血压，心音异常，心率改变，外周阻力降低，心排血量减少，发绀，车轮样杂音以及心脏骤停。无论气体侵入的体积或速率如何，VAE 在控制通气期间最突出的现象是肺动脉压增高。气体进入肺循环的速率越快，肺动脉压升高就越快而且越严重。如果急剧上升的肺动脉压突破了生理屏障，则可能通过隔膜缺损（如 PFO）导致从右向左的分流，使气体进入左心引起反常性栓塞。气体栓塞导致的心电图变化不一，包括快速型心律失常，不同程度的房室传导阻滞，右心室劳损和 ST 段改变。侵入的气体体积过大可导致右心室后负荷严重增加，右心室缺血并急剧衰竭。大量气体栓塞后的右心衰竭是急性低血压，心排血量减少和心脏骤停的主要原因。车轮样杂音意味着大量气体已进入右侧心腔，出现这个体征，说明即将心脏骤停。由气体导致的搅动声是心脏骤停前的最后征象之一。

除体征和症状外，其他用于检测术中气体栓塞的方法可按灵敏度排序为：经食管超声心动图（transesophageal echocardiography，TEE），心前区多普勒超声检查，$ETCO_2$，肺动脉导管，脉搏血氧饱和度和直接观察手术部位。TEE 可检测静脉气体栓塞和反常性气体栓塞，检测灵敏度可达 0.02 ml/kg 气体。但是 TEE 很昂贵，并且在某些手术时很难同时操作 TEE，另外由于没有警报声音，因此难以单人独立使用，尤其是在麻醉科医师忙于急症患者处理的时候。定位良好的心前区多普勒超声检查是非侵入性检查，可探测到循环中 0.05 ml/kg 的气体，能同时向麻醉科医师和外科医师发出警报。如上所述，虽然肺动脉导管可以早期和明确地显示气体栓塞征象，但是有创程度高且不及心前区多普勒超声敏感。

$ETCO_2$ 的突然降低是监测气体栓塞最便捷和广泛使用的无创方法。$ETCO_2$ 下降的幅度及持续时间与侵入血流的气体体积密切相关，并且可在任何全身麻醉中进行监测。相反，脉搏氧测定法不及 $ETCO_2$ 敏感，因为动脉血氧饱和度的降低通常迟于动脉氧分压的下降。此外，手术区域经常被忽视，特别是在高危手术中。其实临床医师很容易注意到创面是否无静脉出血，如果无静脉出血提示静脉压低于大气压。在高风险手术中，应当将心前区多普勒超声和 $ETCO_2$ 监测结合应用：多普勒超声音调改变伴随 $ETCO_2$ 下降意味着气体侵入循环。如果能从中心静脉导管吸出气泡，则可确诊 VAE。

风险评估

VAE 的发病率尚不确定，主要是因为 VAE 的诊断标准不一。尽管如此，我们已经取得了坐位神经外科手术时 VAE 的发生率以及与其相关的病残率和死亡率。VAE 总发生率约为 25%，范围为 2% ～ 60%。在超过 5000 名患者的 10 项研究中，任何单个研究报告的死亡率均未超过 1%。至于并发症发病率，即使在神经外科坐位手术病例中也难以确定。Albin 及其同事曾报道在 400 例坐位手术中有 100 例发生了 VAE。这些患者只有在多普勒超声音调报警并且从中心导管抽出可见的气体时才会被诊断为 VAE。在该标准下，100 名被诊断 VAE 患者中有 25 名出现了从严重低血压到心脏骤停的各种症状。反常性气体栓塞（气体通过未闭的卵圆孔或经肺通道进入左心）的病例报告较少，但可造成患者死亡。令人吃惊的是，大多数 VAE 相关的死亡病例似乎发生于非神经外科手术病例，这可能是因为麻醉科医师未意识到这些病例可能发生 VAE，并且未对 VAE 行充分监测。对 VAE 认识的不足是医学法律中的“恐惧因素”，这可能导致医学文献中对 VAE 的报道不足。剖宫产术、脊柱手术、全髋关节置换术、胃肠内镜手术和玻璃体视网膜切除术中涉及气 / 液交换时均存在巨大的 VAE 风险。

由于气泡会在血液-气泡界面处聚结和成膜，气体进入右心房后会妨碍甚至阻止静脉血液回流到右心。由于心排血量被严重抑制，结果出现低血压、心律失常、甚至循环停止，右心室中“气闸”的出现被认为是导致严重 VAE 血流动力学衰竭的原因。然而，最近的研究表明右心室功能障碍更可能是后负荷急性增加的结果。大量气体连续侵入和通过可能使得肺无法将气体充分经肺循环排出。这引起血-气体界面血管活性物质的释放，导致肺灌注受损。

通气-血流比例失调源于肺循环血流的重新分布，死腔样通气和通气血流比值升高导致 $ETCO_2$ 下降以及动脉 CO_2 张力增加。缺氧则是源于变化的肺内分流，即肺血流重新分布到灌注相对过度但通气相对不足的区域（低通气-血流比），形成混合静脉血。这些通气-灌注受损可以是变化的，因为肺血管中气体的分布受浮力和局部肺灌注共同影响。虽然通气-血流比例失调可能在 VAE 后 30 min 内消失，但由于血管腔对气体的炎症反应，这种失调也可能进行性恶化。连续侵入大量气体可导致进行性肺损伤、肺毛细血管渗漏和急性呼吸窘迫综合征。足够大体积的气体也可能达到或超过其经肺排出的阈值，使得气体得以进入左心和冠状窦并且侵入大脑，导致冠状动脉闭塞和心脏骤停，引起脑栓塞、脑卒中和相关的功能障碍。

管理与预防

由于 VAE 的后遗症特别严重，因此预防和早期发现远远较事后处理重要。预防 VAE 的关键是要了解其风险因素。患者拟行的手术可能出现重力或压力梯度，手术可能有显著失血，或者手术部位血管丰富的情况均易于发生气体侵入和 VAE。文献报道的典型病例包括耻骨后前列腺根治性切除术和俯卧位的腰椎或胸椎椎板多次切除术。对 VAE 的最佳监测应包括心电图、血压、脉搏血氧饱和度、$ETCO_2$、心前区多普勒超声、动脉测压管和尖端超过右心房与上腔静脉交界处 1 ～ 2 cm 的多孔导管。最后一项措施的重要作用虽是治疗，但从中心导管吸出气体毫无疑问具有确诊的能力。此外，右心房导管的换能器可以放置在手术部位水平，以确定是否存在负压梯度。对于存在 VAE 风险并且拟行有创监测的患者，还建议使用动脉留置导管以进行动脉血压监测和血气分析。

针对 VAE 的预防措施有限，并且在某些患者中可能是禁忌的。如果患者能够耐受右心室前负荷增加，那么可以通过水化来降低右心和手术部位之间的压力梯度，但是许多有颅内病变的患者不适用。虽然曾经提出给予呼气末正压以增加胸腹腔内压，但该方法可能增加心室前负荷，另外引起争议的是该方法可能升高跨心房的压力梯度并且打开 PFO，从而使得气体进入左心和大脑。对于颅内手术，手法压迫双侧颈静脉可暂时升高颅内静脉压，从而防止大脑气体栓塞的进展，并且可以帮助定位气体入口。这种操作安全有效，但只可轻柔和短暂地应用于无颈动脉疾病的患者。

如果出现多普勒超声报警或 $ETCO_2$ 降低，或两者同时出现，就必须立即抽吸中心导管（用连接到旋塞上的 50ml 注射器抽吸），因为即使迟疑数秒也能有大量气体侵入。同时，吸入气体中的 N_2O 或空气必须替换为 100% 氧气，并且应该通知外科医师用水浸没手术区域并寻找任何开放的静脉。由此引起的所有低血压或心律失常都应采用正性肌力药和升压药进行对症治疗，以改善血管收缩性并维持血液循环。肾上腺素是大量 VAE 复苏的首选药物。如果短期内无法恢复到 VAE 发生前的生理水平，或者如果气体继续侵入，那么患者应恢复至无压力梯度的体位。

如果怀疑有 VAE，同时术后患者持续昏迷或者存在与外科手术无关的神经缺陷，则需进行神经病学或神经外科咨询，并且应行磁共振检查以诊断是否存在颅内气体。如果发现气体，应考虑行高压氧治疗。

胃肠内镜手术中的 VAE

在胃肠内镜手术中，有关 VAE 的主要问题集中于对特定血管的侵犯，视野有限，以加压气体为介质的环境，手术患者通常为低危人群，所用仪器可能对组织血管造成破坏。这些因素结合在一起意味着气体可以异常迅速地侵入循环，而且因为侵入 100 ml 气体可能致命，这使得人们思考通过以下预防措施应对：

1. **气体**。回顾以往文献似乎表明，在许多病例报告中，空气被用作主要的加压介质。这令人震惊，因为使用 CO_2 代替空气往往可以避免 VAE，因 CO_2 具有可吸收性，而且如果患者无严重肺部疾病，其对人体无害。Derouin 等用 TEE 对 16 例接受腹腔镜胆囊切除术的患者行超声心动图检查，探究术中将 CO_2 作为加压气体的应用情况。经过一系列心肺检查，他们在 16 位患者中发现 11 位出现气体栓塞，但未发现心肺功能衰竭，这表明 CO_2 吸收迅速。
2. **在麻醉混合气中使用 N_2O**。许多研究已经证实，在 O_2 : N_2O 为 50% : 50% 混合气中，由于溶解度的原因，气泡体积会增加一倍。

3. **气体输注压**。压力梯度对于气体侵入循环系统至为重要。高压输入气体能导致压力梯度上升并达到气体被迫进入静脉开口的程度。遗憾的是，所回顾的 30 篇文献中关于气体输注压很少被提及。似乎确保使用限压阀很有临床意义。
4. **对 VAE 的监测**。早期预警设备和技术如下：
   a. 心前区多普勒超声（precordial Doppler，PCD）（图 186.2 和 186.3）应用便捷，能够实时提供数据，价格相对低廉，可靠性高且假阴性率低至 3%，同时与 TEE 相关性良好，*K* 值 =1。
   b. TEE 与 PCD 尽管处于同一级别，但前者灵敏度更高。它的缺点是使用依赖于专业知识，另外价格相对昂贵，并且在启用 TEE 的时间内可能已有大量气体侵入循环。
   c. PA 导管也具有很高的灵敏度，但其较小的内腔和其心房端口的窄径限制了其抽取大量气体的能力。
   d. $ETCO_2$ 监测是一种有效且实用的方法，但其灵敏度低于 PCD（见图 186.2 和 186.3）。
   e. 经 Bunegin-Albin 多孔中心导管抽吸可以确定气泡存在，一般在 PCD 的心音发生变化后进行。

PCD 和 $ETCO_2$ 模块的组合是检测 VAE 的强大工具。在麻醉开始时加用 Bunegin-Albin 多孔中心气体抽吸管可用于中心静脉压监测及气体抽吸，这三种监测方式可应用于高风险患者和接受高危手术的患者。

Donepudi 及其同事的综述文章揭示了气体栓塞并发症的严重程度（表 186.1），其中有 26 例内镜逆行胰胆管造影术（endoscopic retrograde cholangiopancreatography，ERCP），这些造影术都被诊断为发生了气体栓塞事件。26 位患者中，12 位是 60 岁或以上的患者，有 1 人的年龄未知，13 位年龄在 60 岁以下，最小的患者是 8 岁。其中 12 名患者死亡，14 名存活。令人感兴趣的是，作者将气体栓塞分为静脉、脊柱、肺、心脏和大脑 5 类，大脑气体栓塞在 26 例中有 12 例（占比 46%）。该分类方法是基于所涉及的终末器官，但却忽略了整体的病理生理学。当气体或者通过 PFO 或者由于体积过大超过肺的应对

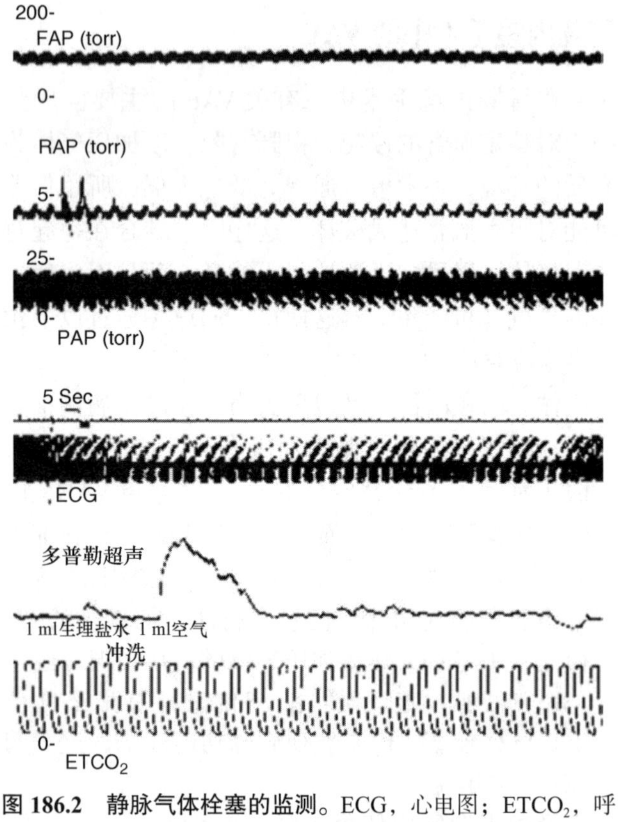

图 186.2 静脉气体栓塞的监测。ECG，心电图；$ETCO_2$，呼气末二氧化碳；FAP，股动脉压；PAP，肺动脉压；RAP，右心房压力

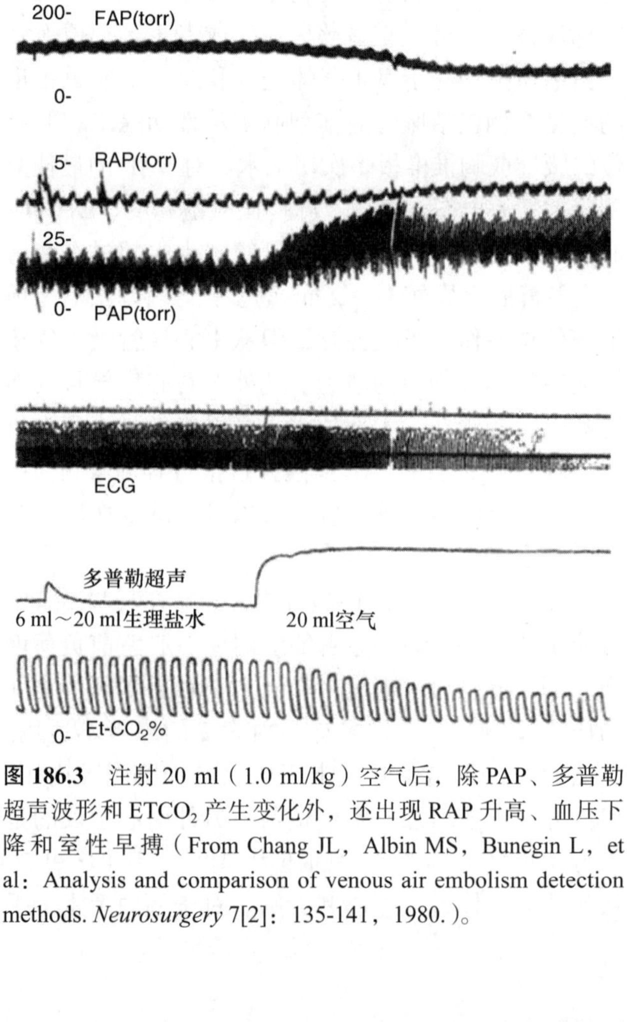

图 186.3 注射 20 ml（1.0 ml/kg）空气后，除 PAP、多普勒超声波形和 $ETCO_2$ 产生变化外，还出现 RAP 升高、血压下降和室性早搏（From Chang JL，Albin MS，Bunegin L，et al：Analysis and comparison of venous air embolism detection methods. *Neurosurgery* 7[2]：135-141，1980.）。

表 186.1 内镜逆行复杂胰胆管造影术中气体栓塞的病例报道

病例	文献	年龄 / 性别	风险因素	诊断	结果
1	Bisceglia 等 [7]	78/ 男	胃十二指肠切除术	肺气体栓塞	死亡
2	Rabe 等 [12]	87/ 男	金属支架置入术	脑气体栓塞	存活
3	Rabe 等 [12]	54/ 男	"毕Ⅱ"式手术，金属支架置入	心脏气体栓塞	死亡
4	Jow 等 [38]	65/ 男	胆道结石 / 炎症	心脏气体栓塞	死亡
5	Maccarone 等 [1]	45/ 男	经皮肝胆管引流术	脑气体栓塞	存活
6	Siddiqui 等 [37]	43/ 女	胆道括约肌切开术，肝活检	静脉气体栓塞	死亡
7	Nayagam 等 [39]	57/ 男	—	脑气体栓塞	死亡
8	Kennedy 等 [8]	63/ 女	胆道括约肌切开术	静脉气体栓塞	死亡
9	Stabile 等 [6]	65/ 男	胆道括约肌切开术，PTC	脑气体栓塞	死亡
10	Mohammedi 等 [4]	27/ 男	胆道括约肌切开术，钝性肝损伤	心脏气体栓塞	存活
11	Romberg[40]	53/ 男	胆道结石	心脏气体栓塞	存活
12	Rangappa 等 [41]	50/ 女	胆道结石	脑气体栓塞	死亡
13	Bechi 等 [33]	79/ 女	胆道括约肌切开术	脑气体栓塞	存活
14	Goins 等 [16]	72/ 女	胆管癌	脑气体栓塞	存活
15	Cha 等 [42]	50/ 女	胆道结石，肝脓肿，胆总管十二指肠吻合术	心脏气体栓塞	死亡
16	Di Pisa 等 [13]	8/ 男	脾前庭门静脉分流术	静脉气体栓塞	存活
17	Giuly 等 [43]	60/ 女	胆道括约肌切开术，胆总管扩张	静脉气体栓塞	存活
18	van Boxel 等 [44]	82/ 男	—	脑气体栓塞	存活
19	Tan 等 [45]	82/ 女	金属支架置入术	脑气体栓塞	死亡
20	Nern 等 [46]	58/ 女	胆管癌	脑气体栓塞	死亡
21	Simmons[47]	未知	胆道括约肌切开术	静脉气体栓塞	存活
22	Merine 等 [48]	39/ 女	胆道括约肌切开术	静脉气体栓塞	存活
23	Barthet 等 [49]	31/ 男	胆道括约肌切开术	静脉气体栓塞	存活
24	Efthymiou 等 [11]	62/ 女	胆道镜检查	脑气体栓塞	存活
25	Donepudi 等 [50]	66/ 男	金属支架置入术	脑气体栓塞	死亡
26	Donepudi 等 [50]	51/ 女	Whipple 手术	脊髓气体栓塞	存活

表中的参考文献见原文

PTC，经皮肝穿刺胆管造影术

From Donepudi S，Chavalitdhamrong D，Pu L，et al：Air embolism complicating gastrointestinal endoscopy：a systematic review. *World J Gastrointest Endosc* 5（8）：359-365，2013.

能力而侵入到左心时，会发生反常性气体栓塞。这种情况下，气体越过了肺床，此后机体不得不面对其进入冠状血管、脑和脊髓的血管的危险（见表186.1）。

总之，PCD 是可以确保快速识别气体栓塞的预防措施，使用 CO_2 作为扩张气体可能引起压缩气体进入脆弱的和（或）受损器官的血管。PCD 和 $ETCO_2$ 模块的组合是高效预警系统的基础。

虽然已有许多关于胃肠内镜下诊断和手术的历史回顾和病案报告，但这些文献本质上是回顾性的，缺乏前瞻性研究。从文献综述中发现的唯一例外是 Crutchley 及其同事的前瞻性观察试验，他们的关注点之一是应用 PCD 和 $ETCO_2$ 监测早期发现 VAE，另一个目的是对 528 名接受 ERCP 的手术患者进行危险分级。528 位患者中有 3 位被发现有 VAE，最重要的是，3 位发生 VAE 的患者都在高风险组

（n=180）。高风险组是指患者可能接受过括约肌切除术、支架手术、组织活检、胆道镜检查或坏死组织切除术中的任一种或多种。由于该报告只是一项涉及 1000 名患者的持续性研究的一部分，因此查看其最终报告会很有意思。但用二氧化碳取代了空气以改善内镜医师的视野后，再未发生 VAE 事件。

玻璃体视网膜手术中的 VAE

第四个病案描述的是一名患有脉络膜黑色素瘤的患者于全身麻醉下接受玻璃体切除术，术中为了稳定视网膜进行了气 / 液交换（air/fluid exchange，AFX），期间发生了致命的 VAE。死后对患者尸体进行 X 线检查和法医学解剖检查后，Rice 及其同事们证实患者死因就是这次 VAE 事件。迄今为止，麻醉学文献中已报道了 6 例眼部发生 VAE 的事件。检索 ASA 内部索赔项目数据库（Posner K，个人通信）发现了视网膜脱落患者接受巩膜搭扣术进行修复时在玻璃体切除期间发生 VAE 的更多病例。

最早的三个病例报道（Ledowski、Ruest 和 Dermigny）发表后，Lim 及其同事以及 Gamulescu 及其同事均向眼科医师发出过该术中并发症可能致命的警告。然而，眼科医师对眼部的 AFX 可导致近乎致命或致命的 VAE 表示怀疑，因为他们认为涡旋静脉系统无法允许大量气体的侵入。然而，Morris 及其同事证实了使用现代玻璃体切除机能够提供高达 120 mmHg 的气体输注压力，这使得发生致命 VAE 变得容易。作者在 40 mmHg 压力下对玻璃体切割术中用的 25 号输气管检测后发现，其每分钟可输送 350 ml 气体，这远高于引起致命 VAE 的气体体积（100 ml）（图 186.4）。他们预测，目前玻璃体切割术中用的较小的、无缝线的输气管可能很容易从玻璃体腔中滑出，这将使加压气体易从受损脉络膜中侵入涡旋静脉，再进入中心静脉循环，由此可能增加 VAE 的发病率。最近，Shin 及其同事还有 Wu 及其同事报告了另外两例眼部 VAE 病例，虽然发生后迅速启动了心肺转流，但最终仍然有一例死亡。

如果患者需要行视网膜填塞，那么手术医师于玻璃体切割术结束时可有多种选择。如前所述，大约 15% 的玻璃体切割术中使用空气，其在被吸收之前的 5 天中能将视网膜保持在适当位置。大约 50% 的玻璃体切割术中使用六氟化硫（SF_6），约 1.5 ml 的 SF_6 被注入玻璃体腔，它能保持 10 天至 2 周，在

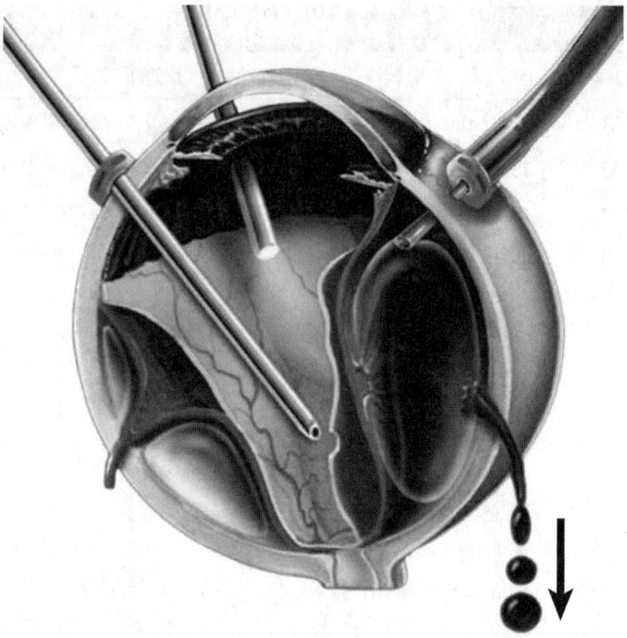

图 186.4 玻璃体切除术中标准的眼内三个导管。中央导管具有摄像头和光源，左侧导管抽吸玻璃体，右侧第三个是注射管，从玻璃体腔脱出后允许注射物通过涡旋静脉进入静脉循环（（From Morris，RE，Sapp MR，Oltmanns MH，et al：Presumed air by vitrectomy embolisation [PAVE] a potentially fatal syndrome. *Br J Ophthalmol* 98[6]：765-768，2014.）

此期间，务必不要用 N_2O 进行麻醉，因为它会明显增加眼中气泡的体积进而导致失明。在此期间，航空旅行也属禁忌。另一种气体，全氟丙烷（C_3F_8）在眼中可持续长达 2 个月，与 SF_6 一样期间应避免用氧化亚氮进行麻醉以及禁止航空旅行。剩余 1/4 需行视网膜固定的玻璃体切割术中会使用硅油。作为更复杂玻璃体切割术中的保留方法，硅油被用于包括糖尿病增生性视网膜病变手术，特别是牵拉性视网膜脱落，巨大撕裂，下部脱落以及其他困难的手术中。置入的硅油需要另外经手术取出。许多玻璃体切割术在结束时不需要进行视网膜填塞，例如玻璃体积血或漂浮物清除。因此，在玻璃体视网膜手术中使用加压气体输注的比例不到 10%。

既往有脉络膜损伤的玻璃体切割术中的 AFX 似乎比大多数常规玻璃体切割术中的 AFX 具有更高的 VAE 风险。所有报道发生 VAE 的手术患者均有明显脉络膜损伤，这些手术包括眼内异物取出术、脉络膜肿瘤切除术和视网膜脱落修复中的巩膜搭扣术。此外，所有报道的眼科 VAE 病例均在全身麻醉下进行，这掩盖了 VAE 的早期症状。幸运的是，需要在全身麻醉下进行的玻璃体切除手术越来越少，当前，

笔者所在的单位得益于小型化导管带来的技术进步，需要全身麻醉的比例仅为 20%。的确，由于新型的 27 号导管被应用于玻璃体切割术，诸如眼内漂浮物清除或者其他不必行视网膜激光或者气体充填的患者，该手术的麻醉方式逐渐趋向于局部麻醉。

由 Morris 及其同事倡议的预防玻璃体视网膜手术中 VAE 的关键步骤是：①再次确认气体输注导管位于玻璃体腔内；②如果在 AFX 期间发生脉络膜抬升，应立即停止气体输注。

对麻醉从业人员而言，无论是在 MAC 麻醉还是全身麻醉中，目前应用于所有麻醉方法的 $ETCO_2$ 是评估 AFX 期间 VAE 发生的宝贵工具。在 AFX 期间，麻醉提供者的注意力应始终关注 $ETCO_2$ 波形，另外务必与眼科医师保持密切沟通。

最后，我们认为，对于有较高 VAE 风险的眼科手术患者（如先前存在脉络膜创伤的患者接受全身麻醉）在需要输注加压气体时，麻醉从业人员应使用 PCD，如此一来，玻璃体切割术中已经很低的 VAE 发生率将更加罕见。知道在手术关键环节有发生 VAE 可能性，那么眼科医师会尽力预防它，麻醉从业人员可以通过观察 $ETCO_2$ 波形和监听 PCD 的声音变化从而显著降低其严重程度，尤其是在高风险患者接受加压气体的时候。俗话说“有备无患”就是这个道理。

（李金泰　译　刘　毅　校）

延伸阅读

综合

Albin MS: Air embolism, *Anesthesiol Clin North Am* 11:1–24, 1993.

Albin MS, Wills J, Schwend RM: Patent foramen ovale and unexplained stroke, *N Engl J Med* 354:1753–1755, 2006.

Bunegin L: Monitoring technology—capnography, intracranial pressure, precordial Doppler. In Albin MS, editor: *Textbook of neuroanesthesia with neuroscience perspectives*, New York, 1997, McGraw-Hill, pp 277–324.

Mirski MA, Lele AV, Fitzsimmons L, et al.: Diagnosis and treatment of vascular air-embolism, *Anesthesiology* 106:164–177, 2007.

法医病理学

Hagen PT, Scholz DG, Edwards WD: Incidence and size of patent foramen ovale during the first 10 decades of life: an autopsy study of 965 normal hearts, *Mayo Clin Proc* 59:17–20, 1984.

Start RD, Cross SS: Pathological investigation of deaths following surgery, anesthesia and medical procedure, *J Clin Path* 52:640–652, 1999.

胃肠内镜手术

Bastovonsky A, Stolilberger C, Finsterer J: Fatal cerebral air embolism due to a patent foramen ovale during endoscopic retrograde cholangiopancreatography, *Clin Endosc* 47:275–280, 2014.

Bisceglia M, Simeone A, Forlano R, et al.: Fatal air embolism during endoscopic retrograde cholangiopancreatography, *Adv Anat Pathol* 16:255–262, 2009.

Crutchley MD, Phillips M, Jones KA, et al.: Venous air embolism during advanced endoscopic pancreatico-biliary procedures (AEPBP): the sound of catastrophe, *Anesth Analg* 118:217–218, 2014.

Derouin M, Couture P, Boudreault D, et al.: Detection of gas embolism by transeophageal echocardiography during laparascopic cholecystectomy, *Anesth Analg* 82:119–124, 1996.

Di Pisa M, Charamonte G, Tarantino I, et al.: Air embolism in a pediatric patient: a very rare complication of endoscopic retrograde cholangiopancreatography. In Hayat MA, editor: *Pediatric cancer, volume 4: diagnosis, therapy, and prognosis*, Dordrecht, 2013, Springer, pp 331–335.

Donepudi S, Chavalitdhamrong D, Pu L, et al.: Air embolism complicating gastrointestinal endoscopy: a systematic review, *World J Gastrointest Endosc* 5:359–365, 2013.

Duca B, Bălă O, Al-Hajjar N, et al.: Laparoscopic cholecystectomy: incidents and complications. A retrospective analysis of 9542 consecutive laparoscopic of operations. *HPB (Oxford)* 5(3):152–158.

Goins KM, May JM, Hucklenbruch C, et al.: Unexpected cardiovascular collapse from massive air embolism during endoscopic retrograde cholangiopancreatography, *Acta Anaesthesiol Scand* 54:385–388, 2010.

Ng WS, Rosen M: Carbon dioxide in the prevention of air embolism during open-heart surgery, *Thorax* 23:194–196, 1968.

Nyagan J, Hok K, Liang J: Fatal systemic air embolism during endoscopic retrograde cholangiopancreatography, *Anaesth Intensive Care* 31:260–264, 2004.

Traiki TB, Baaj J, Al Boukae A, et al.: Fatal air embolism during sigmoidoscopy performed under spinal anaesthesia, *Anesth Essays Res* 6:210–212, 2012.

玻璃体视网膜手术

Dermigny F, Daelman F, Guinot PG, et al.: Fatal air embolism during open eye surgery, *Ann Fr Anesth Reanim* 27:840–842, 2008.

El-Annan J, Barr CC: Does venous air embolism occur during air/fluid exchange? *Arch Ophthalmol* 129:1244, 2011.

Gamulescu M, Helbig H, Bartz-Schmidt U: Air embolisation during vitrectomy? *Kilin Monatsbl Augenheilkd* 227:185–186, 2010.

Ledowski T, Kiese F, Jeglin S, et al.: Possible air embolism during eye surgery, *Anesth Analg* 100:1651–1652, 2005.

Lim LT, Somerville GM, Walker JD: Venous air embolism during air-fluid exchange: a potentially fatal complication, *Arch Ophthalmol* 128:1618–1619, 2010.

Morris RE, Sapp MR, Oltmanns MH, et al.: Presumed air by vitrectomy embolisation (PAVE) a potentially fatal syndrome, *Br J Opthalmol* 98:765–768, 2014.

Rice JC, Liebenberg L, Scholtz RP, et al.: Fatal air embolism during endoresection of choroidal melanoma, *Retin Cases Brief Rep* 8:127–129, 2014.

Ruest P, Aroichane M, Cordahi G, Bureau N: Possible venous air embolism during open eye surgery in a child, *Can J Anaesth* 54:840–844, 2007.

Shin S, Nam B, Soh S, Koo BN: Percutaneous cardiopulmonary support to treat suspected venous air embolism with cardiac arrest during open eye surgery: a case report, *Korean J Anesthesiol* 67:350, 2014.

Wu CC, Chen KY, Hsieh YJ: Fatal air embolism and ocular shrinkage during vitrectomy, *J Anesth* 29:318, 2015.

第六部分

小儿围术期事件

第 187 章 小儿苏醒延迟

Alexandra Szabova，*John B. Rose*

病例概要

患儿，女，2 岁，14 kg，患有 21 三体综合征，因阻塞性睡眠呼吸暂停行腺样体扁桃体切除手术，停用麻醉药 35 min 后，患儿仍无反应并且未拔管。术中给予丙泊酚 2 mg/kg，吗啡 0.1 mg/kg 以及顺阿曲库铵 0.2 mg/kg。采用氧气和空气混合气（FiO_2 0.6），2.5% 七氟烷维持全身麻醉。给予格隆溴铵 0.01 mg/kg 和新斯的明 0.05 mg/kg 拮抗神经肌肉阻滞。

问题分析

定义

苏醒延迟定义为停止全身麻醉后在合理的时间内（大多数情况下少于 30 min）无法恢复意识。恢复意识所需的时间并不确定，取决于几个因素，例如手术的时长，使用的药物剂量和技术以及患者术前身体和精神状态。

识别

患者评估

药物作用、生理紊乱、代谢异常、中枢神经系统（central nervous system，CNS）损伤和既往存在的 CNS 疾病都可能导致全身麻醉苏醒延迟（框 187.1）。应迅速完成初步评估，可能包括以下部分或全部内容：

- 回顾患者的病史和麻醉记录；
- 体格检查包括生命体征和体温评估；气道通畅度；通气充足，氧合和循环以及神经系统检查（瞳孔大小和反应性，反射，对言语和触觉刺激的反应，咽反射存在）；
- 用神经刺激仪评估神经肌肉功能；
- 血糖、电解质、血尿素氮、肌酐、动脉血气分析；
- 头部的计算机断层扫描，神经科医师会诊。

对于病例概要中的患者，她的气道通畅，并且通气和氧合充足。在呼出气体中没有七氟烷。她的生命体征、体温、呼气末 CO_2 和血氧饱和度均正常。用神经刺激仪评估，发现神经肌肉阻滞被充分拮抗。有人指出，她在术前有长时间的禁食（15 h），并且在手术期间接受了无葡萄糖的静脉输液。通过血糖测试（血糖 =42 mg/dl）考虑并确认为低血糖。通过对症治疗，患者恢复了意识并且完全康复。

框 187.1 苏醒延迟的鉴别诊断

药物效应
药物过量（意外或判断错误）
多种 CNS 抑制剂或药物相互作用
用药错误（准备或给药中）
药物代谢受损（消除或蛋白结合减少；敏感性增加）
残余神经肌肉阻滞

生理失衡或代谢紊乱
缺氧；高碳酸血症
电解质失衡（低钠血症、低钙血症、低镁血症）
体温过低或高热
脓毒症
低血糖

CNS 损伤或未确诊的已经存在的疾病
颅内出血或高血压
脑缺血、水肿或栓塞（空气或微粒）
癫痫发作（特别是发作后状态）
脑肿瘤
卒中（例如镰状细胞病、高凝状态）
脑梗死（例如镰状细胞病，高凝状态）

CNS，中枢神经系统

Adapted and modified from Denlinger JK：Prolonged emergence and failure to regain consciousness. In Gravenstein N，Kirby RR，editors：*Complications in anesthesiology*. Philadelphia，Lippincott-Raven，1996，pp 441-450.

药物作用

苏醒延迟的常见原因是麻醉药物的作用延长。虽然意外过量使用一种药物可能是造成这种情况的原因，但更常见的是多种药物合用。药物单独使用可以给予适当的剂量，但是如果联合使用，而不进行剂量调整，相对过量的剂量可能会造成 CNS 抑制作用的增强。在全身麻醉复合区域麻醉的情况下尤其明显。数项研究调查了术前用药对儿科门诊手术恢复的影响。虽然一些研究显示术前用药（口服咪达唑仑）会造成苏醒延迟，但其他研究表明没有影响或影响很小（例如经直肠给予地西泮，口服咪达唑仑和经鼻腔给予咪达唑仑）。

药物代谢和消除的减少可能导致苏醒延迟，特别是早产儿和足月新生儿。阿片类药物和镇静剂引起的呼吸抑制和通气不足可以延缓吸入麻醉药的消除，并延缓婴幼儿自主呼吸恢复的时间。极端体重如病态肥胖青少年，可能导致丙泊酚麻醉后苏醒延迟。

家庭药物治疗方案可能包括几类药物之间潜在的相互作用，与麻醉药相克或发生特异性反应，可表现为苏醒延迟（例如接受氯氮平治疗的精神分裂症儿童）。在成人患者中有大量异常情况的病例报告，但在儿科患者中则较少，限制了对这些异常情况的概括。中成药和非处方药可以影响麻醉苏醒。父母和监护人对这些药物的使用情况报告不足。

术中使用阿片类药物和恩丹司酮可在使用某些抗抑郁药和抗精神病药治疗的患者中引起 CNS 5- 羟色胺水平增高，诱发 5- 羟色胺综合征，这可能会导致苏醒延迟。类似的，中枢抗胆碱能综合征可能是由家庭药物和麻醉药之间的药物相互作用引起。与非麻醉患者相比，麻醉患者临床表现为心动过速、瞳孔散大、皮肤干燥或发热的可能性减少，导致诊断和治疗延迟。Tzabazis 及其同事总结了已发表的病例报告。在接受麻醉的儿科患者中，5- 羟色胺综合征和中枢抗胆碱能综合征的发病率尚不清楚。

在婴儿和儿童中，能够发现他们对麻醉药物催眠效果反应的生物学变异性。如果是这样，对这些反应的敏感性增加可能会导致一些儿童苏醒延长。然而，这必须作为既往无认知障碍或发育迟缓史的健康儿童中的排除诊断。

生理不平衡或代谢紊乱

各种术前状态的存在（如长期禁食、脱水、营养不良、肾或肝病、利尿或抗酸治疗、严重贫血、镰状细胞病、糖尿病和癫痫症）或术中不良事件的发生（如通气不足、低血压、灌注不足、伴有大量血液和液体复苏的大量失血）增加了生理失衡或代谢紊乱导致苏醒延迟的可能性。

脉搏血氧饱和度和二氧化碳描记图的常规使用极大地提高了麻醉科医师监测和治疗与低氧血症和高碳酸血症相关的危及生命疾病的能力。对于经历过低血压或低灌注期的儿童，或者那些大量失血，需要用大量晶体液，胶体液和血液制品进行液体复苏的儿童，应考虑代谢性酸中毒。对术前长期禁食的儿童应该怀疑低血糖，特别是如果他们在术中接受了非葡萄糖的静脉输液，或者是胰岛素依赖性糖尿病患者并且围术期接受了胰岛素治疗。

代谢紊乱是儿童某些综合征的主要特征，如果存在则可能导致苏醒延迟。

中枢神经系统损伤或疾病

儿童麻醉期间 CNS 损伤很少见，但可能导致苏醒延迟。患有右向左分流的先天性心脏病患者，即使仅有少量空气通过静脉输注进入循环系统，也会面临脑空气栓塞的风险。此外，空气或颗粒物质所致的脑栓塞是体外循环的已知并发症。已有报道在早产和足月新生儿的清醒喉镜检查和气管插管过程中，出现脑出血或脑室内出血，这也是脑室腹腔分流术和其他神经外科手术的并发症。输送低氧混合气体、低灌注引起的长期低血压和定位不当引起的颈动脉受压损伤都能引起脑缺血。在青少年颈椎手术后有发生双侧幕上血肿的报导。

未确诊的已存在的 CNS 疾病也可能导致苏醒延迟。迟发性中枢低通气综合征是一种神经系统疾病，可表现为儿童在麻醉后出现术后呼吸系统并发症和苏醒延迟。颅内高压可能存在于脑室腹腔分流功能不良的患者或以前未被发现的脑肿瘤或枕骨大孔狭窄的患者；高碳酸血症、低氧血症或颈部过度伸展可加重颅内高压。在麻醉状态和瘫痪的患者中癫痫发作很难被发现。它们可能发生在全身麻醉期间，发作后状态可以表现为苏醒延迟。最后，未识别的肌肉无力或瘫痪会使患者表现为无意识。必须通过仔细评估神经肌肉功能来与前面描述的疾病进行区分。

转化障碍、嗜睡症和睡眠麻痹已被报导是成人苏醒延迟的罕见原因。有报道使用毒扁豆碱成功治疗了 1 例睡眠麻痹。

风险评估

苏醒延迟的发生率尚不清楚。根据对婴幼儿麻醉并发症的调查，其发病率似乎较低。在一项针对 29 220 名婴儿和儿童的麻醉并发症研究中，没有报告出现苏醒延迟或昏迷的病例。在对 40 240 名婴儿和儿童的并发症进行回顾时，报告了 1 例昏迷病例；其发生在一名 13 岁男孩给予 N_2O –阿片类药物–神经安定药物进行麻醉后。在另一项研究中，10 000 例儿科门诊手术患者中有 2 例由于过度嗜睡在手术后住院治疗。

对这种并发症的报告不足可能是主要原因。全身麻醉后苏醒所需的时间变化很大，因此每位麻醉科医师必须确定是否出现苏醒延迟并报告并发症。如果大多数苏醒延迟的病例与药物作用延长有关并且最终结果良好，许多医师可能不愿意报告看似无关紧要的事件。

启示

当由于药物作用延长导致苏醒延迟时，如果采取合理措施支持气道并确保充分的氧合、通气和血流动力学稳定，患者的长期预后良好。然而，当苏醒延迟是由于代谢异常或 CNS 损伤引起时，必须认识到存在的问题，确定根本原因，并迅速采取纠正措施以避免灾难性结果。

除了对患者预后的影响外，苏醒延迟还会对预期的治疗质量、家长满意度、手术室（operating room，OR）效率和医疗保险费用产生显著影响。即使是短暂苏醒延迟，如果频繁发生，也可能会扰乱干扰 OR 日程安排，消耗 OR 和恢复室时间和人员，并使麻醉科医师不能按时开始其他安排的病例。

管理

苏醒延迟的管理需要以下步骤：

- 确保气道通畅，充分氧合和通气；
- 回顾病史和麻醉管理；
- 药物拮抗试验；
- 排除代谢和电解质异常；
- 排除中枢神经系统损伤。

苏醒延迟的处理首先需要确保患者气道通畅，并确保患者氧合和通气充分。其次，回顾患者的病史和麻醉管理，以确定潜在原因并决定需要采取哪些进一步措施。通常，不能排除阿片类药物或苯二氮革类药物过量的情况，并需要进行纳洛酮、氟马西尼或两者的诊断和治疗试验（框 187.2）。当苏醒延迟是由于吸入麻醉药、东莨菪碱、氯胺酮、吩噻嗪或三环类抗抑郁药引起的，非特异性拮抗剂毒扁豆碱可能有效。需要强调的是，这些拮抗剂中的任何一种都可能只会产生短暂的意识恢复。如果不怀疑麻醉药物作用延长，应对血液进行取样以测定动脉血气、电解质、葡萄糖、钙和镁浓度。如果在初步回顾和检查后未发现明确的原因，可能需要进行神经科会诊、CNS 影像学检查或脑电图检查。

预防

苏醒延迟通常可以预防。用药错误、患者观察或监测不力以及体位性损伤，特别是当手术涉及头颈部或患者处于俯卧位或侧卧位时，是苏醒延迟并发症的一些常见可预防原因。

致谢

感谢 Hector Nicodemus 博士对本章上一版的贡献。

（薛改改　译　范晓华　校）

延伸阅读

Araki H, Fujiwara Y, Shimada Y: Effect of flumazenil on recovery from sevoflurane anesthesia in children premedicated with oral midazolam before undergoing herniorrhaphy with or without caudal analgesia, *J Anesth* 19(3):204–207, 2005.

Bennett T, Allford M: Delayed emergence from anesthesia in a child with congenital generalized lipodystrophy (Berardinelli-Seip syndrome), *Paediatr Anaesth* 22(3):299–300, 2012.

框 187.2　逆转麻醉药镇静作用的拮抗剂

纳洛酮：1 ～ 4 μg/kg 静脉注射至起效；最大剂量，10 μg/kg

氟马西尼：2.5 ～ 5 μg/kg 静脉注射至起效；最大剂量，10 μg/kg

毒扁豆碱：25 ～ 50 μg/kg 静脉注射；最大剂量，2 mg

Bouw J, Leendertse K, Tijssen MA, et al.: Stiff person syndrome and anesthesia: case report, *Anesth Analg* 97(2):486–487, table of contents 2003.

Brosius KK, Bannister CF: Oral midazolam premedication in preadolescents and adolescents, *Anesth Analg* 94(1):31–36, 2002.

Chidambaran V, Sadhasivam S, Diepstraten J, et al.: Evaluation of propofol anesthesia in morbidly obese children and adolescents, *BMC Anesthesiol* 13:8, 2013.

Cohen MM, Cameron CB, Duncan PG: Pediatric anesthesia morbidity and mortality in the perioperative period, *Anesth Analg* 70(2):160–167, 1990.

Crowe S, McKeating K: Delayed emergence and St. John's wort, *Anesthesiology* 96(4):1025–1027, 2002.

Geeraerts T, Moghrabi Z, Benhamou D: Delayed recovery after short-duration, general anesthesia in a patient chronically treated with clozapine, *Anesth Analg* 103(6):1618, 2006.

Hinkle AJ: Neonatal sepsis presenting as delayed emergence from general anesthesia, *Anesthesiology* 57(5):412–414, 1982.

Kreidstein A, Boorin MR, Crespi P, et al.: Delayed awakening from general anaesthesia in a patient with Hunter syndrome, *Can J Anaesth* 41(5 Pt 1): 423–426, 1994.

Li ZJ, Sun P, Dou YH, et al.: Bilateral supratentorial epidural hematomas: a rare complication in adolescent spine surgery, *Neurol Med Chir (Tokyo)* 52(9):646–648, 2012.

Mahmoud M, Bryan Y, Gunter J, et al.: Anesthetic implications of undiagnosed late onset central hypoventilation syndrome in a child: from elective tonsillectomy to tracheostomy, *Paediatr Anaesth* 17(10): 1001–1005, 2007.

Matsuda C, Tachibana K, Fujii M, et al.: Ultrasound guided transversus abdominis plane block in early infancy, *Masui* 62(8):924–928, 2013.

Otsuka Y, Yusa T, Higa M, et al.: Intranasal midazolam for sedation before anesthesia in pediatric patients, *Masui* 43(1):106–110, 1994.

Patel RI, Hannallah RS: Anesthetic complications following pediatric ambulatory surgery: a 3-yr study, *Anesthesiology* 69(6):1009–1012, 1988.

Tiret L, Nivoche Y, Hatton F, et al.: Complications related to anaesthesia in infants and children. A prospective survey of 40240 anaesthetics, *Br J Anaesth* 61(3):263–269, 1988.

Tzabazis A, Miller C, Dobrow MF, et al.: Delayed emergence after anesthesia, *J Clin Anesth* 27(4):353–360, 2015.

Uchiumi R, Hidaka T, Miyagawa A, et al.: Clinical evaluation of diazepam suppository for premedication in children, *Masui* 43(1):102 -105, 1994.

Viitanen H, Annila P, Viitanen M, et al.: Premedication with midazolam delays recovery after ambulatory sevoflurane anesthesia in children, *Anesth Analg* 89(1):75–79, 1999.

第 188 章 儿科困难气道

Herodotos Ellinas

病例概要

患儿，3 岁，拟择期行扁桃体切除术和腺样体切除术。主要病史为 Treacher Collins 综合征（图 188.1），预计会出现困难气道。患儿在自主呼吸下行吸入诱导后，通过声门上装置使用纤维支气管镜成功进行气管插管。

问题分析

定义

困难气道是指存在中重度困难的面罩通气、直接喉镜检查或两者兼有。困难气道可能由解剖（先天性或后天性）或生理缺陷引起。

识别

完整的病史询问和详尽的体格检查，是识别和预测儿科困难气道的最佳方法。了解儿童和成人气道的显著差异，是成功管理儿科困难气道的关键（图 188.2）。气道直径、形状和位置以及气道上皮及其支撑结构存在解剖学差异。新生儿和成人呼吸系统的生理差异，是由解剖学和呼吸控制机制的差异所致。

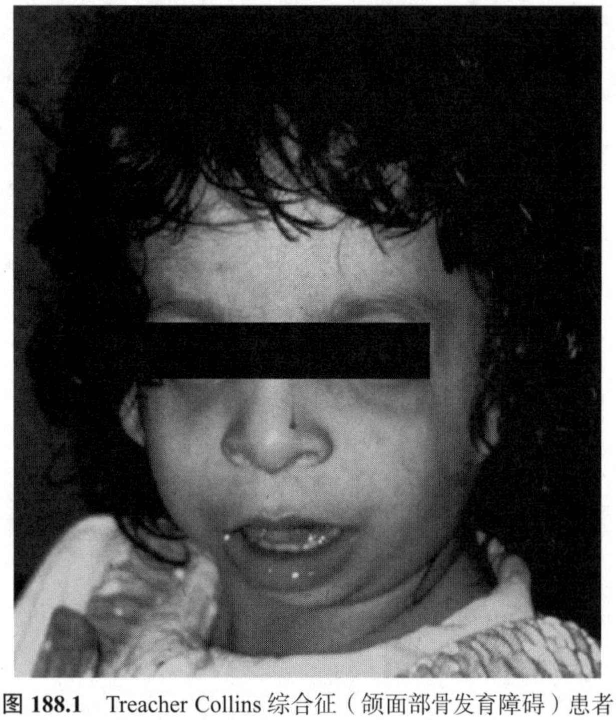

图 188.1 Treacher Collins 综合征（颌面部骨发育障碍）患者的气道管理相关异常包括下颌骨和颧骨发育不全、小口畸形和后鼻孔闭锁

上呼吸道

新生儿的上呼吸道十分特别。其舌体相对较大，完全占据口腔和咽腔。这可能会使在尝试气管插管期间，操纵喉镜和气管导管尤为困难。新生儿直至 6 月龄前，均通过鼻进行呼吸。这是由于位于咽部高处的会厌几乎与软腭相抵，使其难以经口呼吸。

淋巴组织

与年龄较大的婴儿或儿童不同，新生儿几乎没有上呼吸道淋巴组织。扁桃体和腺样体于 1 岁后出现，在 4 ～ 7 岁时体积达到最大，之后逐渐退去。尝试经鼻气管插管时，增大的扁桃体和腺样体可能会增加出血。

会厌

婴儿会厌大，呈 U 形，并以 45° 角突向喉部。使用直柄喉镜片，可直接挑起会厌，有助于直接暴露声带。

喉

新生儿的舌骨体位于 C3 ～ C4 水平。随着婴儿的生长发育，声门逐渐向尾端移动并最终稳定在 C5 ～ C6 水平。会厌和高位喉部使婴儿能同时呼吸和吞咽。同样，随着甲状软骨和环状软骨向尾端移动，环甲膜开始形成。

气流

上呼吸道的气道为湍流，即使在平静呼吸时亦

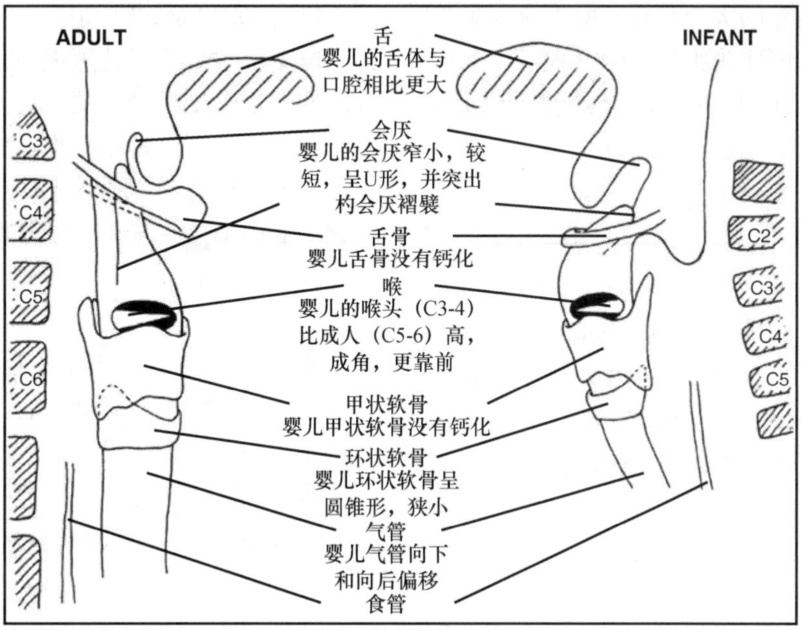

图 188.2 成人和儿童气道对比（From Ho M：The pediatric airway. In Bell C，Hughes C，Oh T，editors：*The pediatric handbook*. St Louis，Mosby-Year Book，1991，p 130. Adapted from Coté CJ，Todres ID：The pediatric airway. In Ryan JF，Todres DI，Coté CJ，editors：*A practice of anesthesia for infants and children*. Orlando，FL，Grune & Stratton，1986.）

如此。层流开始于第四和第五级气管分支的水平，此处气道横截面积的快速增加降低了气流速度。湍流气流的阻力与气道半径的五次方成反比。因此，气管内 1 mm 水肿（半径从 2 mm 减小到 1 mm），可使气流阻力增加约 32 倍。

呼吸力学

幼儿胸壁顺应性高，可减少呼吸做功。顺应性增加是由于较软的非钙化肋，其与脊柱和胸骨呈直角相连。婴儿通气主要依靠膈肌。与成人相比，婴儿的膈肌中 I 型（慢）肌纤维更少，故其效率较低且易于疲劳。

风险评估

儿科困难气道通常可以预期，成功管理困难气道患者需要完整的病史询问和体格检查。病史应关注下述方面：

- 翻阅既往医疗记录，尤其是有关困难气道证据的麻醉记录；
- 先天或后天的气道异常证据；
- 气道梗阻或阻塞性睡眠呼吸暂停的证据。

框 188.1 列出了与围术期气道管理最相关的体格检查的特征。偶尔可能需其他检查（如清醒喉镜、影像学成像、流量-容积环）以充分评估潜在的困难气道。

框 188.1 儿科气道检查

- 头部大小和形状
- 面貌变形和面部不对称
- 下颌骨大小和位置（如下颌后缩）
- 舌头大小
- 上腭形状（如高拱形的上腭）
- 上切牙突出
- 下颌、头部和颈部的活动度

启示

若无法或不能良好地进行面罩通气，且如果确定患者不能气管插管，则患者的病情将变为紧急状况。必须立即恢复患者的气体交换，以避免发生缺氧性脑损伤和死亡。

管理

术前用药

术前用药应该个性化。应谨慎给予镇静剂（如苯二氮䓬类药物、阿片类药物）；这些药物可致肌张力丧失，加重原有气道梗阻或引起呼吸抑制。对部分考虑清醒气管插管的大龄儿童，由具有困难气道丰富管理经验的医师实施镇静较为合理。可考虑使用抗胆碱能药物，因其既具有抗胆碱酯酶的作用，在气道操作期间还可防止迷走神经反应。

诱导

新近指南得到大不列颠和爱尔兰儿科医师协会（Association of Pediatric Anaesthetists of Great Britain and Ireland，APA）和困难气道协会（Difficult Airway Society，DAS）支持，概述了 1 ～ 8 岁儿童困难气道的管理步骤。本文介绍三种情况：

1. **面罩通气困难**
   a. 呼叫寻求帮助。
   b. 给予纯氧。
   c. 确保良好的头部体位。
      i. 小于 2 岁的儿童，使用肩垫。
      ii. 年龄较大的儿童，头后仰提下颌，或将头偏向一侧。
   d. 考虑双手挤皮球面罩通气（bag-mask ventilation，BMV）。
   e. 使用口咽（oropharyngeal，OP）或鼻咽（nasopharyngeal，NP）通气道；选择合适的尺寸有助于改善通气，而不阻塞气道（OP：嘴唇到同侧下颌角；NP：鼻孔到同侧耳屏）。
   f. 检查设备是否故障，并考虑使用充气皮球。
   g. 喉痉挛在儿童中十分常见，应提供有效的麻醉深度（采用吸入或静脉麻醉确保达到麻醉第 3 期）。
   h. 使用口胃（orogastric，OG）或鼻胃（nasogastric，NG）管进行胃减压。
   i. 使用丙泊酚（1 ～ 2 mg/kg 静脉注射）或琥珀胆碱（1 ～ 2 mg/kg 静脉注射或 2 ～ 4 mg/kg 肌内注射）治疗完全性喉痉挛以解除持续性低氧血症。
   j. 使用声门上气道装置或尝试气管插管。
2. **择期手术困难气管插管-非预期**
   a. 呼叫寻求帮助。
   b. 给予纯氧。
   c. 限制所有参与人员尝试气管插管的次数应≤4 次。
      i. 3 岁以下儿童使用 Miller 镜片（直柄），大龄儿童使用 Mac 镜片（弯柄）。
      ii. 考虑较小尺寸的气管导管（endotracheal tube，ETT）。
      iii. 考虑环状软骨压迫。
      iv. 若条件允许，使用视频喉镜或间接喉镜。
   d. 使用声门上装置，或者使用纤维支气管镜进行气管插管，为外科手术提供氧合，通气。
   e. 考虑苏醒患者并推迟手术。
3. **已予肌肉松弛的患者发生困难通气和困难插管**
   a. 呼叫寻求帮助。
   b. 给予纯氧。
   c. 考虑上述措施，包括调整头位，放置口咽 / 鼻咽通气道，双手 BMV，放置 OG/NG 管胃减压，使用声门上装置，唤醒患者（可考虑使用肌松逆转药物）。
   d. 若耳鼻喉科医师在场，可进行经皮环甲膜切开术和高频喷射通气，或选择硬支气管镜 / 外科气管切开术。

绝大多数困难气道的患儿需要全身麻醉。在麻醉诱导期间，应尽一切努力保留其自主呼吸。

气道辅助工具

成功的儿科困难气道管理，需要必要的设备和专业的知识。标准设备包括各种尺寸的面罩、口咽 / 鼻咽通气道、喉镜片、气管导管和引导导丝。其他设备也必须易于获得（如存放在指定的困难气道车内）。

声门上装置

喉罩自 20 世纪 80 年代后期引入临床，声门上装置（泛指放置在喉上方进行通气的装置）不断发展，其中一类（第二代）还能用于胃减压。当气管插管或面罩通气困难时，它们可能是唯一的气道装置。尽管大量的数据已证明老一代喉罩安全性，但新型喉罩已被证明可成功改善特定的困难气道；一旦放置到位且通气良好（$ETCO_2$ 描记），此类装置适用于光纤引导下带套囊气管导管的插管（图 188.3）。

Bullard 喉镜

Bullard 喉镜适用于小儿和成人，可间接观察喉部结构，对张口度或颈部活动度要求较小。使用该喉镜时，无需口咽和喉三条轴线成一条直线。与成人喉镜相比，Bullard 小儿喉镜片更窄且末端角度更小。导管管芯固定在喉镜片上，通过推进事先插入管芯的气管导管完成气管插管。随着视频喉镜的出现，且掌握 Bullard 喉镜用法的学习曲线较长，该喉

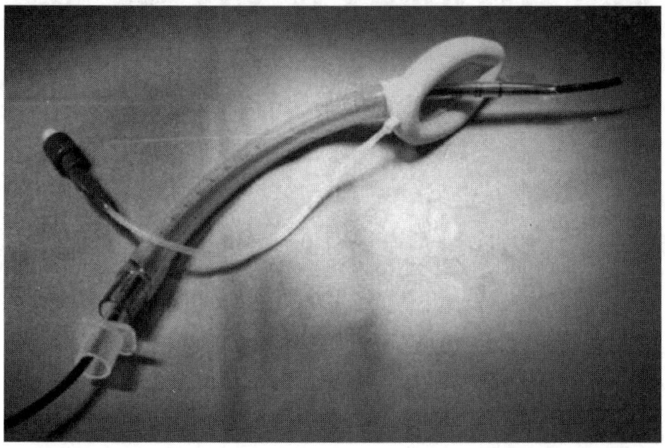

图 188.3　喉罩的使用可有助于盲插或纤支镜引导下气管插管

镜的运用越来越少。

视频喉镜（如 Glidescope）

此类装置为麻醉科医师提供“直接喉镜检查”的同时，也为插管期间其他在场人员提供了充分的气道观察视野。此类装置用于经口气管插管，具有与直接喉镜相似的局限性（如血液、分泌物、张口度小）。

纤维支气管软镜

适用于儿童的纤维支气管软镜，其外径从 2.2 mm 至 4.9 mm 不等。具有 2.2 mm 或 4.9 mm 外径的纤维支气管软镜，可分别通过 2.5 mm 和 5.5 mm 气管导管。2.2 mm 超薄纤维支气管软镜具有灵活的尖端，但没有吸引口，在低龄儿童困难气道的管理中具有非常宝贵的作用。

预防

研究表明，儿童麻醉相关罹病率风险较成人更高，不良呼吸事件是主要原因。全面理解和熟悉儿科气道解剖和生理，有助于降低这一风险。术前及时识别困难气道的儿童，配备充足的人员和设备确保气道安全，避免出现危及生命的事件。通过在病案记录中标注，向患儿家长充分告知，让患儿佩戴 Medic-Alert 手环等，当患儿未来需全身麻醉时，困难气道事件的信息能向医护人员得到有效的传递。

致谢

感谢 Hernando De Soto 博士对本章上一版的贡献。

（耿长振　译　薄禄龙　校）

延伸阅读

Belanger J, Kossick M: Methods of identifying and managing the difficult airway in the pediatric population, *AANA J* 83:35–41, 2015.

Black AE, Flynn PE, Smith HL, et al.: Development of a guideline for the management of the unanticipated difficult airway in pediatric practice, *Pediatr Anaesth* 25:346–362, 2015.

Fiadjoe J, Stricker P: Pediatric difficult airway management: current devices and techniques, *Anesthesiol Clin* 27:185–195, 2009.

Harless J, Ramaiah R, Bhananker SM: Pediatric airway management, *Int J Crit Illn Inj Sci* 4:65–70, 2014.

Heinrich S, Birkholz T, Ihmsen H, et al.: Incidence and predictors of difficult laryngoscopy in 11,219 pediatric anesthesia procedures, *Pediatr Anaesth* 22:729–736, 2012.

Jagannathan N, Ramsey MA, White MC, et al.: An update on newer pediatric supraglottic airways with recommendations for clinical use, *Pediatr Anaesth* 25:334–345, 2015.

Jain RR, Rabb MF: The difficult pediatric airway. In Hagberg CA, editor: *Benumof and Hagberg's airway management*, ed 3, Philadelphia, 2013, Elsevier, pp 723–760.

McNiece WL, Dierdorf SF: The pediatric airway, *Semin Pediatr Surg* 13:152–165, 2004.

Muraika L, Heyman JS, Shevchenko Y: Fiberoptic tracheal intubation through a laryngeal mask airway in a child with Treacher Collins syndrome, *Anesth Analg* 97:1298–1299, 2003.

Nykiel-Bailey SM, McAllister JD, Schrock CR, et al.: Difficult airway consultation service for children: steps to implement and preliminary results, *Pediatr Anaesth* 25:363–371, 2015.

第 189 章 苏醒期躁动和苏醒期谵妄

Tyson Olds，*B. Craig Weldon*

病例概要

4 岁男童，既往体健，全身麻醉下行包皮环切术。手术进行顺利。患儿转入麻醉后恢复室（postanesthesia care unit，PACU）时出现了焦躁不安、易激惹、哭泣的表现，常规的镇静措施无效。随后其激动不安的行为升级为语无伦次的尖叫、肢体拍打和间歇性的攻击。

问题分析

定义

苏醒期躁动（emergence agitation，EA）是指小儿麻醉苏醒期出现哭闹、不安和易激惹等症状，而苏醒期谵妄（emergence delirium，ED）是一种分离的意识状态，患儿表现为多动且语无伦次，并伴有无法安慰的哭喊、尖叫、踢打和拍打。EA 和 ED 很可能是同一认知状态的两种表现。

识别

EA 在幼儿、学龄前儿童和学龄儿童中常见，即使小手术也有可能发生。EA 可能持续 20 ～ 30 min，并且常规的安慰措施无效。5% ～ 10% 的患儿表现为类似谵妄的严重症状。青少年和年轻患者在 PACU 中发生谵妄的比例高于单纯的躁动。

风险评估

生长发育因素

幼儿缺乏成熟的适应能力，所以他们无法接受在一个陌生的地方与父母分离，无法调整疾病或手术所导致的心理应激，也不能接受麻醉及苏醒过程中精神状态的改变。父母的焦虑或缺乏对围术期的认识也可能对孩子的行为产生负面影响。

术前焦虑和性格基础

术前存在严重焦虑的患儿通常在面罩通气的诱导过程中配合也较差，PACU 中 EA 发生率较高，发作的严重程度也较高。同样，在使用面罩麻醉诱导过程中处于高度焦虑状态的患儿，苏醒过程中发生躁动的可能性更大。儿童的性格基础可影响其术后的行为，父母常可预测他们的孩子在应对手术当天的事件时是否存在问题。无论是在父母的陪伴下进行麻醉诱导，还是麻醉前予以口服咪达唑仑镇静，都不能降低 EA 的风险。

原有的精神障碍

患有自闭症、智力障碍、双相情感障碍或破坏性行为（如对立违抗性障碍或其他行为障碍）的儿童和青少年在术后出现行为问题的可能性更大。这些患者应接受常规抗精神病药物治疗至术日。此外，麻醉前镇静也有可能获得较好的效果。

术后镇痛不足

未识别出的术后疼痛是所有年龄组 EA 的常见原因。对于不会说话的婴儿和发育迟缓的儿童，用主观疼痛评分系统评估比较困难。并众所周知，大多数儿童对疼痛强度的自我描述能力较差。当患者在疼痛中麻醉苏醒，通常表现出烦躁甚至精神错乱的行为，但他们不会表现出这种疼痛。其他引起不适的因素也必须排除，如胃或膀胱的扩张、伤口引流、绑带或敷料过紧等。

潜在内科疾病

以下潜在的危及生命的病情，在 PACU 中也可能表现为苏醒期躁动或谵妄：

- 低氧血症或高碳酸血症；
- 休克状态或严重低血压时脑血流减少；
- 低血糖、甲状腺功能亢进或甲状旁腺功能亢进；
- 低钠血症；
- 癫痫发作或颅内压升高。

如果找不出苏醒期躁动或谵妄的原因，或者躁动发作的时间延长或伴随意识水平下降，应根据患者相应的病情予以考虑上述诊断。

抗胆碱能类

东莨菪碱和阿托品（影响程度稍小）与术后精神障碍有关。由于乙酰胆碱介导的神经抑制通路被阻断，这些药物通过血脑屏障引起中枢抗胆碱能危象（或综合征）。完全型中枢抗胆碱能综合征的特点是皮肤温暖、泛红、干燥；视觉障碍；发热和谵妄。用于产生散瞳的眼科用药、多种抗组胺药和非专利药物，均具有中枢抗胆碱能作用，可能导致患者麻醉后行为失常。这些药物多数为叔胺和季胺类药物，更容易透过血脑屏障。

麻醉药物

血溶性低的挥发性麻醉剂（环丙烷、地氟烷、七氟烷）与儿童 EA 有关。这种现象的机制尚不清楚，但可能与血溶性低的这些药物可使患者从麻醉中迅速苏醒有关。然而，接受丙泊酚麻醉的患儿 EA 的发生率明显低于接受七氟烷麻醉的患儿，尽管两种药物都有相似的快速苏醒的特点。镇痛效果迅速消失（地氟烷的镇痛作用大于七氟烷），可能导致术后镇痛不足，引发或加重苏醒期躁动。

长期以来一直认为氯胺酮与青少年和成年人的术后躁动和不安的心理反应有关。然而，在低龄儿童中，有证据表明在七氟烷麻醉期间给予氯胺酮可降低 EA 的发生率。

启示

对于出现 EA 的患儿来说，最大的即刻隐患是自我伤害的风险增加。有严重 EA/ED 的患儿可能存在攻击性或自主体动增多，须防止意外地伤害自己或护理人员。静脉通路（intravenous，IV）、监测管道线路、手术引流 / 敷料等的拔除或移位也会给术后治疗带来不便。在 PACU 中，这些孩子经常会出现各种状况，护士和麻醉科医师需要从其他患者身上转移注意力到他们身上，因而减少了对非躁动的 PACU 患者的监控和治疗。谵妄患者的治疗具劳动密集性，可延长 PACU 停留时间并增加成本。大多数患有严重焦虑症的患儿父母都认为这种经历很可怕，并使他们情绪低落。

管理

对于患有轻度到中度 EA 的儿童，初始治疗方案包括以下内容：①减少日常舒适所需以外的环境刺激，②尽快让孩子的父母参与到他或她的照顾中来，③应认真考虑到镇痛不足的可能性，并予以静脉阿片类药物。

做好对情绪极度激动、易攻击的儿童的保护，避免身体伤害，立刻保护好静脉和其他血管通路，必要时予以身体上的束缚。如果怀疑镇痛效果不佳，应给予快速起效的静脉阿片类药物充分镇痛，如芬太尼。如果仍然存在躁动，可予以右美托咪定（0.2 ～ 0.5 μg/kg）。可使用毒扁豆碱 0.025 mg/kg 拮抗阿托品、东莨菪碱等药物的中枢抗胆碱能作用。

如果术后镇痛充分，但右美托咪定仍不能减轻躁动的严重程度，可予以 0.1 ～ 0.5 mg/kg 丙泊酚直至患儿失去知觉，必要时可重复。可以小剂量持续输注丙泊酚以维持这种状态，直到患儿能够慢慢地重新苏醒。

严重躁动或谵妄的较大的儿童或青少年若已拔除静脉通路，可迅速肌内注射氟哌啶醇 1 ～ 2 mg 予以镇静，对于较小的儿童可使用 0.2 ～ 0.3 mg/kg 氯胺酮滴鼻。然后可以在不进一步刺激患者的情况下重新建立静脉输液通路。

严重 EA 的治疗流程如图 189.1 所示：

预防

考虑患者的发育水平。

- 通过术前宣教减轻父母的焦虑；
- 评估孩子术前焦虑水平；
- 对高危儿童年龄组（1 ～ 6 岁）和术前焦虑水平

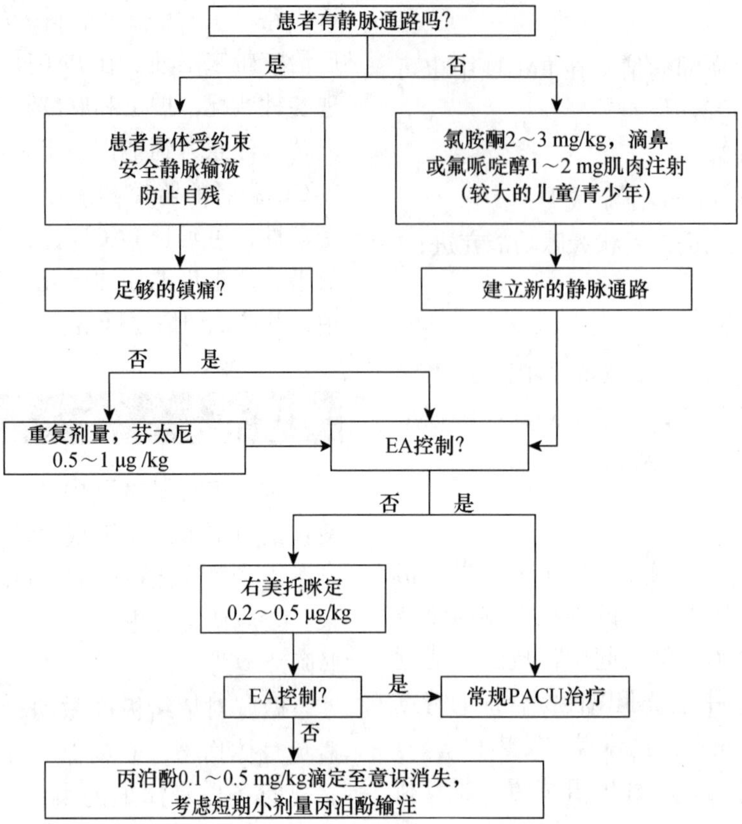

图 189.1 严重苏醒期躁动 / 谵妄的处理

高的儿童实施麻醉前镇静；

- 实施多模式镇痛方案，对术后镇痛不足保持高度怀疑；
- 对于有 EA 风险的患者，考虑术中予以右美托咪定、氯胺酮、静脉用阿片类药物、丙泊酚（连续输注或初期大剂量）或在苏醒之前应用可乐定；
- 迅速让孩子与父母在 PACU 团聚。

（陈 君 译 王晓琳 校）

延伸阅读

Abu-Shahwan I, Chowdary K: Ketamine is effective in decreasing the incidence of emergence agitation in children undergoing dental repair under sevoflurane general anesthesia, *Paediatr Anaesth* 17:846–850, 2007.

Aono J, Ueda W, Marniya K, et al.: Greater incidence of delirium during recovery from sevoflurane anesthesia in preschool boys, *Anesthesiology* 87:1298–1300, 1997.

Cohen IT, Finkel JC, Hannallah RS, et al.: Rapid emergence does not explain agitation following sevoflurane anaesthesia in infants and children: a comparison with propofol, *Paediatr Anaesth* 13:63–67, 2003.

Costi D, Ellwood J, Wallace A, et al.: Transition to propofol after sevoflurane anesthesia to prevent emergence agitation: a randomized controlled trial, *Paediatr Anaesth* 25:517–523, 2015.

Dahmani S, Stany I, Brasher C, et al.: Pharmacological prevention of sevoflurane- and desflurane-related emergence agitation in children: a meta-analysis of published studies, *Br J Anaesth* 104:216–223, 2010.

Kain ZN, Caldwell-Andrews AA, Weinberg ME, et al.: Sevoflurane versus halothane: postoperative maladaptive behavioral changes: a randomized, controlled study, *Anesthesiology* 102:720–726, 2005.

Kain ZN, Wang SM, Mayes LC, et al.: Distress during the induction of anesthesia and postoperative behavioral outcomes, *Anesth Analg* 88:1042–1047, 1999.

Lerman J, Davis PJ, Welborn LG, et al.: Induction, recovery and safety characteristics of sevoflurane in children undergoing ambulatory surgery, *Anesthesiology* 84:1332–1340, 1996.

Malviya S, Voepel-Lewis T, Ramamurthi RJ, et al.: Clonidine for the prevention of emergence agitation in young children: efficacy and recovery profile, *Paediatr Anaesth* 16:554–559, 2006.

Patel A, Davidson M, Tran MC, et al.: Dexmedetomidine infusion for analgesia and prevention of emergence agitation in children with obstructive sleep apnea syndrome undergoing tonsillectomy and adenoidectomy, *Anesth Analg* 111:1004–1010, 2010.

Reduque LL, Verghese ST: Paediatric emergence delirium, *Contin Educ Anaesth Crit Care Pain* 13(2):39–41, 2013.

Sato M, Shirakami G, Tazuke-Nishimura M, et al.: Effect of single-dose dexmedetomidine on emergence agitation and recovery profiles after sevoflurane anesthesia in pediatric ambulatory surgery, *J Anesth* 24:675–682, 2010.

低血糖与高血糖 第 190 章

Ari Y. Weintraub

病例概要

患儿，男，4 岁，既往体健，拟行腹股沟疝修补术。患儿术前一天下午 5 点晚餐，晚 9 点进食饼干和牛奶。术日清晨 5：30 提供苹果汁给患儿饮用（术前 2 h），但患儿拒绝。因急诊手术加台，患儿手术被推迟 4 h。麻醉诱导前，患儿生命体征平稳，神志淡漠，诱导后患儿血浆葡萄糖浓度为 64 mg/dl。

问题分析

定义

临床上，低血糖定义为血浆葡萄糖浓度过低并出现脑功能受损的症状或体征。低血糖通常定义为婴儿及儿童血糖浓度小于 55 mg/dl（3 mmol/L），早产儿或足月新生儿血糖浓度小于 35 mg/dl（2 mmol/L），但这些标准是根据统计学结果得出的，不能脱离临床而单纯应用此标准（**注：**单位换算 mg/dl=mmol/L × 18）。

高血糖通常定义为血糖浓度高于 200 mg/dl（11 mmol/L）。

识别

低血糖

低血糖儿童大部分无症状，部分表现为昏睡、躁动、紧张不安。婴儿及大龄儿童在血糖浓度低于 75 mg/dl 时出现症状，低于 35 mg/dl 时意识消失。对于新生儿，慢性低血糖可能与躯体感觉诱发电位（somatosensory evoked potentials，SEP）及神经发育结局的不良改变相关。低血糖的临床迹象（心动过速、高血压）可能会被术前镇静、全身麻醉、β 受体阻滞剂所掩盖。

高血糖

手术、麻醉的应激反应引起短暂的术中血糖升高，术中麻醉药物应用及局部镇痛通过降低儿茶酚胺的释放减轻应激反应，从而减缓血糖浓度的升高。临床上，很难在手术麻醉中发现高血糖的征象，除非发生渗透性利尿。对疑似高血糖患者，有必要进行血糖浓度测定。

风险评估

对健康婴儿、儿童而言，术前禁食 4 ～ 19 h 后术中低血糖发生率很低。而且，在此类人群中，血糖浓度与禁食时间并无明显相关性。麻醉诱导前 2 h 摄入含葡萄糖液体可明显降低术中低血糖的发生率。

术前禁食引起低血糖的高危人群：

- 早产婴儿、体型小的新生儿；
- 母亲为糖尿病患者的新生儿和婴儿，患糖尿病或胰岛素瘤的儿童；
- 摄食减少（如喂养厌恶、呕吐）或液体过度流失（如腹泻、结肠镜检查肠道准备）的患者；
- 营养不良的患者；
- 严重肝衰竭患者；
- 脂类分解或氨基酸代谢异常患者；
- 肌肉疾病、线粒体疾病或糖原存贮疾病患者；
- 服用某些药物（如普萘洛尔、酒精）的患者；
- 接受静脉营养液或葡萄糖输液（10% 或 12.5%）患者，尤其当突然停止输液时。

导致术中高血糖的因素：

- 外源性高血糖（例如，≥ 20 ml/kg/h）或大量输液；
- 外源性皮质类固醇（长期或临时性 / 术中）；
- 激素水平改变影响血糖调控（例如应激）；
- 外周葡萄糖利用率降低；

- 以术前的速度持续应用 10% 或 12.5% 葡萄糖液。

启示

低血糖

未识别的低血糖可导致神经损害，引起神经功能损伤的低血糖绝对值尚不清楚，但似乎与低血糖持续时间（以时间或天数计算）相关。大脑发育过程中葡萄糖代谢明显增加，与成年人大脑缺血不同的是,，新生儿的大脑能够使用其他底物如乳酸或糖原供能。

20 世纪 80 年代，葡萄糖液是婴幼儿术中常规应用的推荐液体。然而，出于高血糖发生风险越来越多的关注，大多数临床医师已避免常规使用葡萄糖液，除外新生儿、发育体型小于同龄的婴儿、有特殊问题的儿童。值得注意的是，对接受心脏直视手术的婴儿和儿童，大剂量的糖皮质激素、外源性儿茶酚胺、含糖血液制品的联合应用，这些患者静脉液体不再使用葡萄糖似乎与低血糖发生无关。

高血糖

对于非常小的新生儿，高血糖可引起多尿、脱水、电解质紊乱，可能增加脑出血发生率。对于成人，发生缺血或缺氧事件之前出现高血糖，可能增加神经损伤。有假设认为，不管是缺血还是缺氧，均会导致葡萄糖氧化代谢障碍和糖酵解增加，产生过量的乳酸。细胞内乳酸过量蓄积，细胞内 pH 降低，可能导致细胞功能受损或细胞死亡。

对新生儿，中至重度的高血糖可能通过几种机制保护大脑免受缺血性损伤，包括增加糖原储备、脑高能量储备、葡萄糖吸收及代谢较成人缓慢使得乳酸累积减缓，加快乳酸清除。小儿心脏手术期间，高血糖（若存在）对神经系统损伤尚不清楚。事实上，一项新生儿接受动脉调转手术研究发现，高血糖与远期神经性和发育性结局无必然联系。

高血糖与成人脓毒症患者的不良预后相关，对于脓毒症患儿的血糖控制并不明确，但大多数临床医师还是减少了脓毒症患儿术中 1/3 ～ 1/2 的 10% 或 12.5% 葡萄糖溶液输注。

管理

术中液体管理目标是提供适量的肠外液体（水和电解质）维持充足的血容量、心排血量、尿量，以及在某些情况下，提供充足的葡萄糖预防低血糖或减少围术期高血糖的发生。为避免术中发生低血糖或高血糖，一些学者建议使用 2.5% 的葡萄糖-乳酸林格液，同时给予其他无糖液体（例如，乳酸林格液或生理盐水）来补充血液和第三间隙的损失。由于 2.5% 葡萄糖-乳酸林格液尚无现成的商业成品，需要由医师或药剂师临时配制。血糖浓度监测可从中心静脉、动脉导管、指尖或足跟采血。血糖监测通常可以床旁完成，如果不行，则需要送至实验室检测血气结果，此外，还可以根据连续血糖监测结果来调整静脉葡萄糖用量。

预防

预防低血糖和高血糖，需要实施患者个体化的风险-效益分析。一些值得特别注意的事项如下：

- 关注低血糖或高血糖高风险的患者；
- 有发生低血糖风险的患者合理应用含糖溶液；
- 必要时应避免使用含糖溶液；
- 经常监测血糖浓度。

致谢

感谢 D. Ryan Cook 博士对本章上一版的贡献。

（李荣岩 译 薄禄龙 校）

延伸阅读

Aun CD, Panesar NS: Paediatric glucose homeostasis during anaesthesia, *Br J Anaesth* 64:413–418, 1990.

Datta PK, Pawar DK, Baidya DK, et al.: Dextrose-containing intraoperative fluid in neonates: a randomized controlled trial, *Pediatr Anesth* 26:599–607, 2016.

Ferranti SD, Gaureau K, Hickey PR, et al.: Intraoperative hyperglycemia during infant cardiac surgery is not associated with adverse neurodevelopmental outcomes at 1, 4, and 8 years, *Anesthesiology* 100:1345–1352, 2004.

Leelanukrom R, Cunliffe M: Intraoperative fluid and glucose management in children, *Paediatr Anaesth* 10:353–359, 2000.

Loepke AW, Spaeth JP: Glucose and heart surgery: neonates are not just small adults (editorial), *Anesthesiology* 100:1339–1340, 2004.

Pereira GR: Nutrition care of the extremely premature infant, *Clin Perinatol* 22:61–75, 1995.

Steven J, Nicolson S: Perioperative management of blood glucose during open heart surgery in infants and children, *Pediatr Anesth* 21:530–537, 2011.

Welborn LG, Hannallah RS, McGill WA, et al.: Glucose concentration in routine intravenous infusion in pediatric outpatient surgery, *Anesthesiology* 67:427–430, 1987.

Welborn LG, McGill WA, Hannallah RS, et al.: Perioperative blood glucose concentrations in pediatric outpatients, *Anesthesiology* 65:545–547, 1986.

小儿低体温

第 191 章

Barbara M. Dilos

病例概要

患儿，女性，3 月龄，孕 32 周时出生，现需要在镇静状态下接受脑部磁共振成像（magnetic resonance imaging，MRI）检查。女婴体重 4.2 kg，已禁食 6 h，目前没有服用任何药物。她接受了全身麻醉，MRI 在 1 h 内完成。完成检查被送入麻醉后恢复室后，发现她的体温是 35℃，很难苏醒并进食。

问题分析

定义

核心体温是生命体征，正常核心体温为 37 ± 0.2℃。当人体暴露在不同的环境温度下时，其核心体温可以在一定范围内保持稳定。但这样严密的体温调节系统容易被麻醉和手术破坏，特别是在儿科患者人群，最为常见的是新生患儿。最近的研究表明，年龄在 12 ～ 18 岁之间的大龄儿童发生术后低体温的风险也很大。这可能与对该年龄组所实施的手术类型有关，或可能由于年龄稍大，患儿对维持其正常体温所受到的关注有所减少。1 ～ 2℃的轻度体温降低常见于接受全身麻醉的儿科患者。在麻醉过程中维持核心–外周温度梯度是至关重要的，从而避免核心热量通过外周组织分布和丢失。新生儿患者因体温调节系统尚未成熟，对低体温非常易感，因其缺乏可以作为绝热体的皮下脂肪，且无法依靠寒战产热。

启示

麻醉期间与麻醉后低体温在儿科患者中会引起一系列紊乱。对于较大的儿童，术后寒战可使耗氧量增加 400% ～ 600%。低体温对酸碱平衡和麻醉药物的代谢有影响。它可以延长肌肉松弛剂的作用时间，降低吸入麻醉剂的最小肺泡浓度。低体温增加耗氧量，破坏凝血因子，并影响伤口愈合。轻度核心低体温已被证明可损害免疫系统功能，从而直接损害中性粒细胞功能。低体温也会引起血管收缩，进而产生组织缺氧，影响伤口愈合并导致伤口感染。轻度低体温与失血风险增加和输血发生率增加相关。在中重度病例中，低体温可导致心律失常。

识别

热量损失机制

散热的第一步是将热量从核心传递到外周。第二步是热量从外周（皮肤）传递到环境中。麻醉诱导后，第一小时内的核心温度通常下降 1.0 ～ 1.5℃。在婴儿中，热损失发生得更快，通常发生在第一个 10 min 内。婴儿和儿童发生低体温的风险更高，这主要是由于他们体表面积占比大，尤其是躯干和头部。为了防止麻醉后儿科患者出现低体温，我们必须了解在麻醉时，甚至在麻醉诱导前，儿科患者体温调节受影响的机制。影响儿科患者热量损失的四个因素为：辐射、对流、传导和蒸发。

辐射

辐射是两个不同温度物体之间的红外能量传递。能量从较热的物体转移到较冷的物体上。在儿科患者中，由于皮肤表面积相对其体重占比较大，辐射热的损失也成比例增加。辐射占儿科患者热损失的 39%。

对流

对流是由于空气分子在患者周围运动而产生的能量转移。如果患儿周围有冷空气流动，就会有更多的热量散失到环境中。对流与室外温度下的“寒风”效果相当。当患者躺在手术台上没有任何遮盖时，对流将造成30%的热量损失。

传导

传导是当物体相互接触时，热量从一个物体直接传递到另一个物体。例如，即使在麻醉诱导前，患者躺在冰冷的手术台上也会通过台面丧失热量。伤口或体腔中的冷冲洗液也会通过传导导致热量损失。静脉输注冷藏血液和制品也会通过传导产生热量损失的有害影响。

蒸发

蒸发是热量通过皮肤、体腔和手术切口散失到环境中造成的热量损失。蒸发损失的热量用于将液体转化为气体。开放性伤口，尤其是大的伤口，会因蒸发造成大量热量损失。例如，在腹裂畸形患儿中，即使在麻醉诱导前，蒸发热损失也是一个主要问题。

管理

麻醉期间的温度监测

体温调节是指身体尽管受环境因素影响仍保持正常体温的过程。在全身麻醉和区域麻醉期间，机体的体温调节机制受到破坏。此外，手术的应激加剧了这种破坏。因此，持续的体温监测非常重要，尤其是在儿科患者中，以便及时监测体温变化并积极解决出现的问题从而维持正常体温。美国麻醉科医师协会要求体温监测成为最低基本监测标准的一部分。

人体各个部位的体温是不一样的。核心温度通常比四肢高2～4℃，皮肤的温度甚至更低。Sessler认为，核心温度是人体体温状态的最佳监测指标。

麻醉期间，可在身体几个不同位置进行核心温度监测：

- 食管温度是通过食管探头在心脏后方的隆突水平上测量获得。儿童在食管和气管之间没有太多的隔热层，因此吸入气体的温度会对食管温度读数有影响。
- 鼻咽温度是通过经鼻探头在软腭水平测量获得。因其离大脑非常近，故而是测量核心温度的好方法。
- 鼓膜和肺动脉温度也被认为是核心温度。鼓膜非常靠近颈动脉和下丘脑。然而，这些位置并不容易监测。鼓膜温度探头有损伤鼓膜的危险，如果使用，必须覆盖外耳道，以防其中的空气流动导致读数不准确。耵聍也可能造成阻塞，导致温度读数不准确。
- 被认为接近核心温度的部位是直肠、膀胱、腋窝和口腔。只有当尿量足够时，膀胱温度才是准确的。
- 口腔温度取决于患者的合作度，并受摄入食物或饮料的温度影响。
- 皮肤温度是衡量体温最不可靠的指标。

热调节机制

众所周知，下丘脑是哺乳动物的主要体温调节系统，来自机体不同组织的信号被传输到下丘脑。处理这些信息有三种不同的方式：传入热感受器、中央调节和传出效应器。自主控制集中在下丘脑前部，行为控制如增减衣物和改变体位则集中在下丘脑后部。体温调节的中枢控制主要位于下丘脑。大多上行的热信号沿着前脊髓丘脑束传播，传出反应包括出汗、非寒战产热、寒战、血管扩张或血管收缩。自主神经控制包括前毛细血管扩张、四肢末梢动静脉分流处的血管收缩和寒战。非寒战产热是婴儿的主要反应。棕色脂肪组织被去甲肾上腺素转化为热量，其过程是去甲肾上腺素将一种蛋白质解偶联，产生有氧呼吸，进而产生热量。这种褐色脂肪组织存在于肾上腺、前纵隔和颈部的血管周围。因含有大量的线粒体故而颜色为浅棕色。由于婴儿和低龄儿童几乎没有寒战的能力，他们主要依靠非寒战产热来生成热量，非寒战产热可使婴儿产生的热量加倍。

寒战是一种肌肉活动，它通过增加代谢率来提高温度。在年龄较大的儿童和成人，当血管收缩不能维持正常体温时寒战开始发挥作用。

在提高核心温度方面，寒战并不像以前认为的那样有效。因为肌肉运动所需的血管扩张会与防止热量从外周流失所需的血管收缩相抵消。

麻醉和体温调控

全身麻醉和椎管内麻醉对儿科患者的体温调节有很大影响。全身麻醉完全消除了机体的行为性体温调节，并且麻醉药物可以引起剂量依赖性的血管收缩和寒战功能受损。挥发性麻醉药、静脉麻醉药和阿片类药物均无法触发机体体温调节防御机制，因此麻醉患者的核心温度波动幅度可达 4℃，而非麻醉患者仅有 0.2℃的波动。吸入麻醉药和静脉麻醉药（如丙泊酚）对非寒战产热有负面影响。全身麻醉可使代谢产热减少约 30%。全身麻醉诱导后，热量再分配进入第一阶段，即吸入麻醉剂引起血管扩张，核心温度随着热量散失到周围组织而下降。在第二阶段，由于代谢率降低而产热减少，从外周向环境散失的热量也增加。在第三阶段，产热超过散热，体温趋于稳定。

在椎管内麻醉期间，自主神经的阻断影响了体温调节。对同时接受全身麻醉和椎管内麻醉的儿科患者，体温调节效应不会相叠加。

预防

在儿科患者中，围术期体温管理极具挑战性，但必须非常积极地推进。对患者进行预热不会增加核心温度，但会增加外周温度，从而降低核心-外周组织间温度梯度。应在术中尽可能减小和阻止作为热量损失机制的辐射、对流、传导和蒸发的影响。

将手术室温度提高到 23℃或以上是防止小儿患者麻醉中出现低体温的理想选择。这可能会使外科医师感到不舒适，不过只要将患者准备好并铺单，就可以采用其他保温方法。

减少热量损失的方法主要是通过被动和主动加热。手术室温度对防止辐射和对流产生的热损失非常重要。被动加热是通过用绝热体（如棉床单或塑料罩）覆盖患者的暴露区域来完成的。

主动加热最常使用的是加压空气装置，由于外科手术需要更好的体表暴露，通常将这种装置放置于儿科患者身体下方。在过去，人们使用带有循环温水的床垫，然而它们并没有那么有效。此外，与床垫接触部位的组织因局部组织灌注减少加上热的叠加作用，会使患者易患压力性热坏死。

当快速输液时，将液体加热至 37℃非常重要。这相当于成年患者 1L/h 的速度。冲洗液也必须加热，以减少传导性热损失。给呼吸回路的空气加湿对于减少经气管支气管蒸发的热量损失也很重要。

对所有用于防止低体温的设备，使用时必须非常小心，以避免对患者组织（如皮肤或气道黏膜）造成热损伤。已有使用这些设备造成严重烧伤的报道，必须严格按照制造商的建议使用，不得擅自更改。在儿科患者中，预防和及时识别低体温至关重要，因为即使是轻微的低体温也能造成紊乱。关键是要尽一切可能预防低体温，而不是待发现低体温后再行升温。

（张程程　译　包　睿　校）

延伸阅读

Bissonnette B: Temperature monitoring in pediatric anesthesia, *Int Anesthesiol Clin* 30:63–76, 1992.

Dalal PG, Porath J, Parekh U, et al.: A quality improvement project to reduce hypothermia in infants undergoing MRI scanning, *Pediatr Radiol* 46:1187–1198, 2016.

De Witte J, Sessler DI: Perioperative shivering: physiology and pharmacology, *Anesthesiology* 96:467–484, 2002.

Görges M, West NC, Cheung W, et al.: Preoperative warming and undesired surgical and anesthesia outcomes in pediatric spinal surgery—a retrospective cohort study, *Paediatr Anaesth* 26:866–875, 2016.

Kim P, Taghon T, Fetzer M, et al.: Perioperative hypothermia in the pediatric population: a quality improvement project, *Am J Medl Qual* 28(5): 400–406, 2013.

Kurz A: Thermal care in the perioperative period, *Best Pract Res Clin Anaesthesiol* 22(1):39–62, 2008.

Pearce B, Christensen R, Voepel-Lewis T: Perioperative hypothermia in the pediatric population: prevalence, risk factors and outcomes, *J Anesth Clin Res* 1:102, 2010.

Sessler DI: Temperature monitoring and perioperative thermoregulation, *Anesthesiology* 109:318–338, 2008.

Sun Z, Honar H, Sessler DI, et al.: Intraoperative core temperature patterns, transfusion requirement, and hospital duration in patients warmed with forced air, *Anesthesiology* 122:276–285, 2015.

Torossian A: Thermal management during anaesthesia and thermoregulation standards for the prevention of inadvertent perioperative hypothermia, *Best Pract Res Clin Anaesth* 22(4):659–668, 2008.

第 192 章 小儿低氧血症

Lori A. Aronson，*Jennifer E. Lam*

病例概要

患儿，女性，5 岁，因反复感染继发腺样体扁桃体肥大在全身麻醉下行扁桃体和腺样体切除术，拔管后送至苏醒室。苏醒室护士汇报说患者出现喘鸣、肌肉回缩、发绀、心动过速，动脉氧饱和度（SpO_2）降至 60% 以下。

病例分析

定义

低氧血症指血液中氧浓度低于正常水平。低氧血症与**缺氧**不同，缺氧是一种组织氧供不足的状态，导致无法维持正常的细胞有氧代谢。年龄相关的动脉血氧分压正常值见表 192.1。血红蛋白对氧的亲和力随年龄增长而变化，从新生儿到成年其血红蛋白血氧蛋白饱和度逐渐变化，2,3- 二磷酸甘油酸酯（2,3-DPG）水平逐年降低（表 192.2）。

启示

根据 2013 年美国小儿围术期心脏停搏登记署（Pediatric Perioperative Cardiac Arrest，POCA）统计，27% 的患儿心搏骤停是呼吸系统原因所致，主要为喉痉挛，最常发作于术后恢复期。小儿术中低氧血症常与低龄相关（图 192.1）。患儿麻醉过程中需及时发现呼吸系统不良事件并及时处理低氧血症。

表 192.1　婴幼儿正常动脉氧分压（PaO_2）

年龄	PaO_2（mmHg）
早产儿	60
足月儿	70
1 月	95
1 岁	93
12 岁	98

表 192.2　年龄相关的血红蛋白氧饱和度（P50）

年龄	PaO_2（mmHg）[a]
新生儿	20
婴儿（>3 月）	30
成人（>18 岁）	27

[a] 成年前，新生儿氧亲和力最高，婴儿最低

识别

应用脉搏血氧仪监测氧饱和度已经成为术中标准监测，临床医师应能更早发现并处置患者的缺氧状态，提高患者麻醉的安全性。脉搏血氧监测可有效地监测患者的氧合状态，但仅在未吸氧的情况下评估患者的通气功能，即使少量吸氧也会减轻 PaO_2 下降程度，从而掩盖患者通气不足（$PaCO_2$ 升高），因此监测二氧化碳同样重要（图 192.2）。

低氧血症的临床表现随年龄而变化，也必须加以识别。早产儿和新生儿对低氧血症的反应表现为呼吸抑制、心动过缓；而婴幼儿对低氧血症的反应表现为呼吸急促伴心动过速或心动过缓；其他更为普通的临床体征包括发绀、苍白、烦躁不安、精神状态改变等，麻醉状态下大多症状被掩盖。上呼吸道梗阻的体征包括喘鸣、呼噜音、肌肉回缩、鼻翼扩张、呼吸困难、无气体运动的通气努力等；下呼吸道梗阻的体征包括喘息、肺部啰音、呼吸音降低等；上下呼吸道梗阻都会导致气流不畅，难以鉴别。

低氧血症的病因确定，对制定治疗策略至关重要，必须采取系统性的方法确定病因。除体格检查外，在实验室检查前还可采取“从墙壁到肺泡”的方法评估供氧装置、麻醉机及回路以及气道。此外，

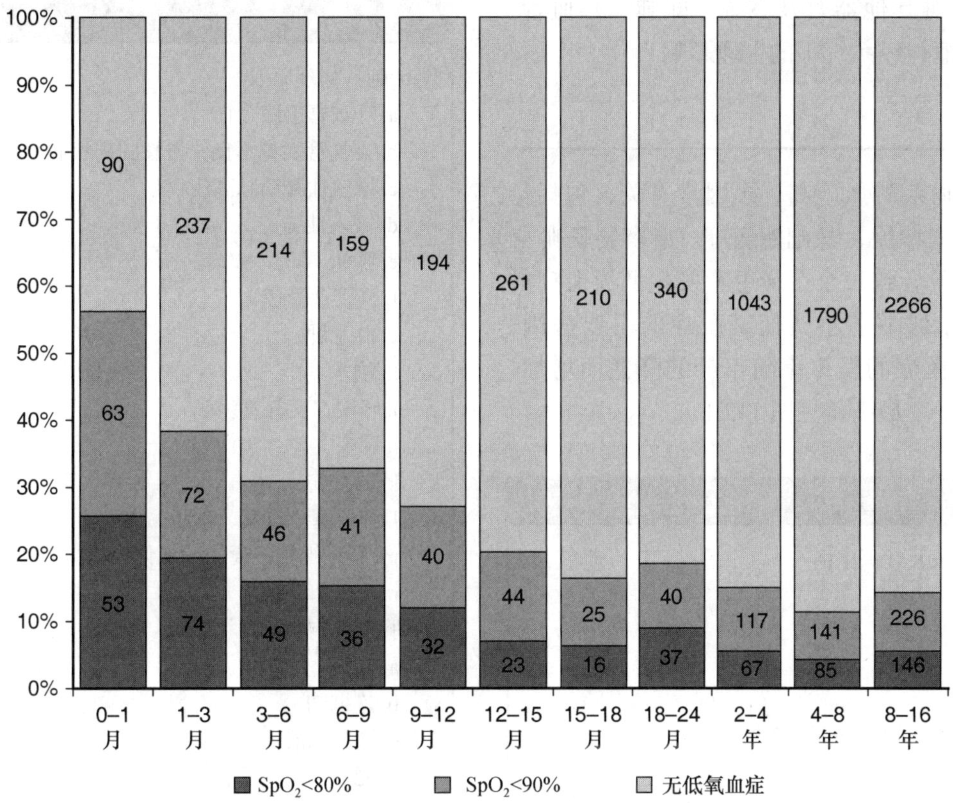

图 192.1 儿童术中低氧血症发生率与年龄关系。回顾队列研究：至少发生 1 次持续 1 min 以上低氧血症病例数占各年龄组的百分比（*n*=8277）（From de Graaff JC，Bijker JB，Kappen TH，et al：Incidence of intraoperative hypoxemia in children in relation to age. *Anesth Analg* 117[1]：169-175，2013.）

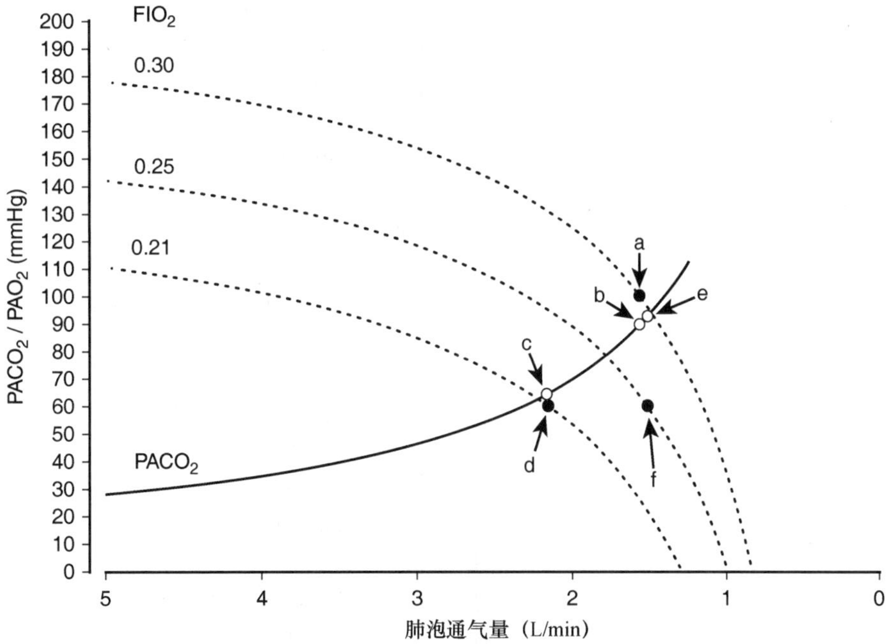

图 192.2 补充 O_2 对 PaO_2 及 $PaCO_2$ 的影响。FiO_2 对肺泡通气量影响建模（气血交换系数 0.8，无生理性分流，生命体征平稳），PaO_2 闭合虚线；$PaCO_2$ 开放实线。FiO_2=0.3，$PaCO_2$ 90 mmHg（b）时，PaO_2 100 mmHg（a）。FiO_2=0.21，$PaCO_2$ 65 mmHg（c） 时，PaO_2 60 mmHg（d）。FiO_2=0.25，$PaCO_2$ 100 mmHg（e） 时，PaO_2 60 mmHg（f）（From Fu ES，Downs JB，Schweiger JW，et al：Supplemental oxygen impairs detection of hypoventilation by pulse oximetry. *Chest* 126[5]：1552-1558，2004.）

还应评估低氧对其他器官及系统（即肺、心血管、血液系统及中枢神经系统）的生理影响。

风险评估

小儿低氧血症的风险与许多因素有关，包括年龄、解剖及生理特征、基础疾病等。麻醉科医师必须评估这些风险导致每个个体患者发生低氧血症的程度。框 192.1 列举了小儿低氧血症的主要病因。事实上，低氧血症的发生率随年龄的降低而增加，在新生儿中发生率最高（见图 192.1）。

框 192.1　小儿低氧血症常见病因

Ⅰ. 中枢神经系统及呼吸中枢
- a. 窒息
- b. 颅脑外伤
- c. 脑肿瘤
- d. 癫痫
- e. 大脑髓质灌注损伤 / 颅内高压
- f. 麻醉药物
  - 1. 阿片药物过量
  - 2. 吸入麻醉药
  - 3. 巴比妥类，其他镇静药
  - 4. 联合用药

Ⅱ. 呼吸道
- a. 会厌炎，格鲁布性喉头炎
- b. 气管软化，喉软骨软化病
- c. 咽后脓肿
- d. 血管环
- e. 小儿喘鸣
- f. 喉痉挛
- g. 淋巴系统疾病
- h. 纵隔肿瘤
- i. 异物，气管导管堵塞
- j. 气管灼伤（烧伤）
- k. 声门下狭窄
- l. 上呼吸道感染

Ⅲ. 呼吸肌
- a. 残余神经肌肉阻滞
- b. 衰弱 / 营养不良
- c. 重症肌无力
- d. 肌肉萎缩症
- e. 膈神经损伤
- b. 气管导管弯曲

Ⅳ a. 肺：生理原因
- a. V/Q 比例失调
  - 1. 分流
  - 2. 死腔通气
- b. 弥散障碍（少见）

框 192.1　小儿低氧血症常见病因

Ⅳ b. 肺：病理原因
- a. 呼吸窘迫综合征
- b. 支气管发育不良，慢性肺部疾病
- c. 原发性肺动脉高压
- d. 吸入性肺炎
- e. 膈疝
- f. 气管食管瘘
- g. 肺水肿
- h. 溺水
- i. 哮喘，支气管痉挛
- j. 肺炎
- k. 肺挫伤
- l. 肺栓塞（空气、脂肪、血栓）
- m. 肺纤维化，囊性纤维化
- n. 支气管扩张

Ⅴ. 胸壁及胸膜
- a. 气胸
- b. 连枷胸
- c. 胸膜积液
- d. 肥胖
- e. 脊柱侧弯
- f. 腹部肿块

Ⅵ. 心血管
- a. 先天性心脏病
- b. 充血性心力衰竭
- c. 动静脉畸形
- d. 低血容量，出血

Ⅶ. 血液系统
- a. 贫血
- b. 镰状细胞贫血
- c. 地中海贫血

Ⅷ. 氧供
- a. 气管插管误入一侧主支气管
- c. FiO_2 降低，低氧气体混合
- d. 呼吸机脱开
- e. 麻醉机故障
- f. 气管导管误入食管

Ⅸ. 氧耗增加
- a. 寒战（低体温）
- b. 持续高热（脓毒症）
- c. 恶性高热
- d. 甲状腺功能亢进

Ⅹ. 其他方面
- a. 体位
- b. 一氧化碳中毒
- c. 氰化物中毒（硝普钠过量）
- d. 肝功能衰竭

了解婴幼儿独特的解剖结构和生理特征对麻醉管理至关重要，包括以下内容：

解剖结构

- 婴头部相对较大，颈部较短，舌体较大，使得上呼吸道易发生梗阻。因此垫高肩部可有益处。此外婴儿扁桃体较大，进一步容易导致呼吸道梗阻。
- 婴儿颈部（C3 ～ C4 椎体）高于成人（C4 ～ C5 椎体），喉部更靠前，声带更偏向头部，气管导管（ETT）尖端角度更大。此外，由于婴儿会厌组织松软、肥大，直片喉镜更加适用于气管插管。
- 婴儿气道解剖最狭窄部位是喉部，功能上最狭窄部位是环状软骨。婴儿气道上皮容易损伤，气管插管时需选择大小合适的 ETT。
- 婴儿气管较成人短，两侧主支气管分叉角度几乎相同（约 45°），气管内插管时避免误入一侧主支气管。成人右主支气管分叉角度（约 30°）小于左主支气管，因此较大的儿童和成人气管内插管时误入右主支气管风险较高。
- 婴儿喉部、气管和支气管顺应性强，容易因扩张、受压，导致气道动态塌陷（喉软化、气管软化、支气管软化）。胸外气管在梗阻部位以下的气管塌陷时常伴有吸气性喘鸣音。患有气道高反应性疾病的婴儿常可导致严重胸内气管塌陷。
- 新生儿胸壁顺应性强，吸气时常向内凹陷。肋骨角度更平，进一步限制吸气时胸部扩张。因此婴儿在吸气时常依赖其腹部肌肉。
- 婴儿腹胀（过度的正压通气或哭闹）明显阻碍膈肌运动。
- 新生儿肺部发育不完善，肺泡数量在 3 周岁时达成人水平，但肺泡大小持续发育至 7 ～ 8 周岁。某些新生儿疾病使气道成分减少或表面活性物质分泌不足，导致肺泡塌陷、顺应性降低和低氧血症。

生理功能

- 由于呼吸系统发育不完善，婴儿及新生儿低氧血症首先表现为短暂的呼吸急促，随后呼吸抑制。婴儿膈肌和肋间肌 I 型纤维较少，容易出现呼吸疲劳、缺氧和低氧血症。此外，由于呼吸与口咽活动及感觉传入发育不成熟，使得婴幼儿只能经鼻强制呼吸。
- 足月儿和早产儿出现周期性呼吸（呼吸暂停持续 ≤ 10 s）是正常现象，12 月龄后发生率明显下降。
- 婴儿呼吸暂停（呼吸暂停超过 20 s，或低于 20 s 并伴有心动过缓、发绀、苍白或肌张力减退）可分为中央性、梗阻性或混合性，较多常见于早产儿。孕妇初潮过早、怀孕年龄过小、贫血是新生儿术后呼吸暂停的高危因素。
- 婴儿耗氧量和肺泡通气量是成人的 2 倍 [7 ml/（kg · min）vs. 4 ml/（kg · min），130 ml/（kg · min）vs. 60 ml/（kg · min）]，然而功能残气量只有成人的一半（25 ml/kg vs. 40 ml/kg）。婴儿肺闭合容量较成人大，呼吸频率较快。婴幼儿氧气储备有限，所以耗氧量增加后，低氧血症很快发生。
- 新生儿出生时随着呼吸开始及脐带血管夹闭，肺血管阻力（pulmonary vasculature resistance，PVR）降低，全身血管阻力（systemic vasculature resistance，SVR）增加，导致卵圆孔功能性闭合，动脉导管分流逆转。在卵圆孔和动脉导管解剖闭合前，婴儿在酸中毒、缺氧、高碳酸血症或低血压情况下易继发血液循环逆转及低氧血症。
- 先天性心脏病血液右向左分流引起 PVR 及 SVR 失衡易导致低氧血症。真性右向左分流型患儿随着 SpO_2 增加对氧气无反应。此外，充血性心力衰竭也易导致低氧血症。
- 新生儿通过增加血红蛋白水平、血容量及心排血量代偿胎儿血红蛋白对氧的高亲和力（FiO_2 不变的情况下，组织释放氧较少）。3 ～ 6 月龄时胎儿血红蛋白向成人血红蛋白转变过程中会导致生理性贫血。新生儿通过代偿性增加 2，3-DPG，氧离曲线右移，提高组织氧供。10 ～ 12 周岁后，2,3-DPG 降至成人水平，氧离曲线稍左移（表 192.2）。

管理

低氧血症的初始处理通过旨在提高 FiO_2 至 1.0 改善氧合，保持呼吸道通畅改善通气。可采用气囊面罩通气、口咽或鼻咽通气道、喉面罩气道、气管插管、环甲膜切开或气管切开保持呼吸道通畅。由于婴幼儿的解剖特点，合适的通气设备及最佳插管体位可有利于气道管理：垫高肩部对于优化喉部视野很有必要，口咽通气道可缓解梗阻，新生儿和婴儿气管插管首选直片喉镜。

进一步治疗则是纠正低氧血症的潜在病因。快速诊断病因可及时逆转低氧血症，避免进一步并发症。持续低氧血症可能需要高级生命支持。

预防

低氧血症及其不良预后的预防始于对患者的全面评估，熟知抢救预案，并在麻醉和手术前检查所有设备。术前评估包括了解患者的急慢性病史、是否急诊手术以及手术风险，确定术前进一步治疗能否降低患者风险。

降低低氧血症发生率的麻醉操作包括：合适的体位，气管插管和拔管前适当预充氧气或去氮气，拔管之前拮抗神经肌肉阻滞药物，婴儿和新生儿谨慎应用阿片类镇痛药，咖啡因易导致早产儿呼吸暂停，麻醉维持和术后转运阶段给患者吸氧，避免寒战，应用脉搏血氧仪、二氧化碳监测及 FiO_2 监测仪等设备提高患者麻醉安全性。尽管麻醉科医师术中密切监护，严重低氧血症仍有可能发生，及早发现和治疗低氧血症，可以最大程度降低不良预后。

（谢 韬 译 吴 倩 校）

延伸阅读

Adewale L: Anatomy and assessment of the pediatric airway, *Pediatr Anesth* 19(Suppl 1):1–8, 2009.

American Academy of Pediatrics: Committee on Fetus and Newborn: Apnea, sudden infant death syndrome, and home monitoring, *Pediatrics* 111: 914–917, 2003.

Bhananker SM, Ramamoorthy C: Anesthesia-related cardiac arrest in children: update from the Pediatric Perioperative Cardiac Arrest Registry, *Anesth Analg* 105:344–350, 2007.

Coté CJ, Zaslavsky A, Downes JJ, et al.: Postoperative apnea in former preterm infants after inguinal herniorrhaphy. A combined analysis, *Anesthesiology* 82:809–822, 1995.

Davidson JA, Hosie HE: Limitations of pulse oximetry: respiratory insufficiency—a failure of detection, *Brit Med J* 307:372–373, 1993.

de Graaff JC, Bijker JB, Kappen TH, et al.: Incidence of intraoperative hypoxemia in children in relation to age, *Anesth Analg* 117:169–175, 2013.

Fu ES, Downs JB, Schweiger JW, et al.: Supplemental oxygen impairs detection of hypoventilation by pulse oximetry, *Chest* 126:1552–1558, 2004.

Givan DC: Physiology of breathing and related pathological processes in infants, *Semin Pediatr Neurol* 10:271–280, 2003.

Keidan I, Gravenstein D, Berkenstadt H, et al.: Supplemental oxygen compromises the use of pulse oximetry for detection of apnea and hypoventilation during sedation in simulated pediatric patients, *Pediatrics* 122:293–298, 2008.

Kurth CD, LeBard SE: Association of postoperative apnea, airway obstruction, and hypoxemia in former premature infants, *Anesthesiology* 75:22–26, 1991.

Litman RS, Weissend EE, Shibata D, Westesson PL: Developmental changes of laryngeal dimensions in unparalyzed, sedated children, *Anesthesiology* 98:41–45, 2003.

Motoyama EK, Finder JD: Respiratory physiology in infants and children. In Davis PJ, Cladis FP, Motoyoma EK, editors: *Smith's anesthesia for infants and children*, ed 8, Philadelphia, 2011, Elsevier, pp 22–79.

Pang LM, Mellins RB: Neonatal cardiorespiratory physiology, *Anesthesiology* 43:171–196, 1975.

Welborn LG, Hannallah RS, Luban NL, et al.: Anemia and postoperative apnea in former preterm infants, *Anesthesiology* 74:1003–1006, 1991.

小儿术中心脏停搏　第193章

Lizabeth D. Martin，Jeremy M. Geiduschek

病例概要

患儿，9个月，美国麻醉科医师协会（ASA）Ⅱ级，在2.5%七氟烷复合氧及芬太尼全身麻醉下行颅缝早闭症修复术。患儿气管插管位置良好，并固定于凝胶卷上。颅骨切除期间，心电图（electrocardiogram，ECG）波形显示心动过速，动脉波形表现为新发低血压，脉搏氧饱和度和呼气末二氧化碳波形消失，未触及脉搏。

问题分析

定义

术中心脏停搏被定义为需启动心肺复苏（cardiopulmonary resuscitation，CPR）或判定为死亡的情况。通常为意外事件，尽管在处理危重患者时可以预见。当可触及的脉搏和可测得的血压消失时，或当脉搏可触及，但心排血量不足以提供器官灌注（例如，婴儿心动过缓心率<60次/分）时应实施CPR。

识别

麻醉下患者病情恶化的早期体征通常可经电子监测信号检测到。不幸的是，电子监护仪报警可能因多种原因错误地激活。尽管如此，当报警响起时，在将报警归因于伪像干扰前必须对患者进行评估。脉搏氧饱和度信号消失、二氧化碳波形突然消失或波幅减小或测不到血压可能表示即将发生心脏停搏。

风险评估

所有接受麻醉的患者都有术中心脏停搏的风险。1954年，Beecher和Todd报道，与成人相比，小儿麻醉的病残率较高。1961年，Rackow及其同事报道，这一增高现象是由于小于1岁的麻醉幼儿心脏停搏发生率较高。1988—1990年间发表的瑞典、法国和加拿大的后续研究进一步支持了这一发现。小儿围术期心脏停搏（pediatric perioperative cardiac arrest，POCA）数据登记库已成为该主题近期数据的主要来源。一项193例麻醉相关心脏停搏的综述提示，与早期数据相比，ASA Ⅰ级患者和年龄小于1岁的患者心脏停搏的比例相应减少。这可能与小儿麻醉中氟烷使用减少有关，伴随着挥发性麻醉药所致的心血管抑制相关的病例较少。

POCA最终更新数据是对397例围术期心脏停搏的回顾分析，其中193例（49%）判定为与麻醉管理有关。心血管系统（41%）和呼吸系统（27%）的病因最常见，合计占所有心脏停搏的68%。明确的最常见的单一病因是与血液丢失有关的低血容量，主要发生于脊柱融合术或开颅术中。麻醉维持期间，50%的心脏停搏是由于心血管病因，术后阶段50%的心脏停搏是呼吸因素。常见的呼吸系统病因包括喉痉挛、支气管痉挛、缺氧/通气不足和过早拔管。只有4例（1%）心脏停搏归因于困难插管。在发生心脏停搏的患者中，28%死亡，5%受到永久性损害，61%无后遗症。ASA Ⅲ～Ⅴ级和急诊手术与死亡率升高有关。年龄不是死亡率的危险因素。心脏病患儿心脏停搏分析显示死亡率较高（33%与23%）。单心室是先天性心脏病患儿中罹患麻醉相关心脏停搏最常见的病变（19%）。

管理

心脏停搏前

早期识别和干预心脏停搏至关重要，因为延误治疗可导致严重的病残和死亡。住院小儿心脏停搏延误使用肾上腺素与存活率降低和神经系统不良预后相关。

多年来，紧急状况模拟已被用于高度可靠的机构如航空和核能，直到最近才用于医学。在 2003 年的声明中，国际复苏委员会建议培训包括采用人体模型和训练模块及经常更新的课程进行更多的动手实践。模拟手术室心脏停搏可使团队实践强调高质量心肺复苏的美国心脏协会共识建议（特别是胸外按压的足够深度和频率，以及减少按压的中断）和早期除颤。用以改善培训的操作系统应确保及时获取设备，实时反馈可改善心脏停搏的结果。所有工作人员必须了解抢救车和除颤仪的位置以及如何使用它们。

心脏停搏中

突发的心脏停搏（如病例中描述的情况）最好采用正规预案处理危及生命的事件。麻醉科医师应遵循最新的小儿高级生命支持（pediatric advanced life support，PALS）方案。

Ⅰ. 沟通与团队协作

- 保持冷静和专注。
- 保持与术中团队的良好沟通（医师、护士、技师）。清楚地解释你在监护仪上看到的内容和患者的生命体征。询问最近是否存在可以解释患者血流动力学的突然恶化的操作。用语言向团队说明情况；例如，“这是心脏停搏；患者处于无脉电活动（pulseless electrical activity，PEA）中。”
- 尽早呼叫帮助。应配备有呼叫系统并可迅速获得帮助。了解该系统如何在每个位置运作非常重要。例如墙上的“抢救”按钮或内部紧急电话系统。
- 需要麻醉和手术护理团队全体成员有序地应答以增加患者获得良好预后的机会。必须指定的角色包括：①团队负责人（指导复苏工作，但不承担任何具体任务）；②气道管理者（负责用 100% 氧手控通气和气管插管）；③被指定实施胸外按压的人；④确认专用静脉（IV）通道和给药的人（根据 PALS 指南）；⑤授权负责抢救车和除颤仪的人；⑥提供事件书面记录的记录员。大多数麻醉记录单不是设计用于全面记录心脏停搏期间的事件和治疗。即便有电子麻醉记录，推荐在单独的标准化表格上手动记录术中心脏骤停，以便清楚地记录事件的顺序和时间，并在之后可以进行清楚的回顾（图 193.1）。
- 团队负责人在控制外部响应者进入正在进行的抢救方面发挥着重要作用，确保所有指定的抢救角色有人担任，优先处理和指导团队行动，对现场状况保持清醒，并向团队成员提供有关复苏方案的明确指示。当恐慌、无序和随时缺乏领导力时，必须要有这样的人存在。
- 人员因素如培训和领导技能有助于团队实施高质量的 CPR，具有更好的技术性能、更短的休克前处理中断和更早的除颤。

Ⅱ. PALS：建立循环、气道以和呼吸

- 评估循环，低龄儿童和婴儿的肱动脉或股动脉搏动是可靠的部位，而较大龄儿童和青少年的颈动脉搏动最佳。
- 如无脉搏，立即开始高质量胸外按压。限制胸外按压的中断。研究表明，除颤之前和除颤过程中持续和充分的心脏按压可大大提高自主循环恢复的可能性。
- 关闭麻醉药，经手控通气给予 100% 氧气。
- 给患者手控通气时，通过听诊器听诊呼吸音评估气道通畅情况。
- 如果尚未建立气道，应予以气管插管。
- 准备好急救车和除颤仪。放置除颤电极板和除颤器充电期间应持续高质量胸外按压。按压停顿超过 10 s 与除颤成功率降低相关。
- 呼气末二氧化碳监测、按压节拍声和压力感应反馈装置可用于改善心肺复苏期间胸外按压的时间和质量。
- 根据心电图判断心脏节律。
- 根据当前的 PALS 方案治疗心律失常。
- 如果静脉通道不佳或 90 s 后仍无法建立，则必须放置骨内针（图 193.2），用于给予急救

抢救记录单188

日期__________

心脏停搏地点__________

心脏停搏估计时间__________

发现者__________

观察到心脏停搏 ❐ 是 ❐ 否

心肺复苏开始时间__________

心脏停搏的初始体征：
- ❐ 呼吸停顿
- ❐ 心动过缓
- ❐ 发绀/氧饱和度低下
- ❐ 低血压
- ❐ 无脉搏
- ❐ 其他__________

体重：

心脏停搏前的病史：

初始心律：

静脉通道	部位	在原位	抢救期间	放置时间
外周：				
中心：				

气道

通气：气囊/面罩______时间______

插管：经口______经鼻______

导管尺寸______时间______

插管和固定

经__________确认

经鼻胃管插入和固定

经__________确认

签字：

负责医师__________

用药注册护士__________

记录注册护士__________

	生命体征								其他				药物剂量路径						输注							
	心肺复苏（是否）	心率	心律	血压/平均压	脉搏（有无）	氧饱和度	通气频率	体温	除颤（同步、功率）	心内或心外起搏（速率、毫安）	血气\实验室检查送检	血糖\化学检查试剂片	肾上腺素	阿托品	碳酸氢钠（浓度）	利多卡因			多巴胺___mg/___ml	肾上腺素___mg/___ml	利多卡因___mg/___ml	___mg/___ml	___mg/___ml	平衡液\生理盐水	血制品	患者的反应： • 实验室结果 • 操作（导尿、腹腔穿刺、胸部X线） • 外观/活动度（颜色、精神状态、神经系统检查、瞳孔、癫痫等） • 尿量
时间			circle one							circle one			Include mg, μg, mEg/IV, ET, IO						Include μg/kg/min or mL/hr/totals							

图 193.1 用于心脏停搏（术中或其他）的标准化机构记录单样表。可用于大多数医疗紧急情况，其中有频繁的干预和给药情况

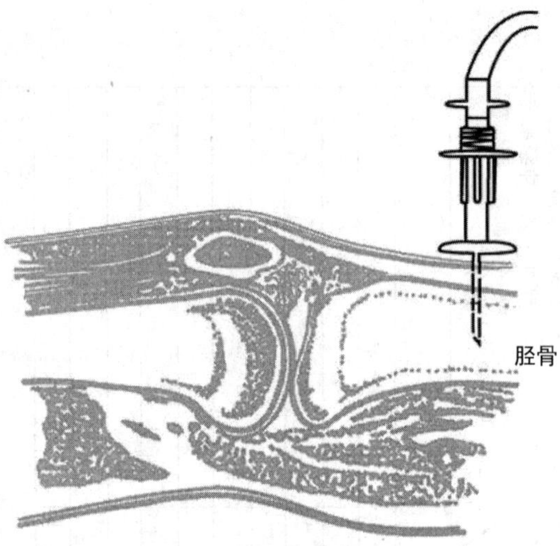

图 193.2 带有电池供电动力驱动的骨内血管通路系统的示例。骨内针可插入胫骨进行液体和药物治疗。穿刺点位于胫骨表面平坦部分的胫骨内侧结节远端约 2.5 cm（1 英寸）处，针与骨表面成直角定向。其他可穿刺部位包括胫骨远端和股骨远端。应注意防止插入骨髓以外。穿刺期间，不用于推动针前行的手应抓住针插入点远端的腿，尽量减少操作者受伤的可能。由于针头移位和筋膜间隙综合征的风险，应定期评估穿刺部位

药物和快速输液，包括输血。早期应用肾上腺素可以挽救生命。

Ⅲ. PALS：评估潜在病因

对气道、呼吸和循环进行评估并实施相应的治疗后，必须要关注心脏停搏的原因判断。气管插管患者始终要考虑张力性气胸。如果有怀疑，用针进行左侧和右侧胸腔穿刺术。胸部 X 线片可能有帮助，应在复苏期间尽早申请。床旁超声是一种新兴技术，有助于气胸的诊断。

尽快抽血行实验室检查，包括动脉血气、电解质（钠、钾、氯、碳酸氢盐、钙）、血糖和红细胞比容。

CPR 的持续时间根据每例患者的具体情况处理。无法重建灌注应提出以下问题：

- 所有麻醉药都停了吗？
- 是否正确实施了 CPR？
- 所有团队角色是否就位并正有效开展工作？
- 患者是否存在导致心脏停搏的潜在问题？
- 患者是否因液体或血液丢失产生严重低血容量？
- 患者是否有过敏反应？
- 患者是否有张力性气胸？
- 患者是否有心脏压塞？
- 患者是否低体温？
- 是否存在用药过量或错误用药？

如果灌注恢复后再次丢失，考虑以下医源性原因：

- 与闭合心脏按压有关的创伤，包括肋骨骨折所致的气胸或肝脾破裂。
- 尝试建立中心静脉通路或机械通气过度充气引起的气胸或血胸。
- 心包压塞（如果存在给予心内药物或血管导管置入右心房的情况）。

心脏停搏后

复苏后，执行以下事项极其重要：

- 使用家属能理解的语言与家属讨论这一意外事件。解释已知的情况，但如果病因不确定不妄加推测。告知家属接下来将发生的情况。
- 允许家属提问。
- 允许家属单独或与指定的辅助人员一起表达悲痛。
- 如果需要进行调查，应隔离设备和废弃材料（尤其是开封的药瓶）。
- 不重复使用设备（包括麻醉机），除非已明确术中心脏停搏的原因。
- 在医疗记录中描述整个事件。
- 如果患者意外死亡，大多数情况下应通知验尸员。
- 向抢救团队汇报。确保团队成员获得情感支持。术中突发心脏停搏伴不良结局对抢救团队成员以及患者家人和朋友来说都是情感上的重大打击。
- 通知机构的风险管理办公室。

预防

许多小儿术中心脏停搏是由患者的基础病情决定的，这些病情可能不易逆转。其他原因可能源于多种因素，包括人为错误、判断错误或警惕性不足、设备故障和原因不明事件。对于许多麻醉中患儿心脏停搏明确的原因而言，警惕性和预防措施可降低其发生率。术中心脏停搏发生前及早发现问题并采取纠治性干预措施逆转患者病情的进一步恶化可降低严重疾病或死亡的发生率。

（姜 静 译 朱文忠 校）

延伸阅读

Anderson L, Berg K, Saindon B, et al.: American Heart Association Get with the Guidelines—Resuscitation Investigators. Time to epinephrine and survival after pediatric in-hospital cardiac arrest, *JAMA* 314(8):802–810, 2015.

Bahananker S, Ramamoorthy C, Geiduschek J, et al.: Anesthesia-related cardiac arrest in children: update from the Pediatric Perioperative Cardiac Arrest Registry, *Anesth Analg* 105:344–350, 2007.

Becker LB, Aufderheide TP, Graham R: Strategies to improve survival from cardiac arrest: a report from the Institute of Medicine, *JAMA* 314(3):223–224, 2015.

Beecher HK, Todd DP: A study of deaths associated with anesthesia and surgery, *Ann Surg* 140:1–35, 1954.

Chamberlain DA, Hazinski MF, et al.: Education in resuscitation, *Resuscitation* 59:11–43, 2003.

Cohen MM, Cameron CB, Duncan PG, et al.: Pediatric anesthesia morbidity and mortality in the perioperative period, *Anesth Analg* 70:160–167, 1990.

Gaba DM, Fish KJ, Howard SK, et al.: *Crisis management in anesthesiology*, New York, 1994, Churchill Livingstone.

Hazinski MF, editor: *Pediatric advanced life support provider manual*, American Academy of Pediatrics–American Heart Association, 2011.

Ollson GL, Hallen B: Cardiac arrest during anesthesia. A computerized study in 250,543 anesthetics, *Acta Anaesthesiol Scand* 32:653–664, 1988.

Morray JP: Cardiac arrest in anesthetized children: recent advances and challenges for the future, *Pediatr Anesth* 21:722–729, 2011.

Morray JP, Geiduschek JM, Ramamoorthy C, et al.: Anesthesia-related cardiac arrest in children: Initial findings of the Pediatric Perioperative Cardiac Arrest (POCA) Registry, *Anesthesiology* 93:6–14, 2000.

Morrison L, Neumar R, Zimmerman J, et al.: Strategies for improving survival after in-hospital cardiac arrest in the United States: 2013 consensus recommendations, *Circulation* 127:1539–1563, 2013.

Rackow H, Salatire E, Green LT: Frequency of cardiac arrest associated with anesthesia in infants and children, *Pediatrics* 28:697–704, 1961.

Ramamoorthy C, Haberkern C, Bhananker S, et al.: Anesthesia-related cardiac arrest in children with heart disease: data from the Pediatric Perioperative Cardiac Arrest (POCA) Registry, *Anesth Analg* 110:1376–1382, 2010.

Steen S, Liao Q, Pierre L, et al.: The critical importance of minimal delay between chest compressions and subsequent defibrillation: a haemodynamic explanation, *Resuscitation* 3:249–258, 2003.

Tiret L, Nivochey Y, Hatton F, et al.: Complications related to anesthesia in infants and children, *Br J Anaesth* 61:263–269, 1988.

Weick KE, Sutcliffe KM: *Managing the unexpected: assuring high performance in an age of complexity*, San Francisco, Jossey-Bass, 2001.

第 194 章 乳胶变态反应

Mahmoud I. Wagih

病例概要

患者，女性，25 岁，有脊柱裂病史，经耻骨上导管行膀胱软镜检查。既往接受过数次泌尿生殖系统手术，并且十年来一直自行导尿。麻醉诱导和气管插管后均非常顺利，20 min 后患者氧饱和度开始下降，躯干上满布皮疹，但血压一直维持在诱导前的水平。

问题分析

定义

乳胶采集于橡胶树（*hevea brasiliensis*）。从乳胶中可分离出 200 多种多肽。蛋白质含量随产地和生产工艺的不同差异很大。从马来西亚、印度尼西亚、泰国和南美洲新鲜收割乳胶，经过氨和其他防腐剂的处理，防止在运输过程中变质。Halstead 于 1890 年首次使用乳胶外科手套。一个世纪以来，由于人们认识到人类免疫缺陷病毒和其他血源性病原体对医护人员具有传染风险，乳胶手套的使用量因此急剧增加。乳胶是麻醉过程中引起过敏反应的第二大常见原因。1984 年，Turjanmaa 及同事报道了第一例与乳胶相关的术中过敏反应。到 1996 年，乳胶大约占麻醉后过敏反应的 20%；据悉截止到 2000 年，乳胶导致的过敏反应在所有人群中占 17%，在小儿中占 27% ～ 76%。

皮肤和黏膜是乳胶抗原进入人体最常见的途径。除此之外，当采用玉米淀粉作为手套润滑剂时，淀粉粉末可存在于空气中长达 5 h，乳胶蛋白附着于其上并随之沉积在呼吸道中。其他的暴露途径包括导尿管、止血带、注射器的橡胶活塞，药瓶的橡胶帽以及静脉导管等。伤口接种、摄入及静脉注射也可能是暴露途径。

乳胶过敏可在临床和免疫学上表现为两种不同的反应（可同时存在）：即Ⅰ型超敏反应（过敏反应）和Ⅳ型超敏反应（接触性皮炎）。刺激性皮炎是一种非免疫介导的乳胶反应。

乳胶过敏的病理生理学过程始于医疗或非医疗情况下与乳胶的首次接触。在人体再次接触乳胶时，抗原与效应细胞、肥大细胞和嗜碱性粒细胞上的特异性免疫球蛋白 E（immunoglobulin E，IgE）发生交联，释放胞内的过敏介质，如组胺、类胰蛋白酶和羧肽酶 A（早期介质），再激活下游的磷脂酶 A2（phopholipase A2，PLA2），继而激活环氧酶和脂加氧酶，产生前列腺素、白三烯、细胞因子（IL-4、IL-13 和肿瘤坏死因子 α）等晚期介质（表 194.1）。

识别

现在的麻醉过程中，大量药物的使用增加了诊断的难度，特别是最近的证据否定了以往认为的乳胶与引起过敏反应的药物之间存在时间轴的说法。

法国过敏反应研究组（Groupe d'Etudes des Réactions Anaphylactoïdes Peranesthésiques，GERAP）调查了 467 例麻醉过程中发生过敏反应的相关病例，其中特应性皮炎 121 例（25.4%），哮喘 41 例（8.6%）。发病率随年龄的增长而逐渐增加，女性 40 岁、男性 50 岁是发病高峰。女性患者占过敏反应病例的 74%。血管性水肿均是伴发的临床特征，不会单独出现。近 10% 的病例出现了心脏停搏。有支气管哮喘病史或使用 β 受体阻滞剂的患者常出现支气管痉挛。过去 15 年中乳胶过敏的发病率持续下降，与其他原因引起的过敏反应相比，乳胶过敏的临床表现较为温和，且预后良好。

麻醉过程中过敏反应的临床表现如下：

- 低血压或循环衰竭（75%）；

表 194.1 过敏反应的介质

介质	效应
组胺	H1：促进黏液分泌，组织水肿，心脏抑制，冠状动脉收缩，肾素释放 H2：促进胃酸分泌，诱导 NO 合成，扩张血管，心动过速 H3：降低去甲肾上腺素水平 H4：趋化作用，介导炎症反应
肝素	抗凝，激活前激肽释放酶和接触系统，释放缓激肽
类胰蛋白酶	激活前激肽释放酶和补体，释放缓激肽、过敏毒素
糜蛋白酶	促进肾素合成，代偿性去甲肾上腺素分泌，引起心律失常
羧肽酶 A	促进前列腺素和白三烯合成，介导炎症反应
血小板激活因子	引起支气管收缩，减少冠状动脉血流和降低心脏收缩力，诱导 NO 合成，扩张血管，低血压，血小板聚集，募集中性粒细胞和嗜酸性粒细胞，双相迟发反应，抗凝
白三烯 LTC4	引起支气管收缩，气道重塑，血管性水肿，诱导 NO 合成，增加血管通透性，低血压
前列腺素 D2	引起支气管收缩，收缩肺动脉和冠状动脉，引起周围血管扩张、血管通透性增加，低血压，面部潮红，荨麻疹
激肽释放酶	促进肾素合成，激活补体，纤维蛋白溶解，促进血液凝固
肿瘤坏死因子	促进中性粒细胞活化，释放趋化因子、细胞因子，募集效应细胞

Data from Stone KD，Prussin C，Metcalfe DD：IgE，mast cells，basophils，and eosinophils. *J Allergy Clin Immunol* 125（2 Suppl 2）：S73-S80，2010.

- 支气管痉挛或哮鸣（44%）；
- 皮疹或荨麻疹（70%）；
- 血管性水肿和喘鸣（11.7%）。

不幸的是，由于全身麻醉和手术铺单可掩盖早期征象，手术室（operating room，OR）中过敏反应可能直接以循环衰竭为首发症状。支气管痉挛可能是哮喘恶化的一种表现，心电图改变可反映心肌缺血或低血压所致的冠状动脉血流减少。大多数麻醉药物都会引起低血压，而当采用椎管内麻醉时，情况可能会变得更加复杂。手术铺单可掩盖皮肤的征象，而多种症状掺杂在一起可能会产生各种临床表现。难以预测从乳胶暴露到症状出现到底需要多长时间，可能是 5 ～ 150 min 不等。

风险评估

以下几类患者容易发生乳胶过敏：

- 具有特异反应性体质的患者。
- 多次接受外科手术（如脊柱裂手术）的儿童，或婴幼儿手术。
- 双手患有严重皮炎的患者。
- 医护人员。
- 对水果过敏的患者，最常见的是香蕉、栗子和鳄梨。
- 使用防护装备的产业工人。

乳胶过敏可见于多达 70% 的脊柱裂患者，暴露于过敏原的混杂因素包括反复的导尿、多次外科手术和手法清除干结的粪便等。

启示

乳胶过敏反应表现的多样化给其及时诊断带来了困难，目前尚无体内检测可以预测其发生。其临床特征可能是典型的类过敏反应或者是Ⅳ型超敏反应，并可能在症状出现后的数小时内变得愈发明显。麻醉过程中过敏反应的全因死亡率约为 4%。

管理

过敏反应的治疗方法如下：

- 第一步：
  - 去除过敏原；
  - 静脉推注肾上腺素（1 ～ 10 μg/kg）；
  - 快速输注晶体液（50 ml/kg）。
- 第二步：
  - 肾上腺素持续输注，0.05 ～ 0.1 μg/（kg·min）；
  - 吸入或静脉推注 β 肾上腺素能受体激动剂（如：沙丁胺醇）；
  - 缓慢静脉注射苯海拉明 0.5 ～ 1 mg/kg 及雷尼替丁 1 mg/kg；
  - 皮质类固醇（如：静脉注射氢化可的松 5 ～ 10 mg/kg）。

留意手术室中所有可能的乳胶来源，包括手套、导尿管、静脉输液器、药瓶塞、注射器活塞、口罩和胶带。要特别注意含粉手套中的玉米淀粉在空气中形成的气溶胶，它可吸附手套中及衣服上的乳胶抗原。

既往有乳胶暴露史的患者再次暴露时仍有可能

发生过敏反应。

检测

由于患者在术前接触过大量过敏原，故应采取一种通用的方法来检测过敏反应。在麻醉科的过敏反应责任医师完成标准化的转诊流程后，负责围术期过敏反应的专科医师应主导展开相关检测。使用的主要测试如下。

肥大细胞类胰蛋白酶（mast cell tryptase，MCT）在过敏反应发生后 1 h 达到高峰，半衰期为 2 h。因其血浆的基础值存在较大的生理性差异，故 MCT 的相对变化比绝对水平更有意义。缺氧或心肌缺血等应激也可导致 MCT 升高。MCT 水平的高低并不能反映过敏反应的严重程度，甚至在过敏反应发生后仍可能正常，而且也会因静脉补液扩容被稀释。在复苏开始就应尽早抽取初始血样查 MCT，在过敏反应症状出现后的 1 ～ 2 h 抽取第二份血样，在 24 h 后或恢复期抽取第三份血样（某些流程还包括暴露后 6 h 的血样）。这可以提供 MCT 的基础水平。

血液中过敏原特异性 IgE 检测（过去称 RAST）是直接针对乳胶 IgE 的体外检测。它在乳胶过敏反应中具有很高的特异性，但其灵敏度差异较大（65% ～ 85%）和成本偏高使得它难以作为一种筛查实验。结果正常并不能排除乳胶过敏。但当患者全面性地表现出过敏反应时，这却是一种可靠的初步检测，而且比下面提到的直接暴露测试更为安全。

皮肤针刺试验（skin-prick testing，SPT）：目前还没有美国食品和药物管理局批准的商品化的试剂盒。国际免疫学会联合会已确认有 14 种与人类 IgE（Hev b 1 ～ Hev b 14）结合的乳胶过敏原，这可以解释欧洲批准的 7 种 SPT 检测液在敏感性和特异性上存在的巨大差异。该实验是先将含乳胶抗原的溶液滴在前臂内侧皮肤上，然后用针轻柔地刺入滴有该溶液的皮肤，同时设立对照。对乳胶过敏的患者测试区皮肤会出现风团，这是一种非常轻的但是具有确切风险的过敏反应。

皮内试验与 SPT 类似，但却是在皮内注射抗原。该实验导致全身反应的风险较高，因此必须在医院中进行，且需要相关的专业技术保障。这项实验不常规用于乳胶过敏的检测，但可作为乳胶过敏检测一部分的麻醉药物的检测。

部分医院会采用支气管激惹实验。它虽然具有较高的敏感性和特异性，但诱发支气管痉挛的风险也非常高。其他类似的黏膜激惹试验具有不同程度的敏感性和特异性。

预防

- 仔细的术前评估是发现潜在乳胶过敏患者的关键。除了识别上文列出的危险因素外，还应注意接触乳胶（如橡胶手套、玩具、气球、牙科检查）后是否出现过手或嘴唇瘙痒肿胀的病史。
- 对上述阳性病史或具有高危因素的患者行术前免疫学检查。
- 避免在诊疗过程中对脊柱裂患者使用乳胶制品，可有效减少致敏作用的发生，该规范已使其发生率在过去的 20 年逐渐下降。
- 每个麻醉部门都应该有治疗乳胶过敏患者的预案。例如包含以下方面的内容：
  - 在手术当天，乳胶过敏患者应被安排在第一台（因需要数次层流循环才能去除手术室空气中的乳胶微粒）。
  - 患者应在手术室中苏醒，将暴露于过敏原的机会降至最低。
  - 应备好不含乳胶的制品随时可用。
  - 尽量减少手术室工作人员数量，且避免人员变动。
- 所有乳胶过敏患者应使用医学警示腕带和自动注射的肾上腺素。
- 对患者和陪护人员的宣教仍是所有预防措施的重要组成部分。
- 家长和医师均可致电脊柱裂协会（1-800-621-3141）或在线获取相关信息，包括医疗及非医疗用品的乳胶含量和代替品。
- 目前尚无预防性使用抗组胺药和（或）皮质类固醇的相关证据。

（魏　玲　译　潘　科　校）

延伸阅读

Anderson J, Rose M, Green S, et al.: The utility of specific IgE testing to chlorhexidine in the investigation of perioperative adverse reactions, *Ann Allergy Asthma Immunol* 114(5):425–426.e1, 2015.

Caballero ML, Quirce S: Identification and practical management of latex allergy in occupational settings, *Expert Rev Clin Immunol* 11(9):977–992, 2015.

Dippenaar JM, Naidoo S: Allergic reactions and anaphylaxis during anesthesia, *Curr Allergy Clin Immunol* 28(1):18–22, 2015.

Geier J, Lessmann H, Mahler V, et al.: Occupational contact allergy caused by rubber gloves—nothing has changed, *Contact Dermatitis* 67(3):149–156, 2012.

Gibbs NM, Sadleir PH, Clarke RC, et al.: Survival from perioperative anaphylaxis in Western Australia 2000–2009, *Br J Anaesth* 111(4):589–593, 2013.

Gurrieri C, Weingarten TN, Martin DP, et al.: Allergic reactions during anaesthesia at a large United States referral center, *Anesth Analg* 113(5):1202–1212, 2011.

Kannan JA, Bernstein JA: Perioperative anaphylaxis: diagnosis, evaluation, and management, *Immunol Allergy Clin North Am* 35(2):321–334, 2015.

Laxenaire M, Mertes PM: Groupe d'Etudes des Réactions Anaphylactoïdes Peranesthésiques: Anaphylaxis during anaesthesia: results of a 2 year survey in France, *Br J Anaesth* 87(4):549–558, 2001.

Mertes PM, Alla F, Tréchot P, et al.: Anaphylaxis during anesthesia in France: an 8-year national survey, *J Allergy Clin Immunol* 128(2):366–373, 2011.

Ogawa Y, Grant JA: Mediators of anaphylaxis, *Immunol Allergy Clin North Am* 27(2):249–260, 2007.

Stone KD, Prussin C, Metcalfe DD: IgE, mast cells, basophils, and eosinophils, *J Allergy Clin Immunol* 125(2 Suppl 2):S73–S80, 2010.

Turjanmaa, K, Reunala, T, Tuimala, R, et al.: Severe IgE mediated allergy to surgical gloves, *Allergy* 39:S-2, 1984.

第 195 章 恶性高热

Herodotos Ellinas

病例概要

患者，男性，12 岁，平素体健，拟行肱骨骨折复位术。七氟烷诱导 15 min 后，呼气末二氧化碳突然升高超过 70 mmHg。患者出现了心动过速，心率超过 150 次 / 分，体温从 36.7℃升高至 39.4℃。

问题分析

定义

恶性高热（malignant hyperthermia，MH）是一种罕见但可能致命的亚临床肌肉疾病。在易感个体暴露于如挥发性吸入麻醉药、琥珀胆碱等触发麻醉药之前，MH 处于潜伏状态。MH 以骨骼肌调节失控导致肌质网钙离子增加为特点。其临床症状为代谢增加、肌肉僵硬和体温升高。

某种类的猪暴露于应激后也会出现类似症状（猪应激综合征）。此类猪暴露后也会经历高代谢、酸中毒、发热和死亡，和人类出现 MH 一样。1996 年霍尔报告说琥珀胆碱和氟烷可诱导这些动物发生恶性高热。这些猪很快成为研究恶性高热的动物模型。6 号染色体上的单点突变导致了猪应激综合征，导致了类似于人类 MH 一样的疾病，该疾病表现出显著的遗传异质性。30 多种不同基因的异常导致了类似的最终症状。人类 MH 有一半被认为是常染色体显性疾病（主要由男性表达），另一半的 MH 则被认为与新的基因突变相关。

MH 的病理生理学表现为骨骼肌的兴奋-收缩偶联紊乱。正常情况下，动作电位沿着肌膜和 T 小管传播，导致钙离子从肌浆网释放，然后钙离子与肌钙蛋白结合，使肌动蛋白结合位点暴露，从而导致肌肉收缩。这个过程因钙离子主动转运至肌质网而终止。

肌质网是钙离子调控的胞内细胞器。当动作电位传导引起 T 小管电压变化时，二氢吡啶受体的 α 亚单位发生构象变化，这可激活雷诺丁受体（ryanodine receptor，RYR1），从而导致 RYR1 开放，钙离子流出引发肌肉收缩。

恶性高热时，钙离子释放缺陷在接触诱发因素时就表现出来了。这种缺陷导致 RYR1 长时间开放，钙离子向肌质外流增加，从而引发肌动蛋白和肌球蛋白长时间相互作用（挛缩），促使肌肉代谢增强。该缺陷已知的两个位点为 *PYR1* 和 *CACNA1S*（电压依赖性钙离子通道，二氢吡啶受体）基因。

识别

理解 MH 的病理生理学有助于掌握其临床表现（框 195.1）。肌肉最初是有氧代谢增加，导致氧耗量增加、高碳酸血症、呼吸性酸中毒以及体温升高。随着 ATP 消耗，代谢转为无氧代谢，从而产生乳酸，并导致代谢性酸中毒，并进一步产生热量。高体温、酸中毒和 ATP 缺乏的情况下，细胞丧失维

框 195.1 恶性高热的临床表现

早期
- 心动过速
- 高碳酸血症
- 肌肉强直
- 呼吸急促
- 心率失常

晚期
- 体温快速上升
- 皮肤出现斑纹
- 肌红蛋白尿
- 高钾血症
- 肌酸激酶升高
- 混合型呼吸和代谢酸中毒

持细胞膜完整性的能力。横纹肌溶解导致钾、肌红蛋白和肌酸激酶释放。高碳酸血症是最早也是最敏感的 MH 的症状，全身性肌肉强直是最特别的症状。MH 的及时诊断和有效治疗是非常必要的，这有助于避免其相关并发症（框 195.2）。MH 初始体征和症状呈非特异性，因此须考虑更广泛的差异以预防长期发病率和死亡率（框 195.3）。

风险评估

由于人类 MH 的罕见性，难以精确预估，儿童的发病率为 1∶30 000，成人的发病率为 1∶1 000 000，其中 1∶2000 的患者因遗传异常导致了 MH 易感。

术前访视时应仔细询问以明确患者发生 MH 的风险。既往麻醉期间发生过 MH 或是有家族病史的患者应多加关注。此外，意外的术中死亡或心脏停搏家族史应高度怀疑 MH。MH 的临床评分系统有助于评估患者发生 MH 事件的可能性。尽管有许多不同疾病患者出现 MH 发作的病例报告，但唯一与 MH 持续相关的疾病是中枢性疾病和 King-Denborough 综合征。

框 195.2 恶性高热的并发症

- 心率失常
- 大面积心肌梗死
- 充血性心力衰竭
- 急性呼吸窘迫综合征
- 肺水肿
- 急性肾衰竭
- 肝功能不全
- 严重的肌肉疼痛 / 全身无力
- 肌肉痉挛
- 昏迷
- 死亡

框 195.3 恶性高热的鉴别诊断

- 过敏反应
- 脓毒症
- 甲状腺功能亢进
- 嗜铬细胞瘤
- 兴奋性药物
- 麻醉 / 镇痛不足
- 抗精神病药物恶性综合征
- 中暑

目前已确定的 MH 诊断试验是咖啡因-氟烷挛缩试验（caffeine-halothane contracture test，CHCT）和欧洲的相对应体外挛缩试验（in vitro contracture test，IVCT）。尽管 CHCT 始于 19 世纪 70 年代，但它仍旧是金标准，具有 97% 的敏感性和 78% 的特异性。肌肉活检必须是新鲜采集的肌肉，且检测必须在指定的美国 CHCT 中心进行。虽然活检是在门诊进行，但美国检测点的减少可能会给一些需要进行活检的患者造成障碍。

行 CHCT 时需取新鲜的大腿肌条，纵向解剖成 6 条，然后在肌肉的两端缝上缝合线，在将肌肉组织放入组织浴。一端连接固定钩，另一端连接传感器。通过直列式蒸发器将氟烷与新鲜气流一起加往其中三个浴槽中，而另外的三个浴槽中则逐步加入咖啡因。如果接触这些药物后肌肉出现了挛缩或是张力增高，则可诊断为 MH 综合征。

虽然 CHCT 仍旧是诊断 MH 的金标准，但近些年来基因诊断技术已被纳入医疗中。为了成功获得基因图谱，需对患者的 DNA 的 PYR1 基因进行已知突变的检测，如果有突变，还需对家庭成员进行因果突变检测。已知这个基因存在多种突变，也包括二氢吡啶受体的 α 亚基的基因突变。随着对 MH 基因构成的更多了解，基因检测可成为筛查高危患者的手段，从而可避免开放性肌肉活检的需要。

启示

MH 是一类严重的潜在致命性疾病。若未经治疗，其死亡率高达 70% ～ 80%；若使用丹曲林治疗，这个比例可下降至 5% ～ 10%。因此，麻醉科医师在诊断和及时治疗 MH 患者以避免其并发症方面具有至关重要的作用（见框 195.2）。

与任何遗传性疾病一样，MH 的诊断对患者及其家庭成员都有意义。美国恶性高热协会作为患者和医生的宝贵资源库，成立于 1981 年，以向患者和医疗保健机构提供 MH 信息，帮助个人诊断并降低其发病率和死亡率为目标。其 MH 咨询热线每周 7 天，且 24 h 都可以为医生提供咨询服务（1-800-MH-HYPER；1-800-644-9737）。

北美恶性高热登记处是美国恶性高热协会的分支机构，可获取并分析 MH 患者特殊的临床和实验室数据。它是 MH 高危患者的中心储存库，收集了

MH 的流行病学资料，并帮助转诊中心标准化诊断测试。卫生保健专业人员无论何时怀疑 MH 相关事件，都可以通过填写麻醉不良代谢反应表格注册。

最近一个令人关注的话题是，当患者未麻醉或未暴露于已知的麻醉触发剂时，也会发生“清醒触发”MH 的可能。回到病例简介中的患者，该男孩在术中被诊断为 MH，并及时接受了丹曲林治疗，且顺利恢复。然而他在 8 个月后的一场足球比赛后出现了肌无力和强直的症状，随后他的病情发展到出现痉挛和呼吸抑制。当医护人员到达时，心电图显示窦性心动过速，并且由于牙关紧闭而导致插管失败。到达医院后患者插管成功，此时体温已经高于 42.2℃。患者出现了心室颤动，行持续心肺复苏，纠正高钾血症并给予丹曲林治疗，但复苏失败。随后的 DNA 检测发现 *RYP1* 基因序列改变，与 MH 的诊断一致。

众所周知，有或无 MH 综合征的人都有可能出现高代谢状态。虽然这种情况罕见，但发作却可能是致命的。卫生保健专业人员建议，MH 综合征的患者只有在出现了严重的肌肉痉挛或有高代谢状态的症状时才会导致其活动受限。尽管在中暑患者中因清醒触发 MH 导致死亡者所占比例很小，但鉴别诊断时应考虑到 MH，并提示可能需要丹曲林治疗。

有趣的是，心脏 *RYR2* 基因突变与儿茶酚胺介导的室性心动过速及 2 型右心发育不良致心率失常患者的猝死相关。*RYR2* 是心肌细胞肌质网主要的钙离子释放通道，*RYR2* 突变导致运动时钙离子调节紊乱或交感神经系统应激激活。因此，*RYR1* 和 *RYR2* 突变分别导致骨骼肌和心肌钙离子代谢紊乱。新的数据表明心脏事件和死亡也有可能与肌肉体积较大有关系。

管理

患者一旦被诊断为 MH，则必须将情况的严重性告知手术团队，并向手术室寻求额外的帮助。美国外科医师学会和儿科麻醉学会的核查表分别为成人和儿童手术室事件提供了简明的管理指南；其中一个关键事件就是 MH。治疗包括：

- 停止接触触发剂（任何挥发性吸入麻醉药，琥珀胆碱）；
- 纯氧过度通气。
- 使用丹曲林。
- 监测动脉血气酸碱度、碱剩余和血钾；检查一系列的肌酸激酶和凝血指标。
  - 使用碳酸氢钠治疗酸中毒。
  - 使用钙剂、葡萄糖和胰岛素治疗高血钾症。
- 放置 Foley 导尿管，使用呋塞米或甘露醇利尿。
- 使用冰袋、冷盐水冲洗体腔和手术部位使核心体温冷却；考虑体外循环。
- 拨打 MH 热线（1-800-MH-HYPER）。
- 填写 AMRA 表格。

丹曲林是直接的骨骼肌松弛剂，通过与 RYR1 受体结合，从而降低其开放状态的概率，阻止钙离子从肌浆网释放。丹曲林首先以 2.5 mg/kg 静脉推注；每 5 min 重复一次，直到高代谢状态消失，最大剂量不超过 30 mg/kg。旧制剂的丹曲林需要花费很长时间稀释，但新的配方制剂制备时间不超过 1 min，这使得给药时更加迅速。丹曲林的维持剂量为每 6 h 静脉注射 1 mg/kg，持续 24 h，以防止高代谢状态复发。因此，患者在 MH 发作后至少要在加强医疗病房监护 24 h。

如果患者在接受大量丹曲林治疗后病情仍未好转，则必须考虑其他诊断（见框 195.3）。某种药物可能与丹曲林及非去极化肌松药发生相互作用；丹曲林已被证明可增强维库溴铵对神经肌肉的阻断作用，同时给予丹曲林和维拉帕米后，麻醉状态的猪发生了心血管衰竭。因此，禁止给予钙离子通道阻断剂。

预防

易感或高危患者进入手术室后，麻醉团队必须仔细计划使用安全的麻醉药：

- 麻醉机必须配备新的一次性回路和新的二氧化碳吸收剂。
- 应禁用蒸发器，并按照机器建议冲洗机器。
- 预防 MH 时，活性炭过滤装置应置于呼气回路和吸气回路的末端并使用 12 h，可在较短时间内有效去除麻醉机中的挥发性麻醉药；若在发生急性 MH 事件中，活性炭过滤装置的有效性只有 1 h。

尽管这些患者应避免使用触发药物，但仍有许多安全的麻醉药可以使用（框 195.4）。丹曲林不建

框 195.4 恶性高热患者的安全药物

巴比妥类（如美索比妥）
苯二氮䓬类药物
右美托咪定
依托咪酯
氯胺酮
局部麻醉药
氧化亚氮
非去极化肌松剂
阿片类药物
丙泊酚

议在患者围术期预防性使用。术后应连续监测心电图至少 4 h，并同时监测核心体温。如果恢复期平安无事，那么在门诊手术后患者返回病房甚至家中都是安全的。

致谢

感谢 Karen M. Van Tassel 和 Scott R. Schulman 博士对本章上一版的贡献。

（郭 玉 译 赵珍珍 校）

延伸阅读

Allen GC, et al.: The sensitivity and specificity of the caffeine-halothane contracture test, *Anesthesiology* 88:579–588, 1998.

Denborough MA: Malignant hyperthermia, *Anesthesiology* 108:156–157, 2008.

Hayes J, Veyckemans F, Bissonnette B: Duchenne muscular dystrophy: an old anesthesia problem revisited, *Paediatr Anaesth* 18:100–106, 2008.

Krause T, Gerbershagen MU, Fiege M, et al.: Dantrolene: a review of its pharmacology, therapeutic use and new developments, *Anaesthesia* 59:364–373, 2004.

Larach MG, Brandom BW, Allen GC, et al.: Cardiac arrest and deaths associated with malignant hyperthermia in North America from 1987 to 2006: a report from the North American Malignant Hyperthermia Registry of the Malignant Hyperthermia Association of the United States, *Anesthesiology* 108:603–611, 2008.

Larach MG, Brandom BW, Allen GC, et al.: Malignant hyperthermia deaths related to inadequate temperature monitoring, 2007–2012: a report from the North American Malignant Hyperthermia Registry of the Malignant Hyperthermia Association of the United States, *Anesth Analg* 119:1359–1366, 2014.

Larach MG, Gronert GA, Allen GC, et al.: Clinical presentation, treatment, and complications of malignant hyperthermia in North America from 1987 to 2006, *Anesth Analg* 110:498–507, 2010.

Malignant Hyperthermia Association of the United States. Available at www.MHAUS.org. Accessed September 27, 2016.

Nelson P, Litman RS: Malignant hyperthermia in children: an analysis of the North American Malignant Hyperthermia Registry, *Anesth Analg* 118:369–374, 2014.

Riazi S, Larach MG, Hu C, et al.: Malignant hyperthermia in Canada: characteristics of index anesthetics in 129 malignant hyperthermia susceptible probands, *Anesth Analg* 118:381–387, 2014.

Rosenberg H, Antognini JF, Muldoon S: Testing for malignant hyperthermia, *Anesthesiology* 96:232–237, 2002.

Rosenberg H, Davis M, James D, et al.: Malignant hyperthermia, *Orphanet J Rare Dis* 2:21, 2007.

Timmins MA, Rosenberg H, Larach MG, et al.: Malignant hyperthermia testing in probands without adverse anesthetic reaction, *Anesthesiology* 123:548–556, 2015.

第 196 章 眼科问题及并发症

Scott D. Cook-Sather

病例概要

患者，女童，5 岁，无眼科病史，全身麻醉下行甲状舌管囊肿切除术。苏醒时，主诉眼睛疼痛。虽然眼睛内没有明显异物，但可以看到过度流泪。气管插管后，其双眼贴上胶布保护。怀疑有角膜擦伤，并请了眼科专家会诊。

引言

对于非眼部手术，麻醉相关眼睛损伤的发生率估计为 0.06%；这占美国麻醉科医师协会（American Society of Anesthesiologists，ASA）非牙科结案索赔案件的 3%。围术期眼部损伤的危险因素包括全身麻醉、长时间手术、头颈部手术和侧卧位。在眼科手术中，麻醉相关的眼睛损伤是非常罕见的。当它发生时，可能与围术期咳嗽或严重的术后呕吐有关，并伴有眼压（intraocular pressure，IOP）的突然升高。与小儿麻醉相关的重要眼科并发症包括角膜磨损、术后失明、早产儿视网膜病变、穿透性眼外伤、眼心反射、术后恶心呕吐。40% ～ 90% 的儿童在斜视手术后发生恶心呕吐。

角膜擦伤

问题分析

定义

角膜擦伤是最常见的眼部并发症，发生率为 0.1% ～ 44%。据报道，在 20 世纪 70 年代，未实施眼睛保护或润滑的麻醉患者的发生率更高。大多数角膜损伤是由于全身麻醉过程中眼睑未闭角膜干燥引起的。

识别

角膜擦伤的症状包括畏光、疼痛和异物感。多泪和瞳孔缩小是典型的体检发现。荧光染色显示钴蓝色光下的绿色磨损区（图 196.1）。

风险评估

虽然角膜擦伤的诱发因素并不明确，但诸如俯卧位或侧卧位、眼球突出等因素会增加患病风险。全身麻醉增加了这种风险，部分原因是由于失去了角膜的保护反射，消除了 Bell 现象（在睡眠中眼球向上转动），以及减少了泪液的产生和稳定性。

启示

大部分在术中角膜擦伤的儿童在接受适当治疗后 24 h 内完全恢复。大面积损伤或延迟治疗导致永

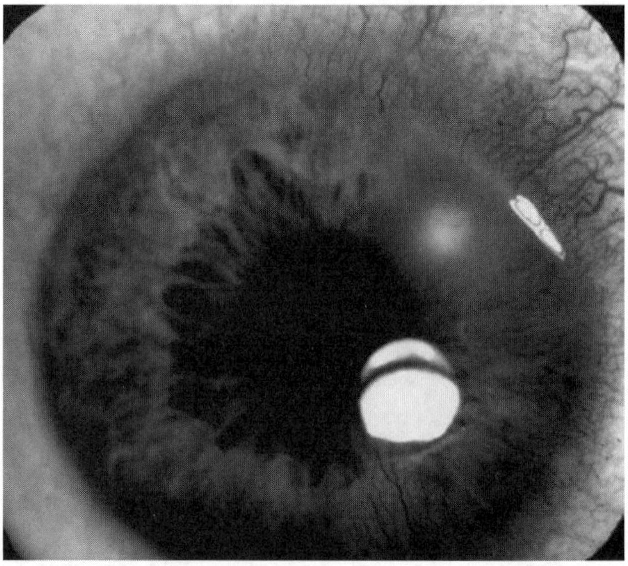

图 196.1 虹膜上 2 点钟位置的不透明区域是角膜擦伤和周围水肿。荧光素染色最容易发现这些病变

久性损伤的发生率为 16%。永久性瘢痕通常与继发性角膜感染或慢性擦伤有关。

管理

角膜擦伤的患者应该由眼科医师进行评估，记录损伤程度并开始治疗。常规建议包括润滑，局部抗生素或睫状肌麻痹剂（或两者兼有）的应用，以及覆盖闭合。

预防

为了防止角膜擦伤，必须避免眼睛与面罩、听诊器、姓名标签、插管设备、床单和填充物接触。在使用喉镜前，应及早采取眼睛保护措施。应使用胶布保持眼睑闭合，较长时间的手术需要使用眼部润滑剂。油性眼膏比水溶性的眼膏更容易在术后引起异物感和视力模糊。将一次性脉搏血氧仪探头置于儿童无名指而不是示指上，可减少术后无意的眼接触和潜在的角膜损伤。

术后失明

问题分析

定义

术后失明（postoperative visual loss，POVL）是最严重的眼科手术并发症，可表现为部分视野丧失或完全失明。一般非眼科手术人群中 POVL 的发生率为 1/125 000 ～ 1/61 000，但在俯卧位脊柱手术中发生率为 1/1100。在开胸心脏手术和头颈部手术中发生率也较高。从 1999 年 7 月 ASA 术后失明登记开始，到 2004 年 7 月报告了 3 例 POVL 儿童病例，年龄从 5 岁到 18 岁不等。

识别

术后即刻可感觉到视力变化，但如果将这种改变错误地认为是麻醉后滴入眼内润滑剂导致的正常反应，可能会导致诊断延迟。在一项 28 例 POVL 病例研究中，50% 的患者在恢复室中发现视觉变化，80% 在术后第 2 天发现。一些患者最初视力正常，但在 1 ～ 12 天后出现症状。儿童患者难以表达症状。当受影响的眼睛周围出现局部淤斑或眶周麻木时，应怀疑有压迫性损伤。

风险评估

与俯卧位脊柱手术相关的缺血性视神经病变（ischemic optic neuropathy，ION）占 ASA POVL 登记处的大多数病例。3 例小儿患者在俯卧位长时间（>8 h）手术后出现 ION，2 例为脊柱侧弯，1 例为颅骨重建。术中发生的事件包括大量失血和低血压。一种损伤机制认为这涉及短暂性贫血、动脉血压低、中心静脉压高和俯卧位 IOP 升高的复杂相互作用，从而导致视神经灌注压力降低和视神经通路血流动力学储备受限。

伴有高血压、吸烟、糖尿病或周围血管疾病的成年患者出现 ION 风险增加。发生 ION 不需要直接的眼眶受压（例如，患者头枕错位）。然而，这种压迫可通过视网膜中央动脉闭塞导致 POVL，在这种情况下，POVL 可归因于 ION。POVL 也可能是围术期皮质缺血的结果。

启示

大多数的术后视力缺陷不会随时间显著改善。那些完全没有光感的患者不太可能恢复视力。

管理

对于明确的视力缺陷（缺乏光感、单侧视力丧失）、眼眶周围淤血或明显外伤，以及麻醉和手术后最初几小时内视力症状未改善的情况，必须进行早期眼科会诊。通常需要视力检查、眼底检查和头部磁共振成像来确诊；然而，目前几乎没有有效的治疗方法。因此，在术后确保足够的血流动力学、血红蛋白浓度和氧合，即便不能逆转最初的损伤，但可以防止进一步的伤害。

预防

虽然直接受压不是 POVL 的常见原因，但保护眼睛不受外部压力至关重要。麻醉从业人员必须仔细摆放患者体位，并时刻监测其体位，因为患者在手术过程中可能会改变与头垫和其他设备的位置关系。带有镜子的特殊头垫可即时评估俯卧位患者的眶周区域。轻度反屈氏体位可降低眶静脉压力，并在不同的平均动脉压下提供更好的灌注。

虽然控制性降压有助于减少术中出血，但它可能增加 POVL 的风险。控制性降压已安全用于数万例，但 ASA POVL 登记的 3 例小儿病例中有 2 例涉及控制性降压技术。我所在机构目前的做法是避免后路脊柱融合术中使用控制性降压，因为正常血压下，躯体感觉和运动诱发电位得到更好的保留。

减少 POVL 风险的精确输血指标尚未明确，但应避免严重贫血。目前的建议还包括尽量减少患者俯卧的时间。如果手术总时间预计超过 8 h，应考虑分期进行。

早产儿视网膜病变

问题分析

定义

50% 以上体重不足 1500 g 早产儿会发生早产儿视网膜病变（retinopathy of prematurity，ROP）。它是由血管组织异常增生，伴视网膜毛细血管床破坏所致。ROP 的严重程度从可逆的新生血管形成到视网膜完全脱离并伴有永久性失明。虽然多种相关因素导致 ROP 的发生，但未成熟的视网膜似乎更容易受到高浓度氧（O_2）和伴随的自由基的影响。

识别

眼科检查可以记录 ROP 的发展或恶化。ROP 的各阶段如下：

- 后部带血管的视网膜与前面无血管的部分呈线性分离；
- 分界线明显并形成高脊；
- 视网膜下新生血管组织增生；
- 部分视网膜脱离；
- 视网膜完全脱离，也称为晶状体后纤维增生。

风险评估

ROP 与低出生体重（<1500 g），低胎龄（≤ 32 周），出生时发生出血性休克、贫血和输血，长时间暴露在高氧环境中有关。视网膜的颞部要到孕后期 40 ～ 44 周才发育成熟，因此，相当于孕后期 44 周的需要手术的新生儿，被认为有 ROP 发生或已有疾病恶化的风险。

启示

虽然大约 85% 的急性 ROP 患者可以自愈，但预后仍取决于分期。存在纤维组织牵拉和视网膜脱离患者预后较差。90% 的患者选择激光光凝治疗。另外可能需要冷冻治疗、巩膜扣带术或玻璃体切割术。

管理与预防

ROP 是新生儿重症监护病房的主要问题，长期暴露于 O_2 可能会使婴儿处于危险之中；因而，努力降低术中 O_2 浓度可能会使患儿受益。早期的研究表明，动脉氧分压（arterial O_2 tension，PaO_2）为 150 mmHg 持续 1 ～ 2 h 会影响未成熟视网膜。最近的数据表明，甚至更低的 PaO_2 也可能导致 ROP。仅数天的高氧接触即可发生此类损伤。因此，需要谨慎处置，包括使用最低氧浓度（fraction of inspired O_2，FiO_2）达到经皮动脉氧饱和度 90% ～ 95%（$PaO_2 \approx 70$ mmHg）。然而，有严重肺病的新生儿需要高 FiO_2 来维持足够的组织氧合，这种情况高 FiO_2 应被允许。

穿透性眼外伤和玻璃体挤压伤

问题分析

定义

穿透性眼外伤，伴眼球内容物挤压风险时，历来给儿科麻醉科医师带来麻醉管理的挑战。患者表现为急危重症，往往不配合治疗，通常需要快速麻醉诱导以减少胃内容物反流肺误吸的风险。然而，麻醉过程中，特别是诱导期间 IOP 的突然升高，可能会增加玻璃体挤压的风险。由于麻醉管理而导致眼内容物缺失非常罕见，仅见于少数非正式报道。

识别

患者的病史可能包括被尖锐物体碰触或撞击，随后出现眼睛疼痛、肿胀、红斑、明显眼裂或原位异物。眼球膨胀不佳和玻璃体外露是玻璃体挤压的征象。

风险评估

对于有严重缺陷的儿童和持续哭泣、咳嗽、恶心或呕吐的儿童，穿透性眼睛损伤更可能导致玻璃体挤压。

启示

眼内容物的挤压是灾难性的且需要立即闭合伤口，有可能需要后路巩膜切开术以释放脉络膜上血液。大部分患者预后极差，受伤侧眼睛失明。

管理与预防

儿童穿透性眼外伤的评估和管理策略见框 196.1。最重要的问题是防止胃内容物的误吸和预防眼压的突然增加，如咳嗽。咳嗽可短暂增加眼压 30 ～ 40 mmHg，并可引起玻璃体挤压、虹膜或晶状体脱垂或脉络膜出血。眼压的小幅度增加也可能导致玻璃体挤压，尽管导致这种挤压所需的最小眼压增加值是未知的；显然这取决于原发损伤的程度。

框 196.1　穿透性眼外伤患者的麻醉评估与管理

受伤的性质，紧急程度，以及预计的手术时间
小损伤：挤压的风险较小
简单损伤：短小手术
复合伤：视网膜复位延长
铜：引起早期玻璃体浑浊
异物突出：真正的眼科急症
眼球不能存活：可以等待数小时

肺误吸的风险
饱胃
胃肠功能受损
创伤严重程度
阿片类药物的使用
胃食管反流，食管裂孔疝

气道评估
困难气道：考虑采用光纤引导插管方法
正常或未预期困难：快速序贯诱导

麻醉管理选择
尽可能延后饱胃患者诱导：固体 8 h 后；清流质 2 h 后
快速序贯诱导：利多卡因 1.5 ～ 2 mg/kg；瑞芬太尼 1 μg/kg 或芬太尼 1 ～ 2 μg/kg；硫喷妥钠 4 ～ 6 mg/kg 或丙泊酚 2 ～ 3 mg/kg；琥珀胆碱 1.5 ～ 2 mg/kg（± NDMR）；若手术时间延长则用大剂量 NDMR（罗库溴铵 1.2 mg/kg）代替琥珀胆碱
监测：通过四个成串刺激确定插管的最早时间和持续肌肉松弛时间

在快诱导插管过程中，琥珀胆碱可通过眼外、面部和眼眶平滑肌的去极化使眼压增加 6 ～ 8 mmHg 持续 5 ～ 10 min。没有明确的病例报告表明琥珀胆碱给药后玻璃体挤压；然而，人们的担忧仅限于一则轶事报道。去肌颤剂量的非去极化肌肉松弛剂（nondepolarizing muscle relaxant，NDMR）可降低琥珀胆碱相关的眼压升高。预处理剂量的 NDMR 可促进麻醉诱导后插管充分条件的实现，但也有干预性乏力、呼吸困难、躁动甚至误吸的报道。一般来说，小儿患者不易耐受与 NDMR 预处理相关的潜在问题；而且理论上，这些也会增加眼睛进一步受伤害的风险。大剂量（ED95 的 2 ～ 3 倍）NDMR，如顺阿曲库铵、米库氯铵、罗库溴铵或维库溴铵，可在 60 ～ 90 s 内插管，但可延长阻滞恢复时间。最后，在整个手术过程中，应保持充分的神经肌肉松弛，并给予足够的阿片类药物，以避免苏醒期呛咳。

眼心反射

问题分析

定义

心率下降与眼球压力或眼外肌肉牵拉有关，这在儿童中很常见。在斜视手术中，眼心反射（oculocardiac reflex，OCR）的报告发生率为 20% ～ 90%。OCR 的传入支通过睫状长神经和睫状短神经。后者首先在睫状神经节聚集；这两个输入神经汇合形成三叉神经的眼神经分支（图 196.2）。OCR 的传出支是迷走神经，发挥心脏抑制神经的作用。

识别

OCR 导致心率减慢或不规则。它可以通过胸前心音、脉搏血氧饱和度仪或心电图监测来检测。窦性心动过缓是最常见的心律失常。窦性停搏、短暂性心脏停搏、游离性心房起搏、房室交界性心律、

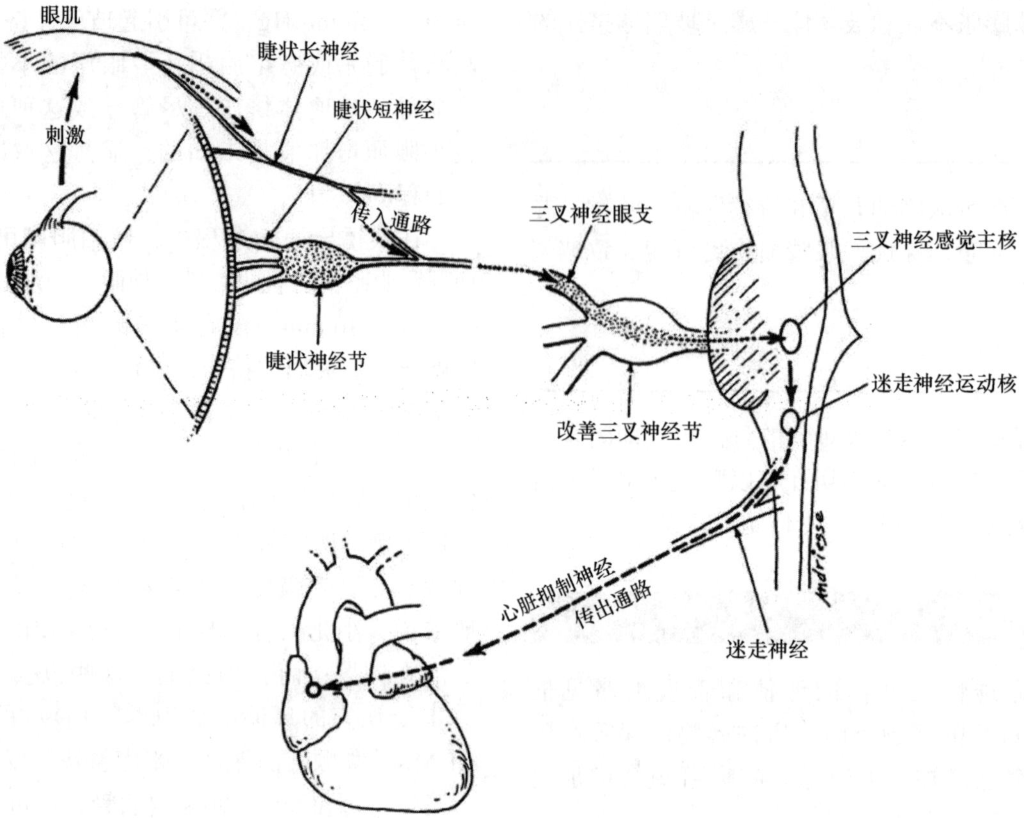

图 196.2 眼心反射（OCR）。通过睫状长神经和睫状短神经刺激三叉神经眼支（传入支）。传入的脉冲到达三叉神经节和三叉神经感觉 y 核。之后它们被传送到迷走神经传出（运动）核。传出通路包括迷走神经和心脏抑制神经。（From Vassallo SA，Ferrari LR：Anesthesia for ophthalmology. In Coté CJ，Ryan JF，Todres ID，et al，editors：*A practice of anesthesia for infants and children*，2nd ed. Philadelphia，WB Saunders，1993，p 325.）

房室传导阻滞和室性心律失常（期前收缩，二联律，逸搏）也可能发生。尽管室性心动过速和心房颤动已有报道，他们最有可能发生在长时间的心脏停搏后（可能是由于心肌缺氧）或使用抗胆碱能类 / β - 肾上腺素能受体激动剂治疗相关，特别是在使用致敏性吸入麻醉剂如氟烷麻醉的患者中。

风险评估

由于迷走神经张力的相对增加，在斜视手术中，较易发生 OCR。对眼外肌肉的突然且强有力牵引是最常见的刺激，但也有其他原因（框 196.2）。预防性应用阿托品和其他变时性药物不能消除 OCR，但可降低其发生率和相关心动过缓的严重程度。然而，正如刚才所述，使用抗胆碱能类或 β - 肾上腺素能受体激动剂进行预防有可能会加重心律失常，尤其是使用早期的吸入麻醉剂如氟烷。高碳酸血症和低氧增加了 OCR 导致心律失常的风险，不合理的麻醉深度与 OCR 有关。

框 196.2 眼心反射的围术期刺激因素

- 牵拉任何眼外肌
- 牵拉结膜或眼眶结构
- 眼外伤或球后血肿
- 眼眶顶端球体或组织的压力（眼球摘除术后）
- 球后阻滞的表现

启示

OCR 通常较短暂，随着牵拉的放松而缓解。术中 OCR 与术后恶心呕吐有显著相关性。事实上，术中 OCR 发作的儿童术后出现恶心呕吐的概率是无此类发作儿童的 2 ～ 3 倍。

管理

虽然 OCR 是斜视手术中心律失常的常见原因，但查找和治疗其他主要原因也很重要，包括低氧、高碳酸血症和麻醉深度不足。所有这些都有可能使 OCR 恶化。然而，如果心律失常持续存在，外科医师应该放松眼部肌肉的张力。不建议在刺激消除和正常节律恢复之前使用拮抗剂；这只会增加更严重心律失常的风险。一般而言，通过反复轻柔的牵拉 OCR 会发生疲劳反应，不需要变时性药物的治疗。

预防

推荐在斜视手术中使用控制性轻度过度通气来预防高碳酸血症。与氟烷相比，七氟烷可降低儿童自主和控制通气时的 OCR 发生率和心动过缓程度。虽然在眼肌牵拉前 30 min 静脉注射阿托品可能降低 OCR 发生率或减弱其幅度，但并不能保证对严重心律失常有预防保护作用。由于阿托品对 OCR 预防并非普遍有效，且严重 OCR 导致血流动力学损害的发生率普遍较低，因此不再推荐常规抗胆碱能药物预防。使用 1 ～ 3 ml 1% ～ 2% 利多卡因球后阻滞可预防成人 OCR，但在儿童中很少使用。

致谢

特别感谢眼科中心主席，宾夕法尼亚大学费城儿童医院 Monte D. Mills 博士，对这一章节的修订和改进。

（徐 航 译 李斌本 校）

延伸阅读

Allison CE, De Lange JJ, Koole FD, et al.: A comparison of the incidence of the oculocardiac and oculorespiratory reflexes during sevoflurane and halothane anesthesia for strabismus surgery in children, *Anesth Analg* 90:306–310, 2000.

Blanc VF, Hardy JF, Milot J, et al.: The oculocardiac reflex: a graphic and statistical analysis in infants and children, *Can Anaesth Soc J* 30:360–369, 1983.

Gild WM, Posner KL, Caplan RA, et al.: Eye injuries associated with anesthesia: a closed claims analysis, *Anesthesiology* 76:204–208, 1992.

Gregory GA: Anesthesia for premature infants. In Gregory GA, editor: *Pediatric anesthesia*, 4th ed, Philadelphia, 2002, Churchill Livingstone, pp 352–353.

Haberer JP: Ophthalmic surgery: anesthetic considerations and postoperative management. In Bissonette B, Dalens B, editors: *Pediatric anesthesia principles and practice*, New York, 2002, McGraw-Hill, pp 1277–1290.

Lee LA, Lam AM: Unilateral blindness after prone lumbar spine surgery, *Anesthesiology* 95:793–795, 2001.

Myers MA, Hamilton SR, Bogosian AJ, et al.: Visual loss as a complication of spine surgery: a review of 37 cases, *Spine* 22:1325–1329, 1997.

Roth S, Thisted RA, Erickson JP, et al.: Eye injuries after nonocular surgery, *Anesthesiology* 85:1020–1027, 1996.

Siffring PA, Poulton TJ: Prevention of ophthalmic complications during general anesthesia, *Anesthesiology* 66:569–570, 1987.

Vachon CA, Warner DO, Bacon DR: Succinylcholine and the open globe, *Anesthesiology* 99:220–223, 2003.

Vassallo SA, Ferrari LR: Anesthesia for ophthalmology. In Coté CJ, Ryan JF, Todres ID, et al.: *A practice of anesthesia for infants and children*, ed 2, Philadelphia, 1993, WB Saunders, pp 323–335.

Warner ME, Warner MA, Garrity JA, et al.: The frequency of perioperative vision loss, *Anesth Analg* 93:1417–1421, 2001.

White E, Crosse MM: The aetiology and prevention of peri-operative corneal abrasions, *Anaesthesia* 53:157–161, 1998.

第 197 章 小儿高热

Kate E. Balbi，*Ronald S. Litman*

病例概要

患者，男性，12 岁，在全身麻醉下行乳突切开鼓室成形术，既往身体健康。麻醉采用七氟烷混合空气加氧气，辅以芬太尼。术中给予地塞米松、昂丹司琼和头孢唑啉。手术进行约 2 h 时，食管温度显示 38.1℃，心率 120 次 / 分，血压 122/78 mmHg。除其姑母 25 年前在手术中不明原因死亡，无其他麻醉相关的家族史。

问题分析

定义

麻醉药物及阿片类药物对体温调控能力的影响导致患者出现体温波动十分常见，但高热可能会引起严重的并发症，麻醉科医师必须能够识别其潜在的原因。

严格地说，核心体温一旦升高就可判定为体温过高，但通常广义的高热定义是核心体温高于 38℃。人体体温根据下丘脑体温调定点进行调节，该调定点会与当前核心体温进行持续比较。当下丘脑的调定点升高，而出汗或血管扩张等体温调节反馈受损，或者过度热暴露时，就会发生高热。不管原因如何，高热都是一种代谢性应激，严重时会影响终末器官的功能（框 197.1）。

美国麻醉科医师协会（American Society of Anest-hesiologists）的基本麻醉监测标准规定，"当临床需要、预计或怀疑体温发生显著变化时，每位接受麻醉的患者都应该进行体温监测。"美国恶性高热协会（Malignant Hyperthermia Association of the United States，MHAUS）建议所有接受全身麻醉超过 30 min 的患者均需进行核心体温监测，因为缺乏温度监测与急性恶性高热发生相关的死亡率增加有关。

框 197.1　严重高热的不良反应

心血管
- 心排血量增加
- 传导缺陷（QT 和 ST 变化，T 波异常）

呼吸系统
- 肺水肿

肾
- GFR 降低
- 肾灌注不足导致急性肾损伤

肝
- 肝细胞损伤导致 AST 和 ALT 升高
- 凝血障碍

血液系统
- 血小板减少症
- DIC

神经系统
- 认知功能障碍
- 血脑屏障的破坏

胃肠
- 缺血
- 出血

ALT，谷丙转氨酶；AST，谷草转氨酶；DIC，弥散性血管内凝血；GFR，肾小球滤过率

Data from Walter EJ，Hanna-Jumma S，Carraretto M，et al：The pathophysiological basis and consequences of fever. *Crit Care* 20（1）：200，2016.

识别

在肺动脉、食管远端、鼓膜或鼻咽部测得的核心温度是热状态的最佳指标。然而，核心温度测量并不适用于所有外科手术；因此，可使用准确性稍差的口腔、腋窝、直肠、膀胱和皮肤表面温度探头来估计核心温度（表 197.1）。皮肤表面和直肠温度可能不能及时反应核心温度，使用时应注意。

表 197.1 体温监测部位和注意事项

位置	注意事项
核心温度监测部位	
位置	**注意事项**
肺动脉	有创，仅在心脏或类似复杂的手术中使用；插入后存在潜在心脏和肺的并发症
食管远端	食管探头中的温度探头必须放置在心音最强处或更远处，以获得准确的温度读数
鼓膜	难以准确定位；小心穿孔
鼻咽	难以准确定位
近似核心温度的监测部位	
位置	**注意事项**
腋窝	当探头放置在腋动脉上方且手臂保持最大内收时最准确
膀胱	有创性；必须有尿流才能准确
皮肤	无法可靠地追踪核心温度；前额皮肤温度通常比核心温度低 2℃
直肠	难以准确定位；取决于直肠内容物；通常滞后于核心温度

风险评估

医源性高热

因为麻醉患者通常容易出现低体温，所以加热技术通常是麻醉治疗的重要组成部分。然而，有时这些加热方法（例如，升高室温、强制热风、气道加湿器）可能导致医源性高热。其他引起高热的医源性原因包括长时间使用止血带、输血反应和监测仪或探头故障。

药物引起的高热

恶性高热（malignant hyperthermia，MH）是一种遗传性疾病，其特征是吸入挥发性麻醉药或使用琥珀胆碱时发生危及生命的高代谢反应。MH 表现为高碳酸血症、心动过速、肌肉强直、酸中毒和高热。药物引起高热的其他原因包括抗精神病药恶性综合征、抗胆碱能药物的使用、对抗生素的反应、单胺氧化酶抑制剂与阿片类药物（尤其是哌替啶）的相互作用以及血清素综合征。

疾病继发的高热

某些潜在的疾病可能会导致围术期的高热，包括甲状腺功能亢进、嗜铬细胞瘤、急性脑损伤或脑卒中、肾上腺功能不全、深静脉血栓、肺栓塞、帕金森病、吸入性肺炎、癫痫、结缔组织病、脓毒症和下丘脑病变。

术后发热

一旦麻醉对体温调节的影响消失，术后高热十分常见。术后发热的原因包括手术和感染引起的炎症反应或菌血症。硬膜外麻醉不但不能抑制发热，反而与轻度发热有关。

该病例描述了全身麻醉期间的发热反应。最可能的原因是医源性升温过度，在环境温度相对较高，手术中几乎没有血液或液体丢失，且体表暴露面积少散热受限的情况下使用加热装置，从而导致体温过高。然而，其他一些不太常见的可能性也必须牢记在心，例如恶性高热，在患者亲属中有术中不明原因死亡的含糊病史时尤其要考虑这种情况（框 197.2）。

管理

治疗高热的主要目标是治疗其根本病因。当患者的体温超过 39℃时，应考虑积极降温。降温方法包括移除铺单和加热装置；降低环境温度；在腹股沟、腋窝或颈部冰敷；输注冷的静脉注射液；冰水冲洗手术伤口；对于最严重的导致器官损伤的病例，行心肺转流术（框 197.3）。

框 197.2 高热的鉴别诊断

术中

- 感染
- 医源性主动加温
- 止血带使用时间过长
- 恶性高热
- 甲状腺功能亢进
- 嗜铬细胞瘤
- 急性脑损伤或脑卒中
- 肾上腺功能不全
- 深静脉血栓形成
- 肺栓塞
- 帕金森病
- 吸入性肺炎
- 癫痫持续状态
- 结缔组织疾病
- 脓毒症
- 下丘脑病变

术后

- 感染或菌血症（外科操作所致）
- 硬膜外麻醉
- 手术后炎症反应
- 药物引起

框 197.3 降温方法

- 移除铺单和加热设备
- 降低环境温度
- 在腹股沟、腋窝或颈部冰敷
- 冷静脉注射液
- 冰水冲洗手术伤口
- 心肺转流术

预防

监测术中核心温度以及合理使用加热或冷却装置，可以预防医源性高热的发生。一些药物引起的高热反应也可以通过识别已知可引起高热的药物来进行预防，例如对正在服用单胺氧化酶抑制剂的患者应避免使用阿片类药物。

（戴柠宇 译 陈 芳 校）

延伸阅读

American Society of Anesthesiologists: Standards for basic anesthetic monitoring, 2015. Available at https://www.asahq.org/~/media/Sites/ASAHQ/Files/Public/Resources/standards-guidelines/standards-for-basic-anesthetic-monitoring.pdf. Accessed December 13, 2016.

Larach MG, Gronert GA, Allen GC, et al.: Clinical presentation, treatment, and complications of malignant hyperthermia in North America from 1987 to 2006, *Anesth Analg* 110(2):498–507, 2010.

Lenhardt R, Grady M, Kurz A: Hyperthermia during anaesthesia and intensive care unit stay, *Best Pract Res Clin Anaesthesiol* 22(4):669–694, 2008.

Lenhardt R, Negishi C, Sessler DI: Perioperative fever, *Acta Anaesthesiol Scand Suppl* 111:325–328, 1997.

Malignant Hyperthermia Association of the United States: Temperature monitoring during surgical procedures. Available at http://www.mhaus.org/healthcareprofessionals/mhaus-recommendations/temperature-monitoring. Accessed December 13, 2016.

Negishi C, Lenhardt R: Fever during anaesthesia, *Best Pract Res Clin Anaesthesiol* 17(4):499–517, 2003.

Rajek A, Greif R, Sessler DI, et al.: Core cooling by central venous infusion of ice-cold (4 degrees C and 20 degrees C) fluid: isolation of core and peripheral thermal compartments, *Anesthesiology* 93(3):629–637, 2000.

Sessler DI: Perioperative thermoregulation and heat balance, *Lancet* 387(10038):2655–2664, 2016.

Sessler DI: Temperature monitoring and perioperative thermoregulation, *Anesthesiology* 109(2):318–338, 2008.

Walter EJ, Hanna-Jumma S, Carraretto M, et al.: The pathophysiological basis and consequences of fever, *Crit Care* 20(1):200, 2016.

小儿喉痉挛

第 198 章

Nancy B. Samol，Eric P. Wittkugel

病例概要

患儿，5 岁，行扁桃体切除术，手术结束拔除气管导管后开始出现咳嗽，而后发展为高音调吸气性喘鸣音，最后进展为静息的摇摆样胸壁运动，可以观察到胸壁凹陷，呼吸音逐渐减弱，直至听不到。尝试面罩通气没有成功，患儿氧饱和度迅速下降。

问题分析

定义

除其他功能以外，喉部可以保护上呼吸道和肺避免吸入异物。吞咽时声门闭合反射最为明显。喉痉挛是一种应对有害刺激时出现的超常的声门关闭反射。喉痉挛引起的部分或完全气道阻塞即使是在去除刺激后仍可持续存在。喉痉挛是由迷走神经介导，传入神经为喉上神经内支，传出神经为喉返神经。

完全性喉痉挛包括两个阶段：①声门痉挛引起真正的声带收缩，导致部分气道梗阻，其机制是通过“快门”机制，在其后联合处留有一个小腔隙开放；②其次是“球形瓣膜”机制，即声门（会厌喉面）向后方移动，杓状软骨均做腹侧运动，有效地封闭喉部，形成一种收缩室带（假声带）的“球阀”机制。

识别

喉痉挛前兆包括反常胸廓运动、鼻翼扇动、肋间凹陷或气管拖拽、吸气性喘鸣音、呼吸音减弱或消失、低氧血症，继而出现心动过缓和发绀。喉痉挛可分为部分（通常描述为“声门痉挛”）或完全。病例概要描述了从部分喉痉挛到完全性喉痉挛的进展。部分喉痉挛与其他原因所导致的上气道梗阻的鉴别可能比较困难。典型的喉痉挛表现为胸廓运动和声带发出的刺耳的“喘鸣”声，同时通过后联合处的开放腔保持最小的通气。支气管痉挛通过听诊哮鸣音诊断。由舌头或咽部其他软组织引起的阻塞通常与打鼾或喘息有关，而由分泌物引起的阻塞通常伴有咕噜声。

快速识别和及时治疗完全性喉痉挛很有必要，因为闭合的声门不能进行气体交换。从部分喉痉挛发展到完全喉痉挛的过程中，胸外气道阻塞（胸壁收缩、鼻翼煽动、反常呼吸）症状加剧，直至呼吸音随着氧合和高碳酸血症而恶化。

风险评估

喉痉挛在儿童人群中发病率为 0.04% ～ 14%。近年来发病率下降趋势反映了早期识别的改善和麻醉及外科技术的改进。在迄今为止关于儿童喉痉挛的最大的单中心研究中，Burgoyne 和 Anghelescu 回顾了 1999—2002 年期间接受麻醉的 21 452 例患者，发现每 1000 例患者中有 1 例（0.1%）出现喉痉挛。喉痉挛的危险因素可分为三类：患者相关、手术相关和麻醉相关因素。

患者相关因素

与患者相关的最重要的因素是低龄。事实上，全身麻醉后喉痉挛的发生率与年龄成反比。此外，上呼吸道感染（特别是经父母确认的上呼吸道感染）引起的气道易激惹性增加是喉痉挛的有效预测因素，它与活动性哮喘一样，增加了 10 倍的风险。Von Ungern-Sternberg 等证实，手术当天或术前 2 周内出现感冒症状时，因分泌物过多和气道高反应可能导致喉痉挛的风险增加。该相关性得到了 Flick 等研究团队的证实，他们的研究提示喉痉挛与结构性或先天性气道异常之间显著相关。暴露在烟草的烟雾中会导致喉痉挛发病率增加10倍，所以术前病史应包括“被动吸烟”的问题。最后，胃食管反流史是喉痉挛的另一个危险因素。

手术相关因素

气道手术，包括扁桃体切除术（21%～27%的患者）和支气管镜检查，有很高的喉痉挛发生率。气道出血也增加喉痉挛的风险。食管内镜检查容易发生因刺激食管远端传出神经而引起喉痉挛。

麻醉相关因素

麻醉相关危险因素中最重要的是诱导期和苏醒期麻醉深度不足。挥发性麻醉药、黏液或血液、吸引管或喉镜片对气道操作均会刺激气道，诱发或加重喉痉挛。酸诱导的喉痉挛动物模型显示，浅麻醉状态可增加喉内收肌神经元的活跃度。在浅麻醉状态下，常用的一些麻醉方法也可增加儿童气道刺激。在吸入诱导期间，麻醉深度Ⅱ（浅）持续时间比静脉诱导时间长，增加了易感喉痉挛的时间。丙泊酚可以降低气道反应性和抑制喉反射，相较于七氟烷，丙泊酚诱导所致喉痉挛的相关性要小。在诱导期，分泌物或呼吸道管理装置（例如口咽通气道）刺激声门可能引发喉痉挛。文献中关于气道装置的选择和喉痉挛的危险性一直存在争议。最近的研究数据表明，喉罩（laryngeal mask airway，LMA）使用与喉痉挛密切相关，即使针对URI或呼吸道异常进行过调整亦会如此。在达至足够的麻醉深度之前，不使用肌肉松弛剂气管插管极易发生喉痉挛。在深麻醉下拔除气管导管，患者处于麻醉Ⅱ期且气道无保护时有喉痉挛的危险。最后，喉痉挛更有可能发生在由经验较少的麻醉科医师负责的患儿身上。

启示

虽然喉痉挛治疗后通常无后遗症，但严重或治疗无效的喉痉挛可发展为完全气道梗阻伴缺氧、高碳酸血症和心动过缓，并导致严重并发症，包括负压性肺水肿和心脏停搏。在完全气道梗阻情况下，患者为克服闭合性声门梗阻而产生的明显负性胸膜内压力可使液体渗入肺泡。负压性肺水肿可通过吸氧和利尿剂进行治疗。极少数情况下，需要气管插管和呼气末正压通气治疗负压性肺水肿。

在1000名出现喉痉挛的患者中，会有5名出现心脏停搏。如果要避免喉痉挛进展为心脏停搏，应及时识别和采取有效的干预措施。

预防

预防是喉痉挛的最佳治疗方法，通常可以通过确认和尽可能减少危险因素来实现。可采取下列措施：

- 有上呼吸道感染、任何被动吸烟、鼻塞或大量痰、高反应性气道疾病史或睡眠呼吸障碍史的儿童患者推迟2～3周进行择期气道手术。
- 高危患者避免在诱导时使用N_2O，以达到更高的氧储备，以防止在发生喉痉挛时出现早期氧饱和度降低。
- 适当应用肌肉松弛药可有助于气管插管。
- 浅麻醉期间避免有害的气道或手术刺激。
- 当喉痉挛的风险很高且不能缓解时，考虑气管插管，而不是使用喉罩或面罩麻醉。
- 麻醉维持选择七氟烷或异氟烷吸入麻醉，避免使用地氟烷，后者可显著增加围术期呼吸不良事件。
- 气管拔除前彻底吸除口咽部分泌物。
- 患者完全清醒时拔除气管。过早拔管是喉痉挛的主要原因。

此外，以下措施可能有助于预防喉痉挛：

- 拔管前静脉注射利多卡因可通过阻断或减弱中枢反射通路或感觉和运动神经末梢预防或减轻喉痉挛。
- 利多卡因局部应用于口咽后部和声带可抑制喉黏膜感觉神经活动。
- 拔管前，让患者吸入100%氧气3 min，以便在气道梗阻和喉痉挛时提高安全界限。
- Tsui及其同事描述如何避免扁桃体-软骨切除术后喉痉挛，采取“非接触”技术包括吸除口咽部分泌物，将患者头低位偏向一侧以保持声带畅通，停止麻醉，避免刺激直到患者完全清醒拔除气管导管。
- 拔管时，在吸气末暂时挤压呼吸囊以15～20 cmH_2O的正压维持较高的肺容积，这样可以减少喉痉挛。在动物模型中，这种胸腔内正压可抑制声门闭合反射，降低喉部内收肌的反应。同时，拔除气管导管时使肺部膨胀可有助于排出分泌物，从而减少了喉痉挛和分泌物误吸的可能性。

患者是否应在深麻醉状态下或清醒时拔除气管

插管和 LMA 以减少喉痉挛，仍有争议。在过去 20 年中，有十多项研究未能就最佳实践达成共识，但研究证据倾向于在深麻醉下拔除喉罩，清醒后拔出气管插管。识别儿童发生喉痉挛的风险非常重要。虽然不可能改变所有的术前危险因素，但谨慎选择麻醉技术和药物可以减少喉痉挛发生。

管理

如果预防失败，对喉痉挛的处理取决于气道梗阻是部分性还是完全性，喉痉挛的严重程度以及病因。任何情况下，及时识别和立即积极处理对于预防和逆转低氧血症至关重要。因此，喉痉挛的治疗成功很大程度上取决于麻醉科医师的经验。如果识别和处理延迟，可能会因为心排血量下降从而降低药物治疗效果而使治疗复杂化。很多研究者建议首先进行气道处理，首先去除刺激物，然后必要时给予药物治疗。图 198.1 和 198.2 分别介绍了喉痉挛引起的完全或部分气道梗阻的处理流程。初始治疗包括以下几个方面：

- 使用脉搏血氧饱和度仪、心电图和心前区听诊器持续监测。
- 二氧化碳描记图确认通气是否有效。
- 通过密封良好的面罩输送 100% 的氧气行持续正压通气（continuous positive airway pressure，CPAP）。
- 张口同时使下颌前移。

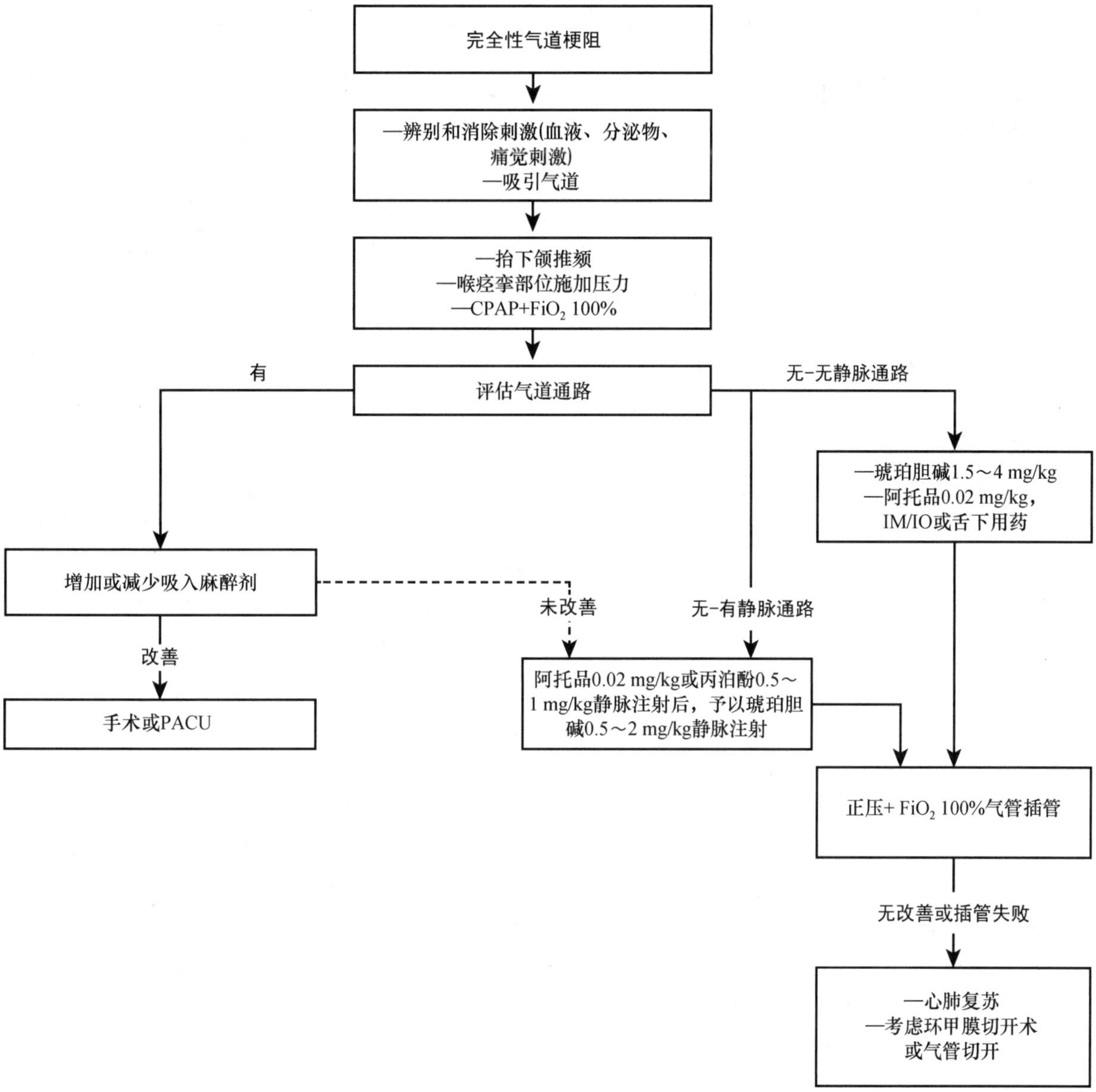

图 198.1　完全气道梗阻的治疗流程。CPAP，持续气道正压通气；FiO_2，吸入氧浓度；IM，肌内注射；IV，静脉注射；IO，骨内注射；PACU，麻醉后恢复室

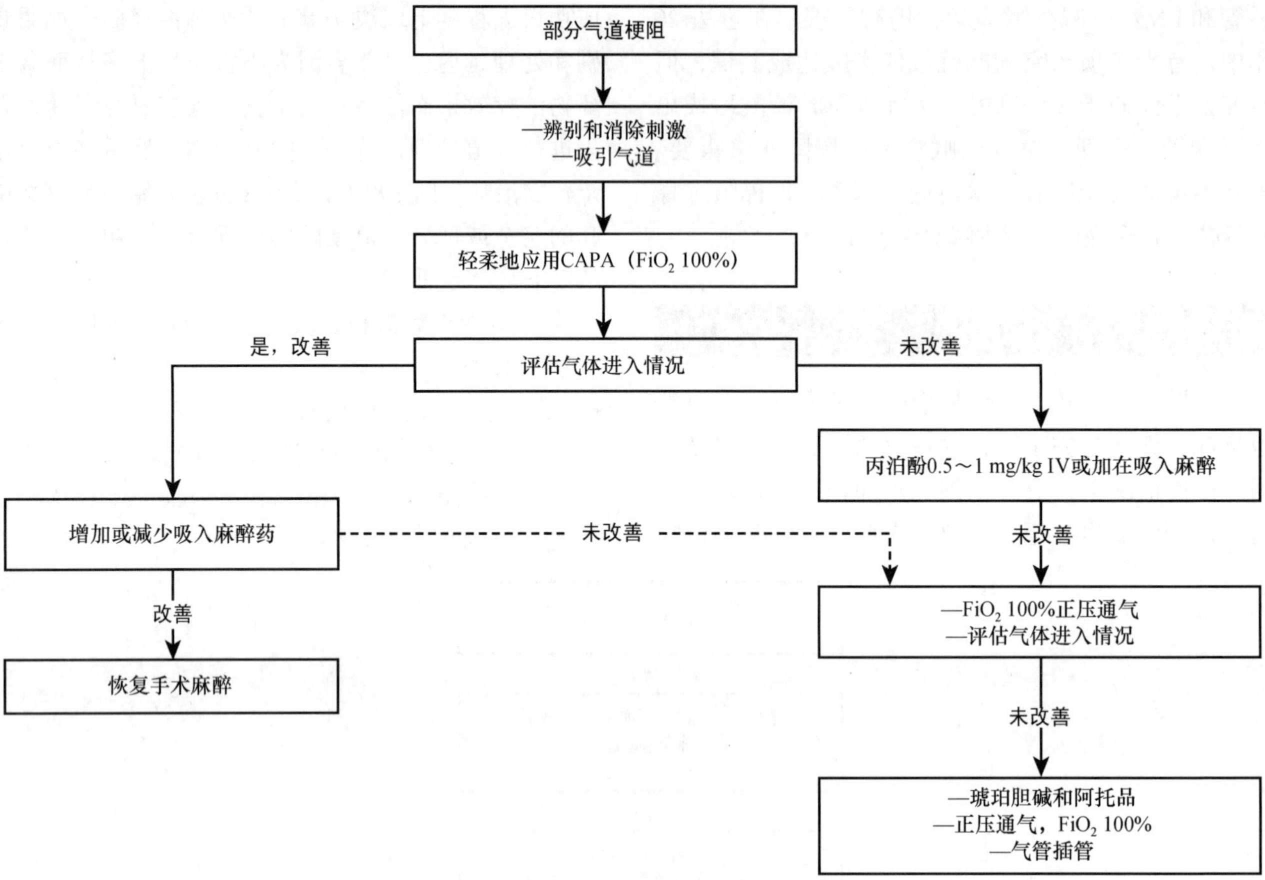

图 198.2 部分气道梗阻的治疗流程。CPAP，持续气道正压通气；FiO_2，吸入氧浓度；IV，静脉注射

- 清除有害气道刺激物（例如，吸除血液和分泌物，移除气道装置）。
- 在喉痉挛部位维持恒定持续气道内压力。
- 使用静脉或挥发性麻醉药减轻或加深麻醉。
- “呼吸球囊扑动”——手动高频通气。
- 对其他措施无效的完全性梗阻，使用肌松药。

在多数情况下，部分性喉痉挛可通过球囊面罩实施正压通气得到有效的治疗。吸气时，喉部经常会有短暂的相对松弛，这时用力挤压麻醉球囊通气，可为患者的呼吸活动提供“压力支持”。该技术可为患者提供维持氧合所需的最低气体交换，并有助于加深或减轻麻醉以缓解喉痉挛。但应尽量避免过度CPAP，因其可能会导致胃胀气，从而进一步限制通气或引起反流，必需插入胃管进行减压。值得注意的是，在完全性喉痉挛和球阀阻塞的情况下，应用正压通气可以加重气道阻塞，因为气道正压可使喉两侧梨状窝肿胀，并加重杓状会厌皱襞的相互挤压。

下颌前移（即抬下颌推颏动作）可引起疼痛性刺激，使颏骨肌伸展而开放部分喉部，这对完全性喉痉挛尤其有益，同时可以确保不会因软组织阻塞而加重喉部闭合导致的气道阻塞。喉痉挛通常由反流或残留的上呼吸道分泌物刺激所诱发。因此，即使在紧急情况下也要吸引咽部分泌物以防止进一步刺激喉上神经。

Larson 研究团队对位于耳后的“喉痉挛切迹”施加压力的简单技术做了描述。该点在髁状突旁下颌升支前方，后缘以乳突为界，与颅底相连。Larson 的方法是用两个手指向颅底施加稳定的压力，同时伴有下颌骨前移，使骨膜产生疼痛，引起自主神经系统反射和声带松弛，“呼吸球囊扑动（Fluttering the bag）”是一种手动高频通气技术，是以类似于心房扑动的间断节奏快速地挤压和释放呼吸球囊。最近，有人提出一种新的技术，即应用 100% 氧气，同时轻柔按压胸部，以替代缓解喉痉挛的标准做法（100% 氧气加 CPAP）。

由于喉痉挛经常发生于浅麻醉，因此加深麻醉或唤醒患者可能会缓解，这取决于喉痉挛是否发生于诱导、维持或苏醒期。丙泊酚（0.5 ～ 0.8 mg/kg）

可迅速加深麻醉水平，可缓解 75% 以上的喉痉挛。只要心排血量足够，丙泊酚缓解喉痉挛的作用可能优于琥珀胆碱（一种去极化剂肌肉松弛药），其优点包括与之前使用的非去极化药物无相互作用，减少延长肌肉松弛的风险，且可安全用于烧伤、肌肉萎缩症、脊髓横断或高钾血症的患者。

如果上述操作不能改善气道梗阻，刚有使用肌肉松弛药的指征。由于琥珀胆碱起效快、作用时间短，成为治疗喉痉挛最常用的肌肉松弛药。琥珀胆碱的另一个优点是，如果无法静脉注射，可以通过肌肉或在舌下途径给药。因其对患儿具有迷走神经过敏的特性，应与阿托品合用。阿托品也可以治疗持续低氧血症引起的心动过缓。静脉注射琥珀胆碱的剂量为 0.5 ～ 2 mg/kg，肌内注射需要更高的剂量（高达 4 mg/kg）。较小剂量的琥珀胆碱可以有效地治疗喉痉挛，但如果需要紧急插管，则需要更大剂量的琥珀胆碱。

如果喉痉挛持续，且患儿长时间低氧血症危及生命，可能必须在无肌肉松弛药的情况下直接插管。如果并列的声带影响气管插管，局部应用利多卡因可以使喉部松弛，可有助于气管插管。如果这些措施和插管后仍不能改善气体交换，则可能需要行环状软骨切开或紧急气管切开。

（鲁 璐 译 余喜亚 校）

延伸阅读

Al-Alami AA, Ayoub CM, Baraka AS: Laryngospasm: review of different prevention and treatment modalities, *Pediatr Anesth* 18:281–288, 2008.

Al-Alami AA, Zestos MM, Baraka AS: Pediatric laryngospasm: prevention and treatment, *Curr Opin Anesthesiol* 22:388–395, 2009.

Badgwell JM: Laryngospasm. In *Clinical pediatric anesthesia*, Philadelphia, 1997, Lippincott-Raven, pp 39–40.

Burgoyne LL, Anghelescu DL: Intervention steps for treating laryngospasm in pediatric patients, *Pediatr Anesth* 18:297–302, 2008.

Flick RP, Wilder RT, Pieper SF, et al.: Risk factors for laryngospasm in children during general anesthesia, *Pediatr Anesth* 18:289–296, 2008.

Hampson-Evans D, Morgan P, Farrar M: Pediatric laryngospasm, *Pediatr Anesth* 18:303–307, 2008.

Johnstone RE: Laryngospasm treatment—an explanation, *Anesthesiology* 91:581–582, 1999.

Larson PC: Laryngospasm—the best treatment, *Anesthesiology* 89:1293–1294, 1998.

Mihara T, Uchimoto K, Morita A, et al.: The efficacy of lidocaine to prevent laryngospasm in children: a systematic review and meta-analysis, *Anaesthesia* 69:1388–1396, 2014.

Orestes MI, Lander L, Verghese S, et al.: Incidence of laryngospasm and bronchospasm in pediatric adenotonsillectomy, *Laryngoscope* 122:425–428, 2012.

Orliaguet GA, Olivier G, Savoldelli GL, et al.: Case scenario: perianesthetic management of laryngospasm in children, *Anesthesiology* 116:458–471, 2012.

Skolnick ET, Vomvolakis MA, Buck KA, et al.: Exposure to environmental tobacco smoke and the risk of adverse respiratory events in children receiving general anesthesia, *Anesthesiology* 88:1144–1153, 1998.

Suzuki M, Sasaki CT: Laryngeal spasm: a neurophysiologic redefinition, *Ann Otol Rhinol Laryngol* 86:150–157, 1977.

Tait AR, Malviya S, Voepel-Lewis T, et al.: Risk factors for perioperative adverse respiratory events in children with upper respiratory tract infections, *Anesthesiology* 95:299–306, 2001.

Tsui BC, Wagner A, Cave D, et al.: The incidence of laryngospasm with a “no touch” extubation technique after tonsillectomy and adenoidectomy, *Anesth Analg* 98:327–329, 2004.

Von Ungern-Sternberg BS, Boda K, Chambers NA, et al.: Risk assessment for respiratory complications in paediatric anaesthesia: a prospective cohort study, *Lancet* 376:773–783, 2010.

Von Ungern-Sternberg BS, Ramgolam A, Hall GL, et al.: Peri-operative adverse respiratory events in children, *Anaesthesia* 70(4):440–444, 2015.

第199章 围术期吸入性肺炎

Marc Mecoli，Joseph Previte

病例概要

患者，男性，5岁，因患嗜酸细胞性胃肠炎致长期吞咽困难及呕吐，影像学表现提示胃肠排空延迟，拟行食管、胃、十二指肠镜检查。既往内窥镜检查提示，即便患者遵循适当的禁食指南，胃内容物依然存在。

问题分析

定义

吸入性肺炎被定义为气管及支气管树部位发现胆汁分泌物或颗粒物。最常发生于胃内容物被动反流或主动呕吐，但误吸血液或咽部分泌物也可引起严重的肺炎。在接受麻醉时发生误吸的儿童患者中，40%为主动呕吐，其余为胃内容物被动反流。在发生误吸的麻醉患者中，80%发生在诱导期，14%在苏醒期，4%在术中，2%在术后发生。

识别

当发生严重的误吸后，体格检查可发现患者有发热、呼吸急促、呼吸暂停、心动过速、顽固性喉痉挛、支气管痉挛、喘鸣或咳嗽。此外还可听到湿啰音和干啰音，可观察到患者发绀。胸部X线片可显示肺泡浸润影，少数情况下可见网状浸润。影像学表现可为局部，但通常较为广泛，且频发于双侧肺。误吸6～24 h后，胸部X线片才能显示出完全的改变。90%的严重误吸患者在1 h内出现症状，几乎所有患者在2 h内出现症状。反流物pH测定可用于预测肺损伤的严重程度。

风险评估

每1万例小儿麻醉中，发生1～10例误吸。与成人相比，儿童患者的误吸率更高，且严重肺损伤的风险更高。当然，现有文献结果并不一致。与成人患者相比，小儿患者具有独特的吸入性肺炎风险（框199.1和框199.2）。

框199.1　儿童吸入性肺炎的特有危险因素

新生儿暂时性咽部无力
新生儿气管食管瘘（修复后常见胃肠道反流）
慢性肺部疾病（哮喘、哮吼、支气管肺发育不良、囊性纤维化）
早产
脑瘫、发育迟缓（吞咽功能障碍）
外伤性儿童患者的急性胃扩张

导致儿童发生误吸风险的胃内容物临界pH和胃内容物体积尚不清楚，但根据未发表的恒河猴实验数据来推断，胃pH（<2.5）和胃残余体积（>0.4 ml/kg）的阈值可应用于人类。根据这些限制，儿童吸入性肺炎的风险将比成人更高。因为76%的儿童患者胃内容物pH小于2.5，体积大于0.4 ml/kg，而成人却只有32%～55%的患者符合以上标准。

婴儿发生肺部误吸的风险最高。胃食管反流病（gastroesophageal reflux disease，GERD）发生在近50%的足月新生儿，这在刚出生后的前6个月被认为是正常的。胃内压力低至23 cmH_2O时亦易发生GERD。如果气管插管时胃底食管角减小，胃内压更低时也会发生GERD。婴幼儿患者由于胃较小，哭闹时吞咽了空气，横膈呼吸，其在静息期胃内压高于较大的儿童或成人，因而导致发生GERD的风险增加。

对于择期手术中的健康患者，使用喉罩发生吸入性肺炎的概率可能不会更高。然而，喉罩并未在喉周围形成紧密的密封。此外，它由于咽部肌肉扩张引起食管下括约肌反射性松弛，如吞咽食团时。使用喉罩时，由于正压通气致胃扩张，导致胃内容

框 199.2 成人和儿童吸入性肺炎的危险因素

身体状况 ASA Ⅲ或Ⅳ级
在正常工作时间以外的手术[a]
急诊手术[a]
肥胖、腹水、腹部巨大肿块
胃炎、溃疡史
胃瘫
自主神经病变（家族性、获得性）
肌肉疾病
长效的全身麻醉药
声带麻痹
糖尿病
电解质紊乱、代谢失衡
麻醉深度不足
困难气道
既往胃食管反流病史
食管和上腹部手术
颅内压升高
退行性神经病变
黄嘌呤类、β-受体激动剂
阿片类药物、甲基
意识水平降低
喉功能障碍或痉挛
胶原血管疾病
肾、盆腔、膀胱或子宫扩张

[a] 增加 5 ～ 6 倍的风险
ASA，美国麻醉科医师协会

物反流至喉部，从而发生吸入性肺炎的可能性增加。因此，对于存在反流高风险的患儿应使用气管导管保护气道。

喉反射是一种重要的防止肺误吸的保护机制，其可被麻醉诱导药、喉部和气管局部麻醉以及超过浓度超过 50% 的氧化亚氮抑制。在成人中，在气管拔管后的 2 ～ 8 h 内，喉反射会受到抑制，即使患者已处于警醒状态。儿童的喉反射也可出现类似的抑制。喉反射能力下降是气管插管的机械作用所致，与麻醉药的残余作用有所不同。

启示

吸入性肺炎的发生和严重程度更多地取决于胃内物的 pH 而非容量。pH 小于 1.8 的少量误吸即可导致严重肺炎，而 pH 大于 2.5 的较多量的误吸（>2 ml/kg）对肺的损伤可能很小。

肺部误吸通过引起上皮细胞水肿和脱落，导致气管和主支气管黏膜保护屏障的丧失。受损组织后续容易受到病毒或细菌感染。高酸性液体反流后可在 12 ～ 18 s 内造成肺损伤，3 min 内即可造成广泛肺不张。发生肺部误吸后 1 h，肺损伤进展为支气管上皮变性、肺水肿、出血。随后肺毛细血管渗漏增加，继之中性粒细胞发生反应。由于肺泡细胞损伤，液体和蛋白质进入肺泡和肺间质，肺表面活性物质的活性下降。由于肺表面活性物质的活性降低，气道阻力增加，肺顺应性下降，导致严重缺氧。此外，患者还可能出现严重的低血压，可能是由于血管内容积减少（由于液体渗漏入肺泡），以及为满足足够的通气所需的高气道压力导致的静脉回流受损。

颗粒状物体的误吸，可使低氧血症发生得更早、更严重。虽然液体渗漏的程度不如吸入酸性胃液广泛，但动脉二氧化碳分压增加得更高，动脉血 pH 降低得更大。临床典型的肺误吸死亡率为 5% 或更低。

管理

治疗包括立即吸引气道或予以鼻导管或面罩吸氧。这通常即已足够，但严重的病例可能需要气管插管和机械通气。

酸性物质误吸不推荐行支气管肺灌洗，因为肺损伤发生在 12 ～ 18 s 内。此外，由于酸性误吸物扩散到肺的较低级的区域，可能会造成更广泛的肺损伤。

颗粒物质误吸的直接危害是机械性阻塞。在这种情况下，应通过支气管镜清除颗粒物。在肺误吸后应用糖皮质激素并没有降低发病率或死亡率的作用，也不建议使用，因为糖皮质激素可使患者易发生革兰氏阴性菌性肺炎。

应根据气管抽吸物微生物培养结果给予抗生素。对于吸入严重污染物质（如粪便、脓）的患者可经验性用药。白细胞增多、肺浸润、稠痰和发热都是化学性肺炎的非特异性反应，这并不是应用抗生素治疗的充分理由。体位引流和应用支气管扩张药呼吸治疗可能有效。大多数患者在 2 周内临床症状消失。

预防

预防和改善肺误吸有赖于传统的抗酸剂和药物

的使用，其可促进胃排空，增加食管下段括约肌张力（促动力剂），减少胃容量（H_2 受体阻滞剂），或增加胃内容物的 pH（H_2 受体阻滞剂，质子泵抑制剂）。表 199.1 概述了这些药物的剂量、用法和主要作用。

对于拟行需要麻醉的手术或操作的健康儿童，表 199.2 中列出了明确的禁食指南。最近，更宽松的禁食指南，包括在术前允许饮用清亮的液体，2015 年 Andersson 及其同事对行择期手术的健康儿童进行了研究，并没有得出该人群发病率增加的证据。目前尚无针对肺误吸风险增加的儿童的禁食指南发布。对于这些患者，建议在诱导前清除胃内容物。如果术前无法从胃腔抽吸，则应行快速序贯诱导，气管插管后立即吸引胃内容物，以减少麻醉苏醒和拔管过程中发生肺呼吸的风险。

为了防止反流，快速序贯诱导可以缩短意识丧失至气道获得保护之间的时间，此段时间内患者易发生误吸。无论有无留置鼻胃管，压迫环状软骨历来是快速序列诱导的重要组成部分，其可有效预防婴幼儿和成人胃液的被动反流。在意识消失之前，对环状软骨的压力（20 牛顿，相当于 2 kg 重）必须在意识消失前施加。这种压力对于清醒患者会有不适感。在静脉麻醉诱导后，意识消失之前，所有年龄组患者均会出现食管上段屏障压力丧失。对于无意识的患者压迫环状软骨的力量应增加到 40 牛顿（此力量对于清醒患者较痛苦）。较高的压力可能使气管和上气道扭曲变形或阻塞，并可能使插管颇具挑战性。对于正在呕吐的患者，压迫环状软骨有可能导致食管破裂。

表 199.1　预防肺误吸的药物

药物	剂量和用法	胃容量	pH	食管下段括约肌张力
制酸剂				
Alka-Seltzer 苏打水	2 汤匙 /30 ml 水（1 h BS）	↑	↑	0
柠檬酸钠	0.5 ～ 1 ml/kg（最多 30 ml；1 h BS）	↑	↑	0
抗胆碱药物				
格隆溴铵	7.5 ～ 10 μg/kg（1 h BS）	?	?	0
H_2 受体阻滞剂				
西咪替丁	7.5 mg/kg（PM/AM）	↓	↑	0
法莫替丁	0.5 mg/kg（PM/AM）	↓	↑	0
雷尼替丁	1.5 ～ 2 mg/kg（1 ～ 2 h BS）	0	↑	0
促动力药物				
甲氧氯普胺	0.1 mg/kg IV 或 PO（1 h BS）	↓	0	↑
质子泵抑制剂				
兰索拉唑	1.5 mg/kg（PM/AM）	↓	↑	0
奥美拉唑	0.3 mg/kg（PM/AM）	↓	↑	0
泮妥拉唑	1.4 mg/kg QID	↓	↑	0

BS，术前；IV，静脉注射；PM/AM，术前晚和术日晨；PO，口服；QID，一日 4 次

表 199.2　行择期手术的健康儿童禁食指南

年龄	固体食物	清水[a]	配方
0 ～ 6 个月	6 h	2 h	6 h
6 个月～ 2 岁	6 h	2 h	6 h
>2 岁	6 h（便餐）[b]	2 h	不适用
>2 岁	8 h(含有脂肪的食物）	2 h	不适用

[a] 某些人把早餐奶当成清水

[b] 根据美国麻醉科医师协会（American Society of anesthesiologists）的指南，清淡的便餐通常包括烤面包和清亮的液体。含有油炸或高脂肪食物或者肉类的食物可能会延长胃排空时间。在确定合适的禁食时间时，必须考虑摄入食物量和食物种类。

在诱导过程中，由于麻醉深度不够或未使用肌肉松弛药，大多数误吸发生于气道操作过程中发生的咳嗽或作呕。喉镜置入前应确保肌肉完全松弛，以减少发生反流的可能性。插管前轻柔的面罩通气及可控的快速序贯诱导可减少缺氧，且不增加肺误吸的发生率（Neuhaus 及其同事，2015）。儿童在长时间插管（如加强治疗病房患者）中使用带套囊的气管导管可减少被动反流引起的隐匿性误吸的发生。

对于发生肺误吸的高危患者，拔管应在患者完全清醒且神经肌肉功能完全恢复的情况下进行。儿童应表现为张口、髋关节屈曲以及吞咽、咳嗽和作呕反射的恢复。患者应保持 10 ～ 15° 头低足高位（Trendelenburg）的侧位，这样任何分泌物或反流物都可以堆积在脸颊下并被动引流。最后，在拔管前即刻应使用 15 ～ 20 cmH_2O 的呼气末正压，以诱导患者的反射性咳嗽，从而将分泌物或误吸物推离喉部。

致谢

感谢 Mark Meyer 博士对本章上一版的贡献。

（魏 玲 译 卞金俊 校）

延伸阅读

Andersson H, Zaren B: Frykholm: Low incidence of pulmonary aspiration in children allowed intake of clear fluids until called to the operating suite, *Pediatr Anesth* 25:770–777, 2015.

Borland LM, Woelfel SK, Saitz EW, et al.: Pulmonary aspiration in pediatric patients under general anesthesia: frequency and outcome, *Anesthesiology* 83:A1150, 1995.

Coté CJ, Goudsouzian NG, Liu LMP, et al.: Assessment of risk factors related to the acid aspiration syndrome in pediatric patients: gastric pH and residual volume, *Anesthesiology* 56:70–72, 1982.

Goudsouzian N: Aspiration in children: practical implications, *Anesthesiol Rev* 11:6–16, 1984.

Neuhaus D, Schmitz A, Gerber A, et al: Controlled rapid sequence induction and intubation—an analysis of 1001 children. Pediatr Anesth 23:734–740.

Orenstein DM: Aspiration pneumonias and gastroesophageal reflux–related respiratory disease. In Behrman RE, Kliegman RM, Arvin AM, editors: *Nelson's textbook of pediatrics*, Philadelphia, 1996, WB Saunders, pp 1213–1217.

Salem MR, Wong AY, Fizzotti GF, et al.: Efficacy of cricoid pressure in preventing aspiration of gastric contents in paediatric patients, *Br J Anaesth* 44:401–404, 1972.

Warner MA, Warner ME, Warner DO, et al.: Perioperative pulmonary aspiration in infants and children, *Anesthesiology* 90:66–71, 1999.

第200章 插管后哮吼

Barbara M. Dilos

病例概要

患儿，女，4 岁，在全身麻醉下行腹腔镜脐疝修补术。进入麻醉后恢复室几分钟后，患儿被发现出现吸气性喘鸣。

问题分析

定义

插管后哮吼（croup）是全身麻醉气管插管的并发症之一。表现为术后期间的吸气性喘鸣，这是声门下水肿导致呼吸阻力增加的表现。气管插管导管被认为是造成插管后气管黏膜损伤的主要原因。

根据拔管后出现的气管水肿程度，插管后哮吼的严重程度不同。插管后哮吼主要是小儿而不是成人并发症的主要原因是两者气道的解剖差异。

小儿气道解剖学

小儿气道与成人气道不同。大约 8 岁时发育的和成人气道相类似。小儿的舌头相对于嘴巴较大，其喉比成人喉位置更高，位于约 C2 水平，而成人喉处于约颈椎前 C5 水平。会厌更像 Ω 形而不是 U 形，与气道成角比成人更小。过去认为小儿喉是圆锥形和圆形的，而最新数据显示是椭圆形的。小儿气道的最窄处位于喉下的环状软骨环，而成人则位于声带处。由于小儿气道口径狭窄，轻微的周围水肿可对层流气流阻力产生很大影响。在层流条件下，阻力与气管半径的四次方成反比。1 mm 的周围水肿对直径仅为 3 ～ 4 mm 的气道阻力的影响大于直径 7 ～ 8 mm 的气道。

风险评估

过去的几年中，小儿全身麻醉声门上气道装置的使用大大增加。当使用这些装置时，插管后哮吼不会出现，但是在许多情况下，麻醉期间需要用气管插管保护气道。

多年来一直认为 8 岁以下的儿童使用带套囊的气管导管插管是发生插管后哮吼的危险因素。套囊压力对气管黏膜的影响，特别是在狭窄的环状软骨环上可导致水肿和插管后哮吼。最近的研究表明，不管是带套囊还是无套囊，气管导管尺寸的选择很重要。选择有套囊的应比无套囊的气管导管小半号，因为气道必须容纳套囊。

使用有套管或无套囊的导管气管插管后，检查 20 ～ 30 cmH_2O 压力是否有气体泄漏是非常重要的，因为这是导管没有对气道黏膜施加压力的一个标志。然而，没有泄漏并不能确定插管后是否会出现哮吼。研究表明，高容量低压套囊不容易引起黏膜水肿。此外，套管在气道中的放置很重要。套囊应该在气管下方，避开狭窄的环状软骨环。这在一定程度上是一个挑战，因为小儿气管很短，因此导管的大小和位置不当时，套囊可能无法避开环状软骨环和阻塞气管隆突。

插管后哮吼风险较高的病例是存在气管内装置和颈部不处于中立位置的病例。此外，患者如有上呼吸道感染并接受插管麻醉，发生插管后哮吼的风险更高。唐氏综合征的患者由于气道特殊的解剖学差异（例如声门下狭窄），插管后哮吼的发生率更高。长时间的手术和反复插管也会增加插管后喘鸣的风险。

识别

插管后哮吼的诊断通过观察得出。如果患者具有前面描述的任何危险因素，则应高度怀疑其发生。喘鸣音是当空气通过胸外梗阻时产生的一种高音调吸气噪声。梗阻是由声门下黏膜水肿引起的。喘鸣可能在拔管后立即发生或者推迟至患者在麻醉后复苏室的时候。可表现为轻度至重度的气道梗阻，伴随或不伴氧饱和度下降。如果水肿严重可能累及呼吸辅助肌肉，此时若不及时识别和治疗，则可能进展为完全梗阻和需要重新插管的呼吸衰竭。

已有一些不同的量表来量化病毒性哮吼和插管后哮吼的严重程度。其中之一是 Westley 系统评分，将临床表现分为五个评分标准：意识水平、发绀、喘鸣、气体进入和胸壁回缩。总共有 17 分，轻度哮吼为 0 ～ 2 分，中度为 3 ～ 5 分，重度为 6 ～ 11 分，即将发生呼吸衰竭的为 12 ～ 17 分。值得注意的是许多标准取决于临床观察。肺活量测定法和食管测压法是可以获得实际测量值的方法，但在临床条件下，这些测量值不易获得。

一旦发现喘鸣，应立即采取治疗措施，以便在气道完全梗阻前阻止气管水肿的进展。

管理

在插管后轻微喘鸣的病例中，湿化氧气已被证明有效。中度至重度病例中，外消旋肾上腺素雾化是首选治疗方案。儿科患者中，外消旋肾上腺素雾化已广泛应用于治疗病毒性哮吼。L 和 D 肾上腺素的外消旋混合物被认为是减轻 L 肾上腺素的肾上腺素能心脏不良反应的方法。研究表明，L 肾上腺素外消旋液是否用于治疗喘鸣的雾化剂，在治疗和不良方面没有差异。治疗后 30 min 内，症状减轻。雾化的肾上腺素使受气道水肿影响的组织的局部血管收缩。目前还没有关于其在插管后喘鸣中应用的正式研究。然而，它已在麻醉后治疗病房和儿科重症监护病房成功使用多年。它可以用雾化器给药，也可以在无创正压通气时输送给药。停止使用后作用消退，尽管水肿可能不会恢复到基线，但可能需要进行再次治疗。发生插管后喘鸣接受肾上腺素雾化治疗的患者至少应严密监测 8 ～ 12 h，以确保气道水肿不会复发。

氦氧混合气体或氦氧混合物作为一种增加层流的方法可用于治疗病毒性哮吼，且对插管后哮吼可能具有益处。

静脉注射类固醇如地塞米松也可以起作用，但药物起效时间需要几个小时。至于预防性应用类固醇，尚无研究表明在儿科患者中常规使用预防性类固醇可以防止插管后哮吼。如果对治疗没有反应并且呼吸衰竭恶化，必须决定是否重新插管。

预防

预防措施对插管后喘鸣至关重要。了解风险因素并确保将这些风险因素降至最低，可有效地预防插管后喘鸣。早期识别和及时治疗减少气管水肿以及治疗后观察是避免完全呼吸衰竭和再插管的基础。

（胡琍琍　译　王　薇　校）

延伸阅读

Anene O, Meert KL, Uy H, et al.: Dexamethasone for the prevention of postextubation airway obstruction: a prospective, randomized, double-blind, placebo-controlled trial, *Crit Care Med* 24(10):1666–1669, 1996.

Kemper KJ, Ritz RH, Benson MS, Bishop MS: Helium-oxygen mixture in the treatment of postextubation stridor in pediatric trauma patients, *Crit Care Med* 19(3):356–359, 1991.

Khemani RG, Hotz J, Morzov R, et al.: Evaluating risk factors for pediatric post-extubation upper airway obstruction using a physiology-based tool, *Am J Respir Crit Care Med* 193:198–209, 2016.

Khemani RG, Randolph A, Markovitz B: Corticosteroids for the prevention and treatment of post-extubation stridor in neonates, children and adults, CD001000 *Cochrane Database Syst Rev*(3), 2009.

Koka BV, Jeon IS, Andre JM, et al.: Postintubation croup in children, *Anesth Analg* 56(4):501–505, 1977.

Lee C-H, Peng M-J, Wu C-L: Dexamethasone to prevent postextubation airway obstruction in adults: a prospective, randomized, double-blind, placebo-controlled study, *Crit Care* 11(4):R72, 2007.

Markovitz BP, Randolph AG, Khemani RG: Corticosteroids for the prevention and treatment of post-extubation stridor in neonates, children and adults, CD001000 *Cochrane Database Syst Rev*(2), 2008. [update of *Cochrane Database Syst Rev* (2):CD001000, 2000].

Miller RL, Cole RP: Association between reduced cuff leak volume and postextubation stridor, *Chest* 110(4):1035–1040, 1996.

Rimenberg PC: *Pediatric and neonatal ventilation: from basics to clinical practice*, New York, 2015, Springer, pp 981–997.

Suominen P, Taivainen T, Tuominen N, et al.: Optimally fitted tracheal tubes decrease the probability of postextubation adverse events in children undergoing general anesthesia, *Pediatr Anesth* 16:641–647, 2006.

Tobias JD: Pediatric airway anatomy may not be what we thought: implications for clinical practice and the use of cuffed endotracheal tubes, *Paediatr Anaesth* 25(1):9–19, 2015.

von Ungern-Sternberg BS, Davies K, Hegarty M, et al.: The effect of deep vs. awake extubation on respiratory complications in high-risk children undergoing adenotonsillectomy: a prospective, randomised, controlled trial, *Eur J Anaesthesiol* 30:529–536, 2013.

Westley CR, Cotton EK, Brooks JG: Nebulized racemic epinephrine by IPPB for the treatment of croup: a double-blind study, *Am J Dis Child* 132(5):484–487, 1978.

第201章 小儿阻塞后肺水肿

Lourdes Al Ghofaily

病例概要

患儿，5 岁，肥胖，发育迟缓，同时存在哮喘和阻塞性睡眠呼吸暂停，拟行扁桃体切除术。吸入麻醉诱导开始后出现间歇性气道部分阻塞，直至插入鼻咽和口腔通气道后缓解。手术结束时，气管导管内可见粉红色、泡沫状液体。行胸部 X 线片检查（图 201.1）并将患儿转移到重症监护病房行呼气末正压通气（positive end-expiratory pressure，PEEP）治疗。次日上午胸部提示结果正常（图 201.2），拔管顺利。

问题分析

定义

阻塞后肺水肿（postobstruction pulmonary edema，POPE），也称为负压性肺水肿（negative pressure pulmonary edema，NPPE），是肺水肿的一种非心源性形式，由肺泡水平的静水压力的急剧变化所诱发。目前认为存在两种类型的 POPE，1 型是在上呼吸道发生梗阻时用力吸气所致，如喉痉挛、会厌炎、喉炎或异物吸入，2 型是在慢性梗阻缓解后发生，如阻塞性睡眠呼吸暂停（obstructive sleep apnea，OSA）患者、切除扁桃体或腺样体解除慢性上呼吸道梗阻后的患者。在 2 型 POPE 中，跨肺压力梯度的变化主要发生在呼气相。

在两种类型的 POPE 中，肺泡内外压力平衡的变化则会导致渗出液体进入肺泡腔，引起肺水肿。

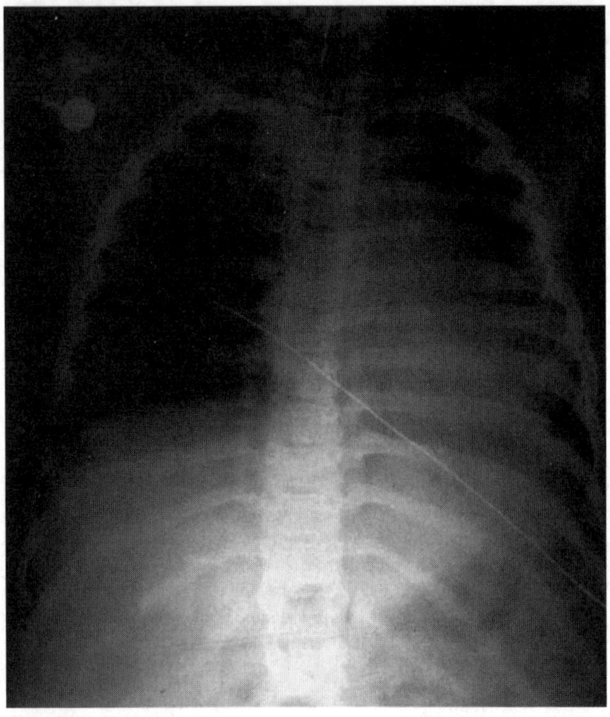

图 201.1　手术结束时胸部 X 线片。注意肺门周围绒毛浸润呈蝴蝶状，与肺水肿一致。左肺下叶不张也可见

识别

POPE 的识别涉及对其病理生理学的理解。正常情况下，肺泡和周围组织之间的静水压力和胶体

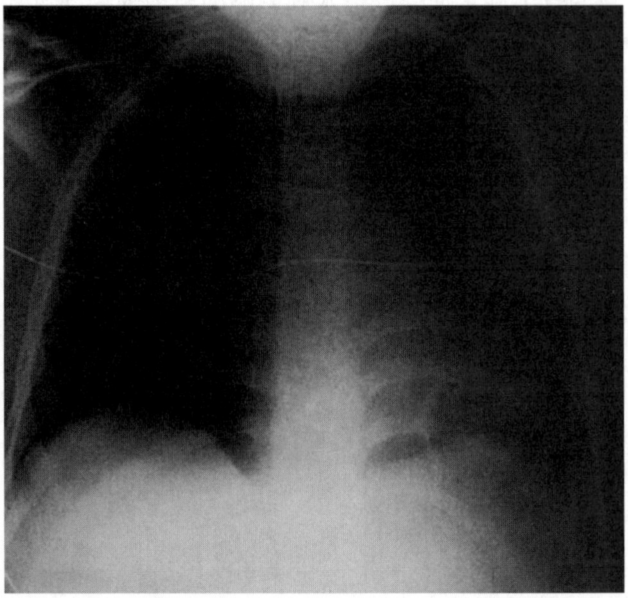

图 201.2　次日上午胸部 X 线片。注意肺门周围浸润的消退

渗透压之间存在平衡，如 Starling 方程所述。

$$液体滤过率=K_f[（P_c-P_i）-\sigma（\pi_c-\pi_i）]$$

方程式中 K_f 为毛细血管通透性，P_c 为肺毛细血管静水压，P_i 为肺间质静水压，σ 为蛋白质的反射系数，π_c 为肺毛细血管渗透压，π_i 为肺间质渗透压。压力平衡可防止液体在肺泡-毛细血管膜上的净流动。其结果是只有少量的液体进入肺间质，且一旦进入肺间质，迅速被肺淋巴管清除。

在 1 型 POPE 中，患者产生极高的胸腔内负压力，右心房静脉回流增加，进而增加肺血容积和毛细血管静水压。与此同时，肺间质静水压显著降低，导致液体进入间质增加。如果淋巴清除机制不堪重负，就会出现肺水肿的体征和症状。气道梗阻常伴发的低氧血症和交感神经张力增高也会增加肺动脉血管压力和左室后负荷，促进肺水肿形成（图 201.3 和 201.4）。急性左心室功能障碍可导致肺水肿进一步发展。然而，这种功能障碍通常极其短暂，事实上，在阻塞性事件后测量中心静脉、肺动脉和肺毛细血管楔压是正常或接近正常的。

在 2 型 POPE 中，慢性上气道阻塞会在肺泡内产生一定基础的 PEEP。当 PEEP 降低时，肺泡内压力降低，按照 Starling 定律有利于净流量从肺间质流入肺泡。

例如，保持正常流体过滤速率的相对压力（假

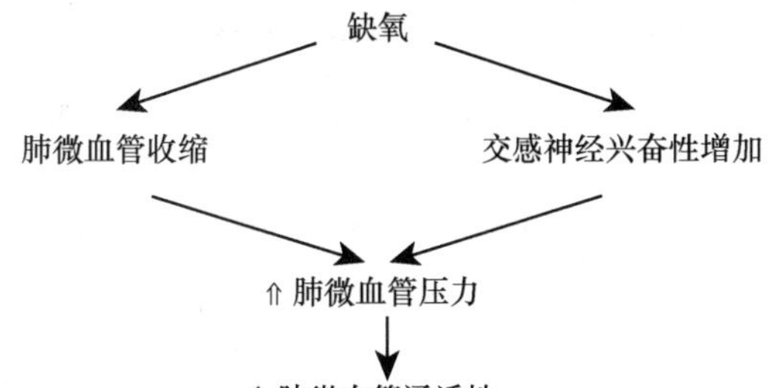

图 201.3　缺氧在梗阻后肺水肿发生中的作用

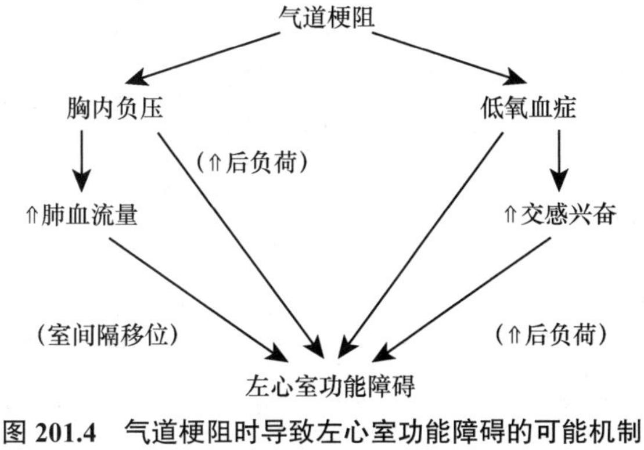

图 201.4　气道梗阻时导致左心室功能障碍的可能机制

设 kf 和 σ 为常量）如下：

$$P_c=12\ mmHg，P_i=4\ mmHg，\pi_c=23\ mmHg，\pi_i=9\ mmHg \approx 2\ mmHg$$

促进流体过滤速度提高和 POPE 发生的相对压力如下：

$$P_c=22\ mmHg，P_i=50\ mmHg，\pi_c=23\ mmHg\ \pi_i=9\ mmHg \approx 58\ mmHg$$

P_c 升高反映肺毛细血管血容量和左心室后负荷增加；P_i 升高反映胸膜腔内压降低。

POPE 多发于年轻健康的个体中。通常在梗阻解除后很快出现水肿，但也可能延迟至 24 h。患者肺泡-动脉氧分压梯度升高，表现为需要吸氧，同时伴发肺水肿，这些现象通常在 36 h 内消失。胸部听诊与肺水肿一致，可为湿啰音，偶尔为干啰音和喘鸣音。胸部 X 线片及 CT 显示肺水肿，支气管周围主要累及肺门周围和更多的中央肺实质，而周围肺组织无明显肺泡水肿，从而形成“蝴蝶”样改变。心脏轮廓正常。通常 POPE 的胸部 X 线片改变迅速。

下列可能引起肺水肿的诱因还应考虑并排除：

- 吸入性肺炎；
- 医源性容量超负荷；
- 肺动脉栓子；
- 原发性心脏异常；
- 继发于缺血的心肌功能障碍；
- 过敏反应；
- 哮喘。

至少在最初阶段，吸入性肺炎是最难排除的鉴别诊断。大量误吸胃内容物可产生与 POPE 相同的影像学图像，但更多累及右上肺叶或后段。此外，由于化学性肺损伤导致临床病程较长。急性胃内容物误吸引起的影像学改变通常滞后于患者的临床病程。

风险评估

尽管自 20 世纪 70 年代中期以来有临床报告描述了这一现象，但 POPE 的总发病率尚不清楚。风险因素一般包括：

- 喉痉挛；
- 肥胖和 OSA；
- 会厌炎；
- 哮吼；

- 异物造成部分气管阻塞；
- 上呼吸道的病变或外科手术（如气管软化、声带麻痹）；
- 食管异物造成部分气管阻塞；
- 气管导管或喉罩的阻塞；
- 困难插管。

目前还没有证据显示特定的麻醉药能增加 POPE 的发病率。然而，可能增加喉痉挛或上气道阻塞发生的麻醉药物或操作有增加 1 型 POPE 发生的潜在风险。

随着对上气道阻塞扁桃体切除术患儿 2 型 POPE 认识的不断深入，回顾性研究显示，该类儿童群体 2 型 POPE 的发病率为 1.2% ～ 1.4%，这类人群所有肺部并发症的危险因素包括：

- 年龄小于 2 岁；
- 呼吸暂停或减慢指数大于 24；
- 在 PACU 吸空气 SpO_2<90%；
- PACU 停留时间超过 100 min。

无论是否有喉痉挛发作，对这一人群可能发生肺部并发症的高度警惕有助于早期识别和治疗这两种类型的 POPE。

启示

POPE 的临床病程通常是自限性的。儿科人群的病例报告描述了治疗机构等级的提高、住院时间的延长、利尿剂的使用和呼吸支持，呼吸支持包括氧疗、持续气道正压通气或双水平气道正压通气、气管插管和重症监护病房治疗。

管理

POPE 的治疗包括重建和维持气道通畅及后续的支持。氧疗很有必要，大多数患者需要气管插管一段时间，在某些情况下最短只需几个小时。许多患者接受气道正压通气，无论是持续气道正压通气还是加用 PEEP 的正压通气，很少有人报告急性上呼吸道阻塞后出现咯血和明显的肺出血。两者都需要有效的通气和心血管支持。除非发现其他引起肺水肿的原因，不建议进行积极的有创血流动力学监测，如肺动脉导管置入术。利尿剂的使用是有争议的，因为水肿不是由于过多的血管内容量（如正常的肺毛细血管楔压测量所支持的那样），而且水肿的消退通常很快。另外，除了利尿作用外，呋塞米还能增加静脉容量，可能在 POPE 的治疗中发挥一定的作用。糖皮质激素和抗生素在 POPE 的治疗中没有作用，除非存在其他原因的适应证。临床症状和影像学的改善通常很快，一般在 2 ～ 3 天内。

预防

POPE 的预防包括①识别可能发生上气道阻塞的临床情况；②制订麻醉管理计划以避免潜在的梗阻。后者包括以下内容：

- 使用面罩或喉罩通气时，确保有足够的麻醉深度。
- 考虑使用“牙垫”以确保麻醉苏醒时人工气道通畅。
- 在患者完全清醒时拔管，以避免喉痉挛或软组织阻塞气道。
- 在已知存在气道异常时，使用纤维支气管镜插管。

麻醉科医师经常面对无法避免的情况，例如麻醉一名患有会厌炎的儿童。在这种情况下，如果发生气道阻塞，应能采取或获得多种策略和措施来避免气道阻塞并发症，包括手术干预。

（常馨宁 译 许 华 校）

延伸阅读

Austin AL, Kon A, Matteucci MJ: Respiratory failure in a child due to type 2 postobstructive pulmonary edema, *Pediatr Emerg Care* 32(1):23–24, 2016.

Broccard AF, Liaudet L, Aubert JD, et al.: Negative pressure post-tracheal extubation alveolar hemorrhage, *Anesth Analg* 92:273–275, 2001.

Devys JM, Balleau C, Jayr C, et al.: Biting the laryngeal mask: An unusual cause of negative pressure pulmonary edema, *Can J Anaesth* 47:176–178, 2000.

Guinard JP: Laryngospasm-induced pulmonary edema, *Int J Pediatr Otorhinolaryngol* 20:163–168, 1990.

Herrick IA, Mahendran B, Penny FJ: Postobstructive pulmonary edema following anesthesia, *J Clin Anesth* 2:116–120, 1990.

Hill CA, Litvak A, Canapari C, et al.: A pilot study to identify pre- and perioperative risk factors for airway complications following adenotonsillectomy for treatment of severe pediatric OSA, *Int J Pediatr Otorhinolaryngol* 75(11):1385–1390, 2011.

Konstantinopoulou S, Gallagher P, Elden L, et al.: Complications of adenotonsillectomy for obstructive sleep apnea in school-aged children, *Int J Pediatr Otorhinolaryngol* 79(2):240–245, 2015.

Lang SA, Duncan PG, Shepard DAE, et al.: Pulmonary oedema associated with airway obstruction, *Can J Anaesth* 37:210–218, 1990.

Mehta VM, Har-El G, Goldstein NA: Postobstructive pulmonary edema after laryngospasm in the otolaryngology patient, *Laryngoscope* 116(9):1693–1696, 2006.

Oswalt CE, Gates GA, Holmstrom MG: Pulmonary edema as a complication of acute airway obstruction, *JAMA* 238:1833–1835, 1977.

Ruffle J, Gleason M, Domino KB, et al.: Pulmonary edema and transient cardiomyopathy in a previously healthy adolescent after general anesthesia, *J Cardiothorac Vasc Anesth* 8:463–470, 1994.

Schwartz DR, Maroo A, Malhotra A, et al.: Negative pressure pulmonary hemorrhage, *Chest* 115:1194–1197, 1999.

婴儿术后呼吸暂停 第202章

Benjamin B. Bruins，C. Dean Kurth

病例概要

一名 2.5 kg，4 个月大的男婴，因巨大、不可复位回纳的腹股沟疝需要做修补术。有重要意义的病史是：该婴儿为妊娠 26 周的早产儿，既往有脑室内出血及因肺未发育成熟需要机械通气 3 周。3 个月时出院。腰硬联合麻醉是该手术采取的单一的麻醉技术。坐位下于 L3 ～ L4 间隙，使用 1 mg/kg 等比重布比卡因进行蛛网膜下腔阻滞，然后进行下肢静脉置管。超声引导下将硬膜外导管从骶骨裂孔（尾部）置入至 L1 水平。将安抚奶嘴浸入蔗糖溶液中，并允许婴儿在手术期间吮吸安抚奶嘴。手术 75 min 时，通过硬膜外导管缓慢推注 0.25% 布比卡因 1.5 mg/kg，持续阻滞以维持 2 h 的外科手术。在新生儿急症监护病房 3 h 后，患儿出现呼吸暂停。静脉注射 20 mg/kg 的咖啡因以防止呼吸暂停进一步发作。

问题分析

定义

术后呼吸暂停的定义是麻醉和手术后恢复期间没有通气，通常发生在有早产病史的婴儿或足月新生儿中。这与早产儿呼吸暂停和婴儿期呼吸暂停不同，后两者分别发生未行麻醉或手术的早产儿和足月儿中。

术后呼吸暂停的特征是持续时间和分型。气流停止持续时间超过 15 s 是诊断呼吸暂停的一种方法。或者，如伴有心动过缓或低氧血症，则较短周期的呼吸暂停（>6 s）也被认为是呼吸暂停。就类型而言，呼吸暂停分为中枢性、阻塞性或混合性（图 202.1）：

- 中枢性呼吸暂停，无呼吸用力。
- 阻塞性呼吸暂停，伴有呼吸运动，但无通气。
- 混合性呼吸暂停，偶有呼吸运动，无通气。

识别

术后呼吸暂停发生率取决于检测方法。使用连续记录装置（呼吸描记图），包括流量和胸壁传感器的研究的检出率为 31% ～ 49%，而依赖于护士观察或床边心肺监测警报的检出率为 5% ～ 10%。

风险评估

术后呼吸暂停的发生率受患者、手术和麻醉因素的影响。其中，早产史最为重要。生物年龄（postconceptual age，PCA）<60 周的早产儿有发生术后呼吸暂停的风险，出生后年龄 <4 周的足月婴儿也有发生术后呼吸暂停的风险。在以前有过早产史的患儿中，影响术后呼吸暂停发生率的因素包括以下几点。

生物年龄

生物年龄（postconceptual age，PCA）的定义为产后年龄和孕龄的总和，是术后呼吸暂停最重要的决定因素。术后呼吸暂停的发生率与 PCA 呈负相关（图 202.2）。PCA<40 周的早产儿发病率很高。此后，发病率急剧下降，直到婴儿 PCA 50 周。术后呼吸暂停的发生率在该点较低，此后逐渐降低。

孕龄

婴儿的孕龄可影响术后呼吸暂停的发生率。图 202.2 显示了妊娠 32 周出生的婴儿术后呼吸暂停发生率与 PCA 的关系，其术后呼吸暂停的发生率约为

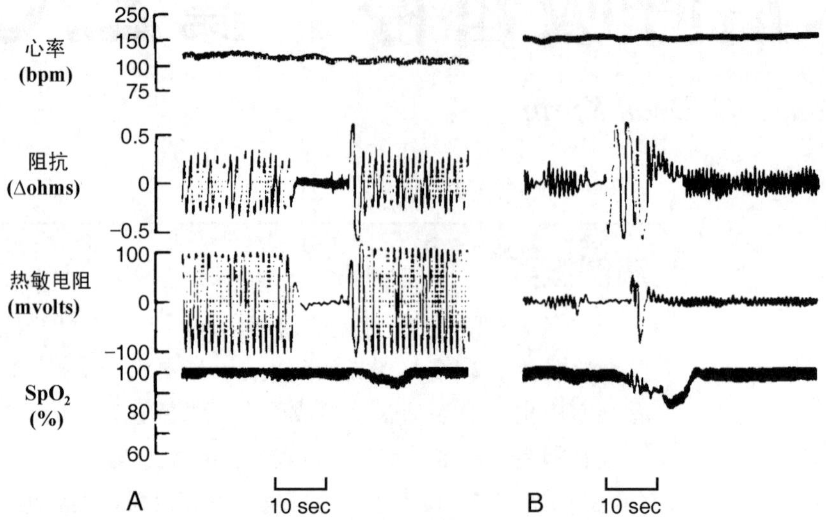

图 202.1 吸入全身麻醉腹股沟疝修补术后婴儿的心率、胸壁运动（阻抗）、鼻气流（热敏电阻）和氧饱和度（SpO_2）记录。 **图 A，**麻醉后恢复室获取的记录描绘了短暂的中枢性呼吸暂停。这表示胸壁无运动和气流不足。注意呼吸暂停后轻度动脉失饱和。**图 B，**麻醉后恢复室另一份记录显示混合性呼吸暂停。在呼吸暂停的最初 6 s 内，没有胸壁运动或气流（短暂的中枢性呼吸暂停），然后是 6 s 的胸壁运动，没有气流（阻塞性呼吸暂停）。注意，图 B 动脉失饱和比对应图 A 中枢性呼吸暂停更严重。

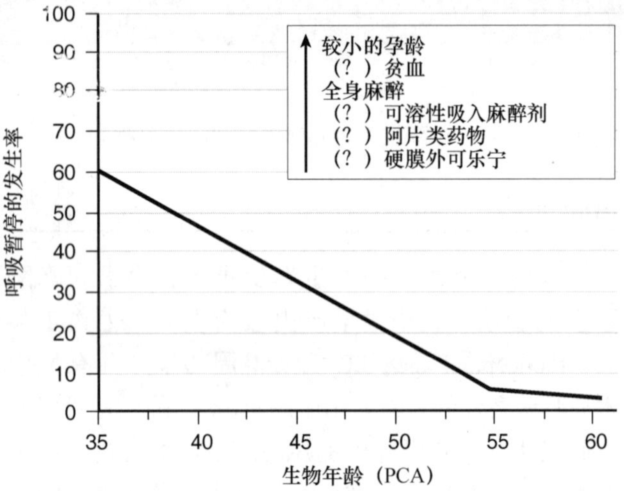

图 202.2 有早产史的患儿术后呼吸暂停的发生率与 PCA 成反比。婴儿的发生率曲线上移①孕龄更小的婴儿；②术后贫血或与早产有关的伴随疾病（如支气管肺发育不良）；③与单纯区域麻醉相比，全身麻醉后；④与不溶性吸入气体相比，可溶性吸入气体全身麻醉后。硬膜外应用可乐定或静脉注射阿片类药物也可使曲线上移

85%。随着孕龄的减少，发生率 -PCA 曲线上移。相反，随着孕龄接近足月，曲线下移。因此，对于任何既定的 PCA 中，妊娠 26 周出生的婴儿术后呼吸暂停发生率高于妊娠 32 周出生的婴儿。

贫血

贫血（血细胞比容 <30%）也会影响有早产病史患儿术后呼吸暂停的发生率。发生率 -PCA 曲线随贫血程度上移（见图 202.2）。之前人们认为贫血是独立危险因素，但最近的研究并未证实这一点，它可能只是有早产病史患儿一般医疗状况的特征。

早产相关并存疾病

如今，极低出生体重婴儿（孕龄 24 ～ 28 周）的存活非常普遍。极低出生体重的幸存者常出现支气管肺发育不良、早产儿视网膜病变、脑积水、癫痫发作和脑性瘫痪。对于既定的 PCA，患有早产残存疾病的有早产史的患儿术后呼吸暂停的风险更大。

外科手术

虽然术后呼吸暂停甚至可以发生在没有进行手术（例如在 MRI 之后）的麻醉后，但手术因素似乎在发病机制中起作用。大手术（例如剖腹手术）后，术后呼吸暂停的风险增加。与幽门狭窄慢性呕吐相关的中枢神经系统碱中毒可能会加剧幽门括约肌切开术后呼吸暂停的风险。表面麻醉下视网膜病变冷冻治疗或脊椎麻醉下腹股沟疝修补术的早产儿可能会出现术后呼吸暂停。

麻醉管理

术后呼吸暂停可能发生在全身麻醉、区域麻醉或全身麻醉联合区域麻醉之后。一项评估新生儿腹股沟疝修补术后呼吸暂停发生率的随机试验指出：进入麻醉后恢复室（postanesthesia care unit，PACU）30 min 内，脊椎麻醉出现呼吸暂停的频率低于全身麻醉。然而，脊椎麻醉具有相当高的失败率

（19%），需要使用镇静药或改为全身麻醉以完成疝气修补手术。区域麻醉加静脉镇静药术后呼吸暂停的发生率与全身麻醉相近，但低于全身麻醉。区域麻醉加面罩吸入七氟烷可能比加静脉镇静药的呼吸暂停发生率更低。此外，脊椎麻醉后的呼吸暂停发作出现低氧血症的概率低，且不太可能需要比触觉刺激更大的干预。作为全身麻醉方案的一部分，使用肌肉松弛药或插管似乎并不会改变术后呼吸暂停的发生率。

值得注意的是，早产性呼吸暂停的病史**并非**术后呼吸暂停的预测因素。之前没有呼吸暂停史但有早产史的患儿可能会出现术后呼吸暂停。相反，既往有呼吸暂停病史和有早产史的患儿可进行麻醉和手术而不会发生术后呼吸暂停。通常用呼吸心动描记法对早产儿进行睡眠研究来记录是否存在呼吸暂停，以帮助确定婴儿是否需要进行家庭监测。然而，术前睡眠正常（无呼吸暂停）并不能保证婴儿不会出现术后呼吸暂停。

启示

术后呼吸暂停可能危及生命。术后呼吸暂停后有心肺骤停和死亡的报道。术后呼吸暂停与婴儿猝死综合征之间的关系尚不清楚。术后呼吸暂停的特征在于其发作和终止变化与麻醉苏醒相关。约 2/3 发生术后呼吸暂停的婴儿开始于 PACU。其余开始于术后 2 ～ 12 h。通常，其特征在于可变时间内多个事件的叠加，可在术后持续数天。呼吸暂停大多是自限性的。偶有，呼吸暂停的婴儿需要手动刺激，例如轻弹脚底，以恢复通气。有时它们需要皮球和面罩通气。极少情况下必须实施心肺复苏以抢救患儿。最近一项包括 700 多名婴儿的研究显示，早产儿的发病率为 6.1%，足月儿的发病率为 0.3%。与全身麻醉相比，区域麻醉降低了术后早期呼吸暂停（PACU 中的前 30 min）的风险。PACU 后期或在病房，区域麻醉与全身麻醉之间的呼吸暂停发生率无差异。这两种麻醉方式都可能在 PACU 或回病房数小时后发生危及生命的呼吸暂停。

管理

有呼吸暂停风险的年幼婴儿的麻醉管理注意事项包括术前、术中和术后。

术前注意事项

应根据 PCA 推迟非紧急手术，因为术后呼吸暂停的风险在 PCA 40 ～ 50 周之间急剧下降，然后缓慢下降直至 PCA70 周。推迟非紧急手术直至 PCA 至少 50 周，可以最大限度地减少术后呼吸暂停的风险。足月婴儿的择期手术应推迟到至少 4 周龄。

完善的术前评估应重点关注神经系统和呼吸系统并存疾病，因为已知早产后遗症会增加呼吸暂停的风险。另外，麻醉前评估血细胞比容可能是有帮助的。

应设置日间手术的限制条件。用于确定哪些婴儿必须在医院过夜监测术后呼吸暂停的流程图见图 202.3。

术中注意事项

有术后呼吸暂停风险的婴儿，可进行吸入全身

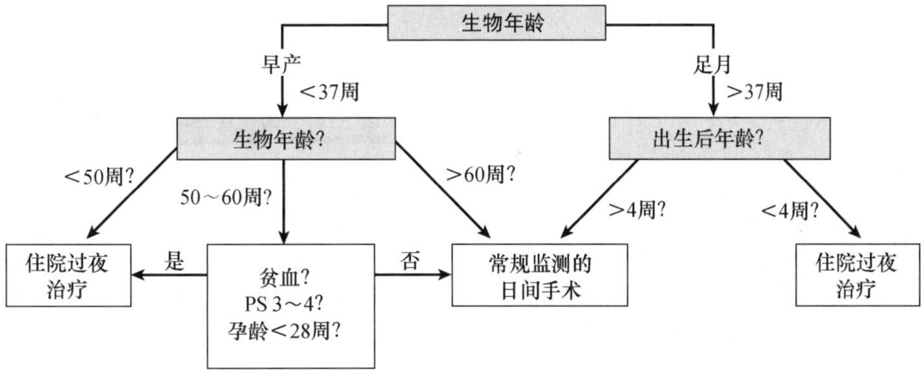

图 202.3　日间手术的可能流程。如果婴儿是足月并且年龄 <4 周，则计划在医院接受过夜监测。如果足月婴儿 >4 周，则可以进行日间手术。PCA>50 周的早产儿，如没有贫血或严重并存疾病的病史，则按计划进行日间手术。PCA>60 周的早产儿，无论是否贫血或有无并存疾病，都按计划进行日间手术。所有早产儿和 PCA<50 周的婴儿都被收治入院进行过夜监测。PS，身体状况

麻醉、脊椎麻醉，骶部硬膜外麻醉或全身麻醉联合区域麻醉。

为降低全身吸入麻醉术后呼吸暂停的发生率，应在麻醉诱导后不久给予枸橼酸咖啡因（静脉注射 20 mg/kg）。咖啡因可降低呼吸暂停的发生率和呼吸暂停时氧饱和度下降的严重程度。虽然即使给予咖啡因也可能发生术后呼吸暂停（咖啡因的有效性受到质疑），但风险-收益比分析更倾向于给药；咖啡因几乎没有副作用，具有极好的安全性。

区域麻醉（蛛网膜下腔或骶部硬膜外麻醉）适用于下肢或腹股沟手术，特别是对于患有慢性肺病的婴儿（例如支气管肺发育不良、气管软化、声门下狭窄）。蛛网膜下腔阻滞可在坐位下进行，通过 22 号 1.5 英寸腰麻针给予 0.6 ～ 1 mg/kg 的等比重或重比重布比卡因。脊椎阻滞的持续时间为 60 min，添加肾上腺素的布比卡因可延长阻滞时间至 90 min。婴儿可能不会保持上肢或躯干不动，或者当他们感到饥饿或麻醉不完全时，可能会哭。尽管静脉镇静会增加术后呼吸暂停的风险，而面罩吸入七氟烷不会增加风险，但静脉给予镇静药或面罩吸入 1% 七氟烷均可提高婴儿依从性。婴儿外科手术通常比较困难，且可能需要比预期更长的时间，使得脊椎麻醉不如骶部硬膜外麻醉或全身麻醉。可进行脊椎麻醉联合骶部硬膜外麻醉以增加麻醉的持续时间。首先进行脊椎麻醉，这样可为随后的骶部硬膜外麻醉置管提供麻醉。应用超声识别导管的尖端达 L1 水平。如果外科手术超过 60 min，可以通过硬膜外导管推注 0.25% 布比卡因以维持麻醉。对于早产儿和小于 4 周龄的足月儿，应避免骶管硬膜外可乐定的使用，因为可能会抑制呼吸。

术后注意事项

有术后呼吸暂停风险的婴儿，心肺监测是最重要的术后监测方法。护士必须熟悉如何应对心肺呼吸警报，包括识别年幼婴儿的呼吸暂停，以及如何治疗呼吸暂停，从手法刺激到心肺复苏。应在护士能听到心肺呼吸警报的位置监测婴儿。因为误报警频繁，所以呼吸或呼吸暂停的视觉确认很重要。采用阻抗技术检测呼吸频率和心率的心肺监护仪灵敏且易于应用。这些监护仪有心率和呼吸频率的高低以及呼吸暂停持续时间的警报。对于年幼的婴儿，呼吸暂停警报设置为 15 s，低心率警报设置为 80 次 / 分（年幼婴儿相对心动过缓）。

术后疼痛控制通常依赖于局部麻醉药和对乙酰氨基酚。通过骶部硬膜外导管连续输注氯普鲁卡因可以在未使用全身阿片类药物的情况下实现良好的镇痛效果，且局部麻醉药毒性风险最小。或者连续输注加入阿片类药物的局部麻醉药也是有效的，但具有阿片类药物全身吸收的风险，尤其是亲脂性药物。

尽管连续骶部硬膜外麻醉与阿片类药物是镇痛的主要手段，但缺乏评估术后区域镇痛与更常规（静脉）镇痛策略比较的随机对照临床试验。

预防

尽管在过去的 20 年里医学快速发展，但婴儿术后呼吸暂停的发生率和危险因素并未发生显著变化。以下推荐可以降低术后呼吸暂停的风险：

- 推迟择期手术直至 PCA 50 ～ 60 周。
- 使用气管插管吸入全身麻醉，并在诱导后给予枸橼酸咖啡因（20 mg/kg 静脉注射）。
- 使用区域麻醉下进行腹股沟和下肢手术：脊椎麻醉或腰硬联合麻醉。如果阻滞不全或失败，通过面罩吸入七氟烷比静脉注射氯胺酮、咪达唑仑或阿片类药物更可取。
- 减少阿片类药物的剂量，或完全避免使用阿片类药物，可静脉注射对乙酰氨基酚。

致谢

感谢 Liana Hosu 博士对本章上一版的贡献。

（王　委　译　陆　军　校）

延伸阅读

Anand KJS, Stevens BJ, McGrath PJ: *Pain in neonates*, 2nd ed., Philadelphia, 2000, Elsevier.

Andropoulos DB, Heard MB, Johnson KL, et al.: Postanesthetic apnea in full-term infants after pyloromyotomy, *Anesthesiology* 80:216–219, 1994.

Coté CJ, Zaslavsky A, Downes JJ, et al.: Postoperative apnea in former preterm infants after inguinal herniorrhaphy: a combined analysis, *Anesthesiology* 82:809–822, 1995.

Craven PD, Badawi N, Henderson-Smart DJ, et al.: Regional (spinal, epidural, caudal) versus general anesthesia in preterm infants undergoing inguinal herniorrhaphy in early infancy, CD003669 *Cochrane Database Syst Rev*(3), 2003.

Davidson AJ, Morton NS, Arnup SJ, et al.: Apnea after awake regional and general anesthesia in infants. The general anesthesia compared to spinal anesthesia study—comparing apnea and neurodevelopmental outcomes, a randomized controlled trial, *Anesthesiology* 123:38–54, 2015.

Fellmann C, Gerber AC, Weiss M: Apnoea in a former preterm infant after caudal bupivacaine with clonidine for inguinal herniorrhaphy, *Paediatr Anaesth* 12:637–640, 2002.

Galinkin JL, Davis PJ, McGowan FX, et al.: A randomized multicenter study of remifentanil compared with halothane in neonates and infants undergoing pyloromyotomy. II. Perioperative breathing patterns in neonates and infants with pyloric stenosis, *Anesth Analg* 93:1387–1392, 2001.

Kurth CD, Cote CJ: Postoperative apnea in former preterm infants. General anesthesia or spinal anesthesia—do we have an answer? *Anesthesiology* 123:15–17, 2015.

Kurth CD, LeBard SE: Association of postoperative apnea, airway obstruction, and hypoxemia in former premature infants, *Anesthesiology* 75:22–26, 1991.

Kurth CD, Spitzer AR, Broennle AM, et al.: Postoperative apnea in preterm infants, *Anesthesiology* 66:483–488, 1987.

Welborn LG, Hannallah RS, Fink R, et al.: High dose caffeine suppresses postoperative apnea in former preterm infants, *Anesthesiology* 74:347–349, 1989.

Welborn LG, Hannallah RS, Luban NLC, et al.: Anemia and postoperative apnea in former preterm infants, *Anesthesiology* 74:1003–1006, 1991.

Welborn LG, Rice LJ, Hannallah RS, et al.: Postoperative apnea in former preterm infants: Prospective comparison of spinal and general anesthesia, *Anesthesiology* 72:838–842, 1990.

William JM, Stoddart PA, Williams SA, et al.: Postoperative recovery after inguinal herniotomy in ex-premature infants: comparison between sevoflurane and spinal anaesthesia, *Br J Anaesth* 86:366–371, 2001.

Wolf AR, Lawson RA, Dryden CM, et al.: Recovery after desflurane anaesthesia in the infant: comparison with isoflurane, *Br J Anaesth* 76:362–364, 1996.

第203章 儿童术后恶心呕吐

Ravish Kapoor，*Mehernoor F. Watcha*

病例概要

患儿，女，10岁，有晕动病史，拟行腺样体扁桃体切除术。这是她的第三次全身麻醉手术。尽管术中使用了止吐药预防，在前两次手术（牙齿修复术和斜视矫正术）后，她发生了多次术后恶心呕吐（postoperative nausea and vomiting，PONV）。斜视手术后，她甚至因顽固性呕吐引起的脱水症状住院。她的母亲在妇科手术后出现了类似的严重PONV。患儿和其父母都非常焦虑，并询问可以做些什么来避免类似的经历。

问题分析

识别

虽然**术后恶心呕吐**（PONV）被称为麻醉中的不大不小的"问题"，但它会降低患者对麻醉的满意度，延长出院时间，并可能增加因计划外住院而导致的费用。在成人中，术后恶心发生率为50%，呕吐发生率为30%，出院后恶心和呕吐（post-discharge nausea and vomiting，PDNV）发生率为37%，各种亚组发生率高达80%。许多年幼的儿科患者无法表达主观感受，但他们有恶心的主观症状。因此，术后呕吐（postoperative vomiting，POV）常被用作儿科研究的终点指标。POV的发病率在儿童中高于成人。

PONV越来越多地被用作医疗质量的标志。2014年出版了一套修订的PONV管理共识指南。这些指南（表203.1）得到了全球许多专业麻醉学协会的认可。指南的第一个推荐是根据确定的风险因素评估个体患者的PONV风险，然后使用各种策略降低基线风险。指南指出，成人和儿童预防性止吐药的使用应根据个体患者的预估风险，风险最低的患者不需进行预防，对中风险进行1～2种药物预防，以及多模式联合治疗（对于风险最高的受试者，进行≥2种干预）。对于那些未接受过预防性治疗的患者，对已发生的PONV进行补救性治疗的建议与使用预防治疗失败的患者有所不同。在后一种情况下，推荐使用预防性药物以外的药物用于补救治疗。最后，指南提倡采取一定措施以助于这些建议的推广实施。

表203.1 术后恶心呕吐的处理指南与共识

指南编号	名称
1	识别患者PONV风险
2	降低PONV的基础风险
3	对PONV中度风险的成人使用1～2中预防PONV的干预手段
4	对PONV高风险的患者使用联合用药（≥2）或多模式方法进行预防性治疗
5	对POV风险较高的儿童预防性使用止吐药，对于成人，联合用药更为有效
6	对未预防性使用或预防失败的PONV患者给予止吐药
7	确保PONV的预防与治疗作为临床常规之一
8	将多模式预防手段纳入PONV的常规医疗之中

PONV，术后恶心呕吐

Data from Gan TJ，Diemunsch P，Habib AS，et al：Consensus guidelines for the management of postoperative nausea and vomiting. *Anesth Analg* 118（1）：85-113，2014.

风险评估

虽然许多因素与PONV增加有关，但共识指南注重于那些在大型队列研究中明确的独立因素，而不是混杂因素。例如，接受腹部手术的成人PONV增加可反映出混杂因素的影响，例如手术持续时间或阿片类药物使用增加。儿科和成人危险分层评分具有不同的独立危险因素。成人中最重要的独立危险因素是女性，PONV/ 晕动病的既往病史，术后应用阿片类药物和不吸烟状态，每个因素使 PONV 的相对风险增加约 20%。儿童的独立危险因素为①手术时间超过 30 min；②年龄大于 3 岁；③患者、其父母或兄弟姐妹既往 POV 病史；④斜视手术。如果存在 0、1、2、3 或 4 个这些因素，则患者 POV 风险分别约为 9%、10%、30%、55% 和 70%。Eberhart 及其同事的这一评分在另一儿科患者人群中得到了验证。

一项对 2392 名儿童的研究提出了简易的儿童术后呕吐（vomiting in the postoperative period，VPOP）6 分评分新方法，根据年龄、POV 易感性、麻醉持续时间超过 45 min、手术类型和使用大剂量的阿片类药物（表 203.2）。儿童 POV 的年龄相关风险在 3 岁以下者中最低，6 ～ 13 岁最高，3 ～ 6 岁或 13 岁以上人群中度。POV 的易感性被定义为 POV 的既往病史、晕动病或 POV 家族史。除了斜视手术外，该研究还将扁桃体切除术和鼓室成形术确定为独立的危险因素。作者认为风险评分为 0 ～ 1 的患者为低风险，2 ～ 3 为中风险，4 ～ 6 为高风险。与 Eberhart 及其同事的早期评分相比，这一新评分在受试者手术特征曲线下面积更大，这表明 VPOP 评分可用于指导儿童 POV 的管理。

与 POV 风险增加无关的患者相关因素

术前焦虑并未显示与儿童 POV 增加有关。虽然成年吸烟者的 PONV 率较低，但二手烟对儿童 POV 的影响尚不清楚。

管理

降低 POV 基线风险的策略

共识指南推荐采用以下策略来降低基线风险和 POV 发生率（框 203.1）：

1. 通过使用区域麻醉以避免全身麻醉；
2. 使用丙泊酚诱导和维持麻醉；
3. 避免使用挥发性麻醉药；
4. 避免使用氧化亚氮；
5. 尽可能减少围术期阿片类药物使用；
6. 充足的水化。

区域麻醉与全身麻醉

无论儿童或成人，区域麻醉 PONV 发生率均低于全身麻醉。在儿科患者群体中，通常在全身麻醉诱导后进行区域麻醉以减少与置针相关的患者应激。研究表明，与未充分镇静的低配合度的儿童患者实施阻滞相比，诱导后实施神经阻滞不会增加神经创伤。全身麻醉和区域阻滞麻醉联合应用的主要优点是减少围术期阿片类药物和挥发性麻醉剂的需求，从而减少 POV。

丙泊酚输注

许多手术不能通过单纯区域麻醉来完成，需要进行单纯的全身麻醉。在这些情况下，使用丙泊酚诱导和维持麻醉可以降低术后最初 6 h 内 POV 的发生率。然而，单次诱导剂量的丙泊酚对 POV 没有

表 203.2 术后呕吐的临床风险评分：VPOP 评分

	得分		
	0	1	2
年龄	3 岁以下	3 ～ 6 岁或大于 13 岁	6 ～ 13 岁
POV 易感体质	不易感	易感体质	
既往 POV、晕动病史、家族 POV 病史			
麻醉时间大于 45 min	否	是	
高风险手术（扁桃体切除术，鼓室成形术，斜视手术）	非高风险手术	高风险手术	
多次阿片类药物使用	否	是	

低风险：总得分 0 ～ 1；中风险：总得分 2 ～ 3 分；高风险：总得分 4 ～ 6 分。

POV，术后呕吐

Modified from Bourdaud N，Devys JM，Bientz J，et al：Development and validation of a risk score to predict the probability of postoperative vomiting in pediatric patients：the VPOP score. *Pediatr Anesth* 24（9）：945-952，2014.

框 203.1 降低术后恶心呕吐基线风险的策略

尽可能使用区域麻醉
使用丙泊酚诱导和维持全身麻醉
充分的水化
避免使用氧化亚氮
避免使用挥发性吸入麻醉剂
尽量减少术中和术后阿片类药物的使用

Adapted from Gan TJ，Diemunsch P，Habib AS，et al：Consensus guidelines for the management of postoperative nausea and vomiting. *Anesth Analg* 118（1）：85-113，2014.

影响。儿童接受术中丙泊酚的亚催眠剂量［推注量为 1 mg/kg，然后以 20 μg/（kg·min）输注］与地塞米松或托烷司琼联合应用于扁桃体切除术相比，其呕吐程度低于仅接受地塞米松或托烷司琼治疗的患者。

避免 N_2O 的使用

丙泊酚和空气/氧气（全凭静脉麻醉）的联合使用具有累加效应，使成人的 PONV 风险降低约 25%。当 PONV 的基线风险较低时，N_2O 的影响很小，但在高危成人和儿童患者中，避免使用 N_2O 与 POV 降低直接相关。

减少阿片类药物的使用

通过辅以非阿片类药物的应用，可减少吗啡用量，从而也可以降低 POV 的基线风险。这些包括非甾体抗炎药（nonsteroidal antiinflammatory drugs，NSAIDs）、环氧合酶-2（cyclooxygenase-2，COX-2）抑制剂，α_2-受体激动剂如可乐定和右美托咪定、对乙酰氨基酚和氯胺酮。一项纳入 928 名儿童的含 12 项研究的系统评价显示，与安慰剂组相比，接受 NSAIDs 治疗组的呕吐较少（优势比 0.49，95% 置信区间 0.29 ～ 0.83）。

水化作用

充足的水化作用是减少呕吐的简单且廉价的策略。与标准的 10 ml/kg 补液治疗相比，接受手术时间短、出血量小的手术患儿使用宽松静脉输液方案（30 ml/kg）呕吐较少。

未见起效的策略

常规胃减压和限制术后口服摄入对减少儿童 POV 无效。通过耳机术中传递有效治疗性建议也不起作用。吸氧和小剂量新斯的明最初被认为有效，但后来证实影响较小或没有影响。

POV 高风险的儿童预防性止吐治疗

儿童 POV 率约为成人的 2 倍，表明该人群更需要 POV 预防。使用 5-HT_3 拮抗剂、类固醇、抗组胺药、抗胆碱能药和多巴胺拮抗剂可以实现有效的 POV 预防（表 203.3）。

昂丹司琼及其他 5-HT_3 拮抗剂

系统评价显示，儿科 POV 预防最有效的止吐药是 5-HT_3 拮抗剂和地塞米松。在接受腺样体扁桃体切除术的 557 名儿童中，昂丹司琼比甲氧氯普胺更有效。与安慰剂相比，5-HT_3 拮抗剂和奋乃静均在儿童中有效，5-HT_3 拮抗剂（昂丹司琼或格拉司琼）显示出优异的功效。单一和联合止吐药物的 Bayesian meta 分析指出，使用 5-HT_3 受体拮抗剂或地塞米松单药预防的最低的相对风险降低值（relative risk reduction，RRR）为 50% ～ 60%，并且该组合 RRR 至少为 80%，而氟哌利多为 40%。

昂丹司琼是应用最广泛的止吐药，与其他第一代 5-HT_3 拮抗剂如格拉司琼、多拉司琼和托烷司琼相比，昂丹司琼有相似的功效和不良反应，可用性更高，成本更低。第二代 5-HT_3 拮抗剂如帕洛诺司琼和雷莫司琼是否具有更高疗效需在不同的儿科患者群体中进行验证，以证实其是否可替代昂丹司琼而成为 POV 预防的首选用药。

儿童的推荐用药时机相关数据很少。短小手术扁桃体切除术为例，诱导后立即给药或在手术结束时给予托烷司琼，其 POV 没有差异。

表 203.3 儿童 POV 预防用止吐药剂量

药物	剂量	最大剂量
地塞米松	150 μg/kg	5 mg
茶苯海明	0.5 mg/kg	25 mg
氟哌利多[a]	10 ～ 15 μg/kg	1.25 mg
5-HT_3 拮抗剂		
• 昂丹司琼	50 ～ 100 μg/kg	4 mg
• 托烷司琼	0.1 mg/kg	2 mg
• 格拉司琼	40 μg/kg	0.6 mg
• 多拉司琼	350 μg/kg	12.5 mg

[a] 美国食品和药物管理局（Food and Drug Administration，FDA）的黑匣子警告呼吁，在服用氟哌啶醇之前，应使用 12 导联心电图排除 QT 间期延长综合征的可能性，并在服用氟哌啶醇后，至少持续监测心电图 2 ～ 3 h。

Adapted from Gan TJ，Diemunsch P，Habib AS，et al：Consensus guidelines for the management of postoperative nausea and vomiting. *Anesth Analg* 118（1）：85-113，2014.

地塞米松

皮质类固醇在预防儿童 POV 方面非常有效，建议在诱导时给药，而不是在麻醉结束时给药。类固醇可通过消耗色氨酸（一种 5- 羟色胺前体）起作用。其他可能的机制包括减少肠道 5- 羟色胺释放和增加血清素受体对其他拮抗剂的致敏作用。大多数用类固醇预防 POV 的研究都是用地塞米松 0.5 mg/kg 进行的，但甲泼尼龙 2.5 mg/kg 已被证明具有非劣性功效。然而，地塞米松在 POV 预防中的剂量-效应关系尚不清楚，有学者对儿童扁桃体切除术进行了研究，术中接受 0.0625 mg/kg、0.125 mg/kg、0.25 mg/kg、0.5 mg/kg 或 1 mg/kg 地塞米松的儿童的 POV 或次要结果没有差异，另一项研究表明，与 0.05 mg/kg 和 0.15 mg/kg 剂量相比，0.5 mg/kg 可获得最佳效应。对扁桃体切除术患者使用类固醇的 Cochrane 最新综述指出："合理剂量仍无答案，最终建议必须等待随机化的剂量对照试验。"

类固醇对扁桃体切除术后出血率的影响是有争议的，最近的一项系统评价得出结论，出血的整体风险没有增加，但再次手术率随地塞米松剂量的增加而增加。美国耳鼻喉-头颈外科学会得出的结论是，接受扁桃体切除术的儿童中使用单次剂量的地塞米松是有益的。

经典药物

许多老药在 POV 治疗方面也很有效（表 203.4）。这些药物包括抗组胺药（苯海拉明），多巴胺拮抗剂如丁酰苯类（例如氟哌利多、氟哌啶醇），吩噻嗪类（异丙嗪、丙氯拉嗪和奋乃静），苯甲酰胺（甲氧氯普胺）和抗胆碱能药（东莨菪碱）。但这些药物的剂量范围和药效数据有限。此外，5-HT_3 拮抗剂更加有效，且不良反应较低。氟哌利多对心律的影响导致的黑框警告可能不完全合理，因为其他止吐药（包括抗血清素类药物）对心律也有类似的影响。甲氧氯普胺和吩噻嗪的不良反应包括锥体外系症状（见表 203.4）。由于昂丹司琼具有更高的可用性和有效性以及较低的价格和不良反应，经典老药现在仅限于在其他药物无效或 5-HT_3 拮抗剂禁忌时，作为补救疗法的二线选择。

非药物性疗法

两项 meta 分析显示针灸和针刺疗法均可有效降低儿童 POV，两种方法无统计学差异。

表 203.4　作为二线用药的药物

药物	剂量（mg/kg）	最大单次剂量	副作用
苯海拉明	1.0	25	镇静，口干，视力模糊，尿潴留
甲氧氯普胺	0.25[b]	10	锥体外系反应多见于儿童；不建议在 1 岁以下
吩噻嗪类			镇静，低血压（特别是在低血容量患者中），锥体外系反应
奋乃静	0.07	2.0	
丙氯拉嗪[c]	0.1 ~ 0.2	2.5	
异丙嗪[d]	0.25 ~ 0.5	25	2 岁以下儿童禁用异丙嗪；静脉注射刺激性强，有严重组织损伤的风险
东莨菪碱（IM，IV，SC）[e]	0.006	0.3	嗜睡，口干，视力障碍，头晕

[a] 这些经典药物的剂量范围和疗效研究很少。这些药物可在 5-HT_3 拮抗剂失败后用于挽救治疗，并且通常不用于常规预防。

[b] 虽然更高的剂量可能更有效，但副作用的发生率也更高。

[c] 对于 2 岁以下或体重 10 kg 以下的儿童，不建议使用丙氯拉嗪。

[d] 异丙嗪在美国食品和药物管理局有两项黑框警告：①由于潜在的致命性呼吸抑制风险，2 岁以下不得使用；②血管周围渗出或无意的动脉内注射时会导致严重组织损伤和坏疽。适宜的给药途径是深部肌内注射，并且禁止皮下注射。

[e] 东莨菪碱贴片不应剪开使用；该贴片不应用于 12 岁以下的儿童。

联合疗法

使用作用于不同受体位点的药物联合预防 POV 可能更为有效，但这是一种叠加效应而不是协同效应。低风险患者可能不需要预防性止吐药，但中度至高度 POV 风险的儿童和可能因呕吐产生后遗症的儿童（如伤口裂开，线性颌骨）应使用 2 ~ 3 种不同类别的止吐药预防性联合治疗。对于 POV 风险最高的大多数患儿，除非有禁忌证，强烈建议预防性使用地塞米松和昂丹司琼。

东莨菪碱

儿童东莨菪碱贴剂并发症的发生率可能高于成人。因为贴剂中药物的分布难以统一，所以很难控制分片时的剂量。此外，即使在去除贴剂后药物也可能持续吸收。这些担忧导致许多医师避免在幼童中使用东莨菪碱贴剂。

对未接受预防疗法或预防疗法无效的患者的补

救治疗一些未接受预防的低风险患者和接受预防性治疗的高风险患者仍可能出现 POV。如果未使用预防措施，应该优选使用 5-HT_3 拮抗剂进行补救治疗。接受预防性治疗无效的 POV 患者中，补救治疗应使用来自不同类别的止吐药。这可能需要给予较老的药物，如甲氧氯普胺、苯海拉明或吩噻嗪，而这可能与镇静和更长的麻醉后恢复室（PACU）停留时间相关。如果在前一次给药后超过 6 h 需要进行补救治疗，可以重复使用预防药物（地塞米松或透皮东莨菪碱除外）。虽然这些推荐来源于成人数据，但将这种方法推广到儿童是合理的。

尽管关于这一问题的文献量很大，但关于儿科患者 POV 治疗的知识中仍具有相当大的差距。未来的研究方向应侧重于提供支持临床实践的证据。一个仍未解决的重要问题是，在使用类固醇和昂丹司琼的联合预防失败后，该如何进行挽救治疗的建议。此外，还需要进一步研究确定 NK_1 拮抗剂在儿童预防和补救治疗中的作用，因为这类药物的儿科 POV 数据仍然匮乏。

本例患者的麻醉方案

根据所提供的信息，我们可以为术前、术中和术后阶段制订相应麻醉计划。这名患儿的儿科 VPOP 评分为 6 分，表明她具有最高的风险。考虑到这些问题，在手术日期之前与家人沟通非常重要，以便医生通过彻底的讨论和规划建立融洽关系。谈话应强调坚持液体疗法的重要性，一直持续到手术前 2 h 以避免脱水。患者和家属也应接受有关术后阿片类药物镇痛治疗后 POV 风险增加的教育，以及基于个体患者每种疾病的舒服度来滴定药物以实现疼痛和 POV 之间的平衡。

虽然术前焦虑不是与儿童 POV 相关的独立因素，但减少术前焦虑的发生仍然可以提供更好的麻醉体验。有系统评价表明咪达唑仑有助于减少成人的焦虑和 PONV。尽管儿童对咪达唑仑和 POV 的研究有限，但在术前期间合理使用该药可能有益。如果在诱导前能够建立静脉通路，则可静脉给予该药，若建立静脉通路有困难或患者不配合，则可予以口服。患者在清醒时建立静脉通道的额外益处在于，医生可以用丙泊酚诱导并避免使用挥发性麻醉剂和氧化亚氮进行吸入诱导。

在整个手术过程中应使用丙泊酚持续输注以维持麻醉，并且应始终避免使用氧化亚氮。这些步骤将进一步降低 POV 的风险。

气管插管之前可以使用利多卡因对喉–气管区进行局部麻醉以减少气管刺激，并允许使用较低剂量的阿片类药物以降低应激反应。应在诱导后不久即给予类固醇，静脉注射对乙酰氨基酚和不会增加扁桃体术后出血的 NSAIDs（如双氯酚酸），以及右美托咪定可减少阿片类药物的需要量。在手术过程中，应该提供宽松的静脉输液，并给予昂丹司琼。麻醉科医师还可考虑在 P6 穴位使用针灸。

经验丰富的 PACU 护士经常表示，接受阿片类药物治疗的儿童频繁和快速的体位变化（例如，从仰卧到坐直到行走）会增加术后即刻发生 PONV 的可能性。尽管可能没有来自随机试验的数据来证实这些印象，但是通过温和处理和避免快速体位变化并不会带来什么损失。此外，患者在从日间手术中心到出院期间坚持口服液体可能会增加 PONV 的发生，而静脉输液直至出院可能有用。如果这些措施失败，则需要从类固醇和抗 5-HT 药物以外的药物中选择药物进行补救治疗。家长也应该被告知他们的孩子可能有 PDNV，特别在回家的路上。在第一次给药后 6 h 提供第二剂的昂丹司琼（可能在口服分散片剂制剂中）可能是有用的。

治疗儿科 POV 需要多模式方法来达到最佳实践，但也需要进一步研究来解决这一问题。

致谢

感谢 Senthilkumar Sadhasivam 对本章上一版的贡献。

（蒋政宇　译　赵珍珍　校）

延伸阅读

Aouad MT, Nasr VG, Yazbeck-Karam VG, et al.: A comparison between dexamethasone and methylprednisolone for vomiting prophylaxis after tonsillectomy in inpatient children: a randomized trial, *Anesth Analg* 115(4):913–920, 2012.

Apfel CC, Korttila K, Abdalla M, et al.: A factorial trial of six interventions for the prevention of postoperative nausea and vomiting, *N Engl J Med* 350(24):2441–2451, 2004.

Apfel CC, Kranke P, Eberhart LH: Comparison of surgical site and patient's history with a simplified risk score for the prediction of postoperative nausea and vomiting, *Anaesthesia* 59:1078–1082, 2004.

Apfel CC, Kranke P, Katz MH, et al.: Volatile anaesthetics may be the main cause of early but not delayed postoperative vomiting: a randomized controlled trial of factorial design, *Br J Anaesth* 88:659–668, 2002.

Apfel CC, Laara E, Koivuranta M, et al.: A simplified risk score for predicting postoperative nausea and vomiting: conclusions from cross-validations between two centers, *Anesthesiology* 91(3):693–700, 1999.

Apfel CC, Philip BK, Cakmakkaya OS, et al.: Who is at risk for postdischarge nausea and vomiting after ambulatory surgery? *Anesthesiology* 86:475–486, 2012.

Aydogan MS, Ozturk E, Erdogan MA, et al.: The effects of secondhand smoke on postoperative pain and fentanyl consumption, *J Anesth* 27(4):569–574, 2013.

Baugh RF, Archer SM, Mitchell RB, et al.: Clinical practice guideline: tonsillectomy in children, *Otolaryngol Head Neck Surg* 144(Suppl 1):S1–S30, 2011.

Benn J, Arnold G, Wei I, et al.: Using quality indicators in anaesthesia: feeding back data to improve care, *Br J Anaesth* 109(1):80–91, 2012.

Bicer C, Aksu R, Ulgey A, et al.: Different doses of palonosetron for the prevention of postoperative nausea and vomiting in children undergoing strabismus surgery, *Drugs R D* 11(1):29–36, 2011.

Blaudszun G, Lysakowski C, Elia N, et al.: Effect of perioperative systemic α_2 agonists on postoperative morphine consumption and pain intensity: systematic review and meta-analysis of randomized controlled trials, *Anesthesiology* 116:1312–1322, 2012.

Bolton CM, Myles PS, Carlin JB, et al.: Randomized, double-blind study comparing the efficacy of moderate-dose metoclopramide and ondansetron for the prophylactic control of postoperative vomiting in children after tonsillectomy, *Br J Anaesth* 99(5):699–703, 2007.

Bolton CM, Myles PS, Nolan T, Sterne JA: Prophylaxis of postoperative vomiting in children undergoing tonsillectomy: a systematic review and meta-analysis, *Br J Anaesth* 97(5):593–604, 2006.

Bourdaud N, Devys JM, Bientz J, et al.: Development and validation of a risk score to predict the probability of postoperative vomiting in pediatric patients: the VPOP score, *Pediatr Anesth* 24(9):945–952, 2014.

Cardwell ME, Siviter G, Smith AF: Nonsteroidal anti-inflammatory drugs and perioperative bleeding in paediatric tonsillectomy, *Cochrane Database Syst Rev*(7), CD003591, 2013.

Carr AS, Brennan L, Courtman S, et al.: Guidelines on the prevention of post-operative vomiting in children: Association of Paediatric Anaesthetists of Great Britain & Ireland. Available at http://www.apagbi.org.uk/sites/default/files/APA_Guidelines_on_the_Prevention_of_Postoperative_Vomiting_in_Children.pdf, 2009 (Accessed September 13, 2016).

Chukudebelu O, Leonard DS, Healy A, et al.: The effect of gastric decompression on postoperative nausea and emesis in pediatric, tonsillectomy patients, *Int J Pediatr Otorhinolaryngol* 74(6):674–676, 2010.

Czarnetzki C, Elia N, Lysakowski C, et al.: Dexamethasone and risk of nausea and vomiting and postoperative bleeding after tonsillectomy in children: a randomized trial, *JAMA* 300(22):2621–2630, 2008.

De Windt AC, Asehnoune K, Roquilly A, et al.: An opioid-free anaesthetic using nerve blocks enhances rapid recovery after minor hand surgery in children, *Eur J Anaesthesiol* 27(6):521–525, 2010.

Drongowski RA, Lee D, Reynolds PI, et al.: Increased respiratory symptoms following surgery in children exposed to environmental tobacco smoke, *Pediatr Anesth* 13(4):304–310, 2003.

Dune LS, Shiao SY: Metaanalysis of acustimulation effects on postoperative nausea and vomiting in children, *Explore (NY)* 2(4):314–320, 2006.

Eberhart LH, Geldner G, Kranke P, et al.: The development and validation of a risk score to predict the probability of postoperative vomiting in pediatric patients, *Anesth Analg* 99(6):1630–1637, 2004.

Elgueta MF, Echevarría GC, De la Fuente N, et al.: Effect of intravenous fluid therapy on postoperative vomiting in children undergoing tonsillectomy, *Br J Anaesth* 110(4):607–614, 2013.

Elia N, Lysakowski C, Tramèr MR: Does multimodal analgesia with acetaminophen, nonsteroidal antiinflammatory drugs, or selective cyclooxygenase-2 inhibitors and patient-controlled analgesia morphine offer advantages over morphine alone? Meta-analyses of randomized trials, *Anesthesiology* 103:1296–1304, 2005.

Elia N, Tramèr M: Ketamine and postoperative pain—a quantitative systematic review of randomized trials, *Pain* 113:61–70, 2005.

Engelman E, Salengros JC, Barvais L: How much does pharmacologic prophylaxis reduce postoperative vomiting in children? Calculation of prophylaxis effectiveness and expected incidence of vomiting under treatment using Bayesian meta-analysis, *Anesthesiology* 109(6):1023–1035, 2008.

Erdem AF, Yoruk O, Alici HA, et al.: Subhypnotic propofol infusion plus dexamethasone is more effective than dexamethasone alone for the prevention of vomiting in children after tonsillectomy, *Paediatr Anaesth* 18(9):878–883, 2008.

Erdem AF, Yoruk O, Silbir F, et al.: Tropisetron plus subhypnotic propofol infusion is more effective than tropisetron alone for the prevention of vomiting in children after tonsillectomy, *Anaesth Intensive Care* 37(1):54–59, 2009.

Fortier MA, Weinberg M, Vitulano LA, et al.: Effects of therapeutic suggestion in children undergoing general anesthesia: a randomized controlled trial, *Paediatr Anaesth* 20(1):90–99, 2010.

Gan TJ, Diemunsch P, Habib AS, et al.: Consensus guidelines for the management of postoperative nausea and vomiting, *Anesth Analg* 118(1):85–113, 2014.

Gan TJ, Joshi GP, Zhao SZ, et al.: Presurgical intravenous parecoxib sodium and follow-up oral valdecoxib for pain management after laparoscopic cholecystectomy surgery reduces opioid requirements and opioid-related adverse effects, *Acta Anaesthesiol Scand* 48:1194–1207, 2004.

Goodarzi M, Matar MM, Shafa M, et al.: A prospective randomized blinded study of the effect of intravenous fluid therapy on postoperative nausea and vomiting in children undergoing strabismus surgery, *Paediatr Anaesth* 16(1):49–53, 2006.

Grant MC, Kim J, Page AJ, et al.: The effect of intravenous midazolam on postoperative nausea and vomiting: a meta-analysis, *Anesth Analg* 122(3):656–663, 2015.

Gross D, Reuss S, Dillier CM, et al.: Early vs late intraoperative administration of tropisetron for the prevention of nausea and vomiting in children undergoing tonsillectomy and/or adenoidectomy, *Paediatr Anaesth* 16(4):444–450, 2006.

Gupta N, Kumar R, Kumar S, et al.: A prospective randomised double blind study to evaluate the effect of peribulbar block or topical application of local anaesthesia combined with general anaesthesia on intra-operative and postoperative complications during paediatric strabismus surgery, *Anaesthesia* 62(11):1110–1113, 2007.

Gurbet A, Basagan-Mogol E, Turker G, et al.: Intraoperative infusion of dexmedetomidine reduces perioperative analgesic requirements, *Can J Anaesth* 53:646–652, 2006.

Henzi I, Walder B, Tramèr MR: Dexamethasone for the prevention of postoperative nausea and vomiting: a quantitative systematic review, *Anesth Analg* 90(1):186–194, 2000.

Jindal V, Ge A, Mansky PJ: Safety and efficacy of acupuncture in children: a review of the evidence, *J Pediatr Hematol Oncol* 30(6):431–442, 2008.

Kapur PA: The big "little problem", *Anesth Analg* 73(3):243–245, 1991.

Kim MS, Cote CJ, Cristoloveanu C, et al.: There is no dose-escalation response to dexamethasone (0.0625–1.0 mg/kg) in pediatric tonsillectomy or adenotonsillectomy patients for preventing vomiting, reducing pain, shortening time to first liquid intake, or the incidence of voice change, *Anesth Analg* 104(5):1052–1058, 2007.

Kovac AL, Eberhart L, Kotarski J, et al.: A randomized, double-blind study to evaluate the efficacy and safety of three different doses of palonosetron versus placebo in preventing postoperative nausea and vomiting over a 72-hour period, *Anesth Analg* 107(2):439–444, 2008.

Kovac AL, O'Connor TA, Pearman MH, et al.: Efficacy of repeat intravenous dosing of ondansetron in controlling postoperative nausea and vomiting: a randomized, double-blind, placebo-controlled multicenter trial, *J Clin Anesth* 11(6):453–459, 1999.

Kranke P, Eberhart LH, Toker H, et al.: A prospective evaluation of the POVOC score for the prediction of postoperative vomiting in children, *Anesth Analg* 105(6):1592–1597, 2007.

Mehta D, Sanatani S, Whyte SD: The effects of droperidol and ondansetron on dispersion of myocardial repolarization in children, *Paediatr Anaesth* 20(10):905–912, 2010.

Park SK, Cho EJ: A randomized, double-blind trial of palonosetron compared with ondansetron in preventing postoperative nausea and vomiting after gynaecological laparoscopic surgery, *J Int Med Res* 39(2):399–407, 2011.

Plante J, Turgeon AF, Zarychanski R, et al.: Effect of systemic steroids on post-tonsillectomy bleeding and reinterventions: systematic review and meta-analysis of randomised controlled trials, *BMJ* 345:e5389, 2012.

Polaner DM, Taenzer AH, Walker BJ, et al.: Pediatric Regional Anesthesia Network (PRAN): a multi-institutional study of the use and incidence of complications of pediatric regional anesthesia, *Anesth Analg* 115(6):1353–1364, 2012.

Radke OC, Biedler A, Kolodzie K, et al.: The effect of postoperative fasting on vomiting in children and their assessment of pain, *Paediatr Anaesth* 19(5):494–499, 2009.

Schnabel A, Eberhart LH, Muellenbach R, et al.: Efficacy of perphenazine to prevent postoperative nausea and vomiting: a quantitative systematic review, *Eur J Anaesthesiol* 27(12):1044–1051, 2010.

Steib A, Karcenty A, Calache E, et al.: Effects of subtenon anesthesia combined with general anesthesia on perioperative analgesic requirements in pediatric strabismus surgery, *Reg Anesth Pain Med* 30(5):478–483, 2005.

Steward DL, Grisel J, Meinzen-Derr J: Steroids for improving recovery following tonsillectomy in children, *Cochrane Database Syst Rev* (8): CD003997, 2011.

Tramèr M, Moore A, McQuay H: Meta-analytic comparison of prophylactic antiemetic efficacy for postoperative nausea and vomiting: propofol anaesthesia vs omitting nitrous oxide vs total i.v. anaesthesia with propofol, *Br J Anaesth* 78(3):256–259, 1997.

Tramèr M, Moore A, McQuay H: Omitting nitrous oxide in general anaesthesia: meta-analysis of intraoperative awareness and postoperative emesis in randomized controlled trials, *Br J Anaesth* 76(2):186–193, 1996.

Visser K, Hassink EA, Bonsel GJ, et al.: Randomized controlled trial of total intravenous anesthesia with propofol versus inhalation anesthesia with isoflurane-nitrous oxide—postoperative nausea and vomiting and economic analysis, *Anesthesiology* 95(3):616–626, 2001.

Wang SM, Kain ZN: Preoperative anxiety and postoperative nausea and vomiting in children: is there an association? *Anesth Analg* 90(3): 571–575, 2000.

索 引

H

J

K

L

M

N

P

Q

R

S

T

V

W

X

Y

Z